Handbook of
Dietary Fiber

FOOD SCIENCE AND TECHNOLOGY

A Series of Monographs, Textbooks, and Reference Books

1. Flavor Research: Principles and Techniques, *R. Teranishi, I. Hornstein, P. Issenberg, and E. L. Wick*
2. Principles of Enzymology for the Food Sciences, *John R. Whitaker*
3. Low-Temperature Preservation of Foods and Living Matter, *Owen R. Fennema, William D. Powrie, and Elmer H. Marth*
4. Principles of Food Science
   Part I: Food Chemistry, *edited by Owen R. Fennema*
   Part II: Physical Methods of Food Preservation, *Marcus Karel, Owen R. Fennema, and Daryl B. Lund*
5. Food Emulsions, *edited by Stig E. Friberg*
6. Nutritional and Safety Aspects of Food Processing, *edited by Steven R. Tannenbaum*
7. Flavor Research: Recent Advances, *edited by R. Teranishi, Robert A. Flath, and Hiroshi Sugisawa*
8. Computer-Aided Techniques in Food Technology, *edited by Israel Saguy*
9. Handbook of Tropical Foods, *edited by Harvey T. Chan*
10. Antimicrobials in Foods, *edited by Alfred Larry Branen and P. Michael Davidson*
11. Food Constituents and Food Residues: Their Chromatographic Determination, *edited by James F. Lawrence*
12. Aspartame: Physiology and Biochemistry, *edited by Lewis D. Steginth and L. J. Filer, Jr.*
13. Handbook of Vitamins: Nutritional, Biochemical, and Clinical Aspects, *edited by Lawrence J. Machlin*

Handbook of
Dietary Fiber

edited by

Susan Sungsoo Cho
Kellogg Company
Battle Creek, Michigan

Mark L. Dreher
Mead Johnson Nutritionals/Bristol-Myers Squibb Company
Evansville, Indiana

MARCEL DEKKER, INC.   NEW YORK · BASEL

ISBN: 0-8247-8960-1

This book is printed on acid-free paper.

Headquarters
Marcel Dekker, Inc.
270 Madison Avenue, New York, NY 10016
tel: 212-696-9000; fax: 212-685-4540

Eastern Hemisphere Distribution
Marcel Dekker AG
Hutgasse 4, Postfach 812, CH-4001 Basel, Switzerland
tel: 41-61-261-8482; fax: 41-61-261-8896

World Wide Web
http://www.dekker.com

The publisher offers discounts on this book when ordered in bulk quantities. For more information, write to Special Sales/Professional Marketing at the headquarters address above.

Current printing (last digit):
10 9 8 7 6 5 4 3 2 1

PRINTED IN THE UNITED STATES OF AMERICA

Preface

Since the mid-1970s, dietary fiber has been an extremely active area of research because of its complexity and wide-ranging biomedical effects. During this time, hundreds of research papers, review articles, and bulletins, and dozens of books have been published on the subject; in addition, scores of seminars and conferences have been held. With active research activities conducted over the past two or three decades demonstrating the health benefits of dietary fiber, the Food and Drug Administration has now mandated that dietary content be declared on food labels. In 1984, the Kellogg Company and the National Cancer Institute (NCI) carried out a joint campaign to educate consumers that wheat bran fiber may lower the incidence of certain types of cancers, such as colon cancer. This opened a new avenue for nutraceuticals and functional foods for consumers throughout the world to lower their risk of chronic diseases by consuming foods formulated with functional ingredients.

The campaign provoked more active research in linking diet and nutrition to chronic diseases to improve public health. Such continuing research efforts have led to health claims made by food manufacturers to help the public choose foods wisely. Numerous patents have been filed and approved for purposes such as functionality improvement and health benefits. Enough information is now available to address the needs of clinicians, dieticians, food scientists, food regulators, and marketers. Because of the great public interest in dietary fiber, there was a need to provide this applied group with a handbook that can bridge the gap between basic research and applied interest. This handbook will help the audience understand key issues and improve the consistency and accuracy of the dietary fiber information used in their work, such as the development of new food products, the regulation of these food products, and the dietary fiber recommendations to patients by health professionals.

The *Handbook of Dietary Fiber* has significantly expanded the scope of dietary fiber applications, such as marketing perspectives, health claims, and patent literature. Each chapter offers contemporary thoughts on dietary fiber.

We would like to thank all the dietary fiber researchers who designed experiments, collected data, and published results that made this book possible.

Susan Sungsoo Cho
Mark L. Dreher

Contents

IV. Functional Dietary Fiber Ingredients

Contributors

Eva Arrigoni   Institute of Food Science, Swiss Federal Institute of Technology, Zurich, Switzerland

Katrine I. Baghurst   CSIRO, Adelaide, South Australia, Australia

Peter A. Baghurst   Women's and Children's Hospital, North Adelaide, South Australia, Australia

Elżbieta Bartnikowska   Food Monitoring, Meat and Fat Research Institute, Warsaw, Poland

James N. BeMiller   Department of Food Science, Purdue University, West Lafayette, Indiana

Anthony R. Bird   Department of Health Sciences and Nutrition, CSIRO, Adelaide, South Australia, Australia

Marguerite C. Bollella   Department of Pediatrics, New York Presbyterian Hospital, New York, New York

Laura Bravo   Department of Metabolism and Nutrition, Instituto del Frío, Consejo Superior de Investigaciones Científicas, Madrid, Spain

Stephen P. J. Brooks   Nutrition Research Division, Health Protection Branch, Health Canada, Ottawa, Ontario, Canada

Isabel Goñi Cambrodón   Nutrition Department, Faculty of Pharmacy, University Complutense of Madrid, Madrid, Spain

David Cameron-Smith   School of Health Sciences, Deakin University, Melbourne, Victoria, Australia

Susan Sungsoo Cho   Kellogg Company, Battle Creek, Michigan

Faye I. Chow   Cereal Product Utilization, Western Regional Research Center, Agricultural Research Service, U.S. Department of Agriculture, Albany, California

Celeste Clark   Kellogg Company, Battle Creek, Michigan

Gregory R. Collier   School of Health Sciences, Deakin University, Melbourne, Victoria, Australia

Paul Coussement   ORAFTI Active Food Ingredients, Tienen, Belgium

Christian Demigné   Laboratoire des Maladies Metaboliques et Micronutriments, INRA de Clermont-Ferrand/Theix, Saint-Genès-Champanelle, France

Mark L. Dreher   Mead Johnson Nutritionals/Bristol-Myers Squibb Company, Evansville, Indiana

Peter Rory Ellis   Biopolymers Group, Division of Life Sciences, King's College London (University of London), London, England

Christine E. Fastnaught   Castle Dome Foods, Inc., Fargo, North Dakota

Lynnette R. Ferguson   Faculty of Medicine and Health Sciences, The University of Auckland, Auckland, New Zealand

Maria Luz Fernandez   Department of Nutritional Sciences, University of Connecticut, Storrs, Connecticut

Anne Franck   ORAFTI Active Food Ingredients, Tienen, Belgium

Janette Gelroth   Nutrition and Analytical Labs, American Institute of Baking, Manhattan, Kansas

F. Guillon   Unité de Recherche sur les Polysaccharides, leurs Organisations et Interactions, Institut National de la Recherche Agronomique, Nantes, France

Barbara F. Harland   Department of Nutritional Sciences, College of Pharmacy, Nursing, and Allied Health Sciences, Howard University, Washington, D.C.

Philip J. Harris   School of Biological Sciences, The University of Auckland, Auckland, New Zealand

Robert Havenaar   Department of Nutritional Physiology, TNO Nutrition and Food Research, Zeist, The Netherlands

Alan Henshall   Dionex Corporation, Sunnyvale, California

Mazda Jenab   University of Toronto, Toronto, Ontario, Canada

Talwinder S. Kahlon   Cereal Product Utilization, Western Regional Research Center, Agricultural Research Service, U.S. Department of Agriculture, Albany, California

Dorit Nitzan Kaluski   Department of Nutrition, Ministry of Health, Jerusalem, Israel

Franco Maria Lajolo   Department of Food and Experimental Nutrition, Faculty of Pharmaceutical Sciences, University of São Paulo, São Paulo, Brazil

Alistair James MacDougall   Division of Food Materials Science, B. B. S. R. C. Institute of Food Research, Colney, Norwich, England

Zecharia Madar   Faculty of Agricultural, Food and Environmental Quality Sciences, Institute of Biochemistry, Food Science and Nutrition, The Hebrew University of Jerusalem, Rehovot, Israel

Yrjö Mälkki   Cerefi Ltd., Espoo, Finland

Judith A. Marlett   Department of Nutritional Sciences, University of Wisconsin, Madison, Wisconsin

Elizabete Wenzel de Menezes   Department of Food and Experimental Nutrition, Faculty of Pharmaceutical Sciences, University of São Paulo, São Paulo, Brazil

Frank J. Miskiel   New Product Development, CP Kelco, San Diego, California

Roger Mongeau   Nutrition Consultant, Ottawa, Ontario, Canada

Christine Morand   Laboratoire des Maladies Metaboliques et Micronutriments, INRA de Clermont-Ferrand/Theix, Saint-Genès-Champanelle, France

Gurleen Narula   Department of Nutritional Sciences, College of Pharmacy, Nursing, and Allied Health Sciences, Howard University, Washington, D.C.

Adam Niegodzisz   Meat and Fat Research Institute, Warsaw, Poland

David Oakenfull   Ingredient Innovation Program, Food Science Australia, North Ryde, New South Wales, Australia

Merete Olesen   Department of Medicine and Gastroenterology, KAS, Gentofte, Copenhagen, Denmark

Edvar Onsøyen   Pronova Biopolymer a.s., Drammen, Norway

Nelly Pak   Center of Nutrition, Faculty of Medicine, University of Chile, Santiago, Chile

G. O. Phillips   Centre for Water Soluble Polymers, North East Wales Institute, Wrexham, Wales

Kenneth J. Pienta   University of Michigan, Ann Arbor, Michigan

Gur S. Ranhotra   Nutrition Research, American Institute of Baking, Manhattan, Kansas

Phillippa Rayment   Biopolymers Group, Division of Life Sciences, King's College London (University of London), London, England

Christian Rémésy   Laboratoire des Maladies Metaboliques et Micronutriments, INRA de Clermont-Ferrand/Theix, Saint-Genès-Champanelle, France

Yilong Ren   Biopolymers Group, Division of Life Sciences, King's College London (University of London), London, England

C. M. G. C. Renard   Unité de Recherche sur les Polysaccharides, leurs Organisations et Interactions, Institut National de la Recherche Agronomique, Nantes, France

Sharon E. Rickard   University of Toronto, Toronto, Ontario, Canada

Marcel Roberfroid*   Department of Pharmaceutical Sciences, Catholic University of Louvain, Brussels, Belgium

Jorge L. Rosado   Department of Nutritional Physiology, National Institute of Nutrition, Mexico City, and School of Natural Sciences, University of Queretaro, Queretaro, Mexico

Simon B. Ross-Murphy   Biopolymers Group, Division of Life Sciences, King's College London (University of London), London, England

Fulgencio D. Saura-Calixto   Department Metabolism and Nutrition, Instituto del Frío, Consejo Superior de Investigaciones Científicas, Madrid, Spain

Eric D. Schwab   Section of Urology, Department of Surgery, University of Michigan, Ann Arbor, Michigan

Robert Rasiah Selvendran‡   B. B. S. R. C. Institute of Food Research, Colney, Norwich, England

Joanne L. Slavin   Department of Food Science and Nutrition, University of Minnesota, St. Paul, Minnesota

Aliza H. Stark   Faculty of Agricultural, Food and Environmental Quality Sciences, The Hebrew University of Jerusalem, Rehovot, Israel

Jean-François Thibault   Unité de Recherche sur les Polysaccharides, leurs Organisations et Interactions, Institut National de la Recherche Agronomique, Nantes, France

Laura Boccia Tolosi   Division of Nutritional Carcinogenesis, American Health Foundation, Valhalla, New York

---

*Professor Emeritus.
‡Retired.

David L. Topping   Division of Human Nutrition, Department of Health Sciences and Nutrition, CSIRO, Adelaide, South Australia, Australia

Raymond C. Valli   Food Applications R&D, CP Kelco, San Diego, California

Ellen van den Heuvel   Department of Nutritional Physiology, TNO Nutrition and Food Research, Zeist, The Netherlands

Wim van Dokkum   Department of Nutritional Physiology, TNO Nutrition and Food Research, Zeist, The Netherlands

Guangya Wang   Department of Food Chemistry, Institute of Nutrition and Food Hygiene, Chinese Academy of Preventive Medicine, Beijing, China

Qi Wang   Biopolymers Group, Division of Life Sciences, King's College London (University of London), London, England

Christine L. Williams   Department of Pediatrics and Institute of Human Nutrition, Babies and Children's Hospital, Columbia University, New York, New York

P. A. Williams   Centre for Water Soluble Polymers, North East Wales Institute, Wrexham, Wales

Fumio Yotsuzuka   Marketing Department, Takeda Chemical Industries, Ltd., Tokyo, Japan

1
Dietary Fiber Overview

Mark L. Dreher
Mead Johnson Nutritionals/Bristol-Myers Squibb Company, Evansville, Indiana

I. INTRODUCTION

In 1953, Hipsley first used "dietary fiber" to designate nondigestible plant cell wall constituents. Between 1972 and 1976, dietary fiber's role was expanded to be used in conjunction with a number of health-related hypotheses. The dietary fiber hypothesis implies that a high intake of fiber-containing foods is directly related to, or is associated with, a low incidence of many disorders and diseases common with a Western lifestyle (e.g., chronic bowel disease, diabetes, coronary heart disease, and colon cancer). Research continues to explore the validity of the hypothesis, and many questions require answers. How much does it explain? Is it overrated? Does it really work in everyday nutrition, especially in interethnic populations? How does it compare with other well-known disease hypotheses (Walker, 1993)?

The passing years have not lessened the significance of dietary fiber in human health and disease. There are over a dozen major identifiable beneficial effects of increased dietary fiber consumption on human health and body function. These attributes range from fiber's contribution to lowering caloric intake to its increase in the water content and mass of human solid waste. Although there is an enormous database to support the health benefits of dietary fiber, the data is not without mixed results. Nevertheless, collectively, dietary fiber contributes to a fascinating story about foods, nutrition, and health which will be examined throughout this book.

While a diet high in fiber-containing foods is associated with health benefits, the extent of the benefits can be enhanced or diminished by the influence of various nondietary factors (e.g., genetic factors, physical activity, stress), and more needs to be known about the health effects of dietary fiber in different food forms such as the metabolic effects of high-fiber whole foods (e.g., whole wheat bread), fiber concentrates (e.g., modified bran), and bioactive isolates (e.g., pectin).

Increased concern about the relationship between diet and chronic disease has led to an increased interest in functional food products for risk reduction. This functional food paradigm was ushered in by the vigorous marketing of bran and fiber-enhanced products. It started in the mid-1980s with the success of a Kellogg's All-Bran campaign that linked colon cancer risk reduction to increased bran intake. Studies from the scientific community and recommendations about dietary fiber from the government and consumer organizations have kept dietary fiber "on the radar screen" for health promotion. In fact, dietary fiber is now a mandatory component of U.S. food labels. It consists of two major fractions—insoluble and soluble—but reporting this distribution is only voluntary on food labels. Five food labeling health claims are currently allowed, which reflect the health significance of dietary fiber. Generally stated, these are: (1) fiber containing grain products, fruits, and vegetables, help reduce the risk of cancer; (2) fruits, vegetables and grain products that contain fiber, particularly soluble fiber, help reduce the risk of heart disease; (3) oat bran helps reduce the risk of heart disease; (4) psyllium helps reduce the risk of heart disease; and (5) whole grains help reduce the risk of heart disease and certain types of cancers.

II. WHAT IS DIETARY FIBER?

Dietary fiber is an umbrella term for a heterogeneous mixture of plant food components that are indigestible in the small intestine. The working definition of dietary fiber over the last few decades is: "Dietary fiber consists of the remnants of edible plant cell, polysaccharides, lignin, and associated substances resistant to digestion by the alimentary enzymes of humans" (Gordon, 1999). It is the term generally used to describe the supporting structures of plant cell walls and the substances intimately associated with them. The typical components of dietary fiber include cellulose, hemicellulose, lignins, pectins, and a variety of gums and mucilages. All of these except lignins are polysaccharides. The heterogeneity of dietary fiber is the primary reason for the diversity of its physiological effects.

Is this definition satisfying the consumer, food and health professionals, food processors and ingredient suppliers, and regulatory agencies (Gordon, 1999)? The American Association of Cereal Chemists is leading an effort to explore updated changes in what the term dietary fiber represents. Now questions must be addressed: How should synthetic polymers be considered? Is dietary fiber only obtained from edible plant cells? Should the definition include both a chemical and physiological component? Recent surveys show that scientists in the area of dietary fiber prefer the inclusion of oligosaccharides, which are not recovered with the current Association of Official Analytical Chemists method for measuring total dietary fiber.

Dietary fiber is available in the human diet through a wide variety of food sources, such as both raw and processed cereals, vegetables, legumes, and fruits. The composition of dietary fiber varies with the type of plant tissue (Table 1). The proportions of different dietary fiber constituents found in plant foods depend on the maturity of the plants. In typical plant cell walls, the percentage of cellulose, lignin, and ash tend to be higher and the percentage of noncellulosic polysaccharides, waxes, and protein tend to be lower in mature than in immature plants. The portion of the plant consumed and its relative maturity, as well as storage and ripening, may influence the dietary fiber composition of plant foods, and food-processing techniques may also alter the native fiber composition. Vegetables and cereals tend to be good sources of cellulose. Lignin is highest in fruits with edible seeds such as strawberries or in mature vegetables such as carrots or other root vegetables. Whole grain cereals and bran are rich in hemicellulose. Pectin is found in fruits such as apples and oranges. Oats and dried beans contain a good source of soluble dietary fiber.

Total dietary fiber is the analytical term for dietary fiber that includes both water-insoluble dietary fiber and water-soluble dietary fiber. Insoluble fiber consists mainly of cell wall components such as cellulose, lignin, and hemicellulose present mainly in wheat, most grain products, and vegetables. Insoluble fiber shortens bowel transit time, increases fecal bulk, and renders feces softer. Soluble fiber consists of noncellulosic polysaccharides such as pectin, gums, and mucilages found in fruits, oats, barley, and legumes. Soluble fiber delays gastric emptying, slows glucose absorption, enhance immune function and lowers serum cholesterol levels. It is to a large degree fermented in the colon into short-chain fatty acids, which may inhibit hepatic cholesterol

Table 1 Influence of Source on Dietary Fiber Composition

Food group	Type of tissue	Major polymers
Cereals	Endosperm	Arabinoxylans
	Seed coats	β-D-Glucans
		Cellulose
		Lignin
Vegetables and fruit	Parenchymatous flesh	Pectic substances
	Vascular tissue	Xyloglucans
	Epidermal tissue	Cellulose
		Lignin
		Cutin
		Waxes
Seeds other than cereals	Cotyledons	Pectic substances
	Endosperm walls	Galactomannans
		Xyloglucans
		Cellulose
Polysaccharide food additives	Amorphous	Gums
	Soluble	Algal polysaccharides
	Dispersible	Sulfated galactans
		Cellulose esters/ethers

Source: Pilch, 1987.

synthesis. About 75% of the dietary fiber in foods is found in the insoluble fraction. Products frequently referred to as soluble or insoluble fibers are often sources of both of these types of fibers.

III. HISTORICAL OVERVIEW

A. Paleolithic Nutrition

Experts in paleolithic nutrition have theorized that primitive diets contained high levels of dietary fiber (Eaton et al., 1988; Eaton, 1990). This stems from the fact that about 65% of the Stone Age diet was comprised of uncultivated fruits and vegetables. Of course, there were wide regional and secular variations in the subsistence patterns of Stone Age living conditions, but a number of similar nutritional patterns have been identified (Eaton, 1990). These contrast strikingly with the nutrition of people living in today's affluent Western culture.

The differences between today's diet and the Stone Age diet are numerous. First, our ancestors ate the meat from wild game. The nutritional composition of wild game is notably different than that of today's domesticated animal products: it has only one fifth as much fat, a higher proportion of unsaturated fatty acids, less than half the calories, and more protein. Second, Stone Age humans had not domesticated dairy animals. Dairy products are now a major component of our diet. Third, Stone Agers consumed uncultivated fruits and vegetables, which were high in dietary fiber (12.6 g/100 g). Our preagricultural ancestors probably consumed in excess of 100 grams of dietary fiber daily. Fourth, the uncultivated plants consumed by our ancestors contained a high level of micronutrients relative to their calorie content. Fifth, sodium content of the Stone Age diet is estimated to have been about 250 mg daily, which is less than one twentieth of our current intake.

B. Evolution of Dietary Fiber in the Food Supply

Interest in fiber-rich foods has a colorful and long history. In 430 B.C. Hippocrates described the laxative effects of whole wheat in comparison with refined wheat. The earliest recorded clinical trial with fiber-rich foods is described in the Bible (Daniel 1:8–16) (Kritchevsky, 1988). The passages explain that Daniel and three of his friends after eating vegetables (pulses) and water for 10 days appeared healthier than others who had partaken of Nebuchadnezzar's feast during the same period. As for early food patterns, in Mesopotamia, Greece, and Rome and in European countries during the Medieval and Middle Ages—indeed, up to the nineteenth century—in general the diet was high in fiber-containing cereals, legumes, vegetables, and fruit and relatively low in dairy products and meat; i.e., the typical diet was low in fat and high in fiber.

At the turn of the century, a marked change took place in the pattern of the Western diet (Walker, 1993). The intake of cereals and of potatoes fell. The intake of fat, sugar, fruit and vegetables, and indulgence items (e.g., ice cream, chocolate) rose. Characteristically, the diet became high in fat and low in fiber. At about this time, Graham (of graham cracker fame) denounced the harmful effects of refined carbohydrate foods, and the Kellogg and Post cereals owe their start to an increased interest in the bran content of the diet. In the 1920s, J. H. Kellogg published extensively on the benefits of bran, claiming that it increased stool weight, promoted laxation, and prevented disease. Bran was researched throughout the 1930s and then forgotten.

The modern era of dietary fiber research began in the 1950s, and interest in it has steadily gained momentum. In 1956, British Surgeon Captain Cleave hypothesized that most diseases of civilization were caused by an overconsumption of sugar and a lack of dietary fiber. This hypothesis caught the attention of Drs. Trowell and Burkitt, who are usually credited with popularizing the idea that dietary fiber may be protective against the development of Western diseases, including diabetes, hypercholesterolemia, heart disease, diverticular disease, and colon cancer. Interest in dietary fiber research began slowly. From 1953 to 1968, there was an average of six publications on dietary fiber per year. *Index Medicus* did not include a dietary fiber subject category until 1982. Today dietary fiber is one of the most widely researched food components.

Table 2 Dietary Guidelines for Americans (2000)

Fiber containing food groups	Number of servings[a]		
	Children ages 2 to 6 years, women, some older adults (about 1,600 calories)	Older children, teen girls, active women, most men (about 2,200 calories)	Teen boys, active men (about 2,800 calories)
Bread, cereal, rice, and pasta group (grain group) especially whole grain	6	9	11
Vegetable group	3	4	5
Fruit group	2	3	4

[a] Dietary Guidelines for Americans (2000).

IV. GENERAL DIETARY GUIDELINES AND RECOMMENDATIONS

The Dietary Guidelines for Americans (2000) calls for Americans to choose a variety of grains, especially whole grains, fruits, and vegetables daily. These food group guidelines are summarized in Table 2.

Eating foods with dietary fiber is important for proper bowel function and may reduce symptoms of chronic constipation, diverticular disease, and hemorrhoids. Populations with diets low in dietary fiber and complex carbohydrates and high in fat, especially saturated fat, tend to have more heart disease, obesity, and some cancers. Just how dietary fiber is involved is still being studied.

Some of the benefits from high fiber diets come natural from the non-dietary fiber components such as natural antioxidants. For this reason, it is best to get most dietary fiber from foods. However, since food consumption of dietary fiber tends to be only half the recommended level, the consumption of fiber supplements may be beneficial when used in moderation.

Dietary fiber intake should range from 20 to 35 grams per day or 10–13 g per 1000 kcal for optimal benefits but the usual intake in developed countries such as the United States is only about half this level (Pilch, 1987; Butrum, 1988; Health and Welfare Canada, 1985). The lower value was selected with special consideration of health benefits such as intestinal function, and the upper value was chosen to avoid possible deleterious effects.

V. SOURCES OF DIETARY FIBER

Most dietary fiber comes from plant products such as fruits, vegetables, legumes, nuts, and whole grains. Because of their higher water content, fruits and vegetables provide less dietary fiber than the whole grains per ounce consumed. The most concentrated sources of dietary fiber are whole grains and cereal brans. Refining processes decrease the fiber content in grains.

The most common form of dietary fiber is insoluble fiber. Composed of cellulose, lignin, and some hemicellulose, it promotes regularity and is being studied for its potential to reduce the risk of colon/rectal cancers. In addition to cereal brans and whole grain cereals, other good sources of insoluble fiber are dried beans, peas, vegetables, and nuts.

Although soluble fiber is less common in foods than insoluble fiber, it is believed to have important effects in the digestive and absorptive processes. A growing number of studies show that soluble fiber as part of a low-fat, low-cholesterol diet may help lower blood cholesterol in those individuals with elevated blood cholesterol levels. It has also been shown to help control blood glucose levels in individuals with diabetes mellitus. Good sources of soluble fiber are whole grain oats and barley, oat bran, some fruits, dried beans, and other legumes.

When changing from a low-fiber diet (typical American diet) to a high-fiber diet, it is best to start by gradually substituting foods with more fiber for low fiber foods. As a result of the diversity of effects of various components of dietary fiber, it is important that the dietary fiber consumed come from a wide variety of foods that provide a broad spectrum of these components. Table 3 provides a comprehensive list of the total dietary fiber content and insoluble/soluble levels found in common foods.

The use of dietary fiber supplements to achieve an increase in dietary fiber intake in the general population should be done prudently (Slavin, 1987; Pilch, 1987). Effects of isolated dietary fibers are likely to be different than their effects in native foods.

Table 3 Dietary Fiber Content of Foods

Food	Moisture (g/100 g edible portion)	Dietary fiber (g/100 g edible portion)		
		Total	Insoluble	Soluble
Baked products				
Bagels, plain	31.6	2.1	1.5	0.6
Biscuits, baking powder	16.7	2.1	1.6	0.5
Breads:				
Boston brown	47.2	4.7	—	—
Bran	39.1	5.4	4.6	0.8
Corn	36.1	3.0	2.8	0.2
Cracked wheat	35.9	5.3	4.5	0.8
French	29.2	2.7	1.9	0.8
Hollywood-type, light	37.8	4.8	4.2	0.6
Italian:				
Plain	26.9	3.8	2.9	0.9
Sesame seeds	34.6	3.4	2.5	0.9
Multigrain	38.6	5.6	4.6	1.0
Oatmeal	37.8	4.3	3.3	1.0
Pita:				
White	32.1	1.6	0.8	0.8
Whole wheat	30.6	7.4	6.6	0.8
Pumpernickel	38.3	5.9	4.3	1.6
Reduced-calorie, high-fiber:				
Multigrain	39.3	13.6	12.7	0.9
White	44.3	12.8	12.3	0.5
Rye (German)	36.8	8.3	6.8	1.5
Sourdough	36.4	3.0	2.0	1.0
White	37.1	1.9	1.3	0.6
Toasted	—	2.5	—	—
Whole wheat	39.7	8.1	7.0	1.1
Toasted	—	8.9	—	—
Bread crumbs, plain or seasoned	5.7	4.2	3.0	1.2
Bread sticks	4.6	3.0	1.8	1.2
Bread stuffing, flavored from dry mix	65.1	2.9	2.0	0.9
Cakes, prepared:				
Angel food	35.5	0.8	0.5	0.3
Chocolate	33.3	2.4	1.8	0.6
Coffeecake				
Crumb topping	22.3	3.3	2.6	0.7
Fruit	31.7	2.5	1.5	1.0
Devil's food	30.4	2.5	1.8	0.7
Fruitcake	22.0	3.7	2.5	1.2
Yellow	26.9	1.4	1.1	0.3
Cheesecake	44.6	2.1	1.5	0.6
Cookies:				
Brownies	12.8	2.5	1.7	0.8
Butter	4.7	2.4	1.6	0.8
Chocolate chip	4.1	2.6	1.9	0.7
Chocolate sandwich	2.2	2.9	2.2	0.7
Fig bar	16.7	4.6	4.0	0.6

Table 3 Continued

Food	Moisture (g/100 g edible portion)	Dietary fiber (g/100 g edible portion)		
		Total	Insoluble	Soluble
Fortune	8.0	1.6	1.2	0.4
Ginger snaps	4.8	1.8	1.2	0.6
Oatmeal	4.9	2.6	1.5	1.1
Peanut butter	6.7	1.8	1.3	0.5
Shortbread	3.3	1.8	0.9	0.9
Sugar	3.3	1.1	0.7	0.4
Vanilla wafers	5.5	1.5	0.7	0.8
Crackers:				
Cheese	3.5	2.5	1.4	1.1
Crispbread	7.2	15.9	13.0	2.9
Flatbread	4.9	16.5	13.2	3.3
Graham	4.4	2.7	1.9	0.8
Honey grahams	3.0	3.0	1.7	1.3
Melba toast				
White	5.1	6.2	4.7	1.5
Whole wheat	5.9	8.9	7.1	1.8
Matzo, plain	6.1	2.9	2.2	0.7
Saltines	3.0	2.3	1.1	1.2
Snack-type	3.3	2.0	1.0	1.0
Soda	4.0	2.7	1.3	1.4
Wheat	1.7	4.1	3.0	1.1
Whole wheat	1.9	10.9	9.1	1.8
Croissants	20.4	2.3	1.4	0.9
Croutons	5.6	4.7	4.0	0.7
Doughnuts				
Cake	19.7	1.7	1.1	0.6
Yeast, glazed	26.7	1.2	0.7	0.5
Hamburger buns	35.0	2.6	1.7	0.9
Ice cream cone:				
Sugar	3.0	4.6	3.4	1.2
Wafer	5.3	4.1	3.0	1.1
Muffins:				
Blueberry	37.3	3.6	3.1	0.5
Bran-raisin	26.7	6.3	4.9	1.4
English	38.0	3.0	2.4	0.6
Oat bran	35.0	7.5	5.0	2.5
Plain	27.1	1.5	1.0	0.5
Wheat bran	23.3	3.3	2.5	0.8
Pastries:				
Plain	19.3	1.3	0.9	0.4
Fruit	27.6	1.9	1.0	0.9
Pie Crust	14.9	2.3	1.8	0.5
Pies:				
Apple	44.9	1.6	1.0	0.6
Cherry	46.2	0.8	0.5	0.3
Pecan	19.8	3.5	3.0	0.5
Pumpkin	58.1	2.7	2.1	0.6

Table 3 Continued

Food	Moisture (g/100 g edible portion)	Dietary fiber (g/100 g edible portion)		
		Total	Insoluble	Soluble
Rolls:				
Brown and serve	23.5	3.0	1.9	1.1
Cinnamon	26.4	2.2	1.6	0.6
Dinner	30.4	3.8	3.0	0.8
French	30.8	3.2	2.2	1.0
Taco shells	4.2	6.3	5.4	0.9
Toaster pastries	8.9	1.0	0.6	0.4
Tortillas:				
Corn	49.0	5.1	4.4	0.7
Flour	29.3	2.3	1.3	1.0
Waffles, frozen	45.0	2.4	1.6	0.8
Breakfast cereals				
Bran	2.9	35.3	32.8	2.5
Bran, extra fiber	3.1	51.2	48.6	2.6
Bran flakes				
Plain	3.2	19.5	17.5	2.0
Raisins	7.6	13.5	15.1	2.4
Cornflakes				
Plain	2.8	2.0	1.7	0.3
Sugar frosted	1.9	2.2	1.8	0.4
Cream of wheat, cooked	87.9	0.7	0.6	0.1
Crispy rice	2.4	1.9	1.4	0.5
Fruit and bran	3.0	14.8	12.0	2.8
Granola	3.3	10.5	—	—
Grapenuts	3.1	10.4	7.3	3.1
Hominy, cooked	85.0	0.6	0.6	0.0
Muesli	5.0	12.0	—	—
Oat bran, uncooked	7.4	17.0	10.5	6.5
Oatmeal, cooked	84.2	1.9	1.2	0.7
Psyllium and bran	3.0	21.2	10.6	10.6
Puffed wheat	6.9	7.5	5.1	2.4
Puffed rice	6.5	1.4	1.0	0.4
Shredded wheat	7.1	12.5	9.9	2.6
Toasted oats	3.5	7.0	4.2	2.8
Wheat flakes	2.4	11.4	9.6	1.8
Cereal grains				
Amaranth	9.8	15.2	—	—
Amaranth flour, whole grain	10.4	10.2	—	—
Arrowroot flour	11.4	3.4	—	—
Barley	9.4	17.3	—	—
Barley, bran	3.5	70.0	67.0	3.0
Barley, pearled	10.1	15.6	—	—

Table 3 Continued

Food	Moisture (g/100 g edible portion)	Dietary fiber (g/100 g edible portion)		
		Total	Insoluble	Soluble
Bulgur, dry	8.0	18.3	—	—
Corn, bran	6.5	82.4	80.4	2.0
Corn, flour, whole grain	10.9	13.4	—	—
Cornmeal:				
Whole grain	11.0	11.0	—	—
Degermed	10.3	5.3	—	—
Cornstarch	12.0	0.9	—	—
Millet, hulled	8.2	8.5	—	—
Oat, bran	10.0	22.2	11.7	10.5
Oat, flour	7.8	9.6	—	—
Oats, rolled, or oatmeal, dry	8.8	10.3	6.5	3.8
Rice:				
Wild	8.4	5.2	—	—
Brown, long-grain:				
Raw	11.7	3.9	—	—
Cooked	73.1	1.7	—	—
White:				
Long-grain:				
Dry	8.7	1.3	1.0	0.3
Cooked	77.5	0.7	0.7	0.0
Short grain	11.1	2.8	—	—
Medium grain	11.7	1.7	—	—
Parboiled rice:				
Dry	10.4	2.2	—	—
Cooked	77.0	0.5	—	—
Instant:				
Dry	8.1	1.6	—	—
Cooked	76.4	0.8	—	—
Rice-a-Roni	71.5	2.5	—	—
Rice bran	6.1	21.7	—	—
Rice flour:				
Brown	12.0	4.6	—	—
White	11.9	2.4	—	—
Rye:				
Dark	11.1	32.0	—	—
Medium	8.8	14.7	—	—
Light	10.6	14.6	—	—
Semolina	12.7	3.9	—	—
Triticale	11.2	18.1	—	—
Triticale, flour, whole grain	9.4	14.6	—	—
Wheat, bran	11.6	42.4	40.3	2.1
Wheat, flour				
White, all-purpose	11.2	2.7	1.7	1.0
Whole-grain	11.5	12.6	10.2	2.3
Wheat germ	2.9	14.0	12.9	1.1

Table 3 Continued

Food	Moisture (g/100 g edible portion)	Dietary fiber (g/100 g edible portion)		
		Total	Insoluble	Soluble
Fruit and fruit products				
Apples:				
Red Delicious:				
Unpeeled	83.6	2.0	1.8	0.2
Peeled	84.6	1.5	1.3	0.2
Granny Smith, unpeeled	83.8	2.7	2.4	0.3
Apple juice, unsweetened	87.9	0.1	0.1	0.0
Applesauce:				
Sweetened	79.6	1.2	1.0	0.2
Unsweetened	88.4	1.5	1.3	0.2
Apricots, dried	31.1	7.8	6.0	1.8
Apricot nectar	84.9	0.6	0.5	0.1
Bananas	75.7	1.7	1.2	0.5
Blueberries:				
Fresh	85.4	2.7	2.4	0.3
Frozen	83.5	3.2	2.5	0.7
Cherries, canned	78.8	1.0	0.4	0.6
Figs, dried	28.4	9.3	—	—
Fruit cocktail	—	1.5	—	—
Grapefruit:				
Fresh	87.8	1.8	0.7	1.1
Juice	90.1	0.5	0.0	0.5
Grapes	80.6	1.2	0.7	0.5
Kiwifruit	83.0	3.4	—	—
Melons	90.1	0.7	0.4	0.3
Nectarine	89.7	1.2	0.8	0.4
Oranges:				
Fresh	86.0	1.8	0.7	1.1
Juice	89.4	0.4	0.1	0.3
Peaches:				
Fresh	87.1	1.9	1.0	0.9
Canned	83.0	1.2	0.7	0.5
Pears:				
Fresh	84.5	3.0	2.0	1.0
Canned	84.1	2.3	1.5	0.8
Pineapple, canned	84.2	0.9	0.7	0.2
Plums:				
Fresh	85.4	1.6	0.7	0.9
Canned	75.8	2.4	1.1	1.3
Prunes, dried	26.2	7.3	3.1	4.2
Prune juice	81.2	1.0	—	—
Raisins, seedless	12.6	3.7	2.4	1.3
Strawberries:				
Fresh	90.5	2.2	1.3	0.9
Frozen	75.0	1.6	0.9	0.7
Jam	31.8	0.9	0.7	0.2

Table 3 Continued

Food	Moisture (g/100 g edible portion)	Dietary fiber (g/100 g edible portion)		
		Total	Insoluble	Soluble
Tangerine:				
Fresh	85.1	1.8	1.4	0.4
Canned	84.5	0.4	0.1	0.3
Watermelon	90.1	0.4	0.3	0.1
Legumes and pulses				
Baked beans, canned:				
B-BQ	—	5.8	—	—
Sweet or tomato sauce:				
Plain	72.6	7.7	—	—
With franks	69.3	6.9	—	—
Black-eyed peas, canned	65.0	3.9	3.5	0.4
Lentils:				
Dried, raw	9.9	11.4	10.3	1.1
Dried, cooked	66.5	5.3	4.7	0.6
Garbanzo beans, canned	65.6	3.5	3.1	0.4
Lima beans, canned	74.5	4.2	3.8	0.4
Kidney beans, canned	70.4	6.3	4.7	1.6
Peas, black-eyed, canned	78.6	3.1	2.7	0.4
Peas, green:				
Canned	81.5	4.3	4.0	0.3
Frozen	82.3	3.5	3.2	0.3
Pinto beans:				
Dried, raw	8.2	19.5	12.1	7.4
Dried, cooked	71.2	8.0	5.8	2.2
Canned	73.3	5.2	4.0	1.2
Soybeans:				
Dry	8.0	15.0	—	—
Tofu	84.6	1.2	—	—
White beans:				
Dried, raw	3.6	17.7	13.4	4.3
Dried, cooked	71.2	5.4	3.9	1.5
Canned	73.6	5.6	3.9	1.7
Nuts and seeds				
Almonds, roasted	3.3	11.2	—	—
Cashews, oil-roasted	5.4	6.0	—	—
Coconut:				
Raw	47.0	9.0	8.5	0.5
Shredded	18.5	6.6	6.2	0.4
Hazelnuts, oil-roasted	1.2	6.4	—	—
Peanuts:				
Dry-roasted	1.6	8.0	7.5	0.5
Oil-roasted	2.0	8.8	8.0	0.8
Peanut butter:				
Chunky	1.1	6.6	6.0	0.6
Smooth	1.4	6.0	5.5	0.5

Table 3 Continued

Food	Moisture (g/100 g edible portion)	Dietary fiber (g/100 g edible portion)		
		Total	Insoluble	Soluble
Pecans	4.8	6.5	—	—
Pistachio nuts	3.9	10.8	—	—
Sesame seeds:				
Dry	24.6	15.4	—	—
Roasted	5.8	11.6	—	—
Walnuts	3.5	3.8	3.7	0.1
Miscellaneous				
Avocado	77.3	3.9	2.6	1.3
Beer	92.3	0.5	—	—
Candy:				
Caramels, vanilla	7.6	1.2	—	—
Milk chocolate	0.8	2.8	—	—
Carob powder	1.2	32.8	—	—
Chili powder	9.1	34.2	—	—
Chocolate, baking	0.7	15.4	—	—
Cocoa, baking	1.3	29.8	—	—
Curry powder	8.7	33.2	—	—
Jelly, apple	32.3	0.6	—	—
Pancake mix	8.3	4.5	3.5	1.0
Pepper, black	9.4	25.0	—	—
Pickles	93.4	1.1	0.7	0.4
Preserves:				
Peach	32.4	0.7	—	—
Strawberry	31.7	1.2	—	—
Olives:				
Black	80.5	2.2	2.1	0.1
Green, with pimento	76.5	2.0	1.8	0.2
Soup:				
Chicken noodle	86.5	0.5	—	—
Vegetable	84.9	1.3	—	—
Yeast, active, dry	6.8	31.6	—	—
Pasta				
Macaroni				
Dry	8.5	4.3	4.1	0.2
Cooked	69.6	2.0	1.7	0.3
Noodles:				
Dry:				
Spinach	8.5	6.8	—	—
Chow-mein	0.7	3.9	—	—
Somen	11.3	4.3	—	—
Egg	9.5	4.0	—	—
Cooked	67.3	1.8	1.3	0.5

Table 3 Continued

Food	Moisture (g/100 g edible portion)	Dietary fiber (g/100 g edible portion)		
		Total	Insoluble	Soluble
Spaghetti:				
Dry:				
Regular	9.2	3.6	2.1	1.5
Whole wheat	7.1	11.8	—	—
Spinach	8.7	10.6	—	—
Cooked	60.7	1.5	1.1	0.4
Snacks				
Corn chips	1.1	4.3	3.9	0.4
Corn puffs	1.5	1.0	—	—
Granola bars, crunchy:				
Chocolate chip	—	4.4	—	—
Cinnamon	—	5.0	—	—
Popcorn:				
Air-popped	—	15.1	—	—
Oil-popped	—	10.0	—	—
Potato chips	2.4	3.8	1.9	1.9
Pretzels				
Hard	3.5	3.7	2.8	0.9
Soft	32.7	2.5	1.6	0.9
Tortilla chips	2.0	6.5	—	—
Vegetables and vegetable products				
Artichoke	84.4	7.6	4.4	3.2
Artichoke, globe	82.5	7.9	4.7	3.2
Asparagus				
Fresh, cooked	90.5	2.1	1.6	0.5
Canned	93.3	1.6	1.2	0.4
Bamboo shoots, canned	97.4	1.5	1.4	0.1
Beans, green				
Canned	91.8	2.1	1.4	0.7
Boiled	91.8	2.5	1.5	1.0
Bean sprouts	96.2	1.2	1.1	0.1
Beets, canned	92.4	1.7	1.3	0.4
Broccoli:				
Raw	88.5	3.3	3.0	0.3
Cooked	90.2	3.5	3.1	0.4
Brussels sprouts	87.2	4.1	3.6	0.5
Cabbage:				
Raw	90.9	1.8	1.1	0.7
Boiled	94.0	1.7	1.1	0.6
Carrots:				
Raw	88.5	2.4	1.1	1.3
Cooked	90.5	2.7	1.2	1.5

Table 3 Continued

Food	Moisture (g/100 g edible portion)	Dietary fiber (g/100 g edible portion)		
		Total	Insoluble	Soluble
Cauliflower:				
Raw	92.6	1.8	1.1	0.7
Cooked	93.3	1.8	1.1	0.7
Celery:				
Raw	94.6	1.5	1.0	0.5
Cooked	95.2	1.4	0.9	0.5
Chives	92.0	3.2	—	—
Corn, sweet:				
Canned:				
Whole	76.7	2.1	1.8	0.3
Cream style	75.6	1.3	1.1	0.2
Fresh:				
Raw	76.0	3.2	3.0	0.2
Cooked	69.6	3.7	3.5	0.2
Frozen, whole	75.8	2.1	2.0	0.1
Cucumbers:				
Peeled	96.2	0.6	0.5	0.1
Unpeeled	95.8	0.9	0.8	0.1
Eggplant	—	6.6	5.3	1.3
Leek	90.3	2.9	2.0	0.9
Lettuce:				
Iceberg	96.0	0.7	0.5	0.2
Romaine	94.9	1.7	—	—
Mushrooms, canned	90.9	2.8	2.6	0.2
Onions, raw:				
Green	92.7	2.2	2.2	0.0
Yellow	90.3	1.7	1.6	0.1
Parsley	88.3	4.4	—	—
Peas, green:				
Canned	80.7	4.5	3.6	0.9
Boiled	76.9	6.7	5.0	1.7
Frozen, boiled	81.6	4.4	3.2	1.2
Peppers, green, raw	93.5	1.9	1.2	0.7
Potatoes:				
Baked, skin	73.3	2.5	1.9	0.6
Boiled,				
without skin	79.5	1.3	1.0	0.3
French fried	48.6	3.0	1.5	1.5
Pumpkin, canned	90.2	2.9	2.4	0.5
Radish, red	94.2	1.4	1.3	0.1
Rutabagas:				
Raw	89.0	2.4	1.2	1.2
Boiled	92.3	2.1	1.2	0.9
Spinach:				
Raw	91.6	2.6	2.1	0.5
Cooked	93.7	2.2	1.8	0.4

Table 3 Continued

Food	Moisture (g/100 g edible portion)	Dietary fiber (g/100 g edible portion)		
		Total	Insoluble	Soluble
Squash:				
Summer:				
Raw	93.7	1.2	—	—
Cooked	93.7	1.4	—	—
Winter:				
Raw	88.7	1.8	—	—
Cooked	89.0	2.8	—	—
Zucchini, raw	94.5	0.9	0.8	0.1
Sweet potatoes:				
Cooked	72.8	3.0	2.5	0.5
Canned	75.6	1.7	1.3	0.4
Tomatoes:				
Raw	94.5	1.2	0.8	0.4
Boiled	93.2	1.5	1.0	0.5
Canned	93.3	1.0	0.7	0.3
Sauce	90.9	1.4	0.8	0.7
Paste	74.1	4.3	—	—
Catsup	66.7	1.2	0.9	0.3
Juice	94.1	0.7	0.4	0.3
Turnip greens:				
Frozen	92.9	2.5	2.4	0.1
Cooked	93.2	3.1	2.9	0.2
Turnips	94.7	2.0	1.5	0.5
Water chestnuts	87.9	2.2	—	—

Based on published values: Am. Assoc. of Cereal Chemists, 1987; Dreher, 1987; Anderson and Bridges, 1988; Cardozo and Eitenmiller, 1988; Del Toma et al., 1988; Mongeau et al., 1989; USDA, 1989; Toma and Curtis, 1989; Ranhotra et al., 1990; Prosky and DeVries, 1992; and Marlett 1991.

REFERENCES

American Association of Cereal Chemists. (1987). Dietary fiber guide. *Cereal Foods World*. 32(8):555–570.

Anderson, J. W. and Bridges, S. R. (1998). Dietary fiber content of selected foods. *Am. J. Clin. Nutr*. 47:440–447.

Block, G., Patterson, B., and Subar, A. (1991). Fruit, vegetables, and cancer prevention: a review of the epidemiological evidence. *Nutr. Cancer* 18(1):1.

Butrum, R. R., Clifford, C. K., and Lanza, E. (1988). NCI dietary guidelines: rationale. *Am. J. Clin. Nutr*. 48:888–895.

Cardozo, M. S. and Ettenmiller, R. R. (1988). Total dietary fiber analysis of selected baked and cereal products. *Cereal Foods World*. 33(5):414–418.

Dietary Guidelines for Americans (2000). *Aim for Fitness, Build a Healthy Base, and Choose Sensibly for Good Health*. USDA and DHHS. Home and Garden Bulletin No. 232.

DeCosse, J. J., Miller, N. H., and Lesser, M. L. (1989). Effect of wheat fiber and vitamins C and E on rectal polyps in patients with familial adenomatous polyposis. *J. Natl. Cancer Inst*. 81:1290–1294.

Del Toma, E., Celemnti, A., Marcelli, M., Cappelloni, M., and Lintas, C. (1988). Food fiber choices for diabetic diets. *Am. J. Clin. Nutr.* 47:243–246.

Dreher, M. L. (1987). Dietary fiber content of food sources. *Handbook of Dietart Fiber: An Applied Approach.* Marcel Dekker, Inc., New York.

Eaton, S. B. (1990). What did our late paleolithic preagricultural ancestors eat? *Nutr. Rev.* 48(5):227–228.

Eaton, S. B., Konner, M. J., and Shostak, M. (1988). Stone agers in the fast lane: chronic degenerative disease in evolutionary perspective. *Am. J. Med.* 84:739–749.

Gordon, D. T. (1999). Defining dietary fiber—a progress report. *Cereal Foods World.* 44(5):336.

Health and Welfare Canada. (1985). *Report of the Expert Advisory Committee on Dietary Fibre to the Health Protection Branch.* Health and Welfare Canada, Ottawa.

International Food Information Council. (1991). How Americans are making food choices. *IFIC Review*, Washington, DC.

Kritchevsky, D. (1988). Dietary fiber. *Ann. Rev. Nutr.* 8:301–328.

Marlett, J. A. (1992). Content and composition of dietary fiber in 177 frequently consumed foods. *J. Am. Diet. Assoc.* 92:175–186.

Mongeau, R., Brassard, R., and Verdier, P. (1989). Measurement of dietary fiber in a total diet study. *J. Food Comp. Anal.* 2:317–326.

Pilch, S. M. (1987). *Physiological Effects and Health Consequences of Dietary Fiber*, Life Sciences Research Office. Federation of American Societies for Experimental Biology. Bethesda, Maryland. Contract Number FDA 223-84-2059, pp. 162, 163.

Prosky, L. and DeVries, J. (1992). Controlling Dietary Fiber in Food Products. Van Nostrand Reinhold, New York.

Ranhotra, G. S., Gelroth, J. A., and Astroth, K. (1990). Total and soluble fiber in selected bakery and other cereal products. *Cereal Chem.* 67(5):499–501.

Siegal, S. W. (1968). Biochemistry of the plant cell wall. *Comprehensive Biochemistry.* M. Florkin and E. H. Stotz (Eds.). Elsevier Publishing Company, Amsterdam, pp. 1–51.

Slavin, J. L. (1987). Dietary fiber: classification, chemical analysis, and food sources. *J. Am. Diet. Assoc.* 87(9):1164–1171.

Walker, A. R. P. (1993). Does the dietary fiber hypothesis really "work?" *Cereal Foods World.* 38(3): 128–134.

2
Dietary Fiber and Cardiovascular Disease

Judith A. Marlett
University of Wisconsin, Madison, Wisconsin

I. INTRODUCTION

The foundation of the recognition of a relationship between diet and cardiovascular disease (CVD) was the demonstration that different fats have significantly different effects on blood lipid levels. These seminal observations were made during two series of classic experiments conducted nearly 35 years ago by Keys et al. (1) and Hegsted et al. (2). These findings have been duplicated often, but rarely with the same rigor shown by these two eminent scientists, and the outcome of all further studies is fundamentally unchanged (3). In the intervening time, several other aspects of dietary fats (e.g., different types of unsaturated and saturated fats and oxidized lipids) were and are being studied for their effects on blood lipid levels (4–7).

Specific nutrients, such as (a) vitamins E and C, cobalamin, pyridoxine, and folate; (b) the minerals potassium, calcium, magnesium, and selenium; (c) specific characteristics of nutrients, (e.g. antioxidants); (d) specific foods, herbs, and spices and other botanical agents; (e) bacteria; and (f) specific components of foods, such as saponins, phytosterols and terpenes, have been explored for their effects on blood lipid levels (8,9). In some cases, unrealistic amounts of these components have been tested. But in many other instances, the component has been shown to lower undesirable concentrations of blood lipids. These nutrients and components in food are generally consumed as part of an incredibly complex mix of chemicals we call a varied diet.

Within this complex milieu, it is surprising that any beneficial response to dietary fiber consumption was identified, particularly since dietary fiber is not a single entity but rather a complex mixture of polysaccharides and lignin (10). In addition, accurate measurement of fiber is difficult (10,11), and interpretation of fiber's effects are confounded by other lipid-altering food components that frequently are part of the fiber source (12).

The role of dietary fiber in the modulation of blood lipid concentrations was initially explored in the 1960s. In fact, one of the earliest demonstrations of the hypocholesterolemic response to dietary fiber was made by Keys et al. (13) in a series of experiments designed to explain why serum cholesterol levels were lower in Italian than in North American populations. They reported that ingestion of 15 g/d of pectin, along with a constant diet, reduced blood cholesterol concentrations by about 5% in healthy adult men. Trowell (14) presented a perspective in nutrition in 1972 to support his hypothesis that "high consumption of natural starchy carbohydrates, taken with their full complement of fiber, is protective against hyperlipidemia and ischemic heart disease."

It is now well established that certain sources of dietary fiber, independent of the fat or carbohydrate content of the diet, can lower serum cholesterol concentrations. Fiber specifically affects the concentration of the major fraction of cholesterol in blood, that carried by low-density lipoproteins (LDL). Blood concentrations of triacylglycerols and high-density lipoproteins are unaffected by these fibers.

The purpose of this chapter is threefold. First, the effects of dietary fibers and high-fiber diets on serum cholesterol levels are reviewed. Second, the kinds and properties of serum cholesterol–lowering sources of dietary fiber are summarized. Third, data are presented to support the conclusion that fibers lower blood cholesterol level only if they are viscous; this viscosity becomes concentrated in the ileum, interfering with bile acid absorption and subsequently stimulating bile acid synthesis from LDL-derived cholesterol (12). This review is based on the generally accepted premise that measuring blood cholesterol levels provides an indication of likely impact on cardiovascular disease. When data are available, the focus is primarily on the results of human studies.

II. EPIDEMIOLOGICAL ASSOCIATIONS

Humble (15) and Anderson (16) summarized the evidence supporting an inverse relationship between CVD and dietary fiber. Interest in this association grew out of the initial observations in Africa by Walker (17), Trowell (14), and Burkitt (18) that ''Western'' diseases were not prevalent among native Africans who consumed high-fiber, low-fat diets and who had very different lifestyles. The results of prospective studies since that time have been variable. In the majority (five of eight) of the prospective studies, the initial inverse correlation between some measure of CVD and dietary fiber intake was retained, although sometimes weakened, after data were adjusted to account for other diet factors (19–23). In three other prospective studies the statistical significance of the associations between CVD and dietary fiber was lost when dietary data were adjusted, usually for energy (24–26). Results of epidemiological studies using ecological case comparisons or cross-sectional population surveys also have not yielded uniform results (16).

III. DIET AND CVD PREVENTION OR REGRESSION

Results of studies that used multiple diet changes to achieve lower fat and higher carbohydrate intakes suggest that diet can have a significant, favorable impact on the incidence and progression of cardiovascular disease. While a reduction in fat intake has a more pronounced effect on blood lipid levels, the higher carbohydrate aspect of these diets undoubtedly increased fiber intake. Such diets resulted in significantly less CVD (27), inhibited progression of CVD (28), and induced actual regression of CVD (29) in clinical trials. Severe changes in diet and lifestyle also induced regression of cardiovascular lesions (30). One study was not able to demonstrate a uniform reduction in mortality rates using a diet expected to lower the frequency of CVD events (31). In one carefully conducted, 8-month study, pectin, compared to cellulose, significantly increased aortic sudanophilia in vervet monkeys (32). It is unlikely that consumption of an isolated fiber supplement without substantial changes in dietary fat intake would affect the results seen when both dietary components are changed.

IV. HYPOCHOLESTEROLEMIC DIETARY FIBER SOURCES

Many sources of dietary fiber have been evaluated for their effects on serum lipid concentrations. The details of most of these studies have been admirably summarized in table form in other

Table 1 Purified and Food Sources of
Hypocholesterolemic Dietary Fibers

Purified sources	Food sources
Beet fiber	Apples
Guar gum	Barley
Gum arabic	Beans and other legumes
Karaya gum	Fruits and vegetables
Konjac mannan	Oatmeal and oat bran
Locust bean gum	Rice hulls
Pectin	
Psyllium seed husk	
Soy polysaccharide	
Xanthan gum	

reviews (33–38). Fibers reported to lower serum cholesterol concentrations significantly in more than one human study are listed in Table 1. Fiber sources having no effect on serum cholesterol levels in humans include purified wood pulp cellulose, wheat bran, and oat hulls.

Responses in humans have been variable after ingestion of a few fibers, such as purified lignin, carrots, corn bran or maize, and diets containing large amounts of fruits and vegetables. For example, blood cholesterol levels significantly decreased in one study when an atypical diet containing less than 20% energy as fat and over 24 g/1000 kcal dietary fiber was modified to contain about one third of the fiber as soluble fiber, compared to 17% soluble in the control diet (39). In another study in which the constant diet was more typical, containing 34% of energy as fat, increasing dietary fiber intake using a mix of foods, from about 5 to 14 g/1000 kcal, which produced a 2.7-fold increase in soluble fiber, had no effect on serum cholesterol concentrations (40). The diet used in the latter study was consistent with the guideline set by the US Food and Drug Administration for adequate dietary fiber intakes, of 12 g total fiber/1000 kcal.

Single reports of lower blood cholesterol concentration after ingestion of a fiber source (e.g., prunes, rhubarb stalk), have not been confirmed (41,42). Much has been written about resistant starch as a dietary fiber source, but few studies have examined its effect on blood cholesterol levels. Asp (43) has concluded that data are too limited to formulate a conclusion about its hypocholesterolemic potential. The variable results from different studies may be explained in part by the use of very different sources of the starch.

The hypocholesterolemic potential of many other fibers have been evaluated in animal models (44,45). Because of the wide range and varying rigor of the experimental designs used in human and animal studies, confirmation of human studies and testing in humans of agents observed to be hypocholesterolemic in animals are important components of developing a hypolipidemic profile for a food or food component.

V. HOW DOES DIETARY FIBER LOWER BLOOD CHOLESTEROL LEVELS?

A. Changing Diet Intake

Sources of dietary fiber may displace some hyperlipidemic agent in the diet or alter the body's sterol pool (Table 2). Human experiments involving a dietary fiber source usually have been conducted in one of two ways. In some studies a ''metabolic'' diet is followed, that is, a diet that is constant in composition and in which intake is rigidly controlled. In other instances

Table 2 Effects of Increased
Dietary Fiber Intake

Change of diet composition
Reduced cholesterol absorption
Reduced bile acid absorption
Change of bile acid synthesis
Reduced cholesterol biosynthesis

---

subjects are counseled to follow specific dietary guidelines, and food intake is assessed one or more times, usually by written questionnaire, during the course of the study to determine whether intake has changed. Clearly, a study using a metabolic diet will generate more accurate results, because sources of diet and nondiet variation have been reduced to a minimum. However, metabolically controlled experiments are costly. When diet is not constant, monitoring adherence to diet guidelines is of critical importance. A good deal of the variation among the studies of hypocholesterolemia with fiber consumption is likely a consequence of subtle changes in the underlying diet which are not detected by most currently used methods of monitoring nutrient intake. This is particularly true for fat and energy intakes, because small changes in both of these diet variables could confound blood lipid responses but not be detected as significant changes in the mean intakes of the study population.

B. Altering Dietary Cholesterol Absorption

Carefully conducted studies that have been repeatedly confirmed have established that a fiber is hypocholesterolemic because it alters the body's total sterol pool. The hypothesis that fibers lower blood cholesterol levels by interfering with absorption of dietary cholesterol is attractive because of its simplicity. However, it is unlikely that fiber-induced hypocholesterolemia is a result primarily of decreased exogenous cholesterol absorption. This is because exogenous cholesterol represents only a quarter to a third of the body's cholesterol, and a substantial change in the proportion absorbed would still represent only a relatively small amount. Some fibers may decrease absorption of dietary cholesterol by altering the composition of the bile acid pool. Pectin (46) and oat bran (47) increased the portion of the total bile acid pool that was deoxycholic acid (DCA). DCA has been reported to decrease the absorption of exogenous cholesterol from 46 to 28 μmol/h during intestinal perfusion in humans (48).

C. Altering Cholesterol Biosynthesis

Demonstrating a reduction in endogenous cholesterol biosynthesis, the major source of the body's cholesterol, is difficult in humans. Many of the data to support such a change are indirect or come from animal experiments. However, data that are available do indicate that endogenous cholesterol synthesis may be affected. Hydroxymethylglutaryl-CoA (HMG CoA) reductase, the rate-limiting enzyme in the cholesterol biosynthesis pathway, is significantly inhibited by DCA, compared to cholic acid (CA) or chenodeoxycholic acid (CDCA) (49). The increase in the proportion of the bile acid pool that was DCA produced by oat bran (47) and pectin (46) supports the hypothesis that part of the hypocholesterolemic action of fiber is a consequence of its inhibitory effect on endogenous cholesterol synthesis. However, cholesterol biosynthesis increased following supplementation of low-cholesterol diets with psyllium (50) or large amounts (40–50 g/d) of pectin (51). When the diet contained typical amounts of cholesterol, psyllium supplementation had no effect on cholesterol synthesis (52). The relative hydrophobicity of the bile acid pool may indicate the extent of the effect on cholesterol metabolism (53,54).

D. Increasing Bile Acid Synthesis

Cholesterol carried by LDL is quantitatively the most important substrate for bile acid synthesis (55). It is estimated that 40–50% of cholesterol is eliminated daily through bile acid synthesis (49,56). Beginning in the early 1970s, Kritchevsky and Story (45,57,58) focused interest on this possible "sink" for blood cholesterol with a series of studies in which the in vitro binding of different bile acids by various fiber sources was examined. Although not all of the in vitro findings have been consistent with subsequent in vivo observations, these important experiments were insightful and ahead of their time.

Two laboratories have unambiguously demonstrated, using stable isotope-labeled bile acids to study bile acid kinetics, that at least two hypocholesterolemic dietary fibers, psyllium (52) and oat bran (47), stimulate bile acid synthesis and alter the composition of the bile acid pool. Oat bran significantly decreased pool size of CA and doubled DCA pool size, whereas psyllium increased CDCA pool size but had no effect on pool sizes of CA or DCA. Neither fiber changed the size of the total bile acid pool (47,52). These studies also revealed that turnover of one or both primary bile acids was increased when bile acid kinetics during fiber supplementation were compared to what was measured during a low-fiber diet control period. The differing effects on the composition of the bile acid pool could be due to the fiber source or to the use of different study populations—normocholesterolemic in the oat bran study and hypercholesterolemic in the psyllium study.

E. Increasing Bile Acid Excretion

Bile acid synthesis reflects fecal losses when total pool size does not change and sterol balance is in steady state. These conditions were met in both of the bile acid kinetic studies (47,52), and thus, it would be predicted from the increased synthesis measured during these studies that fecal sterol excretion also would increase during fiber supplementation. Fecal sterol excretion was increased significantly during the oat bran study (47) but not during the psyllium study (52). Failure to detect a significant increase in fecal excretion when serum cholesterol concentrations are lowered by dietary fiber supplementation has been reported in about half of the studies in which both parameters were measured (36). Forty to fifty percent of bile acids in excreta are microbially produced derivatives, which are not quantitated during gas chromatographic analysis (59,60). It is likely that the inability to account for these bile acid derivatives is responsible for insignificant fecal losses of the bile acids in studies in which serum cholesterol concentrations are significantly lowered by fiber. Increases in ileal bile acid excretion of 40–50% during oat bran (61) or psyllium (62) consumption supports the contention that fecal steroid excretion is an insensitive measure of bile acid loss or synthesis.

VI. HOW DOES FIBER INCREASE BILE ACID EXCRETION?

Two mechanisms have been proposed to explain the hypocholesterolemic properties of some dietary fibers. One is that increased amounts of propionate are produced during microbial fermentation of these fibers and that the propionate inhibits cholesterol biosynthesis (34). The other proposed mechanism is that the viscosity of these fibers becomes concentrated in the ileum and interferes with bile acid absorption (12).

A. Short-Chain Fatty Acids and Fermentation

Most hypocholesterolemic dietary fibers are rapidly fermented and would be expected to create an acute influx of SCFA into the blood. Nonetheless, a wide variety of data from human and animal studies do not consistently support a role for SCFA in the cholesterol-lowering activity of dietary fiber. In vitro hepatic cholesterol biosynthesis from labeled acetate is inhibited by propionate at concentrations of 1.0 mmol (63). However, in the same set of experiments, 2.5 mmol of propionate was needed to inhibit cholesterol biosynthesis from tritiated water or labeled mevalonate (63). These inhibitory effects on cholesterol biosynthesis were not reproduced when physiological concentrations of propionate or acetate were incubated with isolated hepatocytes in the presence of tritiated water (64). Oral propionate had no effect on the blood cholesterol levels in both a rat (65) and a human (66) study, although the activity of HMG CoA reductase activity was slightly depressed in the rat study.

An increase in the concentration of propionate in the cecum occurring with oral β-cyclo-dextrin was accompanied by increased bile acid excretion and microsomal HMG CoA reductase activity, responses that would be consistent with induction of cholesterol biosynthesis (65). However, body weight gain of the test animals was significantly less than that of the control group (65). Surgical removal of the cecum or cecum and colon (67), but not the prevention of coprophagy (68), did negate the hypocholesterolemic response to a beet fiber preparation or oat bran.

In humans, plasma cholesterol levels actually increased when acetate was intrarectally infused (69,70) or rapidly fermented lactulose was consumed (71). Co-infusion of propionate with acetate reduced acetate incorporation into cholesterol, although the small number of subjects prevented the effect from reaching statistical significance (70).

B. Viscosity of Hypocholesterolemic Dietary Fibers

Most viscous dietary fibers are also rapidly fermented to SCFA. Thus, if an independent role for viscosity is to be demonstrated, it is necessary to separate viscosity from SCFA production. Viscosity and SCFA production have been separated by (a) conducting experiments using viscous fibers that are not fermented, (b) using a fermented viscous fiber that has been modified to reduce the viscosity, and (c) employing germfree animals in the experiment.

3-Hydroxylpropyl methylcellulose, a cellulose ether, is not fermented (72). Using this non-fermented synthetic product at three different viscosities, Gallaher et al. (73) demonstrated that the viscosity of the diet or of small bowel digesta was inversely proportional to blood cholesterol levels in hamsters. Lumenal viscosity produced by 3-hydroxypropyl methylcellulose also has been inversely correlated with cholesterol absorption in hamsters (74). In another experiment, methylcelluloses of differing viscosities had no effect on rat blood cholesterol levels (75). Blood cholesterol levels are difficult to perturb in the rat unless they are first elevated (76), which may explain why Topping et al. (75) did not observe a response to the viscous cellulose ester.

Reducing the viscosity of a hypocholesterolemic fiber does appear to lower its effectiveness. Partially hydrolyzed guar gum is not as effective a hypocholesterolemic agent as the unhydrolyzed, more viscous product (77). Isolating some viscous fibers reduces the molecular weight and viscosity, which probably explains why β-glucan isolated from oat bran did not lower blood cholesterol concentrations in one human study (78). Hydrolysis of β-glucans in oat bran eliminated the increased ileal excretion of bile acids that was observed when the unhydrolyzed oat bran was ingested by human ileostomates (79).

Germ-free animals will have no microflora and, thus, do not ferment dietary fiber (80). Guar gum still lowered LDL cholesterol and plasma and hepatic total cholesterol concentrations when germ-free animals were used (81), indicating that SCFA production is not necessary to achieve cholesterol lowering by fiber.

VII. CONFOUNDERS IN HYPOCHOLESTEROLEMIC DIETARY FIBERS

Many natural constituents in plants are being examined for their effects on human metabolism, including lipid metabolism. These botanicals are frequently present in dietary fiber sources. With few exceptions, there has been little research to distinguish the effects of the fiber from those that could be attributed to some other component in the fiber source. Two components of fiber sources that have been studied for their hypocholesterolemic potential are protein and tocotrienols.

A. Plant Protein

Ingestion of soy protein has an established history of lowering blood cholesterol levels in both humans and animal models (82–85). The response differs from that observed when fiber is consumed, as blood triglycerides as well as cholesterol concentrations are usually affected (85). Although the active agent has not been defined, the failure to induce hypolipidemia in female primates fed soy from which the estrogens had been extracted suggest that phytoestrogens, and not the fiber per se, is the active agent (86). Several phytosterols have been shown to lower serum cholesterol levels (87). Three different soy protein preparations had no effect on ileal bile acid or cholesterol excretion in a short-term study in human ileostomates, suggesting that sterol excretion is not involved as the mechanism (88).

Kritchevsky (83) published data from an experiment in rabbits to support his hypothesis that higher ratios of lysine to arginine were more hypercholesterolemic. The experiment used three sources of protein—fish, casein, and whole milk—none of which are known to contain estrogenic compounds. Casein is frequently used as the protein source in the control diets of these experiments, and its hypercholesterolemic effect, at least in rabbits, may be dependent on a high-cholesterol diet (89). As a different approach to exploring the role of protein, doubling protein intake primarily with animal sources, from about 10 to 25% of energy, did reduce serum cholesterol levels in normolipidemic and moderately hyperlipidemic adults when total fat intake was low (25% of energy) (90).

B. Tocotrienols

Tocotrienols are naturally occurring farnesylated analogs of the tocopherols that have been found in the lipophilic fractions of whole oats, oat bran, barley, and rice bran and in palm oil (91–93). Tocotrienols reduce HMG CoA reductase activity and protein levels in HepG2 cells and appear to modulate the mevalonate pathway by suppressing the enzyme posttranscriptionally (94). In humans following the American Heart Association Step I diet, a tocotrienol concentrate from palm oil providing about 250 mg/d of tocos significantly lowered total plasma and LDL cholesterol concentrations and levels of ApoB (95). However, in another study in which oat bran significantly lowered serum cholesterol at one month, no indication of a change in cholesterol biosynthesis could be detected when cholesterol synthesis precursors were measured in the blood (96).

Toco dietary supplements have not uniformly reduced blood cholesterol levels (92,95, 97,98), in part because little attention has been paid to the composition of the supplement. In several experiments, toco mixtures have been used that would not be expected to be effective, had the composition been determined. For example, γ-tocotrienol is the most effective inhibitor of cholesterol biosynthesis, being 30 times more effective than the α-analog (99). Yet, α-tocotrienol is usually the dominant tocotrienol in cereal grains or concentrates (91,100,101). In addition, α-tocopherol, which can be present in grains in significant amounts, has been demonstrated to attenuate the hypocholesterolemic effect of tocotrienols (102).

The concentration of the different toco isomers varies greatly among different genotypes of the same grain (101) and can be further modified by growing (101), storage (103,104), and processing (105) conditions. A third reason for the inability to induce hypocholesterolemia with tocos in animals is the design of the experiment. Available evidence indicates the tocos downregulate endogenous cholesterol synthesis. Many animal models used to study blood cholesterol levels are fed diets supplemented with cholesterol to elevate the normally low blood levels. This exogenous cholesterol overwhelms any effect of the tocos by inhibiting their likely site of action.

VIII. ANALYTICAL MEASUREMENT TO PREDICT HYPOCHOLESTEROLEMIC PROPERTY OF DIETARY FIBER

The most common descripter of hypocholesterolemic fibers is that they are soluble. In reality, not all soluble fibers lower blood cholesterol levels. The data generated over the past 20 years argue convincingly that only those soluble fibers that are also viscous perturb whole body sterol balance. Measuring the active fraction of fiber analytically instead of biologically remains elusive. Many of the viscous fibers are non-Newtonian, making it very difficult and expensive to measure viscosity. The proportion of total fiber measured as the soluble fraction can vary by 100% using methodologies accepted by countries throughout the world (11). Even if viscosity and the proportion of total fiber that is soluble can be accurately measured, few studies have compared analytical results with the biological behavior of the analyzed fiber in the gastrointestinal lumen.

IX. CONCLUSIONS: MECHANISMS OF ACTION FOR HYPOCHOLESTEROLEMIC DIETARY FIBERS

Fiber is the grandparent of the current wave of interest in functional foods and food components. An adequate fiber diet has a variety of specific healthful benefits, the major one of which is optimizing gastrointestinal physiological function. In addition, several therapeutic roles for specific fibers have been identified.

With respect to CVD, only soluble dietary fibers that are also viscous lower blood cholesterol concentrations. Available data support a role for the viscosity in the ileum where it becomes concentrated after most food has been digested and absorbed (12). This lumenal viscosity interferes with bile acid absorption. Actual binding or chelation is probably not required. The resulting loss of bile acids is not always detected, because up to half of fecal steroids are microbially produced metabolites that are not quantitated during fecal steroid analysis (59,60). The increased loss in bile acids stimulates bile acid synthesis, which uses LDL cholesterol as a substrate (47,52).

Bile acid pool size need not be changed, but its composition may be. Though more data are needed, available evidence suggests that increasing the hydrophobicity of the bile acid pool will suppress endogenous cholesterol synthesis (53,54). Suppressing endogenous cholesterol synthesis also promotes lower blood cholesterol levels. Fermentation and its primary product, SCFA, probably have only a minor role, if any, in producing hypocholesterolemia. In fact, a rapid influx of SCFA that would occur with the fermentation of a highly soluble fiber provides substrate for cholesterol synthesis.

Efforts to measure analytically the hypocholesterolemic potential of a fiber remain problematic. It appears that the fiber must be not only soluble, but also viscous.

Because of differences in analytical methodologies, the proportion of a fiber that is analyzed as the soluble component ranges from 15 to 50% of the total fiber (11). Standardization of the methodology for fiber analysis is not really a solution, as the critical measurement is the solubility behavior in the lumen of the gastrointestinal tract.

Similarly, accurate measurement of the hypocholesterolemic property, viscosity, is difficult and expensive if the material is non-Newtonian, as most foodstuffs are. Again, retention of this viscosity in the gut lumen needs to be verified to label the material as hypocholesterolemic. Problems are exacerbated when a fiber fraction is isolated for more definitive studies and analyses. Isolation decreases molecular weight, molecular interaction, and viscosity; the net effect is diminishing hypocholesterolemia.

A diet that prevents CVD or slows its progression is one that is lower in fat ($\sim$25–30% of energy) and higher in complex carbohydrate ($\sim$60% of energy). A higher fiber intake is a natural outgrowth of such a food intake pattern, although the proportion of soluble fiber remains about 25–35% of the total fiber (40). Southgate (106) and Jenkins (107) both recently discussed protective or optimal diets to reduce risk for degenerative diseases. Such diets composed of minimally processed foods undoubtedly also will include other hypocholesterolemic components, including those such as phytoestrogens, vegetable protein, and tocotrienols that have confounded studies of dietary fiber.

REFERENCES

1. Keys A, Anderson JT, Grande F. Prediction of serum-cholesterol responses of man to changes in fats in the diet. Lancet 2:959–966, 1957.
2. Hegsted DM, McGandy RB, Myers ML, Stare FJ. Quantitative effects of dietary fat on serum cholesterol in man. Am J Clin Nutr 17:281–295, 1965.
3. Hegsted DM, Ausman LM, Johnson JA, Dallal GE. Dietary fat and serum lipids: an evaluation of the experimental data. Am J Clin Nutr 57:875–883, 1993.
4. Drevon CA, Nenseter MS, Brude IR, Finstad HS, Kolset SO, Rustan AC. Omega-3 fatty acids—nutritional aspects. Can J Cardiol 11(suppl G):47G–54G, 1995.
5. Katan MB, Mensink RP, Van Tol A, Zock PL. Dietary *trans* fatty acids and their impact on plasma lipoproteins. Can J Cardiol 11(suppl G):36G–38G, 1995.
6. Klör HU, Hauenschild A, Holbach I, Schnell-Kretschmer H, Stroh S. Nutrition and cardiovascular disease. Eur J Med Res 2:243–257, 1997.
7. Hassel CA. Animal models: new cholesterol raising and lowering nutrients. Curr Opin Lipidol 9:7–10, 1998.
8. Mancini M, Parfitt VJ, Rubba P. Antioxidants in the Mediterranean diet. Can J Cardiol 11(suppl G):105G–109G, 1995.
9. Kendler BS. Recent nutritional approaches to the prevention and therapy of cardiovascular disease. Prog Cardiovasc Nurs 12:3–23, 1997.
10. Marlett JA. Analysis of dietary fiber in foods. In: D Kritchevsky, C Bonfield, JW Anderson, eds. Dietary Fiber—Chemistry, Physiology, and Health Effects. New York: Plenum Press, 1990, pp 31–48.
11. Marlett JA. Soluble dietary fiber workshop. In: D Kritchevsky, C Bonfield, eds. Dietary Fiber in Health and Disease. New York: Plenum Press, 1997, pp 311–313.

12. Marlett JA. Sites and mechanisms for the hypocholesterolemic actions of soluble dietary fiber sources. In: D Kritchevsky, C Bonfield, eds. Dietary Fiber in Health and Disease. New York: Plenum Press, 1997, pp 109–121.

13. Keys A, Grande F, Anderson JT. Fiber and pectin in the diet and serum cholesterol concentrations in man. Proc Soc Exp Biol Med 106:555–558, 1961.

14. Trowell H. Ischemic heart disease and dietary fiber. Am J Clin Nutr 25:926–932, 1972.

15. Humble C. The evolving epidemiology of fiber and heart disease. In: D Kritchevsky, C Bonfield, eds. Dietary Fiber in Health and Disease. New York: Plenum Press, 1997, pp 15–26.

16. Anderson JW. Dietary fibre, complex carbohydrate and coronary artery disease. Can J Cardiol 11(suppl G):55G–62G, 1995.

17. Walker ARP. Some aspects of nutritional research in South Africa. Nutr Rev 14:321–324, 1956.

18. Burkitt DP. Some diseases characteristic of modern western civilization: a possible common causative factor. Clin Radiol 24:271–280, 1973.

19. Morris JN, Marr JW, Clayton DG. Diet and heart: a postscript. Br Med J 2:1307–1314, 1977.

20. Khaw KT, Barrett-Connor E. Dietary fiber and reduced ischemic heart disease mortality rates in men and women: a 12-year prospective study. Am J Epidemiol 126:1093–1102, 1987.

21. Humble CG, Malarcher AG, Tyroler HA. Dietary fiber and coronary heart disease in middle-aged hypercholesterolemic men. Am J Prev Med 9:197–202, 1993.

22. Pietinen P, Rimm EB, Korhonen P, Hartman AM, Willett WC, Albanes D, Virtamo J. Intake of dietary fiber and risk of coronary heart disease in a cohort of Finnish men. Circulation 94:2720–2727, 1996.

23. Rimm EB, Ascherio A, Giovannucci E, Spiegelman D, Stampfer MJ, Willett WC. Vegetable, fruit, cereal fiber intake and risk of coronary heart disease among men. JAMA 275:447–451, 1996.

24. Kromhout D, Bosschieter EB, Coulander CD. Dietary fibre and 10-year mortality from coronary heart disease, cancer and all causes. The Zutphen Study. Lancet 2:518–522, 1982.

25. Kushi LH. Re: total energy intake: implications for epidemiologic analyses. Am J Epidemiol 126:981–982, 1987.

26. Fehily AM, Yarnell JWG, Sweetnam PM, Elwood PC. Diet and ischaemic heart disease: the Caerphilly study. Br J Nutr 69:303–314, 1993.

27. Hjermann I, Byre KV, Holme I, Leren P. Effect of diet and smoking intervention on the incidence of coronary heart disease. Report of the Oslo study group of a randomized trial in healthy men. Lancet 2:1303–1306, 1981.

28. Arntzenius AC, Kromhout D, Barth JD, Reiber JHC, Bruschke AVG, Buis B, van Gent CM, Kempen-Voogd N, Strikwerda S, van der Velde EA. Diet, lipoproteins, and the progression of coronary atherosclerosis. The Leiden intervention trial. N Engl J Med 312:805–811, 1985.

29. Watts GF, Lewis B, Brunt JNH, Lewis ES, Coltart DJ, Smith LDR, Mann JI, Swan AV. Effects on coronary artery disease of lipid-lowering diet, or diet plus cholestyramine, in the St. Thomas atherosclerosis regression study (STARS). Lancet 339:563–569, 1992.

30. Ornish D, Brown SE, Scherwitz LW, Billings JH, Armstrong WT, Ports TA, McLanahan SM, Kirkeeide RL, Brand RJ, Gould KL. Can lifestyle changes reverse coronary heart disease? The lifestyle heart trial. Lancet 336:129–133, 1990.

31. Burr ML, Gilbert JF, Holliday RM, Elwood PC, Fehily AM, Rogers A, Sweetnam PM, Deadman NM. Effects of changes in fat, fish, and fibre intakes on death and myocardial reinfarction: diet and reinfarction trial. Lancet 2:757–761, 1989.

32. Kritchevsky D, Davison LM, Goodman GT, Tepper SA, Mendelsohn D. Influence of dietary fiber on lipids and aortic composition of vervet monkeys. Lipids 21:338–341, 1986.

33. Pilch SM, ed. Physiologic effects and health consequences of dietary fiber. Bethesda, MD: Life Sciences Research Office, Federation of American Societies for Experimental Biology, 1987.

34. Anderson JW, Deakins DA, Bridges SR. Soluble fiber: hypocholesterolemic effects and proposed mechanisms. In: D Kritchevsky, C Bonfield, JW Anderson, eds. Dietary Fiber—Chemistry, Physiology, and Health Effects. New York: Plenum Press, 1990, pp 339–363.

35. Truswell AS, Beynen AC. Dietary fibre and plasma lipids: potential for prevention and treatment of hyperlipidaemias. In: TF Schweizer, CA Edwards, eds. Dietary Fibre—A Component of Food. London: Springer-Verlag, 1992, pp 295–332.

36. Jenkins DJA, Spadafora PJ, Jenkins AL, Rainey-Macdonald CG. Fiber in the treatment of hyperlipidemia. In: GA Spiller, ed. CRC Handbook of Dietary Fiber in Human Nutrition, 2nd ed. Boca Raton, FL: CRC Press, 1993, pp 419–438.

37. Lairon D. Dietary fibres: effects on lipid metabolism and mechanisms of action. Eur J Clin Nutr 50:125–133, 1996.

38. Behall KM. Dietary fiber: nutritional lessons for macronutrient substitutes. Ann NY Acad Sci 819: 142–154, 1997.

39. Jenkins DJA, Wolever TMS, Rao AV, Hegele RA, Mitchell SJ, Ransom TPP, Boctor DL, Spadafora PJ, Jenkins AL, Mehling C, Relle LK, Connelly PW, Story JA, Furumoto EJ, Corey P, Würsch P. Effect on blood lipids of very high intakes of fiber in diets low in saturated fat and cholesterol. N Engl J Med 329:21–26, 1993.

40. Haack VS, Chesters JG, Vollendorf NW, Story JA, Marlett JA. Increasing amounts of dietary fiber provided by foods normalizes physiological response of the large bowel without altering calcium balance or fecal steroid excretion. Am J Clin Nutr 68:615–622, 1998.

41. Tinker LF, Schneeman BO, Davis PA, Gallaher DD, Waggoner CR. Consumption of prunes as a source of dietary fiber in men with mild hypercholesterolemia. Am J Clin Nutr 53:1259–1265, 1991.

42. Goel V, Ooraikul B, Basu TK. Cholesterol lowering effects of rhubarb stalk fiber in hypercholesterolemic men. J Am Coll Nutr 16:600–604, 1997.

43. Asp N-G. Resistant starch—an update on its physiological effects. In: D Kritchevsky, C Bonfield, eds. Dietary Fiber in Health and Disease. New York: Plenum Press, 1997, pp 201–210.

44. Shinnick FL, Marlett JA. Physiological responses to dietary oats in animal models. In: PJ Wood, ed. Oat Bran. St Paul, MN: American Association of Cereal Chemists, Inc, 1993, pp 113–137.

45. Kritchevsky D, Story JA. Influence of dietary fiber on cholesterol metabolism in experimental animals. In: GA Spiller, ed. CRC Handbook of Dietary Fiber in Human Nutrition, 2nd ed. Boca Raton, FL: CRC Press, 1993, pp 163–178.

46. Hillman LC, Peters SG, Fisher CA, Pomare EW. Effects of fibre components pectin, cellulose, and lignin on bile salt metabolism and biliary lipid composition in man. Gut 27:29–36, 1986.

47. Marlett JA, Hosig KB, Vollendorf NW, Shinnick FL, Haack VS, Story JA. Mechanism of serum cholesterol reduction by oat bran. Hepatology 20:1450–1457, 1994.

48. Leiss O, von Bergmann K, Streicher U, Strotkoetler H. Effect of three different dihydroxy bile acids on intestinal cholesterol absorption in normal volunteers. Gastroenterology 87:144–149, 1984.

49. Heuman DM, Vlahcevic ZR, Bailey ML, Hylemon PB. Regulation of bile acid synthesis. II. Effect of bile acid feeding on enzymes regulating hepatic cholesterol and bile acid synthesis in the rat. Hepatology 8:892–897, 1988.

50. Miettinen TA, Tarpila S. Serum lipids and cholesterol metabolism during guar gum, plantago ovata and high fibre treatments. Clin Chim Acta 183:253–262, 1989.

51. Miettinen TA, Tarpila S. Effect of pectin on serum cholesterol, fecal bile acids and biliary lipids in normolipidemic and hyperlipidemic individuals. Clin Chim Acta 79:471–477, 1977.

52. Everson GT, Daggy BP, McKinley C, Story JA. Effects of psyllium hydrophilic mucilloid on LDL-cholesterol and bile acid synthesis in hypercholesterolemic men. J Lipid Res 33:1183–1192, 1992.

53. Heuman DM. Quantitative estimation of the hydrophilic-hydrophobic balance of mixed bile salt solutions. J Lipid Res 30:719–730, 1989.

54. Story JA, Furumoto EJ, Buhman KK. Dietary fiber and bile acid metabolism—an update. In: D Kritchevsky, C Bonfield, eds. Dietary Fiber in Health and Disease. New York: Plenum Press, 1997, pp 259–266.

55. Schwartz CC, Berman M, Vlahcevic ZR, Swell L. Multicompartmental analysis of cholesterol metabolism in man. J Clin Invest 70:863–876, 1982.

56. Vlahcevic ZR, Heuman DM, Hylemon PB. Regulation of bile acid synthesis. Hepatology 13:590–600, 1991.

57. Kritchevsky D, Story JA. Binding of bile salts in vitro by non-nutritive fiber. J Nutr 104:458–462, 1974.

58. Story JA, Kritchevsky D. Comparison of the binding of various bile acids and bile salts in vitro by several types of fiber. J Nutr 106:1292–1297, 1976.

59. Tandon R, Axelson M, Sjöval J. Selective liquid chromatographic isolation and gas chromatographic-mass spectrometric analysis of ketonic bile acids in faeces. J Chromatogr 302:1–14, 1984.

60. Setchell KDR, Lawson AM, Tanida N, Sjöval J. General methods for the analysis of metabolic profiles of bile acids and related compounds in feces. J Lipid Res 24:1085–1100, 1985.

61. Zhang J-X, Hallmans G, Andersson H, Bosaeus I, Åman P, Tidehag P, Stenling R, Lundin E, Dahlgran S. Effect of oat bran on plasma cholesterol and bile acid excretion in nine subjects with ileostomies. Am J Clin Nutr 56:99–105, 1992.

62. Gelissen IC, Brodie B, Eastwood MA. Effect of *Plantago ovata* (psyllium) husk and seeds on sterol metabolism: studies in normal and ileostomy subjects. Am J Clin Nutr 59:395–400, 1994.

63. Wright RS, Anderson JW, Bridges SR. Propionate inhibits hepatocyte lipid synthesis. Proc Soc Exp Biol Med 195:26–29, 1990.

64. Nishina PM, Freedland RA. Effects of propionate on lipid biosynthesis in isolated hepatocytes. J Nutr 120:668–673, 1990.

65. Levrat M-A, Favier M-L, Moundras C, Remesy C, Demigne C, Morand C. Role of dietary propionic acid and bile acid excretion in the hypocholesterolemic effects of oligosaccharides in rats. J Nutr 124:531–538, 1994.

66. Todesco T, Rao AV, Bosello O, Jenkins DJA. Propionate lowers blood glucose and alters lipid metabolism in healthy subjects. Am J Clin Nutr 54:860–865, 1991.

67. Nishimura N, Nishikawa H, Kiriyama S. Ileorectostomy or cecectomy but not colectomy abolishes the plasma cholesterol-lowering effect of dietary beet fiber in rats. J Nutr 123:1260–1269, 1993.

68. Jackson KA, Topping DL. Prevention of coprophagy does not alter the hypocholesterolaemic effects of oat bran in the rat. Br J Nutr 70:211–219, 1993.

69. Wolever TMS, Spadafora P, Eshuis H. Interaction between colonic acetate and propionate in man. Am J Clin Nutr 53:681–687, 1991.

70. Wolever TMS, Spadafora PJ, Cunnane SC, Pencharz PB. Propionate inhibits incorporation of colonic [1,2-^{13}C] acetate into plasma lipids in humans. Am J Clin Nutr 61:1241–1247, 1995.

71. Jenkins DJA, Wolever TMS, Jenkins A, Brighenti F, Vuksan V, Rao AV, Cunnane SC, Ocana A, Corey P, Vezina C, Connelly P, Buckley G, Patten R. Specific types of colonic fermentation may raise low-density-lipoproteins-cholesterol concentrations. Am J Clin Nutr 54:141–147, 1991.

72. Braun WH, Ramsey JC, Gehring PJ. The lack of significant absorption of methylcellulose, viscosity 330 cP, from the gastrointestinal tract following single and multiple oral doses to the rat. Food Cosmet Toxicol 12:373–376, 1974.

73. Gallaher DD, Hassel CA, Lee K-J. Relationships between viscosity of hydroxypropyl methylcellulose and plasma cholesterol in hamsters. J Nutr 123:1732–1738, 1993.

74. Carr TP, Gallaher DD, Yang C-H, Hassel CA. Increased intestinal contents viscosity reduces cholesterol absorption efficiency in hamsters fed hydroxypropyl methylcellulose. J Nutr 126:1463–1469, 1996.

75. Topping DL, Oakenfull D, Trimble RP, Illman RJ. A viscous fibre (methylcellulose) lowers blood glucose and plasma triacylglycerols and increases liver glycogen independently of volatile fatty acid production in the rat. Br J Nutr 59:21–30, 1988.

76. Story JA, Tepper SA, Kritchevsky D. Influence of synthetic conjugates of cholic acid on cholesterolemia in rats. J Nutr 104:1185–1188, 1974.

77. Anderson SA, Fisher KD, Talbot JM, eds. Evaluation of the health aspects of using partially hydrolyzed guar gum as a food ingredient. Bethesda, MD: Life Sciences Research Office, Federation of American Societies for Experimental Biology, 1993, pp 1–61.

78. Beer MU, Arrigoni E, Amado R. Effects of oat gum on blood cholesterol levels in healthy young men. Eur J Clin Nutr 49:517–522, 1995.

79. Lia Å. Hallmans G, Sandberg A-S, Sundberg B, Åman P, Andersson H. Oat β-glucan increases bile acid excretion and a fiber-rich barley fraction increases cholesterol excretion in ileostomy subjects. Am J Clin Nutr 62:1245–1251, 1995.

80. Cabotaje LM, Shinnick FL, Lopèz-Guisa JM, Marlett JA. Mucin secretion in germfree rats fed fiber-free and psyllium diets and bacterial mass and carbohydrate fermentation after colonization. Appl Environ Microbiol 60:1302–1307, 1994.

81. Alvarez-Leite JI, Andrieux C, Ferezou J, Riotto M, Vieira EC. Evidence for the absence of participation of the microbial flora in the hypocholesterolemic effect of guar gum in gnotobiotic rats. Comp Biochem Physiol 109A:503–510, 1994.
82. Carroll KK. Hypercholesterolemia and atherosclerosis: effects of dietary protein. Fed Proc 41:2792–2796, 1982.
83. Kritchevsky D. Protein and atherosclerosis. J Nutr Sci Vitaminol 36(suppl):S81–S86, 1990.
84. Carroll KK. Review of clinical studies on cholesterol-lowering response to soy protein. J Am Diet Assoc 91:820–827, 1991.
85. Anderson JW, Johnstone BM, Cook-Newell ME. Meta-analysis of the effects of soy protein intake on serum lipids. N Engl J Med 333:276–282, 1995.
86. Anthony MS, Clarkson TB, Weddle DL, Wolfe MS. Effects of soy protein phytoestrogens on cardiovascular risk factors in rhesus monkeys. J Nutr 125(suppl 3S):803S–804S, 1995.
87. Kritchevsky D. Phytosterols. In: D Kritchevsky, C Bonfield, eds. Dietary Fiber in Health and Disease. New York: Plenum Press, 1997, pp 235–243.
88. Bosaeus I, Sandström B, Andersson H. Bile acid and cholesterol excretion in human beings given soya-bean- and meat-protein-based diets: a study in ileostomy subjects. Br J Nutr 59:215–221, 1988.
89. Lovati MR, West CE, Sirtori CR, Beynem AC. Dietary animal proteins and cholesterol metabolism in rabbits. Br J Nutr 64:473–485, 1990.
90. Wolfe BM. Potential role of raising dietary protein intake for reducing risk of atherosclerosis. Can J Cardiol 11(suppl G):127G–131G, 1995.
91. Barnes PJ. Cereal tocopherols. In: J Holas, Kratochvil, eds. Progress in cereal chemistry and technology, Proc. 7th World Cereal and Bread Congr. Amsterdam: Elsevier, 1983, pp 1095–1100.
92. Qureshi AA, Qureshi A, Wright JJK, Shen Z, Kramer G, Gapor A, Chong YH, Dewitt G, Ong ASH, Peterson DM, Bradlow BA. Lowering of serum cholesterol in hypercholesterolemic humans by tocotrienols (palmvitee). Am J Clin Nutr 53:1021S–1026S, 1991.
93. Elson CE. Tropical oils: nutritional and scientific issues. Crit Rev Food Sci Nutr 31:79–102, 1992.
94. Parker RA, Pearce BC, Clark RW, Gordon DA, Wright JJK. Tocotrienols regulate cholesterol production in mammalian cells by post-transcriptional suppression of 3-hydroxy-3-methylglutaryl-coenzyme A reductase. J Biol Chem 268:11230–11238, 1993.
95. Qureshi AA, Bradlow BA, Brace L, Manganello J, Peterson DM, Pearce BC, Wright JJK, Gapor A, Elson CE. Response of hypercholesterolemic subjects to administration of tocotrienols. Lipids 30:1171–1177, 1995.
96. Uusitupa MIJ, Miettinen TA, Sarkkinen ES, Ruuskanen E, Kervinen K, Kesäniemi YA. Lathosterol and other non-cholesterol sterols during treatment of hypercholesterolaemia with beta-glucan-rich oat bran. Eur J Clin Nutr 51:607–611, 1997.
97. Tan DTS, Khor HT, Low WHS, Ali A, Gapor A. Effect of a palm-oil-vitamin E concentrate on the serum and lipoprotein lipids of humans. Am J Clin Nutr 53:1027S–1031S, 1991.
98. Wahlqvist ML, Krivokuca-Bogetic Z, Lo CH, Hage B, Smith R, Lukito W. Differential serum responses to tocopherols and tocotrienols during vitamin E supplementation in hypercholesterolaemic individuals without change in coronary risk factors. Nutr Res 12:S181–S201, 1992.
99. Pearce BC, Parker RA, Deason ME, Qureshi AA, Wright JJK. Hypocholesterolemic activity of synthetic and natural tocotrienols. J Med Chem 35:3595–3606, 1992.
100. Lasztity R, Berndorfer-Kraszner E, Huszar M. On the presence and distribution of some bioactive agents in oat varieties. In: Inglett GE, Munck L, eds. Cereals for Food and Beverages. New York: Academic Press, 1980, pp 429–445.
101. Peterson DM, Qureshi AA. Genotype and environment effects on tocols of barley and oats. Cereal Chem 70:157–162, 1993.
102. Qureshi AA, Pearce BC, Nor RM, Gapor A, Peterson DM, Elson CE. Dietary α-tocopherol attenuates the impact of γ-tocotrienol on hepatic 3-hydroxy-3-methylglutaryl coenzyme A reductase activity in chickens. J Nutr 126:389–394, 1996.
103. Hakkarainen RVJ, Tyopponen JT, Bengtsson SG. Changes in the content and composition of vitamin E in damp barley stored in airtight bins. J Sci Food Agric 34:1029–1034, 1983.

104. Peterson DM. Oat tocols: concentration and stability in oat products and distribution within the kernel. Cereal Chem 72:21–24, 1995.
105. Peterson DM. Barley tocols: effects of milling, malting, and mashing. Cereal Chem 71:42–44, 1994.
106. Southgate DAT. The diet as a source of dietary fibre. Eur J Clin Nutr. 49(suppl 3):322–326, 1995.
107. Jenkins DJA. Optimal diet for reducing the risk for arteriosclerosis. Can J Cardiol 11(suppl G): 118G–122G, 1995.

3
Dietary Fiber and Colon Cancer

Joanne L. Slavin
University of Minnesota, St. Paul, Minnesota

I. INTRODUCTION

Burkitt is usually credited with popularizing the potential relationship between intake of dietary fiber and colorectal cancer (1). Gastrointestinal diseases, including colon cancer, are common in Western countries but occur rarely in Africa. Burkitt describes the relationship graphically as a link between stool size and the size of the medical treatment facility; in the African world stools are large and health care is taken care of by the witch doctor in a small hut. In the Western world, stool size is small and health care is delivered by a huge medical center. This concept is simple and appealing but is still open to debate.

Intake of dietary fiber is significantly higher in African populations than in the Western world, and ecological data support the correlation of fiber intake and protection from colon cancer. Unfortunately, results of analytical epidemiological studies are not as consistent. Further, mechanistic studies in animals and humans also have yielded inconsistent results. In fact, Wasan and Goodlad (2) recently argued that fiber-supplemented foods may actually damage your health. Most of their argument is based on studies where soluble fibers increase colonic cell proliferation, an intermediate marker of the colon cancer process. They encourage the use of specific fiber supplements only within the scientific context of controlled prospective trials.

Despite the controversies surrounding colon cancer and dietary fiber, the hypothesis that dietary fiber protects against colon cancer remains plausible and attractive. The objective of this review is to summarize the recent studies in this area and describe some of the reasons for the inconsistency of the data.

II. BACKGROUND

Dietary fiber essentially describes the leftovers of digestion. The physiological definition of dietary fiber is plant cellular material resistant to digestion by the endogenous enzymes of humans. According to this definition, starch that resists pancreatic enzyme action and passes to the colon would be considered dietary fiber. Also the disaccharide lactulose would be considered liquid fiber, and lactose escaping digestion in lactase-deficient individuals would be considered dietary fiber. To get around these problems, dietary fiber has been defined as the sum of polysaccharides and lignin not digested by the endogenous secretions of the human gastrointestinal tract (3).

Dietary fiber is not an accurate term because many of its components are not fibrous. Gums and mucilages, for example, are classified as dietary fiber because they are not digested by mammalian enzymes or secretions. Recently, efforts have been made to define fructans such as inulin and fructooligosaccharides as dietary fiber since their physiological effects are consistent with those of dietary fiber. Technically, only one component of dietary fiber, namely cellulose, is truly fibrous; yet dietary fiber is the accepted nomenclature when describing the roughage or residue in the human diet.

III. METHODS TO MEASURE DIETARY FIBER

By accepting a physiological definition for dietary fiber, measurement of dietary fiber becomes problematic. How do you measure dietary fiber except by running it through the digestive tract and measuring the residuals in feces. Despite enormous amounts of scientific interest in dietary fiber, few reliable values exist in the literature for the dietary fiber content of foods (4,5). The values that are available were generated with different analytical methods and are not comparable. Nutrient data bases contain some dietary fiber values, but there are many missing data values.

The difficulty in devising a method for assessing total dietary fiber can be appreciated if one considers the diverse nature of dietary fiber. A simple, reproducible method to remove protein, fat, and soluble sugars and starch from food while retaining both water-soluble and insoluble components of dietary fiber is difficult analytically. Nutrition labels in the United States contain values for total dietary fiber, and these values are generated with the dietary fiber method developed by the Association of Official Analytical Chemists (AOAC). Methods to measure soluble and insoluble dietary fiber are available. Values for dietary fiber vary greatly, depending on the laboratory doing the analysis, sample issues, etc. Dietary fiber values generated with a modified Theander vary from values generated with the AOAC method (6). When the dietary fiber content and composition of different forms of fruits were measured by a modified Theander method and the AOAC method, the two sets of fiber data were significantly different (7). Soluble dietary fiber is difficult to analyze, especially if it has been incorporated into processed foods (8).

Commonly consumed foods are low in dietary fiber. Most commonly consumed foods contain 2 g of dietary fiber or less per serving (9). Generally, the fiber content of foods is quite consistent and can be estimated by multiplying fruit or vegetable servings by 1.5 g of dietary fiber, refined grain servings by 1 g of dietary fiber, and whole grain servings by 2.5 g of dietary fiber. Concentrated fiber sources such as legumes and high-fiber cereals add additional dietary fiber to the diet.

Recommendations for adult dietary fiber intake fall in the range of 20–35 g/day (10) or 10–13 g of dietary fiber per 1000 kcal (11). Usual intakes of dietary fiber in the United States are only 14–15 g/day (12), so few people get the recommended levels of dietary fiber. An obvious reason is that most of the popular foods we consume are not high in dietary fiber. For example, most common servings of grains, fruits, and vegetables contain 1–3 g of dietary fiber (13). Thus, to get the recommended dietary fiber intake you need to consume 10 or more servings of fiber-containing foods per day, assuming your average fiber-containing food contained 2 g of dietary fiber. If consumers were eating according to the USDA Food Guide Pyramid and were choosing whole grain breads and cereals and intact fruits and vegetables, they would be ingesting the recommended levels of dietary fiber.

IV. PHYSIOLOGICAL EFFECTS OF DIETARY FIBER

Dietary fiber affects the digestive tract from mouth to anus and has other important physiological functions. The effect of dietary fiber on the intestinal tract is affected by the type of fiber ingested, the physical state of the subject, previous diet, and other components of the diet. Thus, the confusion in the field of dietary fiber is the result of the many variables that are not controlled in research studies.

When ingested carbohydrates reach the cecum, they are fermented to short-chain fatty acids (SCFAs) and gases, including carbon dioxide, hydrogen, and methane. Gases escape through the lungs or the gastrointestinal tract as flatus. This active fermentation process taking place in the gut is difficult to study in vivo. Dietary fiber fermentation has been estimated by measuring the dietary fiber in food and comparing it to fiber that remains in feces. Researchers have also estimated breath hydrogen and methane production as a means to determine fiber fermentation. SCFA production has been measured by having subjects swallow dialysis bags and collecting these bags in freshly passed feces or measuring SCFA remaining in feces. None of these methods is ideal, and little information is available on the fate of dietary fiber in the body.

Fermentability of dietary fiber is another property linked to physiological effects. It is difficult to measure the fermentation of fibers since fermentation is determined by the breakdown of fiber in the gut and no accepted in vitro methods exist to measure fermentability. Generally, highly soluble fibers such as oat bran, guar gum, and pectin are extensively fermented while insoluble fibers such as cellulose are not well fermented. Unfortunately, hundreds of fiber products are now on the market and their fermentability is not known. This is especially true when fibers are processed that may enhance or limit fermentability. For example, ''oat fiber'' may be mostly insoluble dietary fiber if the fiber is extracted from oat hulls rather than the more soluble oat bran.

Fermentation of carbohydrate in the colon produces SCFAs that help maintain the integrity of the gut (14). It is difficult to measure fermentation in vivo. In vitro methods of determining fermentability of fibers have been developed. Eleven fiber-rich substrates were subjected to in vitro incubation with fecal bacteria and fermentation and SCFA production were measured (15). Citrus pectin was 83% fermentable while oat fiber was about 6% fermentable. SCFA production was correlated to fermentability in the in vitro system. In a similar study (16), the most rapid fermentation rate was with pectin followed by psyllium gum, tragacanth gum, guar gum, soy fiber, and finally cellulose.

It is generally thought that more than 75% of dietary fiber in an average diet is broken down in the large intestine, resulting in the production of carbon dioxide, hydrogen, methane, and SCFAs including butyrate, propionate, and acetate. Propionate and acetate are thought to be metabolized in colonic epithelial cells or peripheral tissue. Butyrate may regulate colonic cell proliferation and serve as an energy source for colonic cells. Propionate acid is transported to the liver and may suppress cholesterol synthesis, a potential explanation for how soluble dietary fiber lowers serum cholesterol.

According to calculations by Cummings and Macfarlane (17), if approximately 20 g of fiber is fermented in the colon each day, approximately 200 mM of SCFAs will be produced, of which 62% will be acetate, 25% propionate, and 16% butyrate. Colonic absorption of SCFA is concentration dependent with no evidence of a saturable process. The mechanism by which SCFAs cross the colonic mucosa is thought to be passive diffusion of the unionized acid into the mucosa cell. SCFAs are respiratory fuels for the colonic mucosa. In isolated human colonocytes, butyrate is actively metabolized to both CO_2 and ketone bodies, which accounts for about 80% of the oxygen consumption of colonocytes. Butyrate is almost completely consumed by the colonic mucosa, while acetate and propionate enter the portal circulation, extending the effects of dietary fiber beyond the intestinal tract.

Butyrate may be an important protective agent in colonic carcinogenesis (14). Trophic effects on normal colonocytes in vitro and in vivo are induced by butyrate. In contrast, butyrate arrests the growth of neoplastic colonocytes and inhibits the preneoplastic hyperproliferation induced by some tumor promoters in vitro. Butyrate induces differentiation of colon cancer cell lines and regulates the expression of molecules involved in colonocyte growth and adhesion.

The controversial effects of butyrate in different experimental models has been reviewed by Hague et al. (18). The effects of butyrate on colonic tumor cell lines in vitro seem to contradict what has been shown in vivo. Butyrate appears to have two contrasting effects; it serves as the primary energy source for normal colonic epithelium and stimulates growth of colonic mucosa, yet in colonic tumor cell lines it inhibits growth and induces differentiation and apoptosis. Since SCFAs are volatile, they are quickly absorbed from the lumen. Therefore, soluble, fermentable fibers will produce SCFAs at the upper end of the colon, while slowly fermentable fibers such as wheat bran will release SCFAs throughout the gut. Fecal levels of SCFAs may have meaning in that they represent events later in the digestive process. The relevance of in vitro data on SCFAs with various fiber supplements is questionable.

SCFAs acidify the gut, which may affect development of colon cancer because changes in gut pH will affect solubility of metabolites and activities of bacterial enzymes (19). Table 1 lists the many potential mechanisms by which dietary fiber affects colorectal cancer risk. It is important to remember that dietary fibers may affect stool size when given as coarse wheat bran and have less effect when given as fine wheat bran. Thus, it is difficult to generalize about the mechanistic effects of any one fiber, since its effect will be determined by how it is fed, in what form, whether it was processed, etc.

Our laboratory was unable to correlate apparent fiber digestibility to SCFA production, but we did find that propionate and butyrate concentrations were greater in wheat bran than vegetable fiber, supporting the need to carefully pick the dietary fiber source if SCFA production is the desired endpoint (20). Kapadia et al. (21) compared bowel function and SCFA production in healthy subjects consuming diets containing either no fiber or 15 g of soy oligosaccharide fiber or oat fiber or soy polysaccharide. The soy oligosaccharide fiber was associated with higher production of butyrate than the other fibers. Compared with a fiber-free polymeric enteral diet, the daily consumption of an enteral diet supplemented with 30 g of total dietary fiber per day derived from a poorly fermentable oat fiber, a highly fermentable soy oligosaccharide fiber, or a moderately fermentable soy polysaccharide fiber had little impact on bowel function measures.

The relationship among famine, fiber, fatty acids, and failed colonic absorption has been reviewed by Roediger (22). Another review by Scheppach and Bartram (23) concludes that the results in clinical studies with dietary fiber have been disappointing, although the model pro-

Table 1 Mechanisms by Which Fiber Can Protect Against the Development of Colorectal Cancer

Increased stool bulk
  Decreased transit time
  Dilution of carcinogens
Binds with bile acids or other potential carcinogens
Lower fecal pH
  Inhibit bacterial degradation of normal food constituents to potential carcinogens
Changes in microflora
Fermentation by fecal flora to short-chain fatty acids
  Decrease in colonic pH
  Inhibition of carcinogens
Increase in lumenal antioxidants
Peptide growth factors

posed—that fiber is fermented, generating SCFAs, which serve as nutrition for colonic mucosal cells—is correct. To study the physiological effects of dietary fiber in vivo is extremely difficult. Studies have been too short, measurements are semi-quantitative, and methods, such as measuring dietary fiber and SCFAs, are not well developed. In vivo, researchers are dependent on feces as a source of SCFAs or must have subjects swallow dialysis bags and retrieve the bags in feces and measure SCFAs in the dialysate. It is not clear that results from in vitro fermentation studies have direct application to the in vivo setting.

A recent cell experiment (24) examined the effects of acetate, butyrate, and propionate on the proliferation, adhesion, and motility of the human intestinal Caco-2 cell line as well as the effects of these SCFA on alkaline phosphatase and dipeptidyl dipetidase specific activity (common laboratory markers of differentiation). All three SCFAs slowed proliferation, promoted brush border enzyme activity, and inhibited adhesion to and motility across a type 1 collagen matrix substrate. Butyrate was uniformly more potent than an equimolar concentration of acetate, while propionate was similar to butyrate in proliferation but intermediate between butyrate and acetate in modulation of cell-matrix interactions. The authors conclude that SCFAs are not equipotent in their effects on human Caco-2 colon cancer cell biology.

V. COLON CANCER BACKGROUND

Cancers of the gastrointestinal tract represent the second most common cancer type in the United States and are second only to cancer of the respiratory tract as a cause of cancer-related mortality in the United States (25). The development of colon cancer involves a complex interplay between environmental and genetic factors. As the colorectal epithelium progresses from normal histology to one that is hyperproliferative, adenomatous, and finally malignant, multiple molecular alterations, including the activation of proto-oncogenes, the inactivation of tumor suppressor genes, and mutations in mismatch repair genes, occur (26). Environmental factors are also intimately involved in the process, and many represent risk factors that can be altered, unlike genetic risk factors. Dietary factors are particularly relevant in the process, with estimates that 35% of all cancers are attributable to diet and that up to 90% of colorectal cancer in the United States could be avoidable with alterations in diet (27). Dietary treatments have been tested as chemopreventive measures in the process of colorectal cancer. However, establishing a cause-and-effect relationship between diet and colorectal cancer is a difficult task.

Studies in diet and cancer include ecological studies in which dietary variables are compared across populations. Case-control studies can examine differences in diet between people who have colon cancer compared to those who do not. A serious limitation of retrospective studies is the accuracy with which intakes of dietary factors can be established. It is difficult to recall dietary intakes in former years, and disease tends to alter diet. A stronger epidemiological design is the cohort study in which subjects exposed to a particular agent are followed over time and their cancer incidence is compared with those who have not been exposed. These studies are costly and require large numbers of subjects. Intervention studies allow investigators to make a dietary change and then follow the course of disease. Intervention studies are limited by the slow progressive nature of the cancer process and the large number of subjects needed for statistical power.

Strategies to avoid these problems include studying individuals who are at high risk for developing cancer to determine whether a chemopreventive agent can prevent the development of cancer. Second, studies use intermediate biomarkers of the cancer process as the endpoint rather than waiting for the cancer to occur. Some intermediate biomarkers of colorectal cancer are listed in Table 2. All these intermediate biomarkers have limitations and have not been

Table 2   Intermediate Biomarkers of Colorectal Cancer

Adenoma
Proliferation markers
   Labeling indices (tritiated-thymidine, bromodeoxyuridine, PCNA)
   Enzymes (ornithine decarboxylase)
Mitotic index
Aberrant crypts
Genetic markers
   DNA methylation
   Alterations of APC, k-ras, p53, and DNA repair genes

clinically validated. Except for colorectal adenomas, modulation of these intermediate biomarkers has not led to a reduction in colorectal cancer occurrence and mortality. Despite these limitations, chemoprevention trials with high-risk individuals with measurement of intermediate biomarkers is commonly used to determine the role of dietary ingredients in colon cancer causation.

Many more studies exist that use animal models to study the relationship between dietary fiber and colon cancer. Animal studies offer greater control of variables, allow for a broader range of interventions, and are generally less expensive than human studies. They suffer from species differences, which for dietary fiber are particularly problematic since the gastrointestinal tract of the rat varies significantly from the human. Other research in dietary fiber and colon cancer is conducted in in vitro systems or with colon cancer cell lines. Mechanistic studies of dietary fiber and its potential role in colon cancer prevention are also conducted in healthy human subjects.

The difficulty in synthesizing all the data into a public health message can be appreciated in attempting to make sense of the role of butyrate in colon cancer. It is well known that butyrate is a preferred substrate for the colonocyte and therefore should play an important role in the healthy colon. Trophic effects on normal colonocytes in vitro and in vivo are induced by butyrate (14). In contrast, butyrate arrests the growth of neoplastic colonocytes and inhibits the preneoplastic hyperproliferation induced by some tumor promoters in vitro (14). Generally, the most fermentable fibers are associated with highest levels of butyrate in vitro. In vivo, it is likely the slowly fermented fibers will release butyrate throughout the gut, rather than the high amounts seen at the cecum, which would be expected with readily fermented fibers. The difficulty in measuring these phenomena in human subjects makes it impossible to answer these issues.

Studies on dietary fiber and colon cancer are also severely limited because of problems in defining, measuring, and quantitating dietary fiber. Because fiber has a physiological definition, it is difficult to agree on a chemical method to measure dietary fiber. Epidemiological studies generally rely on food frequency instruments, which estimate dietary fiber. As argued by Hill, these estimates are woefully inadequate if we are trying to estimate fermentable carbohydrate that reaches the colon (28). He suggests that we return to foods for epidemiological studies rather than attempting to measure dietary fiber, which obviously is problematic. His own research finds that cereals are consistently protective against colon cancer (29). We have reported that whole grain intake also is associated with lower risk of colon cancer (30). Data summarized from Italian case-control studies of whole grain intake and cancer risk support that whole grain intake protects against colon cancer (31).

Despite these limitations and frustrations, we need to move ahead in the area of dietary fiber and colon cancer. This review will summarize the epidemiological evidence, animal and cell studies, and human intervention studies that have been conducted on this topic. Although meant to be inclusive, the number of studies conducted on this topic is overwhelming, so review articles are included to represent the state of the field when that review was written.

VI. EPIDEMIOLOGICAL EVIDENCE LINKING DIETARY FIBER AND COLON CANCER

The relationship between dietary fiber and colon cancer has been studied extensively by epidemiologists since the hypothesis linking fiber to colon cancer was popularized by Denis Burkitt. Besides looking for relationships between dietary fiber and colon cancer, researchers have looked for relationships between colon cancer and foods high in dietary fiber, including vegetables, fruits, grains, and legumes. The majority of descriptive, case-control, and cohort epidemiological studies support an inverse relationship between consumption of vegetables and fruits and colorectal cancer risk (32). Besides dietary fiber, fruits, vegetables, and grains contain a variety of anticarcinogenic compounds (Table 3) (33,34).

Few well-designed cohort studies have examined the relationship between intake of high-fiber foods and colorectal cancer. The relationship between fruit and vegetable intake and colorectal cancer was examined in the Iowa Women's Health Study (35). This study is a prospective cohort study of 98,030 postmenopausal women who were asked to complete a questionnaire on health and diet. The cohort was followed for 4 years. Dietary intake was assessed with the Willett semiquantitative food frequency questionnaire. The occurrence of colorectal cancer was documented and a total of 212 cases and 35,004 noncases remained for analysis. Total intake of both vegetables and fruits did not reduce the relative risk of colorectal cancer. Garlic consumption was linked to reduced risk of colorectal cancer, perhaps because garlic is a good source of

Table 3 Potential Anticarcinogens in Fruits, Vegetables, and Grains

Dietary fiber
Lignans
Isoflavones
Coumarins
Phytates
Dithiothiones
Carotenoids
Tocopherols
Ascorbate
Folate
Isothiocyanates
Indoles
Glucosinolate
Plant sterols
Protease inhibitors
Allium compounds
Flavonoids
Other phenolic compounds

Source: Refs. 33, 34.

glutathione-S-transferase, which has been shown to inhibit experimentally induced carcinogenesis in animals.

Epidemiological evidence that whole grains protects against colorectal cancer is also strong. In an expanded meta-analysis, odds ratios were <1 in 9 of 10 mentions of studies of colorectal cancers and polyps and the relationship to whole grain intake (30). Whole grain intake was estimated by intake of whole grain bread, brown rice, and intake of whole grain cereals. Odds ratios for the highest category of consumption of whole grains was 0.5 in the Italian study (31). Again, intervention studies to test this hypothesis are lacking.

Extensive epidemiological evidence supports the theory that dietary fiber may be protective against large bowel cancer. Correlation studies that compare colorectal cancer incidence or mortality rates among countries with estimates of national dietary fiber consumption suggest that fiber intake may be protective against colon cancer (36). Case-control studies are considered stronger than population-based correlation studies since individual exposure to dietary variables can be related to individual outcome. Case-control studies reviewed by both Bingham (36) and Willett (37) support the protective role of dietary fiber in colorectal cancer.

Two analyses, conducted as meta-analysis, have summarized the observational and case-control epidemiological studies on dietary fiber and colorectal cancer. Trock et al. (38) analyzed 37 epidemiological studies that examined the relationship between colorectal cancer and fiber, vegetables, grains, and fruits, either alone or in combination. Overall, 80% of the studies reported up to that time supported the protective role of dietary fiber in colorectal cancer. Howe et al. (39) conducted a combined analysis of data from 13 case-control studies in populations with different colorectal cancer rates and dietary practices. The risk of colorectal cancer decreased incrementally as dietary fiber intake increased. Consumption of more than 31 g of fiber per day was associated with a 50% reduction in risk of colorectal cancer compared to diet incorporating <11 g/day. The authors estimate that the risk of colorectal cancer in the U.S. population could be reduced by about 31% from an average increase in fiber intake from food sources of about 13 g/day.

Other recently published case-control studies also support the relationship between fiber intake and risk of colorectal cancer (40,41). Marchand et al. (42) report a protective role of fiber from vegetables against colorectal cancer, which appears independent of its water solubility property and of the effects of other phytochemicals. High intake of vegetables, fruits, and grains was associated with decreased risk of polyps in a case-control study (43). Lubin et al. (44) found no significant protection against adenomatous polyps in a case-control study. They did find a significant interaction between water and fiber intake. They suggest that fiber and water increase the volume of colonic contents, which dilutes and adsorbs exogenous and endogenous toxic compounds present in the colonic contents. Also, the increased volume of bowel contents promotes peristalsis, reducing the duration of the contact of colonic contents with the mucosa.

Slattery et al. (45) examined eating patterns and risk of colon cancer in a population-based case-control study. The prudent patterns, which included vigorous exercise, smaller body size, and higher intakes of dietary fiber and folate, were associated with lower risk of colon cancer. In contrast, the western style was associated with increased risk of colorectal cancer.

The data from large cohort studies are not consistent. In the Health Professional Follow-Up Study (46), dietary fiber was inversely associated with risk of colorectal adenoma in men. All sources of fiber (vegetables, fruits, and grain) were associated with decreased risk of adenoma. The Nurses' Health Study found no protective effect of dietary fiber on the development of colorectal cancer in women (47). In the Iowa Women's Health Study, a weak and statistically nonsignificant inverse association was found between dietary fiber intake and risk of colon cancer (35). Thus, evidence from prospective, large epidemiological studies for the protective effect of dietary fiber on colorectal cancer is not strong.

Few epidemiological studies have collected biomarkers of dietary fiber intake. Cummings et al. (48) collected data from 20 populations in 12 countries and found that average stool weight varied from 72 to 470 g/day and was inversely related to colon cancer risk. Unfortunately, laxation data has been collected in few studies of colorectal cancer and fiber intake. It is known that different dietary fibers have different effects on stool weight. As summarized by Cummings (49), wheat bran is most effective in increasing stool weight with each gram of fiber fed, as it increases stool weight by 5.4 grams. In contrast, soluble fibers like pectin only increase stool weight by 1.2 g per gram of fiber fed as pectin. Yet psyllium, a fiber that is at least 70% soluble, increases stool weight by 4.0 g per gram fiber fed as psyllium. Thus, the laxation properties of a fiber source cannot be predicted based on the solubility of the fiber. The relationship between stool weight and protection from colorectal cancer could be strong while the relationship between dietary fiber intake and colorectal cancer is weak because of all these inconsistencies in fiber measurement and physiological effect.

VII. RELATIONSHIP OF COLON CANCER TO HORMONALLY DEPENDENT CANCERS

The hypothesis of a protective influence of reproductive factors and exogenous hormones on colorectal cancer was first proposed by McMichael and Potter (50). This followed observations of ecological correlation between breast and colon cancer, higher than expected incidence of colorectal tumors among nuns, and descriptive sex and site-specific data showing a crossover of colorectal cancer rates around age 50 (51). Women have a similar or higher incidence of colorectal cancer than men before age 50 and a lower incidence thereafter. Potter et al. (52) concluded that both parity and age at first pregnancy were likely not associated with colorectal cancer risk, whereas the available evidence suggest risk reduction associated with hormone replacement. Epidemiological findings in this area vary greatly, with a recent meta-analysis of hormone replacement therapy and colon cancer in women concluding a 0–25% risk reduction among ever users of hormone replacement therapy (53).

Few studies have examined the effects of dietary fiber on hormone metabolism, although colon cancer is affected by diet and hormones (54). Rose et al. (55) reported that when wheat bran was added to the diet of premenopausal women, it significantly reduced serum estrogen concentrations, while neither corn bran nor oat bran had an effect on estrogen levels. Dietary fiber intake was increased from about 15 to 30 g/day in this study, an increase similar to that recommended by the National Cancer Institute. Goldin et al. (56) reported that a high-fiber, low-fat diet significantly decreased serum concentrations of estrone, estrone sulfate, testosterone, and sex hormone–binding globulin in premenopausal women. Dietary fiber also caused a lengthening of the menstrual cycle by 0.72 day and a lengthening of the follicular phase by 0.85 day, changes thought to lower overall risk of developing hormonally dependent cancer. Bagga et al. (57) also found that increased intake of dietary fiber significantly decreased serum estradiol and estrone, which should decrease risk of hormonally dependent cancers.

We reported that gender differences in bowel function were more profound than differences caused by increased fiber intake in a study comparing physiological effects of cereal and vegetable fiber (58). Despite consuming identical diets, women had significantly smaller stools and slower transit times than men. Women digested more fiber, and the concentration of secondary bile acids was greater in men than women. Other data support the idea that menstrual cycle affects transit time and that transit slows during pregnancy, which support the relationship of hormonal status and bowel function.

VIII. INSULIN AND COLON CANCER

Giovannucci (59) has proposed that the etiology of insulin resistance and colorectal cancer are related. He suggests that diets high in fat and energy and low in complex carbohydrates and a sedentary lifestyle lead to insulin resistance and that the associated hyperinsulinemia, hypertriglyceridemia, and glycemia lead to increased colon cancer risk through the growth-promoting effect of insulin on the increased availability of energy. La Vecchia et al. (60) examined the relationship between diabetes mellitus and the risk of colorectal cancer in an Italian case-control study. They found that subjects with non–insulin-dependent diabetes mellitus (NIDDM) have a slightly increased risk of colorectal cancer. Allowance for potential confounding factors, including body mass index, diet, and physical activity, could not explain the excess colorectal cancer risk among subjects with diabetes.

Dietary fibers, especially soluble fiber, are known to affect serum glucose and insulin levels. Guevin et al. (61) compared postprandial glucose, insulin, and lipid response when non–insulin-dependent diabetic subjects consumed four different fiber diets. The fiber diets contained two levels of total dietary fiber (10 g vs. 20 g) and two soluble:insoluble fiber ratios (1:4 vs. 2:3). The incremental area under the curve for glucose and insulin was lowered after consuming 20 g as compared to 10 g of dietary fiber but was not affected by the soluble:insoluble fiber ratio. The authors conclude that the proportion of soluble to insoluble fiber in cereal and fruit does not necessarily predict the effect of fiber on glycemic response, while the overall quantity of fiber does appear to affect postprandial glucose metabolism in NIDDM.

High-fiber diets tend to be lower in fat and thus lower in calories and should be appropriate for weight control. High-fiber cereals eaten at breakfast lowered calorie intake when subjects were served a buffet lunch compared to when subjects did not consume a high-fiber breakfast (62). Thus, high-fiber diets may affect satiety, but whether that translates into weight loss is not known. Despite theoretical reasons why high-fiber diets should aid weight loss, results from clinical trials are inconsistent, and long-term clinical trials of dietary fiber's effectiveness as a weight loss aid in weight management have not been supportive.

IX. MECHANISTIC BASIS FOR THE RELATIONSHIP BETWEEN DIETARY FIBER AND COLORECTAL CANCER

Potential mechanisms for the protective nature of dietary fiber against colon cancer are listed in Table 1. These have been well described by Kim and Mason (25) and Klurfeld (63). A large number of animal studies have been conducted on this relationship, and many are supportive of the relationship. Wheat bran has been well studied in colon cancer causation in laboratory rats. Alabaster et al. (64) fed rats a high-fat, low-calcium diet, supplemented with 1, 4, or 8% dietary fiber from wheat bran for 2 weeks prior, one week during, and 22 weeks after injection with azoxymethane. At the completion of the study, there were significant decreases in both tumor incidence and tumor multiplicity as a function of increased dietary fiber. Boffa et al. (65) concluded that wheat bran modulates colonic butyrate levels, which in turn modulate DNA synthesis in the proliferative compartment of colonic crypts.

McIntyre et al. (66) examined the role of butyrate in colonic cell proliferation in rats. They compared the effect of guar gum, oat bran, and wheat bran at 10% of the diet on butyrate production and colon tumor incidence in the rat following administration of dimethylhydrazine. They found significantly fewer tumors and lower tumor mass in rats consuming wheat bran compared to a guar gum, oat bran, or fiber-free diet. All fibers increased SCFAs, but wheat bran resulted in significantly greater SCFA concentrations in fresh feces. The authors concluded that the production of butyrate from fermentable fibers at the site of tumor formation may be a key component in wheat bran's protective effects against colon cancer.

Other mechanisms for the relationship between dietary fiber and colon cancer have been examined in animal models. Reddy et al. (67) reported that the concentration of fecal secondary bile acids and fecal mutagenic activity were significantly lower during wheat bran supplementation compared to control, whereas an oat bran diet supplemented at a level to achieve the same level of fiber had no impact on these measures. Other studies have examined fiber's ability to increase fecal bulk and speed intestinal transit. Dietary fibers differ in their ability to hold water and their resistance to bacterial degradation in the gut. Pectin is effective in holding water but is quickly fermented in the gut and cannot be found in feces. Wheat bran consistently has been found to have the most effect on stool bulk, probably because it is slowly fermented and survives transit through the gut. Milling of wheat bran may affect the laxative properties of the bran, with larger particle sizes causing larger increases in fecal weight.

Dietary fiber sources such as wheat bran are complex matrices, and attempts have been made to isolate the effects of chemical components of wheat bran. In an animal study, rats were fed wheat bran, dephytinized wheat bran, and phytic acid alone, and aberrant crypt foci were measured after treatment with azoxymethane (68). Wheat bran without phytic acid was less protective than intact wheat bran, suggesting that the protective effects of wheat bran include fiber and phytic acid.

Certain components of dietary fiber are more protective against colorectal cancer. Insoluble fibers have consistently been found to decrease cell proliferation, while soluble fibers may even increase cell proliferation. Lu et al. (69) found that lignin, a component of insoluble dietary fiber, is a free radical scavenger. They suggest that the ability of dietary fiber to protect against colorectal cancer may be determined by the amount of lignin in dietary fiber as well as the free radical–scavenging ability of the lignin.

A usual criticism of animal studies in this area is the large amount of dietary fiber that is fed. Dietary fibers have been fed at levels of 30% of the diet and more. These levels of intake have no bearing on typical or recommended intakes in humans. Yet animal studies allow investigators to screen a wide range of different dietary fibers at many doses.

X. INTERVENTION STUDIES

Several randomized intervention studies with high-fiber diets as a component of chemoprevention have been published. Alberts et al. (70) studied the effects of wheat bran fiber (an additional 13.5 g/day as wheat bran cereal) on rectal epithelial cell proliferation in patients with resection for colorectal cancers. They found that the wheat bran fiber cereal inhibited DNA synthesis and rectal mucosal cell proliferation in this high-risk group, which they argued should be associated with reduced cancer risk. They suggested that such a fiber regimen might be used as chemopreventive agent for colorectal cancers. The study is weakened by poor compliance to the intervention over the 4 years of the study.

The Alberts group also conducted a double-blind, placebo-controlled randomized trial with supplements of fiber and calcium and measurement of labeling index in rectal biopsies (71). They conclude that 9 months of high-dose wheat bran fiber and calcium carbonate supplementation in study participants with a history of recently resected colorectal adenomas did not have a significant effect on cellular proliferation rates in rectal mucosal biopsies, comparing 3- and 9-month results to baseline results.

In a randomized trial of intake of fat, fiber, and beta-carotene to prevent colorectal adenomas, patients on the combined intervention of low fat and added wheat bran had zero large adenomas at both 24 and 48 months, a statistically significant finding (72). The Toronto Polyp Prevention trial demonstrated no significant difference between low-fat/high-fiber and high-fat/low-fiber dietary groups with regard to the recurrence of adenomatous polyps (73). Other ongoing polyp prevention trials in the United States and Europe should provide additional data on the effect of fiber supplementation on polyp recurrence (74).

XI. CONCLUSIONS

The relationship between colorectal cancer and dietary fiber remains complex. Although not all data support the relationship, the difficulty in measuring dietary fiber and the poor data bases for dietary fiber content of foods make it a difficult relationship to study. Stronger protective support has been found for whole foods high in dietary fiber, such as vegetables, fruits, and whole grains. Dietary fiber may be just part of the protective puzzle with other components including antioxidants, phenolic compounds, and associated substances also providing protection against colorectal cancer.

Despite many years of research and nutrition education, dietary fiber intakes are not increasing. Our nutrition message must continue to be increase consumption of foods high in complex carbohydrates, including resistant starch, oligosaccharides, and dietary fiber. Because as many consumers depend on processed foods as the mainstay of their diets, efforts should be made to increase the fiber content of popular foods to assist consumers in obtaining recommended levels of unavailable carbohydrate. Differences in fiber composition must be considered since most studies support that it is the insoluble fraction of dietary fiber that is most protective against colorectal cancer.

REFERENCES

1. Burkitt DP. Epidemiology of cancer of the colon and rectum. Cancer 1971; 28:3–13.
2. Wasan HS, Goodlad RA. Fibre-supplemented foods may damage your health. Lancet 1996; 348: 319–320.
3. Trowell H. Definitions of fibre. Lancet 1974; 1:503.
4. Lanza E, Butrum R. A critical review of food fiber analysis and data. J Am Diet Assoc 1986; 86: 732–743.
5. Fredstrom SB, Baglien KS, Lampe JW, Slavin JL. Determination of the fiber content of enteral feedings. JPEN 1991; 15:450–453.
6. Marlett JA. Content and composition of dietary fiber in 117 frequently consumed foods. J Am Diet Assoc 1992; 92:175–186.
7. Marlett JA, Vollendorf NW. Dietary fiber content and composition of different forms of fruits. Food Chem 1994; 51:39–44.
8. Lee SC, Rodriguez F, Storey M, Farmakalidis E, Prosky L. Determination of soluble and insoluble dietary fiber in psyllium-containing cereal products. J AOAC Int 1995; 78:724–729.
9. Marlett JA, Cheung T. Database and quick methods of assessing typical dietary fiber intakes using data for 228 commonly consumed foods. J Am Diet Assoc 1997; 97:1139–1151.
10. Healthy People 2000. Washington, D.C.: U.S. Dept. of Health and Human Services, Public Health Service, 1990.

11. Pilch S. Physiological Effects and Health Consequences of Dietary Fiber. Bethesda, MD: Life Sciences Research Office, Federation of American Societies for Experimental Biology, 1987.
12. Marlett JA, Slavin JL. Position of the American Dietetic Association: health implications of dietary fiber. J Am Diet Assoc 1997; 97:1157–1159.
13. Slavin JL. Dietary fiber: classification, chemical analyses, and food sources. J Am Diet Assoc 1987; 87:1164–1171.
14. Valazquez OC, Lederer HM, Rombeau JL. Butyrate and the colonocyte—implications for neoplasia. Dig Dis Sci 1996; 14(4):727–739.
15. McBurney MI, Thompson LU. In vitro fermentabilities of purified fiber supplements. J Food Sci 1989; 54:347–350.
16. McBurney MI, Thompson LU. Dietary fiber and total enteral nutrition: fermentative assessment of five fiber supplements. JPEN 1991; 15:267–270.
17. Cummings JH, Macfarlane GT. Colonic microflora: Nutrition and health. Nutrition 1997; 13:476–478.
18. Hague A, Singh B, Paraskeva C. Butyrate acts as a survival factor for colonic epithelial cells: Further fuel for the in vivo versus in vitro debate. Gastroenterology 1997; 112:1036–1040.
19. Thornton JR. High colonic pH promotes colorectal cancer. Lancet 1981; i:1083–1087.
20. Fredstrom SB, Lampe JW, Jung HJ, Slavin JL. Apparent fiber digestibility and fecal short-chain fatty acid concentrations with ingestion of two types of dietary fiber. JPEN 1994; 18:14–19.
21. Kapadia SA, Raimundo AH, Grimble GK, Aimer P, Silk DBA. Influence of three different fiber-supplemented enteral diets on bowel function and short-chain fatty acid production. JPEN 1995; 19: 63–68.
22. Roediger WE. Famine, fiber, fatty acids, and failed colonic absorption: Does fiber fermentation ameliorate diarrhea? JPEN 1994; 18:4–8.
23. Scheppach WM, Bartram HP. Experimental evidence for and clinical implications of fiber and artificial enteral nutrition. Nutrition 1993; 9:399–405.
24. Basson MD, Emenaker NJ, Hong F. Differential modulation of human (Caco-2) colon cancer cell line phenotype by short chain fatty acids. PSEBM 1998; 217:476–483.
25. Kim Y, Mason JB. Nutrition chemoprevention of gastrointestinal cancers: a critical review. Nutr Rev 1996; 54:259–279.
26. Fearton EF, Jones PA. Progressing toward a molecular description of colorectal cancer development. FASEB J 1992; 6:2783–2790.
27. Doll R, Peto R. The causes of cancer: quantitative estimates of avoidable risks of cancer in the United States today. J Natl Cancer Inst 1981; 66:1191–1308.
28. Hill MJ. Cereals, dietary fibre, and cancer. Nutr Res 1998; 18:653–659.
29. Hill MJ. Cereals, cereal fibre and colorectal cancer risk—a review of the epidemiological literature. Eur J Cancer Prev 1997; 6:219–225.
30. Jacobs DR, Marquart L, Slavin J, Kushi LH. Whole-grain intake and cancer—an expanded review and meta-analysis. Nutr Cancer 1998; 30:85–96.
31. Chatenoud L, Tavani A, La Vecchia C, Jacobs DR, Negri E, Levi F, Franceschi S. Whole grain food intake and cancer risk. Int J Cancer 1998; 77:24–28.
32. Steinmetz KA, Potter JD. Vegetables, fruit, and cancer. I. Epidemiology. Cancer Causes Control 1991; 2:325–357.
33. Slavin JL, Jacobs D, Marquart L. Whole-grain consumption and chronic disease—protective mechanisms. Nutr Cancer 1997; 27:14–21.
34. Steinmetz KA, Potter JD. Vegetables, fruit, and cancer. II. Mechanisms. Cancer Causes Control 1991; 2:427–442.
35. Steinmetz KA, Kushi LH, Bostick RM, Folsom AR, Potter JD. Vegetables, fruit, and colon cancer in the Iowa Women's Health Study. Am J Epidemiol 1994; 139:1–15.
36. Bingham SA. Mechanisms and experimental and epidemiological evidence relating dietary fibre (non-starch polysaccharides) and starch to protection against large bowel cancer. Proc Nutr Soc 1990; 49:153–171.
37. Willett W. The search for the causes of breast and colon cancer. Nature 1989; 338:389–394.
38. Trock B, Lanza E, Greenwald P. Dietary fiber, vegetables, and colon cancer: critical review and meta-analyses of the epidemiologic evidence. J Natl Cancer Inst 1990; 82:650–661.

39. Howe GR, Benito E, Castelleto R, Cornee J, Esteve J, Gallagher RP, Iscovich JM, Deng-ao J, Kaaka R, Kune GA, Kune S, L'Abbe KA, Lee HP, Lee M, Miller AB, Peters RK, Potter JD, Bivoli E, Slattery ML, Trichopoulos D, Tuyns A, Tzonou A, Whittemore AS, Wu-Williams AH, Shu Z. Dietary intake of fiber and decreased risk of cancers of the colon and rectum: Evidence from the combined analysis of 13 case-control studies. JNCI 1992; 84:1887–1896.

40. Negri E, Franceschi S, Parpinel M, La Vecchia C. Fiber intake and risk of colorectal cancer. Cancer Epid Biomarkers Prev 1998; 7:667–671.

41. Slattery ML, Potter JD, Coates A, Ma KN, Berry TD, Duncan DM, Caan BJ. Plant foods and colon cancer: an assessment of specific foods and their related nutrients (United States). Cancer Causes Control 1997; 8:575–590.

42. Marchard LL, Hankin JH, Wilkens LR, Kolenel LN, Englyst HN, Lyu L. Dietary fiber and colorectal cancer risk. Epidemiology 1997; 8:658–665.

43. Witte JS, Longnecker MP, Bird CR, Lee ER, Frankl HD, Halle RW. Relation of vegetable, fruit, and grain consumption to colorectal adenomatous polyps. Am J Epidemiol 1996; 144:1015–1025.

44. Lubin F, Rozen P, Arieli B, Farbstein M, Knani Y, Bat L, Farbstein H. Nutritional and lifestyle habits and water-fiber interaction in colorectal adenoma etiology. Cancer Epid Biomarkers Prev 1997; 6:79–85.

45. Slattery ML, Boucher RM, Caan BJ, Potter JD, Ma KN. Eating patterns and risk of colon cancer. Am J Epidemiol 1998; 148:4–16.

46. Giovannucci E, Stampfer MJ, Colditz G, Rimm EB, Willett WC. Relationship of diet to risk of colorectal cancer in men. J Natl Cancer Inst 1992; 84:91–98.

47. Willett WC, Stampfer JM, Colditz GA, Rosner BA, Speizer FE. Relation of meat, fat, and fiber intake to the risk of colon cancer in a prospective study among women. N Engl J Med 1990; 323: 1664–1672.

48. Cummings JH, Bingham SA, Heaton KW, Eastwood MA. Fecal weight, colon cancer risk and dietary intake of nonstarch polysaccharides (dietary fiber). Gastroenterology 1992; 103:1783–1789.

49. Cummings JH. The effect of dietary fiber on fecal weight and composition. In: GA Spiller, ed. CRC Handbook of Dietary Fiber in Human Nutrition. Boca Raton, FL: CRC Press, 1993, pp 263–333.

50. McMichael AJ, Potter JD. Reproduction, endogenous and exogenous sex hormones, and colon cancer: a review and hypothesis. J Natl Cancer Inst 1980; 65:1201–1207.

51. Potter JD. Hormones and colon cancer. J Natl Cancer Inst 1995; 87:1039–1040.

52. Potter JD, Slattery ML, Bostick RM, Gapstur SM. Colon cancer: a review of the epidemiology. Epidemiol Rev 1993; 15:499–545.

53. Hebert-Croteau N. A meta-analysis of hormone replacement therapy and colon cancer in women. Cancer Epid Biomarkers and Prev 1998; 7:653–659.

54. Potter JD. Reconciling the epidemiology, physiology, and molecular biology of colon cancer. JAMA 1992; 268:1573–1577.

55. Rose DP, Goldman M, Connolly JM, Strong LE. High-fiber diet reduces serum estrogen concentrations in premenopausal women. Am J Clin Nutr 1991; 54:520–525.

56. Goldin BR, Woods MNL, Spiegelman D, Longscope C, Morrill-LaBrode A, Dwyer JT, Gualtier LJ, Hertzmark E, Gorbach SL. The effect of dietary fat and fiber on serum estrogen concentrations in premenopausal women under controlled dietary conditions. Cancer 1994; 74(3 suppl):1125–1131.

57. Bagga D, Ashley JM, Geffrey SP, Wang H, Barnard J, Korenman S, Heber D. Effects of very low fat, high fiber diet on serum hormones and menstrual function. Cancer 1995; 76:2491–2496.

58. Lampe JW, Fredstrom SB, Slavin JL, Potter JD. Sex differences in colonic function: a randomized trial. Gut 1993; 34:531–536.

59. Giovannucci E. Insulin and colon cancer. Cancer Causes and Control 1995; 6:164–179.

60. La Vecchia C, Negri E, Decarli A, Franceschi S. Diabetes mellitus and colorectal cancer risk. Cancer Epid Biomarkers Prev 1997; 6:1007–1010.

61. Guevin N, Jacques H, Nadeau A, Galibois I. Postprandial glucose, insulin, and lipid responses to four meals containing unpurified dietary fiber in noninsulin-dependent diabetes mellitus (NIDDM), hypertriglyceridemic subjects. J Am Coll Nutr 1996; 15:389–396.

62. Levine AS, Tallman JR, Grace MK, Parker SA, Billington CJ, Levitt MD. Effect of breakfast cereals on short-term food intake. Am J Clin Nutr 1989; 50:1303–1307.

63. Klurfeld DM. Fiber and cancer protection—mechanisms. In: D Kritchevsky, C Bonfield, eds. Dietary Fiber in Health and Disease. New York: Plenum Press, 1997, pp 249–257.

64. Alabaster O, Tang ZC, Frost A, Shivapurkar N. Potential synergism between wheat bran and psyllium: enhanced inhibition of colon cancer. Cancer Lett 1993; 75:53–58.

65. Boffa LC, Lupton JR, Mariani MR, Ceppi M, Newmark HL, Scalmati A, Lipkin M. Modulation of colonic epithelial cell proliferation, histone acetylation, and luminal short chain fatty acids by variation of dietary fiber (wheat bran) in rats. Cancer Res 1992; 52:5906–5912.

66. McIntyre A, Gibson PR, Young GP. Butyrate production from dietary fiber and protection against large bowel cancer in a rat model. Gut 1993; 34:386–391.

67. Reddy B, Engle A, Katsifis S, Simi B, Bartram HP, Perrino P, Mahan C. Biochemical epidemiology of colon cancer: effect of types of dietary fiber on fecal mutagens, acid, and neutral sterols in healthy subjects. Cancer Res 1989; 49:4629–4635.

68. Jenab M, Thompson LU. The influence of phytic acid in wheat bran on early biomarkers of colon carcinogenesis. Carcinogenesis 1998; 19:1087–1092.

69. Lu FJ, Chu LH, Gau RJ. Free radical-scavenging properties of lignin. Nutr Cancer 1998; 30:31–38.

70. Alberts DS, Einspahr J, Rees-McGee S, Ramanujam P, Buller MK, Clark L, Ritenbaugh C, Atwood J, Pethigal P, Earnest D, Villar H, Phelps J, Lipkin M, Wargovich M, Meyskens FL. Effects of dietary wheat bran fiber on rectal epithelial cell proliferation in patients with resection for colorectal cancers. JNCI 1990; 82:1280–1285.

71. Alberts DS, Einspahr J, Ritenbaugh C, Aickin M, Rees-McGee S, Atwood J, Emerson S, Mason-Liddil N, Bettinger L, Patel J, Bellapravalu S, Ramanujam PS, Phelps J, Clark L. The effect of wheat bran fiber and calcium supplementation on rectal mucosal proliferation rates in patients with resected adenomatous colorectal polyps. Cancer Epid Biomarkers Prev 1997; 6:161–169.

72. MacLennan R, Macrae F, Bain C, Battistutta D, Chapuis P, Gratten H, Lambert J, Newland RC, Ngu M, Russell A, Ward M, Wahlqvist ML. Randomized trial of intake of fat, fiber, and beta carotene to prevent colorectal adenomas. J Natl Cancer Inst 1995; 87:1760–1766.

73. McKeown-Eyssen GE, Bright-See E, Bruce WR, Jazmaji V. The Toronto Polyp Prevention Group. A randomized trial of a low fat high fibre diet in the recurrence of colorectal polyps. J Clin Epidemiol 1994; 47:525–536.

74. Lanza E, Schatzkin A, Ballard-Barbash R, Carle D, Clifford C, Paskett E, Hayes D, Bote E, Caan B, Shike M, Weissfeld J, Slattery M, Mateski D, Daston C, Clifford C. The polyp prevention trial. II: Dietary intervention program and participant baseline dietary characteristics. Cancer Epid Biomarkers Prev 1996; 5:385–392.

4

Dietary Fiber and Breast Cancer Risk

Susan Sungsoo Cho and Celeste Clark
Kellogg Company, Battle Creek, Michigan

Sharon E. Rickard
University of Toronto, Toronto, Ontario, Canada

I. INTRODUCTION

Globally, breast cancer is the second most common cancer among women; in developed countries, it is the most common cancer (1). The rise in breast cancer incidence in developing regions (1,2), which typically have lower rates of breast cancer compared to industrialized nations, may be partly related to a trend towards more Westernized diets, i.e., high in fat and low in dietary fiber (3).

The link between dietary factors and breast cancer risk was first apparent in ecological or correlation studies. International comparisons have found positive correlations between estimated per capita fat consumption in different countries and breast cancer incidence or mortality rates (4–9). Few studies have looked at international differences in dietary fiber consumption or intake of fiber-rich foods and breast cancer risk, observing both high inverse correlations (7,10,11) or no association (8). Other studies looking at general carbohydrate intake, which may include dietary fiber, starch, and sugars, have found moderate inverse correlations with breast cancer incidence or mortality (5,6).

Migrant studies have provided further evidence that the correlations observed in the ecological studies were due to environmental rather than genetic factors. Migrants from regions with low breast cancer incidence and mortality rates such as Japan, China, and Latin America acquire the higher rates characteristic of their new location (i.e., the United States and Western European countries) after one or two generations (12). This change in breast cancer risk observed in subsequent generations has been attributed to changes in dietary habits. Using correlation and migrant studies as a basis, Doll and Peto (13) have estimated that 50% of breast cancer deaths may be attributable to diet.

However, the role of specific dietary components in modulating breast cancer risk is not clear. Of all the nutrients, dietary fat has been the most extensively studied in its relationship to breast cancer. Although most international correlation studies have found strong, positive associations between dietary fat intake and breast cancer (14), only 3 out of 25 case-control studies have found a significant increase in breast cancer risk (15). On the other hand, meta-analyses of case-control studies have significant increases in risk with total fat intake (16,17), particularly in postmenopausal women (16). Of the nine cohort studies examining the relationship between total fat intake and breast cancer risk, four have found a positive relationship, but this was only significant in one study (15). A pooled analysis of six prospective cohort studies found no association for overall fat intake (18).

In contrast, much fewer studies have investigated the role of dietary fiber in altering breast cancer risk. The purpose of this review is to examine the epidemiological and experimental evidence that dietary fiber reduces breast cancer risk and to discuss the potential mechanisms through which fiber exerts its protective effects. But before the studies and mechanisms are discussed, it is essential to understand the definition of dietary fiber and the problems that may be encountered in trying to estimate dietary fiber intakes.

II. DIETARY FIBER: COMPONENTS AND ESTIMATION OF INTAKE

Dietary fiber was first defined by Burkitt and Trowell (19) as the sum of polysaccharides and lignin (a complex, noncarbohydrate, three-dimensional polymer of phenyl propane units) that are not hydrolyzed by human alimentary enzymes. In 1982, Southgate (20) proposed that dietary fiber be defined as the sum of lignin and nonstarch polysaccharides (NSP), which consist of cellulose, hemicellulose, β-glucans, pectin, gums, and mucilages. Resistant starches, formed by retrogradation of amylose, have also been included in the definition of dietary fiber because they escape digestion in the small intestine and thus behave like NSP in the gut (21,22). Cho (formerly Lee) and Prosky (23) have proposed including resistant oligosaccharides—oligosaccharides not hydrolyzed by human alimentary enzymes—in the definition of dietary fiber. Since most foods do not contain resistant oligosaccharides, this new definition would not affect most of the dietary fiber values previously determined but would allow for more accurate quantification of total dietary fiber in new food products developed in the future (24).

Dietary fiber can also be broken down into soluble and insoluble forms. This distinction is based on the solubility characteristics of the fiber in hot aqueous buffer solutions (23). Soluble and insoluble fibers have different physiological actions. Soluble fibers (some hemicelluloses, β-glucans, pectins, gums, and mucilages) delay gut transit time, delay gastric emptying, and impede the absorption of certain nutrients such as glucose, cholesterol, and fats (25). Insoluble fibers (cellulose, lignin, other hemicelluloses) tend to speed up or decrease intestinal transit time, increase stool bulk, slow starch hydrolysis, and delay glucose absorption (25). Another major difference between these two types of fibers is that bacteria in the colon can break down soluble fibers, whereas insoluble fibers are largely resistant to degradation (26). Discrepancies in the literature may be partly attributed to these different types of fiber; fruit and vegetable fibers are mainly soluble, and grain fibers are largely insoluble.

A major problem in any epidemiological study is the accurate estimation of nutrient intakes. This is even more apparent in the case of dietary fiber because of the variety of methods available to quantify all or some of the components in the dietary fiber definition.

Ecological or correlation studies (discussed in more detail below) use food balance (per capita disappearance) statistics and household food surveys to estimate intakes. Food balance estimates assume that all foods produced or imported (and not fed to livestock, lost in storage, or exported) are consumed by the population. Consumption tends to be overestimated since losses in home preparation, produce grown at home, food given to pets, and food waste are not fully accounted for (27,28). In addition, per capita consumption data do not account for variability in dietary practices between individuals. Data from household food surveys also need to be corrected for foods consumed outside of the home as well as for household size and composition (28).

The three methods used by case-control and prospective cohort studies in dietary assessments are 24-hour recall, food frequency questionnaires (FFQ), and detailed food records for varying lengths of time, which may or may not include weighing of the food consumed. The 24-hour recall data tends to underestimate nutrient intake and cannot take into account seasonal variation (29). The FFQ are convenient for assessing food intakes on a large number of individuals and are relatively accurate in estimating typical intakes in individuals over long periods of time. Quantitative FFQ, which often include questions on food preparation practices, are more accurate than semi-quantitative questionnaires. Although detailed food records tend to overestimate intake levels (29), weighed food records are highly correlated to chemical analysis methods of food composites (30). Food records are more labor-intensive for large studies and are generally used to validate FFQ using a subsample of the subjects. Food records are more suited for accurate assessment of the relatively shorter randomized intervention studies.

Once intakes of various foods have been estimated using one of the above methods, fiber intakes are then estimated using established tables or databases. Many of the databases used in the 1970s and early 1980s were based on crude fiber values, which can vary from 10 to 50% of the total dietary fiber present in a food (24). Thus, data using crude fiber values should be interpreted with caution. Later food composition tables in the United Kingdom used values derived from the Southgate method, which estimates dietary fiber as unavailable carbohydrate (31). However, this method tends to overestimate dietary fiber values, especially in high-starch foods. The most recent dietary fiber tables use the Englyst NSP methods (32–34) in the United Kingdom or the global methods (35–37) of the Association of Official Analytical Chemists (AOAC) International, in particular AOAC methods 991.43 (35) and 985.29 (36).

III. EPIDEMIOLOGICAL STUDIES EXAMINING THE RELATIONSHIP BETWEEN DIETARY FIBER AND BREAST CANCER RISK

Now that we have a better understanding of what dietary fiber is and the problems inherent in estimating dietary fiber intake, we will now review the different types of epidemiological studies that have been used to assess the relationship between dietary fiber and breast cancer. A better perspective of the validity and strength of the associations found in each type of study will be achieved by first discussing their respective benefits and limitations.

A. Ecological or Correlation Studies

Ecological or correlation studies are the simplest type of epidemiological study to examine the relationship between dietary factors and breast cancer. They are valuable because the differences in intake of dietary components or foods between populations (e.g., industrialized nations vs. developing nations, omnivores vs. vegetarians) are usually wider than those from within a population. This variability in intake is key to observing a relationship between the dietary factor and breast cancer risk. However, as mentioned earlier, per capita disappearance or household surveys used to estimate dietary intakes tend to overestimate nutrient intakes. In addition, the associations obtained are for populations and are not necessarily applicable to individuals within that population (38). Furthermore, incidence and mortality statistics are dependent upon the accuracy and completeness of reporting, diagnostic practices, and availability of medical treatments (1); this undoubtedly differs among countries, particularly developed versus undeveloped nations. Although the relationships observed in these types of studies do not necessarily point to causation, ecological studies do play an important role in the generation of new hypotheses to be tested in more controlled investigations.

Most ecological studies have found a negative relationship between dietary fiber and breast cancer (Table 1). Consumption of fiber-rich foods has been associated with a reduction in breast

Table 1 Ecological/Correlation Studies Examining the Relationship Between Dietary Fiber and Breast Cancer Risk

Study (Ref.)	Subjects	Design and methods	Results	Comments
Blondell, 1988 (39)	White males and females that lived in Kentucky from 1950–1969	Age-adjusted cancer mortality rates were selected for white male and female patients living in Kentucky from 1950–1969. Twenty-six independent variables were chosen to reflect differences between lifestyle, diet and demographics between urban and rural areas in Kentucky.	17 independent variables were chosen for the final analysis. In rural Kentucky lifestyle was the best predictor of female breast cancer, while in the urban setting fertility was as good a predictor as lifestyle. Subsistence farmers, whose diets are based on whole grains and are high in fiber, exhibited the lowest cancer mortality in both sexes.	
Correa, 1981 (11)		Correlation study of 41 countries comparing age-adjusted breast cancer mortality rates in 1973 with diet data published by the Food and Agriculture Organization (FAO) for 1964–1966.	Breast cancer was negatively correlated with the consumption of rice, maize, and beans ($r = -0.50$ to -0.70). A significant but weak positive association was observed between breast cancer mortality and wheat.	There was no direct estimation of fiber intake and author noted potential for estimation error. No adjustments were made for independent variables.
Guo et al., 1994 (45)	6500 adults: 100 men and women in age groups of 35–44, 45–54, and 55–64 recruited from 65 rural counties	Breast cancer mortality rates obtained during 1973–1975 nationwide survey in China were correlated with data on diet, lifestyle, and biochemical markers collected in a survey of 65 counties in 1983. Blood work was collected for serum markers. Interviews were conducted to obtain information on dietary habits and demographic characteristics.	No significant associations were found for breast cancer mortality and intake of fresh fruits and vegetables.	The authors did not look at dietary fiber intakes. One county was omitted from analyses due to an outlying value of mortality. Although some correlations were significant (animal foods), all correlation coefficients observed in the study were very low ($r < 0.4$).

Reference	Description	Results	Comments
Ingram, 1981 (44)	Retrospective correlation study examining age-adjusted breast cancer mortality in relation to dietary habits in England and Wales from 1928 to 1977.	The strongest correlation was the inverse relationship between cereal consumption and breast cancer mortality at a lag interval of 12 years ($r = -0.92$, $p < 0.00001$). No significant correlation was found for fruit and vegetable intake ($r = 0.14$).	Confounding factors may have included the change in overall nutrition during World War II. Data on lag intervals may have been questionable. Author suggested an inherent beneficial effect from the consumption of cereal products themselves.
Ishimoto et al., 1994 (40)	Japanese age-adjusted breast cancer mortality data from 12 districts for 1966–1980 correlated with food/nutrient intake from national nutrition surveys (1966–1980).	Wheat intake was positively associated with breast cancer mortality. Rice and energy from cereals were negatively correlated with mortality. Carbohydrates and pulses were also negatively correlated but were not statistically significant.	The authors suggest that changes from traditional diets in Japan, where rice is a staple, to more westernized diets increases breast cancer risk.
Kolonel et al., 1981 (27)	4657 adults, approx. 45 years, 5 ethnic groups (Caucasian, Japanese, Chinese, Filipino, and Hawaiian). Diet was correlated with ethnic-specific cancer incidences obtained from the population-based Hawaii Tumor Registry. Diet interviews were conducted in 1977–1979 using a FFQ (83 items) designed to cover main sources of fat and protein, less so on carbohydrate and certain vitamins. Four-day measured food records were also obtained from 100 women in each ethnic group.	Complex carbohydrates were negatively correlated ($r = -0.71$) with breast cancer incidence.	Dietary fiber intake was not examined.
Morales and Llopis, 1992 (41)	Breast cancer mortality in Spain (1977–1985) was correlated to dietary intake, including fiber. Breast cancer mortality, morbidity, and demographic data were obtained from the Instituto Nacional de Estadistica (INE). Nutrient and food consumption data were also obtained from INE for the years 1980 and 1981.	Low correlations were observed in relating mean breast cancer mortality rates for the 50 Spanish provinces to dietary components. Dietary fiber and cereals were among the most significant inverse relationships with breast cancer mortality observed.	Although authors tried to compensate for demographic changes, but it may have still been a confounder.

Table 1 Continued

Study (Ref.)	Subjects	Design and methods	Results	Comments
Rose et al., 1986 (10)		Cancer mortality data (1978 and 1979) were obtained from 30 countries. Dietary data were estimated from the per capita supply of food from 1979–1981 published by the Food and Agriculture Organization of the United Nations.	Cereals were negatively correlated ($r = -0.63$) with breast cancer mortality. Very weak correlations were observed with vegetables ($r = -0.11$) and fruits ($r = 0.09$).	The authors mention that per capita supply does not account for wastage, food fed to pets or domestic animals, or nutrient losses due to storage, food preparation, cooking. In addition, dietary differences of special subgroups within a country and seasonal variations would not be detected.
Rosen et al., 1988 (42)	5760 households in 24 counties of Sweden.	Standardized mortality rate ratios for ages 15–74 years were calculated for various cancers during 1969–1978. In 1978, households were asked to keep a record of all food expenditures (excluding outside meals) for 2 weeks.	Breast cancer mortality was negatively correlated with whole grain breads (crisp bread, whole meal rye bread, and thin unleavened bread: $r = -0.65$) and dietary fiber ($r = -0.67$).	
Taioli et al., 1991 (43)		Age-specific mortality rates for breast cancer in 1970 and 1981 (ages 0–74 years) were obtained for the United States and Italy (north and south). The mortality data could be compared since both countries use the same registration techniques. Dietary information was obtained from national household surveys in 1973–1976.	Age-specific mortality rates for breast cancer were higher in the United States than in Italy for women over 35 years of age. White Americans had the highest mortality rate, while southern Italians had the lowest rate. Wheat consumption was negatively correlated with breast cancer mortality.	Although there are no dietary fiber data per se, the authors found a higher consumption of bread, baked goods, fruits, and vegetables in southern Italy.

cancer mortality (10,11,39–43) and incidence (27). Cereals and whole grain foods appear to be consistent in their protective effect (10,39,41,42,44). On the other hand, fruit and vegetable intake has been found to be negatively correlated with breast cancer mortality in some studies (11) and to have no association in others (10,44,45).

B. Case-Control Studies

In case-control studies, patients with a particular disease, in our case breast cancer, are compared to a group of people without the disease from the same population. In contrast to correlation studies, known or suspected confounding variables can be potentially controlled or removed. Weaknesses of case-control studies include alterations in dietary and biochemical variables being investigated by the disease, biased recall of past diets by cases due to their knowledge of having the disease, and smaller ranges of nutrient intakes (38). In many instances, hospital controls are used for convenience but may also have a disease that could affect the dietary variables being measured. Use of healthy community or neighborhood controls circumvents this problem.

As observed in the ecological/correlation studies, intake of dietary fiber or foods rich in dietary fiber was also largely protective (Table 2). Of the studies looking at overall fiber consumption, 10 found a protective effect (16,46–54), 4 found no association (55–58), and 2 found nonsignificant increases in breast cancer risk (51,59). Vegetable or vegetable fiber intake appears to have the most consistent protective effect (47,49,51,53,60–66) with few studies finding no association (56–58) or a potentially adverse effect (51). The role of bread/cereal intake or grain fiber intake on breast cancer risk is less consistent, having protective (47,51,53,65), adverse (49,60,61), or no effect (57,58,64,67). However, many of the studies observing no association or adverse effects with bread/cereal intake on breast cancer risk examined intakes from refined products (49,60,61,67), which are relatively low in dietary fiber and likely high in fat and/or sugar. Similar inconsistencies have been found for fruit or fruit fiber intake with protective effects (49,51,61,67), no effects (57,58,64), or potentially adverse effects (51) on breast cancer risk. It should also be noted that null or adverse results were found in studies that quantified crude fiber intakes only (51,59,67), underestimating the total amount of fiber consumed.

One may speculate that the greater protective effects with vegetables and vegetable fiber may be partially due to the fact that vegetable fibers are mainly soluble and highly fermentable. Yet evidently from the previous paragraph, the largely soluble fruit fiber has yielded inconsistent results with breast cancer risk. In addition, Baghurst and Rohan (46) found similar protective effects for soluble and insoluble fiber against breast cancer. Moreover, three separate studies found that intake of cellulose, a nonfermentable insoluble fiber, significantly reduced breast cancer risk (46,68,69).

Some investigators that have stratified their data according to menopausal status have observed differences between pre- and postmenopausal women with breast cancer, but the effect has not been consistent. In a meta-analysis of case-control studies, Howe et al. (16) observed that the protective effect for dietary fiber was stronger in postmenopausal women and suggested that the mechanisms involved in premenopausal and postmenopausal breast cancer were different. Baghurst and Rohan (46) had a similar finding, with the protective effects of total dietary fiber and its components stronger in postmenopausal women. Zaridze et al. (68) observed that cellulose significantly reduced breast cancer risk in postmenopausal, but not premenopausal, women. Other studies had observed the opposite effect where the protective effects of fiber were stronger in premenopausal women (50,51,52,69). De Stefani and colleagues (47) found similar protective effects in pre- and postmenopausal women. Interestingly, Pryor et al. (51) saw protective effects with overall and fruit and vegetable crude fiber in premenopausal women

Table 2 Case-Control Studies Examining the Relationship Between Dietary Fiber and Breast Cancer Risk

Study (Ref.)	Subjects	Design and methods	Results	Comments
Baghurst and Rohan, 1994 (46)	451 women with breast cancer, 451 population-based controls, aged 20–74 years.	Study in Adelaide, South Australia (1982–1984). Subjects were interviewed in their homes for demographic, reproductive, and medical information. Dietary information was collected through self-administered FFQ (179 items).	Total dietary fiber, total NSP, soluble and insoluble NSP, and cellulose (expressed as g/MJ energy) significantly reduced breast cancer risk (odd ratio, OR = 0.46–0.58, $p \leq 0.005$). The results were stronger in postmenopausal women.	All fiber fractions appear to be equally effective in reducing breast cancer risk. Consumption of foods rich in dietary fiber may be protective against breast cancer
Braga et al., 1997 (60)	2569 breast cancer patients, 2588 hospital controls, aged 20–74 years.	Study in Italy (1991–1994). Subjects were interviewed for reproductive, demographic, and medical information. Dietary data for the two years prior to diagnosis or hospital admission were obtained using a FFQ (78 items).	Raw vegetables were inversely associated with breast cancer risk in premenopausal women, particularly age < 45 years (OR = 0.64, $p < 0.01$). Bread and cereal dishes were associated with increased breast cancer risk (OR = 1.35, $p \leq 0.05$)	Bread and cereal category contained dishes with meat and high in fat (e.g., savory pies, pasta with meat/pesto sauce).
De Stefani et al., 1997 (47)	351 breast cancer patients, 356 hospitalized controls, aged 20–80 years.	Study in Uruguay (1994–1996). Subjects were interviewed for reproductive, demographic, and medical information. Dietary information was collected through a self-administered FFQ (64 items).	Total dietary fiber and NSP (total, soluble, and insoluble) reduced breast cancer risk (RR = 0.45–0.51, $p < 0.001$). This effect appears to be due mainly to grain and vegetable fiber intake. Similar results were observed for pre- and postmenopausal women.	When dietary fiber is analyzed according to its source, cereal and vegetable fiber, but not fruit fiber, were associated with a strong inverse association.
Franceschi et al., 1996 (55)	2569 women with breast cancer, 2588 hospital controls, aged 20–74 years.	Study in Italy (1991–1994). Subjects were interviewed for reproductive, demographic, and medical information. Dietary data for the two years prior to diagnosis or hospital admission were obtained using a FFQ (78 items).	Odds ratios were adjusted for alcohol and energy intake. Dietary fiber had no effect on breast cancer risk.	

Reference	Subjects	Methods	Results	Comments
Franceschi et al., 1997 (61)	2569 women with breast cancer, 2588 hospital controls, aged 20–74 years.	Study in Italy (1991–1994). Subjects were interviewed for reproductive, demographic, and medical information. Dietary data for the two years prior to diagnosis or hospital admission were obtained using a FFQ (78 items).	Odds ratios were adjusted for alcohol and energy intake. Higher bread and cereal consumption was related to a higher breast cancer risk score. In contrast, the breast cancer risk score was reduced with fruit and vegetable intake.	Breads and cereals in the study were refined products and thus likely low in dietary fiber.
Graham et al., 1982 (56)	2024 breast cancer cases and 1463 hospital controls.	Study in Buffalo, New York (1958–1965). Subjects were interviewed to obtain information on reproductive, demographic, medical factors. Dietary data for 2 years prior to hospital admission were obtained using FFQ.	No differences of note for the risk of breast cancer between cases and controls with respect to intake of cruciferous vegetables or fiber.	Authors suggest limitations due to the reliability of FFQ.
Graham et al., 1991 (48)	439 postmenopausal breast cancer patients, 494 community controls, aged 41–85 years.	Study in western New York. Subjects were interviewed for reproductive, demographic, medical, and dietary (FFQ, 172 items) information.	Risk reduction associated with dietary fiber was significant (OR = 0.74, $p \leq 0.01$).	Breast cancer risk was lowest among those ingesting the largest amount of carotenoids (but not retinol), ascorbic acid, alpha-tocopherol, and dietary fiber.
Hislop et al., 1986 (62)	846 breast cancer cases, 862 neighborhood controls (under 70 years of age).	Study in British Columbia, Canada (1980–1982). Subjects were mailed questionnaires that focused on reproductive and medical history and estrogen and vitamin use. The FFQ (31 items) focused on four different age periods (up to 13, 13–19, 20–40, and 40+). Childhood eating practices were determined from the "up to 13" category and recent eating habits from "20–40" or "40+."	An inverse association between breast cancer risk and recent consumption of carrots and nonyellow vegetables "approached significance" around menopause (premenopausal women > 45 years of age, $p \leq 0.08$ and postmenopausal women < 60 years of age, $p \leq 0.10$).	

Table 2 Continued

Study (Ref.)	Subjects	Design and methods	Results	Comments
Howe et al., 1990 (16)	4427 women with breast cancer, 6095 controls.	A meta-analysis of 12 case-control studies using original individual study records.	Dietary fiber reduced breast cancer risk for postmenopausal (RR = 0.83, $p \leq 0.002$) and all women together (RR = 0.85, $p \leq 0.001$). No association was found between dietary fiber and breast cancer risk in premenopausal women.	Although the protective effect of dietary fiber on breast cancer risk was stronger in postmenopausal women, the differences between pre- and postmenopausal women were not significant.
Ingram et al., 1991 (57)	99 women with breast cancer; 91 women with benign epithelial hyperplasia of the breast, 95 women with benign fibrocystic disease; 209 community controls.	Study in Perth, Western Australia (1985–1987). Subjects were interviewed in the home for reproductive, demographic, and medical information. Dietary data were obtained using a self-administered FFQ (179 items).	No associations were observed with dietary fiber intake, cereal products, or fruits and vegetables.	
Iscovich et al., 1989 (49)	150 women with breast cancer, 300 hospital controls, 300 neighborhood controls.	Study conducted in La Plata, Argentina (1984–1985). Interviews for reproductive, demographic, and medical information were conducted by a nutritionist, social worker, or physician. Dietary information about the 5-year period up to 6 months before the interview was obtained using a FFQ (147 items).	There was an increased breast cancer risk with grain intake, which consisted of mainly refined products (rice, noodles, and pasta), using hospital controls. Green vegetables and fruits other than citrus reduced breast cancer risk. Total dietary fiber intake was inversely associated with risk when using the neighborhood controls.	The diet assessment was not sensitive enough to examine individual nutrient intakes. Pre- menopausal and postmenopausal data were not presented separately.
Katsouyanni et al., 1986 (63)	120 breast cancer patients, 120 hospital controls.	Study in Athens, Greece (1983–1984). Subjects were interviewed by a dietitian and a physician for demographic, medical, reproductive, and dietary habit (FFQ, 120 items) information.	Cases reported a significantly lower consumption of fruits and vegetables as a group. Vegetable consumption, particularly cucumber, lettuce, and raw carrots, yielded an odds ratio of 0.12.	The protective effect of vegetables against breast cancer may be due to micronutrients and/or fiber (through reduction of caloric intake).

Reference	Subjects	Study description	Results	Comments
Katsouyanni et al., 1988 (59)	120 breast cancer patients, 120 hospital controls.	Study in Athens, Greece (1983–1984). Subjects were interviewed by a dietitian and physician to obtain sociodemographic and medical information. Dietary data were obtained using a FFQ (120 items).	Crude fiber was positively associated with breast cancer risk (OR = 1.57), but this was not statistically significant.	The focus of the dietary assessment was fat and not fiber.
La Vecchia et al., 1987 (64)	1108 breast cancer patients (aged 26–74), 1281 hospital controls (aged 25–74).	Case-control study conducted in northern Italy. Subjects were interviewed for reproductive, demographic, and medical information. The FFQ focused on major sources in the Italian diet of retinoids (dairy products, meat, fish) and carotenoids (carrots and fruit).	A strong reduced breast cancer risk was seen with consumption of green vegetables (OR = 0.36). No association was found for fresh fruit or whole grain bread/pasta.	The authors suggest that the current findings confirm that various aspects of diet may influence breast cancer risk; due to the limited data available, a cautionary note is made concerning the implementation of a program at the public health level.
La Vecchia et al., 1997 (69)	2569 women with breast cancer (aged 23–74 years), 2588 hospital controls (aged 20–74 years).	Study in Italy (1991–1994). Subjects were interviewed for reproductive, demographic, and medical information. Dietary data for the previous 2 years were obtained using a FFQ (78 items).	Cellulose intake had a weak, but statistically significant protective effect on breast cancer risk (OR = 0.90, $p < 0.05$). The protective effect of cellulose was stronger in premenopausal women.	The stronger protection of dietary fiber in premenopausal women may be related to reductions in estrogen bioavailability.
Levi et al., 1993 (65)	107 breast cancer patients (aged 32–75 years), 318 hospital controls (aged 30–75 years).	Study conducted in Vaud, Switzerland (1990–1992). Subjects were interviewed for reproductive, demographic, and medical information. Dietary data were obtained using a FFQ (50 items).	After adjusting for total energy intake, inverse associations with breast cancer risk were observed for green vegetables (OR = 0.5), cruciferous vegetables (OR = 0.5), onions (OR = 0.6), and pears (OR = 0.5). Whole-grain bread and pasta were associated with reduced risk, but this was not statistically significant.	Frequent intake of vegetables appeared to protect against breast cancer.

Table 2 Continued

Study (Ref.)	Subjects	Design and methods	Results	Comments
Lubin et al., 1986 (50)	818 breast cancer patients, 743 surgical controls, 813 nonsurgical controls.	Study in Israel (1976–1978). Subjects were interviewed for reproductive, demographic, and medical information. Dietary data obtained using a FFQ (260 items).	Breast cancer risk decreased as fiber consumption increased, but pattern was consistent only for younger patients (< 50 years of age). Little differential effect between premenopausal and postmenopausal women.	The authors conclude that a high-fat, high–animal protein, and low-fiber diet is associated with increased cancer risk, but this relationship needs to be studied further.
Pryor et al., 1989 (51)	172 breast cancer patients, 190 community controls, aged 20–54, Caucasian.	Study in Utah (1980–1983). Dietary data on adolescent intakes were obtained over the phone using a modified NCI questionnaire. Reproductive, demographic, and medical information was also obtained.	There was a significant ($p < 0.01$) trend towards a protective effect from crude fiber intake in premenopausal women. In contrast, fiber intake elevated the odds ratio in postmenopausal group, but this was not significant due to large variability. Fiber from grains significantly lowered risk in both pre- and postmenopausal groups. In premenopausal group, fiber from fruits and vegetables, lowered risk, whereas in postmenopausal group, the risk increased (but not significant).	The authors suggest a bias due to low response rate, recall bias, and validity of dietary recalls. Relation of breast cancer to dietary intake, especially during adolescence, is unclear.

Rohan et al., 1988 (52)	451 women with breast cancer, 451 community controls, aged 20–74 years.	Study in Adelaide, South Australia (1982–1984). Subjects were interviewed in their home for reproductive, demographic, lifestyle, medical, and dietary (FFQ, 179 items) information.	The study showed that risk decreased nonuniformly at upper 3 quintiles of fiber intake with a 30% reduction at the highest level of intake. In premenopausal women, intermediate fiber intake led to a 50% risk reduction; in postmenopausal women, there was a 25% risk reduction at the uppermost quintile of intake.	Authors suggested a high intake of fiber-rich cereal would reduce the risk of breast cancer.
Van't Veer et al., 1990 (53)	133 breast cancer patients, 238 community controls, aged 25–44 and 55–64 years.	Study in the Netherlands (1985–1987). Trained dietitians interviewed subjects in their home for reproductive, demographic, lifestyle, medical, and dietary (FFQ, 236 items) information.	Intake of cereal products, but not vegetables or fruit, was associated with a significantly reduced breast cancer risk (OR = 0.42, $p = 0.03$). A decreasing trend in breast cancer risk was observed with the highest quartile of dietary fiber intake.	
Van't Veer et al., 1991 (54)	133 breast cancer patients, 289 community controls, aged 25–44 and 55–64 years.	Study in the Netherlands (1985–1987). Trained dietitians interviewed subjects in their home for reproductive, demographic, lifestyle, medical, and dietary (FFQ, 236 items) information.	After adjusting for total fat intake, the combination of a high dietary fiber intake, high intake of fermented milk products, and low intake of dietary fat conferred a significant protective effect against breast cancer (OR = 0.33).	

Table 2 Continued

Study (Ref.)	Subjects	Design and methods	Results	Comments
Witte et al., 1997 (58)	140 cases and 222 familial matched controls.	Familial matched case-control study in California, Connecticut, and Southern Quebec examining the effect between diet and premenopausal bilateral breast cancer. Subjects completed questionnaires on family history, dietary habits, and risk factors.	No associations were found between energy-adjusted dietary fiber and premenopausal bilateral breast cancer risk. No associations were found for consumption of fruits, vegetables, or grains.	The authors suggest that dietary fiber does not play a role in modulating the risk of premenopausal bilateral breast cancer.
Yuan et al., 1995 (67)	In Shanghai, 534 women with breast cancer (aged 20–69); in Tianjin, 300 women with breast cancer (aged 20–55). Community controls individually matched to cases by age and sex, with a case-control ratio of 1:1.	Studies in Shanghai and Tianjin, China (1984–1985). Subjects were interviewed for reproductive, demographic, lifestyle, medical, and dietary (FFQ, 63–68 items) information.	Shanghai women in the lowest tertile of crude fiber intake and the highest tertile of fat intake had a 2.9-fold increase in breast cancer risk. In Tianjin, the comparable figure of risk was 2.4. Significant protective effects were observed for vegetable/fruit crude fiber but not cereal crude fiber.	This study suggests that a diet high in fiber, beta-carotene, and vitamin C can protect against breast cancer. The FFQ had many fruits and vegetables but not whole-grain products (cereals consisted of refined products such as rice and noodles).
Zaridze et al., 1991 (68)	139 women with breast cancer, 139 community controls.	Study in Moscow, Russia (1987–1989). Subjects were interviewed for reproductive, demographic, and medical information. Dietary data were obtained through a FFQ (145 items) for the year prior to diagnosis or interview. In a subsample of subjects (46 cases, 53 controls), fasting blood samples were taken for fatty acid analysis.	Cellulose consumption, adjusted for energy intake, drastically reduced breast cancer risk in postmenopausal women (OR = 0.04, $p < 0.001$). Protective effects were also observed for beta-carotene and vitamin C. No significant dietary effects were observed in premenopausal women.	The authors concluded that low risk of breast cancer was associated with high intake of fruits and vegetables.

but a tendency to increased breast cancer risk (although not significantly due to large variability) in postmenopausal women. The differences in premenopausal and postmenopausal breast cancer need to be further explored.

C. Prospective Cohort and Case-Control Studies

In prospective cohort studies, the diets of large groups of individuals are monitored over time and eventually related to the incidence of disease (breast cancer) that develops within the cohort. These types of studies remove the bias that is unavoidable in case-control studies, namely knowledge of the presence of disease prior to dietary assessment. In addition, the present diet is assessed over time, improving the validity of individual dietary measurements. Biological samples (e.g., blood, urine, feces) can also be collected over the duration of the study, allowing for the investigation of potential biomarkers of cancer. Often prospective (also called nested) case-control studies are done using the data obtained from the cohort throughout the study period.

There are a few drawbacks to cohort studies (38). A main limitation of the prospective cohort design is expense. Since only a small percentage of subjects will develop disease, thousands or tens of thousands will need to be enrolled in the study in order to obtain sufficient statistical power. Following that large number of subjects for a number of years is costly. Another limitation is that some of the cohorts of people selected tend to be more homogeneous in lifestyle and dietary habits than the general population. Therefore, the range in intake necessary to observe a difference may not be wide enough. Furthermore, the age range chosen for the cohort is critical since too young a cohort will have too low an incidence of breast cancer, and a cohort that is too old may have already changed their dietary habits. Changes in potential biochemical measurements during early stages of carcinogenesis may also be missed in an older cohort.

In contrast to ecological and case-control studies, most prospective studies examining the relationship between dietary fiber and breast cancer have found no association (Table 3). Seven out of 10 studies found no effect (70–76). Of the 3 remaining studies, one found a protective effect of green and yellow vegetables (77), another found a reduced risk with total dietary fiber and cereal fiber (78), and the third observed significant reductions in breast cancer mortality in a population of health-conscious vegetarians (79). A recent meta-analysis of 3 cohort and 9 case-control studies found only a slight reduction (OR = 0.91) in breast cancer risk (15). For a few of the null studies, dietary fat was the primary focus (70,71,73), and thus it is possible that the dietary assessments used may not have accurately quantified dietary fiber intake in the cohort.

IV. INFLUENCE OF DIETARY FIBER ON BENIGN BREAST DISEASE DEVELOPMENT, BREAST TISSUE DENSITY, AND TUMOR CHARACTERISTICS

In addition to looking at incidence of breast cancer as an endpoint, many investigators have explored the relationship between dietary fiber and both early and later stages of breast carcinogenesis. Two potential risk factors that have been identified are the presence of benign breast disease (80) and mammographically dense breast tissue (81). Benign epithelial hyperplasia of the breast, believed to be a premalignant condition (80), increases the risk of breast cancer by twofold (82). Increased breast tissue density is believed to be a consequence of hormonal changes brought about by diet (83). Dietary fiber consumption has also been investigated in relation to altering tumor characteristics, a change that could potentially increase patient survival.

Table 3 Cohort Studies (Including Nested Case-Control Studies), Intervention Trials, and Randomized Trials Examining the Relationship Between Dietary Fiber and Breast Cancer Risk

Study	Subjects	Design and methods	Results	Comments
Clavel-Chapelon et al., 1997 (15)		Meta-analysis of 14 cohort and 33 case-control studies examining the role of diet on breast cancer risk.	Dietary fiber was examined in 3 cohort and 9 case-control studies. The combined analysis resulted in an OR = 0.91 (cohort alone: OR = 0.98; case-control alone: OR = 0.71).	
Giovannucci et al., 1993 (70)	84,494 women (aged 34–59 years); 300 breast cancer cases, 602 population controls.	Nested case-control study from the Nurses' Health study cohort. Subjects were mailed a FFQ to assess current dietary habits in 1986. In 1989, another FFQ was sent to assess retrospective dietary habits in 1985.	No association was found for dietary fiber in prospective or retrospective data, although fiber appeared to be more protective using prospective data. The opposite was true for dietary fat.	The study indicates how bias can influence studies examining dietary factors, particularly fat, and breast cancer risk.
Graham et al., 1992 (71)	18,586 white postmenopausal women (aged 50–107 years), 344 developed breast cancer.	Cohort study in New York State. Dietary FFQ (45 items) were mailed in 1980, and women who completed them were followed until 1987. The New York Tumor Registry was used to ascertain incidence of breast cancer, other cancers, and death.	No association was found between intake of dietary fiber and risk of breast cancer.	Mailed questionnaire is less reliable than a personal interview. Demographic data of the population do not correspond to that of the State of New York since African Americans and those of low socioeconomic status are underrepresented.
Hirayama, 1986 (77)	122,261 men. 142,857 women, aged 40 and over.	Cohort study in Japan (1966–1982). Participants were interviewed at home for information on lifestyle and diet (using a FFQ). A subset of 7,507 individuals was randomly chosen to validate the green-yellow vegetable and meat consumption.	Breast cancer risk was inversely associated with frequent consumption of soybean paste soup containing GYV, which are high in fiber and β-carotene. Increased breast cancer risk with meat consumption was mitigated by concurrent consumption of green-yellow vegetables.	The author concludes by saying that the study clearly underlines the importance of diet and nutrition as potential modifiers of cancer.

Reference	Population	Methods	Results	Comments
Jarvinen et al., 1997 (72)	4697 women (aged approx. 15 years) followed for 25 years.	Cohort study in Finland. Women were interviewed (1967–1972) for dietary habits in previous year and then followed for 25 years. Breast cancer developed in 88 women.	No significant associations were observed between dietary fiber and breast cancer risk.	
Key et al., 1996 (79)	4336 males and 6435 females, vegetarians, and health conscious.	Observational cohort study in the United Kingdom where subjects recorded their consumption of fiber-rich foods. Some subjects were interviewed to assess the validity stability of their dietary patterns. Subjects were followed until death or emigration.	After 16.8 years of follow-up, mortality was lower in this group than in the general population.	Daily consumption of fresh fruit and cereals reduced mortality from breast cancer as well as lung cancer, colorectal cancer, and coronary heart disease.
Kushi et al., 1992 (73)	34,388 postmenopausal women (aged 55–69).	Cohort study in Iowa. Questionnaires on major breast cancer risk factors and dietary habits mailed in 1986. Follow-up questionnaires were mailed in 1987 and 1989. Breast cancer developed in 459 women.	Results were adjusted for total energy and alcohol intakes. Dietary fiber intake had no effect on breast cancer risk.	
Rohan et al., 1993 (78)	56,837 women, 519 women with incident histologically confirmed breast cancer compared to 1,182 who did not develop BC.	Nested case-control study using data from the Canadian National Breast Screening Study cohort (1982–1987). All subjects completed a lifestyle questionnaire and self-administered FFQ (86 items).	Relatively high fiber intake was associated with a 30% reduction in breast cancer. The reduction was greater after adjustment for vitamin C and E intake and was not confined to any menopausal subgroup. A significant inverse association was found with cereal consumption (OR = 0.74, $p \le 0.014$).	The inverse association between risk of breast cancer and dietary fiber intake was due mainly to cereal sources.

Table 3 Continued

Study	Subjects	Design and methods	Results	Comments
Rohan et al., 1993 (74)	412 breast cancer patients followed for a median of 5.5 years.	Cohort study in Adelaide, South Australia, using data initially collected in a case-control study (1982–1984). Subjects were interviewed to obtain demographic, reproductive, and medical information. Dietary information was collected through a self-administered FFQ (179 items).	The study found little increase of death among breast cancer cases associated with dietary factors. No associations noted for fiber.	Dietary habits do not appear to influence breast cancer mortality.
Verhoeven et al., 1997 (75)	62,573 women, aged 55–69 years.	Prospective cohort study in the Netherlands. Subjects completed self-administered questionnaires on dietary habits, demographics, and risk factors for breast cancer	There was an inverse nonsignificant relationship with fruit intake and breast cancer risk. Dietary fiber showed no association with risk.	This study does not support a strong role for intake of vegetables, fruit, potatoes, retinol, beta-carotene, vitamin E, or dietary fiber in the etiology of breast cancer.
Willett et al., 1992 (76)	84,494 women (aged 34–59 years) followed for 8 years.	Cohort study in 1980 as part of the Nurses' Health Study. In 1976 registered nurses completed a mailed questionnaire on suspected risk factors for heart disease and breast cancer. Every 2 years follow-up questionnaires were sent to update information on menopausal status and parity. Dietary data were obtained through a FFQ (121 items). Breast cancer developed in 1439 women.	After adjustment for age and separately for energy intake, no association was found for the risk of breast cancer and intake of dietary fiber regardless of menopausal status.	The authors suggest that the data provide evidence against a protective effect of dietary fiber consumption by middle-aged women on breast cancer incidence.

The epidemiological data suggest that dietary fiber does not play a strong role in the risk of benign breast disease (Table 4). One study observed a significant reduction in risk of benign breast disease with total dietary fiber, total NSP, insoluble and soluble NSP, and cellulose (84). However, two studies observed no association between dietary fiber and risk of benign breast disease (57,85). The protective effect found by Rohan et al. (86) with dietary fiber disappeared after adjusting for energy intake. Nevertheless, a nested case-control study did find an inverse association between proliferative benign breast disease and intake of green vegetables (87).

In contrast to the evidence with benign breast disease, dietary fiber seems to alter breast tissue density (Table 4). Boyd and colleagues (83) have found that after 2 years of a low-fat, high-carbohydrate diet the area of breast tissue density is significantly reduced. In this study, dietary fiber intake (both soluble and insoluble) was significantly increased in the low-fat, high-carbohydrate group. Similarly, lower breast density patterns were found in premenopausal women with higher dietary fiber intakes in another study (88); however, no associations were present in postmenopausal women. In a study on women with breast cancer, Brisson et al. (89) noted that fiber intakes, adjusted for energy levels, were inversely associated with total and nodular density in breast tissue.

In addition to altering breast tissue density, dietary fiber consumption may have a direct effect on breast tumors (Table 4). Investigators have found that dietary fiber intake was inversely related to tumor size (90,91) but positively associated with estrogen receptor content (91,92). The presence of estrogen receptors is a favorable prognosis since tumors respond more readily to treatment (93). However, one study did find a nonsignificant trend towards lower dietary fiber intakes in premenopausal women with estrogen receptor–rich tumors (88). Other beneficial effects noted for dietary fiber consumption were improved tumor differentiation, reduced vascular invasion (92), and reduced nodal development (90).

V. ANIMAL STUDIES ON DIETARY FIBER AND BREAST CANCER

Rodent models of mammary (breast) cancer are useful in gathering evidence on the role of diet in human cancer because of the similarities between rats/mice and humans in mammary gland development and in the process of mammary gland carcinogenesis (94,95). Most animal studies have used wheat bran, which is rich in insoluble dietary fiber, as the fiber source and have exhibited protective effects against mammary cancer development (Table 5). Supplementation of wheat bran at levels of 9–12% reduced chemically induced mammary tumor development in rats and mice (96–99). This level is approximately 24–32 g of total dietary fiber per 2000 kcal. The inhibitory effects of wheat bran were found to be enhanced with the addition of psyllium, a rich source of soluble dietary fiber, at a 1:1 ratio (100). Because the lignin component of wheat bran appears to be important for estrogen binding (101), one may speculate that the lignin plays an important role in mammary carcinogenesis. However, Birt and colleagues (102) found that dietary wood lignin had no effect on serum estradiol or mammary tumorigenesis when fed at the 5% level. The significance of estrogen in breast cancer will be discussed in detail below.

The effectiveness of wheat bran in mammary tumorigenesis may be influenced by many factors. The protective effects of wheat bran are apparent when supplemented to a high-fat (e.g., 20% by weight) but not a low-fat (5% by weight) diet (97). Only one null study on wheat bran and mammary cancer has been published to date, and a low fat diet was used (103). In addition, the timing of wheat bran feeding in relation to carcinogen administration may play a role. Wheat bran feeding during the promotion phase, 2–3 days after carcinogen administration, of carcinogenesis (97–99) inhibited more tumor parameters than when wheat bran was fed during the

Table 4 Studies Examining the Role of Dietary Fiber in Risk of Benign Breast Disease and in Altering Breast Density and Tumor Characteristics

Study	Subjects	Design and methods	Results	Comments
Baghurst and Rohan (84)	354 women with benign proliferative epithelial disorders of the breast, 354 matched community controls, and 189 biopsy-negative controls, aged 18–75 years.	Case-control study in Adelaide, South Australia (1983–1985). Subjects were interviewed for demographic, reproductive, and medical information. Dietary information was collected through a self-administered FFQ (179 items).	Reduced breast cancer risk was observed for total dietary fiber, total NSP, insoluble and soluble NSP, and cellulose using biopsy-negative controls (OR = 0.35–0.45, $p < 0.04$). Results were stronger in premenopausal women.	The authors suggest that if these results can be substantiated, this could lead to a dietary intervention strategy to reduce the incidence of breast cancer.
Boyd et al., 1997 (83)	817 subjects with mammogram taken at baseline and 2 years after random allocation.	Randomized intervention trial in Toronto, Canada. The intervention group received intensive dietary counseling to reduce fat intake to 15% of calories. The control group received general dietary advice but was not taught to change their fat intake. Changes in breast tissue density were monitored by mammogram taken at baseline and 2 years later.	After 2 years, there was a reduction in the area of dense breast tissue in the intervention, but not control, group that was associated with weight loss. The effect of intervention on the area of dense breast tissue was only marginally statistically significant after correcting for confounding variables. Dietary fiber (both soluble and insoluble) intake was significantly higher in the intervention group ($p < 0.001$).	The authors suggest a longer observation of a larger number of subjects will be needed to determine whether these effects are associated with changes in the risk of breast cancer.
Brisson et al., 1989 (89)	290 breast cancer patients, 645 population controls (aged 40–62 years).	Nested case-control study from the Canadian National Breast Screening Study cohort in Quebec, Canada (1982–1984). Subjects had mammographies and were interviewed in their home to obtain information on reproductive, lifestyle, anthropometric, medical, and dietary (FFQ, 114 items) factors.	Energy-adjusted dietary fiber intake was associated with reduced total and nodular density ($p < 0.04$).	The authors suggest that elevated saturated fat intake combined with a reduction in carotenoid and fiber intakes may be related to an increase in breast cancer risk, as seen by the effects on breast tissue morphology.

Reference	Subjects	Study description	Findings	Conclusions
Hebert and Toporoff, 1989 (90)	546 early-stage breast cancer patients, aged 20–80.	Prospective cohort study in New York, New York (1982–1984). Patients were interviewed at time of diagnosis on demographic and lifestyle-related factors, focusing on diet, alcohol intake, and smoking. A FFQ (26 items) was administered to all women and a subset of women completed a 4-day food diary.	Among premenopausal women, calorie-adjusted fiber intake was inversely related to nodal development and tumor size. No such dietary associations were found among postmenopausal women.	The authors note that their population is not representative of the general U.S. population since they are generally better educated, have a higher socioeconomic status, and have fewer pregnancies.
Hislop et al., 1990 (87)	124 patients with benign breast disease defined by subsequent risk of breast cancer and 274 patients with the same disease at no subsequent risk of breast cancer.	Nested case-control study from Canadian National Breast Screening Study cohort in Vancouver, Canada (1983–1985). Each subject completed a self-administered questionnaire that focused on risk factors for breast cancer, benign breast disease, and usual dietary patterns.	Proliferative benign breast disease was inversely associated with vitamin A supplementation and frequent consumption of green vegetables.	The authors conclude that dietary factors may be related to histological types of benign breast disease, and the high risk for subsequent breast cancer.
Holm et al., 1989 (91)	240 women aged 50–65 who had surgery for breast cancer.	Observational study in Stockholm, Sweden (1983–1986). Subjects were interviewed within 4 months of the tumor resection to obtain reproductive, anthropometric, lifestyle, and dietary (FFQ for year prior to diagnosis) information.	Cases with tumors ~20 mm had lower intakes of fiber (in g or g/10 MJ) than cases with tumors ~20 mm. Cases with estrogen receptor (ER)–rich tumors consumed more fiber (g/10 MJ) than those with ER-poor tumors.	Conclusion was that high fat intake and low consumption of fiber affects tumor size and estrogen receptor content of tumors.
Ingram et al., 1991 (57)	99 breast cancer cases; 91 benign epithelial hyperplasia of the breast cases; 95 benign fibrocystic disease cases; 209 community controls.	Case-control study in Perth, Western Australia (1985–1987). Subjects were interviewed in the home for reproductive, demographic, and medical information. Dietary data were obtained using a self–administered FFQ (179 items).	No associations were observed with dietary fiber intake, cereal products, or fruits and vegetables.	

Table 4 Continued

Study	Subjects	Design and methods	Results	Comments
Ingram et al., 1992 (92)	91 women identified with early breast cancer.	Observational study in Perth, Western Australia. Three months after surgery for breast cancer, the women were interviewed at home. A blood sample was taken and a FFQ was completed.	Increasing intake of fiber, fruit, and vegetables was associated with improved tumor differentiation, reduced vascular invasion, and estrogen-receptor positivity.	Increasing consumption of sugar, fiber, fruits, vegetables, and vitamins were associated with favorable tumor growth characteristics.
Lubin et al., 1989 (85)	857 biopsied cases of benign breast disease, 755 surgical controls, 723 neighborhood controls.	Case-control study in Israel (1977–1980). Subjects were interviewed at home to collect information on suspected risk factors for benign breast disease and on dietary habits in previous 6 months using a FFQ (250 items). Biopsy specimens were graded histologically.	Food containing fiber did not affect risk of benign breast disease regardless of degree of ductal atypia.	The category "foods containing fiber" also included some foods that were high in fat and/or protein, making it difficult to determine the role of dietary fiber alone.
Nordevang et al., 1993 (88)	238 women aged 50–65 years who had surgery for stage I-II breast cancer.	Observational study in Stockholm, Sweden (1983–1986). All subjects had diagnostic mammography prior to surgery. After surgery, the women were interviewed by a nutritionist to obtain information on dietary habits as well as demographic, reproductive, lifestyle, and anthropometric factors.	In premenopausal women, dietary fiber intake (adjusted for energy intake) was lower in women with higher breast density patterns ($p < 0.01$). Similar, but nonsignificant trends were also seen in premenopausal women with ER-rich tumors. No associations were observed between fiber and breast density in postmenopausal women.	This study is limited due to misclassification of dietary habits and use of food composition tables. After multivariate regression analysis, the effects observed with dietary fiber were no longer significant.
Rohan et al., 1990 (86)	383 cases of benign proliferative epithelial disorders, 192 biopsy-negative controls, 383 unbiopsied community controls, aged 18–75 years.	Case-control study in Adelaide, South Australia (1983–1985). Subjects were interviewed for reproductive, demographic, and medical information. Dietary data were collected through a self-administered FFQ (179 items).	When community controls were compared, there was a statistically significant inverse association between high fiber intake (OR = 0.7, $p = 0.041$), but this was no longer true after adjustment for energy intake.	Authors concluded that their study provided "qualified support" for fiber's protective effect.

Table 5 Animal Studies Examining the Relationship Between Dietary Fiber and Risk Factors for Breast Cancer: Emphasis on Wheat Bran Fiber

Study	Subjects	Design and methods	Results	Comments
Arts et al., 1991 (96)	62 female F344 rats.	Rats were fed either a high-fiber (HF) diet (11% fiber, wheat bran based) or a low-fiber (LF) diet (0.5% fiber, white wheat flour based). Diets contained 9% lard and 7% sunflower oil as the fat source. A subset of rats ($n = 40$) were injected with the carcinogen methylnitrosourea (MNU, 50 mg/kg BW) after 3 weeks of dietary treatment and followed for 24 weeks post-MNU. Non–carcinogen-treated rats ($n = 22$) were examined for changes in estradiol metabolism.	Although tumor incidence and latency were similar in LF and HF groups, HF has significantly lower tumor weights. In non–carcinogen-treated rats, increased unconjugated estradiol plasma levels were observed during the peak period of the estrous cycle (second day of diestrus and first day of proestrus) with HF; no effect during other stages of cycle ("basal period"). Rats fed HF also had reduced urinary excretion of estrone and nearly 3-fold higher fecal excretion of free and conjugated estrogens. Fecal beta-glucuronidase activity was also increased in the HF group.	Wheat bran interrupted the enterohepatic circulation of estrogens but plasma levels were generally not affected. It is unknown whether the reduction in mammary tumor weight was due to components of wheat bran, a reduction in body weight, or energy restriction.
Arts et al., 1991 (101)	Four intestine-cannulated pigs; in vitro assessment of estrogen binding.	Pigs, fed standard pig chow, were cannulated in the duodenum. One gram of each different fiber source (wheat bran, cereals, seeds, and legumes) were placed in preincubated nylon bags, which were inserted into the cannula and passed with the feces.	Wheat bran fiber was one of the fibers to which estrogens bound with high affinity in vitro. The in vivo apparent digestibility was lowest with wheat bran where binding of estradiol by the digested residue was similar to the undigested source.	Wheat bran, lignin, oats, linseed and soybean seem to be promising compounds to further test in vivo in experiments looking at diminished estrogen exposure.
Arts et al., 1992 (157)	15 male Wistar rats.	Rats were fed a nonfiber wheat starch diet (< 1% dietary fiber), a low-fiber wheat flour diet (2% dietary fiber), or a high-fiber wheat bran diet (11.6% dietary fiber). Rats were injected with radiolabeled estradiol and/or estrone-glucuronide 2 or 20 days after dietary treatments.	Wheat bran supplementation for 2 days increased fecal excretion and decreased urinary excretion of radiolabeled estradiol. After 3 weeks of wheat bran feeding, the rate of fecal excretion of radiolabeled estradiol was accelerated.	The increased fecal excretion of labeled compounds may be attributed to an interruption in the enterohepatic circulation of estrogens, which may in turn lower tissue or plasma levels of estrogens and potentially reduce breast cancer risk.

Table 5 Continued

Study	Subjects	Design and methods	Results	Comments
Arts and Thijssen, 1992 (134)	45 female F344 rats.	Rats were fed ad libitum high-fiber (HF) diet (9.2% fiber, wheat bran based) or a low-fiber (LF) diet (0.5% fiber, white wheat flour based). A third group was fed an energy-restricted LF diet.	Plasma levels of luteinizing hormone (LH) were significantly higher in the HF group compared to the two LF groups. Plasma follicle-stimulating hormone and progesterone levels were unaffected.	Dietary fiber may affect the hormonal process involved in the development of breast cancer. Increased LH levels indicated that estrogen production was increased in the HF group.
Arts et al., 1992 (136)	45 female F344 rats.	Rats were fed ad libitum high-fiber (HF) diet (9.2% fiber, wheat bran based) or a low-fiber (LF) diet (0.5% fiber, white wheat flour based). A third group was an energy-restricted LF diet. Puberty onset, cell proliferation, and mammary tissue development was analyzed.	The onset of puberty was slightly delayed with wheat bran. Although wheat bran did not significantly affect cell proliferation in the mammary gland, it reduced mammary tissue development compared to the low-fiber diet.	Authors speculate that the mechanism of action may be through reduced energy intake with ad libitum dietary fiber intake. However, reduced exposure to estrogen with wheat bran cannot be excluded.
Birt et al., 1998 (102)	140 female Sprague-Dawley rats.	Rats were fed either a low-fat control diet (5% corn oil) or a 2.5% lignin diet until 2 days after injection with the carcinogen MNU (50 mg/kg BW). The treatment group was then given a 5% lignin diet until 20 weeks post-MNU. A group of rats ($n = 40$) were not given the carcinogen. Subset of rats were killed periodically until 20 weeks post-MNU for uterine, tumor, and estrogen measurements.	Dietary lignin did not affect serum estradiol or mammary carcinogenesis.	
Cohen et al., 1991 (97)	120 female F344 rats.	Rats were injected with the carcinogen MNU (37.5 mg/kg BW) and then given low-(5% by wt. corn oil) or high-(23.5%) fat diets with or without 10% wheat bran. Rats were monitored until 15 weeks post-MNU.	MNU tumor incidence, number, and multiplicity was decreased with 10% wheat bran supplementation to the high-fat, but not the low-fat, diet. The low-fat diet alone was equally protective as the low-fat diet with wheat bran.	The protective effects of wheat bran against mammary tumorigenesis are observed when it is supplemented in high-risk (i.e., high-fat) diets.

Cohen et al., 1996 (98)	240 female F344 rats.	Rats were injected with the carcinogen MNU (40 mg/kg BW) and then fed high-fat diets (20% corn oil) with either 9%, 12%, 15%, or 18% wheat bran or 4.5%, 6%, 7.5% or 9% cellulose. Rats were monitored until 25 weeks post-MNU. A subset of rats ($n = 48$) was used for estrogen analyses.	MNU tumor incidence and multiplicity was decreased with 9% wheat bran compared to higher doses of wheat bran and all doses of cellulose. Combined wheat bran groups had reduced serum estradiol levels compared to combined cellulose groups. Changes in serum estradiol within the wheat bran or cellulose groups were not dose-related. However, urinary estrogens decreased and fecal estrogens increased with wheat bran.	Intermediate doses of wheat bran (9–12%) may be more protective than higher doses against mammary tumor development. Wheat bran alters excretory metabolism of estrogen without affecting serum estrogen levels.
Cohen et al., 1996 (100)	150 female F344 rats.	Rats were injected with the carcinogen MNU (40 mg/kg BW) and then given high-fat diets (20% corn oil) supplemented with 12%, 8%, 6%, 4%, or 0% wheat bran supplemented with 0%, 2%, 3%, 4%, or 6% psyllium, respectively. Rats were monitored until 19 weeks post-MNU. A subset of animals ($n = 29$) was used for estrogen and enzyme activity measurements.	The lowest MNU tumor incidence, number, and multiplicity was found with wheat bran:psyllium in a 1:1 ratio (4% by wt each). Fecal estrogens increased with increasing level of wheat bran. Cecal beta-glucuronidase activity was affected more by the dietary content of psyllium, increasing with psyllium dose. No changes in urinary or serum estrogen level were observed with dietary treatments.	Combination of insoluble (wheat bran) and soluble (psyllium) fiber may be more protective against breast cancer than either type of fiber alone.
Kendall and Cohen, 1992 (135)	120 female F344 rats; in vitro assessment of estrogen and lipid binding.	Rats were injected with the carcinogen MNU (37.5 mg/kg BW) and then given low–(5% by wt. corn oil) or high–(23.5%) fat diets with or without 10% wheat bran. At 15 weeks post-MNU, serum, urine, and feces were collected for estrogen/progesterone measurements. Feces also analyzed for lipids.	Although wheat bran did not affect serum estradiol or progesterone measurements, urinary excretion of estrone and estradiol was increased with wheat bran supplementation to the low- or high-fat diets. There was a trend for increased fecal estrogen excretion with wheat bran added to the high-fat, but not the low-fat, diet. Fecal lipid excretion was higher with wheat bran. In vitro binding of radio-labeled triglyceride, estrone, and estradiol was higher for wheat bran vs. cellulose.	Authors state that it is not known whether fiber-induced changes in hormone and lipid bioavailability are causally related to reductions in mammary tumorigenesis.

Table 5 Continued

Study	Subjects	Design and methods	Results	Comments
Vucenik et al., 1997 (103)	200 female Sprague-Dawley rats.	Rats were given either 0, 5, 10, or 20% wheat bran or 0.4% phytic acid supplemented to a low-fat diet 2 weeks before administration of the carcinogen 7,12-dimethyl-benz(a)anthracene (DMBA, 5 mg/rat). Rats were monitored until 29 weeks post-DMBA.	Wheat bran had no effect on DMBA-induced tumorigenesis. However, 0.4% phytic acid (amount in the 20% wheat bran diet) resulted in reduced tumor incidence and multiplicity.	Authors state that phytic acid is more effective than 20% wheat bran against mammary cancer.
Zile et al., 1998 (99)	353 female Sprague-Dawley rats, 450 C₃H/HeOuJ mice.	1. Seven days after administration of DMBA (2.5 mg/100 g BW), rats ($n = 175$) were given 0, 5, 9.6, or 17.5% dietary fiber as wheat bran in a high fat (20% corn oil) diet and monitored until 13 weeks post-DMBA. 2. Three weeks after DMBA and 2 weeks after ovariectomy, rats ($n = 178$) were given 0 or 9.6% dietary fiber as wheat bran and monitored until 29 weeks after DMBA. 3. At 35 days of age, mice ($n = 240$) were given 0 or 9.6% dietary fiber from wheat bran and spontaneous tumors allowed to develop for 10 months. 4. Mice ($n = 210$) were fed diets as in (3) but were injected with mouse tumor cells at 10 months and tumors were allowed to grow for one month.	In the first study, all doses of wheat bran decreased DMBA tumor multiplicity. Dietary fiber at the 9.6% level as wheat bran decreased tumor multiplicity, number, and incidence in ovariectomized rats. Spontaneous tumor incidence and multiplicity and tumor multiplicity of injected mouse mammary tumor cells was reduced with 9.6% dietary fiber in mice.	Wheat bran is protective in a variety of experimental models of mammary tumorigenesis. Wheat bran's inhibition of mammary tumor development in ovariectomized animals suggest that it may also act through a hormone-independent mechanism.

initiation phase, 2–3 weeks prior to carcinogen administration (96,103). Other potential factors are the length of wheat bran treatment in combination with the strain and species of animal, type and dose of chemical carcinogen, and the source of fat (saturated vs. unsaturated).

VI. HOW DOES DIETARY FIBER REDUCE BREAST CANCER RISK?

One of the major mechanisms by which dietary fiber is thought to protect against breast cancer is by altering estrogen metabolism. Other mechanisms involve the cancer-protective effects of fiber-associated substances such as phytic acid and phytoestrogens.

A. Estrogens and Breast Cancer

Early menarche, late menopause, late first pregnancy, and nulliparity are major risk factors of breast cancer and signify the importance of lifetime exposure to the growth-promoting effects of estrogen in breast cancer (104). Early evidence of the role of estrogen in breast cancer development was seen in a Boston cohort study by Feinleib (105) where women undergoing hysterectomy or bilateral oophorectomy prior to age 40 had a 75% reduction in breast cancer risk. Asian women, who have a relatively low risk of breast cancer, appear to have lower circulating estrogen levels in comparison to the higher-risk North American or European women (106–109). Higher levels of blood hormone levels have also been found between African-American women, who are at higher risk, in comparison to Caucasian women in the United States (110). Further evidence comes from case-control (106,111), prospective case-control (112), and prospective cohort (113) studies that have found higher circulating estrogen levels in women with breast cancer.

The enterohepatic circulation of estrogens is important for maintaining plasma levels. The main source of circulating estrogen in premenopausal women is the ovaries, whereas the major tissue sites for estrogen production in postmenopausal women are the adipose and muscle tissues (114,115). The main estrogens in order of biological potency are estradiol, estrone, and estriol (115). Following synthesis, the estrogens circulate in the blood in the unconjugated or free form and are transported to target tissues bound weakly to albumin or strongly to sex hormone–binding globulin (SHBG), rendering them biologically inactive (115,116). In the liver the estrogens are conjugated primarily with glucuronide and sulfate moieties, and 50% of the estrogen metabolites are excreted into the duodenum via the bile duct (116). Reabsorption of the estrogen conjugates from the intestinal tract requires the action of β-glucuronidase, which removes the glucuronide or sulphate moiety (116). Approximately 80% of the estrogen metabolites are reabsorbed, and most are reconjugated in the intestinal mucosa (117). Estrogens that reach the kidney are excreted in the conjugated form. In contrast, estrogens are excreted in the free form in the feces (116). Diet has been shown to affect bacterial β-glucuronidase activity where dietary fat enhances its effect and dietary fiber decreases it (118). Therefore, reductions in β-glucuronidase activity would lead to less estrogen absorbed, lower levels present in the plasma or excreted in the urine, and higher levels found in the feces.

B. Alteration of Estrogen Metabolism by Dietary Fiber

1. Human Studies

Observational studies of different groups of women have shown that dietary fiber intake is correlated with estrogen measurements in plasma, urine, and feces (Table 6). Not surprisingly, vegetarians have been shown to consume significantly more dietary fiber than omnivores (119–

Table 6 Studies Examining the Relationship Between Dietary Fiber and Hormones (risk factors for breast cancer)

Study	Subjects	Design and methods	Results	Comments
Adlercreutz et al., 1986 (119)	23 healthy premenopausal women: 12 omnivores, 11 lactovegetarians.	Observational study on women in Helsinki, Finland. One 72-hour summer and one winter urine sample was collected in the mid-follicular phase of the menstrual cycle. Detailed 5-day diet records were obtained at these times.	Dietary fiber intake was similar in summer and winter for lactovegetarians. In contrast, omnivores consumed significantly less grain, vegetable, and total fiber in the winter vs. the summer. No significant differences in urinary estrogen and its metabolites between omnivores and vegetarians. Significant negative correlations were observed between dietary intake of total or grain fiber/kg body weight and urinary excretion of individual estrogens.	
Adlercreutz et al., 1989 (124)	33 healthy premenopausal women: 10 with breast cancer, 12 omnivores, 11 lactovegetarians.	Observational study in Helsinki, Finland. Subjects were followed for one year where four dietary records (3- or 5-day) and two 72-hour urine samples (midfollicular phase of the menstrual cycle) were obtained.	Grain fiber intake and urinary excretion of 4-hydroxyestrone and was significantly lower in the breast cancer group. Urinary 2-hydroxyestrone to 4-hydroxyestrone ratio, highest in the breast cancer group, was inversely correlated to total and grain fiber intake.	The ratio of 2-hydroxyestrone to 4-hydroxyestrone seems to depend on diet and is the only urinary estrogen parameter separating premenopausal breast cancer patients from omnivorous and lactovegetarian women.

Reference	Subjects	Methods	Results	Conclusions
Bagga et al., 1995 (125)	12 healthy premenopausal women.	Intervention trial in Los Angeles, CA. Subjects served as their own controls and were followed for 3 months. During the first month, subjects consumed a diet that provided 30% of calories from fat and 15–20 g fiber/day. During the next 2 months, subjects consumed a diet that provided 10% calories from fat and 25–35 g fiber/day. Monthly 4-day food records were maintained. Blood was collected every 2 days for hormonal analyses	After 2 months on the low-fat, high-fiber diet, there was a significant reduction in serum estrone and estradiol levels. This reduction did not interfere with ovulation.	A diet low in fat and high in fiber can reduce circulating estrogen levels in healthy premenopausal women, which could in turn play a role in breast cancer prevention.
Barbosa et al., 1990 (120)	24 healthy Seventh-day Adventist postmenopausal women: 12 vegetarian; 12 nonvegetarian.	Observational study where subjects kept 7-day food records and fasting blood samples were taken for plasma hormone measurements. Anthropometric data was also collected.	Vegetarians consumed significantly more crude and total fiber, had lower plasma estradiol levels, and had smaller skinfold-thickness measurements than nonvegetarians. Significant inverse relationships were observed between crude or total dietary fiber and plasma estradiol.	Studies examining the effects of adiposity and dietary fiber on plasma estradiol levels are warranted.
Goldin et al., 1982 (121)	20 healthy premenopausal women, aged 20–30 years: 10 vegetarian and 10 omnivores.	Observational study where subjects were monitored for 3 days (mid-follicular phase of the menstrual cycle) on 4 separate occasions, 4 months apart. Each sample period included the collection of 72-h urine and feces, a 3-day food record, and daily (total of three) blood specimens.	Vegetarians consumed more dietary fiber than the omnivores. Vegetarians had higher fecal excretion of estrogens and lower urinary and plasma estrone and estradiol levels.	Vegetarian women have higher fecal output, which results in a higher fecal excretion and a decreased plasma concentration of estrogen.

Table 6 Continued

Study	Subjects	Design and methods	Results	Comments
Goldin et al., 1994 (126)	48 premenopausal women.	Metabolically controlled study where subjects initially consumed a high-fat (40%), low-fiber (12 g/day) diet. Subjects were then fed metabolic diets with varying levels of fat and fiber. The subjects completed 58 protocols.	A low-fat (20–25%), high-fiber (40 g/day) diet was associated with significant decreases in serum concentrations of estrogen and a modest lengthening of the menstrual cycle. High dietary fiber levels were responsible for a decrease in estradiol and sex hormone–binding globulin.	Risk of developing breast cancer has been positively associated with late menopause. The reduction in the number of cycles with a high-fiber diet could play a role in decreasing breast cancer incidence.
Heber et al., 1991 (127)	13 healthy postmenopausal women.	Short-term effects of a low-fat (less than 10% of calories), high-fiber (35–45 g/1000 kcal/day) diet on estradiol levels in subjects under residential conditions with a cafeteria food service.	Plasma estradiol levels dropped nearly 50% with free access to the low-fat, high-fiber diet.	Women were in negative caloric balance during the study and thus experienced weight loss. This may account for the dramatic decrease in plasma estradiol levels.
Kaneda et al., 1997 (123)	50 premenopausal Japanese women.	Observational study evaluating the relationship between fat or fiber and serum estradiol and sex hormone–binding globulin levels. Blood samples were taken on days 11 and 22 of menstrual cycle. Nutrient intakes during year prior to study were assessed using a FFQ.	After adjustment for age, cycle length, and energy intake, dietary fiber was significantly inversely related to serum estradiol levels on day 11 of the menstrual cycle.	Both fat and fiber affected hormone status.

Study	Subjects	Design	Results	Comments
Lewis et al., 1997 (132)	40 healthy premenopausal women.	Randomized intervention trial that included feeding wheat bran for two menstrual cycles. Four-day diet records were kept at the beginning and end of each intervention period. Stools and blood were taken for analyses.	Wheat bran tended to decrease gut transit time but this was not statistically significant. Wheat bran decreased serum estrone sulfate levels.	Dietary fiber speeds up intestinal transit time, which can lead to lower serum estrogen levels in premenopausal women.
Lewis et al., 1998 (133)	20 healthy postmenopausal women.	Randomized intervention trial that included consumption of wheat bran and bran-shaped plastic flakes, each for 10 days with a minimum 2 week washout period. Prior to and during the last 4 days of each treatment, the absorption of a 1.5 mg dose of estradiol glucuronide as well as various characteristics of bowel movements were measured.	Wheat bran and plastic flakes reduced whole gut transit time, increased defecation frequency, and increased stool form score. Wheat bran reduced the length of time that the absorbed estrogen, particularly estradiol, was detected in the serum.	Decreased gut transit time can reduce serum levels of estrogen in postmenopausal women.
Rose et al., 1988 (122)	155 premenopausal women.	Observational study in comparing dietary intakes of women in Kuopio, Finland (rural area, $n = 61$) and in New York, NY ($n = 94$). Food frequency questionnaires (FFQ) were used to estimate dietary fat and fiber consumption	Finnish women had a considerable higher fiber intake than American women and a higher level of serum growth hormone.	Dietary factors, perhaps related to fiber intake, affect the synthesis of a growth hormone variant that may influence breast cancer risk.
Rose et al., 1991 (129)	62 healthy premenopausal women.	Randomized controlled trial. Subjects first completed 4-day food record and were then randomly assigned to a wheat bran, oat bran, or corn bran supplement for 2 months. The goal was to increase total dietary fiber intake to 30 g/day.	The wheat bran–supplemented group showed significant reductions in serum estrone and estradiol with no change in progesterone or sex hormone–binding globulin. Oat bran and corn bran supplementation did not alter serum estrogen levels.	Dietary fiber may reduce breast cancer risk by decreasing circulating estrogen levels and their bioavailability. Wheat bran is more effective than corn or oat bran on altering serum estrogen levels.

Table 6 Continued

Study	Subjects	Design and methods	Results	Comments
Rose et al., 1997 (130)	58 healthy premenopausal women.	Randomized controlled trial. Subjects kept 4-day records and were given one of three levels of wheat bran supplementation at 5, 10, or 20 g/day (in the form of Kellogg's All-Bran) for 2 months.	At the 10 g and 20 g level of wheat bran supplementation (which resulted in a total dietary fiber intake of 21 g and 35 g/day, respectively), significantly reduced luteal serum estradiol and estrone after 1 or 2 months.	The long-term effect of wheat bran intake may reduce breast cancer risk in Western women.
Schaefer et al., 1995 (128)	22 healthy premenopausal women.	Intervention trial where subjects first consumed a baseline diet for 4 weeks (40% of fat calories, 12 g/day dietary fiber) followed by a low-fat, high-fiber diet for 8–10 weeks (16–18% fat calories, 40 g/day fiber). Blood samples during the follicular and luteal phases of the menstrual cycle at baseline and treatment were taken for lipid and hormone measurements.	The low-fat, high-fiber diet reduced serum estrone sulfate levels significantly during the follicular phase of the menstrual cycle.	
Woods et al., 1996 (110)	21 healthy premenopausal African American women.	Metabolically controlled trial. Subjects consumed baseline diet (40% fat calories, 12 g/day fiber) for 3 weeks, followed by a low-fat, high-fiber (20% fat calories, 40 g/d fiber) for two menstrual cycles. During the follicular phase of the menstrual cycle and in the last week of each study period, serum was collected for hormone measurements.	The low-fat, high-fiber diet significantly reduced serum estradiol and estrone sulfate. Control serum hormone (total and free estradiol, estrone, and androstenedione) levels in African American women were significantly higher than that found in Caucasian women in a previous study ($n = 68$).	African American women appear to have higher serum hormone levels than Caucasian women. A low-fat, high-fiber diet can reduce serum estrogens in this population and potentially reduce breast cancer risk.

121). Comparisons of women in low-risk versus high-risk populations have shown that women at lower risk of developing breast cancer consume higher amounts of dietary fiber (107,122). Consequently, dietary fiber intake was shown to be inversely related to serum or plasma estrogen levels (107,120,121,123), inversely related to urinary estrogen excretion (107,119,121), and positively related to fecal estrogen output (107,121). Adlercreutz et al. (124) found that both grain fiber intake and a particular estrogen metabolite, 4-hydroxyestrone, was significantly lower in breast cancer patients compared to vegetarian and omnivorous controls.

Evidence on the role of dietary fiber in reducing circulating levels of estrogen has been accumulated from randomized intervention trials (Table 6). Feeding of diets high in fiber (25–45 g/day) and low in fat (10–20% of calories) has resulted in significant reductions in circulating estrogen levels (110,125–128). Rose and colleagues have examined the effect of wheat bran in particular (resulting in average daily fiber intakes of 20–32 g/day) in altering estrogen levels in premenopausal women and also found significant reductions in serum estradiol and estrone after 1 or 2 months of feeding (129,130). In contrast, oat or corn bran had no effect on circulating estrogen levels (129). This may be due to the fact that wheat bran inhibits fecal β-glucuronidase activity to a greater extent than either oat or corn bran (131). In addition to inhibiting β-glucuronidase activity, wheat bran has been shown to have greater binding affinity for estrogen than other fibers (101). The ability of wheat bran to decrease intestinal transit time has resulted in lower serum estrogen levels in pre- and postmenopausal women (132,133).

2. Animal Studies: Role of Wheat Bran

Changes in estrogen metabolism have also been studied in animal models (Table 5). In contrast to humans, wheat bran does not appear to affect circulating estrogen levels in rats (96–98,100,134,135), although one study did find an overall reduction in serum estradiol levels after comparing all doses of wheat bran to all doses of cellulose (98). Wheat bran does, however, reduce urinary and increase fecal excretion of estrogens (96,98,100,135), which indicates that wheat bran interrupts the enterohepatic circulation of estrogens in rats. This interruption may be through a reduction in β-glucuronidase activity (96), as seen with wheat bran in humans (131). Alterations in estrogen metabolism by wheat bran may also affect mammary gland development as observed by Arts et al. in one study (136). Delayed mammary gland development has been associated with reduced breast cancer risk (94,95).

Nevertheless, the inhibitory effects of wheat bran in mammary cancer development may not be related to changes in estrogen metabolism. Decreases in serum and/or urinary estrogen levels have not been found to be associated with reduced tumorigenesis (96,98,100). In addition, wheat bran supplementation was shown to reduce mammary tumor number and incidence in ovariectomized rats (99), suggesting an estrogen-independent mechanism.

C. Anticarcinogenic Activity of Phytic Acid

One such estrogen-independent mechanism for wheat bran may be its high content of phytic acid. Phytic acid, also known as inositol hexaphosphate, is a potent antioxidant (137) with strong binding properties due to its highly negative charge. Wheat bran is one of the richest sources of phytic acid, containing levels of 3–6% by weight (138). Diet supplementation with phytic acid at the 1.2% level decreased early markers of mammary tumorigenesis such as cell proliferation and nuclear aberrations of mammary epithelial cells (139). Phytic acid has also been shown to inhibit the growth of cultured estrogen-independent human breast cancer cells in vitro (140) and of mammary tumors in carcinogen-treated rats when supplemented to either the drinking water or diet (103,141,142). Tumor suppression by phytic acid has been related to its ability to enhance natural killer cell activity (143). However, phytic acid may also modulate estrogen metabolism since it has been shown to inhibit β-glucuronidase activity in carcinogen-treated rats (144). This could explain why wheat bran was more effective in reducing fecal β-glucuronidase activity than either oat or corn bran (131).

Despite the evidence for the anticarcinogenic activity of phytic acid, it is difficult to assess whether this plays a role in studies using wheat bran feeding since all studies examining the role of phytic acid on breast carcinogenesis have used the purified compound. Uncooked or unprocessed wheat bran contains endogenous phytases that can hydrolyze phytic acid in the intestinal tract (145). However, hydrolysis products of phytic acid have been shown to inhibit cancer cell growth in rats and in vitro (146). Yet phytic acid and wheat bran fiber may have synergistic or antagonistic effects on cancer development. Studies comparing the effects of untreated wheat bran with that of dephytinized wheat bran and purified phytic acid, alone and in combination, in breast carcinogenesis would result in a better understanding of the role of wheat bran components in cancer prevention and/or treatment.

D. Phytoestrogens and Breast Cancer

Phytoestrogens are plant-derived compounds with weak estrogenic/antiestrogenic activity. The major classes of phytoestrogens consumed by both animals and humans are the isoflavones and lignans (147). The intestinal bacteria play a significant role in the metabolism of phytoestrogen precursors to their active metabolites (148). Most research on the role of phytoestrogens in breast cancer risk has focused on the isoflavones genistein and daidzein and on the mammalian lignans enterodiol (ED) and enterolactone (EL).

Many of the observational studies on the relationship between phytoestrogens and dietary fiber were done by Adlercreutz and colleagues in Finland. Adlercreutz et al. (149) noted that fiber intake was positively related to the urinary excretion of ED and EL. Macrobiotics and vegetarians, who consume higher levels of dietary fiber than omnivores, have much higher urinary levels of the mammalian lignans and the isoflavones (150). In contrast, Japanese men and women excrete low levels of mammalian lignans but high levels of isoflavones, which correlated to their high intake of soy products (151). Thus, lignans are ubiquitous in fiber-rich plant sources, whereas isoflavones are found mainly in soybean products. The richest source of mammalian lignans is flaxseed (152,153).

The first clue that phytoestrogens may have cancer-protective effects was the observation that urinary EL levels were significantly lower in breast cancer patients compared to omnivores or vegetarians (149). The reason for this decrease is still unknown but may be related to the fact that, like estrogens, lignans (and isoflavones) undergo enterohepatic circulation (154), and this may be altered in the disease state. Numerous in vitro and animal studies have indicated that phytoestrogens or the consumption of phytoestrogen-rich foods (e.g., soybeans, flaxseed) significantly reduce mammary cancer cell growth (147,155). A recent case-control study by Lee et al. found that total soya products reduced breast cancer risk by 60% in premenopausal women (156), providing further evidence of the protective effects of phytoestrogens in humans.

VII. CONCLUSIONS

Ecological and case-control studies indicate that dietary fiber consumption reduces breast cancer risk, whereas most prospective studies have found a less consistent relationship. Reasons for these discrepancies are many. Variability in the estimation of dietary fiber intake, use of crude versus total dietary fiber intakes, different physiological effects of the different components of dietary fiber, and use of premenopausal versus postmenopausal women are just a few. Nevertheless, dietary fiber does appear to play a significant role in altering the risk factors for breast cancer, namely breast tissue density and estrogen bioavailability. Dietary fiber may modulate prognostic factors—tumor size, tumor estrogen receptor content, differentiation, vascular invasion—that affect patient survival. In addition, results from human clinical and animal studies on wheat bran and breast cancer are encouraging.

Fiber-associated substances such as phytic acid and phytoestrogens also appear to play a role in breast carcinogenesis. These factors may contribute to some of the inconsistencies observed in epidemiological studies because of the variability of these components in different fiber-rich foods. Future studies should take into account the potential contributory role of these phytochemicals when examining the role of fiber in reducing breast cancer risk.

REFERENCES

1. Forbes JF. The incidence of breast cancer: the global burden, public health considerations. Semin Oncol 24:S1-20–S21-35, 1997.
2. Gjorgov AN. Emerging worldwide trends of breast cancer incidence in the 1970s and 1980s: data from 23 cancer registration centers. Eur J Cancer Prev 2:423–440, 1993.
3. Drewnowski A, Popkin BM. The nutrition transition: new trends in the global diet. Nutr Rev 55: 31–43, 1997.
4. Jones LA, Gonzales R, Pillow PC, Gomez-Garza SA, Foreman CJ, Chilton JA, Linares A, Yack J, Badrei M, Hajeck RA. Dietary fiber, Hispanics, and breast cancer risk? Ann NY Acad Sci 839: 524–536, 1997.
5. Hems G. The contributions of diet and child-bearing to breast-cancer rates. Br J Cancer 37:974–982, 1978.
6. Saxe GA, Rock CL, Wicha M, Schottenfeld D. Diet and risk for breast cancer recurrence and survival. Breast Cancer Res Treat 53:241–253, 1999.
7. Armstrong B, Doll R. Environmental factors and cancer incidence and mortality in different countries, with special reference to dietary practices. Int J Cancer 15:617–631, 1975.
8. Drasar B, Irving D. Environmental factors and cancer of the colon and breast. Br J Cancer 27:167–172, 1973.
9. Stoll BA. Breast cancer and the western diet: role of fatty acids and antioxidant vitamins. Eur J Cancer 34:1852–1856, 1998.
10. Rose DP, Boyar AP, Wynder EL. International comparisons of mortality rates for cancer of the breast, ovary, prostate, and colon, and per capita food consumption. Cancer 58:2363–2371, 1986.
11. Correa P. Epidemiological correlations between diet and cancer frequency. Cancer Res 41: 3685–3690, 1981.
12. Rohan TE, Bain CJ. Diet in the etiology of breast cancer. Epidemiol Rev 9:120–145, 1987.
13. Doll R, Peto R. The causes of cancer: quantitative estimates of avoidable risks of cancer in the United States today. J Natl Cancer Inst 66:1191–1308, 1981.
14. Goodwin PJ, Boyd NF. Critical appraisal of the evidence that dietary fat intake is related to breast cancer risk in humans. J Natl Cancer Inst 79:473–485, 1987.
15. Clavel-Chapelon F, Nivravong M, Joseph RR. Diet and breast cancer: review of the epidemiologic literature. Cancer Detect Prev 21:426–440, 1997.
16. Howe GR, Hirohata T, Hislop TG, Iscovich, JM, Yuan J-M, Katsouyani K, Lubin F, Marubini E, Modan B, Rohan T, Toniolo P, Shunzhang Y. Dietary factors and risk of breast cancer: combined analysis of 12 case-control studies. J Natl Cancer Inst 82:561–569, 1990.
17. Boyd NF, Martin LJ, Noffel M, Lockwood GA, Trichler DL. A meta-analysis of studies of dietary fat and breast cancer risk. Br J Cancer 68:627–636, 1993.
18. Hunter DJ, Spiegelman D, Adami HO, Beeson L, van den Brandt PA, Folsom AR, Fraser GE, Goldbohm RA, Graham S, Howe GR, Kushi LH, Marshall JR, McDermott A, Miller AB, Speiser

FE, Wolk A, Yuan S-S, Willett WC. Cohort studies of fat intake and the risk of breast cancer—a pooled analysis. N Engl J Med 334:356–361, 1996.

19. Burkitt DP, Trowell HC. Refined Carbohydrate Foods and Disease: Implications of Dietary Fiber. London Academic Press, 1975.

20. Southgate DAT. Definitions and terminology of dietary fiber. In: Vahouny GV, Kritchevsky D, eds. Dietary Fiber in Health and Disease. New York: Plenum Press, 1982, pp 1–7.

21. Englyst HN, Cummings JH. Digestion of polysaccharides of potato in the small intestine of man. Am J Clin Nutr 45:423–431, 1987.

22. Berry CS. Resistant starch: formation and measurement of starch that survives exhaustive digestion with amolytic enzymes during the determination of dietary fibre. J Cereal Sci 4:301–314, 1986.

23. Lee SC, Prosky L. International survey on dietary fiber: definition, analysis, and reference materials. J AOAC Int 78: 22–36, 1995.

24. Cho SS, O'Sullivan K, Rickard S. Worldwide dietary fiber intake: recommendations and actual consumption patterns. In: Cho SS, Dreher M, Prosky L, eds. Complex Carbohydrates. New York: Marcel Dekker 1999, pp. 71–111.

25. Orman M. Position of the American Dietetic Association: health implications of dietary fiber. J Am Diet Assoc 93: 1446–1447, 1993.

26. Reddy BS, Cohen LA, McCoy GD, Hill P, Weisburger JH, Wynder EL. Nutrition and its relationship to cancer. Adv Cancer Res 32:237–345, 1980.

27. Kolonel LN, Hankin JH, Lee J, Chu SY, Nomura AMY, Hinds MW. Nutrient intakes in relation to cancer incidence in Hawaii. Br J Cancer 44:332–339, 1981.

28. Cummings JH. Dietary fibre intakes in Europe: overview and summary of European research activities, conducted by members of the Management Committee of COST 92. Eur J Clin Nutr 49:S5–S9, 1995.

29. Bingham S. Dietary fibre intakes: intake studies, problems, methods and results. In: Trowell, HC, Burkitt, DP, Heaton, K, eds. Dietary Fibre, Fibre-Depleted Foods and Disease. London: Academic Press 1985, pp 77–104.

30. Bingham S, Wiggins HS, Englyst H, Seppanen R, Helms P, Strand R, Burton R, Jorgensen IM, Poulsen L, Paerregaard A, Bjerrum L, James WP. Methods and validity of dietary assessments in four Scandinavian populations. Nutr Cancer 4:23–33, 1982.

31. Southgate DAT. Determination of carbohydrates in foods. II. Unavailable carbohydrates. J Sci Food Agric 20:331–335, 1969.

32. Cummings JH, Englyst HN, Wood R. Determination of dietary fibre in cereals and cereal products—collaborative trials. Part I: Initial trial. J Assoc Off Anal Chem 23:1–35, 1985.

33. Englyst HN, Cummings JH, Wood R. Determination of dietary fibre in cereals and cereal products—collaborative trials. Part II: Studies of the modified Englyst procedure. J Ass Publ Analysts 25:59–71, 1987.

34. Englyst HN, Cummings JH, Wood R. Determination of dietary fibre in cereals and cereal products. Part III: study of further simplified procedures. J Ass Publ Analysts 25:73–110, 1987.

35. Lee SC, Prosky L, DeVries JW. Determination of total, soluble, and insoluble dietary fiber in foods-enzymatic-gravimetric method, MES-TRIS buffer: collaborative study. J AOAC Int 75:395–416, 1992.

36. Prosky L, Asp N-G, Schweizer TF, DeVries JW, Furda I. Determination of insoluble, soluble and total dietary fiber in foods and food products: interlaboratory study. J Assoc Off Anal Chem 71: 1017–1023, 1988.

37. Theander O, Aman P, Westerlund E, Graham H. Enzymatic/chemical analysis of dietary fiber. J AOAC Int 77:703–709, 1994.

38. Zaridze DG, Muir CS, McMichael AJ. Diet and cancer: value of different types of epidemiological studies. Nutr Cancer 7:155–166, 1985.

39. Blondell JM. Urban-rural factors affecting cancer mortality in Kentucky, 1950–1969. Cancer Detect Prev 11:209–223, 1988.

40. Ishimoto H, Nakamura H, Miyoshi T. (1994) Epidemiological study on relationship between breast cancer mortality and dietary factors. Tokushima J Exp Med 41:103–114, 1994.

41. Morales M, Llopis A. Breast cancer and diet in Spain. J Environ Pathol Toxicol Oncol 11:157–167, 1992.
42. Rosen M, Nystrom L, Wall S. (1988) Diet and cancer mortality in the counties of Sweden. Am J Epidemiol 127:42–49, 1988.
43. Taioli E, Nicolosi A, Wynder EL. Dietary habits and breast cancer: a comparative study of United States and Italian Data. Nutr Cancer 16:259–265, 1991.
44. Ingram DM. Trends in diet and breast cancer mortality in England and Wales 1928–1977. Nutr Cancer 3:75–80, 1981.
45. Guo W-D, Chow W-H, Zheng W, Li J-Y, Blot WJ. Diet, serum markers and breast cancer mortality in China. Jpn J Cancer Res 85:572–577, 1994.
46. Baghurst PA, Rohan TE. High-fiber diets and reduced risk of breast cancer. Int J Cancer 56:173–176, 1994.
47. De Stefani E, Correa P, Ronco A, Mendilaharsu M, Guidobono M, Deneo-Pellegrini H. Dietary fiber and risk of breast cancer: a case-control study in Uruguay. Nutr Cancer 28:14–19, 1997.
48. Graham S, Hellmann R, Marshall J, Freudenheim J, Vena J, Swanson M, Zielezny M, Nemoto T, Stubbe N, Raimondo T. Nutritional epidemiology of postmenopausal breast cancer in western New York. Am J Epidemiol 134:552–566, 1991.
49. Iscovich JM, Iscovich RB, Howe G, Shiboski S, Kaldor JM. A case-control study of diet and breast cancer in Argentina. Int J Cancer 44:770–776, 1989.
50. Lubin F, Wax Y, Modan B. Role of fat, animal protein, and dietary fiber in breast cancer etiology: a case-control study. J Natl Cancer Inst 77:605–612, 1986.
51. Pryor M, Slattery ML, Robison LM, Egger M. Adolescent diet and breast cancer risk in Utah. Cancer Res 49:2161–2167, 1989.
52. Rohan TE, McMichael AJ, Baghurst PA. A population-based case-control study of diet and breast cancer in Australia. Am J Epidemiol 128:478–489, 1988.
53. Van't Veer P, Kolb CM, Verhoef P, Kok FJ, Schouten EG, Hermus RJJ, Sturmans F. Dietary fiber, beta-carotene and breast cancer: results from a case-control study. Int J Cancer 45:825–828, 1990.
54. Van't Veer P, van Leer EM, Rietduk A, Kok FJ, Schouten EG, Hermus RJJ, Sturmans F. Combination of dietary factors in relation to breast-cancer occurrence. Int J Cancer 47:649–653, 1991.
55. Franceschi S, Favero A, Decarli A, Negri E, La Vecchia C, Ferraroni M, Russo A, Salvini S, Amadori D, Conti E, Montella M, Giacosa A. Intake of macronutrients and risk of breast cancer. Lancet 347:1351–1356, 1996.
56. Graham S, Marshall J, Mettlin C, Rzepka T, Nemoto T, Byers T. Diet in the epidemiology of breast cancer. Am J Epidemiol 116:68–75, 1982.
57. Ingram DM, Nottage E, Roberts T. The role of diet in the development of breast cancer: a case-control study of patients with breast cancer, benign epithelial hyperplasia and fibrocystic disease of the breast. Br J Cancer 64:187–191, 1991.
58. Witte JS. Ursin G, Siemiatycki J, Thompson WD, Paganini-Hill A, Haile RW. Diet and premenopausal bilateral breast cancer: a case-control study. Breast Cancer Res Treat 42:243–251, 1997.
59. Katsouyanni K, Willett W, Trichopoulos D, Boyle P, Trichopolou A, Vasilaros S, Papadiamantis J, MacMahon B. Risk of breast cancer among Greek women in relation to nutrient intake. Cancer 61:181–185, 1988.
60. Braga C, La Vecchia C, Negri E, Franceschi S, Parpinel M. Intake of selected foods and nutrients and breast cancer risk: an age- and menopause-specific analysis. Nutr Cancer 28:258–263, 1997.
61. Franceschi S, La Vecchia C, Russo A, Negri E, Favero A, Decarli A. Low-risk diet for breast cancer in Italy. Cancer Epidemiol Biomarkers Prev 6:875–879.
62. Hislop TG, Coldman AJ, Elwood JM, Brauer G, Kan L. Childhood and recent eating patterns and risk of breast cancer. Cancer Detect Prev 9:47–58, 1986.
63. Katsouyanni K, Trichopoulos D, Boyle P, Xirouchaki E, Trichopoulou A, Lisseos B, Vasilaros S, MacMahon B. Diet and breast cancer: a case-control study in Greece. Int J Cancer 38:815–820, 1986.
64. La Vecchia C, Decarli A, Franceschi S, Gentile A, Negri E, Parazzini F. Dietary factors and the risk of breast cancer. Nutr Cancer 10:205–214, 1987.

65. Levi F, La Vecchia C, Gulie C, Negri E. Dietary factors and breast cancer risk in Vaud, Switzerland. Nutr Cancer 19:327–335, 1993.
66. Yuan JM, Yu MC, Ross RK, Gao YT, Henderson BE. Risk factors for breast cancer in Chinese women in Shanghai. Cancer Res 48:1949–1953, 1988.
67. Yuan J-M, Wang Q-S, Ross RK Henderson BE. Yu MC. Diet and breast cancer in Shanghai and Tianjin, China. Br J Cancer 71:1353–1358, 1995.
68. Zaridze D, Lifanova Y, Maximovitch D, Day NE, Duffy SW. Diet, alcohol consumption and reproductive factors in a case-control study of breast cancer in Moscow. Int J Cancer 48:493–501, 1991.
69. La Vecchia C, Ferraroni M, Franceschi S, Mezzetti M, Decarli A, Negri E. Fibers and breast cancer risk. Nutr Cancer 28:264–269, 1997.
70. Giovannucci E, Stampfer MJ, Colditz GA, Manson JE, Rosner BA, Longnecker M, Speizer FE, Willett WC. A comparison of prospective and retrospective assessments of diet in the study of breast cancer. Am J Epidemiol 137:502–511, 1993.
71. Graham S, Zielezny M, Marshall J, Priore R, Freudenheim J, Brasure J, Haughey B, Nasca P, Zdeb M. Diet in the epidemiology of postmenopausal breast cancer in the New York State cohort. Am J Epidemiol 136:1327–1337, 1992.
72. Jarvinen R, Knekt P, Seppanen R, Teppo L. Diet and breast cancer risk in a cohort of Finnish women. Cancer Lett 114:251–253, 1997.
73. Kushi LH, Sellers TA, Potter JD, Nelson CL, Munger RG, Kaye SA, Folsom AR. Dietary fat and postmenopausal cancer. J Natl Cancer Inst 84:1092–1099, 1992.
74. Rohan TE, Hiller JE, McMichael AJ. Dietary factors and survival from breast cancer. Nutr Cancer 20:167–177, 1993.
75. Verhoeven DT, Assen N, Goldbohm RA, Dorant E, Van't Veer P, Sturmans F, Hermus RJ, van den Brandt PA. Vitamins C and E, retinol, beta-carotene and dietary fibre in relation to breast cancer risk: a prospective cohort study. Br J Cancer 75:149–155, 1997.
76. Willett WC, Hunter DJ, Stampfer MJ, Colditz G, Manson JE, Spiegelman D, Rosner B, Hennekens CH, Speizer FE. Dietary fat and fiber in relation to risk of breast cancer: an 8-year follow-up. JAMA 268:2037–2044, 1992.
77. Hirayama T. A large cohort study on cancer risks by diet—with special reference to the risk reducing effects of green-yellow vegetable consumption. In: Hayashi Y, Nagao M, Sugimura T, Takayama S, Tomatis L, Wattenberg LW, Woga GN, eds. Diet, Nutrition and Cancer. Tokyo: Japan Scientific Societies Press, 1986, pp 41–53.
78. Rohan TE, Howe GR, Friedenreich CM, Jain M, Miller AB, Dietary fiber, vitamins A, C, and E, and risk of breast cancer: a cohort study. Cancer Causes Control 4:29–37, 1993.
79. Key TJA, Thorogood M, Appleby PN, Burr ML. Dietary habits and mortality in 11,000 vegetarians and health conscious people: results of a 17 year follow up. Br Med J 313:775–779, 1996.
80. Cook MG, Rohan TE. The patho-epidemiology of benign proliferative epithelial disorders of the female breast. J Pathol 146:1–15, 1985.
81. Oza AM, Boyd NF. Mammographic parenchymal patterns: a marker for breast cancer risk. Epidemiol Rev 15:196–208, 1993.
82. Page DL, Jensen RA. Evaluation and management of high risk and premalignant lesions of the breast. World J Surg 18:32–38, 1994.
83. Boyd NF, Greenberg C, Lockwood G, Little L, Martin L, Byng J, Yaffe M, Tritchler D. Effects at two years of a low-fat, high-carbohydrate diet on radiologic features of the breast: results from a randomized trial. J Natl Cancer Inst 89:488–496, 1997.
84. Baghurst PA, Rohan TE. Dietary fiber and risk of benign proliferative epithelial disorders of the breast. Int J Cancer 63:481–485, 1995.
85. Lubin F, Wax Y, Ron E, Black M, Chetrit A, Rosen N, Alfandary E, Modan B. Nutritional factors associated with benign breast disease etiology: a case-control study. Am J Clin Nutr 50:551–556, 1989.
86. Rohan TE, Cook MG, Potter JD, McMichael AJ. A case-control study of diet and benign proliferative epithelial disorders of the breast. Cancer Res 50:3176–3181, 1990.
87. Hislop TG, Band PR, Deschamps M, Ng, V, Coldman AJ, Worth AJ, Labo T. Diet and histologic

types of benign breast disease defined by subsequent risk of breast cancer. Am J Epidemiol 131: 263–270, 1990.

88. Nordevang E, Azavedo E, Svane G, Nilsson B, Holm LE, Dietary habits and mammographic patterns in patients with breast cancer. Breast Cancer Res Treat 26:207–215, 1993.

89. Brisson J, Verreault R, Morrison AS, Tennina S, Meyer F. Diet, mammographic features of breast tissue, and breast cancer risk. Am J Epidemiol 130:14–24, 1989.

90. Hebert JR, Toporoff E. Dietary exposures and other factors of possible prognostic significance in relation to tumour size and nodal involvement in early-stage breast cancer. Int J Epidemiol 18:518–526, 1989.

91. Holm LE, Callmer E, Hjalmar ML, Lidbrink E, Nilsson B, Skoog L. Dietary habits and prognostic factors in breast cancer. J Natl Cancer Inst 81:1218–1223, 1989.

92. Ingram DM, Roberts A, Nottage EM. Host factors and breast cancer growth characteristics. Eur J Cancer 28A:1153–1161, 1992.

93. Kaufmann M. Review of known prognostic variables. Recent Results Cancer Res 140:77–87, 1996.

94. Russo J, Gusterson BA, Rogers AE, Russo IH, Wellings SR, van Zweiten MJ. Biology of disease: comparative study of human and rat mammary tumorigenesis. Lab Invest 62:244–278, 1990.

95. Russo IH, Russo J. Mammary gland neoplasia in long-term rodent studies. Environ Health Perspect 104:938–967, 1996.

96. Arts CJM, de Bie ATHJ, van den Berg H, van't Veer P, Bunnik GSJ, Thijjssen JHH. Influence of wheat bran on NMU-induced mammary tumor development, plasma estrogen levels and estrogen excretion in female rats. J Steroid Biochem Mol Biol 39:193–202, 1991.

97. Cohen LA, Kendall ME, Zang E, Rose DP. Modulation of N-nitrosomethylurea-induced mammary tumor promotin by dietary fiber and fat. J Natl Cancer Inst 83:496–501, 1991.

98. Cohen LA, Zhao Z, Zang E, Rivenson A. Dose-response effects of dietary fiber on NMU-induced mammary tumorigenesis, estrogen levels and estrogen excretion in female rats. Carcinogenesis 17: 45–52, 1996.

99. Zile MH, Welsch CW, Welsch MA. Effect of wheat bran fiber on the development of mammary tumors in female intact and ovariectomized rats treated with 7,12-dimethylbenz(a)anthracene and in mice with spontaneously developing mammary tumors. Int J Cancer 75:439–443, 1998.

100. Cohen LA, Zhao Z, Zang EA, Wynn TT, Simi B, Rivenson A. Wheat bran and psyllium diets: effects on N-methylnitrosourea-induced mammary tumorigenesis in F344 rats. J Natl Cancer Inst 88:899–907, 1996.

101. Arts CJM, Govers CARL, van der Berg H, Wolters MGE, van Leeuwen P, Thijssen JHH. In vitro binding of estrogens by dietary fiber and the in vivo apparent digestibility tested in pigs. J Steroid Biochem Mol Biol 38:621–628, 1991.

102. Birt DF, Markin RS, Blackwood D, Harvell DM, Shull JD, Pennington KL. Dietary lignin, and insoluble fiber, enhance uterine cancer but did not influence mammary cancer induced by N-methyl-N-nitrosourea in rats. Nutr Cancer 31:24–30, 1998.

103. Vucenik I, Yang GY, Shamsuddin AM. Comparison of pure inositol hexaphosphate and high-bran diet in the prevention of DMBA-induced rat mammary carcinogenesis. Nutr Cancer 28:7–13, 1997.

104. Bernstein L, Ross RK. Endogenous hormones and breast cancer risk. Epidemiol Rev 15:48–65, 1993.

105. Feinleib M. Breast cancer and artificial menopause: a cohort study. J Natl Cancer Inst 41:315–329, 1968.

106. Bernstein L, Yuan J-M, Ross RK, Pike MC, Hanisch R, Lobo R, Stanczyk F, Gao Y-T, Henderson BE. Serum hormone levels in pre-menopausal Chinese women in Shanghai and white women in Los Angeles: results from two breast cancer case-control studies. Cancer Causes Control 1:51–58, 1990.

107. Goldin BR, Adlercreutz H, Gorbach SL, Woods MN, Dwyer JT, Conlon T, Bohn E, Gershoff SN. The relationship between estrogen levels and diets of Caucasian American and Oriental immigrant women. Am J Clin Nutr 44:945–953, 1986.

108. Key TJA, Chen J, Wang DY, Pike MC, Boreham J. Sex hormones in women in rural China and in Britain. Br J Cancer 62:631–636, 1990.

109. Shimizu H, Ross RK, Bernstein L, Pike MC, Henderson BE. Serum oestrogen levels in postmeno-

pausal women: comparison of American whites and Japanese in Japan. Br J Cancer 62:451–453, 1990.

110. Woods MN, Barnett JB, Spiegelman D, Trail N, Hertzmark E, Longcope C, Gorbach SL. Hormone levels during dietary changes in premenopausal African-American women. J Natl Cancer Inst 88: 1369–1374, 1996.

111. Jones LA, Ota DM, Jackson GA, Jackson PM, Kemp K, Anderson DE, McCamant SK, Bauman DH. Bioavailability of estradiol as a marker for breast cancer risk assessment. Cancer Res 47:5224–5229, 1987.

112. Berrino F, Muti P, Micheli A, Bolelli G, Krogh V, Sciajno R, Pisani P, Panico S, Secreto G. Serum sex hormone levels after menopause and subsequent breast cancer. J Natl Cancer Inst 88:291–296, 1996.

113. Toniolo PG, Levitz M, Zeleniuch-Jacquotte A, Banerjee S, Koenig KL, Shore RE, Strax P, Pasternack BS. A prospective study of endogenous estrogens and breast cancer in postmenopausal women. J Natl Cancer Inst 87:190–197, 1995.

114. Miller WR, O'Neill JS. The significance of steroid metabolism in human cancer. J Steroid Biochem Mol Biol 37:317–325, 1989.

115. Witt BR, Thorneycroft IH. Reproductive steroid hormones: generation, degradation, reception and action. Clin Obstetr Gynecol 33:563–575, 1990.

116. Gorbach SL, Goldin BR, Diet and the excretion and enterohepatic cycling of estrogens. Prev Med 16:525–531, 1987.

117. Adlercreutz H, Hockerstedt K, Bannwart C, Bloigu S, Hamalainen E, Fotsis T, Ollus A. Effect of dietary components, including lignans and phytoestrogens, on enterohepatic circulation and liver metabolism of estrogens and on sex hormone binding globulin (SHBG). J Steroid Biochem 27: 1135–1144, 1987.

118. Rose DP. Dietary fiber and breast cancer. Nutr Cancer 13:1–8, 1990.

119. Adlercreutz H, Fotsis T, Bannwart C, Hamalainen E, Bloigu S, Ollus A. Urinary estrogen profile determination in young Finnish vegetarian and omnivorous women. J Steroid Biochem 24:289–296, 1986.

120. Barbosa JC, Shultz TD, Filley SJ, Nieman DC. The relationship among adiposity, diet, and hormone concentrations in vegetarian and nonvegetarian postmenopausal women. Am J Clin Nutr 51:798–803, 1990.

121. Goldin BR, Adlercreutz H, Gorbach SL, Warram JH, Dwyer JT, Swenson L, Woods MN. Estrogen excretion patterns and plasma levels in vegetarian and omnivorous women. N Engl J Med 307: 1542–1547, 1982.

122. Rose DP, Boyar AP, Kettunen K. Diet, serum, breast fluid growth hormone, and prolactin levels in normal premenopausal Finnish and American women. Nutr Cancer 11:179–187, 1988.

123. Kaneda N, Nagata C, Kabuto M, Shimizu H. Fat and fiber intakes in relation to serum estrogen concentration in premenopausal Japanese women. Nutr Cancer 27:279–283, 1997.

124. Adlercreutz H, Fotsis T, Hockerstedt K, Hamalainen E, Bannwart C, Bloigu S, Valtonen A, Ollus A. Diet and urinary estrogen profile in premenopausal omnivorous and vegetarian women and in premenopausal women with breast cancer. J Steroid Biochem 34:527–530, 1989.

125. Bagga D, Ashley JM, Geffrey SP, Wang HJ, Barnard RJ, Korenman S, Heber D. Effects of a very low fat, high fiber diet on serum hormones and menstrual function. Implications for breast cancer prevention. Cancer 76:2491–2496, 1995.

126. Goldin BR, Woods MN, Spiegelman DL, Longcope C, Morrill-LaBrode A, Dwyer JT, Gualtieri LJ, Hertzmark E, Gorbach SL. The effect of dietary fat and fiber on serum estrogen concentrations in postmenopausal women under controlled dietary conditions. Cancer 74:1125–1131, 1994.

127. Ferguson LR, Harris PJ. Does wheat bran or wheat dietary fibre protect against breast cancer? Int J Cancer 78:385–386, 1988.

128. Schaefer EJ, Lamon-Fava S, Spiegelman D, Dwyer JT, Lichtenstein AH, McNamara JR, Goldin BR, Woods MN, Morrill-LaBrode A, Hertzmark E, et al. Changes in plasma lipoprotein concentrations and composition in response to a low-fat, high-fiber diet are associated with changes in serum estrogen concentrations in premenopausal women. Metabolism 44:749–756, 1995.

129. Rose DP, Goldman M, Connolly JM, Strong LE. High-fiber diet reduces serum estrogen concentrations in premenopausal women. Am J Clin Nutr 54:520–525, 1991.
130. Rose DP, Lubin M, Connolly JM. Effects of diet supplementation with wheat bran on serum estrogen levels in the follicular and luteal phases of the menstrual cycle. Nutrition 13:535–539, 1997.
131. Reddy BS, Engle A, Simi B, Goldman M. Effect of dietary fiber on colonic bacterial enzymes and bile salts in relation to colon cancer. Gastroenterology 102:1475–1482, 1992.
132. Lewis SJ, Heaton KW, Oakey RE, McGarrigle HH. Lower serum oestrogen concentrations associated with faster intestinal transit. Br J Cancer 76:395–400, 1997.
133. Lewis SJ, Oakey RE, Heaton KW. Intestinal absorption of oestrogen: the effect of altering transit-time. Eur J Gastroenterol Hepatol 10:33–39, 1998.
134. Arts CJM, Thijssen JHH. Effects of wheat bran on blood and tissue hormone levels in adult female rats. Acta Endocrinol 127:271–278, 1992.
135. Kendall ME, Cohen LA. Effect of dietary fiber on mammary tumorigenesis, estrogen metabolism, and lipid excretion in female rats. In Vivo 6:239–246, 1992.
136. Arts CJM, Govers CARL, van den Berg H, Thijssen JHH. Effects of wheat bran and energy restriction on onset of puberty, cell proliferation and development of mammary tissue in female rats. Acta Endocrinol (Copenh) 126:451–459, 1992.
137. Ferguson LR, Harris PJ. Protection against cancer by wheat bran: role of dietary fiber and phytochemicals. Eur J Cancer 8:17–25, 1999.
138. Graf E. Application of phytic acid. J Am Oil Chem Soc 60:1861–1867, 1983.
139. Thompson LU, Zhang L. Phytic acid and minerals: effect on early markers of risk for mammary and colon carcinogenesis. Carcinogenesis 12:2041–2045, 1991.
140. Shamsuddin AM, Yang GY, Vucenik I. Novel anti-cancer functions of IP6: growth inhibition and differentiation of human mammary cancer cell lines in vitro. Anticancer Res 16:3287–3292, 1996.
141. Vucenik I, Yang GY, Shamsuddin AM. Inositol hexaphosphate and inositol inhibit DMBA-induced rat mammary cancer. Carcinogenesis 16:1055–1058, 1995.
142. Hirose M, Hoshiya T, Akagi K, Futakuchi M, Ito N. Inhibition of mammary gland carcinogenesis by green tea catechins and other naturally occurring antioxidants in female Sprague-Dawley rats pretreated with 7,12-dimethylbenz[a]anthracene. Cancer Lett 83:149–156, 1994.
143. Baten A, Ullah A, Tomazic VJ, Shamsuddin AM. Inositol-phosphate-induced enhancement of natural killer cell activity correlates with tumor suppression. Carcinogenesis 10:1595–1598, 1989.
144. Nielsen BK, Thompson LU, Bird RP. Effect of phytic acid on colonic epithelial cell proliferation. Cancer Lett 37:317–325, 1987.
145. Thompson LU. Nutritional and physiological effects of phytic acid. In: Kinsella JE, Soucie WG, eds. Food Proteins. Champaign, IL: AOCS 1989, pp 410–431.
146. Rickard SE, Thompson LU. Interactions and biological effects of phytic acid. In: Shahidi F, ed. Antinutrients and Phytochemicals in Foods. Washington, DC: American Chemical Society 1997, pp 294–312.
147. Rickard SE, Thompson LU. Phytoestrogens and lignans: effects on reproduction and chronic disease. In: Shahidi F, ed. Antinutrients and Phytochemicals in Foods. Washington, DC: American Chemical Society 1997, pp 273–293.
148. Setchell KDR, Adlercreutz H. Mammalian lignans and phytoestrogens: recent studies on their formation, metabolism and biological role in health and disease. In: Rowland IR, ed. Role of the Gut Flora, Toxicity and Cancer. London: Academic Press, 1988, pp 315–345.
149. Adlercreutz H, Fotsis T, Heikkinen R, Dwyer JT, Woods M, Goldin BR, Gorbach SL. Excretion of the lignans enterolactone and enterodiol and of equol in omnivorous and vegetarian postmenopausal women and in women with breast cancer. Lancet 2:1295–1299, 1982.
150. Adlercreutz H, Fotsis T, Bannwart C, Wahala K, Makela T, Brunow G, Hase T. Determination of urinary lignans and phytoestrogen metabolites, potential antiestrogens and anticarcinogens, in urine of women on various habitual diets. J Steroid Biochem 25:791–797, 1986.
151. Adlercreutz H, Honjo H, Higashi A, Fotsis T, Hamalainen E, Hasegawa T, Okada H. Urinary excretion of lignans and isoflavonoid phytoestrogens in Japanese men and women consuming a traditional Japanese diet. Am J Clin Nutr 54:1093–1100, 1991.

152. Axelson M, Sjovall J, Gustafsson BE, Setchell KD. Origin of lignans in mammals and identification of a precursor from plants. Nature 298:659–660, 1982.
153. Thompson LU, Robb P, Serraino M, Cheung F. Mammalian lignan production from various foods. Nutr Cancer 16:43–52, 1991.
154. Axelson M, Setchell KD. The excretion of lignans in rats—evidence for an intestinal bacterial source for this new group of compounds. FEBS Lett 123:337–342, 1981.
155. Adlercreutz H, Mazur W. Phytoestrogens and western diseases. Ann Med 29:95–120, 1997.
156. Lee HP, Gourley L, Duffy SW, Esteve J, Lee J, Day NE. Risk factors for breast cancer by age and menopausal status: a case-control study in Singapore. Cancer Causes Control 3:313–322, 1992.
157. Arts CJM, Govers CARL, van den Berg H, Blankenstein MA, Thijssen JHH. Effect of wheat bran on excretion of radioactively labeled estradiol-17B and estrone-glucuronide injected intravenously in male rats. J Steroid Biochem Mol Biol 42:103–111, 1992.

5
Dietary Fiber and Breast Cancer Epidemiology

Peter A. Baghurst
Women's and Children's Hospital, North Adelaide, South Australia, Australia

Katrine I. Baghurst
CSIRO, Adelaide, South Australia, Australia

I. INTRODUCTION: ESTROGENS AND BREAST CANCER

Estrogens are central to the vast majority of mechanisms proposed to explain the epidemiology of breast cancer. A cornerstone of the unifying theory proposed by Pike and coworkers is that cumulative exposure to proliferative stimuli (primarily estrogen and progesterone) is a major determinant of breast cancer risk (1,2). The vast majority of cancers originate in tissues where active cell division may occur before repairs to DNA damage can be effected, and the epithelial cells of the breast ducts are subject to a monthly proliferative stimulus as a result of the cyclic variations in estrogen and progesterone. The pattern of increasing risk with age (decelerating after a naturally occurring, or surgically induced menopause—see Fig. 1) and decreased risks associated with late age of menarche, early onset of menopause, irregular (less frequent) menses, and early child-bearing are all consistent with this theory (3).

The fact that ovariectomy has long been recognized as an effective means of slowing the progression of breast cancer (4) and that around a third of all breast cancers have estrogen receptors (and cell cultures grown from them are stimulated by estradiol) has further implicated estrogens in this hormone-dependent cancer. Endogenous estrogens are not of themselves carcinogenic, although there is some discussion as to whether the metabolism of estradiol can be preferentially channeled, by dietary manipulation, through the less bioactive 2-hydroxy derivative instead of the 16-hydroxy derivative or the so-called catechol estrogens (5,6).

Speculation that dietary fiber may impact on the risk of breast cancer is comparatively recent. The term dietary fiber will be used in this chapter to encompass all those components of food that reach the large bowel undigested. The major chemical entities included under this rubric are the poly- and oligosaccharides, although materials such as lignin (a component of cell walls in plants) and mineral "ashes" are also included under this definition. This definition would also include substances referred to collectively as phytoestrogens, because of their ability to agonize or antagonize the effects of endogenously synthesized sex hormones.

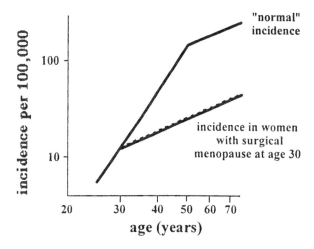

Fig. 1 Relationship between age and risk of breast cancer. (Adapted from Ref. 2.)

II. NONSTARCH POLYSACCHARIDES—PROPOSED MECHANISMS AND EPIDEMIOLOGY

A. Effect of Dietary Fiber on the Enterohepatic Cycling of Endogenous Estrogens

Naturally synthesized, or endogenous, estrogens are excreted partly via the urine and partly in the bile. In order to facilitate this excretion, the estrogens are conjugated with glucuronic acid, which also serves to make them less available for reabsorption further down the alimentary tract. The bacterial flora possess the enzymic machinery (specifically a β-glucuronidase), which can remove the conjugated group and thereby promote reabsorption of estrogens, leading to the establishment of an enterohepatic cycle and reduced overall excretion of endogenous estrogens. Although high-fiber diets increase the bacterial population inhabiting the large bowel, there are qualitative changes in the species profile of the flora, and growth of bacteria with low β-glucuronidase activity appears to be favored. The net effect of a high-fiber diet is, therefore, arguably, to decrease the deconjugating activity in the large bowel and reduce enterohepatic cycling, leading to increased fecal excretion of estrogens and decreased plasma levels and urinary excretion. Data broadly consistent with this hypothesis were reported in a small intervention study of just 10 vegetarian and 10 nonvegetarian women by Goldin et al. (7). Similar observations were made in a later study from the same group (8), but other studies have not been in such agreement. Woods et al. observed significant decreases in serum levels of estrone sulfate (but not estrone or estradiol) when women were placed on a low-fat, high-fiber diet (9), whereas Bagga et al. found significant reductions in estrone and estradiol but not in estrone sulfate (10). A complicating factor in the interpretation of the data from these latter two studies was the simultaneous manipulation of both dietary fat and fiber intakes. Dorgan et al. failed to find any association between fiber intake and plasma concentrations of estrogens in a cross-sectional study of 90 premenopausal women after taking fat and energy intakes into account (11), but in an intervention study Rose et al. significantly reduced the plasma levels of serum estrone and estradiol in premenopausal women with wheat bran, but not corn or oat bran (12).

Animal studies designed to test aspects of the enterohepatic cycling theory have not been conclusive. Cohen and coworkers (13,14) demonstrated striking reductions in the glucuronidase activity in the rat caecum with psyllium fiber, but, curiously, the lower deconjugating capacity was not accompanied by reductions in the circulating levels of estrogens or by increases in fecal estrogens. The further observation that wheat fiber did not affect the deconjugating activity in the anticipated direction, and yet a 4%:4% mixture of psyllium and wheat bran fibers was effective in inhibiting mammary tumor development following administration with N-methylnitrosourea (MNU), would appear to indicate that another mechanism may be dominant in this animal model (13,14).

B. Absorptive Properties of Dietary Fiber

Meats cooked at very high temperatures (e.g., by grilling, broiling, or barbecuing) contain minute amounts of heterocyclic amines (HCAs), which have proved to be carcinogenic in studies involving the administration of purified HCAs to laboratory animals. In vivo studies of the effect of concomitant administration of dietary fiber and parsley with HCA have found reduced mutagenicity of fecal or urine samples (15,16).

Schultz and Howie also reported in vitro binding capacities of a number of natural and purified fibers in support of the hypothesis that the direct binding of steroid hormones may be one of the mechanisms by which dietary fiber can influence the excretion of and hence net exposure to these promoters of hormone-dependent cancers (17). The physiological relevance of these properties of dietary fiber, given that much of it is ultimately fermented in the large bowel, requires further investigation.

C. Effects of Dietary Fiber on Insulin Resistance

Hyperinsulinemia and insulin resistance have been associated with increased levels of bioavailable estrogen and elevated breast cancer risk in the Netherlands (18). The etiology of insulin resistance is still poorly understood, but the general consensus that it is less common in individuals consuming diets rich in dietary fiber has led to growing speculation that a synergistic effect on both bioavailable estrogen and insulin sensitivity may be an important mechanism by which dietary fiber affords protection against breast cancer (19).

D. Epidemiological Studies of Fiber and Breast Cancer

Human studies of fiber and breast cancer are more supportive of a fiber effect than not (Table 1), but discrepancies need to be resolved before these findings are embraced too enthusiastically. Meaningful reductions in risk were associated with high fiber intakes in case-control studies conducted in Australia, the Netherlands, Singapore, Uruguay, and the United States. A meta-analysis by Howe et al. of 12 case-control studies (many of which did not publish any fiber data separately) also found a statistically significant reduction in risk with increasing dietary fiber (20). Although a large and apparently well-conducted case-control study in Italy failed to find any association of breast cancer risk with total fiber intake, a subsequent reanalysis of the data found a statistically significant, if rather modest decrease in risk among the top consumers of the cellulose component of dietary fiber (21). Of the five cohort studies that have addressed this question (three in the United States, one in Canada, and one in the Netherlands), only the Canadian study found a significant inverse association. Authors of the Dutch study reported risk estimates of 0.75 and 0.83 in the second-highest and highest consumption categories, respectively, but the trend statistic had an associated p-value of 0.16. The study of U.S. nurses is interesting for the low levels of dietary fiber consumed (see Table 1), and it is conceivable that if there is a true causal relation between fiber and breast cancer risk, the consumption levels in this population were simply too low to achieve a meaningful effect. The failure of the prospective

Table 1 Studies Reporting Breast Cancer Risk as a Function of Total Dietary Fiber Intake

	Age group	Relative risk/odds ratio	Consumption cut-points (g)	p-value	Ref.
Retrospective (case-control) studies					
Argentina	All	0.41		0.05	2
Australia	All	1 0.77 0.57 0.69 0.48	14 18 23 28	0.003	23
	<50	1 1.37 0.56 0.84 1.19		0.61	
	≥50	1 0.63 0.64 0.65 0.42		0.023	
	All	1 1.09 0.71 0.97 0.71		0.11	
		0.85 (95% CI 0.70–1.04)	per 12 g		
Italy		1 1.02 0.99 0.93 0.94	17 21 24 29	0.30	24
		0.95	per 11.7 g	—	
Netherlands	All	1 1.34 0.98 0.55	Not stated	0.10	25
		1 0.75 (95% CI 0.51–1.19)	≤26 26		
Spain	All	1 0.6 1.38		ns	26
Sweden	All	1 0.7 0.7 0.6	11 15 17	0.09	27
		0.8	per 4.4 g	ns	
Uruguay	All	1 1.15 0.69 0.51	21 26 32	<0.001	28
	<50	1 0.83 0.70 0.53	21 27 32	0.003	29
	≥50	1 1.05 0.96 0.74	19 25 32	0.01	30
Prospective (cohort) studies					
Canada	All	1 0.78 0.72 0.76 0.68	13 16 20 25	0.093	31
Netherlands	All	1 0.94 1.05 0.75 0.83	17 21 25 29 35[a]	0.16	32
	≥50	1 1.15 1.28 0.94 1.07	15 20 25 32	ns	33
	≥50	1 1.15 1.02 0.99	14 18 21 27[a]	0.72	34
U.S. nurses	All	1 0.95 0.93 1.02 1.02	11 14 17 21	0.62	35
	<50	1 0.86 0.80 0.86 1.06		0.95	
	≥50	1 0.97 1.00 1.03 0.96		0.98	
U.S. nurses	All	1 0.76 0.94 1.04 0.62	Means 19.5 cases 20.5 cont	0.38	36

[a] Values are group medians, not cut-points.

studies to find an association between dietary fiber and breast cancer (with the exception of one conducted in Canada) must temper the enthusiasm generated by the case-control studies, which are less sound methodologically, and until satisfactory answers to these discrepancies have been provided, the epidemiological evidence for a protective effect of dietary fiber must be regarded as equivocal.

Since dietary fiber is a collective term for a heterogeneous group of substances derived from fruits, vegetables, and cereals, it is extremely likely that the sources of dietary fiber in one study population will be rather different from the sources in other populations or cultures. And it is becoming increasingly clear that the components of dietary fiber vary considerably in terms of their abilities to affect factors associated with breast cancer etiology. The findings of Rose et al. that wheat bran (but not corn or oat bran) could significantly reduce the plasma levels of serum estrone and estradiol in premenopausal women is a pertinent example (12). Notwithstanding the existence of plausible mechanisms, the possibility that fiber is simply acting as a surrogate marker for other chemopreventive substances present in plant foods has not been eliminated, and to the extent that it may be a much better marker in some studies than in others, this might explain why the studies conducted so far have varied so much in their findings.

III. PHYTOESTROGENS

A. Introduction

Rose has argued that some of the health benefits associated with high-fiber diets may be a consequence not of the polysaccharide component of dietary fiber, but of micromolar quantities of substances known as phytoestrogens (37). Phytoestrogens have recently been defined in terms of their ability to interact with the estrogen signal transduction pathway. Clarke et al. defined them as "plant derived compounds that can regulate gene expression that is mediated by an estrogen response element, in a manner either comparable or apparently antagonistic to 17β-estradiol, as a result of binding to the estrogen receptor" (38). Such a definition would seem to be unnecessarily restrictive and preclude interactions with other aspects of steroid hormone synthesis and metabolism, which, while not involving the signal transduction pathway, are nevertheless dependent on structural or functional similarities to endogenous estrogens and are becoming increasingly associated in the literature with the term "phytoestrogenic."

Major classes of phytoestrogenic substances include bioflavonoid compounds (flavones, isoflavones, flavanones), lignans, coumestrol from legume sprouts, and zearalenone, a mycotoxin derived from fungal molds. While bioflavonoid compounds are widespread in foods of plant origin, the most significant compounds with estrogenic activity in this class are genistein and daidzein, found in largest amounts in the soybean (39), and formononetin from clovers. Lignans, which are characterized chemically by a 2,3-dibenzylbutane structure, are also widespread in plant foods, although flaxseed contains concentrations two orders of magnitude higher than any other known source (40). Phytoestrogens are often co-located (within the plant) with other components of dietary fiber, and in common with nonstarch polysaccharides their biologically activity is critically dependent on the metabolism of their precursor compounds by the microflora in the large bowel (or the forestomach of ruminants), where daidzein may be either generated from formononetin or metabolized to equol (41,42), and the "mammalian lignans" enterolactone and enterodiol are generated from less estrogenic precursors such as matairesinol and secoisolariciresinol (43).

A phytoestrogen that is sufficiently similar to endogenous estrogens to occupy an estrogen-binding site, but which has only limited ability to induce the event that normally ensues when natural estrogen binds, is called an estrogen antagonist. However, when estrogen is either absent or present only in very low concentrations (postmenopausally, for example), the limited ability of a phytoestrogen to induce the secondary event may still be biologically meaningful and warrant its reclassification as an agonist.

B. Effects of Phytoestrogens on Breast Cancer Cell Lines

Given the demonstration in Figure 1 of an increasing risk of breast cancer with increasing cumulative estrogen (and progesterone) exposure, it is perhaps not surprising that historically our interest in the relevance of phytoestrogens to breast cancer stemmed from a supposed ability to act as antagonists of estradiol. However, studies of the growth responses of breast cancer cell lines to phytoestrogens have contributed to a more recent understanding that some of their anticarcinogenic properies may not be mediated by their estrogenic properties. The emerging consensus appears to be that several phytoestrogens do not act as direct antiestrogens in their effects on cell growth (44), and in some situations they actually appear to promote growth. The report by Welshons et al. of the lignan enterolactone and the isoflavonoid metabolite equol stimulating growth of breast cancer cells in vitro is one example (45). However, in competition studies with mixtures of phytoestrogens and estradiol, antiestrogenic effects are often observed, and Adlercreutz et al. found that estradiol and the lignan enterolactone stimulated the growth of MCF-7 cells on their own (i.e., the lignan alone was apparently estrogenic), but when they were mixed together in the growth medium, enterolactone completely inhibited the response to estradiol (46). A number of studies have found genistein to be an effective growth inhibitor of cell lines, but the observation that it is equally effective in both MCF-7 cells, which are estrogen dependent, and MDA-468 cells, which are not, adds further support to the notion that these effects are not necessarily mediated via direct competition with estradiol for an estrogen growth receptor. In cell lines derived from non–hormone-dependent cancers at other sites, genistein has been found to be an effective inducer of differentiation and the expression of the mature phenotype (see Ref. 47).

C. Effects of Phytoestrogens on Breast Cancer—In Vivo Animal Studies

Messina et al. (47) identified eight studies involving soy products and experimental mammary cancer. One study used x-ray irradiation; the others all used dimethylbenz[a]anthracene or N-methyl-N'-nitrosourea as the carcinogenic agent. Five of these studies reported a protective effect, which is not overwhelming evidence for soy foods being anticarcinogens, although the same review article also summarized additional studies that observed protective effects at several other sites. Very little work has been done with lignans, although Thompson et al. reported favorable effects of a linseed-enriched diet on cell proliferation and nuclear aberrations in rats and on mammary tumor initiation and promotion in weanling rats given dimethylbenz[a]anthracene (48).

D. Some Proposed Mechanisms for the Protective Effects of Phytoestrogens

1. Inhibition of Angiogenesis

Angiogenesis, the process by which new capillaries develop from preexisting vessels and on which ''solid'' cancers are critically dependent for growth, has been shown to be sensitive to phytoestrogens, especially genistein (49). Estrogen stimulates the production of vascular endothelial growth factor during the extensive vascular remodeling that accompanies the normal cycle-specific changes in the human female reproductive tract (50), and although the ability of genistein to inhibit angiogenesis is often discussed separately from its more obviously estrogenic properties, it is interesting to speculate, that this ability to inhibit angiogenesis may also be an antiestrogenic effect.

2. Increased Synthesis of Sex Hormone–Binding Globulins

Sex hormone–binding globulins (SHBGs) are circulating proteins which are synthesized in the liver, and which exhibit a high affinity for both estradiol and testosterone (51). Since the biological activity of steroid hormones bound to SHBG is very low, their bioavailability is determined to a significant extent by circulating levels of SHBG. Indeed SHBG concentrations increase in response to rising levels of either sex hormone and hence appear to be acting as regulators. The notion that phytoestrogens might stimulate synthesis of SHBG and thereby significantly reduce the bioactivity of endogenous estrogens has been championed by Adlercreutz and coworkers (52,53), but their human work was based on very heterogeneous groups of participants, and other studies, including unpublished work of our own, have failed to observe any dietary dependence of SHBG (54). A finding by Mousavi and Adlercreutz that genistein effectively stimulates SHBG synthesis in human liver cancer cells (Hep-G2) and suppresses their growth is a much stronger argument for an SHBG-mediated effect of phytoestrogens (55).

3. Inhibition of Protein Kinases and Topoisomerase II

The observation that some phytoestrogens can inhibit growth in tumors with and without estrogen receptors underscores the potential importance of these mechanisms in the prevention of malignancy. Genistein, for example, appears to be able to inhibit the tyrosine-protein kinase intimately involved in determining the activity of proteins that regulate cell proliferation (56), to inhibit topoisomerase II whose activities are crucial in the manipulation of DNA during cell division (57), and to arrest the cell division cycle around the G2 to M phases (58).

4. Effects on Steroid Hormone Synthesis and Metabolism

Within the context of breast cancer, an important property of phytoestrogens may be their ability to inhibit the cytochrome P450 aromatase, which catalyzes the final step in the synthesis of estrogen and estrone from testosterone and androstenedione, respectively (59,60).

E. Human Epidemiological Studies of Phytoestrogens and Breast Cancer

Descriptive studies examining urinary excretion or plasma levels of phytoestrogens in groups with different experiences of hormone-dependent cancers have been summarized by Adlercreutz and Mazur (61). While phytoestrogen intakes are highest in the populations with the lowest cancer risk, this evidence remains circumstantial, and experience with the correlational studies of per capita fat consumption and breast cancer should have taught us to be especially suspicious of this kind of evidence.

To date, only a few human studies have directly investigated the dietary intake of phytoestrogen-rich foods in relation to breast cancer risk. An extremely large cohort study in Japan reported a ''dose-dependent'' decrease with increasing consumption of soybean paste (miso) soup (62). While this early study failed to collect data on ancillary risk factors, the sheer weight of numbers (142,857 women) would require some extreme biases of a systematic nature (e.g., large age-related differences in consumption of miso) for this trend to be nullified. Another cohort study, which used diets of 6860 Japanese men in Hawaii as surrogate measures of the dietary habits of their wives, found that reduced risks of breast cancer in the wives were associated with high intakes of miso and tofu by their husbands during the years 1971–75 but not during the earlier years of 1965–68 (63). A case-control study in Singapore reported significantly reduced risks of breast cancer with increasing dietary intakes of ''soy protein,'' the ratio of soy to total protein, and total soy products (64). Another case-control study in Japan found no association, but the emphasis of this study was more on the consumption of fat (oil) from soy rather than soy itself (65). A case-control study conducted in western Australia by Ingram et al. found substantially reduced risks of breast cancer associated with high urinary excretion of phytoestrogens (66).

IV. CONCLUSION: DIETARY RECOMMENDATIONS

Despite the equivocality of our knowledge relating the risk of breast cancer to dietary fiber intakes, the recommendation to increase the proportion of fiber in the diet could still be regarded as highly prudent. Such advice would be totally compatible with programs aimed at reducing obesity and cardiovascular disease and improving diabetic control and various aspects of gut health.

Current knowledge is also insufficient to specify recommended daily intakes. Dietary fiber is not ''toxic'' in any known sense, and there is very little reason to suggest that the amount of fiber consumed by healthy women should be constrained to lie within any kind of upper limit. Concerns about possible adverse effects of excess dietary fiber have been centered on mineral metabolism and osteoporosis. Although the ability of dietary fiber to reduce circulating levels of estrogens remains arguable (as discussed above), the authors of a cross-sectional study in which high fiber intakes were found to depress circulating estradiol levels in 55 young women in New Zealand have sounded a warning that this effect may impact adversely on bone mass (67).

Historically there has also been a preoccupation with claims (based initially on a study of just two subjects [68]) that mineral absorption could be adversely affected by dietary fiber. There is no doubt that phytate, associated with the chemical matrix described as dietary fiber, remains a potent chelator of minerals, but there is little evidence that even strict vegetarianism leads to problems of mineral absorption (69) (although it is widely appreciated that such diets may be intrinsically low in zinc and bioavailable iron and that vegetarians need to pay special attention to ensure an adequate intake of these nutrients). Knox and coworkers have suggested that calcium absorption may be affected by high-fiber diets in the elderly (70), but recent work suggests that calcium entrapped by fiber in the small intestine may be absorbed with short-chain fatty acids in the large bowel (71).

REFERENCES

1. Pike MC, Spicer DV, Dahmoush L, Press MF. Estrogens, progestogens, normal breast cell proliferation and breast cancer risk. Epidemiol Rev 15:17–35, 1993.
2. Spicer DV, Pike MC. Hormonal manipulation to prevent breast cancer. Scie Am Sci Med (July/August):58–67, 1995.
3. Kelsey JL, Gammon MD, John EM. Reproductive factors and breast cancer. Epidemiol Rev 15:6–47, 1993.
4. Beatson DG. On the treatment of inoperable cases of carcinoma of the mamma: suggestions for a new method of treatment with illustrative cases. Lancet ii:104–107, 1896.

5. Bradlow L, Telang NT, Osborn MP. Estrogen metabolites as bioreactive modulators of tumor initiators and promoters. Adv Exp Med Biol 387:285–296, 1996.
6. Adlercreutz H, Gorbach SL, Goldin BR, Woods MN, Dwyer JT, Hamalainen E. Estrogen metabolism and excretion in Oriental and Caucasian women. J Natl Cancer Inst 18:1076–1082, 1994.
7. Goldin BR, Adlercreutz H, Gorbach SL, Warram JH, Dwyer JT, Swenson L, Woods MN. Estrogen excretion patterns and plasma levels in vegetarian and omnivorous women. N Engl J Med 307:1542–1547, 1982.
8. Goldin BR, Gorbach SL. Effect of diet on the plasma levels, metabolism and excretion of estrogens. Am J Clin Nutr 48:787–790, 1988.
9. Woods MN, Gorbach SL, Longcope C, Goldin BR, Dwyer JT, Morrill-Labrode A. Low fat, high fiber diet and serum estrone sulfate in premenopausal women. Am J Clin Nutr 49:1179–1183, 1989.
10. Bagga D, Ashley JM, Geffrey SP, Wang HJ, Barnard RJ, Korenman S, Heber D. Effects of a very low fat, high fiber diet on serum hormones and menstrual function. Implications for breast cancer prevention. Cancer 76:2491–2496, 1995.
11. Dorgan JF, Reichman ME, Judd JT, Brown C, Longcope C, Schatzkin A, Forman M, Campbell WS, Franz C, Kahle L, Taylor PR. Relation of energy, fat, and fiber intakes to plasma concentrations of estrogens and androgens in premenopausal women. Am J Clin Nutr 64:25–31, 1996.
12. Rose DP, Goldman M, Connolly JM, Strong LE. High fiber diet reduces serum estrogen concentrations in premenopausal women. Am J Clin Nutr 54:520–525, 1991.
13. Cohen LA, Zhao Z, Zang E, Rivenson A. Dose-response effects of dietary fiber on MNU-induced mammary tumorigenesis, estrogen levels and estrogen excretion in female rats. Carcinogenesis 17:45–52, 1996.
14. Cohen LA, Zhao Z, Zang E, Winn TT, Simi B, Rivenson A. Wheat bran and psyllium diets: effects on N-methylnitrosourea-induced mammary tumorigenesis in F344 rats. J Natl Cancer Inst 88:899–907, 1996.
15. Lindeskog P, Overvik E, Nilsson L, Lord C-E, Gustafsson J-A. Influence of fried meat and fiber on cytochrome P450 mediated activity and excretion of mutagens in rats. Mutat Res 204:553–563, 1988.
16. Ohyama S, Kitamori S, Kawano H, Yamada T, Inamasu T, Ishizawa M, et al. Ingestion of parsley inhibits the mutagenicity of male human urine following consumption of fried salmon. Mutat Res 192:7–10, 1987.
17. Schultz TD, Howie BJ. In vitro binding of steroid hormones by natural or purified fibers. Nutr Cancer 8:141–147, 1986.
18. Bruning PF, Bonfrer JMG, van Noord PAH, Hart AAM, Bakker M. de Jong, Nooijen WJ. Insulin resistance and breast cancer risk. Int J Cancer 52:511–516, 1992.
19. Stoll BA. Can supplementary dietary fibre suppress breast cancer growth. Br J Cancer 73:557–559, 1996.
20. Howe GR, Hirohata T, Hislop TG, Iscovitch JM, Yuan JM, Katsouyanni K, Marubini E, Modan B, Rohan T. et al. Dietary factors and risk of breast cancer: combined analysis of 12 case-control studies. J Natl Cancer Inst 82:561–569, 1990.
21. La Vecchia C, Ferraroni M, Franceschi S, Mezetti M, Decarli A, Negri E. Fibers and breast cancer risk. Nutr Cancer 28:264–269, 1997.
22. Iscovich JM, Iscovich RB, Howe G, Shiboski S, Kaldor JM. A case-control study of diet and breast cancer in Argentina. Int J Cancer 44:770–776, 1989.
23. Baghurst PA, Rohan TE. High fiber diets and reduced risk of breast cancer. Int J Cancer 567:173–176, 1994.
24. Franceschi S, Favero A, Decarli A, Negri E, La Vecchia C, Ferraroni M, Russo A, Salvini S, Amadori D, Conti E, et al. Intake of macronutrients and risk of breast cancer. Lancet 347:1351–1356, 1996.
25. Van't Veer P, Kolb CM, Verhoef P, Kok FJ, Schouten EG, Hermus RJ. Dietary fiber, beta-carotene and breast cancer: results from a case-control study. Int J Cancer 45:825–828, 1990.
26. Landa MC, Frago N, Tres A. Diet and the risk of breast cancer in Spain. Eur J Cancer Prev 3:313–320, 1994.
27. Holmberg L, Ohlander EM, Byers T, Zack M, Wolk A, Begstrom R, Thufjell E, Bruce A, Adami

HO. Diet and breast cancer risk. Results from a population based, case-control study in Sweden. Arch Int Med 154:1805–1811, 1994.

28. De Stefani E, Correa P, Ronco A, Mendilaharsu M, Guidobono M, Deneo-Pelligrini H. Dietary fiber and risk of breast cancer: a case-control study in Uruguay. Nutr Cancer 28:14–19, 1997.

29. Freudenheim JL, Marshall JR, Vena JE, Laughlin R, Brasure JR, Swanson MK, Nemoto T, Graham S. Premenopausal breast cancer risk and intake of vegetables, fruits and related nutrients. J Natl Cancer Inst 88:340–348, 1996.

30. Graham S, Hellmann R, Marshall J, Freudenheim J, Vena J, Swanson M, Nemoto T, Stubbe N, Raimondo T. Nutritional epidemiology of postmenopausal breast cancer in western New York. Am J Epidemiol 134:552–566, 1991.

31. Rohan TE, Howe GR, Friedenreich CM, Jain M, Miller AB, Dietary fiber, vitamins A, C, and E, and risk of breast cancer: a cohort study. Cancer Causes Control 4:29–37, 1993.

32. Verhoeven DTH, Assen N, Goldbohm RA, Dorant E, van't Veer P, Sturmans F, Hermus RJJ, van den Brandt PA. Vitamins C and E, retinol, beta-carotene and dietary fibre in relation to breast cancer risk: a prospective cohort study. Br J Cancer 75:149–155, 1997.

33. Graham S, Zielezny M, Marshall J, Priore R, Freudenheim J, Brasure JH, Nasca P, Zdeb M. Diet in the epidemiology of postmenopausal breast cancer in the New York State Cohort. Am J. Epidemiol 136:1327–1337, 1992.

34. Kushi LH, Sellers TA, Potter JD, Nelson CL, Munger RG, Kaye SA. Dietary fat and postmenopausal breast cancer. J Natl Cancer Inst 84:1092–1099, 1992.

35. Willett WC, Hunter DJ, Stampfer MJ, Colditz G, Manson JE, Spiegelman D, Rosner B, Hennekens CH, Speizer FE. Dietary fat and fiber in relation to breast cancer. An 8 year follow-up. JAMA 268: 2037–2044, 1992.

36. Giovannucci E, Stampfer MJ, Colditz G, Manson JE, Spiegelman D, Rosner B, Speizer FE, Willett WC. A comparison of prospective and retrospective assessments of diet in the study of breast cancer. Am J Epidemiol 137:502–511, 1993.

37. Rose DP. Dietary fiber, phytoestrogens and breast cancer. Nutrition 44:945–953, 1992.

38. Clarke R, Hilakivi-Clarke L, Cho E, James MR, Leonessa F. Estrogens, phytoestrogens and breast cancer. Adv Exp Med Biol 401:63–85, 1996.

39. Reinli K, Block G. Phytoestrogen content of foods—a compendium of literature values. Nutr Cancer 26:123–148, 1996.

40. Thompson LU, Robb P, Serraino M, Cheung FF. Mammalian lignan production from various foods. Nutr Cancer 16:43–52, 1991.

41. Nilsson A, Hill JL, Lloyd-Davies H. An in vitro study of formononetin and biochanin A metabolism in rumen fluid from sheep. Biochim Biophys Acta 148:92–98, 1967.

42. Axelson M, Kirk DN, Farrant RD, Cooley G, Lawson AM, Setchell KDR. The identification of the weak estrogen equol [7-hydroxy-4-(4-hydroxyphenyl)-chroman] in human urine. Biochem J 201: 353–357, 1982.

43. Borriello SP, Setchell KDR, Axelson M, Lawson AM. Production and metabolism of lignans by the human fecal flora. J Appl Bacteriol 58:37–43, 1985.

44. Makela S, Santii R, Salo L, McLachlan JA. Phytoestrogens are partial estrogen agonists in the adult male mouse. Environ Health Perspect 103:123–127, 1995.

45. Welshons WV, Murphy CS, Koch R, Calaf G, Jordan VC. Stimulation of breast cancer cells in vitro by the environmental estrogen enterolactone and the phytoestrogen equol. Breast Cancer Res Treat 10:169–175, 1987.

46. Adlercreutz H, Mousavi Y, Loukavaara M, Hamalainen E. Lignans isoflavones, sex hormone metabolism and breast cancer. In: Hochberg R, Naftolin F, eds. The New Biology of Steroid Hormones. New York: Raven Press, 1991, pp 145–154.

47. Messina MJ, Persky V, Setchell KDR, Barnes S. Soy intake and cancer risk: a review of the in vitro and in vivo data. Nutr Cancer 21:113–131, 1994.

48. Thompson LU, Orcheson L, Rickard S, Jenab M, Serraino M, Seidl M, Cheung F. Anticancer effects of flaxseed lignans. In: J Kumpulainen, J Salonen, eds. Natural Antioxidants and Food Quality in Atherosclerosis and Cancer Prevention. Cambridge, UK: Royal Society of Chemistry, 1996, pp 356–364.

49. Fotsis T, Pepper M, Adlercreutz H, Fleischmann G, Hase T, Montesano R, Schweigerer L. Genistein, a dietary-derived inhibitor of in vitro angiogenesis. Proc Natl Acad Sci USA 90:2690–2694, 1993.

50. Gordon JD, Shifren JL, Foulk RA, Taylor RN, Jaffe RB. Angiogenesis in the human female reproductive tract. Obstet Gynecol Surv 50:688–697, 1995.

51. Selby C. Sex hormone binding globulin: origin function and clinical significance. Ann Clin Biochem 27:532–541, 1990.

52. Adlercreutz H, Hockerstedt K, Bannwart C, Bloigu S, Hamalainen E, Fotsis T, Ollus A. Effects of dietary components, including lignans and phytoestrogens, on enterohepatic circulation and liver metabolism of estrogens and on sex hormone binding globulin (SHBG). J Steroid Chem 27:1135–1144, 1987.

53. Adlercreutz H. Diet, breast cancer and sex hormone metabolism. Ann NY Acad Sci 595:281–290, 1990.

54. Field AE, Colditz GA, Willett WC, Longcope C, McKinlay JB. The relation of smoking, age, relative weight, and dietary intake to serum adrenal steroids, sex hormones, and sex hormone-binding globulin in middle-aged men. J Clin Endocrinol Metab 79:1310–1316, 1994.

55. Mousavi Y, Adlercreutz H. Genistein is an effective stimulator of sex hormone-binding globulin production in hepatocarcinoma human liver cells and suppress proliferation of these cells in culture. Steroids 58:301–304, 1993.

56. Akiyama T, Ishida J, Nakagawa S, Ogawa H, Watanabe S, Itou N, Shibata M, Fukami Y. Genistein, a specific inhibitor of tyrosine-specific protein kinase. J Biol Chem 262:5592–5595, 1987.

57. Okura A, Arakawa H, Oka H, Yoshinari T, Monden Y. Effect of genistein on topisomerase activity and on the growth of (val 12) Ha-ras-transformed NIH 3T3 cells. Biochem Biophys Res Commun 157:183–189, 1988.

58. Matsukawa Y, Marui N, Sakai T, Satomi Y, Yoshida M, Matsumoto K, Nishino H, Aoike A. Genistein arrests cell cycle progression at G_2-M. Cancer Res 53:1328–1331, 1993.

59. Adlercreutz H, Bannwart C, Wahala K, Makela T, Brunow G, Hase T, Arosemena PJ, Kellis JT Jr, Vickery LE. Inhibition of human aromatase by mammalian lignans and isoflavonoid phytoestrogens. J Steroid Biochem Mol Biol 44:147–153, 1993.

60. Wang C, Makela T, Hase T, Adlercreutz H, Kurzer MS. Lignans and flavonoids inhibit aromatase enzyme in human preadipocytes. J Steroid Biochem Mol Biol 50:205–212, 1994.

61. Adlercreutz H, Mazur W. Phyto-estrogens and western diseases. Ann Med 29:95–120, 1997.

62. Hirayama T. A large scale cohort study on cancer risks by diet—with special reference to the risk reducing effects of green-yellow vegetable consumption. In: Hayashi Y, et al., eds. Diet, Nutrition and Cancer. Utrecht, The Netherlands: Tokyo/VNU Sci Press, 1986, pp 41–53.

63. Nomura A, Henderson BE, Lee J. Breast cancer and diet among the Japanese in Hawaii. Am J Clin Nutr 31:2020–2025, 1978.

64. Lee HP, Gourley L, Duffy SW, Esteve J, Day NE. Dietary effects on breast-cancer risk in Singapore. Lancet 337:1197–1200, 1991.

65. Hirohata T, Shigematsu T, Nomura AMY, Nomura Y, Horie A et al. Occurrence of breast cancer in relation to diet and reproductive history: a case-control study in Fukuoka, Japan. Natl Cancer Inst Monog 69:187–190, 1985.

66. Ingram D, Sanders K, Kolybaba M, Lopez D. Phytoestrogens and breast cancer—a case control study. Lancet 350:990–994, 1997.

67. Feng W, Marshall R, Lewis-Barned NJ, Goulding A. Low follicular oestrogen levels in New Zealand women consuming high fibre diets: a risk factor for osteopenia? NZ Med J 106:419–422, 1993.

68. Reinhold JG, Faradji B, Abadi P, Ismail-Beigi F. Decreased absorption of calcium, magnesium, zinc and phosphorus by humans due to increased fiber and phosphorus consumption as wheat bread. J Nutr 106:493–503, 1976.

69. Gordon DT, Stoops D, Ratliff V. Dietary fiber and mineral nutrition. In: Kritchevsky D, Bonfield C, eds. Dietary Fiber in Health and Disease. St. Paul, MN: Eagan Press, 1995.

70. Knox TA, Kassarjian Z, Dawson-Hughes B, Golner BB, Dallal GE, Arora S, Russell RM. Calcium absorption in elderly subjects on high and low fiber diets: effect of gastric acidity. Am J Clin Nutr 53:1480–1486, 1991.

71. Trinidad TP, Wolever TMS, Thompson LU. Effect of acetate and propionate on calcium absorption from the rectum and distal colon of humans. Am J Clin Nutr 63:574–578, 1996.

6
Dietary Fiber and Prostate Cancer

Eric D. Schwab and Kenneth J. Pienta
University of Michigan, Ann Arbor, Michigan

I. INTRODUCTION

Prostate cancer is the most diagnosed neoplasm in American males. Approximately 185,000 men will be diagnosed with the disease in the current year, and 39,000 will die from the disease (1). Approximately 18% of all men will develop invasive prostate cancers during their life. Most of these men will be over the age of 60 years when diagnosed. With the advent of prostate specific antigen (PSA) screening, it is likely that the average age at diagnosis will decrease.

The fact that most men who are diagnosed with prostate cancer are over the age of 60 is compounded by the fact that the population in the United States is aging. Table 1 shows the probabilities of developing invasive cancer for men at all organ sites and the prostate. The U.S. Census Bureau projects that by the year 2030, 21% of the population will be age 65 or older and 2.8% will be over the age of 85 (2). In 1980, these percentages were 11% and 1%, respectively. In addition, those 65 or older account for 31% of the nation's personal health care expenses (3). As the population ages, this percentage will also increase. With this increase will be a concomitant increase in the cost of treating older men with prostate cancer.

Prostate cancer can be divided into two broad categories—localized and metastatic. Currently, radiation therapy and surgery are potentially curative strategies for cancer that is confined to the organ, while treatment for metastatic disease remains largely palliative (4). Hormone ablation therapy causes regression or stabilization of the disease in approximately 80% of patients but often fails to prevent disease progression. Until recently, hormone ablation therapy was the last line of defense for men with metastatic disease, and those who fail this therapy have a median survival of 6–9 months (5). New chemotherapeutic agents are now in clinical trials, but no consistently effective therapy for metastatic prostate cancer exists.

It is evident from the above facts that prostate cancer will become a greater and greater public health problem. PSA screening will result in more men being diagnosed with prostate cancer. As the age of the population increases, a greater percentage of the male population will have prostate cancer and will require treatment. Finally, the cost of medical care is rising. While treatment for localized prostate cancer—radiation and surgery—will rise, a greater increase in cost is likely to come from the use of chemotherapy to treat metastatic disease. Prostate cancer, therefore, is becoming an increasingly important public health concern. To help reduce this problem, the progression of prostate cancer from a localized disease to one with metastatic potential must be elucidated. This will allow patients to be treated when the disease is still localized and treatment is less expensive. Ideally, however, one would like to determine how

Table 1 Percentage of Men Developing Invasive Cancers at Certain Ages, United States, 1992–1994

	Birth to 39	40 to 59	60 to 79	Lifetime
All sites	1.68	8.23	36.69	46.64
Prostate	<0.01	1.74	16.40	18.85

to prevent the development of prostate cancer before medical intervention is necessary. One possible strategy is by determining how diet and dietary supplements (e.g., vitamins, fiber) influence prostate carcinogenesis. In this chapter, we will examine the relationship of dietary fiber to prostate cancer.

II. DIET AND PROSTATE CANCER

Extensive efforts have been undertaken to study the pathogenesis of prostate cancer. Despite these efforts, however, the origins of prostate cancer and factors that promote its progression have not been well established (6). Still, evidence exists that suggest that this disease is the result of genetic and environmental interactions. One widely accepted risk factor for prostate cancer is race-ethnicity background (7,8). Chinese and Japanese men have the lowest rates of prostate cancer globally, whereas African-American men have the highest rates (8). While the etiology of prostate cancer is poorly understood, several epidemiological studies have suggested that dietary factors, in addition to ethnic background, may play a role in the development and progression of prostate cancer (9–13). Other evidence that diet may play a role in the development of prostate cancer comes from the geographical variation of clinical disease. While the incidence of latent prostate cancer varies little in countries around the world (14), men in the United States can have as much as a 120-fold increase in clinical disease when compared to Asian men (15). An increase in clinical prostate cancer is also seen among Japanese men who have moved to the United States; this trend continues when first-generation Japanese immigrants are compared to second-generation Japanese-American men (16,17). The primary reason given for the increased incidence of prostate cancer in American men, and in the immigrants, is the "western" high-fat/low-fiber diet. To date, however, no study has established a firm link between dietary fiber and prostate carcinogenesis and progression. The same is not true for other organ-confined cancers.

III. DIETARY FIBER AND HORMONE-DEPENDENT CANCER

The development of prostate and breast cancers are generally thought to be dependent on the continuous exposure of tissue to serum hormones—androgens for prostate cancer and estrogens for breast cancer. In many ways, cancers of the breast and prostate mimic each other. This parallelism is also seen in the sex hormones—estrogen and testosterone. It can be educational, therefore, to look at the effect of dietary fiber on estrogen metabolism and breast cancer.

Epidemiological data suggest that increased dietary fiber may lead to a reduced risk of breast cancer (18,19). Another study, however, showed no correlation (20). Goldin and Gorbach (21) looked at estrogen metabolism in pre- and postmenopausal women and found that estradiol and estriol fecal excretion were higher in vegetarians when compared to omnivores. The diet of vegetarians is generally higher in fiber content than omnivores. Another study showed that wheat bran (but not corn or oat bran) reduced the level of circulating estrogens in the plasma

(22). More significantly, these changes were accomplished without attempting to reduce dietary fat intake. Finally, multiple studies show that pre- and postmenopausal Western women have higher circulating and excretion levels of total estrogens than do low-risk Asian women (23). This difference may be related to the high fiber/fat ratio of the Asian diet (24). The correlation between dietary fiber and estrogen levels may be spurious, however, without a mechanism for this reduction.

Dietary fiber may result in the alteration of the enterohepatic cycling of estrogens (25,26). Briefly, wheat bran minimizes the deconjugation of β-glucuronidase enzymes when conjugated estrogens are secreted in the bile. This deconjugation process is a necessary digestive process for the reabsorption of estrogens from the hepatic circulation. Wheat bran may prevent the enzymes from binding with the conjugated estrogens (27). It is also possible that wheat bran directly inhibits the enzymes. The net result is a decrease in circulating estrogen levels in the plasma and an increase of estrogens excreted in the feces (28).

The development of breast cancer is thought to be the result of the exposure, over the course of years, to high levels of circulating estrogens (29). It has also been shown that women with breast cancer have higher levels of circulating estrogens and higher levels of bio-available estrogens than do women who are breast cancer free (30). Reducing levels of estrogens, therefore, may reduce the lifetime risk of developing breast cancer. By increasing the intake of dietary fiber, the incidence of breast cancer may be reduced. It is evident, therefore, that dietary fiber can effect the development of one hormone-dependent cancer by reducing the circulating levels of sex hormones.

IV. ANDROGENS, DIETARY FIBER, AND PROSTATE CANCER

Studies have demonstrated a positive correlation between prolonged exposure to androgens and the development of prostate cancer (31–35). As mentioned earlier, those populations (e.g., American men) whose diets have a lower proportion of dietary fiber also have a higher incidence of prostate cancer. Another study demonstrated that the ratio of dihydrotestosterone to testosterone was highest in African-American men, intermediate in whites, and lowest in Asian-American men; this also correlates to the incidence of prostate cancer in these three groups (36). As in breast cancer, it is reasonable to conjecture that dietary fiber may decrease the levels of circulating androgens, which would reduce the risk for developing prostate cancer.

Several lines of evidence exist to strengthen the correlation between dietary fiber and the reduction of serum testosterone. Using an animal model, Dorgan et al. found that dietary factors can reduce the plasma concentrations of sex steroids and prolactin (37). Similar results have been found in human studies (38). These studies, however, looked at several dietary/environmental factors and did not focus on fiber intake.

Studies looking specifically at the influence of dietary fiber on prostate cancer and/or serum androgen levels are few. Two investigations, however, attempted to correlate the intake of dietary fiber and steroid hormones in selected groups of men. Both studies, by the same group, evaluated the levels of steroid levels between nonvegetarians, lactoovovegetarians, and vegans (39,40). They analyzed both diet and feces for fiber content and levels of sex hormones in the plasma and excreted in the feces. They found that vegans consumed an average of two to four times more crude and dietary fiber than the other two groups. Plasma concentrations of sex hormones did not differ significantly between the groups; however, vegans excreted approximately twice the amount of sex hormones than the other groups. Another study attempted to assess the effect of dietary fat and fiber on the Dunning R3327-H transplantable prostate adenocarcinoma (41). The Dunning rat tumors are a well-characterized model of prostate cancer (42,43). The effects of dietary fiber, however, were inconclusive. These data combined with the breast cancer data indicate that androgens may be removed from the enterohepatic circulation in a similar manner to estrogens. Further studies, however, will be needed to confirm this hypothesis.

V. DIETARY FIBER AND OTHER PROTECTION MECHANISMS

The above discussion demonstrated that dietary fiber may reduce the risk of prostate cancer by decreasing the amount of androgens available to the body by removing them from the enterohepatic circulation. Other dietary factors (e.g., fat, soy proteins, vitamin E, selenium) may also have effects, both positive and negative, on the development of prostate cancer, but these are beyond the scope of this discussion. Dietary fiber, however, may have several mechanisms of protection.

The primary mechanism is known as the bulking effect. By consuming more fiber, the concentration of a particular carcinogen, including androgens, becomes diluted and reduces the availability of the substance to the body (44). Second, a higher fiber content may change the bacterial composition of the gut, thus preventing the conversion of procarcinogens into active agents by bacterial enzymes (45). Finally, some evidence suggests that a high-fiber diet may increase the transit rate of the stool through the colon, thus reducing mucosal exposure (46). Again, further studies specific to prostate cancer are needed.

VI. CONCLUSIONS

Prostate cancer is becoming an increasing important public health problem. With the aging of the population and the lack of suitable treatment for advanced disease, prostate cancer is likely to become costlier and more burdensome to a society whose resources, both medical and financial, are severely taxed. To combat an increase in the incidence of prostate cancer, a mechanism is required that either identifies all disease before it metastasizes or prevents its occurrence. With PSA screening, more prostate cancers are being diagnosed earlier in their progression, but it is still too early to tell if this will significantly reduce the occurrence of advanced disease. A better strategy would be to adopt a plan of action that would reduce the risk of developing prostate cancer. Increasing the amount of dietary fiber consumed by the male population, while a tremendous undertaking, may prove more beneficial in the long term than additional screening modalities. The cost of such a strategy would also be far less than the development of new therapies and prolonged treatment regimens. While the data correlating a diet high in fiber to a reduced risk of developing prostate cancer are not extensive enough evidence exists to warrant further investigations.

ACKNOWLEDGMENTS

This work was supported by a NIH SPORE for Prostate Cancer P50 CA69568. Eric Schwab was also supported by a fellowship from the American Foundation for Urologic Disease (Hoechst Marion-Roussel Scholar).

REFERENCES

1. Landis SH, Murray T, Bolden S, Wingo PA. Cancer Statistics, 1998. CA Cancer J Clin 47:6–29, 1998.

2. Siegel JS, Davidson M. Demographics and socioeconomic aspects of aging in the United States. In: US Bureau of the Census. Current Population Reports. Washington, DC: US Bureau of the Census, 1984:9–15.
3. Parson PE, Liu BM. Vital Health Statistics 3:76–79, 1987.
4. Panvinchian R, Pienta KJ. Hormonal and chemotherapeutic systemic therapy for metastatic prostate cancer. Cancer Control 3:493–500, 1996.
5. Kantoff PW. New agents in the therapy of hormone-refractory patients with prostate cancer. Semin Oncol 22:32–34, 1995.
6. Carter HB, Coffey DS. The prostate: an increasing medical problem. Prostate 16:39–48, 1990.
7. Ross RK, Henderson BE. Do diet and androgens alter prostate cancer risk via a common etiologic pathway? J Natl Cancer Inst 86:252–254, 1994.
8. Waterhouse J, Muir C, Shanmugaratnam K, et al. Cancer incidence in five continents. In: Cancer Incidence. Vol 6; Lyon, France: IARC Publ. No. 42, 1982.
9. Gann PH, Hennekens CH, Sacks FM, Grodstein F, Giovannucci EL. Prospective study of plasma fatty acids and the risk of prostate cancer. J Natl Cancer Inst 86:281–286, 1994.
10. Rose DP, Connolly JM. Dietary fat, fatty acids and prostate cancer. Lipids 27:798–803, 1992.
11. West DW, Slattery ML, Robison LM, French TK, Mahoney AW. Adult dietary intake and prostate cancer risk in Utah: a case-control study with special emphasis on aggressive tumors. Cancer Causes Control 2:85–94, 1991.
12. Giovannucci E, Rimm EB, Colditz GA, Stampfer MJ, Ascherio A, Chute CC, Willett WC. A prospective study of dietary fat and risk of prostate cancer. J Natl Cancer Inst 85:1571–1579, 1993.
13. Kolonel LN, Yoshizawa CN, Hankin JN. Diet and prostate cancer: a case-control study in Hawaii. Am J Epidemiol 127:999–1012, 1988.
14. Parkin DM, Muir CS, Whelan SL, et al. Cancer Incidence in Five Continents. Vol. 6. IARC Sci Publ No. 120. Lyon: IARC, 1992:970–971.
15. Yatani R, Kusano I, Shiraishi T, Hayashi T, Stemmermann GN. Latent prostatic carcinoma: pathological and epidemiological aspects. Jpn J Clin Oncol 19:319–326, 1989.
16. Haenszel W, Kurihara M. Studies of Japanese immigrants. I. Mortality from cancer and other diseases among Japanese in the United States. J Natl Cancer Inst 40:43–68, 1968.
17. Shimizu H, Ross RK, Bernstein L, Yatani R, Henderson BE, Mack TM. Cancers of the prostate and breast among Japanese and white immigrants in Los Angeles County. Br J Cancer 63:963–966, 1991.
18. Rose DP. Dietary factors and breast cancer. Cancer Surv 5:671–687, 1986.
19. Weisburger JH, Kroes R. Mechanisms in nutrition and cancer. Eur J Cancer Prevent 3:293–298, 1994.
20. Willett WC, Hunter DJ, Stampfer MJ, Colditz G, Manson JA, Spiegelman D, Rosner B, Hennekens CH, Speizer FE. Dietary fat and fiber in relation to breast cancer: an 8 year follow-up. JAMA 268: 2037–2044, 1992.
21. Goldin BR, Gorbach SL. Effect of diet on the plasma levels, metabolism, and excretion of estrogens. Am J Clin Nutr 48:787–790, 1988.
22. Rose DP, Goldman M, Connolly JM, Strong LE. High-fiber diet reduces serum estrogen concentrations in premenopausal women. Am J Clin Nutr 54:520–525, 1991.
23. Bernstein L. and Ross RK. Endogenous hormones and breast cancer risk. Epidemiol Rev 15:48–65, 1993.
24. Aldercreutz H, Mousavi Y, Höckerstedt K. Diet and breast cancer. Acta Oncol 31:175–181, 1992.
25. Gorbach SL. and Goldin BR. Diet and the excretion and enterohepatic cycling of estrogens. Prevent Med 16:525–531, 1987.
26. Gorbach SL. Estrogens, breast cancer, and intestinal flora. Rev Infect Dis 6:85–90, 1984.
27. Arts CJM, Govers C, Van Den Berg H, Wolters MGE, Van Leeuwen P, Thussen JHH. In vitro binding of estrogens by dietary fiber and the in vivo apparent digestibility tested in pigs. J Steroid Biochem Mol Biol 38:621–628, 1991.
28. Black RM. Wheat bran, colon cancer, and breast cancer. In: Dietary Phytochemistry in Cancer Prevention and Treatment. New York: Plenum Press, 1996:221–229.
29. Ota DM, Jones LA, Jackson GL, Jackson PM, Kemp K, Bauman D. Obesity, non-protein-bound estradiol levels, and distribution of estradiol in the sera of breast cancer patients. Cancer 57:558–562, 1986.

30. Toniolo PG, Levitz M, Zeleniuch-Jacquotte A, Banerjee S, Koenig KL, Shore RE, Strax P, Pasternak BS. A prospective study of endogenous estrogens and breast cancer in postmenopausal women. J Natl Cancer Inst 87:190–197, 1995.

31. Clinton SK, Palmer SS, Spriggs CE, Visek WJ. Growth of Dunning transplantable prostate adenocarcinomas in rats fed diets with various fat contents. J Nutr 118:908–914, 1988.

32. Damassa DA, Lin TM, Sonnenschein C, Soto AM. Biological effects of sex hormone-bingin globulin on androgen-induced proliferation and androgen metabolism in LNCaP prostate cells. Endocrinology 129:75–84, 1991

33. Nakhla AM, Rosner W. Stimulation of prostate cancer growth by androgens and estrogens through the intermediacy of sex hormone-binding globulin. Endocrinology 137:4129–4129, 1996.

34. Gann PH, Hennekens CH, Ma J, Longcope C, Stampfer MJ. Prospective study of sex hormone levels and risk of prostate cancer. J Natl Cancer Inst 88:1118–1126, 1996.

35. Henderson BE, Ross RK, Pike MC, Casagrande JT. Endogenous hormones as a major factor in human cancer. Cancer Res 42:3232–3239, 1982.

36. Wu AH, Whittemore AS, Kolonel LN, John EM, Gallagher RP, West DW, Hankin J, Teh CZ, Dreon DM, Paffenberger RS. Jr. Serum androgens and sex hormone-binding globulins in relation to lifestyle factors in older African-American, white and Asian men in the United States and Canada. Cancer Epidemiol Biomarkers Prev 4:734–741, 1995.

37. Dorgan JF, Judd JT, Congcope C, Brown C, Schatzkin A, Clevidence BA, Campbell WS, Nair PP, Franz C, Kahle L, Taylor PR. Effects of dietary fat and fiber on plasma and urine androgens and estrogens in men: a controlled feeding study. Am J Clin Nutr 64:850–855, 1996.

38. Hill P, Wynder EL, Garnes H, Walker ARP. Environmental factors, hormone status, and prostatic cancers. Prev Med 9:657–666, 1980.

39. Ross JK, Pusateri DJ, Shultz TD. Dietary and hormonal evaluation of men at different risks for prostate cancer: fiber intake, excretion, and composition, with in vitro evidence for an association between steroid hormones and specific fiber components. Am J Clin Nutr 51:365–370, 1990.

40. Pusateri DJ, Roth WT, Ross JK, Shultz TD. Dietary and hormonal evaluation of men at different risks for prostate cancer: plasma and fecal hormone-nutrient interrelationships. Am J Clin Nutr 51: 371–377, 1990.

41. Schwab ED, Normolle D, Pacis RA, Cho SS, Pienta KJ. A high-fat diet does not influence the growth of the Dunning R3327-H prostate adenocarcinoma. Anticancer Res 18:3603–3608, 1998.

42. Smolev J, Heston WDW, Scott WW, Coffey DS. Characterization of the Dunning R-3327-H prostatic adenocarcinoma: an appropriate animal model for prostate cancer. Cancer Treat Rep 61:273–287, 1977.

43. Isaacs JT, Isaacs WB, Feitz WFJ, Scheres J. Establishment and characterization of seven Dunning rat prostatic cancer cell lines and their use in developing methods for predicting metastatic abilities of prostatic cancer. Prostate 9:261–281, 1986.

44. Reddy BS, Hedges AR, Laakso K, Wynder EL. Metabolic epidemiology of large bowel cancer: fecal bulk and constituents of high-risk North American and low-risk Finnish populations. Cancer 42: 2832–2838, 1978.

45. Vaughan TL, McTiernan A. Diet in the etiology of cancer. Semin Oncol Nurs 2:3–13, 1986.

46. Glober GA, Nomura A, Kamiyama S, Shimada A, Abba BC. Bowel transit-time and stool weight in populations with different colon-cancer risks. Lancet 2:110–111, 1977.

7
Dietary Fiber and Glucose Metabolism and Diabetes

David Cameron-Smith and Gregory R. Collier
Deakin University, Melbourne, Victoria, Australia

I. INTRODUCTION

Diabetes mellitus is a descriptive term covering a heterogeneous group of chronic metabolic disorders, all characterized by elevated blood glucose concentrations (1). In 1997, an estimated 124 million people worldwide had diabetes, 97% of these having type 2 diabetes, otherwise known as non–insulin-dependent diabetes mellitus (NIDDM) or adult-onset diabetes (2). Type 2 diabetes is most prevalent in the adult population, afflicting approximately 17% of people aged greater than 65 years (2). Diabetes is now the fourth or fifth leading cause of death in these nations, with the total economic burden of type 2 diabetes estimated to be in the order of 8% of the total health care expenditure of the United States (3,4).

Diabetes is a disease with a complex etiology, with the sequential impairment of insulin action, compensated for by elevated insulin secretion, which may be followed by pancreatic beta-cell failure. The onset of beta-cell failure results in chronic hyperglycemia (5). The underlying defect(s) are yet to be adequately characterized, although in recent years there have been enormous advances in our understanding of the cellular mechanisms initiated following the binding of insulin to its receptor. Multiple defects in the varied cellular responses of insulin have been identified, although increasing knowledge of the intricate and complex cellular actions of insulin will undoubtedly result in further discovery (6,7).

II. DIABETES AND GLUCOSE METABOLISM

Impairment of insulin action and eventual loss of insulin secretory capacity impacts on glucose metabolism primarily in the liver and skeletal muscles (5). Diabetics have greatly increased postmeal or postprandial glucose rises, due largely to impaired glucose uptake by the skeletal tissues, which under normal circumstances accounts for around 70% of ingested glucose disposal (8). In the nondiabetic state insulin secretion would normally elicit the activation of insulin-regulated glucose transporters (GLUT4) (9). However, impaired GLUT4 activation in the diabetic state accounts for the majority of the impaired uptake, although recent evidence suggests that impairments in glucose metabolism once glucose enters the muscle cell may be involved (9). Studies examining the intracellular glucose flux using nuclear magnetic resonance (NMR) spectroscopy techniques have revealed that glucose storage, as glycogen, is reduced (10). The liver also has an important role to play in the diabetic state, with excessive liver glucose production the major determinant of plasma glucose concentrations in the fasted state (5).

The maintenance of chronic hyperglycemia in type 2 diabetes is an important determinant of the overall health burden of the disease. Hyperglycemia participates directly in the development of retinopathy, with potential loss of vision; nephropathy, with potential renal failure; peripheral and autonomic neuropathy, increasing the risk of foot ulcer formation and amputation, gastrointestinal, genitourinary, cardiovascular disease, and sexual dysfunction (11).

III. DIABETES AND LIPID METABOLISM

Diabetes cannot be viewed solely as a metabolic disorder of carbohydrate metabolism. Importantly, type 2 diabetics commonly display an atherogenic plasma lipid profile, characterized by elevated plasma triglyceride concentrations and decreased high-density lipoprotein (HDL) cholesterol levels (12). Although total low-density lipoprotein (LDL) cholesterol levels in most cases are unaltered by diabetes, there are often increased numbers of smaller, denser LDL particles (13). Diabetics face a two to four-fold increase in coronary heart disease risk, with prospective studies identifying high total cholesterol and triglycerides, as well as reduced HDL levels the best predictors of subsequent coronary heart disease (CHD) in diabetic populations (14,15). Some authors have also suggested that atherosclerosis is a disease in which the postprandial increase in plasma lipoproteins play an important role. Diabetics typically demonstrate prolonged and elevated postprandial lipemia (16).

IV. GOALS OF NUTRITIONAL THERAPY FOR DIABETES

Dietary therapy in type 2 diabetes remains a cornerstone of treatment and management. The key feature of diabetic nutritional therapy has been in the minimization of plasma glucose concentrations accompanied by increased insulin action. Reductions in plasma glucose levels achieved with more vigorous and aggressive insulin therapy in people with type 1 diabetes, or insulin-dependent diabetes mellitus (IDDM), has clearly demonstrated the effectiveness of glycemic control to prevent or delay the onset of retinopathy, nephropathy, and neuropathy (17). Studies addressing the impact of glycemic control in individuals with type 2 diabetes have explored the impact of using aggressive insulin therapy when added to the current first line of oral therapies and diet. While blood glucose concentrations can normalize with intensive insulin therapy, there is no evidence of improved rates of vascular or cardiovascular disease (18). This apparent conundrum may be due to the persistence of dyslipidemia despite minimization of the abnormality in blood glucose control (19). The goals of dietary therapies in the management of type 2 diabetes must then take into account the impact the dietary prescription has on both blood glucose and lipid levels. This view is reflected in the most recent recommendations issued by the American Diabetes Association (ADA)(20), in which the goals of medical nutrition therapy are outlined in five major points. A summary of these recommendations is provided in Table 1. Importantly, the restoration of near-normal blood glucose and achievement of optimal serum lipids are the first two points in this plan.

The use of diet as a medical therapy in individuals with type 2 diabetes must importantly be a team effort, reflecting the need for a multidisciplined approach. Goal setting and prescription must also involve the individual with diabetes to maximize adherence and allow for cultural, ethnic, and financial constraints (20).

Table 1 Goals of Medical Nutrition Therapy for Individuals with Type 2 Diabetes

1. Maintenance of as near-normal blood glucose levels as possible
2. Achievement of optimum serum lipid levels
3. Provision of adequate calories for maintaining or attaining reasonable weight for adults
4. Prevention and treatment of acute complications, such as hypoglycemia, and long-term complications, such as renal disease, autonomic neuropathy, hypertension, and cardiovascular disease
5. Improvement of overall health through optimum nutrition

Source: Adapted from. Ref. 20.

V. HISTORICAL USE OF DIETARY FIBER IN THE TREATMENT OF DIABETES

For many centuries dietary prescriptions were the most important therapies for the treatment of diabetes. However, traditional recommendations were hampered by a poor understanding of the interactions between dietary ingredients and metabolism. The term diabetes was coined by Areaemus the Greek in the second century A.D., who suggested that the diet of a diabetic should be milk with supplementary cereals, autumn fruits, and sweet wines (21). Over the proceeding centuries many strange diets were prescribed, including diets composed almost entirely of meat (21). The first hint that diabetes is a disease of sugar metabolism was made in 1776 by Dobson, with the observation that diabetics have sweet urine (21). Two schools of thought followed this discovery, with one school proposing that because diabetes was a disease of excess sugar loss, the most appropriate diet is one rich in sugar. However, the second and predominating school advocated the restriction of carbohydrate on the basis that diabetes was a disease of excess production. Carbohydrate-restriction therapies remained in vogue, with doctors prescribing strict carbohydrate avoidance combined with regular periods of fasting, until the landmark discovery of insulin in 1922 (22). The extraction and use of porcine insulin revolutionized the management and life expectancy of diabetics. However, the fear of carbohydrates persisted, with diabetic diets tending to remain low in carbohydrates (10–20% of energy) and high in fat (60–80% of energy). Early concern about the excess risk of diabetic diet in promoting atherosclerosis (21) and the beneficial actions of high-carbohydrate diets on insulin action (23) were largely ignored till the studies of Stone and Conner (24), in which comparison of diets rich in carbohydrates with high-fat diets were made. The surprising result was that the high-carbohydrate diets were not only well tolerated, but that insulin requirements and plasma cholesterol levels were lowered. Dramatic changes in the dietary recommendations for diabetics followed, and in 1971 the American Diabetes Association (ADA) issued recommendations that diabetics should consume a diet containing the same proportion of energy from carbohydrates as the American population as a whole (25). Reports from this era suggest that many diabetic clinics were slow to adopt these recommendations, which in part reflected the failure of subsequent studies to support the use of high-carbohydrate diets (26,27). Yet, despite these findings, the ADA again in 1979 reaffirmed and strengthened the recommendations for carbohydrates to account for 50–60% of total energy intake, protein 12–20%, with fat to make up the remainder (28).

The reinforcement of the 1979 ADA recommendations accompanied the emerging scientific interest in the beneficial actions of dietary fiber. The potential for dietary fiber to protect against the development of noncommunicable diseases began with the hypothesis of a British naval surgeon Dr. Cleave, who postulated that highly refined flour and sugars, lacking dietary fiber, were at the root of many modern ailments (29). This was followed by the classic studies of Burkitt and Trowell in rural Uganda during the 1960s, in which they formed the hypothesis that the low rates of noncommunicable diseases, including diabetes, were linked to consumption of diets rich in dietary fiber (30). This hypothesis was supported by the reduced incidence of diabetes in England during the Second World War, which paralleled the increased consumption of unrefined, high-fiber flour (31). The potential protective role of dietary fiber prompted the investigation of the action of dietary fiber as a component of a high-carbohydrate diet on glucose metabolism in people who already had diabetes.

VI. METABOLIC EFFECTS OF CARBOHYDRATE AND FIBER IN TYPE 2 DIABETES

A. Single Meal Studies

Numerous reports have examined the actions of different test meals on the postprandial blood glucose and insulin profiles of diabetics. A comprehensive analysis of many of these test meal studies is presented elsewhere (32). More recent studies have examined the actions of novel food formulations containing either supplementary dietary fiber (33,34) or plant cultivars or strains with greater concentrations of dietary fiber (35,36). Reduced glycemic responses are most commonly observed with soluble dietary fibers that hydrate rapidly and develop significant viscosity in vitro (37). The inhibition of glucose digestion and absorption is dependent upon the continued actions of the dietary fiber to elevate the viscosity of the gastrointestinal contents, although factors other than the viscosity alone contribute to the resultant glycemia (38).

Closer examination of the factors present in food that were predictive of the resultant glycemia demonstrated that that in vitro digestion rate, to mimic the in vivo actions, only weakly correlated with total dietary fiber content of foods and failed to correlate with soluble fiber (39). Indeed, complex interactions between chemical and physical factors within food were found to modulate digestion rate. Important factors identified included the degree of food refinement, extent of cooking, starch structure, and degree of hydration as well as the cellulose and uronic acid content (39). To account for the complex interaction of many components of foods that contribute to determine the ultimate rate of glucose appearance in the blood stream following the ingestion of a carbohydrate-rich food source, the glycemic index (GI) was developed. The GI has proven to be a robust tool to determine the relative glycemic responses of both single foods and mixed meals (40,41).

Accompanying the liberalization of sucrose intake in diabetic diets has been the analysis of the glycemic impact of foods rich in sucrose and other sugars, including fructose. Interestingly, foods rich in sucrose were found to have GI comparable to those of many starchy foods including bread and many cereal products (41). Indeed, the addition of sucrose to an unsweetened high-GI breakfast cereal lowered the total glycemic response of the meal (41). Fructose, which is sweeter than sucrose, has a lower GI than sucrose, because fructose is slowly absorbed and almost entirely removed from the circulation by the liver. Substitution of starch for either sucrose or fructose has been shown not to alter glucose metabolism (42,43), although there is one report of improvement in insulin action following the substitution of starch for fructose (44). Importantly, the impact of either sucrose or fructose on plasma lipids needs to be considered. To date, the impact of diets rich in fructose, in particular, is controversial, with studies demonstrating either no change (43,45,46) or increased plasma triglyceride concentrations (47,48) in diabetics. Analysis of endogenous very-low-density lipoprotein (VLDL) synthesis has also shown it to be unaltered by fructose-rich diets in five individuals with NIDDM, although considerable variability of responses were observed (49). However, given the marked variability in plasma lipid levels following diets containing considerable amounts of sugar shown in clinical studies and the considerable heterogeneity of postprandial lipid responses in people with NIDDM (50), monitoring and individualized prescription of sugars may be advisable.

1. Mechanisms of Action

It remains a matter of conjecture how slowed carbohydrate absorption might ultimately act to improve insulin sensitivity in diabetics. To date, four distinct mechanisms have been proposed to account for how meals containing increased amounts of dietary fiber may act to improve glucose metabolism at subsequent meals.

   a. Inhibition of Fatty Acid Oxidation.   One hypothesized mechanism for the subsequent improvement in insulin action following the ingestion of a slowly digested and absorbed carbohydrate-rich meal is the inhibitory effect nonesterified fatty acids (NEFAs) have on glucose utilization. Elevated NEFA concentrations have been shown to increase fat oxidation rates, which lead to a commensurate reduction in glucose oxidation, a metabolic relationship known as the glucose–fatty acid cycle, first described by Randle et al. (51). Indeed, the tendency for diabetics to have elevated plasma NEFA levels may contribute to the impairment of insulin action (52). Slowed carbohydrate absorption leads to moderated, although sustained elevations in plasma glucose paralleled by sustained plasma insulin concentrations. The maintained insulin secretion may maximize glucose uptake and oxidation by insulin-sensitive tissues while simultaneously suppressing lipolysis and NEFA availability, thus lowering fat oxidation. Rapid glucose absorption is, however, speculated to rapidly increase plasma insulin concentrations, leading to rebound hypoglycemia and the release of counterregulatory hormones, including the catecholamines. Catecholamine release activates lipolysis and increases plasma free fatty acid (FFA) levels. However, there is limited in vivo evidence for this hypothesis (53). Two studies have reported sustained suppression of NEFA levels and fat oxidation following a high-fiber meal when compared to an isocaloric low-fat meal (54,55). Yet other studies, despite wide variations in blood glucose absorption profiles, have been unable to demonstrate altered substrate oxidation (56,57).

   b. Transient Reductions in Blood Glucose.   Further hypothesized actions of slowed carbohydrate digestion include the impact transient minimization of plasma hyperglycemia and hyperinsulinemia following a meal exerts directly on insulin action. Acute hyperglycemia in vitro rapidly downregulates tyrosine kinase activity of the insulin receptor (58), GLUT4 abundance (59), and potentially dysregulates protein synthesis by modulating gene expression (60). It is well established that chronic hyperglycemia impairs both insulin secretion and sensitivity, a phenomenon known as "glucose toxicity" (11), but evidence that acute postprandial modifications act to improve this glucose toxic effect has yet to be established.

   c. Gastrointestinal Hormone Secretion.   A number of studies have provided evidence of altered gastrointestinal hormone secretion, including glucagon-like peptide 1 (GLP-1), somatostatin, vasoactive intestinal polypeptide (VIP), and insulin-like growth factor 1 (IGF-1), following the ingestion of high-fiber meals (61–64). However, the plasma levels differ significantly between studies, with altered gastrointestinal hormone secretion not observed in all studies (65,66). Most notably, GLP-1 and IGF-1 have crucial roles in regulating insulin secretion and action (67–70), yet it remains to be established if modulated circulatory concentrations can acutely affect insulin action. Further research is required to fully elucidate the impact altered secretion of these gastrointestinal hormones may have on glucose and lipid metabolism in the diabetic.

   d. Short-Chain Fatty Acids.   Colonic fermentation by the resident microflora of malabsorbed starch and undigestible carbohydrates (including, fructo-oligosaccharides, nonstarch polysaccharides, pectins, and gums) has been suggested to affect glucose and lipid metabolism. The major nongaseous by-product of this anaerobic fermentation is short-chain fatty acids (SCFAs), of which acetate, propionate, and butyrate, produced in the approximate molar ratio of 60:25:12, are the predominant products (71). These SCFAs are rapidly absorbed by the colonic epithelia, with significant quantities of acetate and propionate entering the portal blood stream (72). Acetate is the only SCFA found in appreciable concentrations in the peripheral blood (72). Peripheral concentrations of acetate increase in response to a high-fiber diet (73). One study has demonstrated that oral acetate supplementation and cecal infusion may decrease adipose tissue lipolysis, lowering plasma NEFA levels (74), although glucose oxidation or glucose tolerance remained unaltered (75,76).

Propionate is removed from the portal circulation by the liver, where in ruminants it is a major gluconeogenic precursor. In nonruminants, including humans and rats, propionate may act to inhibit gluconeogenesis and stimulate glycolysis (77,78). Oral propionate, supplied in capsules, had no impact on blood glucose levels, although oral glucose tolerance was marginally improved (79). Incorporation of propionate in bread led to improved glucose responses, although this observation may be the result of propionate inhibiting starch digestion (80). The rapid absorption of ingested propionate may fail to mimic the in vivo situation of sustained portal release. Studies utilizing rectal or ileal propionate infusion to better reflect the in vivo situation have been unable to demonstrate any impact of propionate on either liver glucose production or peripheral insulin sensitivity (81–83).

Propionate has also been suggested to regulate the rate of liver cholesterol synthesis in both in vivo and in vitro rodent studies (84–86). While physiologically relevant concentrations of propionate may inhibit cholesterol synthesis in rat hepatocytes, a comparative study has failed to demonstrate inhibition in human hepatocytes, with inhibition of cholesterol synthesis requiring a 100-fold increase in propionate levels (87). Propionate supplementation in human volunteers has tended to show reduced HDL cholesterol and increased triglyceride concentrations (79,80).

There is good evidence from a rodent study, in which cecectomized rats were fed a diet containing guar gum, that the removal of a cecum does not affect glucose metabolism when compared to noncecectomized rats (88). This evidence, combined with the data described above, presents a scenario in which SCFA metabolism is unlikely to significantly affect peripheral carbohydrate or lipid metabolism in nonruminants.

Currently, no clear mechanism has emerged upon which to base dietary strategies to maximize the effectiveness of high-carbohydrate and high-fiber meals. The lack of an acute mechanism can be considered as a factor hampering the design of high-fiber diets, which can be considered to be most effective in improving both carbohydrate and lipid metabolism in type 2 diabetics.

B. High-Carbohydrate Diets

The impact of carbohydrate-rich versus fat-rich diets on insulin action in diabetics has been studied extensively since the early studies of Himsworth (23) and the later studies of Stone and Conner (24). Yet relatively few studies have examined in detail the impact of carbohydrate replacement of saturated fat. Diets in which the carbohydrate content was increased to 85% of daily energy tended to result in largely unaltered or marginally improved glucose tolerance (26,89,90). A similar result has been shown in normal subjects fed either a high-carbohydrate or a high-fat (predominately saturated fat) diet for 3 weeks prior to measurement of in vivo insulin sensitivity using the euglycemic clamp technique (91). These dietary intervention studies are unable to support a marked benefit of high-carbohydrate diets on glycemic control.

Further examination of the actions of high-carbohydrate diets on glycemic control has been made in comparison with diets rich in monounsaturated fatty acids. Clear beneficial actions of diets rich in monounsaturated fatty acids have been reported by a number of differing groups (92–96). The improvements in plasma lipoproteins, particularly reduced plasma triglyceride concentrations and VLDL cholesterol concentrations (93), provide a basis to broaden dietary strategies in diabetes to include diets modeled on the Mediterranean diet.

It is important to note that comparisons between high-fat diets and high-carbohydrate diets have generally not endeavored to select carbohydrate-rich foods on the basis of likely glycemic impact. Of the studies that have examined the action of a low-GI, high-carbohydrate diet in type 2 diabetic subjects, all have demonstrated improved glucose tolerance (97–100). Yet it must be noted that these studies have been restricted to comparisons between high-carbohydrate diets differing only in predicted GI. No comparison has been made to date comparing a high-carbohydrate, low-GI diet with a isocaloric diet rich in monounsaturated fat. Other experimental interventions aimed at slowing carbohydrate absorption have been examined. Slowed or sustained carbohydrate absorption can be achieved with the consumption of many small meals (nibbling) when compared with consuming three regular meals (gorging). Nibbling regimes have been similarly shown to improve glycemic control in type 2 diabetics (101,102). One further technique that has also improved glycemic control is the partial chemical inhibition of α-glucosidase activity at doses that impair and slow carbohydrate digestion while preventing malabsorption (103,104). These studies collectively provide significant evidence that high-carbohydrate diets selected on the basis of slow carbohydrate digestion and absorption have the capacity to improve insulin action. However, there are clear deficiencies in the literature, particularly regarding the adoption of and successful long-term dietary self-management using the GI, although considerable success has been achieved over a 12-week period (98). Clearly the necessity for education, restriction of recipes and food choices, combined with limitation of food options and the inability to determine the likely GI of processed and packaged food limits the widespread adoption of GI in the routine dietary management of diabetics.

C. High-Carbohydrate and High-Fiber Diets

1. Effects on Glucose Metabolism

Given the substantial evidence obtained from studies manipulating GI or glucose absorption profiles, it is surprising that few studies have designed achievable and acceptable high-fiber diets that are likely to impact on postprandial glucose absorption profiles. Fewer dietary interventions have actually measured the glucose and insulin meal responses. Of the dietary interventions examining the actions of a high-fiber diet, there are two distinct modes of dietary modification. The first is to provide supplemental viscous soluble dietary fibers at doses likely to retard glucose absorption. The second broad grouping of studies have utilized very high doses of dietary fiber that at least double daily intake.

Most studies examining the impact on carbohydrate metabolism of dietary interventions containing a single isolated viscous soluble fiber have predominately utilized guar gum, although pectin (105), glucomannan (106), and xanthan gum (107) have been trialed. Guar gum supplementation to a high-carbohydrate diet has in the majority of studies lowered glycosylated hemoglobin (108,109) and glycosurea (110) and improved insulin sensitivity (111). However, the dose of soluble fiber required to achieve these actions is difficult to achieve from food alone. Food products incorporating guar gum (108,112) or that are rich in oat bran (β-glucans) (113) have been trailed with some measure of success, yet commonplace integration into diabetic dietary therapy and widespread acceptance is still lacking.

Evidence supporting the beneficial actions of diets rich in carbohydrate and fiber in diabetic management is, at best, unconvincing. Several studies in diabetics have reported improvements in insulin action of diabetic subjects, but the dietary fiber contents of the diets ranged from 90 to 45 grams daily (114–117). Of these studies, matched carbohydrate and fat intake with either low or high fiber content demonstrated that the beneficial actions on insulin sensitivity were present only following the high-fiber diet (118). Contradicting these studies are the observations that diets in which an approximate daily dose of 40 g of dietary fiber was achieved had no effect on insulin action (119–121). Irrespective of resultant glucose metabolism, these studies are clearly unrealistic and not applicable to the wider diabetic population. Estimates of dietary fiber intake suggest that in westernized nations the average intake is in the order of 10–13 g daily (122). It is clearly uncertain then if realistic longer-term dietary modifications aimed at providing more dietary fiber will be beneficial in the management of blood glucose levels in type 2 diabetes. Of the evidence accrued to date, the more appropriate approach is to modulate both carbohydrate and the soluble dietary fiber fraction to maximize the likelihood that carbohydrate digestion and absorption will be retarded following each meal. However, the impact of high-carbohydrate diets on plasma lipids must also be considered.

2. Effects on Lipid Metabolism

High-carbohydrate diets have been shown to increased plasma triglyceride and lower HDL cholesterol concentrations (119,123–125). Although this finding is not universal (118,126,128), it is clear that high-carbohydrate diets have the capacity to accentuate postprandial hypertriglyceridemia (92,125), due predominantly to increased hepatic secretion of VLDL triglycerides (129). The incorporation of dietary fiber into the high-carbohydrate diet tends to minimize these disturbances of triglyceride metabolism. Indeed dietary fiber, particularly soluble dietary fiber, lowers plasma cholesterol and LDL levels in the majority of studies (130,131). Equally effective in lowering plasma lipids and improving atherogenic risk are diets rich in monounsaturated fats (93). Recent analysis suggests that the combination of monounsaturated fatty acids with dietary fiber, more comparable to a traditional Mediterranean diet, is most effective in improving postprandial plasma lipid profiles (132).

VII. ADDITIONAL BENEFITS OF HIGH-CARBOHYDRATE, HIGH-FIBER DIETS IN DIABETES MANAGEMENT

Despite the uncertainty surrounding the benefit of a high-carbohydrate, high-fiber diet in the management of glucose and lipid metabolism in type 2 diabetes, there remains additional convincing evidence that high-carbohydrate diets have other beneficial attributes. Epidemiological evidence suggests that there is a positive relationship between the amount of dietary fat and body weight (133). Although fat and carbohydrate have equivalent satiation power (134), high-fat foods are likely to result in greater energy intake. Higher-fat foods are in many instances preferred when unrestricted food access is available, with many studies reporting a greater rating of desirability, flavor, and enjoyment with the higher-fat food (135). However, studies comparing intake of identical food products, differing only in fat content, show that consumption is based on volume, rather than energy content, leading to passive energy overconsumption (135).

The capacity of storage and metabolic responses to carbohydrate and fat differ markedly. Carbohydrate stores, primarily as glycogen, are small (200–500 g), and the capacity for synthesis of fats from carbohydrate precursors, de novo lipogenesis, is insignificant in humans (136). The precise maintenance glycogen stores, despite wide variations in daily carbohydrate intake, are achieved by modulating the rate of carbohydrate oxidation. Carbohydrate ingestion elicits an initial repletion of the bodies glycogen stores, followed by compensatory modulation of carbohydrate oxidation to rapidly restoring total body carbohydrate balance. However, unlike carbohydrate, humans possess an enormous capacity for fat storage, predominantly in adipose depots. Fat balance is determined primarily by the difference between total energy expenditure and the energy ingested as carbohydrates or protein (136). Increasing fat intake resulting in paralleled fat storage, rather than a concomitant increase in fat oxidation. There is also little evidence, with respect to energy metabolism, that monounsaturated fatty acids differ from other fatty acid species (137). Deliberate overfeeding of isoenergetic quantities of either carbohydrate or fat results in less weight gain in the carbohydrate-fed group as carbohydrate oxidation and total energy expenditure are increased (138). Yet dietary interventions aimed at increasing the carbohydrate content of the diet lead to reductions in energy intake and body weight (139,140). Clearly then, diets rich in carbohydrates are favorable for adequate weight control in diabetics.

Energy restriction, per se, prior to weight loss may improve insulin action in diabetic individuals (141). With continued energy restriction, weight loss provides marked improvements in glycemic control and diabetes complications (142,143). Diabetic management aimed at aggressively lowering body weight with use of very low calorie diets (VLCD) or gastric restriction surgery is particularly effective in improving insulin action (144). While aggressive weight restriction is appropriate for a small proportion of the adult diabetic population (145), gradual weight loss and, importantly, weight management remains a central priority for many diabetics. The evidence from studies conducted in obese populations suggests that a 10% reduction in fat energy produces on average a 4 to 5 kg weight loss (146). The critical issue is the sustainability of this weight loss with successful, postobese weight management characterized by the continued consumption and enjoyment of a low-fat, high-carbohydrate diet, combined with a regular exercise regime (147,148).

There are currently few data to suggest that diets rich in dietary fiber aid in weight loss and weight maintenance (149). However, whether the dietary fiber is soluble or insoluble may be expected to exert differing effects on postingestive satiety (150). Supplemental soluble fiber has been reported to reduce hunger immediately following meals (151,152), although total daily energy intake may be unaffected (153).

VIII. CONCLUSIONS

Arguments have been strongly made that type 2 diabetics should avoid high-carbohydrate diets, choosing instead a diet rich in monounsaturated fatty acids. This is based on the evidence available that weight-maintaining high-carbohydrate diets chosen without regard for their likely glycemic impact and dietary fiber content may be marginally detrimental to blood glucose and lipid levels. However, minimization of the glycemic impact of the meal combined with the use of low-GI foods or selecting foods rich in dietary fiber may provide some protection. Despite this evidence there is little justification for the selection of diets aimed at providing very high amounts of dietary fiber. While significantly increased dietary fiber may provide some additional health benefit, successful lifestyle adoption is likely to be restricted only to highly motivated individuals.

Nutritional therapy for type 2 diabetes need not focus particular attention on the dietary fiber content of the diet beyond that recommended for the general population. Most appropriate, as described by the American Diabetes Association (1998), is the continued need to emphasize healthful food choices consistent with the dietary guidelines for the general population. Particular focus in type 2 diabetes management should be given to weight loss and/or management. Central to weight management is the selection of high-carbohydrate diets in which diverse meal planning options are provided. Overall, nutritional therapy for type 2 diabetes should continue to focus on personalization, diversity, and sustainability of dietary plans in which a high-carbohydrate diet remains central.

REFERENCES

1. Report of the Expert Committee on the Diagnosis and Classification of Diabetes Mellitus. *Diabetes Care* 21(suppl. 1):S5–S19 (1998).
2. Amos, A. F., McCarty, D. J., and Zimmet, P. The rising global burden of diabetes and its complications: Estimates and projections to the year 2010. *Diabet. Med.* 14:S7–S85 (1997).
3. Songer, T. J. The economic costs of NIDDM. *Diab. Metab. Rev.* 8:389–404 (1992).
4. O'Brien, J. A., Shomphe, L. A., Kavanagh, P. L., Raggio, G., and Caro, J. J. Direct medical costs of complications resulting from type 2 diabetes in the U.S. *Diabetes Care* 21:1122–1128 (1998).
5. Kolaczynski, J. W., and Caro, J. F. Molecular mechanism of insulin resistance in human obesity. *Curr. Opin. Endocrinol. Diabetes* 3:36–43 (1996).
6. DeFronzo, R. A. Pathogenesis of type 2 (non-insulin dependent) diabetes mellitus: a balanced overview. *Diabetologia* 35:389–397 (1992).
7. Heesom, K. J., Harbeck, M., Kahn, C. R., and Denton, R. M. Insulin action on metabolism. *Diabetologia* 40:B3–B9 (1997).
8. Ferrannini, E., Reichard, G. A., and Bjorkman, O. The disposal of an oral glucose load in normal subjects. A quantitative study. *Diabetes* 34:580–588 (1985).
9. Kahn, B. B. Lilly lecture 1995. Glucose transport: pivotal step in insulin action. *Diabetes* 45:1644–1654 (1996).
10. Shulman, R. G. Nuclear magnetic resonance studies of glucose metabolism in non-insulin-dependent diabetes mellitus subjects. *Mol. Med.* 2:533–540 (1996).
11. Yki-Järvinen, H. Acute and chronic effects of hyperglyaemia on glucose metabolism: implications for the development of new therapies. *Diabet. Med.* 14:S32–S37 (1997).
12. Stern, M. P., and Haffner, S. M. Dyslipidemia in type II diabetes. Implications for therapeutic intervention. *Diabetes Care* 14:1144–1159 (1991).
13. Slyper, A. H. Low-density lipoprotein density and atherosclerosis. Unraveling the connection. *J. Am. Med. Assoc.* 272:305–308 (1994).
14. West, K. M., Ahuja, M. M. S., Bennett, P. H., Czyzyk, A., De Acosta, O. M., Fuller, J. H., Grab, B., Grabauskas, V., Jarrett, R. J., and Kosaka K. The role of circulating glucose and triglyceride concentrations and their interactions with other "risk factors" as determinants of arterial disease in nine diabetic population samples from the WHO multinational study. *Diabetes Care* 6:261–369 (1983).
15. Fontbonne, A., Eschwege, E., Cambien, F., Richard, J. L., Ducimetiere, P., Thibult, N., Warnet, J. M., Claude, J. R., and Rosselin G. E. Hypertriglyceridaemia as a risk factor for coronary heart disease mortality in subjects with impaired glucose tolerance or diabetes: results from the 11-year follow-up of the Paris prospective study. *Diabetologia* 32:300–304 (1989).
16. Patsch, J. R., Miesenböck, G., Hopferwieser, T., Muhlberger, V., Knapp, E., Dunn, J. K., Gotto, A. M., Jr., and Parsch, W. Relation of triglyceride metabolism and coronary artery disease. Studies in the postprandial state. *Arterioscler. Thromb.* 12:1236–1345 (1992).
17. The Diabetes Control and Complications Trial Research Group, The effect of intensive treatment of diabetes on the development and progression of long-term complications in insulin-dependent diabetes mellitus. *N. Engl. J. Med.* 329:977–986 (1993).
18. Colwell, J. A. Intensive insulin therapy in type II diabetes: rationale and collaborative clinical trial results. *Diabetes* 45:S87–S90 (1996).
19. Stern, M. P., Mitchell, B. D., Haffner, S. M., and Hazuda, H. P. Does glycemic control of type II diabetes suffice to control diabetic dyslipidemia? A community perspective. *Diabetes Care* 15:638–644 (1992).

20. American Diabetes Association. Nutrition Recommendations and Principles for People With Diabetes Mellitus. *Diabetes Care* 21(suppl. 1):S32–S44 (1998).

21. Stowers, J. M. Nutrition in diabetes. *Commonw. Bur. Animal Nutr.* 33:1–15 (1963).

22. Anderson, J. W. The role of dietary carbohydrate and fiber in the control of diabetes. *Adv. Intern. Med.* 26:67–96 (1980).

23. Himsworth, H. P. The dietetic factor determining the glucose tolerance and sensitivity to insulin of healthy men. *Clin. Sci.* 2:67–94 (1935).

24. Stone, D. B., and Connor, W. E. The prolonged effects of a low cholesterol high carbohydrate diet on serum lipids in diabetic patients. *Diabetes* 12:127–132 (1963).

25. American Diabetes Association. Principles of nutrition and dietary recommendations for patients with diabetes mellitus: 1971. *Diabetes* 20:633–634 (1971).

26. Weinsier, R. L., Seeman, A., and Herrera, M. G. High- and low-carbohydrate diets in diabetes mellitus: study of effects on diabetic control, insulin secretion, and blood lipids. *Ann. Int. Med.* 80: 332–341 (1974).

27. Lewitt, N. S., and Jackson, W. P. U. Trends in the carbohydrate content of diabetic rats. *S. Afr. Med. J.* 2:658–659 (1981).

28. American Diabetes Association. Nutritional recommendations and principles for individuals with diabetes mellitus: 1979. *Diabetes Care* 2:520–528 (1979).

29. Cleave, T. L. The neglect of natural principles in current medical practice. *J. Roy. Nav. Med.* 42: 55–83 (1956).

30. Burkitt, D. P., and Trowell, H. C. *Redefined Carbohydrate Foods and Disease*. London: Academic Press, 1975.

31. Trowell, H. C. Diabetes mellitus deeath-rates in England and Wales 192070 and food supplies. *Lancet* 2:998–999 (1974).

32. Anderson, J. W., and Akanji, A. O. Treatment of diabetes with high fiber diets. In: Spiller GA, ed. *Dietary Fiber in Human Nutrition*. Boca Raton, FL: CRC Press, 1993, pp 443–470.

33. Tappy, L., Gugolz, E., and Wursh, P. Effects of breakfast cereals containing various amounts of beta-glucan fibers on plasma glucose and insulin responses in NIDDM subjects. *Diabetes Care* 19: 831–834 (1996).

34. Fairchild, R. M., Ellis, P. R., Bryne, A. J., Luzio, S. D., and Mir, M. A. A new breakfast cereal containing guar gum reduces postprandial plasma glucose and insulin concentrations in normal-weight human subjects. *Br. J. Nutr.* 76:63–73 (1996).

35. Liljeberg, H. G., Granfeldt, Y. E., and Bjorck, I. M. Products based on a high fiber barley genotype, but not on common barley or oats, lower postprandial glucose and insulin responses in healthy humans. *J. Nutr.* 126:458–466 (1996).

36. Noakes M., Clifton, P. M., Nestel, P. J., Le Leu, R., and McIntosh, G. Effect of high-amylose starch and oat bran on metabolic variables and bowel function in subjects with hypertriglyceridemia. *Am. J. Clin. Nutr.* 64:944–951 (1996).

37. Jenkins, D. J. A., Goff, D. V., Leeds, A. R., Alberti, K. G. M. M., Wolever, T. M. S., Gassull, M. A., and Hockaday, T. D. R. Unabsorbable carbohydrates and diabetes: decreased post-prandial hyperglycaemia. *Lancet* 1:172–174 (1976).

38. Cameron-Smith, D., Collier, G. R., and O'Dea, K. Effect of soluble dietary fibre on the viscosity of gastrointestinal contents and the acute glycemic response in the rat. *Br. J. Nutr.* 71:563–571 (1994).

39. Wolever, T. M. S. Small intestinal effects of starchy foods. *Can. J. Physiol. Pharmacol.* 69:93–99 (1991).

40. Le Floch, J. P., Baudin, E., Escuyer, P., Wirquin, E., Nillus, P., and Perlemuter, L. Influence of non-carbohydrate foods on glucose and insulin responses to carbohydrates of different glycaemic index in type 2 diabetic patients. *Diabet. Med.* 9:44–48 (1992).

41. Brand Miller, J. C. Importance of glycemic index in diabetes. *Am. J. Clin. Nutr.* 59(suppl): 747S–752S (1994).

42. Peterson, D. B., Lambert, J., Darling, P., Carter, R. D., Jelfs, R., and Mann, J. I. Sucrose in the diet of diabetic patients—just another carbohydrate? *Diabetologia* 29:216–220 (1986).

43. Daly, M. E., Vale, C., Walker, M., Littlefield, A., Alberti, K. G. M. M., and Mathers, J. C. Acute

effects on insulin sensitivity and diurnal metabolic profiles of a high-sucrose compared with a high-starch diet. *Am. J. Clin. Nutr.* 67:1186–1196 (1998).

44. Koivisto, V., and Yki-Järvinen, H. Fructose and insulin sensitivity in patients with type 2 diabetes. *J. Intern. Med.* 233:145–153 (1993).

45. Anderson, J. W., Story, L. J., Zettwoch, N. C., Gustafson, N. J., and Jefferson, B. S. Metabolic effects of fructose supplementation in diabetic individuals. *Diabetes Care* 12:337–344 (1989).

46. Crapo, P. A., Kolterman, O. G., and Henry, R. R. Metabolic consequence of two-week fructose feeding in diabetic subjects. *Diabetes Care* 9:111–119 (1986).

47. Bantle, J. P. Clinical aspects of sucrose and fructose metabolism. *Diabetes Care* 12:56–61 (1989).

48. Olefsky, J. M., and Crapo, P. Fructose, xylitol and sorbitol. *Diabetes Care* 3:390–393 (1980).

49. Thorburn, A. W., Crapo, P. A., Beltz, W. F., Wallace, P., Witztum, J. L., and Henry, R. R. Lipid metabolism in non-insulin-dependent diabetes: effects of long-term treatment with fructose-supplemented mixed meals. *Am. J. Clin. Nutr.* 50:1015–1022 (1989).

50. Cavallero, E., Dachet, C., Neufcour, D., Wirquin, E., Mathe, D., and Jacotot, B. Postprandial amplification of lipoprotein abnormalities in controlled type II diabetic subjects: relationship to postprandial lipemia and C-peptide/glucagon levels. *Metabolism* 43:270–278 (1994).

51. Randle, P. J., Garland, P. B., Hales, C. N., and Newsholme, E. A. The glucose fatty-acid cycle. Its role in insulin sensitivity and the metabolic disturbances of diabetes mellitus. *Lancet* 1:785–789 (1963).

52. McGarry, J. D. Glucose-fatty acid interactions in health and disease. *Am. J. Clin. Nutr.* 67:500S–504S (1998).

53. Wolever, T. M. S., Jenkins, D. J. A., Ocana, A. M., Rao, A. V., and Collier, G. R. Second meal effect: low glycemic index foods eaten at dinner improve subsequent breakfast glycemic response. *Am. J. Clin. Nutr.* 48:1041–1047 (1988).

54. Raben, A., Christensen, N. J., Madsen, J., Holst, J. J., and Astrup, A. Decreased postprandial thermogenesis and fat oxidation but increased fullness after a high-fiber meal compared with a low-fiber meal. *Am. J. Clin. Nutr.* 59:1386–1394 (1994).

55. Wolever, T. M., Bentum-Williams, A., and Jenkins, D. J. Physiological modulation of plasma free fatty acid concentrations by diet. Metabolic implications in nondiabetic subjects, *Diabetes Care* 18: 962–970 (1995).

56. Wursch, P., Acheson, K., Koellreutter, B., and Jequier, E. Metabolic effects of instant bean and potato over 6 hours. *Am. J. Clin. Nutr.* 48:1418–1423 (1988).

57. Blaak, E. E., and Saris, W. H. Postprandial thermogenesis and substrate utilization after ingestion of different dietary carbohydrates. *Metabolism* 45:1235–1242 (1996).

58. Bryer-Ash, M. Regulation of rat insulin-receptor kinase by glucose in vivo. *Diabetes* 40:633–640 (1991).

59. Cusin, I., Terrattaz, J., Rohner-Jeanrenaud, F., Zarjevski, N., Assimocopoulos-Jeannet, F., and Jeanrenaud, B. Hyperinsulinemia increases the amount of GLUT4 mRNA in white adipose tissue and decreases that of muscles: a clue for increased fat depot and insulin resistance. *Endocrinology* 100: 1384–1390 (1990).

60. Massillon, D., Chen, W., Barzilai, N., Prus-Wertheimer, D., Hawkins, M., Liu, R., Taub, R., and Rossetti, L. Carbon flux via the pentose phosphate pathway regulates the hepatic expression of the glucose-6-phosphatase and phosphoenolpyruvate carboxykinase genes in conscious rats. *J. Biol. Chem.* 271:9871–9874 (1996).

61. Kok, N. N., Morgan, L. M., Williams, C. M., Roberfroid, M. B., Thissen, J. P., and Delzenne, N. M. Insulin, glucagon-like peptide 1, glucose-dependent insulinotropic polypeptide and insulin-like growth factor I as putative mediators of the hypolipidemic effect of oligofructose in rats. *J. Nutr.* 128:1099–1103 (1998).

62. Gee, J. M., Lee-Finglas, W., Wortley, G. W., and Johnson, I. T. Fermentable carbohydrates elevate plasma enteroglucagon but high viscosity is also necessary to stimulate small bowel mucosal cell proliferation in rats. *J. Nutr.* 126:373–379 (1996).

63. Beck, B., Villaume, C., Bau, H. M., Gariot, P., Chayvialle, J. A., Desalme, A., and Derby, G. Long-term influence of a wheat-bran supplemented diet on secretion of gastrointestinal hormones and on nutrient absorption in healthy man. *Hum. Nutr. Clin. Nutr.* 40:25–33 (1986).

64. Jenkins, D. J., Taylor, R. H., Nineham, R., Goff, D. V., Bloom, S. R., Sarson, D. L., Misiewicz, J. J., and Alberti, K. G. Manipulation of gut hormone response to food by soluble fiber and alpha-glucosidase inhibition. *Am. J. Gastroenterol.* 83:393–397 (1988).
65. Karlander, S., Armyr, I., and Efendic, S. Metabolic effects and clinical value of beet fiber treatment in NIDDM patients. *Diabetes Res. Clin. Pract.* 11:65–71 (1991).
66. Hagander, B., Bjorck, I., Asp, N. G., Efendic, S., Holm, J., Nilsson-Ehle, P., Lundquist, I., and Schersten, B. Rye products in the diabetic diet. Postprandial glucose and hormonal responses in non-insulin-dependent diabetic patients as compared to starch availability in vitro and experiments in rats. *Diabetes Res. Clin. Pract.* 3:85–96 (1987).
67. White, M. F. The IRS-signalling system in insulin and cytokine action. *Philos. Trans. R. Soc. Lond. B. Biol. Sci.* 351:181–189 (1996).
68. Binoux, M. The IGF system in metabolism regulation. *Diabetes Metab.* 21:330–337 (1995).
69. Drucker, D. J. Glucagon-like peptides. *Diabetes* 47:159–169 (1998).
70. Scrocchi, L. A., Marshall, B. A., Cook, S. M., Brubaker, P. L., and Drucker, D. J. Identification of glucagon-like peptide 1 (GLP-1) actions essential for glucose homeostasis in mice with disruption of GLP-1 receptor signaling. *Diabetes* 47:632–639 (1998).
71. Cummings, J. H. Short chain fatty acids in the human colon. *Gut* 22:763–779 (1981).
72. Cummings, J. H., Pomare, E. W., Branch, W. J., Naylor, C. P. E., and Macfarlane, G. T. Short chain fatty acids in human large intestine, portal, hepatic and venous blood. *Gut* 28:1221–1227 (1987).
73. Akanji, A. O., Peterson, D. B., Humphreys, S. and Hockaday, T. D. R. Change in plasma acetate levels in diabetic subjects on mixed high fiber diets. *Am. J. Gastroenterol.* 84:1365–1370 (1989).
74. Akanji, A. O., Bruce, M. A., and Frayn, K. N. Effect of acetate infusion on energy expenditure and substrate oxidation rates in non-diabetic and diabetic subjects. *Eur. J. Clin. Nutr.* 43:107–115 (1989).
75. Akanji, A. O., Humphreys, S., Thursfield, V., and Hockaday, T. D. R. The relationship of plasma acetate with glucose and other blood intermediary metabolites in non-diabetic and diabetic subjects. *Clin. Chem. Acta* 185:25–32 (1989).
76. Scheppach, W., Cummings, J. H., Branch, W. J., and Schrezenmeir, J. Effect of gut-derived acetate on oral glucose tolerance in man. *Clin. Sci.* 75:355–361 (1988).
77. Anderson, J. W., and Bridges, S. R. Short-chain fatty acid fermentation of plant fiber affect glucose metabolism of isolated rat hepatocytes. *Proc. Soc. Exp. Biol. Med.* 177:372–376 (1984).
78. Chan, T. M., and Freedland, R. A. Effects of glucagon on gluconeogenesis from lactate and propionate in the perfused rat liver. *Proc. Soc. Exp. Biol. Med.* 151:372–375 (1976).
79. Venter, C. S., Vorster, H. H., and Cummings, J. A. Effects of dietary propionate on carbohydrate metabolism in healthy volunteers. *Am. J. Gastroenterol.* 85:549–553 (1990).
80. Todesco, T., Roa, A. V., Bosello, O., and Jenkins, D. J. A. Propionate lowers blood glucose and alters lipid metabolism in healthy subjects. *Am. J. Clin. Nutr.* 54:860–865 (1991).
81. Boillot, J. Alamowitch, C., Berger, A. M., Luo, J., Bruzzo, F., Bornet, F. R., and Slama, G. Effects of dietary propionate on hepatic glucose production, whole-body glucose utilization, carbohydrate and lipid metabolism in normal rats. *Br. J. Nutr.* 73:241–251 (1995).
82. Laurent, C., Simoneau, C., Marks, L., Braschi, S., Champ, M., Charbonnel, B., and Krempf, M. Effect of acetate and propionate on fasting hepatic glucose production in humans. *Eur. J. Clin. Nutr.* 49:484–491 (1995).
83. Alamowitch, C., Boillot, J., Boussairi, A., Ruskone-Fourmestraux, A., Chevalier, A., Rizkalla, S. W., Guyon, F., Bornet, F. R., and Slama, G. Lack of effect of an acute ileal perfusion of short-chain fatty acids on glucose metabolism in healthy men. *Am. J. Physiol.* 271(1 Pt1):E199–E204 (1996).
84. Chen, W. J. L., Anderson, J. W., and Jennings, D. Propionate may mediate the hypercholestermic effects of certain soluble fibers in cholesterol-fed rats. *Proc. Soc. Exp. Biol. Med.* 175:215–218 (1984).
85. Demigné, C., Morand, C., Levrat, M.-A., Besson, C., Moundras, C., and Rémésy, C. Effect of propionate on fatty acid and cholesterol synthesis and on acetate metabolism in isolated rat hepatocytes. *Br. J. Nutr.* 74:209–219 (1995).

86. Berggren, A. M., Nyman, E. M., Lundquist, I., and Bjorck, I. M. Influence of orally and rectally administered propionate on cholesterol and glucose metabolism in obese rats. *Br. J. Nutr.* 76:287–294 (1996).

87. Lin, Y., Vonk, R. J., Sloof, M. J. H., Kuipers, F., and Smit, M. J. Differences in propionate-induced inhibition of cholesterol and triacylglycerol synthesis between human and rat hepatocytes in primary culture. *Br. J. Nutr.* 74:197–207 (1995).

88. Nagata, Y., Murase, M., Kimura, Y., and Ebihara, K. Effect of guar gum on glucose metabolism in cecetomized rats. *J. Nutr. Biochem.* 7:303–308 (1996).

89. Brunzell, J. D., Lerner, R. L., Porte, R. L., and Bierman, E. L. Effect of a fat free, high carbohydrate diet on diabetic subjects with fasting hyperglycemia. *Diabetes* 23:138–143 (1974).

90. Anderson, J. W. Effect of carbohydrate restriction and high carbohydrate diets on men with chemical diabetes. *Am. J. Clin. Nutr.* 30:402–408 (1977).

91. Borkman, M., Campbell, L. V., Chisholm, D. J., and Storlien, L. H. Comparison of the effects on insulin sensitivity of high-carbohydrate and high-fat diets in normal subjects. *J. Clin. Endocrinol. Metab.* 72:432–437 (1991).

92. Garg, A., Bonanome, A., Grundy, S. M., Zhang, Z. J., and Unger, R. H. Comparison of a high-carbohydrate diet with a high-monounsaturated-fat diet in patients with non-insulin-dependent diabetes mellitus. *N. Engl. J. Med.* 391:829–834 (1988).

93. Garg, A. High-monounsaturated-fat diets for patients with diabetes mellitus: a meta-analysis. *Am. J. Clin. Nutr* 67(suppl.):577S–582S (1998).

94. Parillo, M., Rivellese, A. A., Ciardullo A. V., Capaldo, B., Giacco, A., Genovese, S., and Riccardi, G. A. A high-monounsaturated-fat/low-carbohydrate, diet improves peripheral insulin sensitivity in non-insulin-dependent diabetic patients. *Metabolism* 41:1373–1378 (1992).

95. Rasmussen, O. W., Thomsen, C., Hansen, K. W., Vesterlund, M., Winther, E., and Hermansen, K. Effects on blood pressure, glucose, and lipid levels of a high-monounsaturated fat diet compared with a high-carbohydrate diet in NIDDM subjects. *Diabetes Care* 16:1565–1571 (1993).

96. Campbell, L. V., Marrnot, P. E., Dyer, J. A., Borkman, M., and Storlien, L. H. The high-monounsaturated fat diet as a practical alternative for NIDDM. *Diabetes Care* 17(3):177–182 (1994).

97. Jenkins, D. J. A., Wolever, T. M. S., and Buckley, G. Low-glycemic-index starchy foods in the diabetic diet. *Am. J. Clin. Nutr.* 48:248–254 (1988).

98. Fontvieille, A. M., Rizkalla, S. W., Penfornis, A., Acosta, M., Bornet, F. R., and Slama, G. The use of low glycaemic index foods improves metabolic control of diabetic patients over five weeks. *Diabet. Med.* 9:444–450 (1992).

99. Frost, G., Wilding, J., and Beecham, J. Dietary advice based on the glycaemic index improves dietary profile and metabolic control in type 2 diabetic patients. *Diabet. Med.* 11:397–401 (1994).

100. Brand, J. C., Colagiuri, S., Crossman, S., Allen, A., Roberts, D. C. K., and Truswell, A. S. Low glycemic index foods improve long-term glycemic control in NIDDM. *Diabetes* 14:95–101 (1991).

101. Jenkins, D. J. A., Wolever, T. M. S., Vuksan, V., Brighenti, F., Cunnane, S. C., and Rao, A. V. ''Nibbling versus gorging'': metabolic advantages of increased meal frequency. *N. Engl. J. Med.* 321:929–934 (1989).

102. Jenkins, D. J. A., Ocana, A., Jenkins, A. L., Wolever, T. M. S., Vuksan, V., Katzman, L., Hollands, M., Greenberg, G., Corey, P., Patten, R., Wong, G., and Josse, R. G. Metabolic advantages of spreading the nutrient load: effects of increased meal frequency in non-insulin-dependent diabetes. *Am. J. Clin. Nutr.* 55:461–467 (1992).

103. Chiasson, J.-L. The effect of acarbose on insulin sensitivity in subjects with impaired glucose tolerance. *Diabet. Med.* 13:S23–S24 (1996).

104. Matsumoto, K., Yano, M., Miyake, S., Ueki, Y., Yamaguchi, Y., Akazawa, S., and Tominaga, Y. Effects of voglibose on glucemic excursions, insulin secretion, and insulin sensitivity in non-insulin-treated NIDDM patients. *Diabetes Care* 21:256–260 (1998).

105. Gardner, D. F., Schwartz, L., Krista, M., and Merimee, T. J. Dietary pectin and glycemic control in diabetes. *Diabetes Care* 7:143–146 (1984).

106. Doi, K., Matsuura, M., Kawara, A., and Baba, S. Treatment of diabetes with glucomannan (Konjac mannan). *Lancet* 1:987–988 (1979).

107. Karlstrom, B., Vessby, B., Asp, N.-P., and Ytterfors, A. Effects of four meals with different kinds

of dietary fiber on glucose metabolism in healthy subjects and non-insulin-dependent diabetic subjects. *Eur. J. Clin. Nutr.* 42:519–526 (1988).

108. Peterson, D. B., Ellis, P. R., Baylis, J. M., Fielden, P., Ajodhia, J., Leeds, A. R., and Jepson, E. M. Low dose guar in a novel food product: improved metabolic control in non-insulin-dependent diabetes. *Diabet. Med.* 4:111–115 (1987).

109. Vaaler, S., Hanssen, K. F., Dahl-Jorgensen, K., Frolich, W., Aaseth, J., Odegaard, B., and Aagenaes, O. Diabetic control is improved by guar gum and wheat bran supplementation. *Diabet. Med.* 3:230–233 (1986).

110. Atkins, T. W., Al-Hussary, N. A., and Taylor, K. G. The treatment of poorly controlled non-insulin-dependent diabetic subjects with granulated guar gum. *Diabetes Res. Clin. Pract.* 3:153–159 (1987).

111. Tagliaferro, V., Cassader, M., Bozzo, C., Pisu, E., Bruno, A., Marena, S., Cavallo-Perin, P., Cravero, L., and Pagano, G. Moderate guar-gum addition to usual diet improves peripheral sensitivity to insulin and lipaemic profile in NIDDM. *Diabetes Metab* 11:380–385 (1985).

112. Fairchild, R. M., Ellis, P. R., Byrne, A. J., Luzio, S. D., and Mir, M. A. A new breakfast cereal containing guar gum reduces postprandial plasma glucose and insulin concentrations in normal-weight human subjects. *Br. J. Nutr.* 76:63–73 (1996).

113. Pick, M. E., Hawrush, Z. J., Gee, M. L., Toth, E., Garg, M. L., and Hardin, R. T. Oat bran concentrate bread products improve long-term control of diabetes: a pilot study. *J. Am. Diet. Assoc.* 96:1254–1261 (1996).

114. Fukagawa, N. K., Anderson, J. W., Hageman, G., Young, V. R., and Minaker, K. L. High-carbohydrate, high-fiber diets increase peripheral insulin sensitivity in healthy young and old adults. *Am. J. Clin. Nutr.* 52:524–528 (1990).

115. Anderson, J. W., Zeigler, J. A., Deakins, D. A., Floore, T. L., Dillon, D. W., Wood, C. L., Oeltgen, P. R., and Whitley, R. J. Metabolic effects of high-carbohydrate, high-fiber diets for insulin-dependent diabetic individuals. *Am. J. Clin. Nutr.* 54:936–943 (1991).

116. Riccardi, G., Rivellese, A., Pacioni, D., Genovese, S., Mastranzo, P., and Mancini, M. Separate influence of dietary carbohydrate and fibre on the metabolic control in diabetes. *Diabetologia* 26:116–121 (1984).

117. Kiehm, T. G., Anderson, J. W., and Ward, K. Beneficial effects of a high carbohydrate high fiber diet on hyperglycemic diabetic men. *Am. J. Clin. Nutr.* 29:895–903 (1976).

118. O'Dea, K., Traianedes, K., Ireland, P., Naill, M., Sadler, J., Hopper, J., and De Luise, M. The effects of diet differing in fat, carbohydrate, and fiber on carbohydrate and lipid metabolism in type II diabetes. *J. Am. Diet. Assoc.* 89:1076–1086 (1989).

119. Coulston, A. M., Hollenbeck, C. B., Swislocki, A. L. M., Chen, Y.-D. I., and Reaven, G. M. Deleterious metabolic effects of high-carbohydrate, sucrose-containing diets in patients with non-insulin-dependent diabetes mellitus. *Am. J. Med.* 82:213–220 (1987).

120. Hollenbeck, C. B., Coulston, A. M., and Reaven, G. M. To what extent does increased dietary fiber improve glucose and lipid metabolism in patients with noninsulin-dependent diabetes mellitus (NIDDM)? *Am. J. Clin. Nutr.* 43:16–24 (1986).

121. Scott, A. R., Attenborough, Y., Peacock, I., Fletcher, E., Jeffcoate, W. T., and Tattersall, R. B. Comparison of high fibre diets, basal insulin supplements, and flexible insulin treatment for non-insulin dependent (type II) diabetics poorly controlled with sulphonylureas. *Br. Med. J.* 297:707–710 (1988).

122. Vinik, A. L., and Jenkins, D. J. A. Dietary fiber in management of diabetes. *Diabetes Care* 11:160–173 (1986).

123. Grundy, S. M. Comparison of monounsaturated fatty acids and carbohydrates for lowering plasma cholesterol. *N. Engl. J. Med.* 314:745–748 (1986).

124. Coulston, A. M., Hollenbeck, C. B., Swislocki, A. L. M., and Reaven, G. M. Persistence of hypertriglyceridemic effect of low-fat, high-carbohydrate diets in NIDDM patients. *Diabetes Care* 12:94–101 (1989).

125. Garg, A., Bantle, J. P., and Henry, R. R. Effects of varying carbohydrate content of diet in patients with non-insulin-dependent diabetes mellitus. *J. Am. Med. Assoc.* 271:1421–1428 (1994).

126. Cominacini, L., Zocca, I., Garbin, U., Davoli, A., Compri, R., Brunetti, L., and Bosello, O. Long-

term effect of a low-fat, high-carbohydrate diet on plasma lipids of patients affected by familial endogenous hypertriglyceridemia. *Am. J. Clin. Nutr.* 48:57–65 (1988).

127. Milne, R. M., Mann, J. I., Chisholm, A. W., and Williams, S. M. Long-term comparison of three dietary prescriptions in the treatment of NIDDM. *Diabetes Care* 17:74–80 (1994).

128. Ullmann, D., Conner, W. E., Hatcher, L. F., Connor, S. L., and Flavell, D. P. Will a high-carbohydrate low-fat diet lower plasma lipids and lipoproteins without producing hypertriglyceridemia? *Arterioscler. Thromb.* 11:1059–1067 (1991).

129. Blades, B., and Garg, A. Mechanisms of increase in plasma triacylglycerol concentrations as a result of high carbohydrate intakes in patients with non-insulin-dependent diabetes mellitus. *Am. J. Clin. Nutr.* 62:996–1002 (1995).

130. Jenkins, D. J., Wolever, T. M., Rao, A. V., Hegele, R. A., Mitchell, S. J., Ransom, T. P., Boctor, D. L., Spadafora, P. J., Jenkins, A. L., and Mehling, C. Effect on blood lipids of very high intakes of fiber in diets low in saturated fat and cholesterol. *N. Engl. J. Med.* 329:21–26 (1993).

131. Ripsin, C. M., Keenan, J. M., Jacobs, D. R. Jr., and Elmer, P. T. Oat products and lipid lowering: a meta-analysis. *J. Am. Med. Assoc.* 267:3317–3325 (1992).

132. Mekki, N., Dubois, C., Charbonnier, M., Cara, L., Senft, M., Pauli, A. M., Portugal, H., Gassin, A. L., Lafont, H., and Lairon, D. Effects of lowering fat and increasing dietary fiber on fasting and postprandial plasma lipids in hypercholesterolemic subjects consuming a mixed Mediterranean-Western die. *Am. J. Clin. Nutr.* 66:1443–1451 (1997).

133. Golay, A., and Bobbioni, E. The role of dietary fat in obesity, *Int. J. Obesity* 21 (suppl. 3):S2–S11 (1997).

134. Rolls, B. J., Kim, S., McNelis, A. L., Fischman, M. W., Foltin, R. H., and Moran, T. H. Time course of effects of preloads high in fat or carbohydrate on food intake and hunger ratings in humans. *Am. J. Physiol.* 260:R756–R763 (1991).

135. Cooling, J., and Blundell, J. Are high-fat and low-fat consumers distinct phenotypes? Differences and the subjective and behavioural response to energy and nutrient challenges. *Eur. J. Clin. Nutr.* 52:193–201 (1998).

135. Rolls, B., and Shide, D. The influence of dietary fat on food intake and body weight. *Nutr. Rev.* 50:283–290 (1992).

136. Flatt, J.-P. Use and storage of carbohydrate and fat. *Am. J. Clin. Nutr.* 61:952S–959S (1995).

137. Awad, A. B., Bernardis, L. L., and Fink, C. S. Failure to demonstrate an effect of dietary fatty acid composition on body weight, body composition and parameters of lipid metabolism in mature rats. *J. Nutr.* 120:1277–1282 (1990).

138. Horton, T. J., Drougas, H., Brachey, A., Reed, G. W., Peters, J. C., and Hill, J. O. Fat and carbohydrate overfeeding in humans: different effects on energy storage. *Am. J. Clin. Nutr.* 62:19–29 (1995).

139. Kendall, A., Levitsky, D. A., Strupp, B. J., and Lissner, L. Weight loss on a low-fat diet: consequence of the imprecision of the control of food intake in humans. *Am. J. Clin. Nutr.* 53:1124–1129 (1991).

140. Thomas, C. D., Peters, J. C., Reed, G. W., Abumrad, N. N., Sun, M., and Hill, J. O. Nutrient balance and energy expenditure during ad libitum feeding of high-fat and high-carbohydrate diets in human. *Am. J. Clin. Nutr.* 55:934–942 (1992).

141. Henry, R. R., Scheaffer, J. M., and Olefsky, J. M. Glycemic effects of intensive caloric restriction and isocaloric refeeding in noninsulin-dependent diabetes mellitus. *J. Clin. Invest.* 61:917–925 (1985).

142. Goldstein, D. J. Beneficial health effects of modest weight loss. *Int. J. Obes.* 16:397–415 (1992).

143. Collins, R. W., and Anderson, J. W. Medication cost savings associated with weight loss for obese non-insulin-dependent diabetic men and women. *Prev. Med.* 24:369–374 (1995).

143. Astrup, A., Toubro, S., Raben, A., and Skov, A. R. The role of low-fat diets and fat substitutes in body weight management: what have we learned from clinical studies? *J. Am. Diet. Assoc.* 97:S82–S87 (1997).

144. Scheen, A. J. Aggresive weight reduction treatment in the management of type 2 diabetes, *Diabetes Metab.* 24:116–123 (1998).

145. Williams, K. V., Mullen, M. L., Kelley, D. E., and Wing, R. R. The effect of short periods of caloric restriction on weight loss and glycemic control in type 2 diabetes. *Diabetes Care* 21:2–8 (1998).

146. Astrup, A., Ryan, L., Grunwald, G. K., Storgaard, M., Saris, W., Melanson, E., and Hill, J. O. The role of dietary fat in body fatness: evidence from a preliminary meta-analysis of ad libitum low-fat dietary intervention studies. *Br. J. Nutr.* 83:S25–32 (2000).

147. Klem, M. L., Wing, R. R., McGuire, M. T., Seagle, H. M., and Hill, J. O. A descriptive study of individuals successful at long-term maintenance of substantial weight loss. *Am. J. Clin. Nutr.* 66: 239–246 (1997).

148. Westerterp-Plantenga, M. S., Kempen, K. P. G., and Saris, W. H. M. Determinants of weight maintenance in women after diet-induced weight reduction. *Int. J. Obes.* 22:1–6 (1998).

149. Pasman, W. J., Westerterp-Plantenga, M. S., Muls, E., Vansant, G., Van Ree, J., and Saris, W. H. The effectiveness of long-term fibre supplementation on weight maintenance in weight-reduced women. *Int. J. Obes. Relat. Metab. Disord.* 21:548–555 (1997).

150. Blundell, J. E., and Burley, V. J. Satiation, satiety and the action of fibre on food intake, *Int. J. Obes.* 11(suppl. 1):9–25 (1987).

151. Saltzman, E., and Roberts, S. B. Soluble fiber and energy regulation. Current knowledge and future directions. *Adv. Exp. Med. Biol.* 427:89–97 (1997).

152. Pasman, W. J., Saris, W. H., Wauters, M. A., and Westerterp-Plantenga, M. S. Effect of one week of fibre supplementation on hunger and satiety ratings and energy intake. *Appetite* 29:77–87 (1997).

153. Delargy, H. J., O'Sullivan, K. R., Fletcher, R. J., and Blundell, J. E. Effects of amount and type of dietary fibre (soluble and insoluble) on short-term control of appetite. *Int. J. Food Sci. Nutr.* 48: 67–77 (1997).

154. Henry, R. R., and Gumbiner, B. Benefits and limitations of very-low-calorie diet therapy in obese NIDDM. *Diabetes Care* 14:802–823 (1991).

8
Resistant Oligosaccharides

Marcel Roberfroid*
Catholic University of Louvain, Brussels, Belgium

Joanne L. Slavin
University of Minnesota, St. Paul, Minnesota

I. INTRODUCTION

Dietary carbohydrates range in molecular size from simple sugars to complex polymers with a degree of polymerisation (DP) of up to 100,000 or more. Oligosaccharides are generally defined as carbohydrates from 2-20 monomeric units long. Oligosaccharides have been dietary staples since antiquity but have received much less attention than other carbohydrates such as simple sugars or dietary fiber. Recently interest in oligosaccharides has increased not only because of properties that include sweetening ability and fat replacement but also, because of resistance to digestion in the upper gastrointestinal tract and fermentation in the large bowel. Thus some oligosaccharides have functional effects similar to soluble dietary fiber such as enhancement of a healthy gastrointestinal tract, improvement of glucose control, modulation of the metabolism of triglycerides. These oligosaccharides are the resistant oligosaccharides.

A. Definition of Resistant Oligosaccharides

Oligosaccharides are carbohydrates with a low degree of polymerization (DP) and consequently low molecular weight (Yun, 1996). They have been variously defined as including anything from 2-20 monosaccharide units (British Nutrition Foundation, 1990; Food and Drug Administration, 1993; IUB-IUPAC, 1982). According to IUB-IUPAC (1982) terminology, the dividing point between oligo- and polysaccharides is 10, there is no rational physiological or chemical reason for this division (Cummings and Roberfroid, 1996).

Moreover, this includes a wide range of substances which, generally, contain mixtures of polymers of different chain lengths (linear or branched) that often cross this artificial oligo/polysaccharide boundary and that vary greatly in chemical composition and physiological effects. Standard oligosaccharide categories do not exist, so it is difficult to compare the many oligosaccharide products on the market. Recently (Englyst and Hudson, 1996) the name ''short-chain carbohydrates'' has been proposed for a new grouping of food carbohydrates that includes the oligosaccharides and the smaller polysaccharides. For analytical purpose, solubility in 80%

References published after 1998 are not included in this chapter.
*Professor emeritus.

(v/v) ethanol has been validated as a practical way of isolating this group of carbohydrates (Cummings and Roberfroid, 1996; Englyst and Hudson, 1996; Van Loo et al., 1998). In practice, therefore, the separation of oligosaccharides from polysaccharides is empirical and does not provide an exact division based on DP (Asp et al., 1992).

The concept of resistant (or nondigestible or unavailable) oligosaccharides originates from the observation that the anomeric C atom (C_1 or C_2) of the monosaccharide units of some dietary oligosaccharides has a configuration that makes their osidic bounds resistant to the hydrolytic activity of the human digestive enzymes. Such a resistance to digestion has been demonstrated in various systems including human ileostomized volunteers (see below). The main categories of resistant oligosaccharides presently available or in development as food ingredients include carbohydrates in which the monosaccharide unit is fructose, galactose, glucose, and/or xylose (Delzenne and Roberfroid, 1994; Cummings and Roberfroid, 1996; Crittenden and Playne, 1997). As interest in oligosaccharides has increased, so has the supply of oligosaccharides on the market. Since large-chain polysaccharides can be hydrolyzed to oligosaccharides, the number of oligosaccharides that may enter the marketplace is great.

From a food science point of view, this may create confusion, especially since chemical and physiological standards for oligosaccharides are not agreed upon. Obvious chemical differences among commercially available oligosaccharides include chain length, monosaccharide composition, degree of branching, and purity. Resistant oligosaccharides are made of one, two, or even three monosaccharides, and the chemical structure of the compounds discussed in the present chapter are described in Table 1. Analytical measurements are accomplished by HPLC, but standard solutions for many oligosaccharide fractions are not available (Yun, 1996). Recently, an analytical method has been developed, validated, and officially accepted by the AOAC for the quantitative analysis of the resistant oligosaccharides composed of fructose, including inulin (Quemener et al., 1994; Hoebregs, 1997), which consequently will be included as soluble dietary fiber. Selected fructooligosaccharides in foods and feeds have been measured by ion exchange chromatography (Campbell et al., 1997).

B. Other Properties of Resistant Oligosaccharides

Resistant oligosaccharides are readily water soluble and exhibit some sweetness, but sweetness decreases with longer chain length; e.g., inulin, with an average DP > 10, does not taste sweet. Depending upon chain length and composition, resistant oligosaccharides may contribute physicochemical properties of the diet, such as water binding, gelling, and thus fat replacement (inulin) value. Since resistant oligosaccharides are not digested and absorbed in the small intestine, they have no caloric value in the traditional sense. However, due to colonic fermentation, they have an energy contribution to food of about 1.5 kcal/g, similar to that of soluble dietary fiber (see below).

C. Preparation of Resistant Oligosaccharides

Three methods are used to prepare the resistant oligosaccharides (Table 1):

1. Hot water extraction form natural sources (e.g., chicory root, Jerusalem artichoke or seeds), such as for inulin, or for the soybean oligosaccharides.
2. Partial enzymatic hydrolysis of oligosaccharides [e.g., oligofructose, the hydrolysate of inulin (Debruyn et al., 1992)] or polysaccharides [e.g., xylooligosaccharides formed by the action of xylanase on xylan polysaccharide (Imaizumi et al., 1991) or pectin hydrolysates (Yamaguchi et al., 1994)].
3. Enzymatic synthesis from one or a mixture of disaccharides using osyl-transferases

Table 1 Resistant Oligosaccharides, Their Chemical Structures, and Methods of Preparation

Resistant oligosaccharides	Chemical structure	Methods of preparation
Galactooligosaccharides	β-D-gal-(1 → 6)-[β-D-gal]$_n$-(1 → 4) α-D-glu	Enzymatic synthesis from lactose
Inulin-type fructans (fructooligosaccharides)	α-D-glu-(1 → 2)-[β-D-fru]$_n$-(1 → 2) β-D-fru and or β-D-fru-(1 → 2)-[β-D-fru]$_n$-(1 → 2) β-D-fru n = 1 up to 60	Extraction from natural sources Partial enzymatic hydrolysis Enzymatic synthesis from sucrose
Isomaltooligosaccharides	[α-D-glu-(1 → 6)-]$_n$ n = 2 to 5	Partial enzymatic hydrolysis + glucosyl-transferase activity on starch
Lactosucrose	β-D-gal-(1 → 4)-α-D-glu-(1 → 2)- β-D-fru	Enzymatic synthesis from lactose + sucrose
Palatinose	[α-D-glu-(1 → 6)-β-D-fru]$_2$ + 1 or 2 branchings through (1 → 2) at fru	Enzymatic synthesis from sucrose
Soybean oligosaccharides	[α-D-gal-(1 → 6)-]$_n$-α-D-glu-(1 → 2)-β-D-fru (n = 1 or 2)	Extraction from natural source
Xylooligosaccharides	β-D-xyl-(1 → 4)-]$_n$ n = 2 to 9	Partial enzymatic hydrolysis of polyxylan

gal: galactose; glu: glucose; fru: fructose; xyl: xylose.

like fructooligosaccharides from sucrose (Spiegel et al., 1994), galactooligosaccharides from lactose, or lactosucrose from a mixture of sucrose and lactose (Fujita et al., 1992).

Polydextrose is a specific case because it is prepared by thermal treatment of solution of glucose in the presence of citric acid. Similarly, pyrodextrins that are (partly) resistant oligosaccharides made of glucose are produced by thermal treatment of starch (Ueno et al., 1976).

Among the resistant oligosaccharides, those composed primarily of fructose occupy a leading position in food science for the following reasons:

They are, historically, among the first products to have been marketed.

They have been, over the last decade, the most studied products.

They can be prepared by the three methods described above, meaning that a wide variety of different commercially available products exist that have different technological properties (from sweetness to fat replacement).

They are recognized in many countries as natural food ingredients as well as dietary fiber.

They occur naturally in many common food products, including banana, rye, garlic, onion, and wheat (Van Loo et al., 1995), and easily available crops like chicory roots and Jerusalem artichoke, which are particularly rich sources (up to 75% on a dry weight basis).

Some controversy exists in the scientific literature concerning the nomenclature of these resistant oligosaccharides. Yun (1996) suggested that fructooligosaccharide is a common name only for fructose oligomers that are mainly composed of 1-kestose (GF2), nystose (GF3), and 1-F-fructofuranosyl nystose (GF4) in which fructosyl units are bound at the β-2-1 position of sucrose (GF). According to this author, this type of FOS, known as Neosugar, NutraFlora, and Actilight, should be distinguished from other kinds of fructose-containing resistant oligosaccharides. Further, he notes that many authors have mingled fructooligosaccharides with fructan, glucofructosan, and inulin-type oligosaccharides. But this view is not shared by most of the other experts in the field who use fructooligosaccharides as a generic name for all resistant oligosaccharides composed mainly of fructose. From a strict point of view of chemical nomenclature, these molecules are "inulin-type fructans," linear β-(2-1)-fructans, which are different from the "levans," β-(2-6), often branched fructans (Waterhouse and Chatterton, 1993; Roberfroid and Delzenne, 1998). Inulin-type fructans are composed of β-D-fructofuranoses attached by β-2-1 linkages. The first monomer of the chain is either a β-D-glucopyranosyl or β-D-fructofuranosyl residue, both of which are in the pyranose configuration. They constitute a series of homologous oligosaccharides derived from sucrose represented by the formulas $G_{py}F_n$ or $F_{py}F_n$. They can be produced by enzymatic conversion of sucrose by different procedures (Yun, 1996). By one method, FOS is produced by the action of a fungal (*Aspergillus niger*) β-fructofuranosidase on sucrose (Spiegel et al., 1994). The product is a mixture of GF2, GF3, GF4, sucrose, glucose, and fructose, and it is not different from the molecules naturally occurring in foods. This product was originally called Neosugar. It has an average DP of 3.8. In this chapter, it will be abbreviated as SFr. Inulin-type fructans also can be isolated from naturally high food components. Generally, the product with DP from 2 to 60+ is labeled as inulin (Raftiline or Fibrulin), abbreviated as INU, while oligofructose is defined as DP < 8 (Raftilose) and is abbreviated as OFr. The inulin from which the small molecular weight oligomers have been eliminated is called inulin HP (Raftiline HP). Other manufacturers of inulin describe their product as having an average DP of 9. Inulin-type fructans are stable to heat and relatively low pH, are mildly sweet, and dissolve readily. Shorter-chain inulin hydrolysates are sweeter than longer-chain inulin products.

D. Worldwide Consumption Patterns of Resistant Oligosaccharides

The only available data are estimates of the consumption of inulin-type fructans. Indeed, Van Loo et al. (1995) have estimated the daily intake of inulin/oligofructose for the United States and Western Europe. According to this publication, an average North American consumes between 0.014 and 0.054 g of inulin or oligofructose per day per kg of body weight. This corresponds to an intake of 1–4 g by a 165 lb person. Wheat, onion, and banana are the most important sources of inulin and oligofructose in the North American diet.

Western Europe intake is estimated at 3.2–11.3 g for a 75 kg person. Consumption will be higher with intake of French onion soup or other concentrated inulin sources such as leeks or garlic. In Western populations, consumption of complex carbohydrates such as resistant oligosaccharides and dietary fiber has decreased and is associated with increased risk of chronic diseases including heart disease and cancer. Despite many years of research and nutrition education, dietary fiber intakes are not increasing. Since dietary fiber and resistant oligosaccharides share many positive physiological properties, it may be more feasible to increase intake of these oligosaccharides than dietary fiber. This is especially true since isolated resistant oligosaccharides from chicory and other natural products are now being incorporated into processed foods.

II. FATE OF RESISTANT OLIGOSACCHARIDES IN THE GASTROINTESTINAL TRACT

A. Nondigestibility in the Upper Gastrointestinal Tract

1. Inulin-Type Fructans

The β configuration of the anomeric C_2 in their fructose monomers make inulin-type fructans resistant to hydrolysis by human digestive enzymes (α-glucosidase, maltase-isomaltase, sucrase), which are mostly specific for α-osidic linkages. Both in vitro and in vivo data support this property. In vitro, SFr is not hydrolyzed to any significant extent by purified rat sucrase-maltase and does not compete with the natural substrates sucrose or maltose (Oku et al., 1984), but yeast invertase hydrolyzes GF_3 (nystose) at about 5% of the rate of sucrose, and that particular oligomer disappears completely within 2 hours (Ziesenitz and Siebert, 1987). When incubated in the presence of an homogenate of different segments (duodenum, jejunum, ileum) of rat or human small intestine, inulin-type fructans remain unchanged for up to 1 or 2 hours (Hidaka et al., 1986; Ziesenitz and Siebert, 1987; Nilsson et al., 1988; Molis et al., 1996). In addition, since the stomach hydrolysis of (inulin-type) fructans is likely to be of limited physiological significance, these products proceed undigested through the upper part of the gastrointestinal tract into the colon (Nilsson et al., 1988).

This has been confirmed by in vivo studies in rats (Nilsson et al., 1988; Nilsson and Björk 1988) and in humans (Bach-Knudsen and Hessov, 1995; Molis et al., 1996; Ellegärd et al., 1997). The most convincing data are those of Bach Knudsen and Hessov (1995) and Ellegärd et al. (1997), who used the ileostomy model which provides a valuable alternative to study digestive physiology in humans. Both studies show that 86–88% of the ingested dose (10, 17, or 30 g) of INU and OFr is recovered in the ileostomy effluent, supporting the conclusion that INU and OFr are practically undigestible in the human small intestine.

Using an intubation technique in human volunteers, Molis et al. (1996) similarly concluded that SFr is unabsorbed in the small intestine (89% recovery). The small but significant loss of inulin-type fructans during the passage through the small intestine could be due to fermentation by the microbial population colonizing the ileum, a population known to be up to 100 times greater in ileostomists than in normal individuals (Drasar and Hill, 1974). Another plausible explanation is acid and/or enzymatic hydrolysis of the low molecular weight fructans. Indeed, Oku et al. (1984), Nilsson and Björck (1988), and Molis et al. (1996) have all reported evidence to show that low molecular weight fructans are more sensitive to stomach and/or small intestinal hydrolysis than high molecular weight components.

2. Other Resistant Oligosaccharides

Published data concerning the resistance of other oligosaccharides to digestion in the upper gastrointestinal tract are rare. Moreover, most of the available evidence either comes from in vitro experiments or are indirectly based on stimulation of growth of specific fecal bacteria or fecal excretion of oligosaccharides in germ-free rats. Human in vivo studies in ileostomy volunteers are not available. Iso-maltooligosaccharides are, at least partly, hydrolyzed by isomaltase in the jejunum (Dahlquist, 1964). The soybean oligosaccharides, raffinose and stachyose, are not hydrolyzed to any significant extent by homogenates of rat intestine, and 90% of the ingested dose are recovered in the feces of germ-free rats (Kato et al., 1991), but only some 50% in the feces of antibiotic-treated rats (Yoshida et al., 1969).

For the galactooligosaccharides the only evidence available is increased breath hydrogen concentration in five human volunteers receiving a dose of 0.5 g/kg (Tanaka et al., 1983). But, as discussed by Ito et al. (1990), ''the absolute amount of galactooligosaccharides reaching the colon without digestion in the small intestina cannot be assessed with certainty.'' For polydextrose, the only data available are derived from studies on caloric value (discussed later) using radiolabeled molecules (Figdor and Rennhard, 1981, 1983; Cooley and Livesey, 1987). But data are controversal and recovery balances are incomplete. Fully convincing data that demonstrate that polydextrose is totally or only partly resistant to digestion in the upper gastrointestinal tract are still missing. The palatinose oligosaccharides or palatinose condensates, but not palatinose itself, resist in vitro hydrolysis by stomach acidity, amylase, and rat intestinal homogenates (Mizutani, 1991).

B. Fermentation in the Large Bowel: The Prebiotic Effect

The large bowel is by far the most heavily colonized region of the gastrointestinal tract, with up to 10^{12} bacteria for every gram of gut content. Through the process of fermentation, colonic bacteria (most of which are anaerobes) produce a wide variety of compounds that may affect gut as well as systemic physiology. The fermentation of carbohydrates reaching the large bowel produces short-chain carboxylic acids (mainly acetate, propionate, and butyrate) and lactate, which allow the host to salvage part of the energy of resistant oligosaccharides and which may play a role in regulating both cellular metabolism as well as cell division and differentiation (for review, see Cummings, 1997).

Evidence for fermentation by bacteria colonizing the large bowel may come from in vitro (both analytical and microbiological) and in vivo studies. In addition, in vitro fermentation experiments are used to confirm the production of lactic and short-chain carboxylic acids as end products of the fermentation. For the demonstration of a prebiotic effect, i.e., the selective stimulation of growth of one or a limited number of bacterial species in the colonic microbiota (Gibson and Roberfroid, 1995), only in vivo data are of real value.

1. In Vitro Fermentation of Resistant Oligosaccharides

The first line of evidence supporting the assumption that resistant oligosaccharides are fermented by the colonic microbiota is the demonstration that these carbohydrates are metabolized when incubated with either pure bacteria strains or fecal samples in anaerobic batch cultures. Since such a fermentation is known to produce various acids, changing the culture pH is an easy way to prove that assumption as well as, by using pure cultures, to identify which bacteria have the potential to perform such a metabolic process. Moreover, by estimating the size of the drop in culture pH over a given period of incubation, it is also possible to compare different substrates on a semi-quantitative basis.

Such data have been reported for inulin-type fructans (Hidaka et al., 1986, 1991; Wang, 1993), and they have been reviewed by Roberfroid et al. (1998). In summary, both INU and OFr are well fermented when incubations are performed using human fecal flora as inoculum. Using adequate analytical methods to quantify INU and OFr, it has furthermore been demonstrated that both resistant oligosaccharides are rapidly and completely metabolized by human fecal microflora and that $G_{py}F_n$ and $F_{py}F_n$ type components disappear from the culture media at a similar rate (Roberfroid et al., 1998). In pure cultures, all strains of bifidobacteria except *Bifidobacterium bifidum* utilize inulin-type fructans, which are as good a fermentation substrate as glucose. Bacteria other than bifidobacteria that also have the potential to ferment inulin-type fructans in pure batch cultures include *Klebsiella pneumoniae*, *Staphylococcus aureus* and *S. epidermidis*, *Enterococcus faecalis* and *E. faecium*, *Bacteroides vulgatus*, *B. thetaiotaomicron*, *B. ovatus*, and *B. fragilis*, *Lactobacillus acidophilus*, and *Clostridium* spp. (mainly *C. butyricum*) (Hidaka et al., 1986, 1991; Wang, 1993; Roberfroid et al., 1998). These studies show that, except for a very few bacteria, the fermentability of OFr and SFr is comparable, but that in most cases INU is, among the three fructans, the least efficient fermentation substrate for bacteria other than bifidobacteria.

When analyzing changes in the composition of both batch and chemostat cultures inoculated with human fecal slurries and INU or OFr, Wang and Gibson (1993) and Gibson and Wang (1994a, 1994b) have demonstrated that both inulin and its hydrolysate selectively stimulate the growth of the bifidobacteria, which, at the end of the incubation, become the predominant species (up to 3 orders of magnitude higher in numbers than bacteroides).

In vitro data are also available for the other resistant oligosaccharides. In pure batch cultures, soybean oligosaccharides (raffinose and stachyose) are fermented by various strains of bifidobacteria, except *B. bifidum*, and to a lesser extent by some strains of lactobacilli, bacteroides, and a few others (Masai et al., 1987). Some strains of *Clostridium perfringens* also ferment soybean oligosaccharides and produce gases (Sachs and Olson, 1979). In one sample of human fecal flora, soybean oligosaccharides have been shown to double the number of total viable bacteria and to increase the number and the relative proportion of bifidobacteria (Saito et al., 1992). But since no other bacteria strain was counted in this experiment, it does not demonstrate any (selective) bifidogenic effect.

For the galactooligosaccharides, the only in vitro data available concern pure batch cultures. They demonstrate that these carbohydrates are readily fermentable by bifidobacteria including *B. bifidum*, some but not all strains of bacteroides, lactobacilli, and enterobacteriaceae, but not by eubacteria, fusobacteria, clostridia, and most strains of streptococci (Tanaka et al., 1983). The palatinose oligosaccharides or palatinose condensates, but not palatinose itself, are also fermented in vitro in pure batch cultures by most bifidobacteria species except *B. bifidum* (Mizutani, 1991).

2. In Vivo Fermentation: The Prebiotic Effect

With the inulin-type fructans and xylooligosaccharides, the selective stimulation of fecal bifidobacteria has been demonstrated in rats fed a diet supplemented with 5% resistant oligosaccharides (Campbell et al., 1997). But resistant oligosaccharides have been used in human volunteer studies with the aim to confirm, in vivo, the selective stimulation of the growth of bifidobacteria anticipated from in vitro data.

The most complete and best protocoled studies have been reported by Gibson et al. (1995). These authors have used adult subjects maintained on strictly controlled diets supplemented with 15 g/day of either OFr or INU, and they have applied validated bacteriological methods to identify and count the major bacteria known to be present in the human feces, which were moreover collected anaerobically and cultured within a maximum of 30 minutes after sampling. These studies show that the intake of 15 g/day of OFr or INU significantly modifies the composition of the fecal microbiota by stimulating the growth of bifidobacteria, which, after 2 weeks of the feeding treatment, become by far the most numerically predominant bacterial group. In addition, feeding OFr significantly reduces the count of bacteroides, fusobacteria, and clostridia. These effects last as long as OFr or INU are consumed, but after 2 weeks on a control unsupplemented diet, the composition of the fecal flora was still different from control, indicating that the changes disappeared progressively.

Similar human studies in adult European, Japanese, and North American populations have been reported for inulin-type fructans using different daily doses (4–40 g), but some of these studies report only the changes in the counts of bifidobacteria, thus questioning the selectivity of the effect (Hidaka et al., 1986, 1991; Mitsuoka et al., 1987; Williams et al., 1994; Bouhnik et al., 1996; Buddington et al., 1996; Kleessen et al., 1997). For most of the other resistant oligosaccharides, human studies have also been performed using doses ranging from 3 to 15 g/day given for 1, 2, or 3 weeks. In most of these studies rather complete bacteriological analysis of fresh fecal samples has been performed. The results of these studies are summarized in Table 2.

With soybean oligosaccharides, a dose of 10 g given twice daily for 3 weeks significantly increased the number of bifidobacteria while slightly decreasing the number of clostridia (Masai et al., 1987); a daily dose of 3 g increased not only bifidobacteria but also bacteroides and eubacteria (Hayakawa et al., 1990; Wada et al., 1992). For the galactooligosaccharides, Tanaka et al. (1983) and Ito et al. (1990, 1993) reported evidence for an increase both in bifidobacteria and lactobacilli for doses ranging from 3 to 10 g/day. Rowland and Tanaka (1993) confirmed

Table 2 Effect of Resistant Oligosaccharides on the Number of Bifidobacteria ($\log_{10}$ of colony-forming units/g) in Human Feces

Resistant oligosaccharides and dose	Log$_{10}$ CFUS/g feces				
	Basal value [A]	After treatment [B]	Increase [B]-[A]	p-value	Ref.
Galactooligosaccharides					
0, 2.5, 5, 10 g/d (anova test)	$10^{9.8}$	$10^{10.1}$	0.3	<0.001	Ito et al., 1990
15 g/d	$10^{10.06}$	$10^{10.31}$	0.25	<0.001	Ito et al., 1993
Inulin-type fructans					
SFr 8 g/d	$10^{8.8}$	$10^{9.7}$	0.9	<0.005	Mitsudra et al., 1987
4 g/d	$10^{8.8}$	$10^{9.6}$	0.8	<0.003	Buddington et al., 1996
OFr 15 g/d	$10^{8.8}$	$10^{9.5}$	0.7	<0.001	Gibson et al., 1995
INU 15 g/d	$10^{9.1}$	$10^{10.1}$	1.0	<0.001	Gibson et al., 1995
20 g/d	$10^{7.9}$	$10^{8.8}$	0.9	<0.001	Kleessen et al., 1997
40 g/d	$10^{7.9}$	$10^{9.2}$	1.3	<0.001	Kleessen et al., 1997
Isomaltooligosaccharides					
13.5 g/d	$10^{9.5}$	$10^{10.0}$	0.5	<0.005	Kohmoto et al., 1988
Lactosucrose					
5, 10 g/d	$10^{9.5}$	$10^{10.1}$	0.6	<0.001	Yoneyama et al., 1992
Palatinose condensates					
11.2 g/d	$10^{9.6}$	$10^{10.2}$	0.5	<0.005	Mizutani et al., 1991
Soybean oligosaccharides					
10 g/d	$10^{9.6}$	$10^{10.0}$	0.5	<0.001	Masai et al., 1987
3 g/d	$10^{9.4}$	$10^{10.3}$	0.9	<0.005	Wada et al., 1992

these data in heteroxenic rats bearing human colonic microflora. A daily dose of galactosylsucrose (5 or 10 g/day) similarly stimulates the growth of bifidobacteria after 1 and 2 weeks (Yoneyama et al., 1992). A dose of 13.5 g/day of isomaltooligosaccharides for 2 weeks significantly increased bifidobacteria in both adult and elderly volunteers (Kohmoto et al., 1988). Finally, confirming the results on resistance to digestibility in the upper intestinal tract, palatinose condensates but not palatinose itself stimulated the growth of bifidobacteria.

In all of the studies reported above, none of the other bacteria species had their number changed during the administration of the resistant oligosaccharide. But it must be underlined that, even though statistically significant, the reported increase in bifidobacteria hardly exceeded 0.5 of a $\log_{10}$ unit in populations in which their average number before the treatment was $10^{9.5}$–10^{10} and increasing up to a maximum of $10^{10.5}$, thus calling into question the physiological significance of the changes. Indeed, as discussed previously (Roberfroid et al., 1998), the dose-effect relationship for the increase in bifidobacteria might not be straightforward. Whatever the dose of resistant oligosaccharide used and whatever its nature, the maximum number of bifidobacteria per g of feces at the end of the feeding period will never exceed $10^{9.5}$–10^{10}, and it is the initial number of bifidobacteria in the feces, before supplementing the diet with the resistant oligosaccharide, that may influence the size of the stimulation (the lower the initial count, the larger the stimulation) more than the daily dose itself.

In conclusion, both in vitro and in vivo studies on the fermentation of resistant oligosaccharides demonstrate that they are metabolized by anaerobic bacteria, which are normal constituents of the colonic microbiota. But even if in pure cultures miscellaneous bacterial species have the capacity to use them as fermentation substrate, in mixed cultures mimicking the large bowel as well as in vivo in human volunteers, they may selectively stimulate the growth of bifidobacteria and thus be ''bifidogenic'' and qualify as ''prebiotics,'' i.e., ''a non-digestible food ingredient that beneficially affects the host by selectively stimulating the growth and/or the activity of one or a limited number of bacteria in the colon and thus improves host health'' (Gibson and Roberfroid, 1995). However, at this stage such a demonstration has convincingly be made only for the inulin-type fructans.

III. PHYSIOLOGICAL EFFECTS IN THE GASTROINTESTINAL TRACT

A. Production of Short-Chain Carboxylic Acids and Related Effects

The colonic fermentation of resistant oligosaccharides produces short-chain carboxylic acids and lactate plus gases. Only part of the energy of these dietary carbohydrates is salvaged, and consequently they qualify as low-energy food ingredients. Indeed, their available energy content is only 40–50% that of a digestible carbohydrate, giving them a caloric value of 1.5–2 kcal/g. The only resistant oligosaccharides for which data have been published to determine a caloric value are INU, OFr, and polydextrose. For INU and OFr the reported values vary between 1 and 2.1 kcal/g (4.2–8.8 kJ/g) (Hosoya et al., 1988; Livesey, 1992; Roberfroid et al., 1993; Molis et al., 1996) and for polydextrose between 1 and 3 kcal/g (4.2–12.6 kJ/g) (Figdor and Rennhard, 1981, 1983; Cooley and Livesey, 1987; Bernier and Pascal, 1990; Livesey, 1992). But, as stated recently by a group of experts, ''all carbohydrates which are more or less completely fermented in human colon, should be given a caloric value of 1.5 Kcal/g (6.3 KJ/g).'' Indeed the daily intake of these dietary carbohydrates is likely to remain relatively small, probably often not more than 5% of total daily calorie intake (Cummings and Frohlich, 1993). Thus, it is scientifically not justifiable to spend much effort in trying to give, for each such carbohydrate, a precise caloric value, the determination of which will often depend on the protocol used (Cummings and Roberfroid, 1997).

Unless very sophisticated studies are performed in humans to measure short-chain carboxylic acids in situ and/or in the portal blood, it is impossible to know their pattern of production precisely. What is excreted in the feces is by no means representative of the in situ situation because up to 95% of the acids produced in the colon are absorbed, most probably in the ascending part of the colon. Data reporting an absence of modification of the fecal pattern of these acids in human volunteers fed inulin-type fructans are by no means relevant. Only in vitro fermentation and animal studies have, up to now, been used to estimate the effect of nondigestible carbohydrates on short-chain carboxylic acids production. From animal in vivo studies, it can be concluded that supplementing diet with resistant oligosaccharides decreases the cecal pH and increases the size of the cecal pool of short-chain carboxylic acids, with acetate being the primary acid followed by butyrate and propionate (Imaizumi et al., 1991; Rowland and Tanaka, 1993; Ito et al., 1993; Hoshi et al., 1994; Campbell et al., 1997).

Possibly related to this increase in the pool of short-chain carboxylic acids is the effect of some resistant oligosaccharides on the intestinal tissue leading to hyperplasia of the mucosa and increased wall thickness in both the small intestine and the cecum (Oku et al., 1984; Hoshi et al., 1994; Campbell, 1997). Additional effects of resistant oligosaccharides in the large bowel relate to the activity of either intestinal or bacterial enzymes, e.g., an increase in cecal wall ornithine decarboxylase (Rémésy et al., 1993), an increase in bacterial β-fructosidase and β-glucosidase (Rowland and Tanaka, 1993; Rowland et al., 1998), a decrease (Rowland and Tanaka, 1993; Buddington et al., 1996; Rowland et al., 1998) or no effect on bacterial β-glucuronidase except for soybean oligosaccharides, which induced an increase (Saito et al., 1992), no effect on reductases (Buddington et al., 1996); to the concentration of metabolites like glycocholic acid (Buddington et al., 1996) and NH_3 (Wada et al., 1992; Ito et al., 1993; Rowland et al., 1998), which are both decreased; and to the mucins, in particular sulfomucin and sialomucin, which are decreased and increased respectively in rats fed INU (Fontaine et al., 1996). Moreover, because of the stimulation of bacterial growth leading to an increase in bacterial biomass, INU, OFr (Roberfroid et al., 1993; Gibson et al., 1995) but not galactooligosaccharides (Ito et al., 1990) have been shown to increase fresh fecal mass either in rats or in humans.

B. Effect on Mineral Absorption

The nondigestible carbohydrates (dietary fiber) have regularly been accused of causing an impairment in the small intestinal absorption of minerals due to their binding/sequestering. Many studies have indicated that nondigestible carbohydrates per se do not affect mineral absorption or mineral balance, an effect which is more likely to be due to the presence of phytate or other mineral complexing agents. However, the minerals that are bound/sequestered and, consequently, are not absorbed in the small intestine reach the colon, where they may released from the carbohydrate matrix and absorbed.

That INU and OFr do not impair mineral absorption in the small intestine has been reported by Ellegärd et al. (1997) in ileostomy patients. Indeed, these authors have demonstrated that the amount of Ca, Mg, and Fe ions recovered in the ileostomate over a 3-day period is not significantly modified after supplementing the diet with 17 g/day of these fructans.

Using growing rats (both males and females), various group have consistently reported that inulin-type fructans enhance Ca^{2+} and Mg^{2+} absorption (Demigné et al., 1989; Delzenne et al., 1995; Ohta et al., 1995) as well as iron ions and Zn^{2+} balance without having significant effect on Cu^{2+} bioavailability (69). Similarly, galactooligosaccharides enhance calcium absorption in rats (Chonan and Watanuki, 1995). Doses of inulin-type fructans in the rat diet varied from 5 to 20%.

The hypotheses most frequently proposed to explain this enhancing effect of resistant carbohydrate on mineral absorption are the osmotic effect; acidification of the colonic content due to fermentation and production of short-chain carboxylic acids; formation of calcium and magnesium salts of these acids; and hypertrophy of the colon wall (Younes et al., 1996; Coudray et al., 1997). But according to Ohta et al. (1994, 1996) different mechanisms may be involved in the increased absorption of Ca^{2+} or Mg^{2+}, the former being absorbed mostly in the cecum and the latter mostly in the colon. In addition to improvement in Ca balance, Ohta et al. (1996) also reported that feeding SFr increases calcium concentration in the femur.

More recently, and based on the consistently repeated observations in rats, in vivo human studies have been performed that confirm the positive effect of INU and OFr on the absorption and balance of dietary calcium but not of iron, magnesium, or zinc. In the first published report, 9 male men (21.5 ± 2.5 years) taking in ±850 mg calcium/day and receiving a dietary supplement of 40 g/day of INU had a significant increase in the apparent absorption (±12%) and balance (+100 mg/day) of calcium without any change in urinary excretion (Coudray et al., 1997). In the second study, twelve 15- to 18-year-old boys consumed 16.8 g of OFr/day, and their calcium balance, measured by the double stable isotope technique, showed an 11% increase ($p = 0.09$) with no effect on urinary excretion (van den Heuvel et al., 1999).

C. Influence of Fructans on Glycemia/Insulinemia

The only resistant oligosaccharides for which published data are available related to their effect on glucose or lipid metabolism are the inulin-type fructans. The only exception is the xylooligosaccharides, for which it has been reported that the octa- and nonasaccharides containing a D-galactose residue at nonreducing terminals inhibit absorption of 3-O-methyl-D-glucose in the rat (Sone et al., 1992) and that in diabetic rats these resistant oligosaccharides improve glycemia (Imaizumi et al., 1991).

The effects of inulin-type fructans on glycemia and insulinemia are not yet fully understood, and available data are sometimes contradictory, indicating that these effects may depend on physiological (fasting vs. postprandial state) or disease (diabetes) conditions. OFr, given at the dose of 10% in the diet of rats for 30 days, reduces postprandial glycemia and insulinemia by 17 and 26%, respectively (Kok et al., 1996a). However, the glycemic response during a glucose-tolerance test after overnight fasting was identical in control and OFr-fed rats (Kok, 1998).

Furthermore, it has been reported that in rats fed 10% SFr for 3 months, the glycemic response to sucrose or maltose load is reduced, most probably as a result of a reduction of dissacharidase activity in the gastrointestinal tract (Oku et al., 1984). Similarly, chronic ingestion of SFr (20 g per day for 4 weeks) does not modify fasting plasma glucose and insulin in healthy human volunteers, even if it lowers basal hepatic glucose production (Luo et al., 1996). However, diabetic subjects taking 8 g/day of SFr for 14 days showed a decrease in fasting blood glucose (Yamashita et al., 1984). Finally, when 10 g of artichoke INU was added to 50 g wheat-starch meal in healthy human subjects, the blood glycemic response was lower, despite no apparent interference of INU with starch absorption. (Rumessen et al., 1990).

IV. SYSTEMIC PHYSIOLOGICAL EFFECTS

A. Effect on Lipid Metabolism

The only reported effects on triglyceridemia concern inulin-type fructans, which have been studied both in human subjects and in animals. In rats, a decrease in serum triglyceridemia (both in fed and fasted state) has consistently been reported in several studies, whereas in healthy humans, only fasting triglycerides have been measured and they are not modified (Rumessen et al., 1990; Luo et al., 1996; Pedersen et al., 1997) except in one study (Canzi et al., 1995). No data have yet been published reporting studies performed in hypertriglyceridemic patients. Data concerning effects of inulin-type fructans on cholesterolemia and/or lipoproteinemia are scarce.

1. Effect on Triglyceride Metabolism

Feeding rats on a diet supplemented with OFr (10%) significantly lowers serum triglycerides and phospholipids concentrations (Fiordaliso et al., 1995) but does not modify free fatty acid concentration in the serum. The hypotriglyceridemia is mostly due to a decrease in the concentration of plasma very-low-density lipoproteins (VLDL) (Fiordaliso et al., 1995). This effect is likely to result from a decrease in the hepatic synthesis of triglycerides rather than from a higher catabolism of triglycerides-rich lipoproteins (Kok et al., 1996b). These data support the hypothesis that a decreased de novo lipogenesis in the liver, through a coordinate reduction of the activity of all lipogenic enzymes, is a key event in the reduction of VLDL-TG secretion in fructans-fed rats. The fact that de novo lipogenesis is the basis for the hypotriglyceridemic effect of fructans in rat liver might explain the lack of effect observed in healthy humans, who eat far fewer carbohydrates than rodents. Some experiments should be performed either in obese patients or in insulin-resistant individuals eating high-carbohydrate, high-calorie diets.

2. Effect on Cholesterolemia

This effect is controversial. SFr has been shown to lower serum total and LDL cholesterol in non–insulin-dependent diabetic patients but not in healthy subjects (Yamashita et al., 1984; Luo et al., 1996). Long-term (16 weeks) administration of OFr also decreases total cholesterol level in the serum of rats (Fiordaliso et al., 1995). Ellegärd et al. (1997) have shown that OFr influence neither the absorption of dietary cholesterol nor the excretion of cholesterol or bile acids in ileostomic subjects. The role of short-chain carboxylic acids in these effects is difficult to establish, because, either in isolation or in mixture, these acids have antagonistic effects on cholesterol metabolism; acetate, being a metabolic precursor of cholesterol, has been claimed to be at the origin of the hypercholesterolemia observed in healthy patients receiving lactulose (Jenkins et al., 1991), whereas propionate, which lowers serum cholesterol when given in the diet of rats, may decrease cholesterol synthesis by inhibiting HMG-CoA reductase (Rodwell et al., 1976). Davidson et al. (1998) reported preliminary data in slightly hypercholesterolemic human volunteers that indicate that INU (18 g/day for 3 weeks) may lower both total and LDL serum cholesterol.

B. Effect on Uremia and Nitrogen/Urea Disposal

Feeding rats a diet supplemented with INU and OFr (10%) for a few weeks decreases uremia in both normal and nephrectomized rats (Delzenne et al., 1995; Younes et al., 1997). Dietary SFr effectively enhances fecal nitrogen excretion and reduces renal excretion of nitrogen in rats (Younes et al., 1996). This occurs because these fermentable carbohydrates serve as an energy source for the intestinal bacteria, which, during growth, also require a source of nitrogen for protein synthesis. In addition, their osmotic effect in the small intestine accelerates the transfer of urea into the distal ileum and the large intestine, where a highly ureolytic microflora may proliferate. As a matter of fact, when fermentable carbohydrates intake is high, the amount of ammonia required to sustain maximal bacterial growth may become insufficient and blood urea is then required as readily source for bacterial protein synthesis in the cecum (Younes et al., 1997). Besides its effect in the gastrointestinal tract and its possible role in modulating lipogenesis, propionate, an important end product of bacterial fermentation of inulin-type fructans, also inhibits ureagenesis in the liver in the presence of ammonia and amino acids. But the direct extrapolation of such results (decreased uremia, shift of N excretion towards the colon) to humans is uncertain due to differences in digestive tract structure or in colonic microflora. In humans, consumption of nondigestible carbohydrates also results in a higher fecal excretion of nitrogen (Stephen and Cummings, 1980; Mortensen, 1982). In addition to increasing total nitrogen transfer to the colon, it is important to limit the formation of ammonia and various end products of protein catabolism, which have been proposed as causative risk factors for colonic carcinogenesis in the distal part of the large bowel (Lupton and Marchand, 1989).

V. SAFETY ISSUES AND ACCEPTABILITY

Being composed of natural monosaccharide units which are hydrolysed and fermented by the endogenous bacteria of the colonic microbiota to produce short chain fatty acids, the resistant oligosaccharides are not of toxicological concern. Moreover, as discussed in this chapter they classify as dietary fiber which are ''generally recognized as safe.'' Such arguments have been taken into consideration by most european health authorities who have classified the inulin-type fructans as natural food ingredients or cleared the SFr as novel food. An extensive toxicological evaluation had previously shown no deleterious effect of these particular resistant oligosaccharides (SFr) in traditional toxicity tests (Clevenger et al 1988).

However, because of their osmotic effect, which may transfer water into the large bowel (an effect inversely related to chain length), and because of their high fermentation rate and production of gases, high doses may cause intestinal discomfort or even diarrhea. This effect is not specific for the resistant oligosaccharides but is common to all nondigested/fermented dietary substrates. The evaluation of an "acceptable dose" is difficult because individual evaluations of "acceptable" and "nonacceptable" intestinal discomfort are subjective.

Data are available concerning the relationship between the intake of inulin-type fructans and gastrointestinal symptoms (Hata and Nakajima, 1985; Stone-Dorshow and Levitt, 1987; Absolonne et al., 1995; Pellier et al., 1995). Based on these data, the following conclusions can be reached:

In liquid form, a single dose of 10 g will cause no effect, whereas 20 g may cause mild transient symptoms.

Except for very resistant individuals, who are probably adapted to a high fruit-vegetable-cereal diet, the single daily dose likely to cause major discomfort or even diarrhea in most people is of the order of 30 g.

If the inulin-type fructans are taken as part of a solid formula, the sensitive dose is relatively higher than in liquid formula.

If the dose is split over the day in a few individual servings, symptoms will be reduced and, in most cases, will disappear even for doses as high as 20–30 g.

A small percentage (1–3%) of the population might have higher than average sensitivity to intestinal discomfort when consuming even relatively small single daily doses, but these highly sensitive individuals are also likely to be very sensitive to the intestinal effects of sugar alcohols or any nondigestible carbohydrates or even fermented dairy products.

VI. RESISTANT OLIGOSACCHARIDES AS FUNCTIONAL FOOD INGREDIENTS: POTENTIAL APPLICATIONS IN RISK REDUCTION OF DISEASES

Resistant oligosaccharides have nutritional properties which, in the present state of scientific knowledge, originate mainly in resistance to the hydrolytic activities in the upper part of the digestive tract of monogastric organisms followed by extensive fermentation in the large bowel. As discussed above, they have the key characteristics of dietary fibers, and a method has recently been approved by AOAC to include the inulin-type fructans in the analysis of complex carbohydrates. In addition, because they selectively stimulate the growth of bifidobacteria in the colonic microbiota, they are model type "prebiotics." Resistant oligosaccharides are obvious candidates to be recognized as functional food ingredients for which health claims may become authorized.

A. Functional Food Ingredients: Definition, Strategy, and Health Claims

In general terms, a functional food ingredient can be defined as "a food ingredient which affects physiological function(s) of the body in a targeted way so as to have positive effect(s) which may, in due course, justify health claims" (Roberfroid, 1995, 1996). A proposed strategy to develop the science base necessary to support such claims involves:

1. The identification of the interaction(s) between the food ingredient and genomic, biochemical, cellular, or physiological function(s) in the body.
2. The demonstration of functional effect(s) in relevant experimental and human models.
3. The investigation, in humans, of the consequence(s) of the functional effect(s), including effects on relevant biomarkers and possible health benefits.

Two different levels of health claims have tentatively been identified (Roberfroid, 1996):

1. A functional claim, which refers to an effect on a specific or a limited number of genomic, biochemical, cellular or physiological function(s) with no proven of fully understood relation to a particular disease. Examples of such claims are bifidogenic effect, increased bioavailability of minerals, hypotriglyceridemic activity, stimulation of a particular immune function.
2. A disease risk reduction claim, which refers specifically to effect(s) on the risk of a particular disease. Examples of such claims are prevention of diarrhea or constipation, reduction of risk of carcinogenesis, cardiovascular disease, diabetes, obesity.

It is the objective of this part of the chapter to put the basic and still mostly experimental scientific information presently available on the effects of resistant oligosaccharides on both gastrointestinal and systemic functions in perspective with potential health claims.

B. Resistant Oligosaccharides: Scientific Evidence for Functional Claims

The available scientific evidence that support or may be used to support functional claims must be critically assessed in terms of "strong," "promising," or "preliminary" evidence (Table 3).

The selective stimulation of growth of bifidobacteria in the fecal flora is demonstrated both in experimental and in human studies for many resistant oligosaccharides. The scientific evidence for a "bifidogenic" effect of inulin-type fructans is "strong" and it can be used to support an application for a functional claim, i.e., "a modification of the composition of the colonic flora." Such a claim has already been officially cleared by the french *Conseil supérieur*

Table 3 Potential Health Claims for Resistant Oligosaccharides: Assessment of Scientific Evidences

Type of health claim	Assessment of evidence	Type of product
Functional claims		
Bifidogenic effect	Strong	Inulin-like fructans
	Preliminary	Other resistant oligosaccharides
Fecal bulking	Promising	Inulin-type fructans
Increased Ca bioavailability	Promising	Inulin-type fructans
	Preliminary	Galactooligosaccharides
Hypotriglyceridemic effect	Preliminary	OFr (INU)
Hypocholesterolemic effect	?	?
Reduction or risk of disease		
Constipation	Preliminary	Inulin-type fructans
Infectious diarrhea	?	?
Osteoporosis	?	?
Atherosclerotic cardiovascular disease	?	?
Obesity	?	?
Colon cancer	Preliminary	Inulin-type fructans

d'Hygiène publique for food products containing OFr or Sfr. For the other resistant oligosaccharides, namely galacto-, soybean, and isomaltooligosaccharides, the evidence is still preliminary and more human studies are needed. Even though the question of dose effectiveness is still debated, the dose-effect relationship for such an effect on a complex ecosystem like colonic microbiota may not be straightforward. It may depend on other factors like the initial number of bifidobacteria (Roberfroid et al., 1998). This could lead to the conclusion that, at the population level, the question of the dose is of low relevance and that, on an average base, taking into account the variability in the number of bifidobacteria in the human colonic flora, doses of a few grams per day are effective in stimulating the growth of these bacteria classified as potentially beneficial for health (Gibson and Roberfroid, 1995). An indirect consequence of the stimulation of growth of bifidobacteria is fecal bulking, for which promising evidence has been published (Roberfroid et al., 1993; Gibson et al., 1995).

A second effect of resistant oligosaccharides worth considering when discussing potential functional claims is increased bioavailability of minerals. If data on the balance of Mg, Fe, or Zn are too preliminary to be taken into consideration, scientific evidences does exist to support effects on Ca. For INU and OFr, such an effect has been reported both in experimental animals and in humans, and the evidence has been assessed as promising. But for SFr and galactooligosaccharides, since only experimental data are presently available, the evidence has been assessed only as preliminary. The effects of resistant oligosaccharides on lipid metabolism are also discussed in this chapter. Experimental data are convincing in supporting the hypothesis that OFr inhibits hepatic lipogenesis in rats and, consequently, induces a significant hypotriglyceridemic effect. The potential mechanisms of this effect include metabolic effects of short-chain carboxylic acids and/or low glycemia/insulinemia. Except for one study, this hypolipidemic effect has, up to now, not been confirmed in human volunteers consuming either INU, OFr, or any other resistant oligosaccharide. The evidence for an effect on cholesterolemia is scarce both in experimental and in human models. When assessing these data, the authors concluded that preliminary evidence exists for a hypotriglyceridemic effect for OFr and possibly INU but that, at the present stage of knowledge, it is impossible to confirm the hypocholesterolemic effect as well as the hypolipidemic effects of SFr or any other resistant oligosaccharides. Because a metabolic link has recently been demonstrated between insulin resistance and the associated risk factors for atherosclerotic cardiovascular disease, especially hypertriglyceridemia, and because of the growing awareness that hypertriglyceridemia itself may be a risk factor in atherogenesis, these potential functional effects need to be carefully studied in humans, especially in conditions known to be associated with hyperinsulinemia and hypertriglyceridemia (Taskinen, 1993; Aarsland et al., 1996).

C. Resistant Oligosaccharides: Scientific Evidence for Disease Risk Reduction Claims

For resistant oligosaccharides, disease risk reduction claims are, based on presently available scientific information, only tentative, and they still need more research to be supported and validated. The most promising areas for the development of such claims are:

1. Constipation relief due to fecal bulking and possibly effects on intestinal motility (Kleessen et al., 1997).
2. Inhibition of diarrhea, especially associated with intestinal infections. This may be directly related to the possible inhibtory effect of bifidobacteria both on gram-positive and gram-negative bacteria, which has been reported by Wang (1993) and Wang and Gibson (1994b).

3. Reduction of risk of osteoporosis if indeed they improve the bioavailability of Ca and if this functional effect is followed by a more physiological change in peak bone density and bone mass.

4. reduction of the risk of atheroclerotic cardiovascular disease associated with dyslipidemia, especially hypertriglyceridemia, and insulin resistance, which, in particular, is known to be associated with hypercaloric high-carbohydrate feeding regimens (Aarsland et al., 1996). The reduction of risk via a hypocholesterolemic effect still needs further investigation as well as sound mechanistic hypothesis to be tested in humans.

5. Reduction of the risk of obesity and possibly non–insulin-dependent diabetes, both of which are known to be associated with insulin resistance.

A last area for further research in the context of disease risk reduction by resistant oligosaccharides is cancer. Indeed, experimental data have been published that demonstrate that feeding rats with inulin-type fructans or galactooligosaccharides significantly reduced the incidence of the so-called aberrant crypt foci induced by colon carcinogens like azoxymethane or dimethylhydrazine (Koo et al 1991; Gallaher et al 1996; Reddy et al 1997; Rowland et al 1998). For this particular effect a symbiotic approach combining resistant oligosaccharides and bifidobacteria was shown to be more active than either the probiotic or the prebiotic approach alone (Gallaher et al 1996; Rowland et al 1998). Furthermore, Pierre et al. (1997) demonstrated that SFr reduces or even suppresses the number of tumors and stimulates the gut-associated lymphoid tissue (number of lymphoid nodules) in transgenic *Min* mice; Taper et al. (1997) reported that supplementing mice diet with INU or OFr slows down the growth rate of two different implanted tumors as compared to control rats; Fontaine et al. (1996) reported that, in heteroxenic rats harboring a human colonic flora, INU stimulates the production of sulfomucin and a reduction in sialomucin, two effects known to be associated with a reduced risk of colon cancer. Moreover, Rowland and Tanaka (1993) reported that feeding rats a diet supplemented with 5% galactooligosaccharides decreases the conversion, by cecal contents, of the dietary carcinogen 2-amino-3-methyl-3H-imidazol [4,5-f] quinoline (IQ) to its genotoxic 7-hydroxy derivative. In the strategy for functional food development described above, these cancer-inhibiting effects in experimental animals correspond to the first step (i.e., identification) of effects that, because of their potential implications in human health, will need careful evaluation including in relevant human studies.

VII. CONCLUSION: DIETARY ROLE FOR RESISTANT OLIGOSACCHARIDES

Besides their positive effects on human health, resistant oligosaccharides offer functional properties to processed food that have increased their use. Many of these products function as soluble dietary fibers. Inulin is known as a fat replacer and texture modifier for processed foods. In low-fat systems, inulin provides a creamy mouthfeel through texture modification. Other applications include salad dressing, baked goods, low-fat cheese, no-fat icings and glazes, chocolate, and confectionery. In meat products, inulin gel binds water, adds freeze-thaw stability, emulsifies, and adds creaminess. Other oligosaccharides such as polydextrose function as dietary fiber and thus can be used to reduce the caloric density of a product. Shorter-chain fructooligosaccharides are actually sweet and can replace other sugars in the product. Our nutrition message must continue to be to increase consumption of foods high in complex carbohydrates, including dietary fiber, resistant starch, and resistant oligosaccharides.

Because many consumers depend on processed foods as the mainstay of their diets, efforts should be made to increase the fiber and resistant oligosaccharide content of popular foods to assist consumers in obtaining recommended levels of carbohydrate.

REFERENCES

Aarsland A, Chinkes D, Wolfe RR. Contribution of de novo synthesis of fatty acids to total VLDL-triglyceride secretion during prolonged hyperglycemia/hyperinsulinemia in normal man. J Clin Invest 98: 2008–2017, 1996.

Abslonne J, Jossart M, Coussement P, Roberfroid M. Digestive acceptability of oligofructose. Proceed. 1st ORAFTI Research Conf., Brussels, January 1995.

Asp N. Nutritional classification and analysis of food carbohydrate. Am J Clin Nutr 59(suppl):679S–681S, 1994.

Asp NG, Schweizer TF, Southgate DAT, Theander O. Dietary fibre analysis. In: TF Schweiser and CA Edwards, eds. Dietary Fibre. A Component of Food. Nutritional Functions in Health and Disease. London: Springer, 57–100, 1992.

Bach Knudsen KE, Hessov I. Recovery of inulin from Jerusalem artichoke (*Helianthus tuberosus* L.) in the small intestine of man. Br J Nutr 74:101–113, 1995.

Bernier JJ, Pascal G. Valeurs énergétiques des polyols (sucres-alcools). Méd Nutr 26:221–238, 1990.

Bouhnik Y, Flourie B, Riottot M, Bisetti N, Gailing, M, Guibert A, Bornet F, Rambaud J. Effects of fructo-oligosaccharides ingestion on fecal bifidobacteria and selected metabolic indexes of colon carcinogenesis in healthy humans. Nutr Cancer 26:21–29, 1996.

British Nutrition Foundation. Complex Carbohydrates in Foods: Report of the British Nutrition's Task Force. London: Chapman and Hall, 1990.

Buddington RK, Williams CH, Chen SC, Witherly SA. Dietary supplement of Neosugar alters the faecal flora and decreases activities of some reductive enzymes in human subjects. Am J Clin Nutr 63: 709–716, 1996.

Campbell JM, Fahey GC, Wolf BW. Selected indigestible oligosaccharides affect large bowel mass, cecal and fecal short-chain fatty acids, ph and microflora in rats. J Nutr 127:130–136, 1997.

Canzi E, Brighenti F, Casighari MC, Del Puppo E, Ferrari A. Prolonged consumption of inulin in ready-to-eat breakfast cereals: effects on intestinal ecosystem, bowel habits and lipid mertabolism. Cost 92, workshop on dietary fiber and fermentation in the colon, Helsinki, 15–17 April, 1995.

Chonan O, Watanuki M. Effect of galactooligosaccharides on calcium absorption in rats. J Nutr Sci Vitaminol 41:95–104, 1995.

Cooley S, Livesey G. The metabolizable energy value of polydextrose in mixed diet fed to rats. Br J Nutr 57:235–243, 1987.

Coudray C, Bellange J, Castiglia-Delahaut C, Rémésy C, Vermorel M, Demigné C. Effect of soluble and partly soluble dietary fibres supplementation on absorption and balance of calcium, magnesium, iron and zinc in healthy young men. Eur J Clin Nutr 51:375–380, 1997.

Crittenden RG, Playne MJ. Production, properties and applications of food grade oligosaccharides. Trends Food Sci Technol 7:353–361, 1997.

Cummings JH. The Large Intestine in Nutrition and Disease. Brussels: Danone Chair Monograph, Institut Danone, 1997.

Cummings JH, Frohlich W, eds. Dietary Fibre Intakes in Europe: An Overview. Brussels: Commission of the European Communinity—DGXII—COST 92, 1993.

Cummings JH., Roberfroid MB, et al. A new look at dietary carbohydrate: chemistry, physiology and health. Eur J Clin Nutr 51:417–423, 1996.

Dahlquist A. Method for assay of intestinal disaccharidases. Anal Biochem 7:18–25, 1964.

Davidson MH, Maki KC, Synecki C, Torri SA, Drennan KB. Evaluation of the influence of dietary inulin on serum lipids in adults with hypercholesterolemia. Nutr Res 18:503–517, 1998.

Debruyn A, Alvarez AP, Sandra P, DeLeenheer L. Isolation and identification of β-D-fructosyl-(2,1)-D-fructose, a product of the enzymatic hydrolysis of the inulin from Cichorium intybus. Carbohydr Res 235:303–308, 1992.

Delzenne N, Roberfroid MB. Physiological effects of non digestible oligosaccharides. Lebensm Wiss Technol 27:1–6, 1994.

Delzenne N, Aertssens J, Verplaetse H, Roccaro M, Roberfroid M. Effect of fermentable fructo-ologosaccharides on mineral, nitrogen and energy digestive balance in the rats. Life Sci 57:1579–1587, 1995.

Demigné C, Levrat AM, Rémésy C. Effects of feeding fermentable carbohydrates on caecal concentration of minerals and their fluxes between the cecum and blood plasma in the rat. J Nutr 119:1625–1630, 1989.

Drasar BS, Hill MJ. The distribution of bacterial flora in the intestine. In: Drasar BS, Hill MJ, eds. Human Intestinal Flora. London: Academic Press, 1974.

Ellegärd L, Andersson H, Bosaeus I. Inulin and oligofructose do not influence the absorption of cholesterol, or the excretion of cholesterol, Ca, Mg, Zn, Fe, or bile acids but increases energy excretion in ileostomy subjects. Eur J Clin Nutr 51:1–5, 1997.

Englyst HN, Hudson GJ. The classification and measurement of dietary carbohydrates. Food Chem 57: 15–21, 1996.

Figdor SK, Rennhard JR. Caloric utilisation and deposition of [^{14}C]-polydextrose in the rat. J Agric Food Chem 29:1181–1189, 1981.

Figdor SK, Rennhard JR. Caloric utilisation and deposition of [^{14}C]-polydextrose in man. J Agric Food Chem 31:389–393, 1983.

Fiordaliso MF, Kok N, Desager JP, Goethals F, Deboyser D, Roberfroid M, Delzenne N. Dietary oligofructose lowers triglycerides, phospholipids and cholesterol in serum and very low density lipoproteins of rats. Lipids 30:163–167, 1995.

Fontaine N, Meslin JC, Lory S, Andrieux C. Intestinal mucin distribution in the germ-free rat and in the heteroxenic rat harbouring a human bacetrial flora: effect of inulin in the diet. Br J Nutr 75:881–892, 1996.

Food and Drug Administration. Food labelling: mandatory status of nutrition labelling and nutrient content revision, format for nutrition label. Fed Reg 58:2079–2228, 1993.

Food Guide Pyramid. Washington, DC: U.S. Dept of Agriculture, Human Nutrition Information Service, 1992.

Fujita K, Kitahata S, Kozo H, Hotoshi H. Production of lactosucrose and its properties. In: MA Clarke, ed. Carbohydrates in Industrial Synthesis. Berlin: Proc. Symp. Div. Carbohydr. Chem. Amer. Chem. Soc., Bartens, 68–76, 1992.

Gallaher DD, Stallings WH, Blessing L, Busta FF, Brady LJ. Probiotics, cecal microflora and aberrant crypts in the rat colon. J Nutr 126:1362–1371, 1996.

Gibson GR, Roberfroid MB. Dietary modulation of the human colonic macrobiota: introducing the concept of prebiotics. J Nutr 125:1401–1412, 1995.

Gibson GR, Wang X. Enrichment of bifidobacteria from human gut contents by oligofructose using continuous culture. FEMS Microbiol Lett 118:121–128, 1994a.

Gibson GR, Wang X. Inhibitory effect of bifidobacteria on other colonic bacteria. J Appl Bacteriol 65: 103–111, 1994b.

Gibson GR, Beatty ER, Wang X, Cummings JH. Selective stimulation of bifidobacteria in the human colon by oligofructose and inulin. Gastroenterology 108:975–982, 1995.

Hata Y, Nakajima K Relationship between fructo-oligosaccharide intake and gastrointestinal symptoms. Geriatr Med 23:817–828, 1985.

Hayakawa K, Mizutani J, Wada K, Masai T, Yoshihara I, Mitsuoka T. Effects of soybean oligosaccharides on human faecal microflora. Microb Ecol Health Dis 3:293–303, 1990.

Hidaka H, Eida T, Takizawa T, Tokunaga T, Tashiro Y. Effects of fructooligosaccharides on intestinal flora and human health. Bifidobacteria Microflora 5:37–50, 1986.

Hidaka H, Tashiro Y, Eida T. Proliferation of bifidobacteria by oligosaccharides and their useful effect on human health. Bifidobacteria Microflora 10:65–79, 1991.

Hoebergs H. Fructans in foods and food products, ion-exchange chromatographic method-collaborative study. J AOAC Int 80:1029–1037, 1997.

Hoshi S, Sakata T, Mikuni K, Hashimoto H, Kimura S. Galactosylsucrose and xylosylfructoside alter digestive tract size and concentration of organic acids in rats fed diets containing cholesterol and cholic acid. J Nutr 124:52–60, 1994.

Hosoya N, Dhorranintra B, Hidaka H. Utilization of [U-14C] fructooligosaccharides in man as energy resources. J Clin Biochem Nutr 5:67–74, 1988.

Imaizumi K, Nakatsu Y, Sato M, Sedarnawati Y, Sugano M. Effects of xylooligosaccharides on blood glucose, serum and liver lipids and cecum short-chain fatty acids in diabetic rats. Agric Biol Chem 55:199–205, 1991.

Ito M, Deguchi Y, Miyamori A, Kikuchi H, Matsumoto K, Kobayashi Y, Yajima T, Kan T. Effect of administration of galcto-oligosaccharides on the human faecal microflora, stool weight and abdominal sensation. Micro Ecol Health Dis 3:285–292, 1990.

Ito M, Kimura M, Deguchi Y, Miyamori-Watabe A, Yajima T, Kan T. Effects of transgalactosylated disaccharides on the human intestinal flora and theri metabolism. J Nutr Sci Vitaminol 39:279–288, 1993.

IUB-IUPAC. Joint Commission on Biochemical Nomenclature & (JCBN): Abbreviated Terminology of Oligosaccharide Chains. Recommendations 1980. J Biol Chem 257:3347–3351, 1982.

Jenkins DJA, Wolever TMS, Jenkins A. Specific types of colonic fermentation may raise low-density-lipoprotein-cholesterol concentrations. Am J Clin Nutr 54:141–147, 1991.

Kato Y, Ikeda N, Iwanami T, Ozaki A, Ohmura K. Change of soybean oligosaccharides in the digestive tract. Nippon Eiyo Shokuryo Gakkaishi 44:29–35, 1991.

Kleessen B, Sykura B, Zunft HJ, Blaut M. Effect of inulin and lactose on faecal microflora, microbial activity, and bowel habit in elderly constipated persons. Am J Clin Nutr 65:1397–1402, 1997.

Kohmoto T, Fukui F, Takaku H, Machida Y, Arai M, Mitsuoka T. Effect of isomalto-oligosaccharides on human fecal flora. Bifidobacteria Microflora 7:61–69, 1988.

Kok N. PhD thesis. Brussels: Université Catholique de Louvain, 1998.

Kok N, Roberfroid M, Delzenne N. Involvement of lipogenesis in the lower VLDL secretion induced by oligofructose in rats. Br J Nutr 76:881–890, 1996a.

Kok N, Roberfroid M, Delzenne N. Dietary oligofructose modifies the impact of fructose on hepatic triacyl-glycerol metabolism. Metabolism 45:1547–1550, 1996b.

Koo M, Rao V. Long term effect of bifidobacteria and Neosugar on precursor lesions of colonic cancer in mice. Nutr Cancer 16:249–257, 1991.

Livesey G. The energy values of dietary fibre and sugar alcohols for man. Nutr Res Rev 5:61–84, 1992.

Luo J, Rizkala S, Alamowitch C, Boussairi A, Blayo A, Barry J, Laffitte A, Guyon F, Bornet FRJ, Slama G. Chronic consumption of short-chain fructooligosaccharides by healthy subjects decreased basal glucose production but had no effect on insulin-stimulated glucose metabolism. Am J Clin Nutr 63: 939–945, 1996.

Lupton JR, Marchand LJ. Independent effects of fiber and pectin on colonic luminal ammonia concentration. J Nutr 119:235–241, 1989.

Masai T, Wada K, Hayakawa K. Effects of soybean oligosaccharides on human intestinal flora and metabolic activities. Jpn J Bacteriol 42:313–329, 1987.

Mitsuoka T, Hidaka H, Eida T. Effect of fructo-oligosaccharides on intestinal microflora. Nahrung 31: 426–436, 1987.

Mizutani T. Properties and use of palatinose oligosaccharides. New Food Ind 33:9–16, 1991.

Molis Ch, Flourié B, Ouarne F, Gailing MF, Lartigue S, Guibert A, Bornet F, Galmiche JP. Digestion, excretion, and energy value of fructooligosaccharides in healthy humans. J Am Clin Nutr 64:324–328, 1996.

Mortensen PB. Effect of oral-administered lactulose on colonic nitrogen metabolism and excretion. Hepatology 16:1350–1356, 1992.

National Research Council. Diet and Health Implication for Reducing Chronic Disease Risk. Washington, DC: National Academy Press, 1989.

Nilsson U, Björck I. Availability of cereal fructans and inulin in the rat intestinal tract. J Nutr 118:1482–1486, 1988.

Nilsson U, Öste R, Jägerstad M, Birkhed D. Cereal fructans: in vitro and in vivo studies on a availability in rats and humans. J Nutr 118:1325–1330, 1988.

Nutrition and Your Health: Dietary Guidelines for Americans. 3rd ed. Washington, DC: U.S. Depts. of Agriculture and Health and Human Services, 1990.

Ohta A, Ohtsuki M, Takizawa T, Inaba H, Adachi T, Kimura S. Effect of fructooligosaccharides on the absorption of magnesium and calcium by cecectomized rats. Int J Vit Nutr Res 64:316–323, 1994.

Ohta A, Ohtsuki M, Baba S, Adachi T, Sakat T, Sakaguchi E. Calcium and magnesium absorption from the colon and the rectum are increased in rats fed fructo-oligosaccharides. J Nutr 125:2417–2424, 1995.

Ohta A, Baba S, Ohtsuki M, Taguchi A, Adachi T. Prevention of coprophagy modifies magnesium absorption in rats fed fructo-oligosaccharides. Br J Nutr 75:755–784, 1996.

Oku T, Tokunaga T, Hosoya H. Nondigestibility of a new sweetener, ''Neosugar,'' in the rat. J Nutr 114: 1574–1581, 1984.

Pedersen A, Sandström B, Van Amelsvoort JMM. The effect of ingestion of inulin on blood lipids and gastrointestinal symptoms in healthy females. Br J Nutr 78:215–222, 1997.

Pellier P, Flourié B, Beaugerie L, Franchiseur F, Bornet F, Rambaud JCI. Symptomatic response to varying levels of fructo-oligosaccharides consumed occasionally or regularly. Eur J Clin Nutr 49:501–507, 1995.

Pierre F, Perrin P, Champ M, Bornet F, Meflah K, Menanteau J. Short-chain fructo-oligosaccharides reduce the occurrence of colon tumors and develop gut-associated lymphoid tissue in Min mice. Cancer Res 57:225–228, 1997.

Quemener B, Thibault JF, Coussement P. Integration of inulin determination in the AOAC method for measurement of total dietary fibre. Lebensm Wiss Technol 27:125–132, 1994.

Reddy BS, Hamid R, Rao CV. Effect of dietary oligofructose and inulin on colonic preneoplastic aberrant crypt foci inhibition. Carcinogenesis 18:1371–1374, 1997.

Roberfroid M, Dietary fiber, inulin, and oligofructose: a review comparing their physiological effects. Crit Rev Food Sci Nutr 33:103–148, 1993.

Roberfroid MB. A functional food: chicory fructooligosaccharides, a colonic food with prebiotic activity. World Ingredients (March-April):42–44, 1995.

Roberfroid MB. Functional effects of food component and the gastrointestinal system: chicory fructooligo-saccharides. Nutr Rev 54:S38–S42, 1996.

Roberfroid MB, Delzenne N. Dietary fructans. Ann Rev Nutr 18:114–143, 1998.

Roberfroid MB, Gibson GR, Delzenne N. Biochemistry of oligofructose, a non-digestible fructo-oligosac-charide: an approach to estimate its caloric value. Nutr Rev 51:137–146, 1993.

Roberfroid MB, Van Loo JAE, Gibson GR. The bifidogenic nature of chicory inulin and its hydrolysis products. J Nutr 128:11–19, 1998.

Rodwell VW, Nordstrom JL, Mitshelen JL. Regulation of HMG CoA reductase. Adv Lipid Res 14:1–74, 1976.

Rowland IR, Tanaka R. The effects of trans galactosylated oligosaccharides on gut flora metabolism in rats associated with human faecal microflora. J Appl Bacteriol 74:667–674, 1993.

Rowland IR, Rumney CJ, Coutts JT, Lievense LC. Effect of *Bifidobacterium longum* and inulin on gut bacterial metabolism and carcinogen-induced aberrant crypt foci in rats. Carcinogenesis 19:281–285, 1998.

Rumessen JJ, Bode S, Hamberg O, Gudmand-Hoyer E. Fructans of Jerusalem artichokes: intestinal transport, absorption, fermentation, and influence on blood glucose, insulin, and C-peptide response in healthy subjects. Am J Clin Nutr 52:675–681, 1990.

Sachs LE, Olson AC. Growth of *Clostridium perfringens* strains on α-galactoside. J Food Sci 44:1756–1760, 1979.

Saito Y, Takano T, Rowland I. Effects of soybean oligosaccharides on the human gut microflora in in vitro culture. Microb Ecol Health Dis 5:105–110, 1992.

Schneeman BO. Carbohydrates: significance for energy balance and gastrointestinal function. J Nutr 124: 1747S–1753S, 1994.

Select Committee on Nutrition and Human Needs, US Senate. Dietary Goals for the Unites States. 2nd ed. Washington, DC: U.S. Government Printing Office, 1977.

Sone Y, Makino C, Misaki A. Inhibitory effect of oligosaccharides derived from plant xyloglucan on intestinal glucose absorption in rat. J Nutr Sci Vitaminol 38:391–395, 1992.

Spiegel JE, Rose R, Karabell P, Frankos VH, Schmitt DF. Safety and benefits of fructooligosaccharides as food ingredients. Food Technol (Jan.): 85–89, 1994.

Stephen AM, Cummings JH. The microbial contribution to human fecal nitrogen. J Med Microbiol 13: 45–56, 1980.

Stone-Dorshow T, Levitt MD. Gaseous response to ingestion of a poorly absorbed fructooligosaccharide sweetener. Am J Clin Nutr 46:1–5, 1987.

Tanaka R, Takayama H, Morotomi M, Kuroshima T, Ueyama S, Matsumoto K, Kuroda A, Mutai M. Effects of administration of TOS and *Bifidobacterium breve* 4006 on the human fecal flora. Bifidobacteria Microflora 2:17–24, 1983.

Taper HS, Delzenne N, Roberfroid MB. Growth inhibition of transplantable mouse tumors by non-digestible carbohydrates. Int J Cancer 71:1109–1112, 1997.

Ueno Y, Izumi M, Kato K. Studies on pyrodextrinization of corn starch. Stärke 28:77–83, 1976.

U.S. Department of Health and Human Services. The Surgeon General's Report on Nutrition and Health. Washington, DC: Public Health Service. DHHS (PHS) Publication no 88-50210, 1988.

van den Heuvel EGHM, Muys T, van Dokkum W, Schaafsma G. Oligofructose stimulates calcium absorption in adolescents. Am J Clin Nutr 69:544–548, 1999.

Van Loo J, Coussement P, De Leenheer L, Hoebregs H, Mits G. On the presence of inulin and oligofructose as natural ingredients in the Western diet. Crit Rev Food Sci Nutr 35:525–552, 1995.

Van Loo J, Cummings JH, Delzenne N, Englyst H, Franck A, Hopkins M, Kok N, MacFarlane G, Newton D, Quigley M, Roberfroid M, van Vliet T, van den Heuvel E. Functional food properties of non digestible oligosaccharides; a consensus report from the 'ENDO' project (DGXII AIRII-CT94-1095). Br J Nutr 81:121–132, 1998.

Wada K, Watabe J, Mizutani J, Tomoda M, Suzuki H, Saitoh Y. Effects of soybean oligosaccharides in a beverage on human fecal flora and metabolites. Nippon Nogeikagaku Kaishi 68:127–135, 1992.

Wang X. Comparative aspects of carbohydrate fermentation by colonic bacteria. PhD thesis. Cambridge, UK: University of Cambridge, 1993.

Wang X. and Gibson, GR. Effect of in vitro fermentation of oligofructose and inulin by bacteria growing in the human large intestine. J Appl Bact 75:373–380, 1993.

Waterhouse AL, Chatterton NJ. Glossary of fructan terms. In: Suzuki M, Chatterton NJ, eds. Science and Technology of Fructans. Boca Raton, Fl: CRC Press, 1–7, 1993.

Williams CH, Witherly SA, Buddington RK. Influence of dietary Neosugar on selected bacterial groups of the human faecal microbiota. Microb Ecol Health Dis 7:91–97, 1994.

Yamaguchi F, Shimizu N, Hatanaka C. Preparation and physiological effect of low-molecular-weight pectin. Biosci Biotech Biochem 58:679–682, 1994.

Yamashita K, Kawai K, Itakura K. Effect of fructo-oligosaccharides on blood glucose and serum lipids in diabetic subjects. Nutr Res 4:961–966, 1984.

Yoneyama M, Mandai T, Aga H, Fujii K, Sakai S, Katayama Y. Effects of 4-β-D-galactosylsucrose (Lactosucre) intake on intestinal flora in healthy humans. Nippon Eiyo Shokuryo Gakkaishi (J. Jpn. Soc. Nutr. Food Sci.) 45:101–107, 1992.

Yoshida A, Umai A, Kurata Y, Kawamura S. Utilization of soybean oligosaccharides by the intact rat. Eiyo Shokuryo 22:262–265, 1969.

Younes H, Demigné C, Rémésy C. Acidic fermentation in the caecum increases absorption of calcium and magnesium in the large intestine. Br J Nutr 75:301–314, 1996.

Younes H, Rémésy C, Behr S, Demigné C. Fermentable carbohydrate exerts a urea lowering effect in normal and nephrectomised rats. Am J Physiol 35:G515–G521, 1997.

Yun JW. Fructooligosaccharides—occurence, preparation, and application. Enzyme Microb Tech 19:107–117, 1996.

Ziesenitz S, Siebert G. In vitro assessment of nystose as a sugar substitute. J Nutr 117:846–851, 1987.

9
Resistant Starches, Fermentation, and Large Bowel Health

Anthony R. Bird and David L. Topping
CSIRO, Adelaide, South Australia, Australia

I. INTRODUCTION

The high socioeconomic costs of noninfectious diseases in westernized countries in Europe, the Americas, and Australia are recognized by nutritionists and health authorities. In common with other major body organs, the human large bowel is subject to a number of these chronic problems. Some of these conditions may only cause discomfort to varying degrees of severity, while others are more serious threats to health and well-being. Thus, it is thought that (at least) 15% of the adult Australian population is affected by irritable bowel syndrome (IBS) (1). This condition is characterized by constipation and/or diarrhea, abdominal pain, cramps, and gas and can cause considerable distress but seems to pose little or no risk of increased mortality (2). This contrasts with cancers of the colon and rectum, which are responsible for approximately 3–4% of total deaths in countries such as the United States, the United Kingdom, and France (3). Moreover, there is evidence that large bowel cancer is becoming an increasing contributor to morbidity and mortality in certain Asian countries (such as Singapore) where previously its incidence was low (4). Between these two extremes of disease impact lie disorders such as constipation and diverticular disease, which result in a relatively limited number of deaths but can contribute substantially to personal discomfort and to health-related expenditure and resource utilization (2). The evidence suggesting an etiological role for diet and supporting dietary change to improve the management and prevention of each of these conditions is variable. In part, this relative lack of consistency of background information may be a reflection of the fact that colonic dysfunction attracts less interest than do more high-profile problems such as those of the coronary circulation. It may also be a consequence of the rapid evolution of knowledge of the relationships between dietary components and colonic physiology and the promotion of large bowel health. This latter possibility seems to be true for complex carbohydrates, particularly nonstarch polysaccharides (NSP, major components of dietary fiber) and starch, which have a major influence on colonic metabolism and, hence, on its health status and risk of disease. One of the major reevaluations that is occurring is of the contribution which starch not digested in the human small intestine makes to the metabolic activity of the human colon. This, so-called, resistant starch (RS) is emerging as a major factor in large bowel physiology and it is the purpose of this review to examine current knowledge and the potential of RS in promoting large bowel health. Particular attention will be given to the potential of processing to modify the RS content of foods so as to enhance their potential to improve colonic health without sacrificing their desirable organoleptic properties.

II. HISTORICAL ASPECTS OF THE RELATIONSHIPS BETWEEN COMPLEX CARBOHYDRATES AND THE RISK OF LARGE BOWEL DISEASE

Any consideration of the role of RS in the etiology of large bowel disease needs to be viewed in the historical context of complex carbohydrates in general. Some of this discussion may be found in other parts of this volume, but a brief review of the literature gives an understanding of the emphasis given to dietary fiber and fiber-rich foods in promoting colonic health and the relative lack of emphasis on RS. Early interest in the potential role of diet in the etiology of noninfectious diseases was stimulated by population studies in Africa by Burkitt, Trowell, Walker, and others, where it was shown that African natives who consumed diets high in unrefined plant foods and low in fat were at substantially lower risk of a number of conditions including constipation than were white Europeans (5). Subsequently it was noted that the incidence of colonic cancer was extremely low in black South Africans in contrast to white South Africans, a difference that was linked to the greater fecal bulk of the former. Further work has lent support to a relationship between stool mass and cancer risk. A more recent meta-analysis of population studies showed a positive relationship between NSP intake and fecal bulk and a negative relationship between the latter and colon cancer risk (6). Controlled studies in humans (see Ref. 7) have shown a positive relationship between the intake of fiber-rich foods (such as wheat bran) and stool output. To a considerable degree these and other findings have tended to obscure the fact that the original concept based on the ecological studies in Africans was of a protective effect of unrefined starchy plant foods of low energy density and not of dietary fiber per se. However, this is not what has eventuated, and most investigations have examined either fiber isolates or fiber-rich foods, especially those high in what has become known as insoluble fiber. Part of the reason for this focus lies in the evolution of the analytical methodology for fiber components. One of the drivers for research and development in fiber chemistry was economic and arose from the need to improve the production of ruminant animals for the production of food and fiber. Plant cell wall polysaccharides are the major substrates for the metabolic activities of rumen microflora. These are substantially insoluble and are relatively stable to enzymic or nonenzymic breakdown. Hence, the techniques to measure them could be relatively robust and destructive to less stable cell wall and non–cell wall constituents. The evolution of fiber chemistry has included the progressive development of more advanced technology to determine dietary fiber, including methodologies to measure NSP (8). These more sophisticated procedures have allowed the development of a fuller understanding of ways in which complex carbohydrates can exert their physiological actions.

III. MECHANISMS OF ACTION OF COMPLEX CARBOHYDRATES IN THE HUMAN COLON

The presence of carbohydrates in ileal effluent means automatically that these polysaccharides have escaped small intestinal digestion and absorption. This is true for NSP and those oligosaccharides not derived from starch, which enter the large bowel almost quantitatively. Some monosaccharides and disaccharides may be malabsorbed in the small intestine due either to relatively inadequate transport (e.g., fructose, sorbitol) or enzyme deficiency in affected individuals, such as those with lactose intolerance (9). Their effects in the colon depend upon both the quantity involved and the degree of polymerization. Excessive consumption of such nonabsorbed saccharides can lead to an osmotic diarrhea. Water-soluble NSP of a higher degree of polymerization (e.g., gum arabic) also can give similar problems, although at much greater levels of intake (10). Generally, such NSP are regarded as laxatives through their softening effect on stool and increase in fecal output and are used practically for this purpose. As has been noted, products high in insoluble NSP also find use as laxative agents. One of the preparations that has been most studied is wheat bran, and there is good evidence to show enhanced fecal bulking in proportion to the quantity consumed. A number of studies (e.g., Ref. 11) have shown prompt and effective relief of simple constipation with this and similar products.

The apparent indigestibility of the major components of wheat bran and similar preparations high in insoluble fiber led to the development of what has been termed the ''roughage model.'' In this model, fiber was postulated to act largely through its physical presence in the gut (12). This concept was adequate for some of the actions of overtly fiber-rich foods, for example, fecal bulking by wheat bran. However, it was quite inappropriate for other products that contained soluble fiber, were not remotely fibrous in appearance, and were not good fecal bulking agents. These preparations had other useful attributes, for example, lowering of plasma cholesterol. The apparent conflict was resolved by the study of Stephen and Cummings (13), who showed in humans that the NSP of fiber preparations such as wheat bran were excreted largely unmodified. However, for others (e.g., cabbage) less of the NSP were excreted but there was an increase in fecal bacterial mass due to fermentation of undigested carbohydrate. The data that have been accumulated show that carbohydrates that enter the colon can affect its physiology directly through their physical presence or indirectly through their metabolism by the microflora. In the case of RS of various types, it appears that most of their actions are mediated through the products of fermentation and not through the physical presence of starch.

IV. HUMAN LARGE BOWEL FERMENTATION, RS, AND SHORT CHAIN FATTY ACID PRODUCTION

The existence of an active bacterial population in the human large bowel has been known for a relatively long time, but only recently has the importance of this colonization to the maintenance of colonic health become appreciated (14,15). In normal adults and children the microbial population of the gut consists of a wide range of species. The main substrates for these organisms are dietary components that have escaped small intestinal digestion (of which the most important are dietary complex carbohydrates) plus endogenous body secretions and sloughed cells. The principal products are short chain fatty acids (SCFA) (chiefly acetate, propionate, and butyrate), gases (H_2, CO_2, and CH_4), energy, and more bacteria. For the fermentation to proceed, the bacteria require a source of nitrogen, which can be provided through the breakdown of dietary and endogenous protein or urea (via the urease reaction).

Under some circumstances simple carbohydrates that are normally digested in the small intestine may enter the large bowel. As has been noted, NSP and oligosaccharides (OS) are essentially indigestible by intrinsic human gut enzymes and pass the ileo-cecal sphincter more or less intact. However, there may be some modification of their physical properties in the upper gut (16). For some time it was thought that NSP were the main fermentative substrates for the large bowel microflora. This supposition is of long standing and is based on numerous in vivo studies showing greater large bowel SCFA when model animals species such as the rat (e.g., Ref. 17) and pig (e.g., Ref. 18) were fed diets high in either fiber-rich foods or purified NSP. In turn, these animal experiments were supported by in vitro studies in which NSP-rich foods or NSP isolates were incubated with human fecal inocula (e.g., Ref. 19). However, examination of the output of feces compared with the intake of NSP showed that there was discrepancy, with greater fecal bulk than would have been expected from the amount of fiber consumed. This difference was called the ''carbohydrate gap'' which was accounted for when it became apparent that a physiologically significant fraction of starch entered the large bowel (20). The term ''resistant starch'' was coined to describe the phenomenon of resistance of certain starches to α-amylase activity in vitro (21). However, it had been noted some time previously in humans that there was an increase in breath H_2 evolution (consistent with increased large bowel bacterial fermentation) following the ingestion of some starches (22). Together with other observations, these data confirmed that RS entered the large bowel of humans consuming normal ''western-type'' diets in meaningful quantities and that its contribution helped to close the carbohydrate gap. In the case of individuals consuming traditional high-starch diets, ecological studies suggest that the quantity of RS appears to be much larger than in people consuming the lower-starch diets considered to be typical of affluent, westernized countries (23). The importance of RS to colonic health in Europe was recognized through EURESTA, a major research and development project funded by the European Community that had health as a major focus and was conducted over the period 1990–1994. The main nutritional outcomes of this project and continuing research of the participants have been reviewed recently (24). One of the interesting aspects of this undertaking was that one of the main programs had food technology as a primary focus. This could be taken as an indicator of the recognition of the importance of the role of food processing in manipulating the RS content of foods and also in determining the nutritional attributes of that starch fraction.

V. FACTORS DETERMINING THE RS CONTENT OF FOODS

RS may be defined as the sum of starch and the products of starch degradation not absorbed in the small intestine of healthy individuals (24). It follows from this definition that RS is a carbohydrate that arises through incomplete small intestinal digestion but has its effects in the large bowel. The resistance of starch to small intestinal digestion has led to the fairly common assumption that the nondigestibility of starch in the upper gut was mirrored by a lowering of the glycemic response of foods that contained RS. In a sense this assumption was warranted, as a lowering of amylolysis would have been expected to limit the amount of glucose released in the small intestine and absorbed via the portal vein. However, Truswell (25) has pointed out that there are a large number of highly individual influences (e.g., small intestinal transit) beyond the rate of starch hydrolysis that bear on glycemic index so that total starch digestibility may be unrelated to excursions in blood glucose. For this reason it is appropriate to subdivide starches into digestible and indigestible starch. The former may be hydrolyzed at a particular rate but nevertheless has an ileal digestibility value of ∼100%. On the other hand, indigestible starches (i.e., RS) have an ileal digestibility of <100%. RS may be subclassified into a number of types (Table 1). RS1 is comprised of physically inaccessible starches found in partly milled grains and seeds. RS2 consists of resistant granules, while RS3 includes retrograded starches formed by cooking and then cooling starchy foods. Until relatively recently there were considered to be three types of RS, but a fourth classification has gained recognition (26). RS4 are the chemically modified starches that are used widely in the food industry for their technological attributes. The modifications include esterification and etherization and lead to a range of products with desirable technological attributes, which may also have beneficial nutritional properties.

Clearly, there are a number of influences on the RS content of a particular food. In addition to what may be termed its ''chemical'' RS content (which is the value obtained by standard analytical procedures), there is an additional component due to other factors. These include the

Table 1 Nutritional Classification of Resistant Starches

Types of resistant starch (RS)	Examples of occurrence
RS1—Physically inaccessible	Partly milled grains and seeds
RS2—Resistant granules	Raw potato, green banana, some pulses, high-amylose starches
RS3—Retrograded	Cooked and cooled potato, bread, cornflakes
RS4—Chemically modified	Etherised, esterified, cross-bounded starches

presence of other food components (such as fat) and also highly individual influences such as chewing and transit. The degree to which food is masticated can be a very important factor for digestibility, as big particles have a more rapid transit and are less accessible for enzymic breakdown than small ones. The variable nature of these influences means that RS determined analytically need not represent the total occurring in vivo. The latter quantity has been termed "physiological" RS to differentiate it from the analytical value (27). In some foods this difference can be quite substantial. For example, animal studies have shown that the feeding of foods such as canned navy (baked) beans (28) or heat-stabilized brown rice (29) leads to increases in large bowel digesta that are much greater than would have been predicted from the analytical fiber value of these foods, and it is assumed that this discrepancy reflects physiological RS. An indication of these differences can be obtained through the use of analytical procedures (30) that take account of the physiological influences on starch digestibility in foods.

VI. SCFA, RS, AND LARGE BOWEL FUNCTION

As has been noted, RS is as a fermentative substrate for the resident colonic microflora with gases (principally CO_2, CH_4, and H_2), energy (both as heat and metabolizable energy for the bacteria), a larger biomass, and SCFA as the major end products. In contrast to fiber-rich foods such as wheat bran (where substantial amounts of unfermented NSP contribute to fecal bulk), very little starch appears in human feces under normal circumstances. Further, RS appears to be only a mild laxative with small (or nonsignificant) increases in fecal bulk (31,32). Thus, it is reasonable to describe the physiological actions of RS in the large bowel in terms of the products of fermentation, i.e., SCFA.

Although the physiological effects of the three major acids (acetate, propionate, and butyrate) will be discussed elsewhere in this volume, it seems useful to summarize them here. Their common actions include a lowering of pH, stimulation of colonic blood flow and motor activity, enhancement of fluid and electrolyte absorption, and stimulation of colonocyte proliferation (33). The lowering of pH is of interest because it appears to be a mechanism whereby fermentation lowers the risk of colonization by acid-sensitive pathogenic bacteria. Additionally, a more acid environment would limit the absorption of basic toxic compounds (such as mutagenic amines) by increasing their ionization. Of the major acids, butyrate continues to attract attention in view of its potential to promote large bowel health. As well as being a preferred substrate for colonocytes, butyrate seems to have a number of specific actions, which encourage the promotion of a normal cell phenotype through enhancing DNA stabilization and repair and inducing apoptosis in potential cancer cells (34). Other studies have shown a direct benefit of butyrate in inducing remission of ulcerative colitis when infused rectally into affected subjects (35). However, a note of caution must be injected at this point. Nearly all of the experimental work on colo-rectal carcinogenesis has been in vitro, and a direct preventative role of butyrate in human large bowel cancer has yet to be shown in vivo. Further, the precise value of butyrate in repairing colitis has to be established. Nevertheless, the potential of butyrate (and the other SCFA) to promote colon health seems to be gaining general acceptance.

RS may have additional benefits in that, as well as altering the colonic environment through SCFA production, there may be other changes that would be considered to be of long-term benefit. Studies in humans have shown that consumption of RS lowers the fecal concentrations of secondary bile acids, especially deoxycholate (32). These acids are produced through bacterial metabolism and are thought to be contributors to colo-rectal tumorigenesis. Studies in pigs have supported this concept with diminished concentrations of this secondary bile acid in gall bladder bile, consistent with lower conversion and exposure of the colon wall to this putative mutagen (36). As seems to be the general case with RS, a cautionary note needs to be sounded, as one recent study has shown limited effectiveness of RS2 or RS3 in lowering putative risk factors for colon cancer in men (37). However, in interpreting these latter data it needs to be recognized that the dietary adaptation period was short relative to comparable studies (1 week vs. 3–4 weeks).

A substantial number of animal trials have shown that feeding diets high in sources of RS as diverse as raw potato (38) or legumes (39), high-amylose starches (40), or canned, cooked beans (28) raises either large bowel digesta mass or total and individual SCFA or both. Some studies suggest that there may be particular benefit of RS from the standpoint of the SCFA produced. Experiments in vitro, in which various fiber preparations were incubated with human fecal inocula, have shown that RS fermentation favored the production of butyrate (41). In view of the putative role for this acid in large bowel health, this is potentially a very important attribute. Studies in humans have confirmed that consumption of RS as high-amylose starches raise the fecal excretion of butyrate but not necessarily total SCFA (31,32). These data are consistent with both an increase in carbohydrate fermentation and a shift to butyrate production. However, earlier animal data suggested that RS from different sources vary in their effects on large bowel SCFA. Studies in pigs have shown substantial differences in the molar proportions of SCFA in colonic contents after the feeding of navy (baked) beans and brown rice with higher levels of butyrate in animals fed the latter (28,29). Further studies in this species have shown that RS2 (but not RS3) reduced ileal and colonic magnesium and calcium absorption (42). Human studies tend to support this idea of differential responses to RS with the large bowel microflora of some individuals seeming to be unable to ferment particular types of RS (43). Similar data have been noted in vitro with slow and incomplete fermentation of RS by fecal inocula from some people (44). Interestingly, there appeared to be no difference in the molar proportions of SCFA produced by the cultures from different individuals, suggesting that some other factor was responsible. One possibility is the supply of protein. Work by Morita and coworkers has shown that, under some circumstances, the supply of nitrogen may be limiting to large RS metabolism both in terms of the rate of fermentation and the products (45). By analogy with starch, these authors have coined the term "resistant protein" for protein that escapes from the small intestine and is fermented in the large bowel. If the supply of nitrogen were limiting, this could be an important regulatory factor. The quality, as well as the absolute amount, may be significant, and both beans and brown rice contain substantial quantities of protein of differing quality. Inter alia, these data raise the possibility that the actual plant source may be important in determining SCFA production from RS. It is of interest that most of the observations of increased butyrate production with feeding of RS have been with maize corn products. A systematic evaluation of the effects of RS from various plant species and food products on SCFA production would seem to be desirable, especially if coupled with an examination of variation between people.

VII. RELATIONSHIPS BETWEEN STARCH, RS, AND HUMAN HEALTH

The sum of the evidence available suggests that RS has beneficial effects on large bowel physiology. Numerous studies in animals have shown improved indices of bowel health (lower pH, higher SCFA, etc.) on feeding of RS. Many of these studies were invasive with measurement of the parameters in question in the large bowel itself. Clearly, such direct measures are not practical in humans for a number of ethical and logistic constraints. For these reasons, most (or all) of the studies in humans have relied on indirect measures such as greater breath H_2 evolution or changes in fecal variables. The former is an index of increased large bowel fermentation but does not necessarily demonstrate an improvement in large bowel function or diminished risk of disease. Thus, consumption of cornflakes (as a source of RS) led to a substantial change in breath H_2 evolution but no change in stool parameters (46). One possibility for this paradox is the speed of fermentation. Studies in pigs suggested that some forms of RS could be fermented rapidly relative to passage of the fecal stream so that SCFA could be raised in the proximal colon but not in the more distal regions (36). This has the potential to be a very important attribute. The distal colon is the site of most large bowel disease. Colorectal cancer predominates in this region of the large bowel (Fig. 1) (47). Studies in pigs have shown that SCFA availability is highest in the proximal large bowel due to greater fermentation. SCFA levels fall towards the distal large bowel through depletion of fermentative substrate and absorption of the acids on passage of the fecal stream. Measurement of SCFA in stomal patients (48) shows a similar decline (Fig. 2) so that limited SCFA availability could be a contributor to the greater prevalence of disease in the distal large bowel.

    While the experimental evidence generally favors a positive role of starch and, by implication, RS in large bowel physiology, it is necessary to show that this translates to improved human health. A direct benefit has been shown in cholera where consumption of a high-amylose starch leads to diminished diarrhoeal water loss (through stimulation of colonic absorption) and more prompt remission of symptoms (49). In the longer term, population studies have given evidence of improved morbidity and mortality from large bowel cancer with greater starch consumption. A connection between consumption of unrefined starchy foods and diminished disease

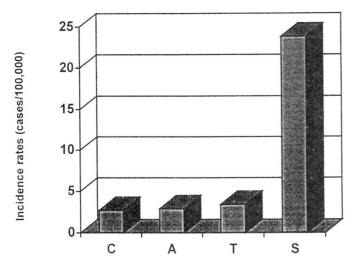

Fig. 1 Cancer incidence rates in the caecum (C) and ascending (A), transverse (T), and sigmoid (S) colon.

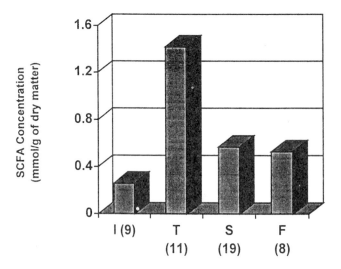

Fig. 2 Concentrations of SCFA in ileostomy (I) and transverse (T) and sigmoid (S) colostomy effluent or normal feces (F).

risk was implicit in the early work in East Africa. That relationship has been extended through a recent meta-analysis of ecological population studies by Cassidy et al. (23). They showed that risk of this malignancy was increased with greater intakes of fat and protein. In keeping with a similar, earlier, analysis (50), fiber (expressed as NSP by Cassidy and coworkers) was only weakly protective, presumably due to its relatively low intakes. However, starch consumption was highly protective with high levels of risk in countries such as Australia where intakes are low. The putative mechanism for the protective effect of starch is through RS, which suggests that increased consumption of this quantity (not necessarily with an increase in total starch intake) should lead to lowering of cancer rates. However, this does beg the question of the comparative effects of fat and protein in increasing risk on the one hand and RS (+ NSP) on the other, so that any change in disease incidence represents a balance between these opposing influences. Clearly, the optimal means of lowering colorectal cancer at the population level is to effect reciprocal changes in both starch and RS on the one hand and fat and protein on the other. It should be noted that there is a human intervention underway in which the effect of RS on large bowel cancer risk are being examined (51). Aspirin, which appears to lower risk of a number of gastrointestinal cancers (including those of the large bowel) by ~40% (52), is being studied in the same trial.

While the balance of the evidence does suggest that RS is beneficial for large bowel function, there are contrary opinions. It has been proposed that increased intakes of RS might not be protective against colo-rectal cancer (53), a numerically important malignancy. This conclusion is based on limited experimental data, all of which are derived from animals. Two of these studies were in animals treated with a carcinogen (dimethylhydrazine). In the first, RS2 (as raw potato starch) enhanced epithelial proliferation and tumor formation, while addition of wheat bran to this diet suppressed tumorigenesis (54). In the second study, dietary cellulose (at 10% of the diet) lowered colonic cancer volume, but diets containing 3 or 10% RS (as corn starch treated with α-amylase) or 3% cellulose did not (55). The lack of effect of RS was despite an increase in large bowel butyrate. Against these should be set other studies in which consumption of RS lowered tumor development compared with sucrose (56,57). Moreover, studies in rats treated with azoxymethane have shown that elevation of large bowel butyrate with a pelletized preparation induced apoptosis but did not alter tumor initiation (58). Clearly there is room for further experimentation in this important area. However, it should be remembered that the many of the studies with RS may not be representative of the situation in humans. Dietary interventions in humans are relatively short term, while only a few of the studies in animals (e.g., with pigs) have been carried out under conditions that approximate the dietary intakes of the population at large. The data from models for colorectal carcinogenesis have been obtained under circumstances that may not necessarily be relevant to the disease process in humans. Moreover, it is possible that effects of RS in rodents differ from those in other species. For example, diets high in RS lower plasma cholesterol in rodents (59), whereas RS does not have the same effects in pigs (36) or humans (32). This discrepancy may be a consequence of the practice of fecal refection in the rat, which could alter large bowel metabolism in a way not seen in pigs or humans. It should be noted that such lowering of cholesterol in rats could enhance bile acid excretion (60), and raised concentrations of these acids in the large bowel may favor tumorigenesis. Clearly, more definitive proof is required from humans, but on balance it appears reasonable to conclude that RS is a net contributor to enhanced bowel health and adds to the beneficial effects of dietary fiber.

VIII. PROCESSED FOODS WITH RAISED RS CONTENT AND HEALTH PROMOTION

In westernized industrial countries the recommended increases in starch consumption and lowering of energy and fat consumption appear to be well based and are to be supported. While targets for fiber and starch consumption have been set by health authorities in these countries, no such figure appears to have been set for RS. However, in these societies starch intakes are low (as are those of dietary fiber) so that any increases should be of benefit. Such benefit may be inferred from the human interventions in which volunteers have consumed foods containing RS to provide about 30–40 g of RS per person per day (31,32). Greater fiber consumption can be effected through the manufacture and consumption of foods relatively high in fiber (e.g., wheat bran), which require relatively small quantities to be consumed to meet desired levels of intake. Alternatively, it is possible to increase consumption through the production of foods (e.g., fiber-enriched breads) that are more modest in fiber content but may be consumed in amounts sufficient to contribute substantially to total intake. A similar situation exists for RS with foods such as pulses, brown rice, etc., which are available to the consumer and appear to be high enough in RS so as to contribute substantially to intakes in their own right. However, to raise the RS content of processed foods that are relatively low in RS without altering their organoleptic properties necessitates the use of alternative technologies. One approach is to use NSP or other additives to alter starch digestion. However, manufacturing processes often involve conditions of heat and moisture that lead to gelatinization and hence greatly increased digestibility, which may oppose the effects of additives. High-amylose starches are one means of achieving this end as they resist gelatinization, and one such starch, containing 70% amylose, has been used to raise the RS content of foods such as white breads and breakfast cereals (26). Experimental studies with these products have confirmed their capacity to improve indices of large bowel health. This starch also has been shown to assist in the management of diarrheal problems and has the potential for incorporation into oral rehydration solutions (49).

While high-amylose starches can find use in food processing, their usefulness is still limited due to the extreme conditions of heat and moisture that may be used, which can cause gelatinization (and loss of resistance). There are also the additional problems of variability, with the microflora of some individuals appearing to be unable to metabolize RS. This problem has

Table 2 Distal Colonic SCFA Pools in Rats Fed Acylated
Starches[a]

Starch	Acetate (mmol)	Propionate (mmol)	Butyrate (mmol)
Control	7	1	1
Acetylated	28	10	5
Propionylated	21	15	3
Butyrylated	18	6	9

[a]Mean of eight observations per group.

been discussed together with the possibility that the supply of nitrogen to the microflora may be an issue. One way to increase the RS content of a food is to exploit the chemically modified starches used in the food industry for their technological attributes. These RS4 starches have defined structures and are also stable to thermal processing. Further, they are resistant to small intestinal amylolysis for chemical reasons, which should be independent of physiological variables such as transit. Thus their capacity to lower the glycemic response may be more predictable than that of other types of RS, and such does seem to be the case. Studies with such modified starches have shown a flattening of the glycemic index with starches modified through acetylation or coupling with β-cyclodextrin (61). Acylation of starches offers the potential to deliver SCFA to the large bowel as they could be labile to bacterial enzymes in that viscus. This hypothesis has been tested in rats fed starches acetylated, propionylated, or butyrylated to 5% (62). The feeding of these acylated starches to rats resulted in an elevation of cecal SCFA and digesta mass (Table 2). This is consistent with the passage of undigested carbohydrate and the release of the esterified acyl groups plus the fermentation of the residual starch. Interestingly, the feeding of these acylated starches raised SCFA availability in the distal colon, the site of greatest disease risk in humans. The capacity of these starches to deliver SCFA to the human colon so as to enhance large bowel health is under current investigation.

REFERENCES

1. Gut Foundation. Irritable Bowel Syndrome. Randwick NSW. 1994.
2. Crowley S, Antioch K, Carter R, Waters A-M, Conway L, Mathers C. The Cost of Diet-Related Disease in Australia. Australian Institute of Health and Welfare, 1992.
3. World Cancer Research Fund and American Institute for Cancer Research. Food, Nutrition and the Prevention of Cancer: A Global Perspective. Washington DC: American Institute for Cancer Research, 1997.
4. Lee HP, Chia KS, Shanmugataram K. Cancer Incidence in Singapore 1983–1987. Singapore Cancer Registry, 1992.
5. Cobiac L, Topping DL. In: Sadler M, Caballero B, Strain S, eds. Encyclopaedia of Human Nutrition. London: Academic Press, 1999.
6. Cummings JH, Bingham SA, KW Heaton KW, Eastwood MA. Gastroenterology 103:1783–1789, 1992.
7. Jenkins DJA, Peterson RD, Thorne MJ, Ferguson PW. Am J Gastroenterol 82:1259–1263, 1987.
8. Baghurst PA, Baghurst KI, Record SJ. Food Aust 48(suppl):S3–S35, 1996.
9. Holtug K, Clausen MR, Hove J, Christiansen J, Mortensen PB. Scand J Gastroenterol 27:545–552, 1992.
10. Topping DL, Mock S, Trimble RP, Storer GB, Illman RJ. Nutr Res 8:1013–1020, 1988.

11. Baghurst KI, Hope A, Down E. Commun Health Studies 8:1054–1061, 1985.
12. Topping DL, Illman RJ. Med J Aust 144:307–309, 1986.
13. Stephen AM, Cummings AJH. Nature 284:283–4, 1980.
14. Cummings JH, Macfarlane GT. J Appl Bacteriol 70:443–459, 1991.
15. Gibson GR, Roberfroid MB. J Nutr 125:1401–1412, 1995.
16. Monro JA. J Food Comp Anal 4:88–99, 1991.
17. Illman RJ, Trimble RP, Snoswell AM, Storer GB, Topping DL, Nutr Rep Int 26:439–446, 1982.
18. Kim KI, Benevenga NJ, Grummer RH. J Anim Sci 46:1648–1657, 1978.
19. Mortensen PB, Norgaard-Anderser I. Scand J Gastroenterol 28:418–422, 1993.
20. Stephen AM. Can J Physiol Pharmacol 69:116–120, 1991.
21. Berry CS. J Cereal Sci 4:301–314, 1986.
22. Anderson IH, Levine AS, Levitt MD. N Engl J Med 304:891–892, 1981.
23. Cassidy A, Bingham SA, Cummings JH. Br J Cancer 69:937–942, 1994.
24. Asp N-G, Amelsvoort van JMM, Hautvast JGAJ. Nutr Res Rev 9:1–31, 1996.
25. Truswell AS. Eur J Clin Nutr 46(suppl 2):S91–101, 1992.
26. Brown IL, McNaught KJ, Moloney E. Food Aust 47:272–275, 1995.
27. Annison G, Topping DL. Annu Rev Nutr 14:297–320, 1994.
28. Topping DL, Illman RJ, Clarke JM, Trimble RP, Jackson KA, Marsono Y. J Nutr 123:133–143, 1993.
29. Marsono Y, Illman RJ, Clarke JM, Trimble RP, Topping DL. Br J Nutr 70:503–513, 1993.
30. Muir JG, O'Dea K. Am J Clin Nutr 57:540–546, 1993.
31. Munster van IP, Tangerman A, Nagengast FM. Digest Dis Sci 39:834–842, 1994.
32. Noakes M, Clifton P, Nestel PJ, Le Leu R, McIntosh GH. Am J Clin Nutr 64:944–951, 1996.
33. Cummings JH. In: Gibson GR, Macfarlane GT, eds. Human Colonic Bacteria, Role in Nutrition, Physiology and Pathology. Boca Raton, FL: CRC Press, 1995, pp. 107–127.
34. Young GP, Gibson PR. In: Cummings JH, Rombeau JL, Sakada T, eds. Physiological and Clinical Aspects of Short-Chain, Fatty Acids. Cambridge: Cambridge University Press, 1995, pp 313–335.
35. Scheppach W, Bartram HP, Richter F. Eur J Cancer 31A:1077–1080, 1995.
36. Topping DL, Gooden JM, Brown IL, Biebrick DA, Mcgrath L, Trimble RP, Choct M, Illman RJ. J Nutr 127:615–622, 1997.
37. Heijnen MLA, Amelsvoort van JMM, Deurenberg P, Beynen AC. Am J Clin Nutr 67:322–332, 1998.
38. Mathers JC, Smith H, Carter S. Br J Nutr 78:1015–1029, 1997.
39. Mathers JC, Dawson LD. Br J Nutr 66:313–329, 1991.
40. Andrieux C, Pacheco ED, Bouchet B, Gallent D, Szylit O. Br J Nutr 67:489–499, 1992.
41. Weaver GA, Krause JA, Miller TL, Wolin MJ. Am J Clin Nutr 47:61–66, 1992.
42. Heijnen ML, Beynen A. Z Ernaehrungswiss 37:13–17, 1998.
43. Cummings JH, Beatty ER, Kingman SM, Bingham SA, Englyst HE. Br J Nutr 75:733–747, 1996.
44. Christl SU, Katzenmaier U, Hylla S, Kasper H, Scheppach WJ Parent Ent Nutr 21:290–295, 1997.
45. Morita T, Oh-hashi A, Takei K, Ikai M, Kasaoka S, Kiriyama SJ Nutr 127:470–477, 1998.
46. Tomlin J, Read NW. Br J Nutr 64:589–595, 1990.
47. Correa P, Haenszel W. Adv Cancer Res 26:1–141, 1978.
48. Mitchell B, Lawson MJ, Davies M, Kerr-Grant A, Roediger WEW, Illman RJ, Topping DL. Nutr Res 5:1089–1092, 1985.
49. Binder HJ, Ramakrishna BS. Gastroenterology 115:512, 1998.
50. Trock B, Lanza E, Greenwald PA. J Natl Cancer Inst 82:650–661, 1990.
51. Burn J, Chapman PD, Mathers J, Bertario L, Bishop DT, Bulow S, Cummings J, Phillips R, Vasen H. Eur J Cancer 31A:1385–1386, 1995.
52. Thun MJ, Namboodri MM, Calle EE, Flanders WD, Heath CW Jr. Cancer Res 53:1322–1327, 1993.
53. Ferguson LR, Harris PJ. J Environ Path Tox Oncol 16:335–341, 1997.
54. Young GP, McIntyre A, Albert V, Folino M, Muir JG, Gibson PR. Gastroenterology 110:508–514, 1996.
55. Sakamoto J, Nakaji S, Sugawara K, Iwane S, Munakata A. Gastroenterology 110:116–120, 1996.
56. Bianchini F, Caderni G, Magno C, Testolin G, Dolara PJ Nutr 122:254–261, 1992.

57. Caderni G, Luceri C, Spagnesi MT, Giannini A, Biggeri A, Dloara P. J Nutr 124:517–523, 1994.
58. Caderni G, Luceri C, Lanconi L, Tessitore L, Dolara P. Nutr Cancer 30:175–181, 1998.
59. Morand C, Levrat MA, Besson C, Demigré C, Rémésy CJ Nutr Biochem 5:138–144, 1994.
60. Younes H, Levrat MA, Demigré C, Rémésy C. Lipids 30:847–853, 1995.
61. Raben A, Andersen K, Karberg MA, Holst JJ, Astrup A. Am J Clin Nutr 66:304–314, 1997.
62. Annison G, Topping DL, Illman RJ, Trimble RP, McGrath I. Proc Nutr Soc Aust 22:91, 1998.

10
Resistant Starches and Lipid Metabolism

Christian Demigné, Christian Rémésy and Christine Morand
INRA de Clermont-Ferrand/Theix, Saint-Genès-Champanelle, France

I. INTRODUCTION

Resistant starch is present in the diet provided in significant amounts by starchy foods after addition as a native form, after modification for technological purposes, or to increase starch availability in the large intestine (1,2). Resistant starch shares some common properties with soluble dietary fibers: it is poorly modified in the small intestine but is extensively broken down by the colonic microflora, which results in the production of short-chain fatty acids (SCFA).

Like fibers *sensu stricto*, resistant starch affects various metabolic processes, such as glycemic control or lipid metabolism. Resistant starch is of interest because it is devoid of some of the drawbacks that limit the use of soluble fibers such as excessive viscosity or problems of palatability, and it can be incorporated into most starchy foods included in the human diet.

II. DIGESTIVE EFFECTS

A. Small Intestine

Certain fibers, especially gel-forming ones, have trophic effects in the small intestine (3). Such alterations are liable to influence the rate of nutrient absorption as well as the quantities of sloughed epithelial cells appearing in the intestinal lumen. Data in this domain about the specific effects of resistant starch are still scarce: a slight increase in small intestine weight has been reported by Younes et al. (4); furthermore, Gee et al. (5) have shown that, in rats adapted to resistant starch diets, the crypt production rate was 66% higher in the ileum than in controls, but there was no significant effect in the jejunum. Meslin et al. (6) also observed that amylomaize starch considerably increased ileal epithelial renewal time in conventional rats.

Fibers such as guar gum may affect the secretion of pancreatic enzymes (7), but this effect is still uncertain for resistant starch. In fact, the effect of undigestible carbohydrates on lipase secretion and activity is equivocal because the presence of bulky materials in the jejunum may dilute the enzyme and its cofacters (hence a lower rate of hydrolysis), but this could also enhance lipase life span in the digestive tract (7).

B. Large Intestine

Most starches are effectively broken down by the colonic microflora. In this part of the digestive tract, resistant starch exerts a potent trophic effect in rats (4,8) and other species (9). The end products of this activity are essentially SCFA, but under some circumstances other organic acids may also be synthesized in noticeable quantities, including lactic acid (especially when large amounts of resistant starch elicit highly acidic fermentations) or succinic acid (overproduction of which may result from nitrogen shortage) (10). Resistant starches have been viewed as butyric-yielding precursors (11,12), nevertheless, in rat model some of these (e.g., amylomaize starch) seem particularly effective in promoting high propionic acid fermentations (8). It must be noted that resistant starch could exert prebiotic effects by promoting the emergence of specific microorganisms such as *Bifidobacteria* in pigs (13) or in rats (14), which should promote propionic acid synthesis.

C. Gastrointestinal Hormones

The presence of resistant starch in the diet tends to enhance the digesta volume, to decrease the energy density, and to promote the digestive absorption of a fraction of the carbohydrate moiety of the diet as SCFA. It has been shown in rats that a high–resistant starch diet blunts the postprandial rise of plasma glucose and insulin (15,16) as well as the insulin/glucagon ratio (17).

In humans it has been shown that postprandial insulin output was significantly reduced compared to controls after a test meal providing 33% of the carbohydrate as high-amylose maize starch (18). Furthermore, it turned out that this type of test meal depressed plasma insulin concentration as well as gastric inhibitory peptide (GIP), glucagon-like peptide-1, and epinephrine (19). The effect on glucose tolerance may require a relatively long period—about 5 weeks (20). Gee et al. (5) failed to obtain a significant change in plasma enteroglucagon in parallel to a rise in crypt cell proliferation rate (CCPR) in the ileum.

III. POSSIBLE MECHANISMS OF INTERFERENCE WITH LIPID DIGESTION

A. Upper Digestive Tract

Soluble fibers undergo various types of interactions with steroids, especially with bile acids ionized at the physiological pH in the small intestine. This implies direct ionic interaction (reminiscent of those established with the $-N(CH_3)_3^+$ of cholestyramine) or indirect interaction with the $(COO \cdots Ca)^+$ of the uronic acid units of pectin. Another important mechanism for lipid lowering is through gel-forming effects, which lead to (a) a dilution of luminal lipids, surfactants, and enzymes, which slow down their interactions and (b) an increase in the unstirred layer, and hence a slower transfer of nutrients to the brush border membrane. With unmodified resistant starch, the above mechanisms are probably irrelevant, except regarding the dilution of the intestinal bulk phase. It has been proposed that helical structures in starch act as binding sites for bile salts (21): the bile salt affinity increased from cholate to deoxycholate (10-fold), then to chenodeoxycholate (another 10-fold), independently of whether bile salt is unconjugated or conjugated with taurine or glycine. However, the authors estimated that the number of binding sites in starch was restricted to 1 per $\sim$300 glucose units (compared to 1 per 7 glucose units for β-cyclodextrin). Cyclodextrin also displays inclusion properties with cholesterol; whether this could be relevant for resistant starch hydrophobic cavities is still uncertain.

B. Large Intestine

Resistant starch and soluble fibers are extensively broken down by the microflora, and molecules trapped on them are thus released in the lumen. Yet a major part of the bile acids is bound, from about 60% with fiber-free diets up to more than 95% with cholestyramine and about 70%

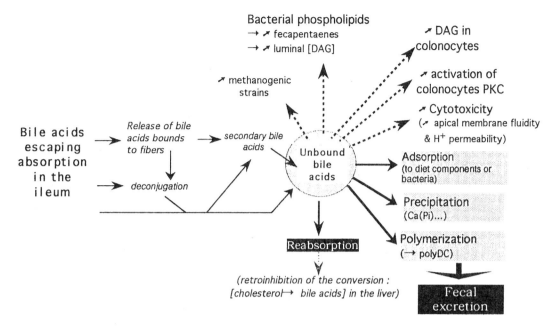

Fig. 1 Factors influencing the concentration of unbound bile acids in the large intestine and some possible biological effects of these compounds on factors affecting cell proliferation in the colon.

with resistant starch diets (4). This point is important since it limits the concentrations liable to interfere with cell proliferation in the colonic mucosa. In fact, several binding processes may contribute to insolubilization of bile acids in the hindgut: acidification, coprecipitation with CaPi complexes (22), polymerization of bile acids (23), and adsorption on bacteria (24). Furthermore, absorption in situ also contributes to the lowering of the soluble bile acid concentration (4,25), but little is known about the influence of resistant starch on the intensity of this reabsorption, which has been shown to increase when some fibers promote active fermentation in the cecum (25) (Fig. 1).

Fermentation of resistant starch and the subsequent acidification of the cecal content may alter the intestinal bile acid profile since low pH tends to depress 7β and 7α dehydroxylation of bile acids (26). Nevertheless, in rat models the fecal excretion of secondary bile acids has frequently been reported to increase (27,28), suggesting that resistant starch is effective in enhancing bile acid fecal excretion but is not always effective in depressing secondary bile acid production in the large bowel. An alternative explanation may be that secondary, apolar bile acids are particularly prone to insolubilization and adsorption in the hindgut and are thus overrepresented in the fecal samples compared to the digestive contents. In contrast, investigations in humans indicate that secondary bile acid excretion is lower during a high–resistant starch period (primary bile acids were not affected) together with a reduction of neutral sterol excretion (29), but this was not found during periods of starch malabsorption (30).

IV. EFFECTS ON FATTY ACID METABOLISM

A. Lipogenesis

It has been shown in a rat model that replacement of a large part of dietary digestible starch by amylomaize-resistant starch elicits dramatic changes in the splanchnic metabolism of glucose

(15): the liver glucose balance was shifted from a net uptake towards a practically nil balance, and most glycogen storage was effected via the indirect (gluconeogenic) pathway, a situation poorly compatible with an active lipogenesis. Accordingly, ^3H_2O incorporation into fatty acids was found to be strongly depressed in rats adapted to a resistant starch diet, together with a coordinate repression of liver lipogenic enzymes (8). In rat adipose tissue, it has been shown that chronic replacement of a high–glycemic index starch by a high-amylose one decreased glucose incorporation into lipids (31) and epididymal fat pads (32). Furthermore, the above effects have generally been investigated during the postprandial period, but resistant starch effects during the postabsorptive period have also been reported both in experimental animals (15) and in humans, where the shift in starch digestion induced by retrogradation leads to a reduction in lipolysis (33).

B. Triglyceride Metabolism

Resistant starch diets have been consistantly shown to depress circulating triglyceride, frequently more effectively than cholesterol itself (4,18,32,34); this action is reminiscent of that of several types of probiotics (35). This triglyceride-lowering effect may be interesting since triglyceride-rich lipoprotein (TGRLP) are supposed to have atherogenic significance (36), all the more so since it has been shown to affect circulating triglycerides not only during the postprandial period but also in the the postabsorptive period. As mentioned above, it is conceivable that the presence of resistant starch in the lumen of the small intestine could alter (a) the rate of release of triglycerides from the complex food matrix, (b) their interaction with surfactants, (c) hydrolytic enzymes (and their cofactors), as well as (d) transfer of lipolysis end products into enterocytes. Nevertheless, it is generally assumed that the overall recovery of dietary fatty acids and monoglycerides from triglycerides by the small intestine is very high, frequently exceeding 95%, except when stearic-rich lipids are present in the food. In fact, the triglyceride-lowering effect might reflect a reduced *de novo* synthesis of fatty acids or fatty acid export as very-low-density lipoprotein (VLDL) by the liver, these processes being under the control of hormones, especially insulin, which is generally depressed by resistant starch feeding (8,16,19,37). Furthermore, as recently stressed by Olson and Schneeman (38), the effect of complex carbohydrates on postprandial lipemia could be lessened by the fact that, although the rate of appearance of triglyceride-rich particles in plasma in reduced, the clearance rate is also altered in parallel with the insulin status and its consequences on extrasplanchnic lipoprotein lipase.

V. EFFECTS ON CHOLESTEROL METABOLISM

A cholesterol-lowering effect of resistant starch is still disputed and has been less consistently reported than the effects on plasma triglyceride (20,39,40); nevertheless, such an effect has been reported in hamsters together with a reduced biliary cholesterol secretion, whereas bile acid secretion was increased (40). In the rat, a significant increase in the biliary secretion of bile acids was also found with dietary resistant starch, but neither biliary cholesterol secretion nor plasma cholesterol was significantly reduced (Table 1). In specific models such as gentically obese Zucker rats, amylomaize starch has been shown to be quite effective in lowering plasma cholesterol levels of obese and lean rats (41). However, in healthy normolipidemic subjects, no significant effect on plasma cholesterol or triacylglycerols was found (42).

It is still unclear whether resistant starch has a capacity to impair cholesterol absorption, as do most of the gel-forming fibers or some sequestrants such as cyclodextrin. Nevertheless, it has been frequently reported that resistant starch diets are effective in enhancing neutral steroid

Table 1 Effects of Replacement of a Part of Dietary Starch (40%) by Amylomaize-Resistant Starch on Lipid Metabolism in the Rat

	Control diet	Resistant starch diet
Plasma cholesterol (mmol/L)	1.94 ± 0.09	1.72 ± 0.10
In d $<$ 1.04 fraction	0.97	0.80
In d $>$ 1.04 fraction	0.99	0.92
Plasma triglycerides (mmol/L)	1.43 ± 0.13	1.13 ± 0.11[a]
Liver total cholesterol (mg/g)	5.3 ± 0.4	4.7 ± 0.6
Liver triglycerides (mg/g)	22.4 ± 1.1	20.4 ± 0.8
Bile flux (mL/h)	1.02 ± 0.09	1.30 ± 0.11[a]
Bile acid secretion (μmol/h)	36.0 ± 6.7	52.1 ± 10.3[a]
Cholesterol secretion (μmol/h)	0.48 ± 0.07	0.54 ± 0.12

[a] Significantly different from rats adapted to the control diet ($p < 0.05$).

excretion (10,28,43), although not systematically (44). Nevertheless, in a hamster model receiving a lithogenic diet, it has been shown that cholesterol excretion was decreased by amylomaize starch (40). It has also been reported in healthy volunteers that resistant starch may decrease fecal sterol excretion, especially the concentration of 4-cholest-3-one, which can be relevant for cancer prevention (45).

VI. EFFECTS OF RESISTANT STARCH ON THE ENTEROHEPATIC CYCLING OF BILE ACIDS

Whether resistant starch affects the rate of bile acid synthesis and secretion from the liver is still uncertain; no changes (40) or significant but relatively limited increases (4) in bile acid production have been reported together with an enlargement of the cecal bile acid pool (Table 2). In humans, some data suggest that bile acid excretion could be decreased by resistant starch diets.

In fact, data are still lacking about the possible changes in the small intestine bile acid pool, representing the major part of the total pool in the rat that is devoid of gallbladder storage

Table 2 Effects of Replacement of a Part of Dietary Starch (40%) by Amylomaize-Resistant Starch on Digestive Steroid Elimination in the Rat

	Control diet	Resistant starch diet
Cholesterol intake (μmol/d)	170 ± 8	186 ± 10
Cecal bile acid pool (μmol)	11.5 ± 1.6	21.9 ± 3.2[a]
Fecal sterol excretion (μmol/d)	65.0 ± 5.2	101.5 ± 7.8[a]
Coprostanol/cholesterol molar ratio	52/48	73/27
Fecal bile acid excretion (μmol/d)	36.2 ± 4.9	41.1 ± 6.8
Total steroid excretion (μmol/d)	101.2 ± 9.7	142.6 ± 18.5[a]
Steroid apparent balance (μmol/d)	68.8 ± 4.6	43.4 ± 9.8[a]
Cholesterol apparent absorption (μmol/d)	105.0 ± 9.0	84.5 ± 11

[a] Significantly different from rats adapted to the control diet ($p < 0.05$).

(46) and also very important in other species. With soluble fibers, such as guar gum, it has been shown that the increase of jejunal and ileal bile acids pool elicited by the presence of fiber probably play a major role in the alteration of the enterohepatic cycling of bile acids (25). The classical concept of an impairment of the ileal reabsorption of bile acids in the presence of complex carbohydrates is questionable, since in fact an enhanced appearance of bile acids in the portal vein was detected (47). Accordingly, measurement of [^{14}C]taurocholate absorption from ileal segments carried out by Riottot and Sacquet (48) showed that the capacity for bile acid reabsorption in the ileum was probably enhanced in rats adapted to a resistant starch diet. The mechanisms are still not known, but it has been reported that the ileal Na-dependent bile acid transporter could be subject to upregulation under the influence of a variety of factors, including bile acids themselves (49,50). In human subjects, data on this point are scarce; some investigations in ileostomized subjects receiving experimental meals containing complex carbohydrates (beet fiber, psyllium) indicate that these compounds may increase neutral sterol excretion while bile acid excretion was unchanged or even slightly depressed (51,52). This observation does not necessarily prove that ileal bile acid reabsorption is increased; it could also reflect a decrease of hepatic bile acid secretion. Nevertheless, this indicates that fermentable carbohydates do not systematically lead to an increase of bile acid transfer into the colon.

The effect of resistant starch on the metabolism of bile acids by the hindgut microflora has been more extensively investigated. Acidification of the proximal large intestine content is likely to inhibit 7α-dehydroxylase activity and, in contrast, to activate bile acid amidate hydrolysis. In fact, Andrieux et al. (26) showed that the effects of resistant starch bile acid bacterial biotransformation are relatively complex, since transformation of β-muricholic acid to hyodeoxycholic is the first to disappear, followed by cholic acid transformation (e.g., to deoxycholic acid). These authors concluded that bacterial transformation of bile acids was modified by at least two mechanisms: inhibition of the bacterial enzyme activities dependent on pH and modification of the microbial flora. A rise in the fecal excretion of lithocholic and muricholic acids has also been found in rats fed retrograded starch (44) and in rats fed potato starch (4), but in this last case the effect was far less potent than that of cholestyramine and there was no synergism between resistant starch and cholestyramine.

In the cecum (or the proximal colon), total bile acid concentrations are frequently in the range of 10–15 mM, mostly unconjugated secondary bile acids, which could represent a threat to control of mucosal cell proliferation (53). In fact, a substantial part is bound and/or insolubilized: about 20% in rats adapted to a resistant starch diet compared to 40–50% in fiber-free controls (4). Furthermore, due to the dilution of the cecal contents with resistant starch, the absolute concentration of free bile acids was in fact depressed four- to fivefold. The factors responsible for bile acid insolubilization are certainly complex: resistant starch itself is unlikely to play a direct role (all the more so since it is readily broken down by the microflora), bulk pH acidification certainly participates in bile acid insolubilization, together with Ca salts (especially CaPi salts), and furthermore, bacteria themselves might constitute effective binding sites for bile acids (24), especially when their proliferation is stimulated. This helps limit the concentrations of potentially cytotoxic bile acids, since the secondary bile acids are more prone to insolubilization in acidic conditions. This could also affect the passive reabsorption of bile acids from the large intestine, which accounts for a large part (more than 20%) of bile acid absorption (54). In the rat, bile acid reabsorption in the cecal vein is somewhat increased by fermentable polysaccharides (in spite of lowered concentrations of soluble bile acids) because physiological factors such a greater surface area of exchange and blood flow improve the cecal capacity of absorption (25). This point has been clearly shown in rats adapted to GG diets, which promote moderately acidic fermentations, but it remains to confirm this adaptive response with acidic fermentations generally encountered with high–resistant starch diets. Whether resistant starch in humans affects bile acid reabsorption from the colon is unknown, although colonic reabsorption is clearly established, as shown by the presence of secondary bile acids in the bile acid pool in humans.

The fact that resistant starch chiefly affects the cholesterol digestive balance and lowers bile acid availability in the large intestine is of interest. First, it suggests that an accelerated transfer of bile acids from the ileum to the large intestine is not the only mechanism whereby fibers stimulate bile acid secretion by the liver, generally in parallel to an induction of cholesterol 7α-hydroxylase (55). Pandak et al. (56) have postulated the existence of a factor able to downregulate the amount of liver cholesterol 7α-hydroxylase, possibly an intestinal peptide secreted or absorbed from the intestine in the presence of bile acids; whether fibers or resistant starch could interfere with such a process awaits further investigation.

VII. ROLE OF SCFA IN THE LIPID-LOWERING EFFECTS OF RESISTANT STARCH

It has been speculated that SCFA could constitute a mediator of the lipid-lowering effect of fibers. This could be particularly relevant for compounds such as resistant starch or oligosaccharides (57). Resistant starches have been frequently considered as butyric acid–yielding substrates, but investigations have shown that large amounts of resistant starch in the diet were also very effective in promoting high–propionic acid fermentations (4,18,25). Nevertheless, under most conditions acetic acid is the major end product of resistant starch fermentation.

Experiments in vitro suggest that acetate can stimulate fatty acid synthesis by rat liver cells while inhibiting cholesterogenesis (58). Furthermore, acetate is anti-lipolytic and tends to decrease the availability of free fatty acids for liver metabolism, which could raise the contribution of acetate to the provision of hepatic acetyl CoA (e.g., for cholesterol synthesis) at the expense of long-chain fatty acids.

In vitro experiments have demonstrated that propionate is an effective inhibitor of both fatty acid and cholesterol synthesis (59,60). On the contrary in vivo investigations with the rat were less consistent (57,61). Nevertheless, investigations in humans have shown a short-term cholesterol-lowering effect of propionate (62). Todesco et al. (63) reported a slight lowering of total serum cholesterol and of low-density lipoprotein (LDL) and high-density lipoprotein (HDL) cholesterol. A significant inhibitory effect of propionate on [^{13}C] acetate recovery in triglycerides, but not in cholesterol, has been observed (64).

A noticeable induction of HMG CoA reductase has been reported in rats fed diets promoting high–propionic acid fermentations in the cecum, such as resistant starch (57). Propionate is a potent inhibitor of acetate utilization by liver cells in vitro and in vivo (65,66), but it is conceivable that propionate exerts a significant inhibition on lipid synthesis only when acetate is a major precursor of cytosolic acetyl CoA (60). In this context, with isolated hepatocytes obtained from rats fed a control or pectin diet, it has been reported that acetate incorporation into cholesterol was considerably enhanced (about ninefold) in rats adapted to the fiber diet (67). Propionate is also liable to inhibit the metabolism of other acetyl CoA precursors, especially lactate or long-chain fatty acids (8,60). It has also been reported that propionate may accelerate the conversion of cholesterol to bile acids in hepatocytes (68). In work performed on rat and human liver cells (69), propionate seemed to be ineffective in inhibiting cholesterogenesis on human hepatocytes; these cells exhibited a very high basal rate of cholesterogenesis— far higher than that reported in rat hepatocytes. Propionate can combine with carnitine to yield propionyl-carnitine, which tends to increase in the liver when high concentrations of propionate are present in the portal vein. It has been suggested that this could, in turn, deliver a signal to transfer carnitine from muscle to the liver (70). Furthermore, some data suggest that L-propionyl carnitine protects cell membranes and circulating lipoproteins from peroxidation (71).

VIII. CONCLUSION

Resistant starch appears intrinsically less effective than viscous fibers (gums, pectins, and some hemicelluloses) at interacting with the digestion and absorption of lipids in the small intestine. Nevertheless, it must be kept in mind that some structural features of resistant starches could give them a certain capacity to form inclusion complexes with acidic steroids. In the large intestine, resistant starch is clearly as effective as other fermentable fibers in promoting acidic fermentation by the microflora. This in turn profoundly affects the production of secondary bile acids and accentuates the insolubilization of bile acids in the hindgut, but little is known about the consequences of bile acid reabsorption from the large intestine. Whether alterations of bile acid metabolism are sufficient to elicit a noticeable cholesterol-lowering effect remains to be assessed, but they are certainly complementary to the action of sequestrants in the small intestine (72).

Various investigations indicate that resistant starch may play a regulatory role in postprandial triglyceridemia and, in a limited number of cases, in plasma cholesterol concentrations. It seems likely that these effects should be chiefly ascribed to the metabolic effects of resistant starch, especially the changes in postprandial glycemia and insulinemia, together with—possibly—some other gastrointestinal hormones. The actual role of SCFA is still a matter of discussion—it probably requires sufficient amounts to be absorbed to exert a significant effect. In fact, the metabolic effects of resistant starch result not only from SCFA production but also from a lower availability of glucose-yielding substrates in the small intestine, which corresponds to some extent to a substitution for glucose of SCFA.

Compared to most fibers, resistant starch is relatively easy to add in substantial amounts to the diet (especially starchy meals) provided that food processing does not convert resistant starch into a more digestible form. There is certainly a permanent supply of undigested starch in the colon; several authors have calculated that, besides dietary fibers, about 40 g daily would be required to account for daily bacterial output (1,70). It has been suggested that 5–10% of starch escapes absorption, with considerable interindividual differences. This indicates that ingestion of high-starch foods (cereals, some vegetables, etc.) should lead to a substantial appearance of resistant starch in the large intestine, and that resistant starch supplementations should then be relatively important to elicit significant changes in lipid metabolism.

REFERENCES

1. Stephen AM. Can J Physiol Pharmacol 69:116–120, 1991.
2. Annison G. Topping DL. Ann Rev Nutr 14:297–320, 1994.
3. Ikegami S. Tsuchihashi F, Harada H, Tsuchuhashi N, Nishide E, Innami S. J Nutr 120:353–360, 1990.
4. Younes H, Levrat M-A, Demigné C, Rémésy C. Lipids 3:847–853, 1995.
5. Gee JM, Faulks RM, Johnson IT. J Nutr 121:44–49, 1991.
6. Meslin JC, Andrieux C, Riottot M. Reprod Nutr Dév 32:73–81, 1992.
7. Poksay KS, Schneeman BO. J Nutr 133:1544–1549, 1983.
8. Morand C, Levrat M-A, Besson C, Demigné C, Rémésy C. J Nutr Biochem 5:138–144, 1994.
9. Topping DL, Gooden JM, Brown IL, Biebrick DA, McGrath L, Trimble RP, Choct M, Illman RJ. J Nutr. 127:615–622, 1997.
10. Morita T, Kasaoka S, Oh-hashi A, Ikai M, Numasaki Y, Kiriyama S. J Nutr 128:1156–1164, 1998.

11. Mathers JC, Dawson LD. Br J Nutr 66:313–329, 1991.
12. Silvester KR, Englyst HN, Cummings JH. Am J Clin Nutr 62:403–411, 1995.
13. Brown I, Warhurst M, Arcot J, Playne M, Illman RJ, Topping DL. J Nutr 127:1822–1827, 1997.
14. Kleeseen B, Stoof G, Proll J, Schmiedl D, Noack J, Blaut M. J Anim Sci 75:2453–2462, 1997.
15. Morand C, Rémésy C, Levrat M-A, Demigné C. J Nutr 122:345–354, 1992.
16. Byrnes SE, Brand Miller JC, Denyer GS. J Nutr 125:1430–1437, 1995.
17. Zhou X, Kaplan ML. J Nutr 127:1349–1356, 1997.
18. Noakes M, Clifton PM, Nestel PJ, Le Leu R, MacIntosh G. Am J Clin Nutr 64:944–951, 1996.
19. Raben A, Tagliabue A, Christensen NJ, Madsen J, Holst JJ, Astrup A. Am J Clin Nutr 60:544–551, 1994.
20. Behall KM, Scholfield DJ, Yuhaniak I, Canary JJ. Am J Clin Nutr 49:337–344, 1989.
21. Abadie C, Hug M, Kübli C, Gains N. Biochem J 299:725–730, 1994.
22. Rémésy C, Levrat M-A, Gamet L, Demigné C. Am J Physiol 264:G855–862, 1993.
23. Benson GM, Haskins NJ, Eckers C, Moore PJ, Reid DG, Mitchell RC, Waghmare S, Suckling KE. J Lip Res 34:2121–2134, 1993.
24. Gelissen I, Eastwood MA. Br J Nutr 74:221–228, 1995.
25. Moundras C, Behr SR, Rémésy C, Demigné C. J Nutr 127:1068–1076, 1997.
26. Andrieux C, Gadelle D, Leprince C, Sacquet E. Br J Nutr 62:103–119, 1989.
27. Verbeek MJ, Deckere De EA, Tijburg LB, Amelsvoort Van JM, Beynen AC. Br J Nutr 74:807–820, 1995.
28. Chezem JC, Furumoto E, Story J. Nutr Res 11/12:1671–1682, 1997.
29. Hylla S, Gostner A, Dusel G, Anger H, Bartram H-P, Christl SU, Kasper H, Sheppach W. Am J Clin Nutr 67:136–142, 1998.
30. Bartram HP, Scheppach W, Heid C, Fabian C, Kasper H. Cancer Res 51:4238–4242, 1991.
31. Kabir M, Rizkalla SW, Champ M, Luo J, Boillot J, Bruzzo F, Slama GJ Nutr 128:35–43, 1998.
32. Deckere De EA, Kloots WJ, Amelsvoort Van JM. Br J Nutr 73:287–298, 1995.
33. Achour L, Flourié B, Briet F, Franchisseur C, Bornet F, Champ M, Rambaud J-C, Messing B. Am J Clin Nutr 66:1151–1159, 1997.
34. Lere-Metzger M, Rizkalla SW, Luo J, Champ M, Kabir M, Bruzzo F, Bornet F, Slama G. Br J Nutr 75:723–732, 1996.
35. Kok NN, Taper HS, Delzenne NJ Appl Toxicol 18:47–53, 1988.
36. Sehti S, Gibney MJ, Williams CM. Nutr Res Rev 6:161–183, 1993.
37. Heijnen ML, Van Amelsvoort JM, Deurenberg P, Beynen AC. Am J Clin Nutr 64:312–318, 1996.
38. Olson B, Schneeman B. J Nutr 128:1031–1036, 1998.
39. Horigome T, Sakagushi E, Kishimoto C. Br J Nutr 68:231–244, 1992.
40. Khallou J, Riottot M, Parquet M, Verneau C, Lutton C. Dig Dis Sci 40:2540–2548, 1995.
41. Mathé D, Riottot M, Rostaqui N, Sacquet E, Navarro N, Lécuyer B, Lutton C. J Clin Biochem Nutr 14:17–24, 1993.
42. Heijnen ML, Amelsvoort Van JM, Deurenberg P, Beynen AC. Am J Clin Nutr 64:312–318, 1996.
43. Cheng H-H, Yu W-W. J Nutr 127:153–157, 1997.
44. Verbeek MJ, Deckere De EA, Tijburg LB, Amelsvoort Van JM, Beynen AC. Br J Nutr 74:807–820, 1995.
45. Hylla S, Gostner A, Dusel G, Anger H, Bartram H-P, Christl SU, Kasper H, Sheppach W. Am J Clin Nutr 67:136–142, 1998.
46. Ide T, Horii M. Agric Biol Chem 51:3155–3157, 1987.
47. Demigné C, Levrat M-A, Behr SR, Moundras C, Rémésy C. Nutr Res 18:1215–1216, 1998.
48. Riottot M, Sacquet E. Br J Nutr 53:307–310, 1985.
49. Lilienau J, Crombie DL, Munoz J, Longmire-Cook SJ, Hagey LR, Hoffmann AF. Gastroenterology 104:38–46, 1993.
50. Stravitz RT, Sanyal AJ, Pandak WM, Vlahcevic ZR, Beets JW, Dawson PA. Gastroenterology 113:1599–1608, 1997.
51. Langkilde AM, Andersson H, Bosaeus I. Br J Nutr 70:757–766, 1993.
52. Sandberg AS, Andersson H, Bosaeus I, Carlsson NG, Hasselblad K, Harrod M. Am J Clin Nutr 60:751–756, 1994.
53. Reddy BS, Engle A, Simi B, Goldman M. Gastroenterology 102:1475–1482, 1992.

54. Juste C, Legrand-Defretin V, Corring T, Rerat A. Dig Dis Sci 33:67–73, 1988.
55. Chiang JYL. Front Biosci 15:D176–D193, 1998.
56. Pandak WM, Heuman DM, Hylemon PB, Chiang JYL, Vlahcevic Z. R. Gastroenterology 108:533–544, 1995.
57. Beynen AC, Buechler K, Van Der Molen AJ. Int J Biochem 14:165–169, 1982.
58. Anderson JW. In: Binder HJ, Cummings JH, Soergel K, eds. Physiological and Clinical Aspects of Short-Chain Fatty Acids. Lancaster: Kluwer Academic Press, 1994, pp. 509–523.
59. Demigné C, Morand C, Levrat M-A, Besson C, Rémésy C. Br J Nutr 74:209–219, 1995.
60. Levrat M-A, Favier M-L, Moundras C, Rémésy C, Demigné C, Morand C. J Nutr 124:531–538, 1994.
61. Berggren AM, Nyman MGL, Lundquist I. Br J Nutr 76:287–296, 1996.
62. Wolever TMS, Spadafora PJ, Eshuis H. Am J Clin Nutr 53:681–687, 1991.
63. Todesco T, Rao A, Bosello O. Am J Clin Nutr 54:860–865, 1991.
64. Wolever TMS, Spadafora PJ, Cunnane SC. Am J Clin Nutr 61:1241–1247, 1995.
65. Gordon MJ, Crabtree B. Int J Biochem 24:1029–1031, 1992.
66. Rémésy C, Demigné C, Morand C. In: Cummings JH, Rombeau JL, Sakata T, eds. Physiological and Clinical Aspects of Short-Chain Fatty Acids. Cambridge: Cambridge University Press, 1995, pp. 171–190.
67. Stark AH, Madar Z. J Nutr 123:2166–2173, 1993.
68. Imaizumi K, Hirata K, Yasni S, Sugano M. Biosci Biotech Biochem 56:557–564, 1992.
69. Lin Y, Vonk RJ, Maarten JHS. Br J Nutr 74:197–207, 1995.
70. Stephen A. In Binder HJ, Cummings JH, Soergel K, eds. Physiological and Clinical Aspects of Short-Chain Fatty Acids. Lancaster: Kluwer Academic Press, 1994, pp. 250–271.
71. Bertelli A, Conte A, Ronca G. Drugs Exp Clin Res XX:191–197, 1994.
72. Luner PE, Amidon GL. Pharm Res 9:670–676, 1992.

11

Critical Review of Hydrogen Breath Test Methods in Resistant Starch and Dietary Fiber Research

Merete Olesen
KAS, Gentofte, Copenhagen, Denmark

I. INTRODUCTION

Dietary fibers (nonstarch polysaccharides, NSP) and resistant starch (RS, the sum of starch and products of starch degradation not absorbed in the small intestine of healthy individuals) are, per definition, indigestible by mammalian digestive enzymes, but not necessarily by microbial enzymes (1). An important aspect of NSP and RS research is therefore the fermentability by the colonic bacterial flora, in terms of both amounts escaping digestion in the small bowel, amounts actually fermented by the colonic bacteria, and pathways of carbohydrate metabolism in the colon. Several techniques in vitro and in vivo have been developed to evaluate these aspects of carbohydrate metabolism. In vitro hydrolysis with pancreatin and amyloglucosidase has been used to identify nondigestible fractions of starches, and the results have been compared with amounts of starch escaping digestion in ileostomates (2). Studies in ileostomates (3–5) and in healthy humans using ileal intubation techniques (6,7) have also contributed to estimating the amounts of carbohydrate escaping digestion in the small intestine. Identification and quantitation of fermentation products have been performed with fecal slurries (8). Quantitative recovery and analysis of fecal contents have helped to quantify the carbohydrates, especially NSP, that are neither absorbed nor fermented. In addition, fecal analysis has been used for semiquantitative estimates of end products of carbohydrate metabolism (9). The advantages and shortcomings of these methods will not be discussed here.

The major end products of carbohydrate fermentation are CO_2, H_2, CH_4, H_2S, and short-chain fatty acids (SCFAs), especially acetate, butyrate, and lactate.

II. THE H_2 BREATH TEST

The fecel content of end products of carbohydrate fermentation only represents the "overflow" of the end products escaping absorption in colon. This has prompted interest in tracing the end products of fermentation in other end organs such as blood (acetate) or expiratory air (H_2 and CH_4).

The presence of H_2 and CH_4 in the gut lumen has been known for a long time (10,11). Measurements of H_2 in expired air was pioneered by Calloway and Murphy in the 1960s (12). The relationship between unabsorbed carbohydrates in the colon and increasing concentrations of H_2 in expired air has been established (13,14). During the 1970s compact and rapid monitors using H_2-sensitive electrochemical cells were developed (15). Use of the H_2 breath test in carbohydrate research has been extensively reviewed (16–18). One major methodological improvement of the test has been published (19).

III. H_2 DISPOSAL

Based on studies by Levitt with intestinal gas perfusion (20), it has been assumed that a constant fraction (14%) of the total H_2 produced in the gut lumen was excreted via the lungs. This raised the hope that measuring expired H_2 would give a quantitative estimate of substrate fermented in the colon. With the nonabsorbable disaccharide lactulose as a standard, several groups have tried to quantitate the malabsorbed fractions of lactose (21) and fructose (22) and the malabsorption of wheat starch (23–25). Several studies addressing standardization of experimental conditions and interpretation of the test results have been published (for an overview, see Ref. 16).

In spite of improvements in the H_2 breath test, discrepancies between the quantitative estimates obtained by the H_2 breath test and ileal intubation techniques have been reported (6,7).

Levitt's original results were challenged by the results of Christl et al. (26). Based on studies in a whole body calorimeter and simultaneous breath gas measurements, this group found that 65% of total H_2 and CH_4 was expired in breath at production rates up to 200 mL/24 h. At higher excretion rates, the proportion decreased to a nadir of 25%. A production rate of 200 mL/24 h and recovery of 65% corresponds fairly well to acute measures of 13–16 ppm. Stimulated H_2 recovery in breath easily exceeds this level, implying that the assumption of linearity between H_2 production and pulmonary excretion only covers the situation of nonstimulated H_2 production.

Another interesting difference between these two studies is the estimate of H_2 production (20,26). Levitt studied the production rate by continuous washout from the intestines, whereas Christl et al. only measured the H_2 that actually escaped into the open air. The two different techniques resulted in very different estimates of basal production rates of H_2. Levitt found a basal rate of 0.24 mL/min (345 mL/24 h), in contrast to 35 ± 6.1 mL/24 h found by Christ et al.

H_2 is eliminated from the colon via three routes: anal excretion, diffusion to the blood with subsequent pulmonary excretion, or metabolization by the colonic bacterial flora to other end products (27). Adaptation to a given substrate may even reduce H_2 production (28). From the figures mentioned above, it seems that 90% of H_2 produced under basal circumstances is metabolized by the colonic bacterial flora. With an accelerated production rate, an increasing fraction of produced H_2 may be disposed of via diffusion to the blood and/or more rapid propulsion through the colon. It seems, therefore, that the H_2 breath test is a measure of "overflow" during colonic fermentation rather than a quantification of carbohydrate fermentation per se.

IV. OUR EXPERIENCE WITH THE H_2 BREATH TEST

A. The H_2 Breath Test and Resistant Starch

Classification of starch as readily digestible, slowly digestible, and resistant starch is based on in vitro analysis of starch (2), with the ileostomy model as an in vivo control. An important aspect of resistant starch is fermentability. Unfortunately, the ileostomy model and ileal intubation techniques are unsuitable for studying colonic starch metabolism. The capacity for fermentation depends on the microbial flora, the microenvironment, and the motility of the bowel—factors that are difficult or impossible to control for in vitro.

The H_2 breath test is convenient in elucidating the human colonic microbial flora's capacity for fermentation of different carbohydrates. As indicated above, the H_2 breath test estimates the "overflow" of H_2 production and an increase in expiratory H_2 signals ongoing fermentation. This information can be used to elucidate the fate of resistant starch in the colon. We have measured the fermentability of three different kinds of RS (29). Raw potato starch (RPS) contains approximately 58% resistant starch (RS_2, resistant starch granules) (2); corn flakes (CF), 4.6% RS (RS_3, retrograded starch) (2); and hylon VII, high-amylomaize starch (HAS), 30% RS (RS_3). We compared the H_2 response patterns to the usual lactulose standard (Fig. 1).

The highest cumulated H_2 response was seen after ingestion of 50 g of RPS containing approximately 29 g of RS_2 (Fig. 1). We found no increase in end expiratory H_2 after ingestion of 75 g of HAS, even during 24-hour recording. This implies that the RS_3 from HAS is fermented to end products other than H_2 or that it may only be fermented to a very limited extent in the human colon or is digested and assimilated in the small intestine. In a study of fecal recovery after ingestion of different sources of RS, it was found that the average digestibility of potato RS_2 was 89%, wheat RS_3 65%, and maize RS3 84%. There were considerable individual differences, recovery of RS_3 in feces from some individuals amounted to nearly 100% of ingested amounts (30).

CF contained far less RS_3 than did HAS (4.6 g vs. 22.5 g per 100 g, respectively). Nonetheless, the H_2 response after CF was significantly higher than after HAS, indicating a difference in fermentation pattern of the two different sources of RS_3 or a difference in fermentable substrate, including carbohydrates other than RS_3 reaching the colon with the two different test meals.

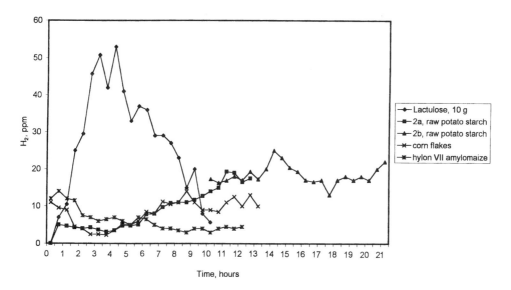

Fig. 1 Increases in end expiratory H_2 after ingestion of different test meals. Results represented as mean values for seven volunteers. Results obtained after ingestion of: 1) lactulose, 10 g; 2a) raw potato starch, 50 g at 8 a.m. or 2b) at 11 p.m. and registration of H_2 response from 8.30 a.m. the following day; 3) corn flakes, 100 g; 4) hylon VII high amylomaize starch 75 g.

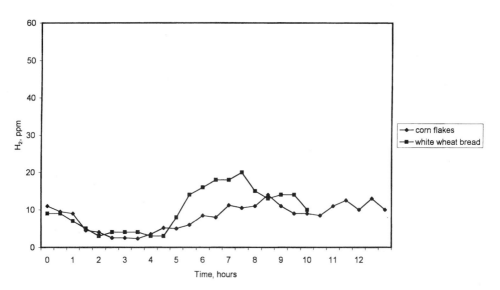

Fig. 2   Increases in end expiratory H_2 after ingestion of 1) corn flakes, 100 g, 4.6 g RS_3, 2) white wheat bread made from 100 g wheat flour, 1–2 g RS_3. Results represented as means values from seven healthy volunteers.

Figure 2 depicts the H_2 response after ingestion of bread baked of 100 g white wheat flour (WWF) (31) compared to the H_2 response elicited by ingestion of 100 g CF. The content of RS in WWF bread is 1–2 g/100 g (2) and 4.6 g/100 g in the CF test meal, but this difference was not mirrored in the cumulative H_2 responses after the two test meals. These results may indicate that in vitro and in vivo resistant starches are not necessarily identical. A lack of appropriate test systems leaves this hypothesis untestable at present.

RS is defined as the sum of starch and starch degradation products not absorbed in the small intestine of healthy individuals (1). Using the H_2 breath test, we found that the amount of starch reaching the colon in healthy individuals also depended on the composition of the total meal. The H_2 responses to test meals consisting of bread made from 100 g wwf + 11 g butter were significantly higher than the H_2 responses to test meals consisting of the bread alone, indicating that absorption in the small intestine depended not only on the nature of the food elements (31) but also on the composition of the total meal.

From the H_2 responses, it seemed that the rate of lactulose fermentation $\gg RS_2 \gg RS_3$. The H_2 breath test is inappropriate to decide if RS_3 and RS_2 are fermented to the same extent as lactulose, but the patterns of fermentation are obviously different. The increase in end expiratory H_2 after lactulose peaked within 1–2 hours after ingestion, followed by a gradual return to basal values. In contrast, the increase in end expiratory H_2 after RPS only started 5–8 hours postingestion, followed by an elevated H_2 level for several hours. In 5 of 7 volunteers, the H_2 excretion had not returned to basal levels 22 hours after ingestion. In this way, the H_2 breath test has shown that fermentation of RS from RPS must be slow compared to fermentation of lactulose and that the colonic bacterial flora can handle a large dose of fermentable substrate without excessive H_2 production.

B.   The H_2 Breath Test and Dietary Fibers (NSP)

Use of the H_2 breath test has been largely unsuccessful in the study of NSP fermentation (32,33). This may reflect a slow and incomplete fermentation, especially of nonsoluble NSP, in the

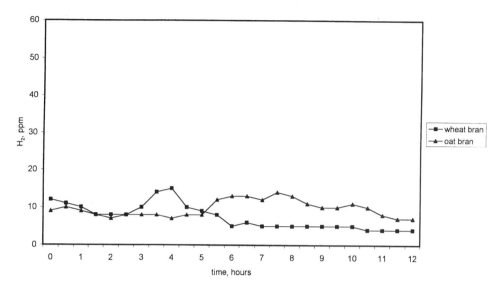

Fig. 3 Increases in end expiratory H$_2$ after ingestion of 1) wheat bran, 20 g (48% NSP), 2) oat bran, 20 g (19% NSP). Results presented as mean values from seven healthy volunteers.

human colon (34). With the modified H$_2$ breath test introduced by Strocchi et al. (19), however, we detected fermentation of wheat bran and oat bran (35). We found these two sources of NSP to result in different patterns of fermentation. Oat bran elicited a significantly higher cumulative H$_2$ response than wheat bran (Fig. 3).

Fermentation of pectin, a viscous, soluble fiber, has also been studied successfully using the H$_2$ breath test (36). The pattern of H$_2$ production after pectin resembles the pattern after ingestion of RPS (RS$_2$) (Fig. 1). In herbal medicine, both pectin (raw apples) and RS$_2$ (raw potato starch) have been used to treat acute diarrhea. RS$_2$ has been found to prolong intestinal transit time (30), and the viscous NSP pectin may exert the same effect. Even though both increase the fecal volume, they may exert a beneficial effect on watery diarrhea. Lactulose, well known for its laxative effect, may accelerate the intestinal transit (37), in addition to its osmotic effect. Wheat bran, a nonsoluble NSP used as a laxative, which has been found to be only moderately fermented by the human colonic flora (34) by the H$_2$ breath test, was found to accelerate intestinal transit (31).

In conclusion, the H$_2$ breath test can provide new information on fermentation and the biological effects of putative fermentation substrates in the human colon.

V. THE H$_2$ BREATH TEST SUPPLEMENTED BY THE CH$_4$ BREATH TEST

Thirty to fifty percent of healthy adults in the western world excrete CH$_4$ in breath (38,39) in addition to H$_2$. Several groups have tried to supplement the information obtained by the H$_2$ breath test with simultanous measurements of expiratory CH$_4$. The degree of fermentation of NSP and RS cannot be predicted by 24-hour records of H$_2$ and CH$_4$ production in a whole body cnnalorimeter (26,40). CH$_4$ is mainly produced in the left-sided human colon, while H$_2$ is produced throughout the colonic length, with a maximum in the right-sided colon (41).

We found three patterns in breath H$_2$/CH$_4$ excretion in response to a lactulose challenge (Fig. 4). The most common pattern is a sustained increase in end expiratory H$_2$ and no CH$_4$ (more than 50% of all cases). In some cases H$_2$ and CH$_4$ increase in parallel. Finally, a small

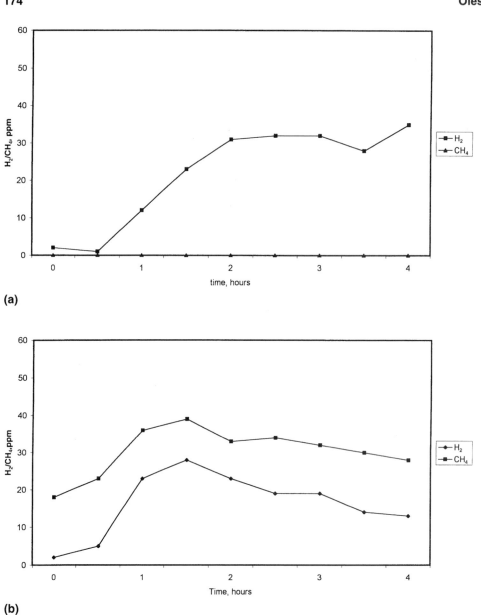

(a)

(b)

Fig. 4 Three principally different H_2/CH_4 responses to a lactulose challenge (10 g): (a) a sustained significant increase in end expiratory H_2, no CH_4; (b) a parallel significant increase in both H_2 and CH_4; (c) a sustained increase in CH_4 and a small, insignificant increase in H_2.

number of subjects respond with no increase in breath H_2. They all have a sustained high CH_4 production. This last pattern may be due to slow bowel transit or a particular colonic bacterial flora (or both).

In our studies of RS and NSP fermentation, we select humans with a significant increase in end expiratory H_2 after a lactulose challenge, whether or not they have a concomittant increase in end expiratory CH_4. The usefulness of CH_4 measurements is still under evaluation.

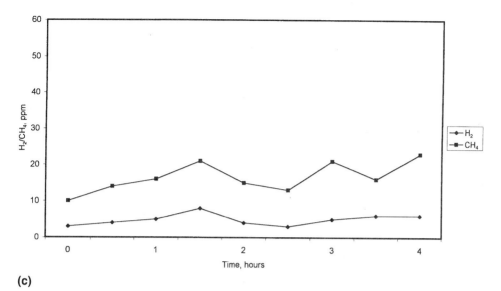

(c)

Fig. 4 Continued.

VI. CONCLUSIONS

1. The H_2 breath test is easy to perform, noninvasive, and involves no health hazards.
2. The H_2 breath test provides a clear qualitative detection of fermentable substrates in the human colon.
3. The H_2 breath test provides an easy and robust estimate of the oro-cecal transit time.
4. The H_2 breath test provides a semiquantitative measure of the influence of different test meals on the oro-cecal transit time and the size of the H_2 response to a given fermentable marker.

REFERENCES

1. Asp NG. Resistant starch. Proceedings from the second plenary meeting of EURESTA: European FLAIR Concerted Action No. 11 on physiological imålications of the consumption of resistant starch in man. Eur J Clin Nutr 1992; 46(suppl 2): S1.
2. Englyst HN, Kingman SM, Cummings JH. Classification and measurement of nutritionally important starch fractions. Eur J Clin Nutr 1992; 46(suppl 2): S33–S50.
3. Chapman RW, Sillery JK, Graham MM, Saunders DR. Absorption of starch by healthy ileostomates: effect of transit time and of carbohydrate load. Am J Clin Nutr 1985; 41:1244–1248.
4. Langkilde AM, Andersson H, Schweizer TF, Würsch P. Digestion and absorption of sorbitol, maltitol and isomalt from the small bowel. A study in ileostomy subjects. Eur J Clin Nutr 1994; 48:768–775.
5. Lia Å, Sundberg B, Åman P, Sandberg AS, Hallman G, Andersson H. Substrates available for colonic fertentation from oat, barley, and wheat bread diets. A study in ileostomy subjects. Br J Nutr 1996; 76:797–808.
6. Stephen AM, Haddag AC, Phillips SF. Passage of carbohydrate into the colon. Direct measurements in humans. Gastroenterology 1983; 85:589–595.
7. Flourié B, Leblond A, Florent Ch, Rautureau M, Bisalli A, Rambaud JC. Starch malabsorption and

breath gas excretion in healthy humans consuming low- and high-starch diets. Gastroenterology 1988; 95:356–363.

8. Barry JL, Hoebler C, MacFarlane GT, MacFarlane S, Mathers JC, Reed KA, Mortensen PB, Nordgaard I, Rowland IR, Rumney CJ. Estimation of the fermentability of dietary fibre in vitro: a European interlaboratory study. Br J Nutr 1995; 74:303–322.

9. MacFarlane GT, Gibson GR. Microbiological aspects of the production of short-chain fatty acids in the large bowel. In: Cummings JH, Rombeau JL, Sakata T, eds. Physiological and Clinical Aspects of Short-Chain Fatty Acids. Cambridge: Cambridge University Press, 1995:87–105.

10. Kirk E. The quantity and composition of human colonic flatus. Gastroenterology 1949; 12:782–794.

11. Ruge E. Beiträge zur Kenntnis der Darmgase. Chem Zentralbl 1862; 7:347–364.

12. Calloway DH, Murphy EL. The use of expired air to measure intestinal gas formation. Ann NY Acad Sci 1968; 150:82–95.

13. Calloway DH, Murphy EL, Bauer D. Determination of lactose intolerance by breath analysis. Am J Dig Dis 1969; 14:811–815.

14. Levitt MD, Donaldson RM. Use of respiratory hydrogen (H_2) excretion to detect carbohydrate malabsorption. J Lab Clin Med 1970; 75:937–945.

15. Bartlett K, Dobson JV, Eastham E. A new method for the detection of hydrogen in breath and its application to acquired and inborn sugar malabsorption. Clin Chem Acta 1980; 108:189–194.

16. Rumessen JJ. Hydrogen and methane breath tests for evaluation of resistant carbohydrates. Eur J Clin Nutr 1992; 46(suppl 2): S77–S90.

17. Strocchi A, Levitt MD. Measurement of starch absorption in humans. Can J Physiol Pharmacol 1991; 69:108–110.

18. McBurney MI. Passage of starch into the colon of humans: quantitation and implications. Can J Physiol Pharmacol 1991; 69:130–136.

19. Strocchi A, Corazza G, Ellis CJ, Gasbarri G, Levitt MD. Detection of malabsorption of low doses of carbohydrate: accuracy of various breath H_2 criteria. Gastroenterology 1993; 105:1404–1410.

20. Levitt MD. Production and excretion of hydrogen gas in man. N Engl J Med 1969; 281:122–127.

21. Bond JH, Levitt MD. Quantitative measurement of lactose absorption. Gastroenterology 1976; 70: 1058–1062.

22. Rumessen JJ, Gudmand-Høyer E. Absorption capacity of fructose in fructose in healthy adults. Comparison with sucrose and its constituent monosaccharides. Gut 1986; 27:1161–1168.

23. Wolever TMS, Cohen Z, Thompson LU, Thorne MJ, Jenkins MJA, Prokipchuk EJ, Jenkins DJA. Ileal loss of available carbohydrate in man: comparison of breath hydrogen method with direct measurement using a human ileostomy model. Am J Gastroenterol 1986; 81:115–122.

24. Levitt MD, Hirsch P, Fetzer CA, Sheahan M, Levine AS. H_2 excretion after ingestion of complex carbohydrates. Gastroenterology 1987; 92:383–389.

25. Flourié B, Florent C, Etanchaud F, Evard D, Franchisseur C, Rambaud JC. Starch absorption by healthy man evaluated by lactulose hydrogen breath test. Am J Clin Nutr 1988; 47:61–66.

26. Christl SU, Murgatroyd PR, Gibson GR, Cummings JH. Production, metabolism, and excretion of hydrogen in the large intestine. Gastroenterology 1992; 102:1269–1277.

27. Gibson GR, Cummings JH, MacFarlane GT, Allison C, Segal I, Vorster HH, Walker ARP. Alternative pathways for hydrogen disposal during fermentation in the human colon. Gut 1990; 31:679–683.

28. Hertzler SR, Savaiano DA, Levitt MD. Fecal hydrogen production and consumption measurements. Dig Dis Sci 1997; 42:348–353.

29. Olesen M, Rumessen JJ, Gudmand-Høyer E. Intestinal transport and fermentation of resistant starch evaluated by the hydrogen breath test. Eur J Clin Nutr 1994; 48:692–701.

30. Cummings JH, Beatty ER, Kingman SM, Bingham SA, Englyst HN. Digestion and physiological properties of resistant starch in the human large bowel. Br J Nutr 1996; 75:733–747.

31. Olesen M, Gudmand-Høyer E. Maldigestion and colonic fermentation of wheat bread in humans and the influence of dietary fat. Am J Clin Nutr 1997; 66:62–66.

32. Ranganathan S, Champ M, Pechard C, Blanchard P, Nguyen M, Colonna P, Krempf M. Comparative study of the acute effects of resistant starch and dietary fibers on metabolic indexes in men. Am J Clin Nutr 1994; 59:879–883.

33. Rosado JL, Lopez P, Morales M, Allen LH. Fiber digestibility and breath-hydrogen excretion in subjects consuming rural and urban Mexican diets. Am J Clin Nutr 1991; 53:55–60.
34. Cummings JH. Dietaty fibre. Br Med Bull 1981; 37:65–70.
35. Olesen M, Gudmand-Høyer E, Norsker M, Kofod L, Adler-Nissen J. Fermentability of an enzymatically modified solubilised potato polysaccharide (SPP). Eu J Clin Nutr 1998; 52:110–114.
36. Pomare Ew, Branch WJ, Cummings JH. Carbohydrate fermentation in the human colon and its relation to acetate concentration in venous blood. J Clin Invest 1985; 75:1448–1454.
37. Wutzke KD, Heine WE, Plath C, Leitzmann P, Radke M, Mohr C, Richter I, Gülzow HU, Hobusch D. Evaluation of oro-cecal transit time: a comparison of the lactose-(^{13}C, ^{15}N)ureide ^{13}CO$_2$- and the lactulose H$_2$ breath test in humans. Eu J Clin Nutr 1997; 51:11–19.
38. Björneklett A, Jensen E. Relationships between hydrogen (H$_2$) and methan (CH$_4$) production in man. Scand J Gastroenterol 1982; 17:985–992.
39. McKay LF, Eastwood MA, Brydon WG. Methane excretion in man-a study of breath, flatus, and faeces. Gut 1985; 26:69–74.
40. Poppitt SD, Livesey G, Faulks RM, Roe M, Prentice AM, Elia M. Circadian patterns of total 24-h hydrogen and methane excretion in humans ingesting nonstarch polysaccharide (NSP) diets and the implications for indirect calorimetric and D$_2$^{18}O methodologies. Eur J Clin Nutr 1996; 50:525–534.
41. Flourié B, Pellier P, Florent C, Marteau P, Pochart P, Rambaud JC. Site and substrates for methane production in human colon. Am J Physiol 1991; 260:G752–757.

12

Lactulose

A Review on Effects, Clinical Results, and Safety Aspects in Relation to Its Influence on the Colonic Environment

Robert Havenaar and Wim van Dokkum
TNO Nutrition and Food Research, Zeist, The Netherlands

I. INTRODUCTION

Lactulose is a synthetic disaccharide [4-O-β-D-galactosyl-D-fructose, molecular weight (MW) = 342.3], which does not occur in nature. It is produced in small amounts during heat treatment of milk. Lactulose can be made on a large scale from lactose by alkaline isomerization during which galactose is linked to fructose by β 1, 4-glycoside. There are five possible isomers of lactulose: α and β-pyranose, α and β-furanose, and the acyclic form (1,2).

Lactulose can be produced as a syrup (50/50% w/w; 67 g lactulose/100 mL syrup) or as crystalline pure lactulose powder. In the text below the lactulose dosage is given in mL or g, indicating the intake of syrup or powder, respectively.

Lactulose is thought to have many potential applications, ranging from stimulation of beneficial bacteria in the intestinal microflora to the treatment of severely ill, chronic hepatic encephalitic patients. This chapter will assess the scientific background for these health-promoting and therapeutic properties of lactulose.

II. INTESTINAL MICROFLORA

A. Intestinal Fermentation of Lactulose

Lactulose is not absorbed from the small intestine. In the cecum and, if still available, in the colon, lactulose is anaerobically fermented by the indigenous microflora, evidenced by the production of hydrogen or methane (3–5), which can be measured in expired breath (see Sec. X) and by the production of short-chain fatty acids (SCFA) (6) and lactic acid (7,8), especially after adaptation (7). After the intake of lactulose an increased concentration of serum acetate has been found (4,5). Peak concentrations of portal blood SCFA were found 15–45 minutes after instillation of 10 g lactulose in the cecum during surgery (acetate, propionate, and butyrate concentrations of 241 ± 142, 39 ± 18, and 27 ± 17 mmol/L, respectively). In peripheral blood the acetate concentration reflected the portal increase, while propionate and butyrate were found in low and very low concentrations, respectively (9). The fermentation of lactulose also resulted in a lower fecal pH, depending on the dose, ranging from pH 6 (20 g/day) (7) to pH 5 (>100 g/day) (10).

The ultimate role of SCFA in the function of the large intestine, such as stimulation of the mucosal proliferation, and their relationship to health aspects, such as the possible antimutagenicity of butyrate, is not completely understood, but clinical evaluation to define their role would be worthwhile (11).

B. Influence of Lactulose on the Ecology of the Intestinal Microflora

It is not known whether lactulose can act as a substrate for beneficial microorganisms in the large intestine, resulting in an increased colonization resistance against potential pathogens. In vitro studies have shown that lactulose can act as a substrate for many lactic acid bacteria, including gastrointestinal genera (*Lactobacillus, Streptococcus, Bacteroides*) and *Bifidobacterium*, and can support their growth (12,13). In rats fed formula milk containing 0.5% lactulose for 3 and 5 weeks, no change in fecal numbers of bifidobacteria was found after 3 weeks, but significantly increased numbers were demonstrated after 5 weeks (14). In a second study in rats this result was confirmed: a bifidogenic effect in combination with a lower fecal pH was found after feeding the animals infant formula with 0.5% lactulose as compared with control milk (15). Besides, a significantly higher phagocytic index of peritoneal macrophages were found in the lactulose group in comparison to the control group, indicating a positive response of the host nonspecific defense system.

The effect of lactulose (1.2 g in infant diet) on *Bifidobacterium* was studied for the first time by Petuely in 1957. The next positive studies were published approximately 10 years later: in 1966 Schneegans studied the combination of freeze-dried *B. bifidum* and lactulose in a diet for healthy and sick children in order to suppress *Escherichia coli*, followed by studies with lactulose in infant nutrition (1.2–1.5%) published by Haenel and coworkers in 1967 and 1968 (reviewed in Ref. 16). These studies showed an increased number of *B. bifidum* in the large intestine in association with lower numbers of gram-negative bacteria and a lower pH value, suggesting intestinal conditions more similar to those in breast-fed children than when formula milk was fed without lactulose. However, the pH was not as low as found in breast-fed babies, and *B. bifidus* type IV, which appeared specific for breast-fed babies, was not found. The bifidogenic effect of lactulose was confirmed by the studies performed by Braun, published in 1971, 1973, and 1974. He questioned, however, the role of bifidobacteria in comparison to immunological factors in the resistance to infections of breast-fed babies (reviewed in Ref. 2). In a study published in 1959 (17) the intake of lactulose in combination with lactose (in total 7.5%) by infants ($n = 38$; 4 months old) did not result in an appreciable decrease in the numbers of *E. coli*. Babies fed formula milk containing 0.5–1.0% lactulose showed an increased level of bifidobacteria and a decreased level of coliform bacteria in comparison to control formula milk (18). Incorporation of 0.5% lactulose resulted in a similar fecal pH and in levels of bifidobacteria similar to those found in breast-fed babies.

In healthy adults ($n = 8$, 18–22 years of age) the intake of 3 g of lactulose per day for 2 weeks resulted in a significantly ($p < 0.01$) increased number of *Bifidobacterium* in fecal samples. The numbers of lecithinase-positive Clostridia, including *C. perfringens*, and Bacteroidaceae as well as the fecal indole, skatol, phenol, β-glucuronidase, nitro- and azoreductase activity decreased significantly ($p < 0.05$), while the fecal pH changed from 7.0 to 6.4 (19).

In a second study by this team the intake of lactulose (3 g/day) by adults ($n = 9$) for 14 days resulted in a decreased number of individuals colonized with lecithinase-positive clostridia and at lower numbers per gram of feces (20): before treatment nine out of nine were colonized with an average of 3.9×10^5 clostridia/g feces; after treatment four out of nine were colonized with an average of 4.2×10^3 Clostridia/g feces. In cirrhotic patients ($n = 21$) the treatment with lactulose or lactitol for 10 days resulted in higher numbers of fecal Lactobacilli (21). Although both products decreased fecal pH, lactulose did not decrease the numbers of enterococci and enterobacteria, in contrast to lactitol.

The treatment of human volunteers infected with *Salmonella* or *Shigella* with lactulose resulted in fecal clearance of both, indicating a reduction of intestinal infections (16). A significant reduction in respiratory tract infections in long-term hospital patients by lactulose has also been described (22). Regular lactulose therapy (30 mL syrup/day) in a 6-month retrospective study with long-term hospital patients ($n = 45$; 66–93 years of age) resulted in a significantly ($p < 0.005$) lower prevalence of urinary tract infections in comparison to a nontreated control group (23), resulting in a significant ($p < 0.005$) lower number of patients requiring antibiotic therapy. These results could not, however, be confirmed in two additional groups treated with low dose of lactulose for 6 months or less than 2 months.

Intensive liver resection in rats without further treatment resulted in a high mortality rate due to endotoxemia, while pretreatment with agents that altered the gut contents, such as lactulose, reduced the level of serum endotoxins and enhanced survival (24). In in vitro studies it has been shown that 55 mg of lactulose inactivated 0.01 mg of endotoxin on limulus lysate, suggesting a direct antiendotoxin effect of lactulose (25). Besides, the authors found a significantly decreased blood endotoxin level ($p < 0.01$) and reduced liver damage in rats after treatment with lactulose, indicating an inhibiting effect of lactulose on endotoxin absorption from the gut. In a rat model of colitis it has been shown that enteral administration of lactulose to rats significantly reduced the systemic concentration of endotoxins from gram-negative bacteria as compared with the control group treated with water (5.4 pg/mL vs. 23.7 pg/mL) (26). The above-mentioned studies support the hypothesis that patients with inflammatory bowel disease may benefit from treatment with lactulose due to the prevention of systemic endotoxemia.

C. Lactulose in Combination with Probiotics

The intake of a yogurt product containing 5 g/L lactulose in combination with *Bifidobacterium longum* for 3 weeks (500 mL/day) by 12 healthy volunteers resulted in an increased number of fecal bifidobacteria as compared to the pretreatment period ($p < 0.02$), but this increase was similar to that found in volunteers after consumption of normal yogurt (27). Salminer et al. (28) reported the beneficial effect of *Lactobacillus acidophilus* in combination with lactulose in the prevention of diarrhea induced by radiotherapy.

D. Lactulose and the Microbial Ecology in Foods

Some food products are preserved by a high sucrose content, such as found in marmalade and syrups. The high osmotic and low water activity (A_w) value inhibits the growth of microorganisms. Lactulose can be used as substitute for sucrose, because it gives similar A_w-lowering effects as sucrose but proves to be more inhibitory for food spoilage and foodborne pathogens (*Pseudomonas aeruginosa*, *E. coli*, *Staphylococcus aureus*, *Salmonella typhimurium*, and *Clostridium botulinum*) (29). Heat-treated lactulose syrups were most inhibitory, whereas non–heat-treated lactulose was only slightly more inhibitory than sucrose.

III. CHRONIC HEPATIC ENCEPHALOPATHY

A. Introduction

The early expression of chronic hepatic encephalopathy leads to paroxysmal neuropsychological episodes (transient attacks of generalized apraxia, anomia, agraphia acalculia). During the disease the frequency and severity of attacks can increase (for review see Refs 30–34). The blood ammonia concentrations are high. In general there is a good response to a low-protein diet in combination with an antibiotic (neomycin, rifaximin) or lactulose. The therapeutic use of lactulose was described for the first time by Bircher and coworkers in 1966 (35). An extended review on therapeutic trials and pharmacokinetic studies was published in 1972 (36) and a short review in 1979 (2). It was concluded that lactulose is effective in the treatment of hepatic encephalopathy (approximately 80% of patients respond satisfactorily) and is more suitable for long-term administration than neomycin due to its nontoxic nature.

The efficacy and safety of lactulose in the treatment of hepatic encephalopathy as well as research to find the mechanism of action, is discussed below.

B. Efficacy of Lactulose in the Treatment of Hepatic Encephalopathy

In a double-blind, double-dummy study, patients (45–72 years of age) suffering a mild hepatic encephalopathy were treated with rifaximin ($n = 20$, 1.2 g/day) or lactulose ($n = 20$, 120 mL/day) during the first 2 weeks of every month for 90 days (37). Both treatments appeared effective in controlling neurological symptoms of hepatic encephalopathy. Although the serum levels of ammonia significantly decreased during the first days of treatment in comparison to the pretreatment period, they returned to "normal" after the tenth day of treatment. The therapeutic efficacy of rifaximin was faster than that of lactulose. In two comparable studies in 40 (38) and 58 (39) patients (42–60 years old) affected by hepatic encephalopathy, lactulose proved as effective as rifaximin in controlling neurological signs and symptoms of hepatic encephalopathy and in reducing serum ammonia levels.

Patients ($n = 55$, 30–86 years of age) suffering hepatic encephalopathy (grades 1–3) were treated with rifaximin (1200 mg/day) in combination with lactulose for 15 days (40). The combined use proved efficient in controlling the majority of signs and symptoms in all patients without any drug-related side effects.

In two studies with liver cirrhotic patients ($n = 20$ and $n = 40$), lactulose in crystalline form (60 g/day in comparison with a nontreated group and a lactitol-treated group, respectively) approved to be effective in the treatment of hepatic encephalopathy (41,42) in combination with a significantly ($p < 0.005$) decreased blood ammonia concentration and a significantly ($p < 0.025$) increased number of natural killer cells (41). The latter finding suggests a cell-mediated immune modulation by lactulose, which can be beneficial for immune depressed cirrhotic patients.

In a Chinese study (43) hepatic encephalopathy patients were treated with lactitol ($n = 21$; mean dose 66 g) or lactulose ($n = 20$; mean dose 57 mL) for 5 days. The neural signs, serum ammonia concentrations, and adverse effects were monitored before and after treatment. All parameters decreased significantly in both groups, although the neural improvements were significantly higher in the lactitol group than in the lactulose group ($p < 0.05$). Similar results have been described by Riggio and coworkers (44,45): lactulose (mean dose 48 mL and 38 g, respectively) and lactitol (mean dose 36 g in both studies) were both effective in the treatment of surgically shunted cirrhotic patients ($n = 31$ and $n = 14$) with recurrent episodes of hepatic encephalopathy. However, side effects (meteorism, flatulence) were reported during the treatment with lactulose; fewer or no side effects were reported during the treatment with lactose.

In a cross-over study in cirrhotic patients ($n = 14$) with subclinical hepatic encephalopathy, the efficacy of treatment with lactulose (mean dose 25 mL) and lactitol (mean dose 26 g) for 2 months (with a wash-out period of 4–6 weeks between the change of sugar) was confirmed. During treatment with either lactitol or lactulose, psychometric performance improved consistently to the same degree. Side effects (flatulence, diarrhea) were mentioned but tended to disappear with continued treatment.

In a meta-analysis study of published randomized clinical trials (46), the efficacy of lactulose in the treatment of chronic hepatic encephalopathy was similar to that of lactitol.

In some patients a lactulose-resistant hepatic encephalopathy was found. In these cases the treatment with vancomycin (2 g/day) appeared to be successful (47).

C. Mechanism of Lactulose in the Treatment of Hepatic Encephalopathy

The literature clearly demonstrates that lactulose (and other fermentable carbohydrates) is effective in the treatment of hepatic encephalopathy. However, its exact mechanism of action is not known (34). It is suggested that the fermentation by the colonic microflora plays an important role, especially in relation to an increased production of (non-toxic) acetate in combination with lower quantities of butyric and valeric acids, and an inhibition of the production of ammonia, as shown in an in vitro study (48,49), and consequently decreased serum ammonia levels. It has also been hypothesized that the beneficial effect of lactulose be exerted by its effect on intermediary glutamine metabolism and/or inhibition of the bacterial production of γ-aminobutyric acid.

In a number of studies lower serum ammonia concentrations were found after treatment with lactulose (38,39,41,43,44), although only temporarily in one study (37). In one reported study (50) no change was observed in blood ammonia, glucose, insulin, or free fatty acid levels in cirrhotic patients ($n = 6$) as compared with healthy volunteers ($n = 6$) after the intake of lactulose (<28 g/d). Plauth et al. (51) found no reduction of ammonia generation by the small intestinal mucosa of rats through a specific effect of lactulose on intermediary glutamine metabolism.

A study by Fernandes et al. (50) showed that the fermentation of lactulose resulted in significantly higher peripheral blood acetate levels in cirrhotic patients as compared to healthy subjects. This was also found in surgery patients after direct instillation of 10 g of lactulose in the cecum (9). Although a significantly higher level of serum acetate was found in cirrhotic patients as compared with healthy subjects ($p < 0.04$), the increase in serum acetate concentration after the intake of lactulose was similar in both groups (50).

In relation to serum ammonia concentrations it can be important to promote fecal nitrogen excretion. In a study with 14 cirrhotic patients (without signs of hepatic encephalopathy) treated with lactitol or lactulose showed that lactitol significantly increased fecal nitrogen output and decreased the urinary nitrogen excretion in contrast to lactulose (52). According to the authors the beneficial effect of lactulose in the treatment of hepatic encephalopathy seems not related to increased fecal nitrogen excretion.

In in vitro experiments and rat studies, Al Mardini et al. (53) tried to find the role of lactulose in the production of γ-aminobutyric acid by E. coli. They could demonstrate a significantly increased production of γ-aminobutyric acid after the addition of proteins, but lactulose did not reduce the synthesis.

IV. LACTULOSE IN THE TREATMENT OF CONSTIPATION

Children with chronic idiopathic constipation ($n = 42$, 8 months to 6 years of age) were treated with lactitol (250–400 mg/kg/day) or lactulose (500–750 mg/kg/day). In both groups a significant increase in stool frequency was found ($p < 0.001$) (54). In another study (55) 77 children (3 months to 12 years of age) suffering chronic constipation (on average for 11.5 months) were treated with lactulose for 6 weeks (9–15 mL/day in the first week and 9–11 mL/day in the following weeks). The stool frequency during treatment significantly increased ($p < 0.001$) from 2.5 to 6.5 stools/week. Also, the consistency of the feces was normalized after 2 weeks of treatment.

In human volunteers the intake of 9.5 g lactulose per day for 7 days did not significantly increase the whole-gut transit times (56). Although the stool form was not affected, the stools were significantly softer ($p < 0.05$) in comparison to after the intake of high- and low-resistant starch (56). Adults ($n = 124$) with a history of constipation for at least 3 weeks were randomized in two parallel groups and treated with lactulose (15 mL/day, increasing to 60 mL/day if necessary) or psyllium (1 sachet of 5 g/day) for 4 weeks. Both treatments showed similar efficacy, but the acceptability of lactulose was higher (57). In adults with chronic constipation ($n = 108$) the treatment with lactulose (2 dd 15 mL syrup) for 12 weeks was compared with the treatment with viable $E.\ coli$ cells (Mutaflor®) in capsules (58). At the end of the trial the stool frequency was 5.5 stools/week in the lactulose group and 6.3 stools/week in the $E.\ coli$ group ($p < 0.026$). Well-being during the treatment was good in both groups, but the incidence of adverse effects was higher in the lactulose group.

The efficacy of lactulose in the treatment of chronic or occasional constipation in pregnant women ($n = 62$, 19–40 years of age) has been shown in a base-line controlled study described by Müller and Jaquenoud (59). The frequency of stools was significantly increased ($p < 0.001$) after 1 week (4.0 stools/week) in comparison to the pretreatment period (2.5 stools/week) and "normalized" after 2 weeks (6 stools/week).

Elderly people are relatively frequently treated with laxatives (20–70% of the population), especially in nursing homes. Lactulose is the most frequently (63%) prescribed laxative in Dutch nursing homes (60).

The treatment of geriatric patients ($n = 30$; 65–94 years of age) suffering chronic constipation with 20.1 g/day lactulose resulted in 2.2–1.9 stools per week, which was significantly lower ($p < 0.05$) than 4.5 stools by 14.8 g/day of bulk laxative containing senna (61). A double-blind crossover study in elderly patients with chronic constipation ($n = 77$) also resulted in a higher efficacy of a fiber-senna combination (10 mL daily) in comparison to lactulose (15 mL syrup daily) in the study conditions (62,63).

In a review studying the results of clinical trials published before 1992, it was concluded that the treatment of constipation with lactulose has a beneficial effect compared with placebo (64). This conclusion is confirmed by the results of recent studies summarized above.

V. LACTULOSE IN THE TREATMENT OF MISCELLANEOUS CLINICAL DISEASES

Children ($n = 24$, 21 months of age) with nonspecific chronic diarrhea (without enteric infection) suspected of an imbalance of intestinal microflora were treated with lactulose for 15 days. After treatment all patients showed complete remission of intestinal disorders and fully formed feces and decreased fecal pH values in the lactulose group (65). The authors claimed a reestablishment of balanced intestinal microflora, although microbial investigation was not included in this study.

In premature babies with disturbance of the large intestinal microflora and high values of blood ammonia and bilirubin levels, the intake of lactulose ($n = 22$; 2 dd 0.5 mL/kg body weight) from day 8 to day 21 resulted in significantly lower levels of ammonia ($p < 0.01$) as compared with a control group without treatment ($n = 18$), while the bilirubin concentrations decreased similarly in both groups (57).

Patients ($n = 23$) with chronic renal failure were treated with lactulose (18 g/day). Only 10 patients were continuously treated for 8 weeks, while 12 patients dropped out because of side effects (nausea, diarrhea) during therapy (66). After 8 weeks the levels of guanidinosuccinic acid (GSA) in plasma were significantly lower than before treatment. Interruption of the lactulose intake resulted in a significant increase of GSA.

The treatment of patients with symptomatic diverticular disease ($n = 43$) with lactulose (15 mL/day) or a high-fiber diet (30–40 g/day) showed both to be effective, with a slight advantage for lactulose (67).

VI. LACTULOSE IN RELATION TO CELL PROLIFERATION AND CANCER

Persons ($n = 38$) at increased risk for developing colorectal cancer because of a family history of the disease ingested 60 mL of lactulose syrup per day for 12 weeks. Rectal mucosal proliferation was determined as crypt cell proliferation rate (CCPR) in biopsies taken before and after treatment (68). The mean CCPR was not significantly decreased by the intake of lactulose (in contrast to the intake of 10.5 g/day of wheat fiber; $p = 0.02$).

Geboes et al. (69) studied the short- and long-term effects of continuous ingestion of lactulose in rats (2, 6, and 12 weeks) in relation to epithelial cell proliferation (BrdUrd labeling technique). It was concluded that the tested "contact" laxatives such as lactulose have no predominant influence on ileal and colonic epithelial cell proliferation. Results of a study in rats described by Hennigan et al. (70) suggested that lactulose significantly reduces tumor yield in the small intestine (not in the colon). The hypothesis behind this study was that lactulose would reduce colonic pH, thus inhibiting the conversion of primary bile acids to carcinogenic secondary bile acids and resulting in a reduced colon cancer risk. However, the tumor-reducing effect was only found in the small intestine and not in the colon.

In in vitro studies it has been shown that lactulose significantly reduced the endotoxin-induced necrosis factor production by monocytes (71). The in vivo significance of this property is unknown.

VII. LACTULOSE AND MINERAL ABSORPTION

Infant milk formula with 0.5–1% lactulose fed to weanling rats for 5 weeks did not significantly increase the absorption and retention of nitrogen, calcium, phosphorus, and iron (72). Studies in rats showed a significantly increased ileal absorption of magnesium, calcium, and phosphate when lactulose in the diet (100 g/kg) was substituted for glucose (73). Substitution of lactose for glucose resulted in an increased absorption of magnesium only. Lactulose reduced the ileal pH in comparison to lactose and glucose (pH 7.0, 7.2, and 7.5, respectively). It is suggested by the authors that these lower pH values resulted in an improved solubility of minerals. This was confirmed in in vitro experiments for magnesium and, to a lesser extent, for calcium and phosphate.

In a rat study with calcium isotopes described by Brommage et al. (74), a significant increase in calcium absorption was found. Lactulose appeared more effective than lactose, but other poorly absorbed sugars (xylitol, arabinose, raffinose, raftulose, sorbitol, gluconate, lactobionate, and pyroglutamate) stimulated calcium absorption to the same extent. The stimulation of calcium absorption by a lactulose-containing diet increased when the dietary calcium concentration was raised. In order to stimulate calcium absorption, lactulose must be present in the same meal as the calcium.

VIII. LACTULOSE AND CHOLESTEROL METABOLISM

In studies by Ebner (1971) and Conte (1977) it was suggested that lactulose (max. 60 mL syrup/day for 1–2 months) could have a serum cholesterol–lowering effect. This has not been supported by more recent human studies (4), although some influence on lipid and bile acid metabolism was found. Schumann concluded (75,76) that the scientific evidence for the effect of lactulose, at an acceptable intake, on serum cholesterol and lipid concentrations is very weak.

IX. LACTULOSE IN PERMEABILITY STUDIES

For studying the permeability of the intestinal mucosa lactulose is generally used in combination with mannitol or rhamnose in humans and animals. The permeability is related to the concentrations and ratio found in urine. In this way the increased permeability of the small intestine can be investigated for the diagnosis of mucosal damage, e.g., during enteric infection (77). Interspecies variation in intestinal permeability can also be demonstrated (78).

    Using this method it was shown that lactulose significantly reduced the absorption of sugars (rhamnose, xylose) in healthy volunteers and ileostomic patients by retention of fluid and electrolyte (79). This could explain the finding that dietary supplementation with biscuits containing fiber and lactulose (intake 10 g dietary fiber, 2 g raw fiber, and 8.25 g lactulose per day) by obese subjects ($n = 10$) resulted in a lower blood glucose and insulin response after a meal as well as during the day (in combination with an increased plasma amino acid response) (80).

X. LACTULOSE IN THE HYDROGEN BREATH TEST

Lactulose is not digested in the stomach and small intestine. Therefore, the ingested dose of lactulose reaches the large intestine. The dense microflora in the cecum and colon can ferment lactulose, resulting in the production of hydrogen in most persons. The produced hydrogen is (partly) excreted by the expiration air and can be analyzed, using a breath-hydrogen analyzer. Due to this property, lactulose can be used to determine in a simple, noninvasive, and reproducible way the oro-cecal transit time in heathy subjects (81) as well as in patients (e.g., diabetics) (82). However, it is important to recognize some side effects, such as significantly increased myoelectrical activity of the small intestine (83) and an accelerated transit through the colon (84) by small quantities (10–20 g) of lactulose, and some important limitations. According to Sciarretta et al. (85) the method with 20 g lactulose is accurate in comparison to a scintigraphic method ($r = 0.90$) if a hydrogen threshold increment of 5 ppm is chosen and if the mean hydrogen concentration in the first 30 minutes of the right colon filling is taken into account. In some studies a high percentage (up to 27%) of non–hydrogen producers are mentioned (82), depending on the level of intake of lactulose: 12 g, 27% nonresponders; 20 g, 14% nonresponders (86).

    The lactulose-hydrogen breath test can also be used to study the malabsorption of carbohydrates by comparing the reaction during more than 6 hours after intake of different carbohydrates (87,88). Even in babies (2–8 weeks of age; $n = 22$) the lactulose-hydrogen breath test has been performed to study the effects of a fiber-containing formula milk (89).

XI. SAFETY OF LACTULOSE

A. In Laboratory Animal Experiments

The toxicological aspects of lactulose has been studied in laboratory animals in acute, subacute, and subchronic studies. The toxicity of lactulose (approximately 25 g/kg) is equivalent to that of sucrose (1).

In weanling rats fed infant formula milk for 5 weeks, lactulose (0.5–1.0%) in the milk did not affect growth, blood composition, or histopathology of the liver (72), indicating that continuous consumption of lactulose by rats has no adverse effects during their growth. The formation of platelet-activating factor (PAF) by duodenal and colon mucosal cells of rats, mouse, guinea pigs, and rabbits was measured ex vivo after in vivo treatment with lactulose (50 mg/ kg body weight). The results showed that lactulose and mannitol have no increasing effect on PAF, in contrast to some other laxatives, indicating that lactulose and mannitol did not impart mucosal damage (90).

B. In the Treatment of Hepatic Encephalopathy

In studies with lactulose in the treatment of hepatic encephalopathy, the safety of lactulose has been demonstrated (37,38) as has its combination with rifaximin (40). However, in some studies side effects of lactulose are mentioned, such as meteorism, flatulence, and nausea (43,44,91). It is suggested that the crystalline form of lactulose induced fewer side effects than the syrup formulation (42).

The use of lactulose in combination with neomycin should not be used in the treatment of acute hepatic encephalopathy because the combination is not well tolerated in a significant number of patients (92). It was found that lactulose treatment in cirrhotic patients may increase fecal fat excretion, which should be taken into account in case of long-term prescription (93).

C. In the Treatment of Constipation

Most laxatives, including lactulose, if used intermittently in the absence of contraindications, are relatively safe (94), even in elderly people (95). However, bulking agents may diminish absorption of some minerals and drugs, but this is not usually clinically significant. Some laxatives can cause serious allergic reaction, such as ispaghula. Induction of epithelial damage, increased cell proliferation (trophic effects of short-chain fatty acids), and release of prostaglandins are also mentioned.

During the processing of milk, such as for the production of infant formula, low to high amounts of lactulose can be formed. Children (<2 years of age) with gastroenteritis were given saline with glucose for 12–24 hours followed by full-strength milk feeds. This treatment resulted in diarrhea in several children (96). Fecal analysis showed the absence of lactose, galactose, and glucose, but the presence of lactulose. The manufacturer's data sheet did not mention the presence of lactulose.

During the treatment of constipation in children ($n = 42$, 0.8–16 years of age) with 500– 750 mg/kg/day of lactulose, the patients complained about abdominal pain and flatus more frequently than during treatment with lactitol ($p < 0.005$). In both groups other side effects, such as vomiting and meteorism, were found (54). In a study with 0.4- to 6-year-old chronically constipated children, daily intake of 9–11 mL of lactulose for 6 weeks was tolerated very well by 87% of the children; 12.5% tolerated lactulose moderately. Only incidentally were flatulence and abdominal pain reported (55).

The ingestion of 60 g of lactulose in 350 mL of water by healthy volunteers ($n = 12$) resulted in (osmotic) diarrhea (97). Prolonged ingestion of 60 g of lactulose for 8 days (20 g, twice daily) resulted in 65% of the subjects in significantly reduced severity of diarrhea ($p <$ 0.05). In the other subjects no changes were observed. It was concluded that changes in colonic function induced by prolonged ingestion of a nondiarrhegenic amount of lactulose (e.g., an increased velocity of bacterial breakdown and a change in metabolic pathways) (7) moderate the severity of diarrhea caused by large doses of lactulose (97). In another study in healthy volunteers a maximum of 80 g/day of lactulose was metabolized by the colon microflora (98) The produced organic acids were only partly absorbed, resulting in an accumulation of inorganic cations in the diarrheal fluid.

The treatment of geriatric patients with chronic constipation using lactulose (20.1 g/day) showed no adverse effects and appeared to be safe (61,62).

During pregnancy constipation is a common problem, which should be relieved without any risk to the developing child. Because lactulose is not absorbed in the small intestine, it is of great significance when treating constipation during pregnancy, as it presents no threat to the fetus (59). It is also asserted by these authors that lactulose does not appear in the breast milk. The treatment of chronic or occasional constipation of 62 pregnant women given lactulose for 4 weeks was without serious side effects (59).

XII. CONCLUSIONS

Three types of health aspects claimed for lactulose are relatively well documented: the influence on the intestinal microflora and the therapeutic significance in chronic hepatic encephalopathy as well as in chronic constipation. The information about other beneficial properties described for lactulose, such as treatment in chronic renal failure, prevention of cell proliferation, and increased mineral absorption, is much too limited for final conclusions.

A. Intestinal Microflora

Lactulose is hardly or not at all absorbed in the small intestine and is relatively easily fermented in the large intestine (cecum, colon) by the dense indigenous microflora. During fermentation short-chain fatty acids, lactic acid, and hydrogen or methane are produced. No one specific type of SCFA is formed; acetic acid, propionic acid and butyric acid are produced and found in increased concentrations in the portal blood after fermentation. In the peripheral blood mainly an increased concentration of acetic acid is found, suggesting liver metabolism of propionic and butyric acid (apart from direct absorption of butyric acid by the mucosal cells). After prolonged ingestion of lactulose, adaptation of the intestinal microflora is found, resulting in a changed fermentation pattern.

The clinical significance of SCFA production in relation to health aspects is not completely understood, but preliminary results stress the importance of further studies, such as mucosal and hepatic cell metabolism, cytotoxicity, and antimutagenicity/carcinogenicity.

The beneficial influence of lactulose on the composition of the intestinal microflora, i.e., stimulation of *Bifidobacterium* and *Lactobacillus* and suppression of gram-negative bacteria (e.g., *E. coli*) and *Clostridium*, has been studied by various research teams. The results should be interpreted carefully, because the conditions under which this aspect has been studied are diverse (age, composition of basic food, concentration of lactulose, rat vs. human studies). Nevertheless, there are strong data showing that lactulose stimulates the numbers of bifidobacteria and suppresses the numbers of gram-negative bacteria (e.g., coliform) and clostridia. This is considered to be an important property to improve the indigenous intestinal balance and subsequently to increase the resistance against the colonization of unfavorable microorganisms and to decrease the production of endotoxins. This property is supported by the finding that pretreatment with lactulose enhances the recovery from severe stress conditions (e.g., intense surgery). An important feature can be the inactivation and inhibited absorption of endotoxins by lactulose as described by some researchers, resulting in decreased levels of endotoxemia. This property can be of clinical significance but needs further research before final conclusions can be made.

The combination of lactulose as prebiotic and lactic acid bacteria or bifidobacteria as probiotic has hardly been investigated. Nevertheless, it would be interesting to use lactulose-fermenting probiotic strains in a lactulose-containing product.

B. Hepatic Encephalopathy

It is very well documented that lactulose proved to be successful in the treatment of chronic hepatic encephalopathy, no matter the age of the patients and without serious adverse effects. It is at least as effective as lactitol and rifaximin. Rifaximin can have a somewhat faster effect on the symptoms, while lactulose is better for long-term therapy than antibiotics for safety reasons. Lactulose can be combined with rifaximin but is not recommended in combination with neomycin.

C. Constipation

Chronic constipation in babies, children, adults, pregnant women, and elderly persons can successfully and safely be treated with lactulose. The effective dose is in general somewhat higher than prescribed by the manufacturers. Individual sensitivity should be recognized, which means that the therapeutic dose should start at a relatively low level and be increased based on the frequency and consistency of the stools. The side effects are limited to flatulence. Abdominal pain, vomiting, and meteorism are reported as incidental, temporary adverse effects, but their frequency may increase at higher doses.

D. Other Health Claims

The use of lactulose in the treatment of some other clinical diseases, such as chronic diarrhea, renal failure, and diverticular disease, are mentioned in the literature in a positive way, but only very incidentally. Therefore, no conclusions can be made regarding these topics. In rat studies investigating the effect of lactulose on intestinal cell proliferation (colon cancer) and mineral absorption, inhibition of cell proliferation could not be demonstrated. The absorption of minerals seems to be increased by lactulose, probably by the indirect effect of an enhanced solubility at a lower intestinal pH due to the production of acid from lactulose by the microflora.

E. Clinical and Diagnostic Tools

Lactulose can be used to determine the oro-cecal transit time by analyzing the breath-hydrogen concentration after lactulose intake. In combination with mannitol, lactulose can be used to determine the permeability of the intestinal mucosa by analyzing the concentrations in urine. In both cases it can be used as a relatively simple, safe, and reliable tool to investigate the normal as well the anomalous conditions of the gastrointestinal tract.

F. Safety

It is demonstrated that the acute and subchronic toxicity of lactulose is extremely low and comparable with sucrose. Lactulose at relatively high doses is tolerated well in rats without intestinal and liver damage.

During therapeutic treatments of patients over long periods lactulose is well tolerated without serious adverse effects. Flatulence and incident abdominal pain, vomiting, and meteorism are reported. High intakes can cause osmotic diarrhea due to the high amount of lactulose and/or short-chain fatty acids in the large intestine. Lactulose can easily be prescribed in an individual dose.

G. Conclusion

Lactulose is an interesting compound with very well documented properties in relation to the intestinal microflora, hepatic encephalopathy and chronic constipation. Besides, it can have some additional therapeutic applications in chronic diseases, such as in renal failure, diverticulum disease and chronic diarrhoea due to disbacteriosis, and it can be beneficial in the absorption of minerals, particularly calcium and magnesium. However, these aspects should be further investigated.

Lactulose is safe in short- and long-term use, no matter the age of the user.

REFERENCES

1. Mizota T, Tamura Y, Okonogl S. Lactulose as a sugar with physiological significance. Bull Int Dairy Fed 212:69–76, 1987.
2. Mendez A, Olano A. Lactulose. A review of some chemical properties and applications in infant nutrition and medicine. Dairy Sci Abstr 41:531–535, 1979.
3. Rulili A, Brusa T, Canzi E, Ferrari A. Human intestinal methanogens and lactulose administration. Microbiologica 16:99–104, 1993.
4. Jenkins DJ, Wolever TM, Jenkins A, Brighenti F, Vuksan V, Rao AV, Cunnane SC, Ocana A, Corey P, Vezina C. Specific types of colonic fermentation may raise low-density-lipoprotein-cholesterol concentrations. Am J Clin Nutr 54:141–147, 1991.
5. Wolever TMS, Robb PA, Ter Wal P, Spadafora PG. Interaction between methane-producing status and diet on serum acetate concentration in humans. J Nutr 123:681–688, 1993.
6. Uribe M, Campollo O, Cote C. Effect of lactulose on the metabolism of short-chain fatty acids. Hepatology 12:1251–1252, 1990.
7. Florent C, Flourie B, Leblond A, Rautureau M, Bernier J-J, Rambaud JC. Influence of chronic lactulose ingestion on the colonic metabolism of lactulose in man (an in vivo study). J Clin Invest 75:608–613, 1985.
8. Hove H, Rye Clausen M, Mortensen PB. Lactate and pH in faeces from patients with colonic adenomas or cancer. Gut 34:625–629, 1993.
9. Peters SG, Pomare EW, Fisher CA. Portal and peripheral blood short chain fatty acid concentrations after caecal lactulose instillation at surgery. Gut 33:1249–1252, 1992.
10. Holtug K, Clausen MR, Hove H, Christiansen J, Mortensen PB. The colon in carbohydrate malabsorption: short-chain fatty acids, pH, and osmotic diarrhoea. Scand J Gastroenterol 27:545–552, 1992.
11. Elsen RJ, Bistrian BR. Recent developments in short-chain fatty acid metabolism. Nutrition 7:7–11, 1991.
12. Hidaka H, Hirayama M, Tokunaga T, Eida T. The effects of undigestible fructooligosaccharides on intestinal microflora and various physiological functions on human health. Adv Exp Med Biol 270:105–117, 1990.

13. Smart JB, Pillidge CJ, Garman JH. Growth of lactic acid bacteria and bifidobacteria on lactose and lactose-related mono-, di- and trisaccharides and correlation with distribution of beta-galactosidase and phospho-beta-galactosidase. J Dairy Res 60:557–568, 1993.

14. Nagendra R, Venkat Rao S. Effects of incorporation of lactulose in infant formulas on the intestinal bifidobacterial flora in rats. Int J Food Sci Nutr 43:169–173, 1992.

15. Nagendra R, Venkat Rao S. Effect of feeding infant formulations containing bifidus factor on in vivo proliferation of bifidobacteria and stimulation of intraperitoneal macrophage activity in rats. J Nutr Immunol 2:61–68, 1992.

16. Liao W, Cui X-S, Jin X-Y, Floren CH. Lactulose—a potential drug for the treatment of inflammatory bowel disease. Medical Hypotheses 43:234–238, 1994.

17. MacGillivray PC, Finlay HVL, Binns TB. Use of lactulose to create a preponderance of lactobacilli in the intestine of bottle-fed infants. Scot Med J 4:182–189, 1995.

18. Nagendra R, Viswanatha S, Kumar SA, Murthy BK, Rao SV. Effects of feeding milk formula containing lactulose to infants on faecal bifidobacterial flora. Nutr Res 15:15–24, 1995.

19. Terada A, Hara H, Kataoka M, Mitsuoka T. Effects of lactulose on the composition and metabolic activity of the human faecal flora. Microb Ecol Health Dis 5:43–50, 1992.

20. Terada A, Hara H, Shou-Tou-Li, Ikegame K, Sasaki M, Mitsuoka T. Lecithinase-positive clostridia isolated from human feces on consumption of lactulose and lactosucrose. Jpn J Food Microbiol 11: 119–123, 1994.

21. Riggio O, Varriale M, Testore GP, Di-Rosa R, Di-Rosa E, Merli M, Romiti A, Candiani C, Capocaccia L. Effect of lactitol and lactulose administration on the fecal flora in cirrhotic patients. J Clin Gastroenterol 12:433–436, 1990.

22. Fulton JD. Infection limitation with lactulose therapy. J Clin Exper Gerontol 10:117–124, 1988.

23. McCutcheon J, Fulton JD. Lowered prevalence of infection with lactulose therapy in patients in long-term hospital care. J Hosp Infect 13:81–86, 1989.

24. Van Leeuwen PA, Hong RW, Rounds JD, Rodrick ML, Wilmore D. Hepatic failure and coma after liver resection is reversed by manipulation of gut contents: the role of endotoxin. Surgery 110:169–174, 1991.

25. Hou RX. Treatment of gut-derived endotoxemia with lactulose. An experimental study. Chin J Surgery 29:248–250, 1991.

26. Gardiner KR, Erwin PJ, Anderson NH, McCaigue MD, Halliday MI, Rowlands BJ. Lactulose as an antiendotoxin in experimental colitis. Br J Surg 82:469–472, 1995.

27. Bartram H-P, Scheppach W, Gerlach S, Ruckdeschel G, Kelber E, Kasper H. Does yoghurt enriched with *Bifidobacterium longum* affect colonic microbiology and fecal metabolites in healthy subjects? Am J Clin Nutr 59:428–432, 1994.

28. Salminen E, Elomaa I, Minkkinen J, Vapaatalo H, Salminen S. Preservation of intestinal integrity during radiotherapy using living *Lactobacillus acidophilus* cultures. Clin Radiol 39:435–437, 1988.

29. Huhtanen CN, Parrish FW, Hicks KB. Inhibition of bacteria by lactulose preparation. Appl Environ Microbiol 40:171–173, 1980.

30. Walter E. Das Leberkoma. Schweiz Med Wochensch 124:1147–1154, 1994.

31. Salvati CA. Reversible hepatic decerebration. Am J Gastroenterol 89:1604–1605, 1994.

32. Weissenborn K. Diagnostik und Therapie der portosystemischen Enzephalopathie. Schweiz Rundschau Med Praxis 83:1059–1064, 1994.

33. Rodes J. Clinical manifestations and therapy of hepatic encephalopathy. Adv Exp Med Biol 341: 39–44, 1993.

34. Evers NAEM, De Knegt RJ, Buurke EJ, Overdiek JWPM. Hepatische encephalopathie. Pharm Weekbl 129:621–625, 1994.

35. Bircher J, Müller J, Guggenheim P, Haemmerli UP. Treatment of chronic portal systemic encephalopathy with lactulose. Lancet 1:890–893, 1966.

36. Avery GS, Davis EP, Brogden RN. Lactulose: a review of its therapeutic and pharmacological properties with particular reference to ammonia metabolism and its mode of action in portal systemic encephalopathy. Drugs 4:7–48, 1972.

37. Giacomo F, Francesco A, Michele N, Oronzo S, Antonella F. Rifaximin in the treatment of hepatic encephalopathy. Eur J Clin Res 4:57–66, 1993.

38. Massa P, Vallerino E, Dodero M. Treatment of hepatic encephalopathy with rifaximin: double blind, double dummy study versus lactulose. Eur J Clin Res 4:7–18, 1993.

39. Bucci L, Palmieri GC. Double blind, double-dummy comparison between treatment with rifaximin and lactulose in patients with medium to severe degree hepatic encephalopathy. Curr Med Res Opin 13:109–118, 1993.

40. Puxeddu A, Quartini M, Massimetti A, Ferrieri A. Rifaximin in the treatment of chronic hepatic encephalopathy. Curr Med Res Opin 13:274–281, 1995.

41. Vendemiale G, Palasciano G, Cirelli F, Altamura M, De Vincentiis A, Altomare E. Crystalline lactulose in the therapy of hepatic cirrhosis. Arzneim Forsch Drug Res 42:969–972, 1992.

42. Grandi M, Sacchetti C, Pederzoli S, Celani MF. Studio clinico di confronto tra lattulosio puro in cristalli e lactitolo puro in polvere nella encefalopatia porto-sistemica del paziente cirrotico. Minerva Gastroenterol Dietol 37:225–230, 1991.

43. Pai C-H, Huang Y-S, Jeng W-C, Chan C-Y, Lee S-D. Treatment of porto-systemic encephalopathy with lactitol versus lactulose: a randomized controlled study. Chin Med J 55:31–36, 1995.

44. Riggio O, Balducci G, Ariosto F, Merli M, Pieche U, Pinto G, Tremiterra S, Ziparo V, Capocaccia L. Lactitol in prevention of recurrent episodes of hepatic encephalopathy in cirrhotic patients with portal-systemic shunt. Dig Dis Sci 34:823–829, 1989.

45. Riggio O, Balducci G, Ariosto F, Merli M, Tremiterra S, Ziparo V, Capocaccia L. Lactitol in the treatment of chronic hepatic encephalopathy; a randomized cross-over comparison with lactulose. Hepato-Gastroenterology 37:524–527, 1990.

46. Camma C, Fiorello F, Tine F, Marchesini G, Fabbri A, Pagliaro L. Lactitol in treatment of chronic hepatic encephalopathy. A meta-analysis Dig Dis Sci 38:916–922, 1993.

47. Tarao K, Ikeda T, Hayashi K, Sakurai A. Successful use of vancomycin hydrochloride in the treatment of lactulose-resistant hepatic encephalopathy. J Gastroenterol Hepatol 4:284–286, 1989.

48. Mortensen PB, Holtug K, Bonnen H, Clausen MR. The degradation of amino acids, proteins, and blood to short-chain fatty acids in colon is prevented by lactulose. Gastroenterology 98:353–360, 1990.

49. Vince AJ, McNeil NI, Wager JD, Wrong OM. The effect of lactulose, pectin, arabinogalactan and cellulose on the production of organic acids and metabolism of ammonia by intestinal bacteria in a faecal incubation system. Br J Nutr 63:17–26, 1990.

50. Fernandes J, Morali G, Wolever TM, Blendis LM, Koo M, Jenkins DJ, Rao AV. Effects of acute lactulose administration on serum acetate levels in cirrhosis. Clin Invest Med 17:218–225, 1994.

51. Plauth M, Raible A, Graser TA, Noeldeke IL, Fuerst P, Doelle W, Hartmann F. Lactulose or paromycin do not affect ammonia generation in the isolated perfused rat small intestine. Zeitschr Gastroenterol 32:141–145, 1994.

52. Riggio O, Zimmatore E, Meddi P, Montagnese F, Ricci G, Merli M, Capocaccia L. Nitrogen excretion in cirrhotic patients during non-absorbable disaccharide administration. Riv Ital Nutr Parenter Enterale 13:130–134, 1995.

53. Mardini Al H, Jumaili Al B, Record CO, Burke D. Effect of protein and lactulose on the production of gamma-aminobutyric acid by faecal *Escherichia coli*. Gut 32:1007–1010, 1991.

54. Pitzalis G, Deganello F, Mariani P, Chiarini-Testa MB, Virgilli F, Gasparri R, Calvani L, Bonamico M. Il lattitolo nella stipsi cronica idiopatica del bambino. Pediatr Med Chirurg 17:223–226, 1995.

55. Müller M, Jaquenoud E. Behandlung der chronische Obstipation bei Kindern mit Lactulose. Ars Medici 84:568–574, 1994.

56. Tomlin J, Read NW. A comparison of the effect of 9.5 gram/day resistant starch and lactulose on colon function. Eur J Clin Nutr 46:S139–S140, 1992.

57. Rouse M, Chapman N, Mahapatra M, Grillage M, Atkinson SN, Prescott P. An open, randomised, parallel group study of lactulose versus ispaghula in the treatment of chronic constipation in adults. Br J Clin Prac 45:28–30, 1991.

58. Bruckschen E, Horosiewicz H. Chronisch Obstipation, Vergleich von mikrobiologischer Therapie und Lactulose. Münch Med Wochensch 136:35–41, 1994.

59. Müller M, Jaquenoud E. Behandlung der Obstipation bei Schwangeren. Eine Multizenterstudie in gynaekologischen Praxis. Schweiz Med Wochenschr 125:1689–1693, 1995.

60. Brouwers JRBJ, Tytgat GNJ. Laxantia bij bejaarden met obstipatie. Keuzecriteria, voorzorgen en complicaties. Pharm Weekb 128:1483–1487, 1993.
61. Kinnunen O, Winblad I, Koistinen P, Salokannel J. Safety and efficacy of a bulk laxative containing senna versus lactulose in the treatment of chronic constipation in geriatric patients. Pharmacology 47:253–255, 1993.
62. Passmore AP, Davies KW, Flanagan PG, Stoker C, Scott MG. A comparison of Agriolax and lactulose in elderly patients with chronic constipation. Pharmacology 47:249–252, 1993.
63. Passmore AP, Wilson-Davies K, Scott ME. Chronic constipation in long stay elderly patients: a comparison of lactulose and senna-fibre combination. Br Med J 307:769–771, 1993.
64. Kot TV, Pettit-Young NA. Lactulose in the management of constipation: a current review. Ann Pharmacother 26:1277–1282, 1992.
65. Roggero P, Volpe C, Ceccatelli MP, Lambri A, Giuliani MG, Donattini T, Garavaglia MC, De Vincentiis A. Lattulosio cristallino e preparazioni orali di microorganismi quale trattamento della diarrea cronica aspecifica dell'infanzia. Studio clinico controllato. Minerva Pediatr 42:147–150, 1990.
66. Miura M, Nomoto Y, Sakai H. Short term effect of lactulose therapy in patients with chronic renal failure. Tokai J Exp Clin Med 14:29–34, 1989.
67. Smits BJ, Whitehead AM, Prescott P. Lactulose in the treatment of symptomatic diverticular disease: a comparative study with high-fibre diet. Br J Clin Pract 44:314–318, 1990.
68. Rooney PS, Hunt LM, Clarke PA, Gifford KA, Hardcastle JD, Armitage NC. Wheat fibre, lactulose and rectal mucosal proliferation in individuals with a family history of colorectal cancer. Br J Surg 81:1792–1794, 1994.
69. Geboes K, Nijs G, Mengs U, Geboes KF, Van Damme A, De Witte P. Effects of 'contact laxatives' on intestinal and colonic epithelial cell proliferation. Pharmacology 47:187–195, 1993.
70. Hennigan TW, Sian M, Matthews J, Allen-Mersh TG. Protective role of lactulose in intestinal carcinogenesis. Surg Oncol 4:31–34, 1995.
71. Greve JW, Gouma DJ, Van Leeuwen PA, Buurman WA. Lactulose inhibits endotoxin induced tumour necrosis factor production by monocytes. An in vitro study. Gut 31:198–203, 1990.
72. Nagendra R, Viswanatha S, Naraimha-Murthy K, Venkat-Rao S. Effects of incorporating lactulose in infant formula on absorption and retention of nitrogen, calcium, phosphorous and iron in rats. Int Dairy J 4:779–788, 1994.
73. Heijnen A, Brink EJ, Lemmens AG, Beynen AC. Ileal pH and apparent absorption of magnesium in rats fed on diets containing either lactose or lactulose. Br J Nutr 70:747–756, 1993.
74. Brommage R, Binacua C, Antille S, Carrie A-L. Intestinal calcium absorption in rats is stimulated by dietary lactulose and other resistant sugars. J Nutr 123:2186–2194, 1993.
75. Schumann C. Herausforderung Lactulose. Teil 1. Zur cholesterinsenkender Wirkung von Lactulose. Z Ärztl Fortbild 86:901–904, 1992.
76. Schumann C. Herausforderung Lactulose. Teil 2. Bedeutung der Regulation des enterischen Gallensaure-Kreislaufs durch pH-Wert-Senkung für die Lithogenese. Z Ärztl Forbild 86:905–908, 1992.
77. Bjarnason I. Intestinal permeability. Gut 1(suppl):S18–S22, 1994.
78. Bijlsma PB, Peeters RA, Groot JA, Dekker PR, Taminiau JAJM, Meer Van der R. Differential in vivo and in vitro intestinal permeability to lactulose and mannitol in animals and humans: a hypothesis. Gastroenterology 108:687–696, 1995.
79. Jenkins AP, Menzies JS, Nukajam WS, Creamer B. The effect of ingested lactulose on absorption of L-rhamnose, D-xylose, and 3-O-methyl-D-glucose in subjects with ileostomies. Scand J Gastroenterol 29:820–825, 1994.
80. Bianchi GP, De Mitri MS, Buganesi E, Abbiati R, Fabbri A, Marchesini G. Lowering effects of a preparation containing fibres and lactulose on glucose and insulin levels in obesity. Ital J Gastroenterol 26:174–178, 1994.
81. Jorge JMN, Wexner SD, Ehrenpreis ED. The lactulose hydrogen breath test as a measure of orocaecal transit time. Eur J Surg 160:409–416, 1994.
82. Sarno S, Erasmus LP, Haslbeck M, Hoelzl R. Orocaecal transit, bacterial overgrowth and hydrogen production in diabetes mellitus. Ital J Gastroenterol 25:490–496, 1993.
83. Bruley des Varannes S, Cherbut C, Schnee M, Delort-Laval J, Galmiche J-P. Effects of lactulose on fasting small intestine myoelectrical activity in humans. Eur J Gastroent Hep 4:539–545, 1992.

84. Barrow L, Steed KP, Spiller RC, Watts PJ, Melia CD, Davies MC, Wilson CG. Scintigraphic demonstration of lactulose-induced accelerated proximal colon transit. Gastroenterology 103:1167–1173, 1992.

85. Sciarretta G, Furno A, Mazzoni M, Garagnani B, Malaguti P. Lactulose hydrogen breath test in orocecal transit assessment. Critical evaluation by means of scintigraphic method. Dig Dis Sci 39: 1505–1510, 1994.

86. Corazza G, Strocchi A, Sorge M, Benati G, Gasbarrini G. Prevalence and consistency of low breath H_2 excretion following lactulose ingestion. Possible implications for clinical use of the H2 breath test. Dig Dis Sci 38:2010–2016, 1993.

87. Strocchi A, Corazza G, Ellis CJ, Gasbarrini G, Levitt MD. Detection of malabsorption of low doses of carbohydrates: accuracy of various breath H_2 criteria. Gastroenterology 105:1404–1410, 1993.

88. Rumessen JJ, Nordgard-Andersen I, Gudmand-Hoyer E. Carbohydrate malabsorption: quantification by methane and hydrogen breath tests. Scand J Gastroenterol 29:826–832, 1994.

89. Treem WR, Hyams JS, Blankschen E, Etienne N, Paule CL, Borschel MW. Evaluation of the effect of fiber-enriched formula on infant colic. J Pediatr 119:695–701, 1991.

90. Izzo AA, Mascolo N, Autore G, Di Carlo G, Capasso F. Increased ex-vivo colonic generation of PAF induced by diphenylmethane stimulant laxatives in rats, mice, guinea-pigs and rabbits. J Pharm Pharmacol 45:916–918, 1993.

91. Morgan MY, Alonso M, Stanger LC. Lactitol and lactulose for the treatment of subclinical hepatic encephalopathy in cirrhotic patients. A randomised, cross-over study. J Hepatol 8:208–217, 1989.

92. Blanc P, Daues JP, Liautard J, Buttigieg R, Desprez D, Pageaux G, Allaz JL, Parelon G, Larrey D, Michel H. Association lactulose-neomycine versus placebo dans le traitement de l'encephalopathie hepatique aigue. Resultats d'un essai controle randomise. Gastroenterol Clin Biol 18:1063–1068, 1994.

93. Merli M, Caschera M, Piat C, Pinto G, Diofebi M, Riggio O. The effect of lactulose and lactitol administration on faecal fat excretion in patients with liver cirrhosis. J Clin Gastroenterol 15:125–127, 1992.

94. Gattuso JM, Kamm MA. Adverse effects of drugs used in the management of constipation and diarrhoea. Drug Safety 10:47–65, 1994.

95. De Looze D. Constipatie en faecale incontinentie bij de bejaarde. Tijdschr Geneeskunde 51:338–342, 1995.

96. Hendrickse RG, Wooldridge MAW, Russell A. Lactulose in baby milks causing diarrhoea simulating lactose intolerance. Br Med J 1:1194–1195, 1977.

97. Flourie B, Briet F, Florent C, Pellier P, Maurel M, Rambaud J-C. Can diarrhea induced by lactulose be reduced by prolonged ingestion of lactulose? Am J Clin Nutr 58:369–375, 1993.

98. Hammer HF, Santa-Ana CA, Schiller LR, Fordtran JS. Studies of osmotic diarrhea induced in normal subjects by ingestion of polyethylene glycol and lactulose. J Clin Invest 84:1056–1062, 1989.

13

Physicochemical Properties of Dietary Fiber: Overview

David Oakenfull
Food Science Australia, North Ryde, New South Wales, Australia

I. INTRODUCTION

As explained in other parts of this book, dietary fiber is a complex mixture of polysaccharides with many different functions and activities as it passes through the gastrointestinal tract. Many of these functions and activities depend on physicochemical properties—some in ways that are obvious, some not so obvious—ranging from the influence of fiber on our food preferences to its effects on laxation.

In this Chapter, I shall outline the physicochemical properties of polysaccharides that seem to be of most relevance and then discuss their role at the various stages in the passage of fiber through the gut.

II. THE RELEVANT PHYSICOCHEMICAL PROPERTIES

A. Solubility

Solubility is a major factor in the nutritional properties of dietary fiber. Soluble fiber influences plasma lipids and protects against cardiovascular disease; insoluble fiber promotes laxation and appears to be protective against colorectal cancer. But solubility is a vague concept and in this context certainly not well defined—particularly because "soluble fiber" is usually a complex mixture of different polysaccarides of different molecular weights. In general we can say that "soluble fiber" is definitely strongly hydrated in water, and if the conditions are right, some or all of the polysaccharide molecules may go into true solution. So what determines whether a particular fiber fraction is soluble or insoluble?

The key to understanding why some polysaccharides are soluble in water and others are not is molecular structure (1). Polysaccharides are composed of linked monosaccharide units, the most common of which is D-glucose. The structure of glucose is shown in Fig. 1. When in solution, the monosaccharide chain takes up a ring form through a reversible intramolecular reaction between the aldehyde group and one of the hydroxyl groups, forming a hemiacetal (see also Fig. 3). Hydroxyl groups from other monosaccharide molecules can react with the hemiacetal, forming a glycosidic link, creating first a disaccharide and ultimately a polysaccharide. In the case of D-glucose, a glycosidic link can be formed between C1 of one glucose molecule and C1, C2, C3, C4, or C6 of another. Thus, many different structures are possible. Polysaccha-

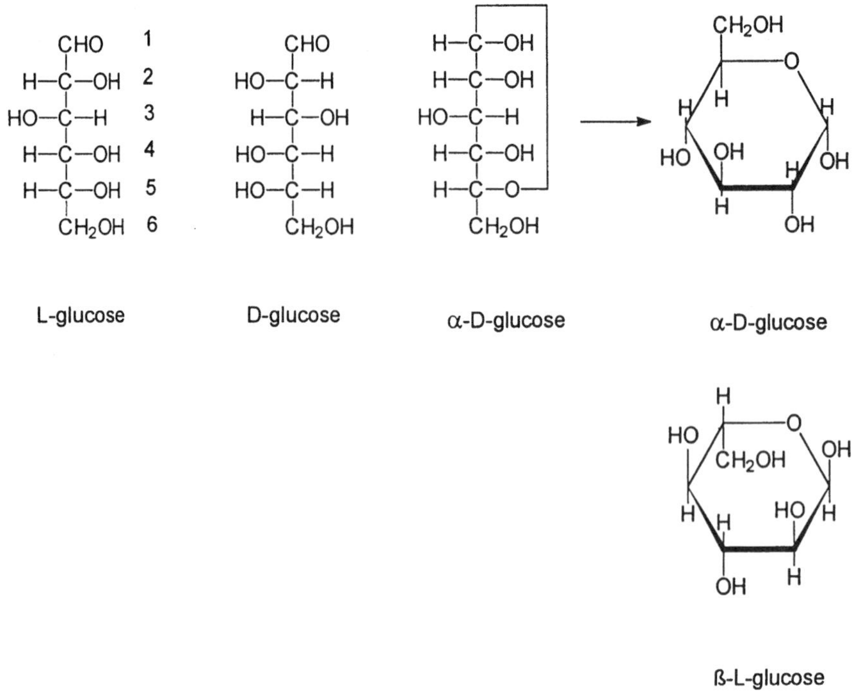

Fig. 1 Representations of D- and L-glucose in open chains and α-D-glucose and β-L-glucose in ring forms.

ride structures are therefore determined both by the nature of the monosaccharide units and by the nature of the linkages between them. But physical properties (such as solubility) are determined more by the linkages than the nature of the monosaccharide units (2).

This is illustrated by comparing two forms of poly-D-glucose—cellulose, which is insoluble, and the water-soluble "β-glucans" from barley and oat bran. Cellulose has exclusively β(1 → 4) linkages, whereas the β-glucans have mixed β(1 → 4) and β(1 → 3) linkages. Cellulose's regularity enables it to adopt ordered crystalline structures of polysaccharide chains held together by hydrogen bonds (3). These ordered structures are insoluble (4). The irregular structure of the β-glucans prevents the formation of ordered crystalline structure, so these polysaccharides tend to be water soluble. Similarly, branched structures, as in the arabinoxylans in wheat, are unable to adopt ordered crystalline structures, and these compounds are also water soluble. Polysaccharides with charged groups (COO^- or SO_3^-), such as the pectins and carrageenans, are again water soluble, in this case, because electrostatic repulsion prevents the molecules from packing close together in ordered structures (4).

B. Viscosity

Almost all water-soluble polysaccharides produce viscous solutions. Viscosity is caused by physical interactions between polysaccharide molecules in solution—in simple terms by the molecules becoming entangled (5,6). We can go a long way towards understanding the properties of polysaccharide solutions by a single unifying concept—the degree of space occupancy by the polymer (7). Most polysaccharides exist in solution as conformationally disordered "random coils,'' their molecules randomly fluctuating in shape under the influence of Brownian motion. At low concentrations the molecules are well separated from each other and free to move independently. When the concentration is increased, the molecules eventually touch, and further molecules can be accommodated only by overlapping and interpenetrating one another—they become entangled (Fig. 2). The critical concentration is usually termed c* and marks a very definite change in the concentration dependence of viscosity, as shown in Fig. 3.

The viscosity of polysaccharide solutions can also be strongly dependent on the rate of shear (this means, in effect, the rate at which the liquid is stirred). They usually show ''shear thinning''—the apparent viscosity decreasing with increasing rate of shear. In dilute solutions, at concentrations below the onset of entanglement (c < c*), viscosity is only slightly dependent on the rate of shear. (The coils are stretched out by the flow and offer little resistance to movement.) However, at concentrations above the onset of entanglement (c > c*), these entanglements have to be ripped apart for the solution to flow. At high shear rate, the rate of reentanglement is slower than the rate of entanglement and the viscosity decreases. It is important to remember that it is totally meaningless to quote the viscosity of a polysaccharide solution without at the same time specifying the conditions under which it was measured.

C. Water-Holding Capacity

Polysaccharides are hydrophilic molecules; they have numerous free hydroxyl groups, which can form hydrogen bonds with water. Consequently soluble and insoluble polysaccharides alike have the ability to hold water. The most obvious demonstration of the ability of soluble polysaccharides to hold water is the phenomenon of gelation. A relatively small amount of polysaccharide, such as 1% agarose, can be enough to entrap the water in which it is dissolved in a three-dimensional network of polysaccharide molecules (Fig. 4). The water is held within the polysaccharide matrix, unable to flow away, and the system has the semisolid properties characteristic of a gel. Insoluble fibers can also adsorb water, but more in the manner of a sponge. They also form a hydrophilic matrix in which water is entrapped, but where the quasi-crystallinity of the polysaccharide remains and water fills the interstices, often causing considerable swelling.

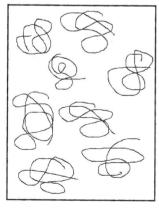 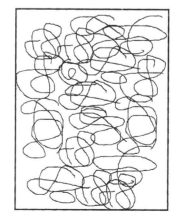

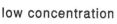 high concentration

Fig. 2 Random coil molecules, showing how entanglement can influence viscosity. At higher concentrations, the effective volumes occupied by the polymer molecules overlap and entanglement occurs.

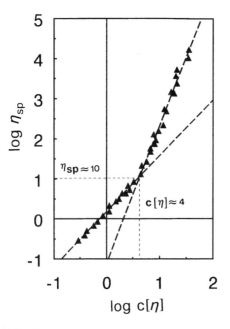

Fig. 3 Generalized concentration dependence of viscosity for conformationally disordered (''random coil'') polysaccharides. The extent of space occupancy by the polymer (x-axis) is characterized by the product of concentration (c, proportional to the number of chains present) and intrinsic viscosity ($[\eta]$, proportional to coil volume). Viscosity measured under low-shear conditions (y-axis) is expressed as specific viscosity (η_{sp}) to remove the solvent contribution. (From Ref. 7.)

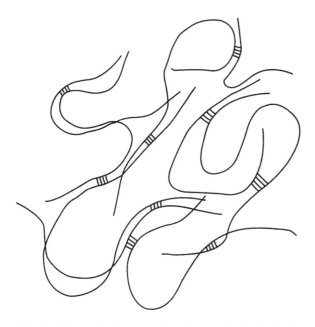

Fig. 4 Schematic diagram of a gel network. The hatched areas represent the junction zones where the polysaccharide molecules are cross-linked.

D. Adsorption of Small Molecules and Ions

In addition to binding water, polysaccharides have the ability to bind other polar molecules and ions. The reduced mineral availability and electrolyte absorption associated with some diets high in fiber appear to be due to binding of metal ions (8). The number of free carboxyl groups and particularly the uronic acid content seem to be the major factors determining the ability of polysaccharides to bind metal ions. It is possible, though, that these ions are subsequently released and absorbed as fiber is broken down in the colon. It has been reported that absorption of zinc and iron are actually enhanced by sugar beet fiber and that the inhibition of absorption observed with wheat bran is caused by phytate (9).

More questionable is the often cited ability of fiber to bind bile acids (10,11). The cholesterol-lowering effect of dietary fiber, it is suggested, can, at least in part, be explained by adsorption of bile acids to fiber in the small intestine. Bile acids are thereby diverted from the enterohepatic cycle, lost by fecal excretion, and the loss made good by conversion of cholesterol into bile acids by the liver (10,11). Although dietary fiber, for example, oat bran, can indeed increase fecal excretion of bile acids, adsorption of bile acids to fiber preparations in vitro is so small as to be trivial when expressed quantitative in terms of μmoles adsorbed per gram of fiber (12). Moreover, pectin also causes increased fecal excretion of bile acids and adsorption of bile acids onto pectin is physically impossible because both molecules are negatively charged at gut pH (13,14).

E. Microstructure—Resistant Starch

Resistant starch (discussed in more detail in Sec. II) behaves functionally as dietary fiber because it resists digestion by the enzymes of the stomach and small intestine. This is a case in which microstructure has a powerful effect on physiological properties. Starch is poly-D-glucose in a complex structure—a mixture of linear amylose and highly branched amylopectin. Amylose has $\alpha(1 \rightarrow 4)$ linkages, which introduce a twist in the molecule, leading to the formation of helical structures; amylopectin has mixed $\alpha(1 \rightarrow 4)$ and $\alpha(1 \rightarrow 6)$ linkages, giving rise to its highly branched structure. In the plant, the starch is mostly "packaged" as starch granules, but the majority of starch-rich foods have been processed by a combination of heat and moisture, which disrupts the native granular structure and causes partial solubilization of the starch polysaccharides. Starch that has been gelatinized by heating in water is readily hydrolyzed by the amylolytic enzymes, but on cooling to room temperature the solubilized polysaccharides can reassociate or "retrograde" (15). Retrograded amylose is more than 70% resistant to amylolysis in vitro (16) and restricts access of the enzyme to the starch substrate as a whole in vivo (17). Gidley and colleagues have investigated the molecular structure of resistant starch in great detail using a combination of physicochemical techniques (18). They showed that resistant starch has substantial segments of the amylose chains in the form of double helices loosely arranged into aggregates. Single-chain material is also present as imperfections in helices or as chains trapped between aggregates. The double-helical conformation appears to be the primary barrier to enzyme action (18).

III. THE INFLUENCE OF PHYSICAL PROPERTIES DURING THE PASSAGE OF FIBER THROUGH THE GUT

A. Food Preferences

Our food preferences depend very much on texture. Many of the texture-modifying agents used in the food industry are nonstarch polysaccharides and as such constitute dietary fiber. Another aspect to which a great deal of attention is currently being paid is the use of polysaccharides to mimic the texture of fat. The appeal of fatty foods is to a large extent due to their attractive texture. We expect sensory gratification in food, and most people are unwilling to sacrifice this for vague health benefits. There are already a number of polysaccharide-based products available that, according to the manufacturers, can be used to formulate low-fat versions of traditionally high-fat products such as ice cream (see also, e.g., Ref. 19). Although a step in the right direction, these products are not yet completely convincing. Fats are very complex substances. Fat melts in a peculiarly complex way that is hard to mimic, and it releases flavor volatiles (governed by Raolt's law) in a way that is also very difficult to replicate. More research is needed in this very difficult area.

Another aspect relating to food preferences may be that foods rich in dietary fiber often require considerable effort to chew. A study comparing breakfast cereals suggested that the energy required to break the product down into small pieces (the comminution energy) increases with its dietary fiber content. Further, the popularity of these products (reflected in sales in supermarkets) was inversely proportional to the comminution energy, as shown in Fig. 5 (20). Apparently we prefer foods that require little chewing!

B. Satiety

Not surprisingly, physical factors are also significant in the influence of dietary fiber on satiety and hence energy intake. Because distension of the stomach is believed to be one of the the signals to stop eating, several investigators have speculated that the bulk associated with high-fiber foods will induce a feeling of satiety and reduce meal size and food intake. Experimentally, however, conflicting results have been reported. Some workers have found that fiber intake decreases energy intake (21,22); others have found that it has no effect (23,24). It now seems that solubility and viscosity are critical factors. A fiber supplement of psyllium gum decreased spontaneous energy intake in a group of 12 women, whereas wheat bran had no effect (25). Studies in experimental animals and in humans have suggested that viscous polysaccharides can slow the rate of gastric emptying (26,27). Blundell and colleagues (28) found that soluble and insoluble fiber behave differently. Soluble fiber reduced appetite a longer time after eating

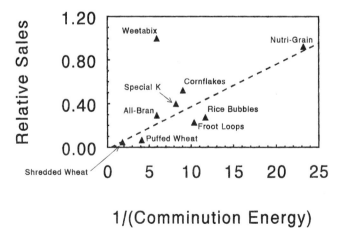

Fig. 5 Relative sales in Australia of breakfast cereals plotted against the reciprocal of the comminution energy as determined from the electrical energy required to grind the cereal to fine particles in a small hammer mill (see text).

Table 1 Effect of Fiber from Different Sources on Plasma Cholesterol Concentrations

Source of fiber	Quantity ingested (g/day)	Change in plasma cholesterol (%)
Cellulose	16	0
Wheat bran	17	+1
Whole oats[a]	15	−11
Oat bran[a]	27	−17
Pectin[a]	25	−13
Guar gum[a]	24	−16
Beans[a,b]	30	−19

[a] Composed of or containing viscous polysaccharides.
[b] Would also contain saponins, which have cholesterol-lowering activity.
Source: Ref. 30.

than soluble fiber, but there was no difference between how the two types affected total energy intake.

C. Absorption of Nutrients from the Small Intestine

Polysaccharides that form a gel matrix may slow absorption by trapping nutrients, digestive enzymes, or bile acids in the matrix and by slowing mixing and diffusion in the intestine. In an in vitro model using dialysis tubing, Johnson and Read (29) showed that guar gum appears to inhibit absorption by resisting the convective effects of intestinal contractions. Polysaccharides that give viscous solutions seem to be the most effective in lowering plasma cholesterol concentrations (Table 1). So it is not unreasonable to suppose that viscous, soluble fiber inhibits absorption of cholesterol and bile acids from the small intestine (31,32). Newman and colleagues (33), for example, have suggested that the cholesterol-lowering observed in rats fed high β-glucan barley fractions is related to the increased viscosity in the small intestine, and Tietyen and colleagues (34) found that reducing the viscosity of oat bran fiber (by treatment with endo-β-glucanase from *Bacillus subtilis*) reduced its ability to lower plasma cholesterol. In a study using everted sacs of rat jejunum, Johnson and Gee (35) found that viscous gums (guar and carboxymethyl cellulose) increased the thickness of the unstirred layer overlying the mucosa (Table 2). But the relevance of the unstirred layer has been questioned (36), and in an experiment in a which rats were fed methylcelluloses of different viscosity grades, no differences between plasma or liver cholesterol concentrations were observed (37). In another study, in which guar

Table 2 Apparent Thickness of Mucosal Unstirred Layer in Jejunal Sacs Preincubated With and Without Guar Gum or Carboxymethylcellulose

Polysaccharide	Unstirred layer thickness (μm)	
	Control	With polysaccharide
Guar gum (viscosity 16 cP)	317 ± 15	468 ± 25
Carboxymethycellulose	346 ± 12	402 ± 12

Source: Ref. 35.

gum, locust bean gum, and fenugreek gum were compared, reduction of plasma cholesterol was again not related to viscosity (Table 3) (38). Viscosity does, however, appear to influence glucose absorption, and guar gum and pectin have proved beneficial in controlling hyperglycemia (39). Ellis and colleagues (40) have shown that guar gum inhibits glucose absorption in inverse proportion to the viscosity of the digesta. Also, high dietary intakes of pectin (6 and 8% of the diet) decrease the availability of vitamin E in rats (41). But in contrast, gum acacia, which is not viscous, also improves glucose tolerance (40), and viscosity is not predictive of glycemic response (43). Eastwood and Morris (44) have concluded that there is in fact little evidence to suggest that viscous polysaccharides inhibit transport across the small intestinal epithelia. This is obviously a complex and controversial area.

D. Fermentation in the Colon

Although by definition fiber is not broken down by the enzymes of the gastrointestinal tract, virtually all fiber fractions are broken down to some extent by the microorganisms in the colon. Pectin, gum arabic, and guar gum disappear almost completely during transit; in humans, about 40% of dietary cellulose is broken down (45). Fermentation depends on the accessibility of the polysaccharide molecules to the microorganisms, which depends, in turn, on chemical structure and physical properties, particularly solubility. The chemical properties of the polysaccharide also appear to influence the types of microbial activity present in the large intestine (46). Soluble fiber fractions are very accessible and ferment rapidly in the proximal colon; insoluble fiber fractions ferment much more slowly in a process that is continuous during transit. The extent of breakdown may also be related to the physical structure of the plant—fiber from fruits and vegetables appears to be more fermentable than that from cereals (47). Thus, physical effects have a profound effect on the kinetics of release of metabolically important metabolites such as short-chain fatty acids. It is often suggested that short-chain fatty acids may be factors in controlling cholesterol metabolism, although some evidence suggests otherwise (38), and short-chain fatty acids, particularly butyrate, may influence the development of colorectal cancer (46,48). In this connection the kinetics of fermentation appears to be a particularly important factor.

Animal studies have shown that readily fermented fiber, such as guar gum and pectin, offer little protection from colorectal cancer. In contrast, slowly fermented fiber, such as wheat bran, has a more protective effect (49). These studies are summarized in Table 4. The explanation seems to be that readily fermented fiber produces a short-lived burst of metabolites, confined

Table 3   Relationship Between Viscosity and Cholesterol Lowering: Comparison of Three Galactomannans and α-Cellulose in the Cholesterol-Fed Rat

Fiber	Viscosity	Total plasma cholesterol (mM)
α-Cellulose	(Insoluble)	4.60 ± 0.34
Guar gum	High	3.26 ± 0.09
Locust bean gum	Medium	3.46 ± 0.12
Fenugreek gum	Low	3.16 ± 0.09

Source: Ref. 38.

Table 4 Summary of Published Reports on Effects of Dietary Fibers on Tumorigenesis in Rat Models of Large Bowel Cancer

Fiber type	Effect on tumorigenisis			Total number
	Protective	Equivocal	Enhanced	
Poorly fermentable				
Cellulose	8	3	0	11
Lignin	2	0	0	2
Slowly fermentable				
Wheat bran	7	9	0	16
Rapidly fermentable				
Guar gum	0	2	1	3
Pectin	0	2	3	5
Oat bran	0	0	1	1

Source: Ref. 49.

to the proximal colon, whereas slowly fermented fiber produces a sustained release of metabolites along the full length, reaching the distal colon (49). The fermentation pattern also seems to be important. In a series of rat studies with partially hydrolyzed guar gum, Weaver and colleagues (50) found that propionate as a fermentation product promotes the development of cancer, whereas butyrate was confirmed as having a protective effect.

E. Laxation

The huge displays of laxatives to be seen in any supermarket or pharmacy testify to the to popular concern with this topic. Feces are approximately 25% water and 75% dry matter. The major components are undigested residues plus bacteria and bacterial cell debris. These form a sponge-like, water-holding matrix, which conditions fecal bulk and consistency (51). Thus, the effect of fiber on laxation depends not only on the undegraded fiber residue, but also on bacterial cell mass. The ability of different fiber types to increase fecal bulk depends on a complex relationship between the chemical and physical properties of the fiber and the bacterial population in the colon. Cereal fibers are highest in pentoses and therefore have the greatest fecal bulking power (52). This is illustrated by comparing the results from studies of increased fecal bulk in response to various fiber supplements (Table 5). The physical form of the fiber is also important. Coarsely ground wheat bran is a very effective fiber source in increasing fecal bulk, whereas finely ground wheat bran has little or no effect, and may even be constipating (53). Additionally, some laxation effects may be due to the short-chain volatile fatty acids produced by fermentation (44,54), and it is probably for this reason that resistant starch has a mild laxative effect (55). Osmotic effects may be important in a way that is not yet well defined. Kinetic effects may also be significant, again with rapidly fermented fiber different in its effects from slowly fermented fiber, which gives a sustained release of low molecular weight (osmotically active) metabolites along the full length of the colon (56).

IV. CONCLUSIONS

The physiological functions of dietary fiber change as it progresses through the gastrointestinal tract. These functions depend to a large extent on physical properties, which also change. Thus,

Table 5 Effect of Fiber Supplements
on Fecal Bulk

Fiber supplement	% increase in fecal wet weight
Oat bran	15
Pectin	16–35
Guar gum	20
Apple	40
Carrot	59
Cabbage	67
Cellulose	75
Wheat bran, coarse	80–127
Wheat bran, fine	24

Source: Ref. 47.

we are dealing with a highly complex kinetic system that is still not well understood. Although the chemistry of dietary fiber is now well defined, it does not in itself predict biological activity. Biological activity depends on physical properties that do not relate in any simple way to crude chemical composition. The polysaccharides of which dietary fiber is mostly composed are complex structures in which the geometry of the linkage between monomer units largely defines physical properties. This means that we cannot assume that any material that falls within the chemical definition of dietary fiber, and analyses as dietary fiber by the usual methods, will necessarily be of significant health benefit to consumers.

REFERENCES

1. Morris ER, Norton IT. Polysaccharide aggregation in solutions and gels. In: Wyn-Jones E, Gormally J, eds. Aggregation Process in Solution. New York: Elsevier, 1983, pp. 549–593.
2. Morris ER. Polysaccharide structure and conformation in solutions and gels. In: Blanshard JMV, Mitchell JR, eds. Polysaccharides in Food. London: Butterworth, 1979, pp. 15–31.
3. Rees DA. Polysaccharide Shapes. London: Chapman and Hall, 1977.
4. Morris ER. Polysaccharide solution properties: origin, rheological characterization and implications for food systems. In: Millane RP, BeMiller JN, Chandrasekaran R, eds. Frontiers in Carbohydrate Research—1: Food Applications. London: Elsevier, 1989, pp. 132–163.
5. Glicksman M. Gum Technology in the Food Industry. New York: Academic Press, 1969.
6. Graessley WW. The entanglement concept in polymer rheology. Adv Polymer Sci 16:1–179, 1974.
7. Morris ER, Cutler AN, Ross-Murphey SB, Rees DA, Price J. Concentration and shear rate dependence of viscosity in random coil polysaccharide solutions. Carbohydrate Polym 1:5–21, 1981.
8. Schneeman BO. Dietary fiber: physical and chemical properties, methods of analysis and physiological effects. Food Technol 40:104–110, 1986.
9. Fairweather-Tait SJ, Write AJA. The effects of sugar beet fibre and wheat bran on iron and zinc absorption in rats. Br J Nutr 64:547–552, 1990.
10. Eastwood MA, Hamilton D. Studies on the adsorption of bile salts to non-absorbed components of diet. Biochim Biophys Acta 152:165–173, 1968.
11. Kritchevsky D, Story JA. Binding of bile salts in vivo by non-nutritive fiber. J Nutr 104:458–462, 1974.
12. Oakenfull DG, Fenwick DE. Adsorption of bile salts from aqueous solution by plant fibre and cholestyramine. Br J Nutr 40:299–309, 1978.

13. Hoagland DD, Pfeffer PE. Role of pectin in binding of bile acids to carrot fiber. In: Fishman ML, Jen JJ, eds. Chemistry and Function of Pectins. ACS Symposium Series, 310, 1986, pp. 266–274.

14. Oakenfull DG, Sidhu GS. Effects of pectin on intestinal absorption of glucose and cholate in the rat. Nutr Rep Int 30:1269–1278, 1986.

15. Miles MJ, Morris VJ, Orford PD, Ring SG. The roles of amylose and amylopectin in the gelation and retrogradation of starch. Carbohydr Res 135:271–281, 1985.

16. Ring SG, Gee JM, Whittam MA, Orford PD, Johnson IT. Resistant starch: its chemical form in foodstuffs and effect on degestibility in vitro. Food Chem 28:97–109, 1988.

17. Botham BL, Morris VJ, Noel TR, Ring SG. A study on the in vivo digestibility of retrograded starch. Carbohydr Polym 29:347–352, 1996.

18. Gidley MJ, Cooke D, Darke AH, Hoffmann RA, Russell AL, Greenwell P. Molecular order and structure in enzyme-resistant retrograded starch. Carbohydr Polym 28:23–31, 1995.

19. Ward FM. Hydrocolloid systems as fat mimetics in bakery products: icings, glazes and fillings. Cereal Foods World 42:386–390, 1995.

20. Parker NS, Oakenfull DG. Comminution energy and the sales of breakfast cereals. Proc Nutr Soc Aust 11:119, 1986.

21. Porikos K, Hagamen S. Is fiber satiating? Effects of a high fiber diet preload on subsequent food intake of normal-weight and obese young men. Appetite 7:153–162, 1986.

22. Mickelsen O, Makdani DD, Cotton RH, Titcomb ST, Colmey JC, Gatty R. Effects of a high fiber bread diet on weight loss in college-age males. Am J Clin Nutr 32:1703–1709, 1979.

23. Bryson E, Dore C, Garrow JS. Wholemeal bread and satiety. J Hum Nutr 34:113–116, 1980.

24. Russ CS, Atkinson RL. Use of high fiber diets for the out-patient treatment of obesity. Nutr Rep Int 32:193–198, 1985.

25. Stevens J, Levitsky DA, van Soest PJ, Robertson JB, Kalkwarf HJ, Roe DA. Effect of psyllium gum and wheat bran on spontaneous energy intake. Am J Clin Nutr 46:812–817, 1987.

26. Leeds AR. Gastric emptying, fibre and absorption. Lancet i:872, 1979.

27. Schwartz SE, Levine RA, Singh A, Schneidecker JR, Track NS. Sustained pectin ingestion delays gastric emptying. Gastroenterology 83:812–817, 1982.

28. Delargy HJ, O'Sullivan KR, Fletcher RJ, Blundell JE. Effects of amount and type of dietary fibre (soluble and insoluble) on short-term control of appetite. Int J Food Sci Nutr 48:67–77, 1997.

29. Johnson IT, Read NW. Do viscous polysaccharides slow absorption by inhibiting diffusion or convection? Eur J Clin Nutr 42:307–312, 1988.

30. Chen W-JL, Anderson JW. Effects of plant fiber in decreasing plasma total cholesterol and increasing high density lipoprotein cholesterol. Proc Soc Exp Biol Med 162:310–315, 1979.

31. Gee JM, Blackburn NA, Johnson IT. The influence of guar gum on intestinal transport in the rat. Br J Nutr 50:215–224, 1983.

32. Superko HR, Haskell WL, Sawrey-Kubicek L, Farquhar JW. Effects of solid and liquid guar gum on plasma cholesterol and triglyceride concentrations in moderate hypercholesterolemia. Am J Cardiol 62:51–56, 1988.

33. Danielson AD, Newman RK, Newman CW, Berardinelli JG. Lipid levels and digesta viscosity of rats fed a high-fiber barley milling fraction. Nutr Res 17:515–522, 1997.

34. Tietyen JL, Nevins DL, Schoemaker CF, Schneeman BO. Hypocholesterolemic potential of oat bran treated with an endo-β-D-glucanase from *Bacillus subtilis*. J Food Sci 60:558–560, 579, 1995.

35. Johnson IT, Gee JM. Effect of gel-forming gums on the intestinal unstirred layer and sugar transport in vitro. Gut 22:398–403, 1981.

36. Smithson KW, Millar DB, Jacobs G, Gray M. Intestinal diffusion barrier: unstirred layer or membrane surface mucous coat. Science 214:1241–1243, 1981.

37. Topping DL, Oakenfull D, Trimble RP, Illman RJ. A viscous fibre (methylcellulose) lowers blood glucose and plasma triacylglycerols and increases liver glycogen independently of volatile fatty acid production in the rat. Br J Nutr 59:21–30 (1988).

38. Evans AJ, Hood RL, Oakenfull DG, Sidhu GS. Relationship between structure and function of dietary fibre: a comparative study of the effects of three galactomannans on cholesterol metabolism in the rat. Br J Nutr 68:217–229, 1991.

39. Jenkins DJA, Leeds AR, Wolever TMS, Goff DV, Alberti KGMM, Gassull M, Hockaday TDR.

Dietary fibres, fibre analogues, and glucose tolerance: importance of viscosity. Br Med J 1:1392–1394, 1978.

40. Ellis PR, Roberts FG, Low AG, Morgan LM. The effect of high-molecular weight guar gum on net apparent glucose absorption and net apparent insulin and gastric inhibitory polypeptide production in the growing pig: relationship to rheological changes in jejunal digesta. Br J Nutr 74:539–556, 1995.
41. Schaus EE, de Lumen BO, Chow FI, Reyes P, Omaye ST. Bioavailability of vitamin E in rats fed graded levels of pectin. J Nutr 115:263–270, 1985.
42. Sharma RD. Hypoglycemic effect of gum acacia in healthy human subjects. Nutr Res 5:1437–1441, 1985.
43. Carrington-Smith D, Collier GR, O'Dea K. Effect of soluble dietary fibre on the viscosity of gastrointestinal contents and the acute glycaemic response in the rat. Br J Nutr 71:563–571, 1994.
44. Eastwood MA, Morris ER. Physical properties of dietary fiber that influence physiological function: a model for polymers along the gastrointestinal tract. Am J Clin Nutr 55:436–442, 1992.
45. Topping DL, Illman RJ. Bacterial fermentation in the human large bowel: time to change from the roughage model of dietary fibre? Med J Aust 144:307–309, 1986.
46. Cummings JH. The Large Intestine in Nutrition and Disease. Brussells: Institut Danone, 1997.
47. Schneeman BO. Dietary fiber: physical and chemical properties, methods of analysis and physiological effects. Food Technol 40:104–110, 1986.
48. Burkitt DP. Dietary fiber and cancer. J Nutr 118:531–533, 1988.
49. Young GP. Dietary fibre and bowel cancer: Which fibre is best? Cereals International. Proceedings of an International Conference held in Brisbane Australia, Royal Australian Chemical Institute, Melbourne, 1991, pp. 379–383.
50. Weaver GA, Tangel CT, Krause JA, Alpern HD, Jenkins PL, Parfitt MR, Stragand JJ. Dietary guar gum alters colonic microbial fermentation in azoxymethane-treated rats. J Nutr 126:1979–1991, 1996.
51. Stephen AM, Cummings JA. Mechanism of action of dietary fibre in the human colon. Nature 284:283–284, 1980.
52. Cummings JH, Southgate DAT, Branch W, Houston H, Jenkins DJA, James WPT. Colonic response to dietary fibre from carrot, cabbage, apple, bran and guar gum. Lancet i:5–9, 1978.
53. Oakenfull D, Topping DL. The nutritive value of wheat bran. Food Tech Aust 39:288–292, 1987.
54. Topping DL. Soluble fiber polysaccharides: effects on plasma cholesterol and colonic fermentation. Nutr Rev 49:195–203, 1991.
55. Cummings JH, Beatty ER, Kingman SM, Bingham SA, Englyst HN. Digestion and physiological properties of resistant starch in the human large bowel. Br J Nutr 75:733–747, 1996.
56. Edwards CA, Bowen J, Eastwood MA. Effect of isolated complex carbohydrates on cecal and fecal short chain fatty acids in stool output in the rat. In: Southgate DAT, Waldron K, Johnson IT, and Fenwick GR, eds. Dietary Fiber: Chemical and Biological Aspects. London: Royal Society of Chemistry, 1990, pp. 273–276.

14
Adsorption of Carcinogens by Dietary Fiber

Lynnette R. Ferguson and Philip J. Harris
The University of Auckland, Auckland, New Zealand

I. INTRODUCTION

Epidemiological studies indicate that diets containing a high proportion of dietary fiber can protect against the development of various cancers, especially those of the colon and breast (1,2). Animal studies provide further evidence for the protective properties of such diets, although these studies indicate that only certain types of dietary fibers, or sources of dietary fibers, are protective (e.g., Ref. 3). One of the various hypotheses that have been advanced to account for the protective properties of dietary fibers is that dietary fiber can adsorb carcinogens in the digestive tract (4). Providing that the dietary fiber is not significantly degraded by bacterial enzymes in the colon, the carcinogen could be carried out of the body adsorbed in this manner. This would lower the concentrations of carcinogens available to initiate or promote cancerous changes in the colonic mucosal cells.

To test the hypothesis that dietary fibers can adsorb dietary carcinogens in the conditions encountered in the human gut, various in vitro model systems have been used (e.g., Refs. 5–7). These experiments indicate that at least in vitro various types of dietary fibers can adsorb dietary carcinogens. However, whether this happens in vivo and its relevance to protection against cancer is much less certain. In this review, we summarize the in vitro evidence and what in vivo evidence is available.

II. DIETARY FIBERS TESTED IN CARCINOGEN ADSORPTION EXPERIMENTS

A. Plant Cell Walls of Fruits and Vegetables

It has been estimated that approximately 95% of the dietary fiber most commonly consumed in western diets comes from plant cell walls (8). The major chemical components of these plant cell walls are nonstarch polysaccharides, and indeed it has been suggested that the definition of dietary fiber should be restricted to nonstarch polysaccharides from plant cell walls (9). Most of the fruits and vegetables in western diets are from dicotyledonous (broad-leaved) plants, and the most common cell type is the parenchyma cell. This cell type has walls composed almost solely of polysaccharides.

It is important to recognize that cell walls vary in composition, depending on cell type. In contrast to parenchyma cell walls, the walls of some cell types that occur in small quantities in food plants contain, in addition to polysaccharides, the hydrophobic polymers lignin or suberin, which make the cell walls hydrophobic. Both lignin and suberin are complex, three-dimensional, hydrophobic polymers (10). Lignin is composed of interconnected phenylpropanoid residues and occurs, for example, in the cell walls of sclerenchyma fibers, sclereids, and xylem vessels. Suberin is believed to have a domain with a structure similar to lignin and a hydrophobic, polyester domain. Suberin, together with associated waxes, occurs in the walls of cork cells which, for example, form the skin of potato tubers.

Cell walls for in vitro carcinogen adsorption experiments have been isolated from various plant tissues. Furthermore, it is sometimes possible to obtain sufficient quantities of cell walls from a particular cell type. For example, we have isolated cell-wall preparations from parenchyma cells of potato tubers for such studies (11,12). However, because of the scarcity in food plants of cells with lignified or suberized cell walls, it is technically much easier to isolate pure preparations of these cell walls from plant material that is not usually eaten by humans. Thus, we have obtained cell wall preparations containing mostly lignified cell walls from wheat straw and from the woody, secondary xylem cylinder of mature cabbage stems. We have also obtained cell wall preparations containing mostly suberized cell walls from commercial cork. This latter material is from the outer bark of cork oak (*Quercus suber*) and consists of cork cells.

The cell walls were isolated from the various plant materials using methods commonly used to obtain cell wall preparations for the study of cell wall chemistry and biochemistry. These methods are intended to minimize changes to the cell wall components as a result of the isolation method, and the principles and details of such methods have been reviewed (13–15). In our experiments (11,12) we isolated cell walls by homogenizing the plant material in buffer containing 10 mM 2-mercaptoethanol at 4°C. The homogenate was centrifuged, the resulting pellet sonicated, and the cell walls recovered by filtering onto nylon mesh (pore size 11 µm). It is important that the cell wall preparation does not contain contaminating components, such as starch, as they may adsorb carcinogens and confound the results (16). Thus, if the plant tissue contained starch, this was removed during the isolation of the cell walls using either an α-amylase preparation or 90% (v/v) aqueous dimethyl sulfoxide (11). Other authors have used similar methods to isolate cell walls for in vitro studies on carcinogen adsorption (e.g., Ref. 6). To obtain sufficient amounts of cell wall preparations to supplement diets in animal experiments, we used simpler methods than we used to isolate cell wall preparations for in vitro studies on carcinogen adsorption. For example, we obtained a large-scale preparation of suberized cell walls by refluxing ground commercial cork with 80% ethanol five times and drying the residue.

In addition to whole cell wall preparations, insoluble dietary fiber preparations obtained from plant cell walls have frequently been used in studies on carcinogen adsorption. For example, we used a commercial α-cellulose preparation, which is readily available in bulk quantities, to develop a model in vitro system for studying the adsorption of carcinogens to dietary fibers (7). α-Cellulose is a cell wall fraction containing principally cellulose and is obtained as a residue after extracting cell walls with a variety of chemicals including aqueous solutions of sodium or potassium hydroxide (17). Kosikova and coworkers (18) also used a variety of lignin preparations obtained from wood and cereal straw to study the adsorption in vitro of nitrosamines.

B. Cereal Brans

Cereal brans are often erroneously described as dietary fibers, but in fact they are simply good sources of dietary fibers. For example, the bran from the hard red spring wheat cultivar Otane contained 41.8% dietary fiber as determined by the AOAC method (19). Nevertheless, the outer bran layers of cereal grains contains a high proportion of the dietary fiber in the whole grain;

wheat bran, for example, contains 70% of the whole grain dietary fiber. Furthermore, in wheat bran some of the cell types have lignified walls. Vikse et al. (20) obtained from this bran a series of dietary fiber preparations which had been treated in various ways to enrich their lignin content.

There is good evidence that whole grain cereals and cereal brans can protect against a range of cancers, including those of the colon, rectum, breast, pancreas, and possibly stomach (21). However, components other than dietary fiber may at least be partially responsible for this protection. From animal studies it has been found that the species from which the bran is derived is important in determining its protective effects. For example, in many experiments, wheat bran and possibly also rice bran protect against various carcinogen-induced cancers, whereas oat and barley brans do not protect and may even enhance cancer development (16,22,23). Furthermore, not only the source of the bran but also the particle size may be important for cancer prevention (19).

C. Soluble Dietary Fibers

Some polysaccharides become soluble in water after they have been extracted from plant cell walls and are referred to as soluble dietary fibers. We have shown that in vitro these polysaccharides can affect adsorption of carcinogens to insoluble dietary fibers. These soluble polysaccharides are widely used as additives (thickeners, stabilizers, emulsifiers, and gelling agents) in the food industry (24,25). These include preparations of pectic polysaccharides (pectins), which are also used medicinally and sold commercially as health foods. Other soluble dietary fibers are obtained from microorganisms (e.g., xanthan gum), from the cell walls of seaweeds (e.g., agar and carrageenans), and from plant sources other than cell walls, such as mucilages produced by the outer layers of some seeds (e.g., ispagula or psyllium from *Plantago* spp.).

III. CARCINOGENS TESTED IN DIETARY FIBER ADSORPTION EXPERIMENTS

A. Mutagenic Carcinogens

A range of different carcinogens have been tested for their abilities to adsorb to different types of dietary fibers; the chemical structures of these carcinogens are illustrated in Fig. 1. However, there is no universal agreement as to which carcinogens, or which groups of carcinogens, are involved in causing these types of human cancers. In part, this uncertainty is a result of there being a number of mutational steps in the pathway to colon cancer in humans (26), and it is likely that several carcinogens are involved. One candidate group of carcinogens is the heterocyclic amines (HCAs), which are known to occur in the human diet. At least in rats, the following members of this group are colon carcinogens: 2-amino-3-methylimidazo[4,5-*f*]quinoline (IQ), 2-amino-3,4-dimethylimidazo[4,5-*f*]quinoline (MeIQ), and 2-amino-1-methyl-6-phenylimidazo[4,5-*b*]pyridine (PhIP) (27). The most abundant of these in human diets is PhIP, which occurs in concentrations consistent with it being one of the human colon carcinogens.

N-nitroso-*N*-methylurea (NMU) and 1,2-dimethylhydrazine (DMH) are two carcinogens that have commonly been used in animal experiments to test the protective effects of dietary fibers. They are convenient for animal experiments because they produce large numbers of tumors. However, they probably do not occur in a normal human diet. Furthermore, they are very much more hydrophilic than the HCAs, and this property appears to reduce considerably their ability to adsorb to dietary fiber and dietary fiber sources (see Sec. VI).

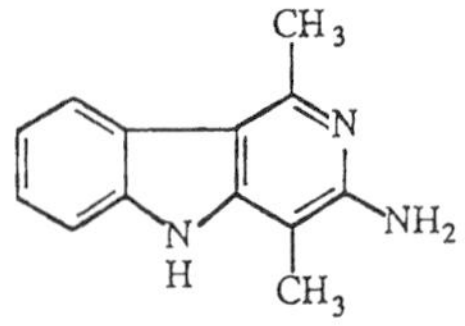

Trp-P-1
3-amino-1,4-dimethyl-5*H*-pyrido[4,3-*b*]indole

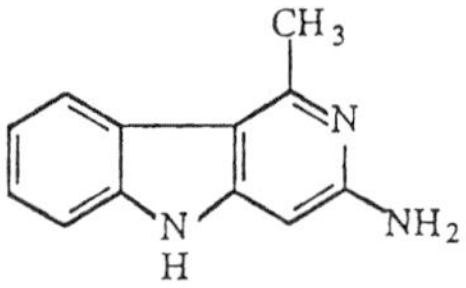

Trp-P-2
3-amino-1-methyl-5*H*-pyrido[4,3-*b*]indole

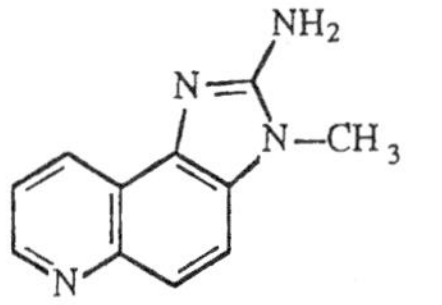

IQ
2-amino-3-methylimidazo[4,5-*f*]quinoline

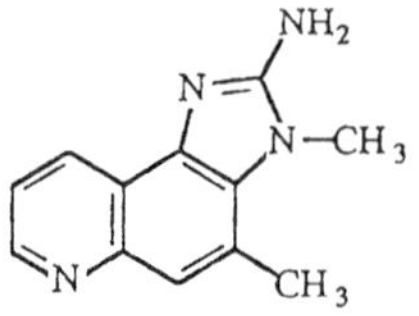

MeIQ
2-amino-3,4-dimethylimidazo[4,5-*f*]quinoline

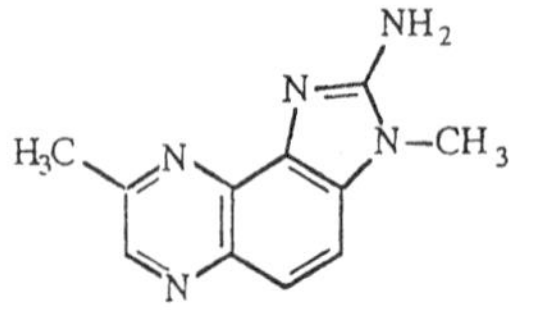

MeIQx
2-amino-3,8-dimethylimidazo[4,5-*f*]quinoxaline

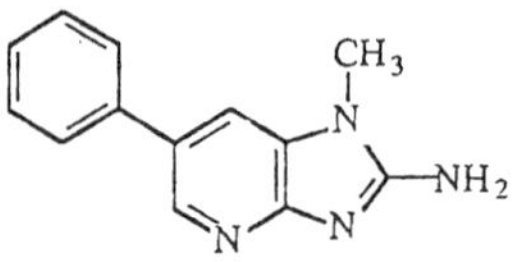

PhIP
2-amino-1-methyl-6-phenylimidazo[4,5-*b*]pyridine

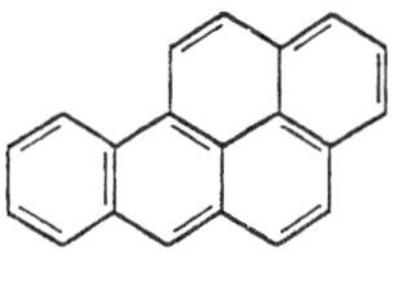

B[*a*]P
Benzo[*a*]pyrene

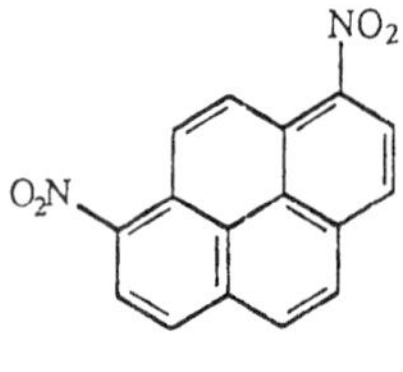

DNP
1,8-dinitropyrene

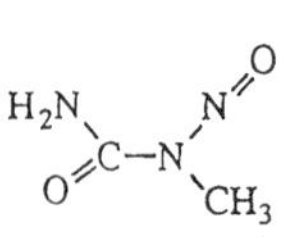

NMU
N-nitroso-N-methylurea

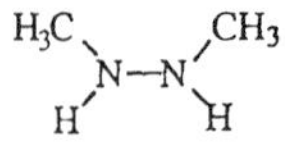

DMH
1,2-dimethylhydrazine

Fig. 1   Structures of various carcinogens.

Benzo[*a*]pyrene (BaP) is an important environmental carcinogen which has been used in in vitro experiments to determine its adsorption to dietary fibers, although it is probably not involved in human colon cancer (5). The carcinogen 1,6-dinitropyrene (DNP) has also been used in similar in vitro experiments.

B.   Bile Acids as Tumor Promoters

A range of in vitro and animal studies have shown co-mutagenic, co-carcinogenic, and tumor-promoting effects of secondary bile acids (e.g., 28, 29). The ability of dietary fibers or dietary fiber sources to adsorb bile acids has been suggested as an important mechanism, not only for reducing the bioavailability of bile acids themselves, but also for modulating cholesterol metabolism in vivo (30,31).

C. Estrogens

It has been accepted for some time that estrogens are involved in the development of uterine endometrial adenocarcinoma in humans (32). More recent epidemiological evidence also implicates these substances in human breast cancer (33). They are also active carcinogens in animal models (34), and Liehr (35) suggested they may act both as hormones and as pro-carcinogens.

Dietary fiber sources, such as wheat bran, can protect against breast cancer in animal models (36). Adlercreutz (37) suggested that dietary fiber could protect against breast cancer by altering the metabolism and excretion of such estrogens. Kendall and Cohen (38) suggested that the ability of conjugated and/or unconjugated estrogens to adsorb to dietary fiber may play a role in this effect.

IV. IN VITRO ADSORPTION EXPERIMENTS

A. Methods

In many of the early experiments on carcinogen adsorption to dietary fibers, the amounts of carcinogen adsorbed by the dietary fibers were calculated from the concentrations of carcinogens in the supernatant after various incubation times. For example, Kritchevsky and Story (30) incubated 5 mL of the substrate solution (a radioactive bile acid in this example) with a known amount of the dietary fiber at 37°C with shaking for 1 hour. After incubation, the dietary fiber was centrifuged down and the amount of radioactivity in the supernatant determined using standard procedures. Although this method may be adequate for some carcinogens, we found that the results can be confounded by carcinogens adsorbing to the wall of the incubating vessel (e.g., Ref. 7). As an example, Fig. 2a shows the effects of increasing amounts of wheat bran on the amount of the hydrophobic carcinogen, DNP, in the supernatant after 1 hour of incubation. Figure 2b illustrates a similar experiment showing the effects of increasing amounts of α-cellulose on the amount of the HCA, 3-amino-1-methyl-5H-pyrido[4,3-b]indole (Trp-P-2) in the supernatant. If carcinogen adsorption had been estimated only by sampling the supernatant, we would have concluded that Trp-P-2 adsorbs to α-cellulose considerably more effectively than does DNP to the wheat bran. In fact, estimating the amount of carcinogen adsorbed to the dietary fiber by washing it off the pellet and quantifying it revealed that the opposite was true: the wheat bran adsorbed the DNP more effectively than the α-cellulose adsorbed the Trp-P-2.

B. Data

1. Plant Cell Walls

In our studies, we have determined the abilities of parenchyma cell walls from the dicotyledonous plants potato and cabbage to absorb a range of carcinogens (11,12,16). These types of cell walls were not very effective in adsorbing carcinogens, no matter what carcinogen was used. Similar, poor adsorptive abilities for a range of different carcinogens were also found by a number of other authors for dietary fiber preparations obtained from dicotyledonous food plants that would be expected to be rich in parenchyma cells. It thus appears that parenchyma cells, from whatever dicotyledonous food plant, are generally ineffective in carcinogen adsorption.

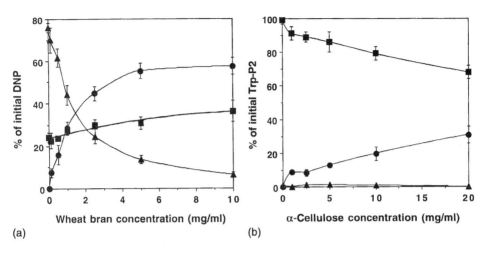

Fig. 2 (a) Effects of increasing concentrations of wheat bran on adsorption of the hydrophobic carcinogen DNP from solution. DNP (100 ng/2 mL) was incubated in phosphate-buffered saline with various concentrations of wheat bran. The concentration of DNP in the supernatant, on the tube walls, and associated with the wheat bran was estimated using mutagenicity assays as previously described (7). (b) Effects of increasing concentrations of α-cellulose on adsorption of the carcinogen Trp-P2 from solution. Samples were taken for mutagenicity assays after a total incubation time of 1 hour. Values represent total numbers of revertant colonies (minus those of negative controls) expressed as a percentage of the numbers seen for a comparable sample of DNP diluted into dimethyl sulfoxide and plated immediately. Filled circle, mutagenic activity associated with wheat bran and α-cellulose; filled square, mutagenic activity in supernatant; filled triangles, mutagenic activity adsorbed to tube walls.

For example, Kada et al. (6) examined the abilities of dietary fiber preparations from seven European and Chinese dicotyledon vegetables to adsorb the carcinogens 3-amino-1,4-dimethyl-5H-pyrido[4,3-b]indole (Trp-P-1) and Trp-P-2, but none of the preparations were very effective. Ryden and Robertson (39) also examined the abilities of dietary fiber preparations from a range of fruits and vegetables to adsorb the carcinogen, 2-amino-3,8-dimethylimidazo[4,5-f]quinoxaline (MeIQx). Dietary fiber preparations from apple, carrot, and sugar beet did not adsorb MeIQx. However, a dietary fiber preparation from cabbage, which contained the highest proportion of lignified xylem cell walls, did adsorb MeIQx, but this was significantly less than a dietary fiber preparation from wheat bran.

In contrast to cell wall preparations containing mainly unlignified parenchyma cell walls, we also examined the adsorptive abilities of cell wall preparations that contained mostly lignified cell walls, which are hydrophobic. We isolated these preparations from the woody, secondary xylem cylinder of mature cabbage stems and from the stem internodes of wheat straw (16). These two model cell-wall preparations had similar adsorptive abilities, but both were less effective than two further cell wall preparations containing mostly suberized cell walls, which were even more hydrophobic. These preparations were obtained from commercial cork and from potato skins. Subsequent work using other types of carcinogens has also shown that lignified and suberized plant cell walls have much better adsorptive abilities than parenchyma cell walls (12). This is probably a consequence of the hydrophobicity of these cell walls. Indeed, Kosikova et al. (18) showed using an in vitro system that various lignin preparations could adsorb nitrosamines.

Lignified cell walls also appear to be effective in adsorbing bile acids. For example, in his summary of in vitro adsorption of bile acids to dietary fiber, Kritchevsky (40) concluded that lignin was highly important to the adsorptive capacity; however, he did not report studies on suberized plant cell walls. Nevertheless, Selvendran (41) claimed that pectic polysaccharides rather than lignin provided the major adsorptive sites for sodium cholate and the adsorption increased as the pH decreased. His evidence was based on studies of the adsorption of radioactive sodium cholate to two cell wall preparations from runner bean pods: one containing mostly parenchyma cell walls and the other mostly lignified cell walls. However, these experiments were complicated by the precipitation of cholic acid at low pH and by the fact that adsorption to the cell walls was measured by quantifying the amount of sodium cholate in the supernatant.

2. Cereal Brans

We have compared the abilities of brans from cereals (barley, oats, maize, rice, and wheat) to adsorb in vitro the carcinogen DNP (23). Although all the brans adsorbed this carcinogen, there were very significant differences among the different brans. The order of effectiveness of the brans were rice (most effective), wheat, maize, barley, and oats. We also measured the adsorption of DNP to total and insoluble dietary fiber preparations from the brans. Although the DNP adsorbed to these preparations and the order of effectiveness was the same as the unextracted brans, our results suggested that dietary fibers were not the only components adsorbing DNP in the unextracted brans. A number of other authors have also shown that a variety of carcinogens can adsorb to brans and bran dietary fibers from different cereal species, especially wheat bran. For example, de Kok et al. (42) showed that fecapentaenes, which are human fecal mutagens, can adsorb effectively to wheat bran. Arts et al. (43) found that various estrogens also adsorbed effectively to wheat bran. Smith-Barbaro et al. (44) showed that DMH adsorbed to wheat and maize brans, and Barnes et al. (5) demonstrated that IQ adsorbed to bran from these two species. Furthermore, Ryden and Robertson (45) showed that dietary fiber from wheat bran adsorbed MeIQx much more effectively than dietary fibers from several fruits and vegetables that contained a high proportion of parenchyma cells. Takeuchi et al. (46) studied refined maize bran, a preparation rich in dietary fiber obtained by mechanically refining maize bran, and found that this effectively adsorbed various mutagenic carcinogens. When this preparation was added at a concentration of 10 mg/mL to an aqueous solution of DNP, 91.6% of the mutagenicity towards *Salmonella* tester strain TA98 disappeared. Under similar conditions, wheat bran and cellulose powder reduced the mutagenicity by only 58.4% and 43.0%, respectively. The maize bran preparation also adsorbed several HCAs such as IQ, Trp-P-1, Trp-P-2, 2-amino-6-methyldipyrido[1,2-α:3′2′-*d*]imidazole (Glu-P-1), and 2-aminodipyrido[1,2α:3′2′-*d*]imidazole (Glu-P-2). Shultz and Howie (47) compared the in vitro adsorption of a number of steroid hormones (estrone, estradiol-17 beta, estriol, testosterone, dihydrotestosterone, and estrone-3-glucuronide) to various cereal brans. Wheat and oat brans each adsorbed 45% of the unconjugated hormones, and maize bran adsorbed 44%. These authors suggested that lignin was an important component in the interaction with steroid hormones. Kendall and Cohen (38) also showed that wheat bran was able to adsorb various estrogens fairly effectively. Good evidence for the importance of lignin in cereal cell walls in determining their abilities to adsorb carcinogens was obtained by Vikse et al. (20). They used a series of dietary fiber preparations from wheat bran that had been treated in various ways to enrich their lignin content and found an increased ability to adsorb MeIQx with increased enrichment in lignin.

Ryden and Robertson (48) showed that in addition to the lignin content of the dietary fiber, the size of the bran particles is also important in determining its ability to adsorb carcinogens. They found that dietary fiber preparations from fine wheat bran adsorbed in vitro MeIQx much better than similar preparations from coarse wheat bran.

3. Soluble Dietary Fibers

Soluble dietary fibers such as pectic polysaccharides affect the abilities of hydrophobic carcinogens to adsorb to insoluble dietary fibers. Our initial studies showed that pectic polysaccharides released during incubation of parenchyma cell walls from potato tubers in aqueous solutions were able to maintain the hydrophobic carcinogen DNP in solution and to decrease its adsorption to insoluble cell wall components (11). We then examined eight commercial preparations of soluble dietary fibers and found all maintained DNP in aqueous solution and decreased its adsorption to α-cellulose. Gum arabic was the most effective and kappa-carrageenan the least (49). We then examined the ability of gum arabic to reduce the adsorption to α-cellulose of three other carcinogens: B[a]P, and the HCAs Trp-P-1 and MeIQx (50). Gum arabic reduced the adsorption of B[a]P to α-cellulose but did not affect the adsorption of Trp-P-1 and MeIQx, which are less hydrophobic than DNP (see Sec. III.A). On the basis of these results, we suggested three possible mechanisms by which soluble dietary fibers may enhance the development of colorectal cancer by hydrophobic carcinogens. First, because they reduce the ability of insoluble dietary fibers to adsorb hydrophobic carcinogens, more carcinogens may enter the colon maintained in solution than adsorbed onto insoluble dietary fibers. Second, if soluble dietary fibers are maintaining hydrophobic carcinogens in solution and these polysaccharides are degraded by bacterial enzymes in the colon, then the carcinogens may come out of solution and be deposited onto the mucosal surface of the colon. Third, soluble dietary fibers may cross the intestinal epithelium and carry with them carcinogens maintained in solution. These studies have important consequences for nutrition, because soluble dietary fibers are a common component of foods. However, a subsequent study by Ryden and Robertson (48) suggested that any harmful effects of soluble dietary fibers in maintaining hydrophobic mutagens in solution can be prevented by the presence of wheat bran.

V. ROLE OF HYDROPHOBICITY IN CARCINOGEN ADSORPTION

In a study of the adsorption of HCAs and other carcinogens to an α-cellulose preparation, Ferguson et al. (51) showed that the adsorptive ability of a carcinogen was strongly related to its hydrophobicity (measured as C log P): the more hydrophobic the carcinogen, the more effectively it adsorbed. These studies were extended by Harris et al. (12), who showed that the abilities of a range of HCAs to adsorb to plant cell walls depended not only upon the hydrophobicity of the HCAs, but also on the hydrophobicity of the cell walls. The more hydrophobic the cell wall preparation, the more effectively a particular carcinogen adsorbed. Cell walls from commercial cork that contained the hydrophobic polymer suberin had the best adsorptive ability and were also more hydrophobic than any other cell walls examined by us or others. Lignin is not as hydrophobic as suberin, and lignified plant cell walls, although effective in adsorbing HCAs, were inferior to suberized cell walls. We also showed that suberized and lignified cell walls were effective in adsorbing the hydrophobic carcinogen DNP (39).

Hydrophilic carcinogens, such as NMU, are commonly used in animal experiments. However, we found it difficult to determine experimentally the adsorption of NMU to various cell wall preparations because it is unstable, especially at 37°C (12,51). Even when the experiments were carried out at 22°C, at which temperature the extent of breakdown was reduced, we found that NMU adsorbed significantly (approximately 9%) only to the cell wall preparation from commercial cork. We also found that NMU was poorly adsorbed by α-cellulose (51). Thus, protection by dietary fibers in animal experiments in which such hydrophilic carcinogens have been used is probably the result of mechanisms other than adsorption and may or may not be relevant to humans.

VI. EFFECTS OF DIGESTION AND FERMENTATION OF THE DIETARY FIBER

If the adsorption of carcinogens to dietary fiber is relevant to protection against cancer, it is essential that the dietary fiber is not substantially degraded before being excreted in the feces. In contrast to humans, ruminant animals have been studied extensively in respect of bacterial degradation of plant cell walls in the gastrointestinal tract. The bacteria in the rumen degrade and ferment structural carbohydrates in forage cell walls, providing short-chain fatty acids and protein to the host animal (52,53). Although microbial colonization of the cell walls is quite rapid, the rate and extent to which they are degraded depends on the chemical composition of the cell walls. The presence of lignin and probably suberin protects the cell wall polysaccharides from degradation.

Except for the studies of Ryden and Robertson (39,45,48), there have been few studies of the effects of dietary fiber degradation and fermentation on carcinogen adsorption. Ryden and Robertson incubated dietary fiber preparations from fruits, vegetables, and wheat bran in vitro using a human fecal inoculum. The dietary fiber preparations from the fruits and vegetables were extensively degraded, and the polysaccharides in the residues were enriched in xylose, which is consistent with them being derived from lignified cell walls. These residues adsorbed the carcinogen MeIQx much more readily than did the corresponding unincubated preparations. Incubation of dietary fiber preparations from coarse and fine wheat bran also resulted in some degradation, but this was much less extensive than for dietary fiber preparations from fruits and vegetables. The residues also adsorbed MeIQx more readily than did the unincubated preparations, which is again consistent with these being enriched in lignified cell walls. However, a dietary fiber preparation from beeswing bran was only degraded to a slight extent by the human fecal inoculum and showed no increase in ability to adsorb MeIQx after incubation. Beeswing bran is from the outermost part of the bran and contains mostly lignified cell walls. All of these results are consistent with lignified cell walls being less degradable and having a greater ability to adsorb MeIQx than unlignified cell walls.

VII. ANIMAL STUDIES

If dietary fibers protect against cancer by adsorbing carcinogens, then we would predict that in animal experiments the bioavailability of exogenous and endogenous carcinogens would be reduced, and more would be excreted in the feces. In experiments in which the carcinogen IQ was administered to Fisher 344 rats, we found that supplementing the diet with wheat bran did increase the amount of IQ excreted (54). However, we were unable to determine whether this was caused by decreased transit time and increased fecal bulk or by the carcinogen adsorbing to the wheat bran or by a combination of these mechanisms.

In all of our in vitro studies, a dietary fiber preparation from commercial cork was consistently superior to anything else in adsorbing a range of dietary carcinogens. A preparation from potato skins also showed excellent adsorption properties. We explored whether these effects had significance in animals by studying the ability of these dietary fiber preparations to protect against the formation of aberrant crypts induced by IQ in Fisher 344 rats (54). As predicted by our in vitro experiments, the dietary fiber preparation from commercial cork showed good protective abilities, that from potato skins was intermediate, and both were superior to wheat bran used as a positive control in the experiments. The magnitude of the effects was too great to be attributed solely to changes in fecal bulk and transit time.

O'Neill et al. (55) showed that total B[*a*]P excreted was increased by the addition of wheat bran to a rat diet. However, their evidence suggested that wheat bran decreased the availability of B[*a*]P metabolites to the intestinal mucosa through its bulking effect, and they found no evidence for carcinogen adsorption.

VIII. HUMAN STUDIES

There is little definitive evidence from human studies that dietary fibers protect against cancer by adsorbing carcinogens. However, de Kok et al. (42) suggested that a high intake of dietary fiber may increase the excretion of fecapentaenes, which are putative initiators of colorectal cancer, by the dietary fiber adsorbing the fecapentaenes. Such adsorption would result in a reduced exposure of the human bowel epithelium to these compounds. In contrast, high concentrations of fecal bile acids may act as fecapentaene-solubilizing factors which increase fecapentaene bioavailability, thereby possibly resulting in increased risk for colorectal cancer. This interpretation appears consistent with their human data.

The ability of conjugated and/or unconjugated estrogens to adsorb to dietary fibers may explain how diets rich in dietary fiber may reduce the risk of breast cancer (38). Rose and coworkers (56) suggested that a high-fiber diet may reduce breast cancer risk at least in part through a reduction in circulating estrogens. They examined the effects of three levels of wheat bran supplementation on the major serum estrogens during both the luteal and follicular phases of the menstrual cycle in several groups of women. They found some decreases in the concentrations of luteal serum estrone and in the serum estradiol and variable effects on the serum estrone or estrone sulfate concentrations, but the serum sex hormone–binding globulin concentrations were unaffected by the wheat bran.

Further data consistent with the adsorption of such hormones by dietary fibers were obtained by Akingbala et al. (57). They investigated 12 healthy premenopausal women with regular ovulatory cycles for 3 months. These women consumed a diet providing 30% of their energy from fat and 15–25 g of dietary fiber per day for one month, followed by a crossover period in which they consumed a very low-fat, high-fiber diet providing 10% of their energy from fat and 25–35 g of dietary fiber per day for 2 months. By the end of the second month of the very low-fat, high-fiber diet, there was a significant reduction in serum estrone and estradiol levels during the early follicular and late luteal phases.

IX. CONCLUSIONS

There is no question that carcinogens can adsorb in vitro to dietary fibers and dietary fiber sources, and this probably also occurs in vivo. However, to what extent this relates to human cancer is still an open question. If the results from in vitro models do fully extend to humans, there are implications for the types of dietary fibers desirable in the human diet. Thus, it may be an advantage to increase the consumption of food plants that contain suberized or lignified cell walls. These types of cell walls are the most effective absorbers of hydrophobic carcinogens. However, in western diets these cell walls usually occur in only small amounts. One of the most important sources of lignified cell walls is wheat bran. Furthermore, sclereids or stone cells, which have thick, lignified cell walls, occur in various fruits including pears (58) and feijoas (59). In some vegetables the walls of specific cell types, such as sclerenchyma fibers, lignify as the vegetables mature. For example, this occurs in developing asparagus shoots giving the shoots a tough, stringy texture and making them less palatable. Cork cells with suberized cell walls also occur in the skins of a variety of tubers and root vegetables in addition to potatoes.

REFERENCES

1. Burkitt D. Lancet 2:1229–1231, 1969.
2. Potter JD, ed. Food, Nutrition and the Prevention of Cancer: A Global Perspective. Washington, DC: World Cancer Research Fund/American Institute for Cancer Research, 1997.
3. Jacobs LR. Advances Exp Med Biol 206:105–118, 1986.
4. Harris PJ, Ferguson LP. Mutat Res 290:97–110, 1993.
5. Barnes WS, Maiello J, Weisburger JH. J Natl Canc Inst 70:757–760, 1983.
6. Kada T, Kato M, Aikawa K, Kiriyama S. Mutat Res 141:149–152, 1984.
7. Roberton AM, Harris PJ, Hollands HJ, Ferguson LR. Mutat Res 244:173–178, 1990.
8. Stevens BJH, Selvendran RR, Bayliss CE, Turner R. J Sci Food Agric 44:151–156, 1988.
9. Englyst HN, Cummings JH. J Assoc Off Anal Chem 71:808–814, 1988.
10. Bacic A, Harris PJ, Stone BA. In: Preiss J, ed. The Biochemistry of Plants, Vol. 14, Carbohydrates. San Diego: Academic Press, 1988, pp. 297–371.
11. Harris PJ, Roberton AM, Hollands HJ, Ferguson LR. Mutat Res 260:203–213, 1991.
12. Harris PJ, Triggs CM, Roberton AM, Watson ME, Ferguson LR. Chem-Biol Interactions 100:13–25, 1996.
13. Harris PJ. In: Hall JL, Moore AL, eds. Isolation of Membranes and Organelles from Plant Cells. London: Academic Press, 1983, pp. 25–53.
14. Fry SC. In: Linskens H-F, Jackson JF, eds. Plant Fibers. Berlin: Springer, 1989, pp. 12–36.
15. Selvendran RR, Ryden P. In: Dey PM, ed. Methods in Plant Biochemistry. London: Academic Press, 1990, pp. 549–579.
16. Roberton AM, Ferguson LR, Hollands HJ, Harris PJ. Mutat Res 262:195–202, 1991.
17. Rogers HJ, Perkins HR. Cell Walls and Membranes. London: E. & F.N. Spon Ltd, 1968.
18. Kosikova B, Mlynar J, Joniak D, Konigstein J, Micko M. Cellulose Chem Technol 28:85–91, 1989.
19. Ferguson LR, Harris PJ. Lebensm-Wiss Technol 30:735–742, 1997.
20. Vikse R, Mjelva BB, Klungsoyr L. Food Chem Toxicol 30:239–246, 1992.
21. Zoran DL, Turner ND, Taddeo SS, Chapman RS, Lupton JS. J Nutr 127:2217–2225, 1997.
22. Ferguson LR, Harris PJ. Int J Cancer 78:385–386, 1998.
23. Harris PJ, Sasidharan VK, Roberton AM, Triggs CM, Blakeney AB, Ferguson LR. Mutat Res 412:323–331, 1998.
24. Glicksman M, ed. Food Hydrocolloids, Vol. 1. Boca Raton, FL: CRC Press, 1982.
25. Glicksman M, ed. Food Hydrocolloids, Vol. 3, Boca Raton, FL: CRC Press, 1986.
26. Vogelstein B, Fearon ER, Hamilton SR, Kern SE, Preisinger AC, Leppart M, Nakamura Y, White R, Smits AMM, Bos JL. N Engl J Med 319:525–532, 1988.
27. Wakabayashi K, Nagao M, Esumi H, Sugimura T. Cancer Res 52 (suppl):2092s–2098s, 1992.
28. Cameron RG, Imaida K, Tsuda H, Ito N. Cancer Res 42:2426–2428, 1982.
29. Wilpart M, Mainguet P, Maskens A, Roberfroid M. Carcinogenesis 4:45–48, 1983.
30. Kritchevsky D, Story JA. J Nutr 104:458–462, 1974.
31. Gallaher D, Schneeman BO. American J Physiol 250:G420–426, 1986.
32. Greenwald P, Caputo TA, Wolfgang PE. Obstet Gynecol 50:239–243, 1977.
33. Henderson BE, Ross RK, Pike MC. Science 244:1131–1138, 1991.
34. Newbold RR, Bullock BC, McLachlan JA. Cancer Res 50:7677–7681, 1990.
35. Liehr JG. Eur J Cancer Prev 6:3–10, 1997.
36. Zile MH, Welsch CW, Welsch A. Int J Cancer 75:439–443, 1998.
37. Adlercreutz H. Gasteroenterology 86:761–764, 1986.
38. Kendall ME, Cohen LA. In Vivo 6:239–245, 1992.
39. Ryden P, Robertson JA. Carcinogenesis 16:1711–1716, 1995.
40. Kritchevsky D. Eur J Clin Nutr 49(suppl 3):S113–115, 1995.

41. Selvendran RR. Chem Ind 428–430, 1978.
42. de Kok TM, van Iersel ML, ten Hoor F, Kleinjans JC. Mutat Res 302:103–108, 1993.
43. Arts CJ, Govers CA, van den Berg H, Wolters MG, van Leeuwen P, Thijssen JH. J Steroid Biochem Mol Biol 38:621–628, 1991.
44. Smith-Barbaro PD, Hansen D, Reddy BS. J Natl Cancer Inst USA 67:495–497, 1981.
45. Ryden P, Robertson JA. Cancer Lett 114:47–49, 1997.
46. Takeuchi M, Hara M, Inoue T, Kada T. Mutat Res 204:263–267, 1988.
47. Shultz TD, Howie BJ. Nutrition Cancer. 8:141–147, 1986.
48. Ryden P, Robertson JA. Carcinogenesis 16:209–216, 1995.
49. Harris PJ, Roberton AM, Watson ME, Triggs CM, Ferguson LR. Nutr Cancer 19:43–54, 1993.
50. Ferguson LR, Roberton AM, Watson ME, Triggs CM, Harris PJ. Chem-Biol Interact 95:245–256, 1995.
51. Ferguson LR, Roberton AM, Watson ME, Kestell P, Harris PJ. Mutat Res 319:257–266, 1993.
52. Akin DE. In: Jung HG, Buxton DR, Hatfield RD, Ralph J, eds. Forage Cell Wall Structure and Digestibility. Madison, WI: American Society of Agronomy, 1993, pp. 73–82.
53. Varga GA, Kolver ES. J Nutr 127(suppl 5):819S–823S, 1997.
54. Ferguson LR, Harris PJ. Chem-Biol Interact 114:191–209, 1998.
55. O'Neill IK, Povey AC, Bingham S, Cardis E. Carcinogenesis 11:609–616, 1990.
56. Rose DP, Lubin M, Connolly JM. Nutrition 13:535–539, 1997.
57. Akingbala JO, Oguntimein GB, Sobande AO, Bagga D, Ashley JM, Geffrey SP, Wang HJ, Barnard RJ, Korenman S, Heber S. Cancer 76:2491–2496, 1995.
58. Sterling C. Food Res 19:433–443, 1954.
59. Harman JE. NZ J Exp Agric 15:209–215, 1987.

15
Dietary Fiber and Mineral Interaction

Barbara F. Harland and Gurleen Narula
Howard University, Washington, D.C.

I. INTRODUCTION

Just 10 years ago B. Harland summarized what was known on this subject (1); 5 years ago, another summary was published with a coauthor (2). A year ago, the American Dietetic Association, in response to expanding research interest and consumer demand, published a position paper on the health implications of dietary fiber (3). What has been learned during those long years of research and study? We are living longer, and for those of us with the proper application of increased health and nutrition–related knowledge, we are living better.

Now there are specific dietary fiber guidelines: recommendations for dietary fiber intakes for adults range from 20 to 35 g/day, or 10–13 g of dietary fiber per 1000 kcal. Americans are not yet living up to the recommendations, averaging only 14–15 g/day. Human research has become more costly and restrictive. Yet there are advances in the use of isotopes for identifying and quantifying specific fiber fractions and their physiological roles.

Other components within the fiber matrix—tannins, oxalates, and phytoestrogens—are being identified and characterized. The primary, pervasive antinutrient, phytate, the compound present in all plant life for which monogastric animals (humans) have no phytase enzyme to lessen its mineral binding effects, is still strongly present. However, safe phytate:mineral dietary ratios are being developed to serve in dietary assessments and diet formulations (4,5).

Most of the recent studies chronicled in this chapter present discouraging data concerning the effect of fiber on mineral absorption and bioavailability. However, many studies are short term, involving selected populations, and examine only a few minerals. There is little evidence that the fiber content of a fiber-rich (20–35 g/day) American diet will cause long-term mineral deficiencies when a balanced diet is consumed. Studies of lowered bone mass densities have been reported among vegetarians (6) whose dietary intakes are not supported by the Food Guide Pyramid (3).

An early negative association of dietary fiber and mineral bioavailability was reported in 1942 by McCance and Widdowson (7). Yet, epidemiological studies rarely indicate concern about an adverse effect of dietary fiber alone on mineral utilization in human populations. Studies dealing with mineral nutrition, especially human nutrition, lack sensitive methods to assess mineral status. In most human studies, mineral absorption has been measured after the consumption of a few foods. In reality, humans consume mixed diets containing a number of dietary factors other than fiber, which can influence mineral bioavailability. Observations from animal studies have relevance for humans, however, direct extrapolation from animals to humans should be done with caution.

Concerns associated with a high intake of dietary fiber and its adverse effects on mineral bioavailability are largely due to the ability of dietary fiber to chelate ions in vitro. The complexities associated with nutrient interactions due to various physical and chemical conditions make it difficult to predict with precision mineral bioavailablity. Dietary fiber rarely affects the absorption of minerals uniformly; it will affect specific minerals or mineral groups.

The site of each mineral's absorption in the gastrointestinal tract is also significant. The soluble and insoluble fractions of dietary fiber behave differently and have a different fate in the alimentary tract. Although most minerals seem to be absorbed from the small intestine, there is some evidence suggesting that copper and selenium are absorbed from the stomach. The magnitude and importance of the colon as a site of mineral absorption is also a controversial issue.

Following are reports of recent studies which exemplify the problems and concerns of investigators working in vitro, in animals, and in humans. It is through their efforts that guidelines for improved health have been formulated.

II. MINERAL INTERACTION WITH DIETARY FIBER IN VITRO

Claye et al. studied the whole fibers of wheat bran (WB), rice bran (RB), oat fiber (OF), apple fiber (AF), and tomato fiber (TF), as well as their isolated, isoluble fiber fractions (8). Copper (Cu) and zinc (Zn) were the minerals of interest. Endogenous Cu concentrations in the foods ranged from 1.0 μg/g for OF to 14 μg/g for WB. Endogenous Zn concentrations ranged from 11 μg/g for OF to 136 μg/g for WB. In all fibers, total bound Cu was significantly greater than total bound Zn. More Cu and Zn were bound by the fiber fractions than by the intact fibers, probably due to the exposure of more binding sites on the polymers formed during the fractionation process. The fiber components of all five fibers bound Cu and Zn in the following decreasing order: hemicellulose A > lignocellulose > lignin > cellulose. Protein content of these fibers enhanced both Cu and Zn binding. The inevitable effects of naturally occurring phytate in these fibers were not discussed.

III. MINERAL INTERACTION WITH DIETARY FIBER IN ANIMALS

A. Calcium

In a 4-week experiment, ground rhubarb stalk fiber containing 74% total dietary fiber (66% insoluble, 8% soluble) was fed at the 0, 1, 3, or 5% level to male, weanling Sprague-Dawley rats (9). Cellulose was added, where warranted, to keep the fiber level constant across groups. The purpose of the experimental design was to test the belief that the oxalate in the rhubarb fiber would bind calcium (Ca). Such was not the case. As the rhubarb content in the diets increased, retention and absorption of Ca increased. However, as dietary cellulose increased, the Ca bioavailability decreased. Added cellulose may have increased intestinal motility, thus decreasing binding opportunities. It was suggested that powdered rhubarb stalk, despite known oxalate-binding ability, when fed up to a level of 5% may not have a negative effect on Ca bioavailability.

Table 1 Composition of the Basal Diet
(Control)

Component	%
Egg albumin	22.2980
Corn oil	4.9820
Vitamin mixture	1.0000
Zinc-deficient mineral mixture	3.5000
Choline bitartrate	0.2000
D,L-Methionine	0.3000
Sucrose	22.6000
Corn starch	45.1731
Zinc acetate	0.0027

Source: Adapted from Ref. 10.

B. Zinc

The influence of dietary fiber on the bioavailability of Zn in young, male albino rats was studied by Kondo and Osada (10). Semipurified diets supplemented with or without 5% purified dietary fiber (cellulose, agar-agar, pectin, chitin, or chitosan) were fed for 31 days. The study was designed to choose fibers with virtually no endogenous phytate, which might cloud interpretation of the results (see Table 1). All test diets contained Zn at a level of 8 ppm from zinc acetate (the minimal recommended level for rats of this age). The apparent absorption of dietary Zn in the control group was approximately 80%. Rats fed the agar-agar diet showed Zn absorption at 70%. Raising agar-agar levels from 5 to 15% did not reduce Zn absorption. Conversely, rats fed the pectin diet showed Zn absorption at 90%.

Table 2 shows the Zn levels in tibias and femurs of rats fed the diets. The total amount of Zn in the tibia and femurs of rats fed the control diet was slightly higher than that in rats fed the experimental diets, but there were no significant differences.

Table 3 depicts the Zn concentration in serum and red cells. Again, the serum Zn concentration of rats fed the control diet was slightly higher than in the experimental groups with no significant differences. However, the red cell Zn concentration was significantly lower in both the agar-agar and the chitosan-fed groups ($p < 0.05$).

In Table 4 liver Zn was significantly less in the pectin-fed group and greater in the chitosan-fed group. The concentrations of Zn in the kidneys were greater in the control group and significantly less in the pectin-fed group. The groups fed pectin and chitosan had lower spleen Zn ($p < 0.05$).

Table 2 Bone Zinc Concentration in Rats Fed
Test Diets

Diet	Tibia (μg/g)	Femur (μg/g)
Control	100 ± 12	91 ± 17
Cellulose	78 ± 8	74 ± 6
Agar-agar	78 ± 16	65 ± 17
Pectin	68 ± 4	67 ± 4
Chitin	86 ± 7	83 ± 6
Chitosan	93 ± 3	90 ± 8

Source: Adapted from Ref. 10. Mean ± standard error.

Table 3 Zinc Concentration in Blood of Rats Fed Test Diets

Diet	Serum (μg/g)	Red cells (μg/g)
Control	1.06 ± 0.31	11.98 ± 0.17[a]
Cellulose	0.31 ± 0.35	10.16 ± 0.89[a]
Agar-agar	0.46 ± 0.19	9.69 ± 0.34[b]
Pectin	0.83 ± 0.15	10.52 ± 0.55[a]
Chitin	0.67 ± 0.17	12.76 ± 4.55[a]
Chitosan	0.71 ± 0.35	9.44 ± 0.70[b]

Mean ± standard error. Values not sharing a common superscript differ significantly ($p < 0.05$).
Source: Adapted from Ref. 10.

Overall, the effect of specific dietary fiber intakes on Zn bioavailability had no effect on tibias, femurs, and serum Zn and only marginal effects on red cell, liver, kidney, and spleen Zn. These results indicate that dietary fiber may decrease the utilization of Zn because of differences in absorbability, hydration qualities, viscosity, or ion exchange action.

C. Multiple Minerals

A comparison of the influence of dietary fiber sources with different proportions of soluble and insoluble fiber on Ca, copper (Cu), iron (Fe), magnesium (Mg), manganese (Mn), and Zn absorption in 50 rats was made in a 6-week study by Gralak et al. (11).

The following fiber preparations were fed at 10% of the diet: high methoxylated citrus pectin, apple pomace, potato fiber, and sugar beet pulp, all at the expense of wheat starch in the control diet. The protein source was casein fed at 11.6%, and soybean oil was fed at 10% of the diet. The investigators had planned to observe mineral absorption during the third and final (sixth) week of the experiment, with 4-day, consecutive fecal collections during those two periods. Feed intake was monitored daily and rats were weighed weekly.

At the end of the experiment, body weights varied only slightly. Despite attempts to keep the experimental diets comparable to the control diet, there was 1½ times the Ca in the apple and beet pulp diets, 1½ times the Mg in the potato diet, 4 times the Fe, and 2 the Zn in the pectin diet compared with the control.

Table 4 Zinc Concentration in Liver, Kidney, and Spleen of Rats Fed Test Diets

Diet	Liver (μg/g)	Kidney (μg/g)	Spleen (μg/g)
Control	26 ± 3[a]	25 ± 2[b]	28 ± 4[a]
Cellulose	24 ± 2[a]	23 ± 1[a]	23 ± 1[a]
Agar-agar	26 ± 2[a]	23 ± 1[a]	24 ± 1[a]
Pectin	24 ± 1[b]	20 ± 1[c]	19 ± 1[b]
Chitin	24 ± 2[a]	23 ± 2[a]	22 ± 1[a]
Chitosan	28 ± 1[c]	23 ± 1[a]	19 ± 1[b]

Mean ± standard error. Values not sharing a common superscript differ significantly ($p < 0.05$).
Source: Adapted from Ref. 10.

There were no negative mineral balances in the control group for either observational period; however, the following negative balances were observed in the first assessment period (at 3 weeks): Mg in the apple-fed group, Fe in the beet-fed group, and Mn in both the citrus pectin and apple-fed groups. During the second observational period (at 6 weeks), Fe and Mg were in negative balance in the beet-fed group and Mn was in negative balance in the apple-fed group. Apparent absorption increased in the control and citrus pectin groups from the third to the sixth week, while it decreased in the potato and beet groups during the same time period.

When comparing the effects of soluble versus insoluble fiber in each experimental diet, soluble fiber had very little effect on apparent absorption at either observational period. Thus, the effects upon mineral absorption in this study may be attributed primarily to the presence of insoluble fiber. Because total dietary fiber includes a range of structural plant compounds with apparent digestibilities varying from 0 (lignin) to 100% (pectin), it is difficult to identify which factor plays the key role and in which part of the GI tract the absorption outcome is determined. Ca absorption in the large intestine made a substantial contribution to the digestive balance of Ca. In rats, Ca is more effectively absorbed in the large intestine when there is active fermentation. The fermentation is amplified when resistant starch or soluble fiber reaches the large intestine, and there may be substances that depress the absorption of Ca in the small intestine. After 6 weeks, the apparent absorption of all minerals determined in this study tended to decrease, and in the case of Ca and Zn, the differences were significant ($p < 0.05$).

IV. MINERAL INTERACTION WITH DIETARY FIBER IN HUMANS

A. Adults—Calcium

A randomized, crossover study in 26 healthy adult women was designed by Weaver et al. (12) to study calcium absorption. In a previous study, the Ca from milk that accompanied regular meals was not fully absorbed; as Ca ingestion increased, less was absorbed. The authors wanted to obtain more information about the Ca absorption mechanism and assess Ca binders such as fiber and phytate. In test meal situations, Ca-carbonate, intrinsically labeled with ^{45}Ca, was ingested with either 40 g of dry, extruded wheat bran cereal or white bread toast. Subjects ingesting the Ca-carbonate load at five levels of Ca showed greater absorption at the lower levels of Ca intake.

In all cases, the impairment of Ca absorption by the addition of wheat bran exceeded that of Ca-carbonate ingestion alone. Perhaps the nature of Ca binding by wheat bran could be through physical entrapment, absorption, or ionic binding. Phytic acid is not the only controlling constituent affecting Ca absorption. There are uronic acid residues, pectin, cellullose, and lignin, all of which might play a role. Although neutral cellulose has little affinity for cations, lignin strongly binds Ca. Pectin can be degraded during digestion, but lignin is indigestible.

B. Adults—Multiple Minerals

Cu, Mg, and Zn absorption and retention from a fiber-rich diet of conventional foods were investigated by Knudsen et al. (13). The diet was designed to provide 29 g of dietary fiber per day. A conventional diet was fed for one day, and the stable isotopes of Ca, Mg and Zn were added to this diet. Apparent absorption, retention, and endogenous losses were estimated for the respective minerals based on fecal and urinary excretion during the last 16 days of a 21-day study. The overall absorption of Cu, Mg, and Zn by the subjects was $44 \pm 7\%$, $46 \pm 6\%$, and $29 \pm 12\%$, respectively. Even so, the fractional absorptions were insufficient to cover urinary losses, resulting in negative balances in all subjects. The interpretation of these results is difficult because the presence of phytate, primarily found in the whole meal bread, clouds the issue. In most studies where phytate is present, it plays the major mineral-binding role, compared with all other endogenous factors. Although the minerals Ca, Mg, and Zn are primarily excreted in feces, it was of interest to learn that in this study, 8% of excreted Zn and 37% of Mg were found in urine, but no Cu was found to be excreted in urine. A baseline concentration of serum Cu, Mg, and Zn did not change during the period of study.

In summary, the fractional absorption of Cu, Mg, and Zn from the fiber-rich diet was not sufficient to cover intestinal and urinary losses of these elements resulting in negative balances.

C. Infants—Multiple Minerals

Davidsson et al. (14) studied the effect of dietary fiber in weaning cereals on the Ca, Fe, and Zn bioavailability in healthy infants 7–17 weeks old. The study had a crossover design, with each infant acting as his or her own control. Since no studies have defined desirable fiber intakes for infants and children younger than 2 years (3), the investigators had some concern when formulating infant cereals, which are the earliest solid food to which infants are exposed.

Two formulations of cereals were tested: a wheat/soy cereal (8.0 and 1.8% dietary fiber, respectively) fed to 34 infants, and a wheat/milk cereal (5.3 and 2.0% dietary fiber, respectively) fed to 23 infants. Absorption of ^{42}Ca and ^{70}Zn was studied by examining fecal excretion; bioavailability of ^{58}Fe was assessed by measuring the amount incorporated into erythrocytes. The investigators found no negative effects on the apparent absorption of energy and nutrients from these experimental cereals when fed to healthy, formula-fed infants.

V. SUMMARY

Dietary fiber is an essential part of the diet, both as a natural food component and as an added ingredient, providing an invaluable contribution to human nutrition and health (15). In spite of the strong evidence of beneficial effects from dietary fiber from fruits, vegetables, legumes, and cereal grains, one must allow for a possible decreased bioavailability of certain minerals. However, the positive effects of consuming a high-fiber diet far outweigh the probable adverse effects of decreased mineral absorption. Nutritionists and health scientists continue to promote a daily intake of 20–35 g of dietary fiber for adults (3).

The various chemical and physical conditions make it virtually impossible to predict the bioavailability of all minerals in a mixed diet since fiber components such as phytate, tannins, and saponins occur together in a food. It is difficult to distinguish between the effect of the chelating components and the fiber fractions themselves. Phytate:mineral ratios are being developed for some of the more vulnerable nutrient minerals, but there is still much work to be done.

REFERENCES

1. Harland BF. Dietary fibre and mineral bioavailability. Nutr Res Rev 2:133–147, 1989.
2. Munoz JM, Harland BF. Overview of the Effects of Dietary Fiber on the Utilization of Minerals and Trace Elements. In: GA Spiller, ed. CRC Handbook of Dietary Fiber. Boca Raton, FL: 1993 pp 245–252.
3. Marlett JA, Slavin JL. Position of the American Dietetic Association: Health Implications of Dietary Fiber. J Am Diet Assoc 97:1157–1159, 1997.
4. Oberleas D. Mechanism of zinc homeostasis. J Inorg Biochem 62:231–241, 1996.

5. Oberleas D. Mild to moderate zinc deficiency. J Pediatr Nutr Dev 79:2–13, 1997.

6. Barr SI, Prior JC, Janelle KC, Lentle BC. Spinal bone mineral density in premenopausal vegetarian and nonvegetarian women: cross-sectional and prospective comparisons. J Am Diet Assoc 98:760–765, 1998.

7. McCance RA, Widdowson EM. Mineral metabolism of dephytinized bread. J Physiol 101:304–308, 1942.

8. Claye SS, Idouraine A, Weber CW. In vitro mineral binding capacity of five fiber sources and their insoluble components for copper and zinc. Plant Foods Hum Nutr 49:257–269, 1996.

9. Goel V, Ooraikul B, Basu TK. Effect of dietary rhubarb stalk fiber on the bioavailability of calcium in rats. Int J Food Sci Nutr 47:159–163, 1996.

10. Kondo H, Osada A. Influence of dietary fiber on the bioavailability of zinc in rats. Biomed Environ Sci 9:204–208, 1996.

11. Gralak MA, Leontowicz M, Morawiec M, Bartinkowska E, Kulasek GW. Comparison of the influence of dietary fibre sources with different proportions of soluble and insoluble fibre on Ca, Mg, Fe, Zn, Mn and Cu apparent absorption in rats. Arch Anim Nutr 49:293–299, 1996.

12. Weaver CM, Heaney RP, Teegarden D, Hinders SM. Wheat bran abolishes the inverse relationship between calcium load size and absorption fraction in women. J Nutr 126:303–307, 1996.

13. Knudsen E, Sandstrom B, Solgaard P. Zinc, copper and magnesium absorption from a fibre-rich diet. J Tr El Med Biol 10:68–76, 1996.

14. Davidsson L, Mackenzie J, Kastenmeyer P, Rose A, Golden B, Aggett PJ, Hurrell RF. Dietary fiber in weaning cereals: a study of the effect on stool characteristics and absorption of energy, nitrogen, and minerals in healthy infants. J Ped Gastro Nutr 22:167–179, 1996.

15. Frolich W. Bioavailability of micronutrients in a fibre-rich diet, especially related to minerals. Eur J Clin Nutr 49:S116–S122, 1995.

16

The Influence of Wheat Fiber and Bran on Mineral Nutriture

Susan Sungsoo Cho and Celeste Clark
Kellogg Company, Battle Creek, Michigan

Mazda Jenab
University of Toronto, Toronto, Ontario, Canada

Current research in nutritional sciences is showing a growing relationship between diet and a large number of diseases. For example, as the western diet has changed from high to low dietary fiber, so has the epidemiology of diseases that afflict humans, causing an increase in a variety of diseases, particularly a large number of cancers (Bennett and Cerda, 1996). The intake of dietary fiber from cereals, fruits, and vegetables and the general composition of the diet may play a role in (a) the etiology of a number of cancers such as those of the breast, kidney, nasopharynx, oesophagus, oral cavity, ovary, pancreas, and particularly, the colon (Committee on Medical Aspects of Food Policy, 1994; Willett, 1996) and (b) a number of other diseases such as diabetes, diverticulosis, coronary heart disease, hypercholesterolemia, irritable bowel syndrome, vericose veins, and obesity (Bennett and Cerda, 1996). In fact, many public health agencies in a large number of nations have formulated dietary cancer and disease prevention strategies and made dietary recommendations to increase fruit, vegetable, and dietary fiber intake to the general public (Cannon, 1992), since dietary modulation is believed to have the greatest potential for impact in the prevention of these diseases (Ames et al., 1995). There have been concerns that increasing dietary fiber intake may have negative effects on mineral nutrition, absorption, balance, and body pool size. However, the Life Sciences Research Office and the National Research Council have both reported that reasonably increased intakes of dietary fiber have no detrimental effects in humans (Pilch, 1987; National Research Council, 1989).

Perhaps the most popular source of dietary fiber has been wheat bran, with widespread recommendations for its use for ailments such as constipation to inclusion in disease and cancer prevention strategies of many national and international health promotion agencies (Bennett and Cerda, 1996). In fact, in the first reference to fiber in the medical literature, Hippocrates wrote the following about wheat bran: ''To the human body it makes a great difference whether the bread be made of fine flour or coarse, whither of wheat; with the bran or without the bran'' (Burkitt, 1995). Wheat bran is now used extensively in breads and cereals and, despite the use and exploitation of a large number of other dietary fibers, remains a major fiber source throughout the world.

Increased intake of dietary fiber or wheat bran in the diet may also have some drawbacks, such as causing changes in the intake volume and energy density of the diet, affecting stool bulk, transit times, and colonic function in general, or its potential effects on mineral availability, which has been regarded as a possible cause for concern in the recommendations of high fiber intakes (Southgate, 1987). Vegetarians, believed to have higher dietary fiber intakes than omnivores (Hardinge et al., 1958; Anderson et al., 1981; King et al., 1981; Treuherz, 1982; Gibson et al., 1983; Davies et al., 1985; Howie and Shultz, 1985), were one of the first populations studied for the effects of fiber on mineral nutriture. In general, vegetarians have been shown to have normal calcium (Levin et al., 1986), copper (Gibson et al., 1983), iron (Anderson et al., 1981; Ganapathy and Dhanda, 1980; Levin et al., 1986), magnesium (Levin et al., 1986), manganese (Gibson et al., 1983), selenium (Gibson et al., 1983; Shultz and Leklem, 1983), and zinc (Freeland-Graves et al., 1980; Anderson et al., 1981; King et al., 1981; Treuherz, 1982; Kies et al., 1983; Levin et al., 1986; Laitinen et al., 1988) parameters. These studies draw from a wide range of vegetarians in different countries, from different age groups, and under different physiological circumstances such as pregnancy. In addition, Walker (1985), in a review of third world mineral deficiencies, concluded that there is little evidence to suggest that observed deficiencies are due to the higher dietary fiber intake of these populations. Thus, it appears that individuals on higher dietary fiber diets do not have a decreased availability of minerals or compromised mineral status.

A key feature of the normal mineral parameters measured in vegetarians is the concept of adaptation whereby individuals can adapt to decreased intakes or lower bioavailability of minerals (Kelsay, 1986). This can be observed in nonvegetarians who are not adapted to regular high dietary fiber consumption and so may respond with decreased mineral utilization when shifted to a vegetarian or high dietary fiber diet while long-term vegetarians consuming similar diets may stay within normal ranges (Freeland-Graves et al., 1981). The effect of adaptation by vegetarians can also be observed in the efficiency of mineral absorption. For example, Kies et al. (1983) reported better utilization of zinc from vegetarian diets by practicing vegetarians than by omnivores. The concept of adaptation is important in comparing and drawing conclusions from short-term versus long-term studies on mineral bioavailability. For example, Morris et al. (1988) show that feeding of wheat bran initially caused a negative apparent absorption of iron, manganese, and zinc. Their apparent absorption became positive after only 5 days, and by the end of the study overall balances were positive for calcium, copper, iron, phosphorus, magnesium, manganese, and zinc. In a smaller study, Campbell et al. (1976) showed that consumption of unleavened whole wheat bread caused initial negative balances for calcium, magnesium, phosphorus, and zinc, with all except calcium becoming positive after 50 days. Thus, in order to adequately study the effect of dietary fiber intake on mineral nutriture, it is necessary to take into consideration the time period of intake and its relevance to real life situations and modes of intake. As a result, in order to determine the mineral-binding effects of dietary fiber that is constantly and uniformly present in the diet, emphasis must be placed on longer-term studies that more adequately reflect levels of intake and other physiological parameters such as the concept of adaptation.

Many papers have been published on the both the short-term (defined as 4 weeks or less; Table 1) and long-term (greater than 4 weeks; Table 2) effects of wheat bran or wheat bran fiber. The short-term studies show very mixed results with either (a) a decrease in balance (McCance and Walsham, 1948; Cummings et al., 1979; Moak et al., 1987; O'Brien et al., 1993), retention (Knox et al., 1991), absorption (McCance and Widdowson, 1942; Björn-Rasmussen, 1974; Simpson et al., 1981; Sandberg et al., 1982; Balasubramanian et al., 1987), availability (van Dokkum et al., 1982) or physiological parameters (Jenkins et al., 1975; McWhinnie et al., 1982) of some minerals, (b) no effect at all on balance, status, or absorption of some minerals (Sandstead et al., 1978; Guthrie and Robinson, 1978; Macleod et al., 1979; Papakyrikos et al., 1979; Sandstrom et al., 1980; Sandberg et al., 1982; van Dokkum et al., 1982; Andersson et al.,

1983; Spiller et al., 1986; Morris et al., 1988; Jahnen et al., 1992), or (c) an increase in balance (Reinhold et al., 1973a; Navert et al., 1985; Moak et al., 1987; Wisker et al., 1990), absorption (Moak et al., 1987), retention (Farah et al., 1984; Fairweather-Tait, 1989), fecal loss (Spiller et al., 1986), and/or physiological parameters (Papakyrikos et al., 1979) of various minerals. These mixed results obtained under a variety of test situations, such as wheat bran supplementation or single test meal administration, using different time periods, parameters of measurement, and experimental procedures, do not allow for the drawing of any firm conclusions other than that wheat bran can either positively or negatively affect mineral nutriture.

In contrast, the longer-term studies, although still showing mixed results, tend to be skewed, with most showing no adverse effects on balance, absorption, or physiological parameters of various minerals (Walker et al., 1948; Brodribb and Humphreys, 1976; Campbell et al., 1976; Persson et al., 1976; Heaton et al., 1976; Weinreich et al., 1977; Sandstead et al., 1979; Anderson et al., 1980; Stasse-Wolthuis et al., 1980; Obizoba, 1981; Rattan et al., 1981; Zoppi et al., 1982; Sandstrom et al., 1983; Vaaler et al., 1985; Hallfrisch et al., 1987; Liu et al., 1989; Mason et al., 1990; Davidsson et al., 1996) and some showing either an increase (Morris et al., 1985; Liu et al., 1989) or a decrease in balance of some minerals (Campbell et al., 1976) or physiological parameters (Persson et al., 1976; Harland et al., 1979). As is evident, a large number of the long-term studies show that under different experimental designs, time lengths, amount, and means of wheat bran or fiber administration there are no adverse effects of increased wheat bran consumption.

Since the trend of increased dietary fiber and wheat bran in the North American diet is most likely a long-term event, studies with shorter experimental periods should be considered less relevant than the longer-term ones. The length of most balance study periods has been 2–4 weeks, and it has been observed that most mineral negative balances improve in study periods ranging from 8 to 18 weeks (Pilch, 1987). In the shorter time periods, the subjects may not have had a chance to adjust to the higher fiber intake. Some have suggested that up to a 4-week period of acclimatization should be required for any dietary fiber test diets (Schwartz et al., 1986). As discussed above, the concept of adaptation may play a significant role in the maintenance of mineral balance and status in vegetarians and those consuming higher-fiber diets. The individual may adapt to the higher dietary fiber intake by way of increased mineral absorption in the colon due to fermentation, which causes both the release of the fiber bound minerals as well as enhancing their absorption with the help of the short-chain fatty acids produced (Trinidad et al., 1993, 1996; Thompson et al., 1991). Thus, the fermentation of dietary fiber in the colon aids mineral absorption in two ways: first by releasing them from the fiber and second by enhancing their uptake with short-chain fatty acids. Thus, a possible inhibition of the small intestinal uptake of minerals by dietary fiber may not necessarily affect overall or absolute absorption or alter the body mineral pool (Frølich, 1990). This, as well as the adaptation data of Morris et al. (1988), emphasizes the importance of considering adaptation and having a sufficiently lengthy study period.

The shorter-term studies often tend to be poorly controlled and similar studies conducted by independent investigators often produce varying or conflicting results (Munoz and Harland, 1993). In addition, as is evident from Tables 1 and 2, most of the short-term studies use small numbers of subjects ranging from 4 (Cummings et al., 1979) to 66 (Sandstrom et al., 1980) with an average number of 16 subjects per study. In contrast, the long-term studies range from 2 subjects (Campbell et al., 1976) to 131 (Rattan et al., 1981), with an average number of 25 subjects per study. Since there are large intra- and interindividual variations in mineral absorption, utilization, balance, and excretion, the use of small numbers of subjects may lead to low statistical power and inaccurate results, particularly on a short timeline. Furthermore, many of the short-term studies with reasonable numbers of subjects (Sandstrom et al., 1980; Simpson

Table 1 Short-Term Clinical Studies on Effects of Whole Wheat, Bran, or Cereal on Mineral Nutriture

Mineral	Ref.	Subjects	Design, methods, background	Duration	Fiber source and amount	Results
Decrease in balance of some minerals:						
Ca	McCance and Walsham, 1948	6	Balance study; no control	11 days	Whole wheat bread, 123 g	Negative Ca balance
Ca	Cummings et al., 1979	4 m	Balance study	21 days	Wheat cereal, bread, crisp bread and bran, 31 g fiber	Adding wheat fiber led to significant negative Ca balance
Mg	Moak et al., 1987	12 m	Balance study	28 days	Wheat bran, 33.1 g TDF, or 16.6 g NDF	Mg balances slightly negative
Ca	O'Brien et al., 1993	7 m	Absorption, balance, and kinetics measured	23 days	31.3 g fiber, including 8.5 g Kellogg's All Bran/d	Reduced apparent absorption of Ca and calcium balance, although balance was on average positive during high- and low-fiber periods; during high-fiber period, subjects had sig. lower bone accretion, resorption and turnover rates, and calcium flow to bone from the exchangeable pool than in low-fiber period
Decrease in retention of some minerals:						
Ca	Knox et al., 1991	Elderly; 9 normal and 8 subjects with achlorhydria	Radioisotope, whole-body counter; controlled diet varying in fiber content and exogenous acid; own controls	Single test meals	23.7 g wheat bran	Ca retention was less for high fiber and high fiber plus acid than for low fiber

Decrease in absorption of some minerals:

Mineral	Reference	Number	Study design	Duration	Source	Results
Ca, Mg, P, K	McCance and Widdowson, 1942	4m, 4w	Balance; controlled diet, with breads of different extraction %; own controls	14–28 days	Whole wheat flour (extraction rate 92%) 40–50% of energy from flour	With whole wheat bread, Ca absorption reduced, but Mg, P, and K balance maintained
Fe	Bjorn-Rasmussen, 1974	34 m	Serum radioisotope; radioiron added to bread dough; subjects divided into groups fed bread with varying bran content, and fed white bread as own controls	10 days	Wheat rolls, 30 g/d, with bran content of 0.3–40%	Even small amounts of bran in bread inhibited iron availability in Bread, possibly due to phytates in bran
Fe	Simpson et al., 1981	60	Serum dual radioisotope measurement; test meals with bran or plain muffins; subjects acted as own controls	Single test meals	Wheat bran, 12 g	Iron absorption decreased with wheat bran
Zn	Sandberg et al., 1982	6 m, 2 w	Balance; bran supplement added to basal meal; ileostomy patients, own controls	10–14 days	Wheat bran, 16 g/day	Absorption of Zn decreased; concluded bran does not impair mineral absorption, except for Zn
Ca	Balasubramanian et al., 1987	5 w, 2m	Balance; self-selected diet plus bran; subjects served as own controls	22 days	Wheat bran 30 g/day	Decreased apparent absorption of Ca

Decrease in availability of some minerals:

Mineral	Reference	Number	Study design	Duration	Source	Results
Ca, Cu, Fe, Mg, Zn	Van Dokkum et al., 1982	12 m	Balance; subjects ate controlled diet, with varying amounts of fiber added; own controls	20 days	Wheat bran, containing 22 or 35 g NDF	Concluded bran does not affect mineral balance but may decrease mineral availability

Table 1 Continued

Decrease in some physiological parameters caused by some minerals:

No adverse effects at all on the balance, status, or absorption of various minerals:

Mineral	Ref.	Subjects	Design, methods, background	Duration	Fiber source and amount	Results
Fe	Jenkins et al., 1975	6 m	Serum; bran added to controlled diet; own controls	21 days	Wheat bran and whole wheat, containing 36 g dietary fiber	Serum Fe reduced during bran period, but Hb unchanged
Fe	McWhinnie and Mack, 1982	20	Serum Fe; 2-part randomized cross-over study; test meals consisted of ferrous sulfate and orange juice, w/ or w/o wheat bran	Single test meals	Wheat bran 7.5 g	Serum Fe levels significantly less after bran
Cu, Fe, Zn	Sandstead et al., 1978	5 m	Balance study; controlled diet; each subject had low-fiber, wheat bran, and corn bran periods	28 days	Wheat bran, 26 g/d	Absorption during wheat bran period not significantly reduced for Zn, Fe, or Cu
Zn	Guthrie et al., 1978	4 w	Balance; subjects consumed normal diet then bran supplement	28 days	Wheat bran, 14 g/day	Bran caused no overall changes on Zn metabolism
Ca	MacLeod and Blacklock, 1979	7 normal 2 calcium stone formers	Radioisotope; own controls; self-selected diet plus glucose or glucose with bran	Single test meals	Wheat bran 15 g	Ca uptake with bran similar to control, less than when glucose added without bran
Mg, Zn	Papakyrikos et al., 1979	7 w	Balance and serum; control and test diets adding varying fiber supplements	7 days	Wheat bran (10–20 g), cellulose, hemicellulose	No significant change in Mg or Zn balance

Mineral	Reference	Subjects	Design	Duration	Fiber source	Results
Zn	Sandstrom et al., 1980	35 w, 31 m	Radioisotope, whole-body, single measurement and serum measurement after test meal; randomized into 3 white bread and 9 whole wheat groups	Single test meals	Whole wheat, 60 g	Absorption lower but bioavailability (absolute amount) higher with whole wheat; concluded whole wheat has no adverse effect on Zn status
Ca, Fe, Mg, P,	Sandberg et al., 1982	6 m, 2 w	Balance; bran supplement added to basal meal; ileostomy patients, own controls	10–14 days	Wheat bran, 16 g/d supp.	Ca, Fe, Mg, and P absorption increased or unaffected by bran
Ca, Cu, Fe, Mg, Zn	Van Dokkum et al., 1982	12 m	Balance; subjects ate controlled diet, with varying amounts of fiber added; own controls	20 days	Wheat bran, containing 22 or 35 g NDF	No significant effect on balance for any mineral between wheat bran at 22 g NDF level and white bread; concluded bran does not affect mineral balance
Ca, Fe, Mg, Zn	Andersson et al., 1983	5 m, 1 w	Balance and serum concentration study; controlled diet; own controls; subjects fed breads with differing amounts of bran but similar amounts of phytate	Three 24-day periods	Whole wheat (DF 16.1, 23.7, or 31.5 g/d)	Increased fiber had no significant effect on Ca, Zn, Fe, or Mg balance; serum Ca, Mg, and Zn unchanged, while serum Fe fell slightly, but not due to bran
Cu, Fe, Mg, Zn	Spiller et al., 1986	36 w	Fecal excretion measured; controlled diet; random block design	21 days	Hard red wheat bran baked in yeast leavened bread, adding 5.7, 17.1, or 28.5 g DF/d	Bran did not increase fecal loss of Zn, Cu, Fe, or Mg

Table 1 Continued

Mineral	Ref.	Subjects	Design, methods, background	Duration	Fiber source and amount	Results
Ca, Cu, Fe, Mg, Mn, P, Zn	Morris et al., 1988	10 m	Balance; randomized crossover; controlled diet, with whole bran muffins or dephytinized bran muffins	30 days	Wheat bran, 36 g	Although balances were negative the first 5 days of whole bran period for Fe, Mn, and Zn, apparent absorption increased the last 10 days and balances overall were positive for Zn, Mg, Ca, P, Fe, Cu, and Mn; absorption greater for dephytinized than whole bran
Ca	Jahnen et al., 1992	15 w	Renal calcium excretion, in study of bran as treatment for hypercalciuria; controlled diet, with bran and calcium supplements; own controls	17 days	36 g wheat bran	Ca excretion decreased with intake of wheat bran, but not statistically significant

Positive or increase in balance of various minerals:

Ca, P, Zn	Reinhold et al., 1973a	3 m	Balance and serum; controlled diet with varying bread types and phytate sources; own controls	32 days	Iranian unleavened whole wheat bread; 350 g/d, Iranian leavened wheat bread, 150 g/d, or white bread, 350 g/d	Whole meal bread resulted in negative Ca and Zn balances; P increased in one subject and fluctuated in others; plasma Zn and serum Fe fell shortly after phytate consumption began, but later rose; whole phytate consumption continued; plasma Ca and serum P fell and remained below normal; concluded phytate inhibits absorption, and body does not fully adapt.
Zn	Navert et al., 1985	17 m, 25 w	Radioisotope, whole-body counter; test meals varied in wheat bran content and leavening	Single test meals	Wheat bran, 10, 16, or 30 g	Percentage Zn absorption reduced by increased wheat bran, although this was partially compensated by high Zn content of bran; leavening reduced phytates and increased absorption
Ca, Cu, Zn	Moak et al., 1987	12 m	Balance; basal diet, plus 1 group fed wheat bran and 1 group oat bran, in high- and low-fiber periods	28 days	Wheat bran, 33.1 or 16.6 g NDF	Cu absorption higher in high wheat bran period; Zn and Ca balances positive with wheat bran

Table 1 Continued

Mineral	Ref.	Subjects	Design, methods, background	Duration	Fiber source and amount	Results
Ca, Fe, Mg, Zn	Wisker, 1990		Balance; controlled diet, differing fiber sources added to basal diet in four 21-day studies	21 days	Whole wheat bread and rolls, adding 29 g/d DF to diet; other fiber sources	Balances of Fe and Zn increased due to tent of whole wheat; balances of Ca and Mg did not decrease
Positive or increase in retention, fecal loss, and/or physiological parameters of various minerals:						
Zn	Farah et al., 1984	23	Radioisotope, whole body monitor; randomized into 3 groups given one test meal plus oral Zn, alone or with Rice Krispies or bran	Single test meals	Wheat bran, 20 g	Retention of Zn reduced by bran; use of ionic Zn does not permit extrapolation to long-term clinical effect
Fe, Zn	Fairweather-Tait et al., 1989	11	Radioisotope fecal excretion and retention; test meals of extruded or nonextruded bran mixture; own control	Single test meals	Wheat bran, 20 g	Extrusion cooking of bran and flour mixture increased Fe retention
Ca	Spiller et al., 1986	36 w	Fecal excretion measured; controlled diet, random block design	21 days	Hard red wheat bran baked in yeast leavened bread, adding 5.7, 17.1, or 28.5 g/d DF	Bran increased fecal loss of Ca
Mg, Zn	Papakyrikos et al., 1979	7 w	Balance and serum; control and test diets adding varying fiber supplements	7 days	Wheat bran (10–20 g), cellulose, hemicellulose	Serum Mg and Zn were significantly increased with bran

et al., 1981; McWhinnie et al., 1982; Navert et al., 1985) based their data only on single test meals, which may not be relevant in the study of mineral interactions and habitual, constant dietary fiber intake and which certainly do not consider the concept of adaptation. In addition, a decrease in mineral balance may not necessarily dictate a negative balance, as was observed by O'Brien et al. (1993), who noticed that although there was a fall in calcium balance with wheat bran supplementation, it still remained positive on average and so may not have affected overall mineral nutriture at all if continued long term. Thus, it is reasonable to place more emphasis on the long-term studies listed in Table 2, since they may be more reflective of the prolonged effects of wheat dietary fiber consumption on mineral bioavailability and may have more statistical power in their conclusions due to the higher numbers of subjects involved.

The largest and longest study (6–48 months) listed in Table 2 (Rattan et al., 1981) found no evidence of mineral or nutrient deficiencies with moderate (10.8 ± 5.9 g of wheat bran as a supplement) or high (50 g/day in long-term vegetarians—much higher than that of the general population) intakes of dietary fiber. This suggests that long-term intake of wheat bran or dietary fiber in general at various levels of intake has little or no effect on human mineral nutriture. Similar results were found for serum calcium, iron, magnesium, and phosphorus at a level of intake of 25–35 g of wheat fiber per 1000 kcal for over 5 months (Anderson et al., 1980), for serum calcium levels with 18–20 g/day intake of wheat fiber for over 4.5 months (Heaton et al., 1976), as well as for serum calcium, inorganic phosphate, iron, magnesium, selenium, and zinc with an intake of 33 g/day of wheat bran fiber for over 3 months (Vaaler et al., 1985). Thus, no deleterious effects on mineral nutriture have been observed at various levels of wheat bran or wheat fiber intake over several different long-term time periods under separate experimental conditions.

In addition to the long-term studies listed in Table 2, there have been four recent long-term clinical trials dealing with the protective effects of wheat bran supplementation on colon cancer (DeCosse et al, 1989; McKeown-Eyssen et al., 1994; MacLennan et al., 1995; Alberts et al., 1996). These studies monitored a number of physiological parameters, including clinical mineral and vitamin measures, and found no detrimental effects of wheat bran supplementation ranging from 13.5 g/day (Alberts et al., 1996) to 35 g/day (McKeown-Eyssen et al., 1994) for periods from 9 months (Alberts et al., 1996) to over 4 years (DeCosse et al., 1989).

Human clinical studies are often difficult to control and, as discussed, have been plagued with problems such as short duration, varying habitual diets of the subjects, and low numbers of subjects. Such problems can be overcome and better controlled in animal studies. Table 3 shows a number of animal studies that have been performed on wheat bran and its mineral interactions. Most of the studies used rats, while some use chicks or pigs. Only three studies listed in Table 3 (Donangelo and Eggum, 1986; Fairweather-Tait and Wright, 1990; Galibois et al., 1994; Shen et al., 1998) show a decrease in the availability or absorption of various minerals. All but one of these studies (Galibois et al., 1994) were short term or involved single test meals and thus are not as reliable as the longer-term studies. The study by Galibois et al. (1994), although by definition longer term, was also only 4 weeks long and discussed only the apparent reduced absorption of iron, zinc, and magnesium with wheat bran consumption. The same study showed no adverse effects on calcium availability or absorption. However, in this study, wheat bran was always used in conjunction with oat bran and never alone, making it difficult to establish the effects of wheat bran without interaction with the oat bran fiber.

A large number of the studies listed in Table 3 (Harland et al., 1978; Ranhotra et al., 1979; Morris and Ellis, 1980; Bagheri and Gueguen, 1981; Morris et al., 1981; Thompson and Weber, 1981; Bagheri and Gueguen, 1982a, 1982b; Caprez and Fairweather-Tait, 1982; Fair-weather-Tait, 1982; Frolich and Lyso, 1983; Ballam et al., 1984; Fairweather-Tait and Wright, 1985; Rockway et al., 1987; Akhtar et al., 1987; Hallmans et al., 1989; Fairweather-Tait and

Table 2 Long-Term Clinical Studies on Whole Wheat, Bran, or Cereal on Mineral Nutriture

Mineral	Ref.	Subjects	Design, methods, background	Duration	Fiber source and amount	Results
No adverse effects at all on the balance, status, absorption or physiological parameters of various minerals:						
Ca, Fe, P, Mg	Walker et al., 1948	4 m	Balance; subjects ate usual diets, then periods of whole wheat bread supp. and white bread supp.	3–19 weeks	Whole wheat bread 1 lb/day	Ca, P, and Mg retention reduced at first with whole wheat, then improved as subjects adapted; no effect on Fe
Ca, Fe	Brodribb et al., 1976	40 diverticulosis patients	Serum concentrations measured before and after bran supplementation period	≥6 months (mean 8 months)	Wheat bran, 24 g/d	No significant change in Ca, Fe, or hemoglobin
P, Mg, Zn	Campbell et al., 1976	2	Balance; no control	59–63 days	Unleavened Iranian whole wheat bread	Balances negative in initial period for Mg, P, Zn, but all became positive after 50 days
Ca	Persson et al., 1976	18 w, 9 m (60–89 y)	Serum concentration; 2 treatment groups; self-selected diet	6 weeks	Wheat bran supplement, 10 g/d, 20 g/d	Serum Ca levels unchanged
Ca	Heaton et al., 1976	19 m	Plasma concentration; own controls	19 weeks	Whole wheat bread, 181 g/d (bread contained 102–112 g DF/kg)	Change from white to wheat bread had no significant effect on Ca concentrations
Ca	Weinreich et al., 1977	25	Serum; own controls; bran added to self-selected diet	5 weeks	Wheat bran, 24 g	No decrease in serum Ca as result of bran
Ca, Cu, Fe, Mg, Zn, P	Sandstead et al., 1979		Balance; subjects fed low-fiber control diet plus diets with various fibers and protein content; mineral requirement calculated by regression	30 days	Wheat bran, 26 g	Bran did not affect Zn, Cu, Fe, or P requirements, increased Ca requirement; concluded modest intakes of fiber do not adversely affect persons consuming Western diet

Minerals	Reference	Subjects	Study design	Duration	Fiber	Results
Ca, Fe, Mg, P, folate, carotene, B$_{12}$	Anderson et al., 1980	15 diabetics	Serum levels and intake measured; controlled diets, own controls	5–51 months (avg. 21 months)	Plant fiber (various sources, including wheat bran) 25–35 g/1000 kcal	No evidence of deficiencies of Ca, Fe, Mg, P, carotene, folate, or B$_{12}$ after high-fiber diets of as long as 51
Cu, Zn	Obizoba, 1981	3 m, 4 w	Balance study; each subject fed control and 4 test diets in Latin square design	32 days	Whole wheat 88 g/d, rice, corn	Cu absorption not affected; Zn balance positive in 3 of 4 test diets containing wheat bran, although lower than control for 3 of 4 test diets; phytate negatively affected balance
Ca, Fe, Mg, P, Zn	Rattan et al., 1981	131	Serum concentrations; self-selected diet; subjects in three groups: control group, test group supplementing regular diet with bran, and vegetarian group	6–48 months	Wheat bran, mean 10.8 ± 5.9 g	Levels of all minerals were within normal range for bran group, and for vegetarians (who ate 50 g/d of dietary fiber); concludes "a moderately and even extremely increased intake of dietary fiber for months and years does not cause detectable mineral and nutrient deficiencies"
Ca, Cu, Fe, Mg, Zn	Zoppi et al., 1982	6 infants	Serum; infants received bran supplement in addition to controlled meal	1 month	Wheat bran, 15 g/d for infants 6–12 months, 30 g/d for infants over 12 months of age	Serum concentrations were less, but not significantly so, after bran period for Ca, Mg, Cu, and Zn; Fe increased after bran
Ca, Mg	Stasse-Wolthuis et al., 1980	40 m, 22 w	Balance; controlled diet; control, and test groups fed supplements of different fibers	5 weeks	Wheat bran, 38 g/d	No deleterious effects on Ca or Mg absorption

Table 2 Continued

Mineral	Ref.	Subjects	Design, methods, background	Duration	Fiber source and amount	Results
Ca, Fe, Mg, Zn	Sandstrom et al., 1983	10 geriatric	Serum concentrations; subjects fed controlled diet plus 2 bran supplements in randomized studies	Two 6 week studies	Wheat bran, 20 or 15 g low-phytate	Bran supplements had no effect on Ca, Fe, Mg, or Zn levels
Ca, Fe, Mg, Se, Zn	Vaaler et al., 1985	28 diabetics	Serum; each patient went through 3 dietary periods of 3 months each in crossover pattern, including self-selected diet period, self-selected diet plus bran, and self-selected diet plus guar	3 months	Bran supplement, 33 g/d in wheat bread	Concentrations of Ca, Fe, Mg, Se, Zn did not differ from control period
Ca, Cu, Fe, Mg, Mn, Zn	Hallfrisch et al., 1987	20 m, 19 premenopausal w, 13 postmenopausal w	Balance; subjects ate high-fiber diet and acted as own controls	12 weeks	40 g neutral detergent fiber from wheat and other sources	After 6-week adaptation period, high-fiber diets had no adverse effects on balances of Zn, Fe, Mn, or Cu; Ca balance was more negative during self-selected than high-fiber diets; Mg balances were negative regardless of diet
Ca, Cu, Mg	Liu et al., 1989	24 diabetics	Balance	4 weeks	Wheat bran 0.4 g/kg/d	Wheat bran had no effect on Ca, Cu, and Mg balance
Fe, Zn	Mason et al., 1990	15 w	Balance, radioisotope, and serum measurements; controlled diets; low-fiber and high-fiber periods	13 weeks	Various sources, 33 g NDF/d	Increase in fiber had no significant affect on isotope Fe or Zn, on Fe or Zn balance, or on serum Fe, hemoglobin, or Zn

Mineral	Reference	N	Design	Duration	Treatment	Results
Ca, Fe, Zn	Davidsson et al., 1996	57 infants	Infants received wheat in addition to formula; Ca and Zn determined by stable isotopes; Fe determined by incorporation into erythrocytes	4 weeks	Wheat or soy mixtures in addition to regular formula; up to 8.0% dietary fiber.	No significant effect of absorption of nutrients with this level of dietary fiber intake in primarily formula fed well-nourished infants

Increase in balance of various minerals:

Mineral	Reference	N	Design	Duration	Treatment	Results
Ca	Morris and Ellis, 1985	Ex. 1: 10 m, Ex. 2: 12 m	Balance; own controls; controlled diet. Ex. 1: whole wheat muffin period and dephytinized period. Ex. 2: different levels of phytate added to dephytinized bran	30 days	Ex. 1: Wheat bran, 36 g. Ex. 2: 8.65 g of insoluble fraction dephytinized bran	Ca balance positive with 36 g bran; no difference in Ca absorption in Ex. 1 between whole and dephytinized bran; in Ex. 2, Ca absorption less with increased phytate
Zn	Liu et al., 1989	24 diabetics	Balance	4 weeks	Wheat bran 0.4 g/kg/d	Wheat bran increased the intestinal absorption and positive balance of Zn

Decrease in balance or physiological parameters of various minerals:

Mineral	Reference	N	Design	Duration	Treatment	Results
Ca, P, Mg, Zn	Campbell et al., 1976	2	Balance; no control	59–63 days	Unleavened Iranian whole wheat bread	Balances negative in initial period for Mg, P, Zn, but all became positive after 50 days; Ca balance negative in initial period, improved in later period but remained negative
Ca, Fe	Persson et al., 1976	18 w, 9 m (60–89 y)	Serum concentration; 2 treatment groups; self-selected diet	6 weeks	Wheat bran supplement, 10 g/d, 20 g/d	Serum Fe and ionized Ca dropped
Zn	Harland et al., 1979	28	Serum; own controls; self-selected diets, measured by 3-day records; 1 group added wheat flake and 1 group added bran products	15 weeks	Wheat bran (2.17 g crude fiber) and wheat flake (0.23 g crude fiber) products	Serum Zn fell in wheat flake and wheat bran groups; both phytate and fiber may be inhibiting factors

Table 3 Animal Studies on Effects of Wheat Bran or Cereal on Mineral Nutriture

Mineral	Ref.	Subjects	Design, methods, background	Duration	Fiber source and amount	Results
Decrease in availability or absorption of various minerals:						
Ca, Zn	Donangelo and Eggum, 1986	Rats: 50 5-week-old and 50 10-week old Wistar rats	Balance, serum and femur levels measured; controlled diet; 4 control and 16 treatment groups fed different levels of wheat bran and barley husk	9 days	Wheat bran 42 g dietary fiber/kg; 52 g DF/kg; 61 g DF/kg; 79 g DF/kg; 116 g DF/kg	Wheat bran decreased absorption of Zn when bran contributed 40 g DF/kg or more, and decreased Ca only when bran contributed 80 g DF/kg; Ca levels in femurs were not significantly reduced by increasing wheat bran; Zn levels were significantly reduced
Zn	Fairweather-Tait et al. 1990	Rats: 140 Wistar	Radioisotope whole body counter; test meals; 2 control and 5 treatment groups	Single test meals	Wheat bran, 1.9 g added to 3 g semi-synthetic diet	Wheat bran reduced Zn absorption by 9%
Fe, Mg, Zn	Galibois et al., 1994	Rats: 50 male Sprague-Dawley	Balance; controlled diet; rats in 1 control group and 4 experimental groups, fed diets containing different fiber sources and amounts	4 weeks	1. (Control) 5 g/100 g cellulose 2. 5 g/100 g cellulose and pectin 3. 10 g/100 g cellulose and pectin 4. 5 g/100 g wheat bran and oat bran 5. 10 g/100 g wheat bran and oat bran	Absorption of Fe, Zn, and Mg less from wheat bran
Ca	Shen et al., 1998	Rats: 16 male Sprague-Dawley	^{45}Ca injection, absorption determined by femur uptake	Single test meals	Wheat bran extruded cereal diet versus AIN76A diet	Ca absorption decreased by wheat bran.

No adverse effects at all of fiber on the balance, status, retention, or absorption of various minerals or growth of animals:

Mineral	Reference	Animal	Experimental design	Duration	Fiber source	Results/Comments
Zn	Harland et al., 1978	Rats: 48	Kidney and femur concentrations, body weight; controlled diet; 1 control (no fiber) and 5 test groups with varying fiber sources; Zn added		Wheat bran, 10% of diet	With feeding of additional Zn, to attain phytate: Zn molar ratio of 6, femur and kidney Zn levels not significantly different in bran group than control group
Fe	Ranhotra et al., 1979	Rats: 112	Hb depletion-repletion technique controlled diet; control group, and 9 test groups fed breads with differing grains	3 weeks	Wheat bran and whole wheat flour	Bioavailability from bran and whole wheat less than inorganic Fe but similar to white bread; interference with availability unrelated to fiber or phytate content
Fe, Zn	Morris and Ellis, 1980	Rats	Fe bioavailability measured by hemoglobin regeneration technique; Zn bioavailability measured by femur concentration and growth response; controlled diet	3–4 weeks for Zn	Wheat bran, 71–142 g/kg in Zn study	No evidence that fiber from bran reduces bioavailability of Zn; wheat bran with phytate/zinc molar ratios of 8 or less equivalent to zinc sulfate as dietary source
Ca, Mg, P, Zn	Bagheri and Gueguen, 1981	Rats: 20	Balance; controlled diet; control and 3 test groups fed different levels of bran	41 days	Wheat bran 0.5%, 10%, or 15% of diet	Bran had no significant effect on retention of Ca, Mg, or Zn; increased bran increased retention of P

Table 3 Continued

Mineral	Ref.	Subjects	Design, methods, back-ground	Duration	Fiber source and amount	Results
Zn	Morris and Ellis, 1981	Rats: 220	Growth response; controlled diet, plus different breakfast cereals	4 weeks	Breakfast cereals with bran, whole wheat, other grains (up to 27.6% wheat fiber)	Wheat bran with phytate-Zn molar ratios below 15 support rat growth, but wheat bran with ratios above 15 depress growth; response not directly correlated with fiber; molar ratio is major factor affecting Zn bioavailability
Cu, Fe, Mg, Mn, Zn	Thompson and Weber, 1981	Chicks: 18	Liver and tibia levels; randomized into basal and 8 test diet groups, differing in fiber added	4 weeks	Wheat bran, 12% of diet	Bran did not reduce chick growth or mineral levels
Ca, Zn	Bagheri and Gueguen, 1982a	Rats: 20	Balance, radioisotope measurement; controlled diet; control group and 3 exp. groups, which were fed diets with differing wheat bran content	47 days	Wheat bran, 0.0, 5.0, 10.0, or 15.0% of diet	Addition of up to 15% wheat bran caused no significant change in Ca or Zn absorption
Ca, Mg, P, Zn	Bagheri and Gueguen, 1982b	Rats: 20	Balance; controlled diet; control and 3 test groups fed bran at different levels, with mineral levels kept constant	6 weeks	Wheat bran, 0.0, 5.0, 10.0, or 15.0% of diet	Ca absorption unaffected by bran level; Mg, P, and Zn absorption reduced by higher bran level, but balance still positive

Mineral	Reference	Animal	Methods	Wheat bran	Duration	Results
Fe, Zn	Caprez and Fairweather-Tait, 1982	Rats	Isotope dilution technique and balance; rats divided into groups receiving semisynthetic diets with different treated brans	Wheat bran, 100–180 g/kg	9 days	Reduction in bran particle size slightly increased Zn, but not Fe, retention; diphytinization signifcantly increased Zn retention but had no effect on Fe retention
Fe	Fairweather-Tait, 1982	Rats: 80 Wistar	Balance and radioisotope studies; controlled diet; rats randomized into control group and 3 groups fed bread with differing bran content but constant phytate	Wheat bran, 60.6–221.2 g DF/kg	14 days balance; single test meal radioisotope	Showed only small difference in absorption among the groups; radioisotope study clearly demonstrated no difference in Fe absorption; concluded that addition of wheat bran to breads has no effect on absorption of Fe
Fe	Frølich and Lyso, 1983	Pigs	Serum iron and Hb measured; anemic pigs divided into 4 groups, fed test diet that varied in bran content and Fe source	Wheat bran, 0.0, 7.0, or 20.0%	6 weeks	Wheat bran up to 20% did not inhibit Fe absorption, even when diet included 20% bran; bioavailability of Fe from bran same as from ferrous sulfate
Ca, Cu, Mg, P, Zn	Ballam et al., 1984	Rats	Serum, liver, and tibia concentrations; controlled diet; rats fed basal diet plus differing fiber sources	Wheat bran (10% of diet)	9 days	Concentrations of Ca, Cu, Mg, P, Zn unaffected by wheat bran

Table 3 Continued

Mineral	Ref.	Subjects	Design, methods, back-ground	Duration	Fiber source and amount	Results
Ca, Fe, Zn	Fairweather-Tait and Wright, 1985	Rats	Radioisotope, whole body counter; rats randomly allocated to 6 groups, given high- or low-fiber test diets, with added Ca, Zn, or Fe; also mineral status measured in blood and organs	7 days 28 days	400 g/kg, including: 72.7 g Kellogg's Bran-flakes, 72.7 g Pre-wett's bran, and 72.7 g Kellogg's All-Bran, in 3 g test meal	Absorption of both Ca and Fe were higher in high-fiber than in low-fiber diet, but no difference in Zn; no significant difference in status between high-fiber and low-fiber groups for plasma Ca, bone Ca, liver Zn, bone Zn, or liver Fe, but liver Fe was lower in high-fiber group; concluded high-fiber diet had no major adverse effect on Fe, Zn, or Ca metabolism in rats
Cu	Rockway et al., 1987	Rats: 50 Mice: 50	Heart and hepatic concentrations; controlled diet, rats and mice divided into 5 groups each with varying fiber and Cu sources	4–5 weeks	Wheat bran, 3% of diet	Cu bound to bran utilized sufficiently to supply Cu requirement
Fe	Akhtar et al., 1987	Rats: 21	Balance; rats fed controlled diet and randomized into control and 6 test groups fed Fe fortified and unfortified white bread, whole wheat bread, or bran	10 days	Whole wheat, 30.64 g/500 g; wheat bran 31.66 g/500 g	No significant difference among bran, whole wheat bread, or white bread, in relative or absolute Fe absorption

	Reference	Subjects	Method	Duration	Diet	Results
Zn	Hallmans et al., 1989	Rats: 36 Sprague-Dawley	Radioisotope retention and absorption; serum, liver, and femur concentrations; after Zn depletion, purified diet, plus different wheat flours, some with added Zn, fed to 6 groups of rats; randomized, own controls	18 days	Whole wheat and wheat bran (DF ranging from 4.8–7.5%)	Retention and absorption of Zn slightly but significantly reduced with bran, but Zn concentrations in serum, blood, liver, and femur not affected; all the supplemented Zn was absorbed, including in the whole wheat and bran-enriched groups; rats ate more of the bran-enriched diet; concluded that factors such as fiber or phytate in wheat bran have little effect on Zn absorption when all Zn is needed for growth and development
Fe	Fairweather-Tait and Wright, 1990	Rats: 140 Wistar	Radioisotope whole body counter; test meals; 2 control and 5 treatment groups	Single test meals	Wheat bran 1.9 g added to 3 g semi-synthetic diet	Wheat bran had no effect on Fe absorption
Ca, Mg, P	Shah et al., 1990	Rats: 140	Balance; rats in 7 groups fed controlled diet plus fiber varying in source and amount	24 weeks	Wheat bran 14% of diet, by weight	Absorption of Ca, Mg, P not significantly affected by wheat bran

Table 3 Continued

Increase in availability or absorption of various minerals:

Mineral	Ref.	Subjects	Design, methods, background	Duration	Fiber source and amount	Results
Fe	Chao and Gordon, 1983	Rats: 91 Long-Evans	Hb regeneration technique measuring relative biological value of iron; rats in 2 control and 11 experimental groups; basal diet, plus varying added fiber and Fe sources	14 days	Wheat bran 21%	Bioavailability of iron in wheat bran significantly greater than in other sources, including $FeSO_4$
Fe	Gordon and Chao, 1984	Rats: 91 Long-Evans	Hb regeneration technique used to measure relative biological value of iron; control and 13 treatment groups; basal diet, plus varying added fiber and Fe sources	14 days	Wheat bran 21%	Bioavailability of iron significantly higher in wheat bran than in spinach
Fe	Zhang et al., 1985	Rats: 59	Hemoglobin regeneration; randomized into control and 5 test groups with different Fe sources	10 days	Wheat bran cereal, 370 g/kg	Bioavailability of Fe better from bran than from $FeSO_4$; concludes bran and other plant foods are excellent sources of dietary iron
Zn	Seal and Mathers, 1989	Rats	Zinc transfer and accumulation were measured by everted-gut-sac technique; rats randomly allocated to control and three treatment groups which differed in fiber content	3 weeks	Wheat bran 200 g/kg Pectin 200 g/kg	Zn transfer with wheat bran slightly higher than with no-fiber diet, less than with pectin diet; concluded that the colon has considerable capacity to absorb zinc

Wright, 1990; Shah et al., 1990) show no adverse effects of wheat bran fiber on the balance, status, retention, or absorption of the various minerals or the growth of the animals. A majority of these studies were longer term, allowing more time for adaptation to the diet and equilibration of body mineral pools and thus mineral balances. In contrast to some of the above-listed studies, some animal studies listed in Table 3 have shown an increase in the availability and absorption of various minerals (Chao and Gordon, 1983; Gordon and Chao, 1984; Zhang et al., 1985; Seal et al., 1989). Surprisingly, all of these studies have been, by definition, shorter term. This is very indicative of the variability and lack of conformity of studies in this subject area, suggesting a need for better, bigger, and longer well-controlled experiments before any definitive conclusions can be drawn.

A number of the studies listed in Tables 1 to 3 used a balance technique to determine mineral availability. The use of balance studies as a means of estimating mineral requirements and availability has been often criticized (Mertz, 1987). Balance studies are based on the theory that the intake of a nutrient less than the sum of the daily losses will result in a deficiency (Mertz, 1987). But observation suggests that despite common negative balance intakes, such deficiencies are very rare in developed countries (Mertz, 1987). In addition, it has been shown that the amount of available nutrient in the diet determines the pool size of that nutrient in the body but may not necessarily indicate a deficiency state. At best, balance studies may be able to indicate changes in existing body mineral pool size with variations in levels of mineral intake until new equilibriums are reached. Depending on the mineral, this may take from months to years, suggesting that long-term balance studies are more effective. As a result, the bioavailability of minerals could be equated with their absorption from the gastrointestinal tract (as is the case in most of the studies listed here), or, in more complex but perhaps better terms, the bioavailability could be determined by changes in the biological function of each mineral in its various body compartments and pools, an option rarely exercised due to the lack of knowledge about the different functions of each mineral. Thus, even if wheat bran is shown to decrease mineral balance in certain studies, there is no credible evidence showing that its intake at any level will produce a state of mineral deficiency. In fact, wheat bran itself is a rich source of a large number of minerals (Morris et al., 1988; Frolich, 1990). So, its increased intake may also increase their ingestion such that a decrease in the percent uptake does not necessarily decrease the total absolute absorption or alter the mineral pool size in the body. Many studies, both human and animal, fail to take into consideration the increased mineral contribution of wheat bran and the roles these minerals play and interactions they may have with other minerals in the test diets, e.g., radiolabeled minerals used in some of the studies. These points need to be addressed effectively in future studies on wheat bran and its mineral interactions.

The biological availability of minerals may be affected by a large variety of general factors such as the chemical form of the mineral in the diet, its valence state, whether it is bound as an inorganic salt or in covalent or noncovalent organometallic complexes, or its interactions with proteins, fats, carbohydrates (including fibers), or charged substances within the lumen (Burk and Solomons, 1985). Wheat bran may be able to affect the intestinal bioavailability of various minerals by either directly binding the mineral or by a dilution effect whereby the concentration and thus absorption of the mineral is lessened due to the increased bulk produced by the bran. Aside from physically being able to bind minerals, wheat bran may also alter other factors that affect mineral bioavailability. For example, the degree of gastric pH buffering by the wheat bran starch may affect the absorption of a pH-sensitive mineral such iron or copper (Burk and Solomons, 1985).

A major complicating issue is components of wheat bran that may be responsible for some of the observed decreases in mineral availability. Compounds such as oxalate, phytic acid (myoinositol-hexaphosphate; phytate), ascorbic acid, and other isolated fiber components could all affect mineral absorption to varying degrees (Burk and Solomons, 1985). Most of the research in this area, however, has focused on the role of phytic acid. Although in vitro studies show that purified fiber components can bind and absorb minerals at pH values found in the small intestine, most of the in vitro studies using cell wall preparations (Reilly et al, 1979; Reddy et al, 1982) are confounded by the presence of phytic acid, which is present at levels as high as 6.4% in wheat bran (Graf, 1983). It consists of a myoinositol ring with six phosphate moieties attached (Graf and Eaton, 1993). In the seed, phytic acid serves as the chief storage form of phosphorus (Graf et al., 1987) and so can bind or chelate divalent minerals (well as starches and proteins), thus altering their solubility and absorption (Rickard and Thompson, 1997). In fact, it is generally thought that the effects of phytate on mineral absorption and balance may be greater than that of fiber, particularly with respect to zinc, for which phytic acid has a very high affinity (Oberleas and Harland, 1977; Davies, 1978) and with which it forms a very stable and insoluble complex (Evans et al., 1988). A number of studies in both animals (Davies and Olpin, 1979; Morris and Ellis, 1980; Lo et al., 1981) and humans (Reinhold et al., 1973; Morris and Ellis, 1989; Turnlund et al., 1984) indicate that phytic acid plays a strong role in inhibiting zinc utilization and growth, particularly at a [PA]/[Zn] molar ratio >15 (Morris and Ellis, 1981), although later studies (Fordyce et al., 1987) have determined that a [PA][Ca]/[Zn] molar ratio >3.5 mol/kg of body weight in rats is a better indicator of compromised zinc status. Increased phytic acid intake may not necessarily lead to decreased absorption of all minerals. For example, by binding zinc, phytic acid may in fact increase the absorption of copper, which competes with zinc at the site of intestinal absorption (Lee et al., 1988). Other factors may also affect the degree of phytic acid mineral binding and decrease mineral bioavailability. For example, the presence of dietary, endogenous, or bacterial phytase may act to hydrolyze phytic acid in the gastrointestinal tract, thereby potentially releasing any bound minerals. Wheat bran contains a large amount of endogenous phytases. In fact, they are used in some of the dephytinization processes for wheat bran (Morris and Ellis, 1980). Thus, it can be hypothesized that if not destroyed by processing or cooking, these phytases could act to hydrolyze phytic acid in the gastrointestinal tract. Also, the presence or lack of absorption enhancers such as ascorbic acid, vitamin D_3, and meat protein may also play a role in affecting mineral bioavailability and absorption particularly in situations of combined high phytic acid and marginal mineral intakes (Rickard and Thompson, 1997). Although phytic acid can by itself affect mineral availability, its role within its natural matrix in the dietary fiber and whether the fiber itself has any inhibitory role is still under debate.

A study by Cook et al. (1983) showed that fiber is not the major determinant of iron availability, suggesting that phytic acid may be responsible for any observed effects. Furthermore, Hall et al. (1989) have shown that percentage reductions of area under plasma zinc time curve (measuring difference between zinc test alone and zinc administered with fiber) were lower with wheat bran, compared to reduced phytate bran and Rice Krispies, concluding that phytate is the main inhibitor of zinc absorption. Similar conclusions on zinc absorption have been drawn by Davies et al. (1977). Studies trying to differentiate the role of fiber from that of phytate have shown that when the amount of phytate is maintained while the level of wheat bran is altered, there is no significant effect on Ca, Zn, Fe, or Mg balance (Andersson et al., 1983) suggesting that the fiber plays little role in the alteration of mineral bioavailability. Similar results have been obtained by Fairweather-Tait (1982) for iron. On the other hand, Morris et al. (1988) have shown no significant difference between whole or dephytinized wheat bran on mineral bioavailability, suggesting that phytate does not play a role. Even other studies have shown that observed interferences with mineral bioavailability are unrelated to either wheat bran fiber or phytate (Ranhotra, 1979). In addition, some early studies show that just as with longer-term intake of dietary fiber and wheat bran, longer-term intake of high–phytic acid diets can lead to adaptation where initial negative balances become positive after several weeks (Walker et al., 1948), suggesting that even if phytic acid had any detrimental effects on mineral nutriture, they would disappear over time and not affect long-term mineral balance and bioavailability. Thus, it is currently not possible to suggest that phytic acid is the wheat bran component fully responsible for any negative mineral bioavailability effects sometimes observed with wheat bran intake.

Although phytate may be a possible antinutrient, it may also serve a very important role as an anticancer phytochemical. In rats, pure phytic acid dissolved in the drinking water has been shown to significantly decrease the number of colon tumors and tumor volume before (Shamsuddin et al., 1988; Ullah and Shamsuddin, 1990; Pretlow et al., 1992) and after carcinogen injection (Shamsuddin and Ullah, 1989). Pure phytic acid added to the diet as well as phytic acid in its natural matrix in the wheat bran, dephytinized wheat bran, and pure phytic acid added to dephytinized wheat bran have been shown to significantly decrease various early biomarkers of colon cancer risk (Jenab and Thompson, 1998), suggesting that both the wheat bran fiber and its phytic acid may play important antipreneoplastic roles. Phytic acid has also been shown to be protective against mammary carcinogenesis both in vitro (Shamsuddin, 1995) and in vivo (Hirose et al., 1994; Vucenik et al., 1995) and in reducing early biomarkers of risk such as cell proliferation (Thompson and Zhang, 1991). Furthermore, Vucenik et al. (1997) have shown that pure phytate may be even more effective in reducing mammary tumorigenesis than wheat bran diets containing equivalent amounts of phytate. In addition to colon and mammary tissues, phytic acid has reduced the growth and promoted the differentiation of erythroleukemia (Shamsuddin et al., 1992) and prostate cancer (Shamsuddin and Yang, 1995) cell lines. Thus, it is important to consider that although phytic acid may somewhat decrease mineral availability in the short term, it may have potentially strong cancer-protective effects, making it an important part of a long-term, high-fiber dietary regimen.

Although in theory wheat bran is capable of decreasing mineral bioavailability, there is little firm evidence to support this. Even if long-term constant intake of wheat bran is shown to strongly decrease mineral bioavailability, there is little potential for development of mineral deficiency in the face of appropriate mineral intake from other sources as well as adaptation over time to maintain body mineral pools. The majority of human and animal studies show that wheat bran intake at normal levels do not compromise mineral status or cause decreased mineral bioavailability or deficiency. This is particularly true in longer-term studies, which are likely more representative of real life wheat bran intake levels and patterns. It is still unclear exactly which component of wheat bran, whether fiber or phytate or their combination, affects mineral bioavailability in either human or animal models. More carefully designed, controlled, performed, and analyzed studies are required to be able to effectively judge the mineral interactions of wheat bran fiber and phytic acid.

REFERENCES

Akhtar D, Begum N, Sattar A. Effect of dietary phytate on bioavailability of iron. Nutr Res 7:833–842, 1987.

Alberts DS, Ritenbaugh C, Story JA, Aickin M, Rees-McGee S, Buller MK, Atwood J, Phelps J, Ramanujam PS, Bellapravalu S, Patel J, Bettinger L, Clark L. Randomized, double-blinded, placebo-controlled study of effect of wheat bran fiber and calcium on fecal bile acids in patients with resected adenomatous colon polyps. J Natl Cancer Inst 88:81–92, 1996.

Ames BN, Gold LS, Willett WC. The causes and prevention of cancer. Proc Natl Acad Sci 92:5258–5265, 1995.

Anderson BM, Gibson RS, Sabry JH. The iron and zinc status of long-term vegetarian women. Am J Clin Nutr 34:1042–1048, 1981.

Anderson JW, Ferguson SK, Karounos D, O'Malley L, Sieling B, Chen WL. Mineral and vitamin status on high-fiber diets: long term studies of diabetic patients. Diabetes Care 3:38–40, 1980.

Andersson H, Navert B, Bingham SA, Englyst HN, Cummings JH. The effects of breads containing similar amounts of phytate but different amounts of wheat bran on calcium, zinc and iron balance in man. Br J Nutr 50:503–510, 1983.

Bagheri SM, Gueguen L. Influence of wheat bran diets containing unequal amounts of calcium, magnesium, phosphorus and zinc upon the absorption of these minerals in rats. Nutr Rep Int 24:47–56, 1981.

Bagheri SM, Gueguen L. Effects of wheat bran on the metabolism of calcium-45 and zinc-65 in rats. J Nutr 112:2047–2051, 1982a.

Bagheri SM, Gueguen L. Bioavailability to rats of calcium, magnesium, phosphorus and zinc in wheat bran diets containing equal amounts of these minerals. Nutr Rep Int 25:583–589, 1982b.

Balasubramanian R, Johnson EJ, Marlett JA. Effect of wheat bran on bowel function and fecal calcium in older adults. J Am College Nutr 6:199–208, 1987.

Ballam GC, Nelson TS, Kirby LK. The effect of phytate and fiber source on phytate hydrolysis and mineral availability in rats. Nutr Rep Int 30:1089, 1984.

Bennett WG, Cerda JJ. Benefits of dietary fiber: myth or medicine? Postgrad Med 99:153–156, 166–168, 171–172, 1996.

Björn-Rasmussen E. Iron absorption from wheat bread. Influence of various amounts of bran. Nutr Metab 16:101–110, 1974.

Brodribb AJM, Humphreys DM. Diverticular disease: three studies. Br Med J 1:424–430, 1976.

Burk RF, Solomons NW. Trace elements and vitamins and bioavailability as related to wheat and wheat foods. Am J Clin Nutr 41:1091–1102, 1985.

Burkitt D. Historical aspects. In: Kritchevsky D, Bonfield C. Dietary Fiber in Health and Disease. St. Paul, MN: Eagan Press, 1995, pp 459–465.

Campbell BJ, Reinhold JG, Cannell JJ, Nourmand I. The effects of prolonged consumption of wholemeal bread upon metabolism of calcium, magnesium, zinc and phosphorus of two young American adults. Pahlavi Med J 7:1–17, 1976.

Cannon G. Food and Health: The Experts Agree. London: Consumers Association Publishers, 1992.

Caprez A, Fairweather-Tait SJ. The effect of heat treatment and particle size of bran on mineral absorption in rats. Br J Nutr 48:467–475, 1982.

Chao LS, Gordon DT. Influence of fish on the bioavailability of plant iron in the anemic rat. J Nutr 113: 1643–1652, 1983.

Committee on Medical Aspects of Food Policy Panel of the World Cancer Research Fund. Diet and Cancers. London: World Cancer Research Fund, 1994.

Cook JD, Noble NL, Morck TA, Lynch SR, Petersburg SJ. Effect of fiber on nonheme iron absorption. Gastroenterology 85:1354–1358, 1983.

Cummings JH, Hill MJ, Jivraj T, Houston H, Branch WJ, Jenkins DJA. The effect of meat protein and dietary fiber on colonic function and metabolism. Am J Clin Nutr 32:2086–2093, 1979.

Davidsson L, Mackenzie J, Kastenmayer P, Rose A, Golden BE, Aggett PJ, Hurrell RF. Dietary fiber in weaning cereals: a study of the effect on stool characteristics and absorption of energy, nitrogen and minerals in healthy infants. J Ped Gastro Nut 22:167–179, 1996.

Davies NT. The effects of dietary fiber on mineral availability. In: Heaton KW, ed. Dietary Fiber, Current Developments of Importance to Health. London: Newman Publishing, 1978, pp 113–121.

Davies NT, Olpin SE. Studies on the phytate:zinc molar contents in diets as a determinant of Zn availability to young rats. Br J Nutr 41:590–603, 1979.

Davies NT, Hristic V, Flett AA. Phytate rather than fibre in bran as the major determinant of zinc availability to rats. Nutr Rep Inc 15:207–214, 1977.

Davies GJ, Crowder M, Dickerson JWT. Dietary fiber intakes of individuals with different eating patterns. Nutr Appl Nutr 39A:139–148, 1985.

DeCosse JJ, Miller HH, Lesser ML. Effect of wheat fiber and vitamins C and E on rectal polyps in patients with familial adenomatous polyposis. J Natl Cancer Inst 81:1290–1297, 1989.

Donangelo CM, Eggum BO. Comparative effects of wheat bran and barley husk on nutrient utilization in rats. 2. Zinc, calcium and phosphorus. Br J Nutr 56:269–280, 1986.

Evans WJ, Martin CJ. Heat of complex formation of Al(III) and Cd(II) with phytic acid. J Inorg Biochem 34:11–18, 1988.

Fairweather-Tait SJ. The effect of different levels of wheat bran on iron absorption in rats from bread containing similar amounts of phytate. Br J Nutr 47:243–249, 1982.

Fairweather-Tait SJ, Wright AJA. The effect of 'fibre-filler' (F-plan diet) on iron, zinc and calcium absorption in rats. Br J Nutr 54:585–592, 1985.

Fairweather-Tait SJ, Wright AJA. The effects of sugar-beet fibre and wheat bran on iron and zinc absorption in rats. Br J Nutr 64:547–552, 1990.

Fairweather-Tait SJ, Portwood DE, Symss LL, Eagles J, Minski MJ. Iron and zinc absorption in human subjects from a mixed meal of extruded and nonextruded wheat bran and flour. Am J Clin Nutr 49: 151–155, 1989.

Farah DA, Hall MJ, Mills PR, Russell RI. Effect of wheat bran on zinc absorption. Hum Nutr Clin Nutr 38:433–441, 1984.

Freeland-Graves JH, Bodzy PW, Eppright MA. Zinc status of vegetarians. J Am Diet Assoc 77:655–661, 1980.

Fordyce EJ, Forbes RM, Robbins KR, Erdman JWJ. Phytate calcium/zinc molar ratios: are they predictive of zinc bioavailability? J Food Sci 52:440–444, 1987.

Frølich W. Chelating properties of dietary fiber and phytate. The role for mineral availability. Adv Exp Med Biol 270:83–93, 1990.

Frølich W, Lysø A. Bioavailability of iron from wheat bran in pigs. Am J Clin Nutr 37:31–36, 1983.

Galibois, I, Desrosiers T, Guévin N, Lavigne C, Jacques H. Effects of dietary fibre mixtures on glucose and lipid metabolism and on mineral absorption in the rat. Ann Nutr Metab 38:203–211, 1994.

Ganapathy S, Dhanda R. Protein and iron nutrition in lacto-ovo-vegetarian Indo-Aryan United States residents. Indian J Nutr Diet 17:45–52, 1980.

Gibson RS, Anderson BM, Sabry JH. The trace metal status of a group of postmenopausal vegetarians. J Am Diet Assoc 82:246–250, 1983.

Gordon DT, Chao LS. Relationship of components in wheat bran and spinach to iron bioavailability in the anemic rat. J Nutr 114:526–535, 1984.

Graf E. Applications of phytic acid. J Am Oil Chem Soc 60:1861–1867, 1983.

Graf E, Eaton JW. Suppression of colonic cancer by dietary phytic acid. Nutr Cancer 19:11–19, 1993.

Graf E, Empson KL, Eaton JW. Phytic acid: a natural antioxidant. J Biol Chem 262:11647–11650, 1987.

Guthrie BE, Robinson MF. Zinc balance studies during wheat bran supplementation (abstr) Fed Proc 37: 254, 1978.

Hall MJ, Downs L, Ene MD, Farah D. Effect of reduced phytate wheat bran on zinc absorption. Eur J Clin Nutr 43:431–440, 1989.

Hallfrisch J, Powell A, Carafelli C, Reiser S, Prather ES. Mineral balances of men and women consuming high fiber diets with complex or simple carbohydrate. J Nutr 117:48–55, 1987.

Hallmans G, Sjöström R, Wetter L, Wing KR. The availability of zinc in endosperm, whole grain and bran-enriched wheat crispbreads fed to rats on a Zn-deficient diet. Br J Nutr 62:165–175, 1989.

Hardinge MG, Chambers AC, Crooks H, Stare FJ. Nutritional studies of vegetarians III. Dietary levels of fiber. Am J Clin Nutr 6:523–525, 1958.

Harland BF, O'Dell RG, Stone CL, Prosky L. Metabolic effects of altered fiber, phytate and increased zinc in wheat bran fractions fed to rats (abstr). Fed Proc 37:756, 1978.

Harland BF, Stringfellow DE, Connor DH, Foster WD, Heggie CM. Lowered plasma zinc in humans ingesting wheat bran products (abstr). Fed Proc Fed Am Soc Exp Biol 38:548, 1979.

Heaton KW, Manning AP, Hartog M. Lack of effect on blood lipid and calcium concentrations of young men on changing from white to wholemeal bread. Br J Nutr 35:55–60, 1976.

Hirose M, Hoshiya T, Akagi K, Futakuchi M, Ito N. Inhibition of mammary gland carcinogenesis by green tea catechins and other naturally occuring antioxidants in female Sprague-Dawley rats pretreated with 7, 12-dimethylbenz[alpha]anthracene. Cancer Lett 83:149–156, 1994.

Howie BJ, Shultz TD. Dietary and hormonal inter-relationships among vegetarian Seventh-Day Adventists and non-vegetarian men. Am J Clin Nutr 42:127–154, 1985.

Jahnen A, Heynck H, Gertz B, Claussen A, Hesse A. Dietary fibre: the effectiveness of a high bran intake in reducing renal calcium excretion. Urol Res 20:3–6, 1992.

Jenab M, Thompson LU. The influence of phytic acid in wheat bran on early biomarkers of colon carcinogenesis. Carcinogenesis 19:1087–1092, 1998.

Jenkins DJA, Hill MS, Cummings JH. Effect of wheat fiber on blood lipids, fecal steroid excretion and serum iron. Am J Clin Nutr 28:1408–1411, 1975.

Kelsay JL. Update on fiber and mineral availability. In: Vahouny GV, Kritchevsky D, eds. Dietary Fiber: Basic and Clinical Aspects. New York: Plenum Press, 1986, pp 361–372.

Kies C, Young E, McEndree L. Zinc bioavailability from vegetarian diets: influence of dietary fiber, ascorbic acid and past dietary practices. In: Inglett GE, ed. Nutritional Bioavailability of Zinc. Washington DC: American Chemical Society, 1983, pp 115–126.

King JC, Stein T, Doyle M. Effect of vegetarianism on the zinc status of pregnant women. Am J Clin Nutr 34:1049–1055, 1981.

Knox TA, Kassarjian Z, Dawson-Hughes B, Golner B, Dallal GE, Arora S, Russell RM. Calcium absorption in elderly subjects on high- and low-fiber diets: effect of gastric acidity. Am J Clin Nutr 53: 1480–1486, 1991.

Laitinen R, Räsänen L, Vuori E. Serum zinc and copper in relation to diet in 3- to 18-year old Finnish girls and boys. Eur J Clin Nutr 42:911–918, 1988.

Lee DY, Schroeder JD, Gordon DT. Enhancement of copper bioavailability in the rat by phytic acid. J Nutr 118:712–717, 1988.

Levin N, Rattan J, Gilat T. Mineral intake and blood levels in vegetarians. Isr J Med Sci 22:105–108, 1986.

Liu ZQ, Chao CS, Wu HW. Investigation of the effect of a diet with wheat bran on the metabolic balances of Zn, Cu, Ca and Mg in diabetics. Chung Hua Nei Ko Tsa Chih 28 (12):741–744, 769, 1989.

Lo GS, Settle SL, Steinke FH, Hopkins DT. Effect of phytate: zinc molar ratio and isolated soybean protein on zinc bioavailability. J Nutr 111:2223–2235, 1981.

MacLennan R, Macrea F, Bain C, Battistutta D, Chapuis P, Gratten H, Lambert J, Newland RC, Ngu M, Russell A, Ward M, Wahlqvist ML, and the Australian Polyp Prevention Project. Randomized trial of intake fat, fiber, and beta carotene to prevent colorectal adenomas. J Natl Cancer Inst 87:1760–1766, 1995.

Macleod MA, Blacklock NJ. The influence of glucose and crude fibre (wheat bran) on the rate of intestinal ^{47}Ca absorption. The influence of glucose and wheat bran on calcium absorption. J R Nav Med Serv 65:143–146, 1979.

Mason PM, Judd PA, Fairweather-Tait SJ, Eagles J, Minski MJ. The effect of moderately increased intakes of complex carbohydrates (cereals, vegetables and fruit) for 12 weeks on iron and zinc metabolism. Br J Nutr 63:597–611, 1990.

McCance RA, Widdowson EM. Mineral metabolism of healthy adults on white and brown bread dietaries. J Physiol 101:44–85, 1942.

McCance RA, Walsham CM. The digestibility and absorption of the calories, proteins, purines, fat and calcium in wholemeal wheaten bread. Br J Nutr 2:26–41, 1948.

McKeown-Eyssen GE, Bright-See E, Bruce WR, Jazmaji V, and the Toronto Polyp Prevention Group. A randomized trial of a low fat high fibre diet in the recurrence of colorectal polyps. J Clin Epidemiol 47:525–536, 1994.

McWhinnie DL, Mack AJ. The interaction of wheat bran and oral iron supplements in vivo. Hum Nutr Clin Nutr 36C:315–318, 1982.

Mertz W. Use and misuse of balance studies. J Nutr 117:1811–1813, 1987.

Moak, S, Pearson N, Shin K. The effects of oat and wheat-bran fibers on mineral metabolism in adult males. Nutr Rep Int 36:1137–1146, 1987.

Morris ER, Ellis R. Bioavailability to rats of iron and zinc in wheat bran: response to low-phytate bran and effect of the phytate/zinc molar ratio. J Nutr 110:2000–2010, 1980.

Morris ER, Ellis R. Phytate-zinc molar ratio of breakfast cereals and bioavailability of zinc to rats. Cereal Chem 58:363–366, 1981.

Morris ER, Ellis R. Bioavailability of dietary calcium. Effect of phytate on adult men consuming nonvegetarian diets. In: Kies C, ed. Nutritional Bioavailability of Calcium. Washington, DC: American Chemical Society, 1985, pp 63–72.

Morris ER, Ellis R. Usefulness of the dietary phytic acid/zinc molar ratio as an index of zinc bioavailability to rats and humans. Biol Trace Elem Res 19:107–117, 1989.

Morris ER, Ellis R, Steele P, Moser PB. Mineral balance of adult men consuming whole or dephytinized wheat bran. Nutr Res 8:445–458, 1988.

Munoz JM, Harland BF. Overview of the effects of dietary fiber on the utilization of minerals and trace elements. In: Spiller GA, ed. Dietary Fiber in Human Nutrition. 2nd ed. Boca Raton, FL: CRC Press, 1993, pp 245–252.

National Research Council. Evidence of Dietary Components and Chronic Diseases: Dietary Fiber: Implications for Reducing Chronic Disease Risk. Washington, DC: National Academy Press, 1989, pp 291–309.

Nävert B, Sandström B, Cederblad Å. Reduction of the phytate content of bran by leavening in bread and its effect on zinc absorption in man. Br J Nutr 53:47–53, 1985.

Oberleas D, Harland BF. Nutritional agents which affect metabolic zinc status. In: Zinc Metabolism, Current Aspects in Health and Disease. New York: A.R. Liss Publishing, 1977, pp 11–27.

Obizoba IC. Zinc and copper metabolism of human adults fed combinations of corn, wheat, beans, rice, and milk containing various levels of phytate. Nutr Rep Int 24:203–210, 1981.

O'Brien KO, Allen LH, Quatromoni P, Siu-Caldera ML, Vieira, Perez A, Holick MF, Yergey AL. High fiber diets slow bone turnover in young men but have no effect on efficiency of intestinal calcium absorption. J Nutr 123:2122–2128, 1993.

Papakyrikos H, Kies C, Fox HM. Zinc and magnesium utilization as affected by graded levels of hemicellulose, cellulose and wheat bran (abstr). Fed Proc Fed Am Soc Exp Biol 38:549, 1979.

Persson I, Raby K, Fønss-Bech P, Jensen E. Effect of prolonged bran administration on serum levels of cholesterol, ionized calcium and iron in the elderly. J Am Geriatr Soc 24:334–335, 1976.

Pilch SM. Physiological effects and health consequences of dietary fiber. Fed. Am. Soc. for Exp. Biol., Prepared for Center For Food Safety and Applied Nutrition, FDA, DHHS, under Contract No. FDA 223-84-2059, 1987.

Pretlow TP, O'Riordan MA, Somich GA, Amini SB, Pretlow TG. Aberrant crypts correlate with tumour incidence in F344 rats treated with azoxymethane and phytate. Carcinogenesis 13:1509–1512, 1992.

Ranhotra GS, Lee C, Gelroth JA. Bioavailability of iron in some commercial variety breads. Nutr Rep Int 19:851–857, 1979.

Rattan J, Levin N, Graff E, Weizer N, Gilat T. A high-fiber diet does not cause mineral and nutrient deficiencies. J Clin Gastroenterol 3:389–393, 1981.

Reddy NR, Sathe SK, Salunkhe DK. Phytates in legumes and cereals. Advances in Food Research, Vol. 28. 1982, pp 1–9.

Reilly C. Zinc, iron and copper binding by dietary fiber. Biochem Soc Trans 7:202–204, 1979.

Reinhold J, Nasr K, Lahimgarzadeh A, Hedayati H. Effects of purified phytate and phytate-rich bread upon metabolism of zinc, calcium, phosphorus, and nitrogen in man. Lancet 1:283–288, 1973a.

Reinhold J, Hedayati H, Lahimgarzadeh A, Nasr K. Zinc, calcium, phosphorus and nitrogen balances of Iranian villagers following a change from phytate-rich to phytate-poor diets. Ecol Food Nutr 2:157–162, 1973b.

Rickard SE, Thompson LU. Interactions and biological effects of phytic acid. In: Shahidi F, ed. Antinutrients and Phytochemicals in Food. Washington, DC: American Chemical Society, 1997, pp 294–312.

Rockway SW, Brannon PM, Weber CW. Bioavailability of copper bound to dietary fiber in mice and rats. J Food Sci 52:1423–1427, 1987.

Sandberg AS, Hasselblad C, Hasselblad K, Hultén L. The effect of wheat bran on the absorption of minerals in the small intestine. Br J Nutr 48:185–191, 1982.

Sandstead HH, Muñoz JM, Jacob RA, Klevay LM, Reck SJ, Logan GM, Dintzis FR, Inglett GE, Shuey WC. Influence of dietary fiber on trace element balance. Am J Clin Nutr 31(suppl):S180–S184, 1978.

Sandstead HH, Klevay LM, Jacob RA, Munoz JM, Logan GM, Reck SJ, Dintzis FR, Inglett FE, Shuey WC.

Effects of dietary fiber and protein level on mineral element metabolism. In: Inglett GE, Falkehag SI, eds. Dietary Fibers: Chemistry and Nutrition. New York: Academic Press, 1979, pp 147–156.

Sandström B, Arvidsson B, Cederblad Å, Björn-Rasmussen E. Zinc absorption from composite meals. I. The significance of wheat extraction rate, zinc, calcium and protein content in meals based on bread. Am J Clin Nutr 33:739–745, 1980.

Sandström B, Andersson H, Bosaéus I, Flakheden BT, Goransson H, Melkersson M. The effect of wheat bran on the intake of energy and nutrients and on serum mineral levels in constipated geriatric patients. Hum Nutr Clin Nutr 37:295–300, 1983.

Schwartz, R, Apgar BJ, Wien BM. Apparent absorption and retention of Ca, Cu, Mg, Mn, and Zn from a diet containing bran. Am J Clin Nutr 43:444–455, 1986.

Seal CJ, Mathers JC. Intestinal zinc transfer by everted gut sacs from rats given diets containing different amounts and types of dietary fibre. Br J Nutr 62:151–163, 1989.

Shah BG, Malcolm S, Belonje B, Trick KD, Brassard R, Mongeau R. Effect of dietary cereal brans on the metabolism of calcium, phosphorus and magnesium in a long term rat study. Nutr. Res. 10: 1015–1028, 1990.

Shamsuddin AM. Inositol phosphates have novel anticancer function. J Nutr 125:725S–732S, 1995.

Shamsuddin AM, Ullah A. Inositol hexaphosphate inhibits large intestinal cancer in F344 rats 5 months after induction by azoxymethane. Carcinogenesis 10:625–626, 1989.

Shamsuddin AM, Yang GY. Inositol hexaphosphate inhibits growth and induces differentiation of PC-3 human prostate cancer cells. Carcinogenesis 16:1975–1979, 1995.

Shamsuddin AM, Elsayed AM, Ullah A. Suppression of large intestinal cancer in F-344 rats by inositol hexaphosphate. Carcinogenesis 9:577, 1988.

Shamsuddin AM, Baten A, Lalwani ND. Effects of inositol hexaphosphate on growth and differentiation in K-562 erythroleukemia cell line. Cancer Lett 64:192–202, 1992.

Shen X, Weaver CM, Martin BR, Heaney RP. Lignin effect on calcium absorption in rats. J Food Sci 63: 165–167, 1998.

Shultz TD, Leklem JE. Selelnium status of vegetarians, non-vegetarians, and hormone-dependent cancer subjects. Am J Clin Nutr 37:114–118, 1983.

Simpson KM, Morris ER, Cook JD. The inhibitory effect of bran on iron absorption in man. Am J Clin Nutr 34:1469–1478, 1981.

Southgate DAT. Minerals, trace elements and potential hazards. Am J Clin Nutr 45:1256–1266, 1987.

Spiller GA, Story JA, Wong LG, Nunes JD, Alton M, Petro MS, Furumoto EJ, Whittam JH, Scala J. Effect of increasing levels of hard wheat fiber on fecal weight, minerals and steroids and gastrointestinal transit time in healthy young women. J Nutr 116:778–785, 1986.

Stasse-Wolthuis M, Albers HFF, van Jeveren JGC, Jong JW, Hautvast JGAG, Hermus RJJ, Katan MB, Brydon MG, Eastwood MA. Influence of dietary fiber from vegetables and fruits, bran or citrus pectin on serum lipids, fecal lipids, and colonic function. Am J Clin Nutr 33:1745–1756, 1980.

Thompson LU, Zhang L. Phytic acid and minerals: effects on early markers of risk for mammary and colon carcinogenesis. Carcinogenesis 12:2041–2045, 1991.

Thompson LU, Trinidad TP, Wolever TMS. Calcium absorption in the colon of man. Trace Elem Man Anim 7:30–35, 1991.

Thompson SA, Weber CW. Effect of dietary fiber sources on tissue mineral levels in chicks. Poultry Sci 60:840–845, 1981.

Treuherz J. Possible inter-relationship between zinc and dietary fiber in a group of lacto-ovo vegetarian adolescents. Plant Foods 4:89–93, 1982.

Trinidad TP, Wolever TMS, Thompson LU. Interactive effects of calcium and short chain fatty acids on absorption in the distal colon of man. Nutr Res 13:417–425, 1993.

Trinidad TP, Wolever TMS, Thompson LU. Effect of acetate and propionate on calcium absorption from the rectum and distal colon of humans. Am J Clin Nutr 63:574–578, 1996.

Turnlund JR, King JC, Keyes WR, Gong B, Michel MC. A stable isotope study of zinc absorption in young men: effects of phytate and α-cellulose. Am J Clin Nutr 40:1071–1077, 1984.

Ullah A, Shamsuddin AM. Dose-dependent inhibition of large intestinal cancer by inositol hexaphosphate in F344 rats. Carcinogenesis 11:2219–2222, 1990.

Vaaler S, Aaseth J, Hanssen KF, Dahl-Jørgensen K, Frølich W, Ødegaard B, Agenæs Ø. Trace elements in serum and urine of diabetic patients given bread enriched with wheat bran or guar gum. In: Int. Symp. Trace Element Metabolism in Man and Animals, TEMA-5 142:446–449, 1985.

van Dokkum W, Wesstra A, Schippers FA. Physiological effects of fibre-rich types of bread. 1. The effect of dietary fibre from bread on the mineral balance of young men. Br J Nutr 47:451–460, 1982.

Vucenik I, Yang GY, Shamsuddin AM. Inositol hexaphosphate and inositol inhibit DMBA-induced rat mammary cancer. Carcinogenesis 16:1055–1058, 1995.

Vucenik I, Yang GY, Shamsuddin AM. Comparison of pure inositol hexaphosphate and high bran diet in the prevention of DMBA-induced rat mammary carcinogenesis. Nutr Cancer 28:7–13, 1997.

Walker A. Mineral metabolism. In: Trowell H, Burkitt D, Heaton K, eds. Dietary Fiber, Fiber-Depleted Foods and Disease. New York: Academic Press, 1985, pp 191–203.

Walker A, Fox FW, Irving JT. Studies in human mineral metabolism. 1. The effect of bread rich in phytate phosphorus on the metabolism of certain mineral salts with special reference to calcium. Biochem J 42:452–462, 1948.

Weinreich J, Pedersen O, Dinesen K. Role of bran in normals. Acta Med Scand 202:125–130, 1977.

Willett WC. Nutrition and cancer: a summary of the evidence. Cancer Causes Control 7:178–180, 1996.

Wisker E, Schweizer TF, Feldheim W. Effects of dietary fiber on mineral balances in humans. In: Waldron K, Johnson IT, Fenwick GR, eds. Dietary Fibre: Chemical and Biological Aspects. Norwich: Royal Society of Chemistry, 1990, pp 203–207.

Zhang D, Hendricks DG, Mahoney AW, Cornforth DP. Bioavailability of iron in green peas, spinach, bran cereal, and corn meal fed to anemic rats. J Food Sci 50:426–428, 1985.

Zoppi G, Gobio-Casali L, Deganello A, Astolfi R, Saccomani F, Cecchettin M. Potential complications in the use of wheat bran for constipation in infancy. J Pediatr Gastroenterol Nutr 1:91–95, 1982.

17

Nondigestible Oligosaccharides and Mineral Absorption

Wim van Dokkum and Ellen van den Heuvel
TNO Nutrition and Food Research, Zeist, The Netherlands

I. INTRODUCTION

Nondigestible oligosaccharides (NDO) are carbohydrates that escape digestion/hydrolysis in the stomach and small intestine, but they are (partly) fermented by the colonic bacterial flora. These oligosaccharides may consist of one moiety of glucose to which, on average, 2 to about 10 fructosyl, galactosyl, or other carbohydrate monomers are bound by a β bond, which means that NDO cannot be digested by the enzymes naturally present in the stomach and small intestine of humans and animals. Fructo-oligosaccharides are present in large amounts in inulin (extracted from, e.g., chicory root) and are present in various natural foods such as leek and onions (1). Galacto-oligosaccharides may be found in soybeans and can be synthesized from lactose. It is estimated that the intake of inulin-type NDO in populations consuming a western-type diet ranges from 1 to 4 g/d (1).

Mostly on the basis of animal experiments, it can be concluded that the effects of NDO are comparable with those of dietary fiber, which means a potential influence on colonic fermentation, with a number of primary and secondary effects on blood lipid concentrations, glucose absorption, and mineral utilization. Generally these effects are evaluated as beneficial for human health. A review by Roberfroid (2) summarizes the findings and hypotheses (see also Chapter 8). Based on the resistance of NDO to (human) intestinal enzymes and the results from animal and human studies, it can be concluded that NDO have physiological properties comparable to dietary fiber.

One of the adverse effects of an increased dietary fiber intake is the decreased availability of minerals and trace elements for absorption. Basically, the mechanisms involved include the possible binding of minerals to dietary fiber during the preabsorption stage. Thus, the influence of dietary fiber on mineral utilization is significant only in this stage and not during the actual absorption of minerals through the intestinal cell wall. Apart from binding of minerals by dietary fiber components of either a chemical or a complex character, dietary fiber might reduce the availability of minerals for absorption by (a) diluting the mineral concentration in the intestinal chyme, (b) trapping minerals within dietary fiber particles, and (c) providing surfaces for mineral adsorption. From the literature and from studies in our laboratory, we concluded that indeed dietary fiber may bind with minerals and trace elements during the preabsorptive stage, but an increased dietary fiber intake often results in a higher intake of several minerals and trace elements; if a mixed diet is consumed with an ample amount of dietary fiber, the net effect on mineral balance and retention is not necessarily negative. (3).

Another route for mineral absorption that did not receive much attention until recently is the possible increase of the soluble mineral pool in the cecum and colon due to fermentation of nondigested food remnants, mostly nondigested carbohydrates. One of the hypotheses is the acidification of the gut contents, which may enhance the availability of minerals to be absorbed by the colon cell wall (4,5). It has also been suggested that short-chain fatty acids (SCFA), which are formed in cecum and colon, may improve mineral absorption through an exchange of intracellular H^+ for Ca^{2+} or Mg^{2+} present in the distal colon (6,7). Apart from the influence of dietary fiber (in general terms) on the availability of minerals and trace elements for absorption in the small and large intestine, the effects may also be applicable to nondigestible oligosaccharides.

In this chapter the emphasis will be placed on the effects of NDO and some related carbohydrates on the absorption of minerals, of which calcium and magnesium have received particular attention, mostly in animal studies.

For a proper understanding of the relative importance of the various factors that may either inhibit or enhance mineral absorption, these factors are summarized in this chapter. Results of various in vitro animal and human studies on the influence of NDO and a few related nondigestible carbohydrates on mineral absorption will be discussed next, and the conclusions will finally give an insight into the significance of NDO for mineral utilization.

II. NONDIGESTIBLE OLIGOSACCHARIDES AND MINERAL ABSORPTION

A. Mineral Absorption

It is well documented that various factors influence the absorption of minerals and trace elements (8). Of particular interest are factors that play a role during the preabsorptive stage, i.e., during the digestion process (9). Various intraluminal interactions occur, such as adsorption of minerals to micronutrients (e.g., attachment of minerals to the surface of fiber particles) and binding of minerals to other components and inclusions (e.g., within fiber particles). In addition, reduction and oxidation of some trace elements, such as Fe, may take place. Thus, the chemical ''environment,'' i.e., the species of minerals and trace elements formed during digestion in the stomach/small intestine and also in the large intestine, will finally influence whether a mineral will become available to be at least taken up by the cell wall. This chemical ''environment'' includes the strength of the mineral-chelate bond, the solubility of the mineral complex, the presence of other (competing) chelating compounds, and gastrointestinal pH and oxidation potential. Competing chelating compounds may desorb minerals from the initial complex to form even stronger mineral-chelate complexes or, as a result of desorption, they may complex minerals into a more soluble form. In general, the strength of a bond of a ligand with minerals and the solubility of the complex contribute to either enhancement or inhibition of mineral absorption. In this respect the molecular weight and the particle size of any mineral precipitate formed will influence the extent to which a mineral species changes into a soluble form, as illustrated for phytate by Wise (10). Moreover, the factor ''time'' should not be underestimated: many reactions in the gastrointestinal tract may be so slow that the transit time through stomach, small intestine, and colon is too short for any change in mineral solubility. Finally, it should be noted that in vivo the dynamic behavior of mineral ions during all stages of digestion and fermentation may alter the availability for absorption considerably, which makes prediction of the absorption on basis of the food intake difficult.

The factors summarized above are also applicable to dietary fiber and NDO, in particular regarding pH and solubility of any NDO-mineral complex formed in the gastrointestinal tract.

B. NDO and Mineral Absorption

Regarding the proposed mechanisms of the influence of NDO on mineral absorption, the effects in the stomach/small intestine are basically different from those in the colon. As discussed above, during digestion of foods various factors may play a role in the interaction with minerals. Based on the structure of NDO with various polar groups, it is conceivable that minerals are (temporarily) bound or complexed to NDO, which may either result in a better availability for absorption or a decreased availability, depending on the strength of the NDO-mineral bond and the solubility of the complex. In the colon, fermentation of the undigested oligosaccharides by the bacterial flora forms the basis of the proposed mechanisms as to mineral availability for absorption by the colonic cell wall. The intestinal microflora use the NDO as a substrate for their metabolism, resulting in various metabolites, including short-chain fatty acids (SCFA). The most important SCFA produced are acetate, propionate, and butyrate. In vitro fermentation of fecal flora has indicated that fructo-oligosaccharides (FO) may increase the production of acetate and butyrate, whereas galacto-oligosaccharides (GO) increase the production of acetate and propionate, and xylo-oligosaccharides prefer produce acetate (11,12). The production of SCFA may result in a decrease of colonic pH (13–15), and as a consequence this may improve the solubility of mineral complexes in the colon, which makes minerals more available to be absorbed (5,16). Moreover, fermentation of fiber and other nondigestible carbohydrates may cause a release of minerals complexed in the small intestine, which may become available to be absorbed from the colon (17). Generally, the role of the colon in the overall absorption of minerals has to be considered, especially for Ca and Mg (5). The large intestine is even considered to be the major site of Mg absorption (18,19). As Mg is mainly present in plant foods that also contain dietary fiber, the microbial digestion of fiber may result in a higher availability of Mg for colonic absorption (5). In fact, nondigestible carbohydrates may shift the major site of mineral absorption towards the large intestine (20). The importance of pH reduction, brought about by the production of SCFA during fermentation, for increasing the availability of Ca for cecal or colonic absorption is also indicated for lactulose, a synthetic, nondigestible disaccharide (21). The evidence for a colonic component of Ca absorption was found in studies by Barger-Lux et al. (22). They investigated the time course of calcium absorption in humans who were given milk extrinsically labeled with radio-calcium. It was estimated that approximately 4% of total Ca absorption takes place in the colon and is completed after about 26 hours.

Scharrer and Lutz (23) reported studies on Mg absorption in ruminants and rats. They emphasized the importance of fermentable carbohydrates in the large intestine for Mg absorption. In the rat large intestine, SCFA, particularly butyrate, enhanced Mg absorption by the distal colon; propionate and acetate were less effective. It is suggested that the effect is due to the function of SCFA as intracellular proton donors for the Mg^{2+}/H^+ exchanger located in the apical membrane of the epithelium in the distal colon.

Lutz and Scharrer (24) used an in vivo luminal perfusion technique to investigate the influence of SCFA on Ca absorption by the rat colon. The distal colon was the major site for Ca absorption, which was increased by acetate and butyrate. They attributed a similar mechanism to this effect, as was suggested for Mg. From the results of studies in humans, in which six healthy subjects were given rectal infusions of $CaCl_2$ together with acetate and propionate, Trinidad et al. (6) concluded that SCFA enhance absorption of Ca from the human distal colon, but that propionate has a greater effect at higher concentrations, which may be due to the fact that propionate is more lipid-soluble than acetate and thus is more rapidly absorbed than acetate. The positive effect of complex carbohydrates and oligosaccharides on Ca digestibility, probably by improving the solubility of Ca in cecal contents of rats, was also found by Levrat et al. (15,25) and Rémésy et al. (16).

It can be concluded that fermentation of nondigested carbohydrates, including NDO, seems to be an important phenomenon accounting for the absorption of minerals from the colon. In the following section scientific evidence is summarized regarding the role of fiber, in particular NDO, in the absorption of minerals, with a focus on the colon as the site for absorption.

C. Fructo- and Galacto-oligosaccharides and Mineral Absorption

Studies on the influence of NDO on mineral absorption have mainly be carried out in animals, mostly rats. Rémésy et al. (16) observed that inulin feeding of rats increased the percentage of soluble Ca. Also, Ca absorption from the cecum was markedly higher in rats fed inulin compared to rats on a fiber-free diet. The authors attribute part of the effects to the fermentation of inulin in the large intestine, yielding a particularly acidic pH in the lumen, which could increase the availability of Ca and of Mg for absorption (15).

From experiments in rats who were given a 5% FO-containing diet, the group of Ohta (26,27) found an increased absorption of Ca and Mg. They suggest two reasons for this effect: a reduction of the pH brought about by fermentation of FO and consequently a better solubility of the minerals and a direct influence on colonic Ca and Mg absorption by SCFA as products of fermentation of FO in the cecum. However, they suggest different mechanisms for the absorption of Ca and Mg from experiments in cecectomized rats (28). The same group of Ohta (29) investigated in rats the influence of 5% FO in the diet on apparent absorption of Ca and Mg. Their results indicated that indigestible and fermentable carbohydrates facilitate colorectal absorption of both minerals. They also determined whether the effects of FO on the absorption of Ca and Mg were altered by prevention of coprophagy in rats. They observed an increased absorption of Ca and Mg and an increased Ca content of the femur in rats on the FO diet when coprophagy was prevented (30). Ohta et al. (31) confirmed the increasing effect of FO on Mg absorption in a study in rats fed Ca- and Mg-free diets, either with or without FO, and in which aqueous suspensions of $CaCO_3$ and MgO were infused into the cecum. Regarding the route for Ca absorption (either in the small or large intestine), they concluded that the chemical form of the Ca source (the Ca species) will determine in what way and to what extent FO may affect the availability of Ca for absorption both in the small and in the large intestine. Results from additional studies in rats by Baba et al. (32) indicate that FO feeding stimulates Mg absorption mainly in the hindgut through a mechanism of increased solubility of Mg by a decrease of luminal pH as a result of fermentation of FO.

In addition to Ca and Mg absorption studies in rats on FO feeding, the effects were also studied for iron in Fe-deficient anemic rats (4). The experimental diets contained two levels of Fe (15 or 30 mg/kg diet) and two levels of FO (0 or 50 g/kg diet). Not only did FO feeding lower pH and raise the solubility of Fe in the cecal contents, but hematocrit and hemoglobin levels in blood samples were also higher on the FO diets as compared with the FO-free diets. Their data suggest that the large intestine is able to absorb Fe. Delzenne et al. (33) assessed the apparent retention of Ca, Mg, Fe, Zn, and Cu in rats receiving a diet supplemented with fermentable FO. They observed that FO feeding improved the absorption of Ca, Mg, Fe, and Zn, mainly by the large intestine through the increase of mineral solubility resulting from a decrease of cecal/colonic pH by the formation of SCFA as a result of FO fermentation.

Vanhoof et al. (34) studied the effect of inulin on Ca, Mg, Fe, and Zn utilization in rats and in ileum-fistulated pigs. They could not, however, confirm the results of Delzenne et al.

(33) and the studies of the group of Ohta: the changes in apparent absorption of the studied minerals were not significant.

Chonan and Watanuki (35) studied the effect of GO, mainly a nondigestible trisaccharide consisting of two galactose units and one glucose unit, on Ca absorption in rats. The apparent Ca absorption and retention were significantly higher in the rats fed GO-containing diets as compared with the GO-free diets. Injecting GO into the cecal lumen of rats also resulted in an apparent increase of Ca absorption. The authors conclude that the stimulatory effect of GO on Ca absorption may be partly associated with the increased solubility of Ca in the intestinal lumen. In ovariectomized rats Chonan et al. (36) studied the effect of GO on Ca absorption and prevention of bone loss. Rats fed a diet containing GO absorbed Ca more efficiently than those on the control diet. Moreover, bone ash weight and tibia Ca content of rats fed the GO diet were significantly higher than those of the control animals. GO fermentation, subsequent production of SCFA, lowering of cecum pH, and increase of Ca solubility are mentioned as important factors accounting for the observed effects which are also dependent on the Ca content of the diet (35).

Until recently only a few human studies have been carried out. Coudray et al. (37) studied the effect of dietary fiber supplementation on absorption and balance of Ca, Mg, Fe, and Zn in healthy young men. Nine men (mean age 21.5 years) were given a control diet or the same diet complemented with either inulin or sugar beet fiber during 28-day periods according to a 3 × 3 latin square design with three repetitions. The experimental fiber sources were incorporated into bread (60%) and liquid foods (40%) up to a maximum of 40 g/d. Ingestion of inulin significantly increased the apparent absorption and balance of only Ca. Although they could not measure separately the absorption of the minerals in the small or large intestine of the human subjects, the authors emphasize the mechanism by which minerals can be absorbed in the colon, as has been described for rats. The different results regarding Mg absorption between rat and human are accounted for by the different tract physiology of the rat versus humans: the cecum segment, absent in human, plays an important role in Ca and Mg absorption in rats. Fe and Zn are mainly absorbed in the small intestine of humans. The possible role of NDO on Fe and Zn absorption in the large intestine, as suggested by Delzenne et al. (33), could not be confirmed in the human study of Coudray et al.

Inulin and oligofructose were not found to influence Ca, Mg, Zn, and Fe absorption in ileostomy subjects (38). In a double-blind crossover study 10 subjects with conventional ileostomy were given three identical control diets with either 17 g of inulin, 17 g of oligofructose, or 7 g of sucrose during three experimental periods of 3 days each. The absorption of the studied minerals were not affected by inulin and oligofructose. The authors concluded that NDO do not affect mineral excretion and hence hardly mineral absorption.

In our laboratory we investigated the effect of NDO on Ca and nonheme iron absorption in young healthy men (39). Twelve healthy nonanemic male subjects (aged 20–30 years) received four treatments consisting of a constant basal diet supplemented with 15 g/d of inulin, FO, or GO and a control treatment without NDO. These four treatments were given for 21 days each according to a randomized crossover design. True intestinal Ca and Fe absorption were measured using a dual stable isotope technique (oral and intravenous administration of the isotopes). None of the differences of mineral absorption between treatments, however, reached statistical significance. It is concluded that intake of amounts up to 15 g/d of NDO does not inhibit or enhance Fe and Ca absorption at normal intakes of the elements by young healthy men with an apparently adequate Ca and Fe status.

In another study we investigated the effect of FO on the absorption of Ca in male adolescents (40). Twelve healthy boys aged between 14 and 16 years received 15 g of FO or sucrose (control treatment) during 9 days. The treatments were given according to a randomized, double-blind, crossover design, separated by a 19-day washout period. True fractional Ca absorption was measured using the double stable isotope technique. A significant increase in fractional Ca absorption was observed due to the intake of FO. From both human studies carried out in our laboratory we may conclude that the FO-induced enhancement of Ca absorption may be dependent on the subject's Ca requirement and may take place predominantly in the large intestine.

D. Nondigestible Disaccharides and Mineral Absorption

Although it is well documented that digestible disaccharides, particularly lactose, may enhance Ca absorption (8), the influence of nondigestible disaccharides on mineral absorption has not been studied extensively until recently.

Lactitol is a nondigestible, fermentable disaccharide, which can be produced by β-galactosidase by reduction of lactose (41). From studies in rats, Yanahira et al. (42) conclude that the observed stimulatory effect of lactitol on Ca absorption may be accounted for by the increased acetic acid concentration produced by intestinal bacteria fermentation in the rat cecum and by the enhancement of the rate of transepithelial Ca transport in the small intestine by modulation of the passive diffusion of Ca. For Mg, the increased absorption seems to be stimulated predominantly by fermentation of lactitol in the rat cecum and influenced by the produced SCFA.

Isomalt or palatinit is a partly digestible disaccharide that can be produced by reduction of isomaltulose or palatinose and used in various food products as a noncariogenic nutritive sweetener (43). Maltitol is an α-linked disaccharide produced by catalytic hydrogenation of maltose. Because they are only partly digestible, they may be classified as low-digestibility or slow-release carbohydrates or even as "resistant sugars" (44).

Both Kishi et al. (44) and Kashimura et al. (45) studied the influence of this type of disaccharide on Ca absorption in rats. Apart from an important effect of the partly digestible compounds on Ca absorption in the small intestine, they attribute part of the observed increased Ca absorption by the primary and secondary effects in the cecum and colon to fermentation of the undigested residues of these disaccharides.

Lactulose is a synthetic β-linked disaccharide consisting of a galactose and a fructose moiety. It can be prepared from lactose by alkaline isomerization in which the glucose moiety is converted into a fructose unit. It is not digestible and may be used as a laxative (for details, see Chapter 12).

Demigné et al. (20) conducted studies in rats to investigate the possible effect of lactulose on cecal concentration of Ca, which was increased on a 10% lactulose intake compared to a fiber-free diet. It is concluded that Ca absorption is probably tightly controlled along the whole digestive tract with some possibilities of compensation for a reduced absorption in the small intestine. From results of rat studies that were fed lactulose and other "resistant sugars," Brommage et al. (46) concluded that these compounds stimulate Ca absorption mostly in the small intestine.

In contrast, Trinidad et al. (17) concluded from their in vitro experiments that lactulose may bind Ca and reduce its availability for absorption in the small intestine. However, in the colon bound Ca may be released for potential absorption due to fermentation of lactulose. Heijnen et al. (47) observed an increased absorption of Ca and Mg in rats which they ascribe to a lowering of ileal pH from 7.5 (control diet) to 7.0 (lactulose diet).

Recently we investigated whether lactulose would affect Ca absorption in postmenopausal women (48). Twelve subjects between 56 and 64 years of age were selected. They were all certified to be in good general health. They were given 5 or 10 g of lactulose or a reference substance dissolved in 100 mL of water at breakfast for 9 days. The three treatments were given according to a randomized, double-blind, crossover design, separated by two 19-day washout periods. On day 8 of each treatment Ca stable isotope administration took place (one isotope orally, another isotope intravenously) and urine was collected until 36 hours after isotope administration. From the isotope ratios measured, true fractional Ca absorption was calculated. A significant difference in Ca absorption was found between the highest dose of lactulose and the reference treatment. Several hypotheses have been proposed to explain the stimulatory effect of lactulose on intestinal Ca absorption. These hypotheses refer to effects on passive, trans- and/or paracellular Ca absorption in the small and/or large intestine. Transcellular transport of Ca may be stimulated by SCFA. In humans, an increased production of SCFA in the large intestine was found (21). The direct effect probably involves diffusion of protonated SCFA across the apical membrane. In the cell the protonated SCFA molecule dissociates, resulting in an increased concentration of intracellular H^+, which is secreted from the cell in exchange for Ca^{2+} from the distal colon. Once outside the cell, H^+ becomes available to protonate a SCFA to diffuse into the cell (6,24). This enhancing effect of SCFA seems to occur in the distal but not in the proximal colon (24). Whether this process involves passive or active transport needs to be further investigated. Paracellular Ca absorption may be stimulated by pH reduction. In humans the fermentation of lactulose (40 g/d) also results in a lower cecal pH (21). The pH reduction is associated with an increased amount of soluble Ca in the cecum of rats given NDO (4,35).

III. CONCLUSIONS

Because nondigestible oligosaccharides have similar physiological effects as dietary fiber, the question is relevant whether one of the adverse effects known for fiber, i.e., inhibition of mineral absorption, might also be applicable to NDO. From the studies reviewed, no such negative effect was observed for NDO. On the contrary, based on the fermentation of NDO in the colon, evidence indicates that absorption of particularly Ca and Mg is even enhanced in the colon after consumption of an ample amount of NDO in the diet. The mechanisms involved probably include the formation of SCFA as a consequence of NDO fermentation, which may lower colonic pH and make the minerals more soluble and available for absorption. In this process an exchange of intracellular H^+ for Ca^{2+} or Mg^{2+} might improve the absorption of both minerals.

The conclusions for NDO regarding mineral absorption also seem to be applicable to nondigestible disaccharides, such as lactitol, maltitol, and lactulose. Because only a few studies have been executed with minerals and trace elements other than Ca and Mg, it is not known whether NDO have positive effects on the availability for absorption of, for example, Fe, Zn, and Cu.

REFERENCES

1. van Loo J, Coussement P, de Leenheer L, Hoebregs H, Smits G. On the presence of inulin and oligofructose as natural ingredients in the Western diet. Crit Rev Food Sci Nutr 35:525–552, 1995.
2. Roberfroid M. Dietary fiber, inulin, and oligofructose: a review comparing their physiological effects. Crit Rev Food Sci Nutr 33:103–148, 1993.
3. van Dokkum W. The relative significance of dietary fibre for human health. Front Gastrointest Res 14:135–145, 1988.
4. Ohta A, Ohtsuki M, Baba S, Takizawa T, Adachi T, Kimura S. Effects of fructo-oligosaccharides on the absorption of iron, calcium and magnesium in iron-deficient anemic rats. J Nutr Sci Vitaminol 41:281–291, 1995.

5. Younes H, Demigné C, Rémésy C. Acidic fermentation in the caecum increases absorption of calcium and magnesium in the large intestine of the rat. Br J Nutr 75:301–314, 1996.
6. Trinidad TP, Wolever TM, Thompson LU. Effect of acetate and propionate on calcium absorption from the rectum and distal colon of humans. Am J Clin Nutr 63:574–578, 1996.
7. Scharrer E, Lutz T. Effects of short chain fatty acids and K on absorption of Mg and other cations by the colon and caecum. Z Ernährungswiss 29:162–168, 1990.
8. Hazell T. Minerals in foods: dietary sources, chemical forms, interactions, bioavailability. Wld Rev Nutr Diet 46:1–123, 1985.
9. van Dokkum W. The significance of speciation for predicting mineral bioavailability. In: DAT Southgate, IT Johnson, GR Fenwick, eds. Nutrient Availability: Chemical and Biological Aspects. Cambridge: The Royal Society of Chemistry, 1989, pp. 89–96.
10. Wise A. Dietary factors determining the biological activities of phytate. Nutr Abstr Rev 53:791–806, 1983.
11. Djouzi Z, Andrieux C. Compared effects of three oligosaccharides on metabolism of intestinal microflora in rats inoculated with a human flora. Br J Nutr 78:313–324, 1997.
12. Campbell JM, Fahey GCJ, Wolf BW. Selected indigestible oligosaccharides affect large bowel mass, cecal and fecal short-chain fatty acids, pH and microflora in rats. J Nutr 127:130–136, 1997.
13. Hidaka H, Eida T, Takizawa T, Tokunaga T, Tashiro Y. Effects of fructo-oligosaccharides on intestinal flora and human health. Bifidobacteria Microflora 5:37–50, 1986.
14. Mitsuoka T, Hidaka H, Eida T. Effect of fructo-oligosaccharides on intestinal microflora. Die Nahrung 31:426–436, 1987.
15. Levrat MA, Rémésy C, Demigné C. High propionic acid fermentations and mineral accumulation in the cecum of rats adapted to different levels of inulin. J Nutr 121:1730–1737, 1991.
16. Rémésy C, Levrat MA, Gamet L, Demigné C. Cecal fermentations in rats fed oligosaccharides (inulin) are modulated by dietary calcium level. Am J Physiol 264:G855–862, 1993.
17. Trinidad TP, Wolever TMS, Thompson LU. Availability of calcium for absorption in the small intestine and colon from diets containing available and unavailable carbohydrates: an in vitro assessment. Int J Food Sci Nutr 47:83–88, 1996.
18. Hardwick LL, Jones MR, Brautbar N, Lee DBN. Site and mechanism of intestinal magnesium absorption. Minerals Electr Metabol 16:174–180, 1990.
19. Lutz T, Wurmli R, Scharrer E. Short-chain fatty acids stimulate magnesium absorption by the colon. In: B Lasserre, J Durlach, eds. Magnesium—A Relevant Ion. London: John Libbey, 1991, pp. 131–137.
20. Demigné C, Levrat MA, Rémésy C. Effects of feeding fermentable carbohydrates on the caecal concentrations of minerals and their fluxes between caecum and blood plasma in the rat. J Nutr 119:1625–1630, 1989.
21. Florent C, Flourie B, Leblond A, Rautureau M, Bernier JJ, Rambaud JC. Influence of chronic lactulose ingestion on the colonic metabolism of lactulose in man (an in vivo study). J Clin Invest 75:608–613, 1985.
22. Barger-Lux MJ, Heaney RP, Recker RR. Time course of calcium absorption in humans: evidence for a colonic component. Calcif Tissue Int 44:308–311, 1989.
23. Scharrer E, Lutz T. Relationship between volatile fatty acids and magnesium absorption in mono- and polygastric species. Magnesium Res 5:53–60, 1992.
24. Lutz T, Scharrer E. Effect of short-chain fatty acids on calcium absorption by the rat colon. Exper Physiol 76:615–618, 1991.
25. Levrat MA, Rémésy C, Demigné C. Very acidic fermentations in the rat caecum during adaptation to a diet rich in amylase-resistant starch (crude potato starch). J Nutr Biochem 2:31–36, 1991.
26. Ohta A, Baba S, Takizawa T, Adachi T. Effects of fructooligosaccharides on the absorption of magnesium in the magnesium-deficient rat model. J Nutr Sci Vitaminol 40:171–180, 1994.
27. Ohta A, Osakabe N, Yamada K, Saito Y, Hidaka H. Effect of fructooligosaccharides and other saccharides on Ca, Mg and P absorption in rats. J Jpn Soc Nutr Food Sci 46:123–129, 1993.
28. Ohta A, Ohtuki M, Takizawa T, Inaba H, Adachi T, Kimura S. Effects of fructooligosaccharides on the absorption of magnesium and calcium by cecectomized rats. Int J Vit Nutr Res 64:316–323, 1994.

29. Ohta A, Ohtsuki M, Baba S, Adachi T, Sakata T, Sakaguchi E. Calcium and magnesium absorption from the colon and rectum are increased in rats fed fructooligosaccharides. J Nutr 125:2417–2424, 1995.

30. Ohta A, Baba S, Ohtsuki M, Taguchi A, Adachi T. Prevention of coprophagy modifies magnesium absorption in rats fed with fructo-oligosaccharides. Br J Nutr 75:775–784, 1996.

31. Ohta A, Baba S, Ohtsuki M, Takizawa T, Adachi T, Hara H. In vivo absorption of calcium carbonate and magnesium oxide from the large intestine in rats. J Nutr Sci Vitaminol 43:35–46, 1997.

32. Baba S, Ohta A, Ohtsuki M, Takizawa T, Adachi T, Hara H. Fructooligosaccharides stimulate the absorption of magnesium from the hindgut in rats. Nutr Res 16:657–666, 1996.

33. Delzenne N, Aertssens J, Verplaetse H, Roccaro M, Roberfroid M. Effect of fermentable fructo-oligosaccharides on mineral, nitrogen and energy digestive balance in the rat. Life Sci 57:1579–1587, 1995.

34. Vanhoof K, de Schrijver R. Availability of minerals in rats and pigs fed non-purified diets containing inulin. Nutr Res 16:1017–1022, 1996.

35. Chonan O, Watanuki M. Effect of galactooligosaccharides on calcium absorption in rats. J Nutr Sci Vitaminol 41:95–104, 1995.

36. Chonan O, Matsumoto K, Watanuki M. Effect of galactooligosaccharides on calcium absorption and preventing bone loss in ovariectomized rats. Biosc Biotechn Biochem 59:236–239, 1995.

37. Coudray C, Bellanger J, Castiglia-Delavaud C, Rémésy C, Vermorel M, Rayssignuier Y. Effect of soluble or partly soluble dietary fibres supplementation on absorption and balance of calcium, magnesium, iron and zinc in healthy young men. Eur J Clin Nutr 51:375–380, 1997.

38. Ellegård L, Andersson H, Bosaeus I. Inulin and oligo-fructose do not influence the absorption of cholesterol or the excretion of cholesterol, Ca, Mg, Zn, Fe or bile acids but increases energy excretion in ileostomy subjects. Eur J Clin Nutr 51:1–5, 1997.

39. van den Heuvel EGHM, Schaafsma G, Muijs T, van Dokkum W. Nondigestible oligosaccharides do not interfere with calcium and nonheme-iron absorption in young healthy men. Am J Clin Nutr 67:412–420, 1998.

40. van den Heuvel EGHM, Muijs T, van Dokkum W, Schaafsma G. Fructo oligosaccharides stimulate calcium absorption in adolescents. In: R Hartemink, ed. Non-digestible Oligosaccharides: Healthy Food for the Colon? Wageningen: Graduate School VLAG, 1997, pp 154.

41. Yanahira S, Suguri T, Yakabe T, Ikeuchi Y, Hanagata G, Deya E. Formation of oligosaccharides from lactitol by *Aspergillus oryzae* β-galactosidase. Carbohydr Res 232:151–159, 1992.

42. Yanahira S, Morita M, Aoe S, Suguri T, Takada Y, Miura S, Nakajima I. Effects of lactitol-oligosaccharides on calcium and magnesium absorption in rats. J Nutr Sci Vitaminol 43:123–132, 1997.

43. Tsuji Y, Yamada K, Hosoya N, Moriuchi S. Digestion and absorption of sugar and sugar substitutes in rat's small intestine. J Nutr Sci Vitaminol 32:93–100, 1986.

44. Kishi K, Goda T, Takase S. Maltitol increases transepithelial diffusional transfer of calcium in rat ileum. Life Sci 59:1133–1140, 1996.

45. Kashimura J, Kimura M, Itokawa Y. The effects of isomaltulose-based oligomers feeding and calcium deficiency on mineral retention in rats. J Nutr Sci Vitaminol 42:69–76, 1996.

46. Brommage R, Binacua C, Antille S, Carrié AL. Intestinal calcium absorption in rats is stimulated by dietary lactulose and other resistant sugars. J Nutr 123:2186–2194, 1993.

47. Heijnen AMP, Brink EJ, Lemmens AG, Beynen AC. Ileal pH and apparent absorption of magnesium in rats fed on diets containing either lactose or lactulose. Br J Nutr 70:747–756, 1993.

48. van den Heuvel EGHM. Application of dual stable isotope techniques to measure absorption of calcium, magnesium and iron in man. PhD dissertation, Maastricht University, The Netherlands, 1998.

18

Enzymatic Modification of Dietary Fiber Sources

Eva Arrigoni
Swiss Federal Institute of Technology, Zurich, Switzerland

I. INTRODUCTION

It is generally agreed that an increase in dietary fiber consumption in western countries would be beneficial to maintaining health. The average fiber intake in Europe has been reported to be in the range of 16–21 g/day (1). Highly variable values are found for Japan [12–24 g/day (2)], whereas in the United States the daily intake is even lower [12–13 g/day (3)]. To reach the recommendations of 20–35 g of dietary fiber per day, or 10–12 g/1000 kcal, it would be necessary to change dietary habits by increasing the intake of fruits, vegetables, and whole grain cereal products. Another possibility is the production of fiber-enriched foods incorporating dietary fiber sources such as cereal brans, pulps, or pomaces, which are mainly used as feed, fertilizers, or fuels (4,5). However, due to their physicochemical properties, which can cause severe functional problems in product development, most of these by-products cannot be added in physiologically relevant amounts. In addition, off-flavors and unpleasant color and texture make incorporation difficult. One way to overcome these technological and organoleptic problems is enzymatic modification.

In this chapter procedures to modify dietary fiber sources by means of enzyme preparations are reviewed. Two different approaches are possible. On the one hand, an increase in dietary fiber content can be achieved by removing digestible compounds. On the other hand, chemical composition as well as physicochemical properties can be altered by enzyme attack of the fiber fraction itself.

II. USE OF ENZYMES TO INCREASE DIETARY FIBER CONTENT

A. Procedures Applying Starch- and Protein-Degrading Enzymes

The principle to increase the dietary fiber content by removing digestible compounds is used in enzymatic-gravimetric fiber determination methods and in approaches to produce undigestible substrates for in vitro fermentation studies. The latter mainly apply enzymes of mammal origin at moderate incubation temperatures to approach physiological conditions as closely as possible. In contrast, bacterial enzyme preparations allowing higher temperatures and shorter incubation times are utilized to determine the dietary fiber content. Similar approaches are used to increase the fiber content of dietary fiber sources, as summarized in Table 1. Starch degradation is carried

Table 1 Procedures to Increase Dietary Fiber Content by Applying Starch- and Protein-Degrading Enzymes

Fiber source	Enzymes applied	Incubation	Ref.
Wheat bran, beet pulp, or corn germ meal	1. Alcalase 2. Termamyl 3. AMG	pH 7.5; 60°C; 2 h pH 6.0; 100°C; 30 min pH 4.5; 60°C; 30 min	6
Wheat bran	1. Termamyl 2. Alcalase 3. AMG	pH 6.0; 95°C; 30 min pH 7.5; 60°C; 30 min pH 4.5; 60°C; 30 min	7
White wheat bran	1. Termamyl 2. Neutrase	90–95°C; 90 min pH 6.0; 40°C; 1 h	8
Potato pulp	1. Amylogal 2. AMG	pH 6.5; 85°C; 2 h pH 4.5; 60°C; 48 h	9
Tapioca fiber[a]	1,4-α-D-glucosidase	25°C–85°C; 3–5 h	5

[a] Patented procedure.

out by means of thermostable α-amylases (Termamyl, Amylogal) and bacterial amyloglucosidases (AMG), whereas proteins are digested by bacterial proteases (Alcalase, Neutrase). In most of the procedures commerical enzyme preparations are utilized, all being produced by Novo Nordisk A/S (Bagsvaerd, Denmark) except for the Polish preparation Amylogal. In a patent (5) it is claimed to apply a 1,4-α-D-glucosidase in general in a very broad temperature range; in the examples provided either endo-enzymes (Termamyl, BAN) or the exo-enzyme amyloglucosidase were applied.

Pretreatments of dry fiber sources involved grinding and defatting, if necessary, prior to incubation (6,7). Potato pulp (9) and tapioca fiber (5), both being by-products of starch production, were utilized as slurries. In order to improve liquefaction of residual starch, the potato product was steamed under pressure before enzyme addition (9), whereas it seemed appropriate to cook the tapioca fiber before the amyloglucosidase incubation (5).

Soluble fibers were precipitated in ethanol after incubation followed by filtration or centrifugation and drying (6,7). In contrast, the soluble fraction was removed by filtration in some experiments, and the insoluble residue was washed and dried (5,8,9). Enzymes are supposed to be inactivated by the drying step. However, the modification of tapioca fiber can include an enzyme deactivation by lowering the pH to 2.0 for 15 minutes (5).

B. Effects of Enzyme Treatment on Composition

Due to the removal of digestible compounds, a distinct increase in total dietary fiber (TDF) content was observed in all experiments, but only a few comments about qualitative changes were made. Hoebler et al. (6) reported complete starch removal with their procedure, but proteolysis rates varied from 23 to 67%. Concerning the fiber fraction, some solubilization and losses, mainly of pectic substances, occurred. It seems likely that they were induced during the proteolysis step, since the authors determined a very low polygalacturonase activity in the Alcalase preparation (10). Shorter Alcalase incubation times, as applied by Oh and Grundleger (7), did not cause a shift from insoluble to soluble fiber. The neutral detergent fiber (NDF) content of white wheat bran could be increased from 47.4 to 74.7% by Termamyl and Neutrase incubation (8). However, taking the overall yield of 53.5% into account, a slight solubilization of fiber components, which were removed by filtration, must have occurred. No comparison can be made for the enzymatically treated potato pulp (9), since different fiber determination methods were applied before and after modification and no recovery data were reported. In tapioca fiber the dietary fiber content was increased from approximately 60% to at least 70% (5). Although the soluble fibers were removed by filtering and washing steps, a proportion of soluble fiber of at least 12% was achieved (calculated as TDF minus NDF).

C. Application Experiments with Fiber-Enriched Sources

The experiments to increase the dietary fiber content of food-processing by-products were carried out for different reasons. Aside from the obtention of cell wall residues for in vitro fermentation studies (6) or fiber enrichment for further enzymatic treatments (7) (see Sec. III.A), mainly application aspects were mentioned. Improving functional properties of the dietary fiber sources was expected to make their incorporation into food products more suitable (5,8,9).

Baking experiments were carried out with wheat bran and potato pulp. Enzymatically modified wheat bran at 10–20% flour substitution levels led to breads of poorer quality than the corresponding breads with untreated bran (8). Significantly higher water-holding capacities but slow water uptake rates as well as the increased fiber content combined with the removal of soluble compounds affected dough development. Moreover, the authors do not exclude a carryover due to incomplete enzyme inactivation, which may have had a negative effect on wheat starch and gluten. An incorporation of 5% of enzymatically treated potato pulp into white bread was found to give suitable and advantageous products, whereas at 10% levels adverse effects on bread quality were observed (9).

Lacourse et al. (5) claimed to incorporate tapioca fiber at levels of 1–43% into food products. Examples of formulations for bread (containing 4.8% of TDF from tapioca), donut (1.7%), extruded wheat flakes (14.1 and 21.2%), and an expanded cereal (14.1%), which led to acceptable products compared to the unmodified control, are provided.

III. ENZYMATIC MODIFICATION OF THE DIETARY FIBER FRACTION

A. Procedures Applying Fiber-Degrading Enzymes

Enzymatic treatments to modify the dietary fiber fraction itself is a demanding and delicate task. A depolymerization to a certain extent leading to a solubilization of polysaccharides is desired, but significant losses due to a more intense enzyme attack have to be avoided. In addition, optimum incubation conditions depend on the composition of the fiber source, the chosen enzymes, the required functional and physicochemical properties, etc. and have therefore to be evaluated for every single purpose. Modification experiments were carried out on different by-products of cereal, fruit, and vegetable processing (Table 2). Although similar dietary fiber sources were investigated by different research groups, limited information about origin and composition make a comparison difficult. Aside from the often utilized sources such as cereal brans, pea fiber, and sugar beet pulp, investigations were made on the residues of apple juice production (13), on a starch- and protein-free insoluble residue prepared from a commercial potato fiber product (16), and on the by-product from olive oil extraction (17). Due to the considerable variation of fiber composition within these substrates, a wide a variety of enzymes and enzyme combinations was applied.

Maceration of plant tissues requires a combination of cellulases, hemicellulases, and pectolytic enzymes, each exhibiting different activities (4). Commercial enzyme preparations, mainly produced from specific *Aspergillus* strains, provide a defined main activity as well as various side activities. They are applied for different purposes in the food industry, depending on their activity spectra. Pectolytic preparations are used to liquefy apple mashes and to produce fruit

Table 2 Optimized Conditions for Enzymatic Modifications of Dietary Fiber Sources

Fiber source	Enzymes applied	Incubation	Ref.
Wheat bran	Cellulase 36	pH 4.0; 21°C; 18 h	11
	Pectinol	pH 4.0; 21°C; 18 h	11
Spelt wheat bran	1. Pectinex Ultra SP-L plus Pulpzyme	pH 3.5–4.5; 50°C; 2 h	12
	2. Celluclast	pH 4.5–5.5; 60°C; 2 h	
Purified wheat bran[a]	Gamanase	pH 5.0; 30°C; 40 min	7
Pea bran	1. Pectinex Ultra SP-L	pH 5.5–6.0; 40°C; 2 h	12
	2. Celluclast	pH 4.5–5.5; 60°C; 2 h	
Pea hulls	Pectinex Ultra SP-L plus Celluclast	pH 5.0; 40°C; 4 h	13
Apple pomace	Pectinex plus Celluclast	pH 5.0; 40°C; 4 h	13
Sugar beet pulp	Viscozyme	pH 4.5; 45°C; 4 h	14
Sugar beet pulp	Betanaza T	Applied during extrusion (mass temp. 85°C)	15
Purified potato fiber	Pectinex Ultra SP-L	pH 4.0; 45°C; 0–4 h	16
	Pectinex Ultra SP-L plus Celluclast	pH 4.0; 45°C; 0–4 h	16
Olive cake	Viscozyme plus Olivex	pH 5.0; 45°C; 3 h	17

[a]For purification conditions, see Ref. 7 as described in Table 1.

and vegetable pulps (18–20). Pectinol (Röhm GmbH, Darmstadt, Germany) as well as Pectinex Ultra SP-L (Novo Nordisk A/S) contain high polygalacturonase activities with pectinesterase, cellulase, and, in the case of Pectinex Ultra SP-L, pectin lyase and hemicellulase side activities (21,22) catalyzing a fast breakdown of pectin. They are suitable for loosening cell wall structures, which contain mainly insoluble pectin in the middle lamella. Pectinex (Novo Nordisk A/S), on the other hand, exhibits higher pectin lyase but lower polygalacturonase activities than Pectinex Ultra SP-L (22), an activity combination known to solubilize mainly dissolved pectins. Olivex (Novo Nordisk A/S), which is also characterized by pectolytic main as well as hemicellulose and cellulase side activities, was designed to increase the oil extractability by breaking down olive fruit cell walls (17). The hemicellulolytic preparations are more heterogeneous. Gamanase (Novo Nordisk A/S), causing a rapid viscosity decrease in galactomannans due to its endo activities (22), turned out to degrade insoluble wheat fiber hemicelluloses to the required extent (7). Pulpzyme (Novo Nordisk A/S), characterized as a xylanase preparation virtually free of cellulase, is utilized by the paper industry (22). Betanaza T (Pliva, Zagreb, Croatia) exhibits β-glucanase and xylanase activity (15). Viscozyme (Novo Nordisk A/S) is described as a multienzyme complex including a wide range of carbohydrases such as arabinanase, cellulase, β-glucanase, hemicellulase, and xylanase activities (22). The cellulases (Cellulase, Miles Laboratories, Elkhart, IL, and Celluclast, Novo Nordisk A/S) used in the examples described in Table 2 seem to be more pure, since various cellulolytic but no hemicellulose or pectolytic side activities were mentioned.

Prior to the incubation step, the fiber sources were ground to a suitable particle size in order to improve the susceptibility to enzymes, if necessary. Whereas most incubations were carried out in excess of water, several experiments were made with paste-like slurries of approximately 25% dry matter (13,15,17). Enzyme activity was stopped after the modification either by autoclaving (13) or by adding sodium hydroxide (14), both procedures causing a slight shift from insoluble to soluble fibers. Moreover, it was presumed that heating to 95°C to inactivate enzymes led to slight structural changes of cellulose and hemicelluloses in wheat bran (11). In small-scale assays inactivation was carried out in a boiling water bath (16). In some experiments the insoluble residues were separated by centrifugation and the soluble fibers precipitated. Oh and Grundleger (7) mixed both fractions after drying, whereas Kofod et al. (16) kept them separate. At a pilot-scale level soluble potato fibers were obtained by ultrafiltration and spray-drying (16). Pechanek et al. (12) removed most of the soluble compounds by decanting the supernatant. Modified products were mainly used as dry additives for fiber enrichment, ground to an appropriate particle size, if necessary. Caprez et al. (13) and Valiente et al. (17) incorporated the resulting pastes directly into different food products.

Aside from the optimized incubation conditions summarized in Table 2, the effects of enzyme concentration, pH, incubation temperature, and time were investigated in several experiments. Moreover, additional enzyme combinations were tested. An incubation with Celluclast alone was found to have a neglectible effect on sugar beet pulp (14). This result was to be expected because of the high content of pectic substances of the fiber source. On the other hand, treating a substrate rich in hemicelluloses and cellulose with pectolytic preparations did not cause any modifications either, as experiments with Pectinex and Pectinex Ultra SP-L on purified wheat fiber showed (7).

B. Effects of Enzyme Treatment on the Fiber Fraction

The effect of enzymatic modifications on the fiber fraction is summarized in Table 3. All figures are based on enzymatic-gravimetric determinations according to the AOAC method (23) or slightly modified procedures (24,25) and the Asp method (26) except for the experiments with purified wheat bran (7). These figures represent the relative recovery of insoluble and soluble dry matter corrected for starch, protein, and fat. The total fiber loss due to the enzyme treatment was reported to be less than 4.1%. In general, enzyme incubations led to a decrease in TDF combined with a shift from insoluble (IDF) to soluble fiber (SDF). The changes are more pronounced for fiber sources high in pectic substances than for substrates rich in cellulose and

Table 3 Effect of Enzymatic Modifications on Dietary Fibers: Decrease in Total Dietary Fiber (g/100 g) and Relative Proportion of Insoluble to Soluble Dietary Fiber (%)

Fiber source	TDF content		Relation IDF:SDF		Determination according to Ref.	Ref.
	Before	After	Before	After		
Purified wheat bran	—	—	84:16	70:30		7
Pea hulls[a]	90.2	85.5–73.7	92:8	85:15–83:17	24	13
Apple pomace[a]	68.0	56.4–52.2	76:24	67:33–64.36	24	13
Sugar beet pulp[a]	67.9	64.1–57.4	79:21	74:26–73:27	23	14
Sugar beet pulp[b]		66.3–47.2		75:25–72:28		
Sugar beet pulp	77.0	—	81:19	71:29–63:37	26	15
Olive cake[a]	80.2	73.5–71.3	92:8	89:11–92:8	24	17
Olive cake[b]		75.5–70.9		88:12–93:7		
Spelt wheat bran[c]	48.1	58.4	94:6	98:2	25	12
Pea bran[c]	89.2	79.0	93:7	94:6	25	12

TDF, Total dietary fiber; IDF, insoluble dietary fiber; SDF, soluble dietary fiber; —, no data reported.
[a] Depending on enzyme concentrations.
[b] Depending on incubation time.
[c] Soluble compounds not recovered.

hemicellulose. The proportion of soluble fiber could be increased to approximately one third in experiments with apple pomace and sugar beet pulp, but losses of total fiber of 23 and 30% respectively occurred. For apple pomace a ratio of 65:35 (IDF:SDF), causing a decrease of 20% of total fibers was considered as an optimum treatment (13), whereas the corresponding values for sugar beet pulp were reported to be 73:27 and 9% (14). Interestingly, enzyme treatment of sugar beet pulp during extrusion cooking did not change the total fiber content significantly (no exact data reported), but a pronounced solubilization occurred (15). Whether this effect was mainly due to the extremely mild extrusion conditions or due to the use of the restricted enzyme activities of Betanaza at a relatively high temperature remains unclear. However, extrusion cooking under increased thermal and mechanical energy inputs but without enzyme led to similar solubilization rates (15).

The solubilization degree of cellulose- and hemicellulose-rich fiber sources is less pronounced (Table 3). Consequently, the losses of total fibers did not exceed 18% even for severe treatments. Optimized values were reported to be a IDF:SDF ratio of 84:16 and a 12% fiber loss for pea hulls (13) and a 89:11 ratio and a 8% loss for olive cake (17). Results obtained with wheat bran (7) as well as spelt wheat bran and pea bran (12) are difficult to compare. Data for wheat bran were not determined analytically, whereas in the investigations with spelt wheat bran and pea bran, soluble compounds were discarded. This led to products with a very low soluble fiber content. For spelt grain, which turned out to be highly resistant even to the hemicellulose preparation Pulpzyme, an increase of 21% of total dietary fiber was observed, which was attributed to the removal of minerals and proteins during the whole procedure (12). An increase in soluble substances of about 20% depending on enzyme concentration and incubation time was reported for insoluble potato fiber (16), but no information about losses due to degradation of soluble fiber was given. However, an increased amount of glucose-containing small fragments indicating a loss of fiber material was detected. Similar decomposition patterns were observed for wheat bran carbohydrate fractions (11). Column chromatographic separation showed a clear disappearance of oligosaccharides, large amounts of glucose, and some xylose and arabinose in the cellulase-treated hydrolysates, whereas the pectinase preparation only led to minor decompositions. Not surprisingly, pronounced degradation mainly occurred in the hemicellulose and cellulose fractions, which are predominant in wheat bran. It could be demonstrated by microscopy, however, that the pectolytic preparation led to some cell wall maceration (11). Similarly, a distinct loosening of the cell wall matrix was observed in pea hulls after the treatment with Pectinex Ultra SP-L and Celluclast (E. Arrigoni, A. Caprez, H. Neukom, and R. Amadò, unpublished results, 1986). Treating potato pulp with a corresponding enzyme combination led to a very intense cell wall degradation in potato pulp, where only starch granules remained as intact structural components (21), whereas incubations with single enzyme preparations turned out to be less effective.

Molecular weight distributions after enzyme treatment resulted in different populations. Kofod et al. (16) determined approximately 75% of solubilized potato fiber to be mainly in a range of slightly above 100,000 and 25% smaller than 15,000. Concerning the soluble fraction of pea hulls and apple pomace, similar degradation patterns were observed independent from fiber source and enzyme combination used (E. Arrigoni, A. Caprez, H. Neukom, and R. Amadò, unpublished results, 1986). The high molecular weight fraction was found to be slightly decreased due to the enzyme treatment with two additional peaks appearing, representing degradation fragments in a molecular weight range of approximately 10,000 and 20,000.

C. Effects of Enzyme Treatment on Physical and Sensory Properties

Altering the fiber fraction quantitatively as well as qualitatively leads to changes in physical properties. Nevertheless, not much data is available in this respect. No changes of water-holding capacity were reported for spelt wheat bran (12). In contrast, a significant decrease from 5.1 to 2.8 g water/g dry matter occurred in the pea bran samples, despite the minor changes in chemical composition (Table 3), pointing to structural changes of the fiber fraction. Caprez et al. (13) measured a reduction from 3.2 to 2.5–1.8 g/g in their experiments with pea hulls. The considerable differences reported for the reference materials are difficult to explain, since both research groups used the same method to determine the water-holding capacity (27). However, variations in particle size could be partly responsible for these differences. Enzymatic modification of apple pomace led to a distinct decrease in water-binding capacity from 4.5 to 2.5–2.2 g/g correlating with the relatively high decrease of IDF (Table 3). Such decreases in water-binding capacities of the dietary fiber sources are of considerable advantage from a technological point of view. In contrast, the water absorption index of extruded sugar beet pulp samples was increased by approximately 50% following the enzyme treatment (15), clearly pointing to an increased gelling ability of the insoluble fraction. Since the considerably increased amount of soluble fibers (Table 3) was not taken into account, the behavior of this product in application can hardly be predicted.

Aside from hydration characteristics, lipid binding can be of importance from a technological point of view. Oil adsorption values were found to be reduced due to the enzyme treatments for pea hulls from 1.7 to 1.5–1.2 g/g dry matter and for apple pomace from 1.9 to 1.7–1.5 g/g, depending on the incubation conditions (13). These measurements are thought to give information about changes in surface characteristics, since oil is mainly adsorbed by mechanical entrapment (28). Soluble potato fiber, obtained from insoluble potato fiber after enzymatic modification, ultrafiltration, and spray-drying, did not exhibit any oil emulsifying ability (16), but the emulsifying capacity of whey proteins was found to be increased in presence of soluble potato fiber, presumably due to a fiber-protein interaction.

Sensory improvements due to enzymatic modifications were reported for pea bran (12). Pea hulls as well as apple pomace were characterized as homogeneous pastes with a softer texture having lost most of the grittiness of the corresponding milled fiber sources (29). These changes were also clearly visible as shown by photographs (13). Similar liquefaction effects were visualized recently on apple pomace modified with a new Pectinex preparation, which was specifically developed for pomace treatments (19).

D. Application Experiments with Enzymatically Modified Fiber Sources

Consumer acceptance is determined to a considerable extent by organoleptic properties of foods. Moreover, changes of functional characteristics can be of technological advantage in product development. Therefore, most of the investigators carried out application experiments to test the suitability of enzymatically modified fiber sources.

It is well known that fiber incorporation into bakery products can impair dough development as well as bread texture. The effect on bread quality was tested with different enzymatically treated dietary fiber sources. Pechanek et al. (12) showed that modified pea bran caused much smaller reductions of the specific bread volume compared to the untreated fiber product at replacement levels of 5–20%. Breads containing 10% of untreated or enzymatically modified pea hulls were evaluated by a test panel (E. Arrigoni, A. Caprez, H. Neukom, and R. Amadò, unpublished results, 1986). A triangle test revealed a significant difference, which was clearly attributed to the improved texture of the enzymatically treated sample. Modified spelt wheat fiber, however, affected bread volume to a greater extent than the corresponding raw material (12). This influence had to be expected, since the enzymatic treatment caused a 10% increase of mainly insoluble fibers without improving physicochemical or sensory properties. The addition of either 2.5% soluble or 2.5% insoluble potato fiber (16) influenced the specific volume of bread differently. No change compared to the control was observed for the soluble product, and neither taste nor appearance was affected. In contrast, a significant volume decrease was observed when the insoluble fraction was added. Italian focaccia bread containing pieces of olives was chosen to test the incorporation of untreated and enzymatically modified olive cake at a 10% replacement level of flour (17). Both additives decreased loaf volume and darkened crumb as well as crust. The bread containing untreated olive cake exhibited an unpleasant gritty texture, which was completely absent in the bread containing enzymatically modified olive cake. Although the chemical composition of the fiber fraction was not altered substantially (Table 3), cellulose and xylose containing hemicelluloses, representing the most important compounds of olive cake IDF, must have undergone relevant structural changes. Baking experiments with different types of pastries showed that apple pomace can easily be added to pastries without influencing their fine texture as long as the pleasant fruity taste of the fiber source corresponded to the end product (E. Arrigoni, A. Caprez, H. Neukom, and R. Amadò, unpublished results, 1986). Extruded rye snacks containing 5–10% raw or treated wheat bran or spelt wheat bran showed good sensory properties and texture (12).

Soluble potato fiber was further tested for applications aside from bakery products (16). An incorporation into sugar-free ice cream as a fat replacer at a 5% replacement level resulted in a higher melting point and a pleasant creamy texture. Addition of 2% to a protein diet drink increased the viscosity of the drink slightly, but no changes in organoleptic quality could be detected by trained panelists.

E. Effects of Enzyme Treatment on Physiological Properties

Modifications of wheat bran with Pectinol or Cellulase 36 were mainly carried out to increase protein digestibility (11). In vitro tests showed that, depending on the incubation conditions, increases of 69–93% were achieved. This effect was confirmed in vivo by rat-feeding trials with a Pectinol-treated wheat bran. Because of the pronounced disintegration of the cell wall matrix shown by microscopy, the susceptibility of digestive enzymes to aleurone cells was improved.

Studies with human volunteers were designed to test the influence of raw and modified pea fiber on defecation habits and blood lipids (12). In a first set-up, a daily intake of 15 g of untreated pea bran over a 4-week period led to a significant increase in stool weight and an even more pronounced decrease in transit time. Twenty grams of modified pea bran administered for 3 weeks to a different collective of volunteers in a second study also caused a significant increase in stool weight, but no change in transit time. Although differences in the study set-up make a comparison difficult, the in vivo water-binding capacity did not seem to be greatly affected by the enzyme treatment despite the considerable decrease found in the in vitro determinations (see Sec. III.C). This is not surprising, since the water-binding capacity can still be considered as high compared to other main constituents of the human diet (28). Neither untreated nor enzymatically modified pea bran affected any blood lipid and cholesterol levels (12).

IV. ENZYME TREATMENTS WITHIN PATENTED PROCEDURES

Enzyme treatments are also carried out as parts of more or less complex, patented procedures for fiber rich materials. Table 4 gives an overview over claims for enzymes and incubation conditions of such inventions. Because of the inclusions of wide variations in the claims and lack of experimental data, a detailed discussion of the influence of enzyme treatment is difficult. Mainly carhohydrases are applied for modifications, with the exeption of a claim for a protease, which is in an additional claim specified as trypsin (30). All enzyme activities mentioned in the claim by Karinen and Lehtomäki (31) are included in the preparation Econase, which is therefore

Table 4 Enzyme and Incubation Condition Claims in Patented Procedures to Modify Dietary Fiber Compounds

Fiber source	Enzyme activities	Conditions	Ref.
Raw materials derived from cereal grains	Protease		30
Fibrous materials	Cellulase, hemicellulase, β-glucanase, pec-tinase, and/or pro-tease	0–70°C; 0.5–4 h	31
Spent grain or oat bran	Hemicellulase and/or cellulase	50–55°C; 4–5 h	32
Apple pomace	SPS-ase and/or cellulase	10–65°C; 10 min to 15 h	33
Soy fiber material	Cellulase and carbohy-drase	pH 3.75–4.25; approx. 49–60°C	34

considered as a suitable product to modify cellulose-containing materials. The SPS-ase preparation applied on apple pomace (33) is described as a soluble polysaccharidase including pectinase, cellulase, and hemicellulase side activities. The carbohydrase to modify soy fiber comprises, according to the claim, a mixture of arabinanase, cellulase, β-glucanase, hemicellulase, and xylanase (34).

In order to increase the content of soluble dietary fiber, such as mixed-linked β-glucans and/or pentosans, of mainly oat, barley, or rye products, the cereals are processed with thermal, enzymatic, and/or osmotic treatments (30). Enzyme treatment is carried out to improve fiber solubility, if necessary. Precipitation at high temperatures with a polar solvent and separation of fine particles (mainly starch) are additional steps. It is stated that, due to a limited proteolysis, fiber solubility is improved by reducing the viscosity of β-glucans without changing their molecular weight. In contrast, enzyme preparations containing β-glucanase activity are applied to eliminate coarseness, unpleasant taste and dusting quality of fibrous materials of any cellulose-containing part of cereal plants (31). The enzymatically modified product, for example, from barley, is homogenized and separated by sieving to produce a fine fiber suitable as raw material in the foodstuff and animal fodder industry, but no application examples are provided. Fiber-containing drinks are produced from cereal dietary fiber sources by incubating spent grain or oat bran suspensions with hemicellulase and/or cellulase preparations (32). The resulting products, which may be homogenized and pasteurized, are claimed to contain up to 30 g/L of total dietary fiber, of which up to 10g/L can be insoluble. A technological reason is given for the enzymatic treatment of apple pomace, comminuted fruits, or vegetables (33). The application of the specified enzyme preparation makes it possible to increase juice yield and to improve pomace separation. A comparison with pectolytic and cellulolytic preparations shows that SPS-ase is approximately twice as effective in reducing juice viscosity. The enzymatic modification of a soy fiber slurry can be followed by a neutralization to pH 6.5–7.0, a jet cooking step, and/or spray-drying (34). This procedure does not cause a substantially reduced dietary fiber content but leads to improved sensory properties including smoothness and mouthfeel. Examples given include enzyme treatments with Celluclast and Viscozyme at pH 4.0 and 50°C for 1 and 2 hours, respectively. Sensory evaluations showed that both incubation times led to a considerable decrease in mouthfeel chalkiness of the products themselves as well as after their incorporation into skim milk. In an additional experiment, the optimum incubation conditions for pea hulls (see Table 2) as reported by Caprez et al. (13) were applied on soy fiber. The incubation with Pectinex Ultra SP-L and Celluclast led to a slightly lower fiber solubilization rate compared to the Celluclast and Viscozyme treatment, which was also reflected in moderately higher chalki-ness. This shows clearly that, depending on chemical composition and physicochemical proper-ties of a dietary fiber source, different incubation conditions have to be applied in order to reach the desired functional changes.

V. CONCLUSIONS AND PERSPECTIVES

The high hydration capacities of dietary fiber components can make an incorporation of fiber sources into food products difficult. Moreover, consumer acceptance is greatly affected by their organoleptic properties. Enzymatic modifications offer a possibility to overcome these draw-backs. An improvement of functional and sensory properties can be achieved by a slight solubili-zation of the fiber fraction by appropriate enzymes. Depending on the chemical composition, different combinations of pectolytic, cellulolytic, and hemicellulolytic preparations have to be applied. Great care is needed to find the optimum conditions leading to the required improve-ments without losing the physiologically beneficial properties. Application experiments, mainly in the field of cereal processing, showed that the substitution level can be increased if enzymati-cally modified fiber sources are incorporated into food products. The removal of digestible compounds due to amylolysis and/or proteolysis, on the other hand, causing a considerable increase in the dietary fiber content but only minor structural changes, did not seem to lead to the desired improvements.

An alternative to the addition of enzymatically modified fiber sources to refined products could be the application of enzymes during processing of fiber-rich foods such as whole grain products. A correspondent set-up was tested recently in wheat breads supplemented with 5% of rye bran (35). The addition of Fermizyme H, an α-amylase preparation containing a standardized hemicellulase activity (Gist Brocades, Delft, The Netherlands), resulted in improved bread qual-ity compared to the fiber-enriched product without enzyme. In addition, the ratio between soluble and insoluble fiber was considerably altered with increased amounts of soluble pentosans. More-over, it was shown that a pure hemicellulase preparation was less effective. It is expected that hemicellulases establish their importance aside from amylases and proteases in cereal processing (36). In addition, endogenous enzymes, which are mainly located in the fiber-rich parts of the grain, could play a role in solubilizing nutrionally important polysaccharides.

Dietary fiber sources may be utilized increasingly as starting materials for the production of functional ingredients or of flavor compounds (e.g., vanillin) by applying cell wall macerating enzymes to improve the extractability of specific compounds. The production of water-soluble arabinoxylans by treating rice or wheat bran with a cellulase preparation has been described in a patent (37). Tailoring of polysaccharides by means of enzymes has been described as a interest-ing new technique to achieve desirable functional properties (38). However, specific enzyme attacks in order to design functional ingredients require detailed information about the polymer structure. Therefore, this technique will be restricted to homogeneous polysaccharides.

Modern biotechnology as well as genetic engineering are the techniques of choice in order to produce enzyme preparations containing specific activity spectra. The exclusion of undesired side activities enabling a better control of breakdown patterns could help to facilitate enzymatic modifications of such complex matrices as dietary fiber.

ACKNOWLEDGMENT

The author wishes to thank Prof. Dr. Renato Amadò for critically reviewing the manuscript.

REFERENCES

1. Cummings JH, Frølich W. Dietary fibre intakes in Europe. Luxembourg: Office for Official Publications of the European Communities, 1993.
2. Mori B, Nakaji S, Sugawara K, Ohta M, Iwane S, Munakata A, Yoshida Y, Ohi G. Proposal for recommended level of dietary fiber intake in Japan. Nutr Res 16:53–60, 1996.
3. Ganji V, Betts N. Fat, cholesterol, fiber and sodium intakes of US population: evaluation of diets reported in 1987–88 Nationwide Food Consumption Survey. Eur J Clin Nutr 49:915–920, 1995.
4. Grohmann K, Bothast RJ. Pectin-rich residues generated by processing of citrus fruits, apples, and sugar beets: enzymatic hydrolysis and biological conversion to value-added products. In: Himmel ME, Baker JO, Overend RP, eds. Enzymatic Conversion of Biomass for Fuels Production. Washington, DC: American Chemical Society, 1994, pp. 372–390.
5. Lacourse NL, Chicola K, Zallie JP, Altieri PA. Dietary fiber derived from cassava. Eur. Patent 552478 (1993).
6. Hoebler C, Barry J-L, David A, Kozlowsi F. Enzymatic preparation and analysis of dietary fibre residues, suitable for in vitro fermentation studies. Food Hydrocoll 5:35–40, 1991.
7. Oh YN, Grundleger ML. Improvement in soluble fiber content of wheat fiber through enzymatic modification. J Agric Food Chem 38:1142–1145, 1990.
8. Rasco BA, Borhan M, Yegge JM, Lee MH, Siffring K, Bruinsma B. Evaluation of enzyme and chemically treated wheat bran ingredients in yeast-raised breads. Cereal Chem 68:295–299, 1991.
9. Nebesny E. Utilization of potato pulp for baking of bread. Starch/Stärke 47:36–39, 1995.
10. Hoebler C, Barry J-L, Kozlowsi F, David A. Study of enzymatic preparation of cell wall residue. Sci Alim 10:255–263, 1990.
11. Saunders RM, Connor MA, Edwards RH, Kohler GO. Enzymatic processing of wheat bran: effects on nutrient availability. Cereal Chem 49:436–442, 1972.
12. Pechanek U, Pfannhauser W, Holler C, Irsliger K, Pintscher H. Chemical and physiological aspects of enzyme-modified fibre. Eur J Clin Nutr 49 (suppl 3):S291–S295, 1995.
13. Caprez A, Arrigoni E, Neukom H, Amadò R. Improvement of the sensory properties of two different dietary fibre sources through enzymatic modification. Lebensm Wiss Technol 20:245–250, 1987.
14. Quaglia GB, Carletti G. Enzymatic treatments for the production of modified dietary fibre. Eur J Clin Nutr 49 (suppl 3):S130–S133, 1995.
15. Jezek D, Curic D, Karlovic D, Tripalo B. Production of soluble fibres from sugar beet pulp with Betanaza T enzyme in the extrusion process. Chem Biochem Eng Q 10:103–106, 1996.
16. Kofod LV, Norsker M, Adler-Nissen J. Enzymatic modification of potato fibre. In: Meuser F, Manners DJ, Seibel W, eds. Progress in Plant Polymeric Carbohydrate Research. Hamburg: Behr's Verlag, 1995, pp. 207–211.
17. Valiente C, Arrigoni E, Esteban RM, Amadò R. Chemical composition of olive by-product and modifications through enzymatic treatments. J Sci Food Agric 69:27–32, 1995.
18. Urlaub R. Advantages of enzymatic apple mash treatment and pomace liquefaction. Fruit Proc 6:399–406, 1996.
19. Stutz C. Enzymatische Verflüssigung: Vision oder Tatsache? Flüssiges Obst 63:371–373, 1996.
20. Siliha H, El-Zoghbi M, Labib A, Askar A. Effect of enzymatic treatment of carrot puree. Fruit Proc 5:318, 320–322, 1995.
21. Dongowski G. Untersuchungen an Kartoffelpülpe als Ballaststoffquelle. Zum Einfluss von pektolytischen und cellulolytischen Enzymen. Starch/Stärke 45:166–171, 1993.
22. Novo Nordisk A/S, Bagsvaerd, Denmark. Different product descriptions (1984–1996).
23. Prosky L, Asp NG, Schweizer TF, DeVries JW, Furda I. Determination of insoluble/soluble and total dietary fiber in foods and food products: interlaboratory study. J Assoc Off Analyt Chem 71:1017–1023, 1988.
24. Arrigoni E, Caprez A, Amadò R, Neukom H. Gravimetric method for the determination of insoluble and soluble dietary fibre. Z Lebensm Unters Forsch 178:195–198, 1984.
25. Swiss Food Manual. Chapter 22, method 8.1. Berne: Eidgenössische Druck- und Materialzentrale, 1991.

26. Asp NG, Johansson CG, Hallmer H, Siljeström M. Rapid enzymatic assay of insoluble and soluble dietary fiber. J Agric Food Chem 31:476–482, 1983.

27. Caprez A, Arrigoni E, Amadò R, Neukom H. Influence of different types of thermal treatment on the chemical composition and physical properties of wheat bran. J Cereal Sci 4:233–239, 1986.

28. Amadò R. Physico-chemical properties related to type of dietary fibre. In: Amadò R, Barry J-L, Frølich W, eds. Physico-chemical Properties of Dietary Fibre and Effect of Processing on Micronutrients Availability. Luxembourg: Commission of the European Communities, 1994, pp. 49–54.

29. Arrigoni E, Caprez A, Amadò R. Influence of enzymic treatment on the physico-chemical and sensory properties of dietary fibre sources. Eur J Clin Nutr 49 (suppl 3):S253, 1995.

30. Mälkki Y, Myllymäki O. A method for enriching soluble dietary fibre. PCT International Patent Application WO 94/28742 (1994).

31. Karinen P, Lehtomäki I. Procedure for producing fine fibre, and fine fibre. PCT International Patent Application WO 90/10392 (1990).

32. Tretzel J. Wässeriges Ballaststoffkonzentrat enthaltend Getreidefasern. German Patent DE 4226245 (1994).

33. Dörreich KA. Enzymatic treatment of pomace. U.S. Patent 4483875 (1984).

34. Wong TM, Singer DA, Lin SHC. Modified soy fiber material of improved sensory properties. U.S. Patent 5508172 (1996).

35. Laurikainen T, Härkönen H, Autio K, Poutanen K. Effects of enzymes in fibre-enriched baking. J Sci Food Agric 76:239–249, 1998.

36. Poutanen K. Enzymes: an important tool in the improvement of the quality of cereal foods. Trends Food Sci Technol 8:300–306, 1997.

37. Shiiba K, Yamada H. Water-soluble arabinoxylan preparation. Jpn. Patent 5219976 (1993).

38. Shirakawa M, Yamatoya K, Nishinari K. Tailoring of xyloglucan properties using an enzyme. Food Hydrocoll 12:25–28, 1998.

19

Chemistry, Architecture, and Composition of Dietary Fiber from Plant Cell Walls

Alistair James MacDougall and Robert Rasiah Selvendran*
B. B. S. R. C. Institute of Food Research, Colney, Norwich, England

I. INTRODUCTION

A.   Dietary Fiber Definition and Measurement

Dietary fiber (DF) was originally defined as ''the skeletal remains of plant cells in our diet that are resistant to hydrolysis by the digestive enzymes of man.'' Later this definition was extended to include polysaccharide food additives. However, these compounds contribute only about 3% of the DF content of most diets, so that the bulk of DF can be said to come from the cell walls of edible plant organs (1,2).

So far, the main emphasis in the measurement of DF has been to determine the actual amount of DF polymers present in the diet. Values for DF can be obtained from a measure of the nonstarch polysaccharides plus lignin in the diet, and methods have been developed to make determinations of DF on this basis for a range of plant foods (3–7). However these values for DF alone are not particularly meaningful, because they do not take into account the architecture of the cell wall in different cell types, the assembly of the cell types in different tissues, and the effects of cooking and processing on the properties and behavior of cell wall polymers. A short review covering these aspects, based mainly on work up to 1992, has been published (18). Early attempts to begin to address this lack of information on the natural state of DF polymers in the plant cell wall suffered from several serious deficiencies. These include (a) the presence of contaminating intracellular polymers in the cell walls analyzed, (b) degradation of polysaccharides during the extraction procedures, (c) little appreciation of the structure of the polysaccharides extracted from the cell walls of various tissue types, and (d) a lack of information on glycoproteins and phenolics. It is only since the early 1980s, when techniques were developed specifically for the isolation of gram quantities of relatively pure cell walls from edible plant organs and for the extraction of polymers from the cell wall material (CWM) with minimal degradation, that significant progress has been possible in this area (9,10). Most of the available information on the cell walls of edible plant organs up to 1984 has been summarized in two reviews (11,12), and additional information was included in a subsequent review (1). These reviews should be consulted for a better appreciation of this chapter. In this chapter we shall

---

*Retired.

attempt to present a view of cell wall polysaccharides and of the cell wall matrix that is emerging from more recent work (1985 onwards), using improved methods for isolating and analyzing cell walls. Particular advances have been made in methods of isolation, fractionation, and analysis of different polysaccharide fractions from cell walls. Important examples include the use of improved techniques of chromatography, gel filtration, ultra-centrifugation, and electrophoresis; the use of highly purified enzymes for specific degradation of polymers; the ability to characterize less than 25 mg of material by GLC-MS and HPLC-MS, MS-MS, and ^{1}H- and ^{13}C-NMR spectroscopy (NMR being particularly of value in determining anomeric configurations). (For a general description of the chemistry of plant cell wall polymers, see Refs. 13–17.) The group at the Complex Carbohydrate Research Center (Athens, Georgia) has used highly sophisticated analytical techniques to unravel the structure of complex plant cell wall polysaccharides. The main purpose of this chapter is to focus on the work done on cell walls of edible plant organs in a DF context. To this end the principles underlying some of the methods of isolation and fractionation and brief descriptions of the methods are given to make the results more meaningful. Where necessary, the results of recent investigations will be compared with earlier work, and most of the comments will be restricted to the cell walls of edible plant organs.

B. Cell Walls in the Diet

The cell walls that make up the DF content of the diet are derived from the wide range of plant organs that provide the fruits and vegetables, and cereals, found in the diet (Table 1). Even if one considers only those foodstuffs that are eaten in sufficient quantity to contribute significantly to the intake of DF, almost all the possible different parts of the plant are found. When less commonly eaten foods are included, for instance, globe artichoke (flower bracts), the list becomes nearly complete. Table 1 shows that both monocots and dicots are well represented in

Table 1 Different Edible Plant Organs and Their Dietary Fiber Content[a]

	Dicots	Monocots
Roots	Carrot (2.5) Turnip (5.7) Sweet potato (2.4) Red beet (2.5)	Palmyra (seedling root)
Tuber, corm, rhizome	Potato (1.2)	Taro Yam (1.2)
Stems	Bean shoots	Asparagus (1.7) Bamboo shoot
Leaves	Cabbage (1.6–3.7) Spinach (1.6)	Leek (2.3) Onion (1.9)
Flowers	Cauliflower (1.7) Calabrese (2.7)	—
Fruits	Tomato (1.0) Bean (3) Apple (1.6–2.0) Mango (2.6)	Pineapple (1.2) Plantain (1.2) Banana (1.1) Date (4.0)
Seeds	Peas (3–5)[b] Pulses (5–16)[b]	Coconut (7.3) Sweet corn (2.7) Barley Oats Rice Wheat

[a] Figures in parentheses are total DF content in g/100 g fresh weight (4).
[b] Soaked for 20 h.

most categories and that the DF content of most vegetables and fruit lies in the range of 1.5–2.5% of fresh weight. It can be seen that there is a large variation in the DF content of soaked legume seeds.

In order to understand the cell wall chemistry of these plant organs, the apparent complexity of cell type in each fruit or vegetable is best viewed as the differentiation of the basic cell type formed by the meristematic cells. Nuclear division of the meristematic cells is followed by formation of a cell plate. Pectic polysaccharides, and in particular their calcium salts, are deposited on this plate by each of the daughter cells to form a layer of intercellular cement known as the middle lamella. This is followed by the deposition of cellulose, hemicelluloses, additional pectic polysaccharides, glycoproteins, proteoglycans, and phenolics to form the primary wall. Deposition of all the polymers within the wall takes place in an organized and controlled manner. The expansion and vacuolation of these cells during organ growth and development give rise to a bulky undifferentiated tissue—the parenchyma. This tissue is characterized by having large cells and thin cell walls, which have a simple appearance under the electron microscope, consisting of a primary cell wall separated from the adjacent cell wall by the middle lamella region. In considering the detailed composition of the cell walls of edible plants later in this chapter, the parenchyma cell wall will be described at some length. In most of the plants eaten, and particularly in fruits, the parenchyma forms the bulk of the organ—indeed it is the predominance of this thin-walled, highly vacuolated tissue that makes these foods succulent and attractive to eat. In vegetables, where lignification tends to occur more commonly, the product is usually eaten in an immature state before the tougher lignified tissues have time to develop, and breeding programs are specifically designed to produce vegetables with reduced lignification (e.g., snap beans). Parenchyma cell walls are therefore the biggest contributor to DF in the diet.

During the development of a plant organ, new cell types are formed from the cambial tissues. These cells differentiate to form vascular tissues (xylem and phloem), epidermal tissues, storage tissues (endosperm), and a variety of other specialized cell types (sclerenchyma, stone cells, endodermis). In almost all of these examples new polymers are laid down, and in some cases the cell wall may be considerably thickened. These alterations can lead to a large change in the properties of the cell wall. The presence of these differentiated cell types in foods contributes significantly to the variation in DF content and properties. In certain instances where extraction procedures or processing methods lead to the enrichment of foods in specialized cell types (e.g., lignified tissues and thick-walled aleurone layer cells in wheat bran), their contribution to DF is increased significantly above that of the parenchyma/endospermous cell wall. And in the extreme case deliberate extraction of certain plant materials such as guar seed or brown algae (which give alginates) yields polysaccharide food additives of defined and specialized origin.

To illustrate the extent of the complexity of cell type that can result in a fully developed plant organ, Figures 1 and 2 show a transverse section through a runner bean pod (dicot) and an asparagus spear (monocot), giving the main cell types and the cell wall polymers particularly associated with each. For runner bean, the inner parenchyma layer is the source of material for the studies described in later sections in this chapter.

II. CELL WALL PURIFICATION AND SEQUENTIAL EXTRACTION OF POLYMERS

A. Cell Wall Purification

In order to carry out chemical analysis of the cell wall to determine its constitution, it is first necessary to obtain pure CWM free from contamination with intracellular compounds. In earlier work contamination with intracellular proteins and starch were particular problems (9). Even

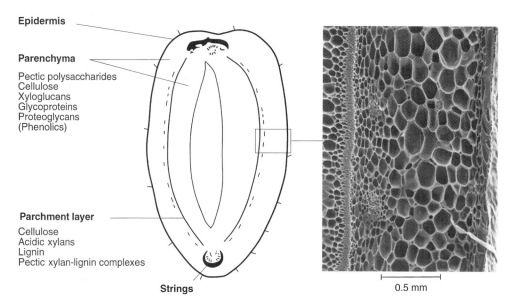

Fig. 1 Line diagram of a cross section of a mature runner bean pod showing the main polymers present in different tissue types. The inset scanning electron micrograph shows the variation in cell size and cell arrangement in the part of the pod from the epidermal cells to the inner parenchyma. The thick-walled cells on the left of the micrograph constitute the parchment layer. (Photograph ML Parker.)

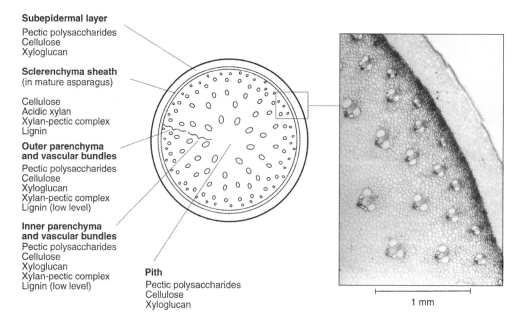

Fig. 2 Line diagram of a cross section of a mature asparagus stem showing the main polymers present in different tissue types. The inset light micrograph shows the variation in cell size and cell arrangement.

low levels of contaminating intracellular protein may prejudice the analysis of the cell wall proteins that play an important role in the wall, but which are present in relatively small amounts. Intracellular protein is effectively solubilized by sodium dodecyl sulfate (SDS) and/or phenol: acetic acid:water (PAW) (9). For protein-rich tissues (e.g., seeds) both treatments are required for complete removal of contaminating intracellular protein (9). PAW is also useful in ensuring the inactivation of cell wall enzymes, which is an especially important consideration in the study of fruit cell walls. Without this precaution the high levels of hydrolytic enzymes can cause degradation of polymers during extraction (18). In more recent work on fruit cell walls, phenol saturated with Tris buffer has been preferred to PAW because the acidity of the PAW leads to calcium depletion of the cell wall and solubilization of ionically bound pectic polysaccharides (19). While the pectic polysaccharides extracted from tomato cell walls prepared with buffered phenol have been shown to be uncontaminated with protein (20), the extent to which buffered phenol is generally effective at removing contaminating protein from plant cell walls is unclear. The high levels of starch present in certain tissues can only effectively be removed by using 90% aqueous dimethyl sulfoxide (DMSO) (9). Particular caution is needed in the use of starch-degrading enzymes, since many commercial preparations contain other activities, which lead to degradation of the cell wall polymers. In Table 2 a typical protocol for the preparation of pure CWM from fruits and vegetables is given. After initial blending of the tissue and filtration or centrifugation, ball-milling is used to completely disrupt the cell structure and enable complete removal of contaminants. Using 50 g fresh weight of starting material one would expect a yield of approximately 0.6 g dry weight CWM. In most vegetables and mature unripe fruits about 6–8% of the CWM is solubilized during the purification process, the bulk of this in step 2. In ripe fruits larger amounts of polymer are solubilized during cell wall preparation, and in this case it is better to use a hot-alcohol–insoluble residue, extracted with PAW (or buffered phenol), and 90% aq. DMSO, for cell wall analysis. Extraction in hot alcohol does not lead to significant degradation by β-elimination because of the low water content of the alcohol solution, but this type of preparation is not suitable for studies on cell wall glycoproteins because co-precipitating proteins in the AIR cannot be solubilized quantitatively.

Table 2 Typical Protocol for Preparation of Purified Cell Wall Material[a]

Step	Treatment	Comment
1.	Homogenize in 1.5% aq sodium dodecyl sulfate (SDS) containing 5 mM $Na_2S_2O_5$ and centrifuge	Removes bulk of intracellular compounds; $Na_2S_2O_5$ prevents oxidation of phenolics
2.	Ball-mill residue in 0.5% SDS containing 3mM $Na_2S_2O_5$ for 15 h at 2°C	Breaks up cells not ruptured in 1; some cold-water-soluble pectic polysaccharides solubilized
3.	Extract twice with phenol:acetic acid:water (2:1:1, w/v/v) and wash thoroughly.	Removes proteins, lipids, SDS, and some starch; inactivates enzymes
4.	Extract twice with 90% aq. dimethyl sulfoxide (DMSO)	Removes starch, quantitatively
5.	Wash thoroughly and dialyze to remove DMSO	

[a] This example is for potato. Between each step, cell wall material is collected by filtration or centrifugation.

B. Sequential Extraction of Cell Wall Polymers

Extraction of polymers under degradative conditions in the past led to misleading results. This problem may be illustrated by the debate over the existence of neutral pectic polysaccharides, which for a long time were thought to exist as separate entities from the galacturonic acid–containing pectic polysaccharides. Using hot water or hot oxalate, galactans (21,22) and arabinans (23) can be obtained from certain vegetable cell walls, and the isolation of these polysaccharides from a number of other plant tissues has been reported (13,24). Through work on apple and sugar beet pectic polysaccharides, these results can be explained as the degradation of highly methyl esterified pectic polysaccharides in which the neutral side chains are clustered into hairy regions (8,25–28). Random cleavage of the methyl esterified galacturonan backbone by β-elimination caused by heat treatment (Fig. 3) leads to the release of short lengths of polysaccharide highly enriched in neutral sugars (12). Careful extraction made under the mild conditions described below yields a range of differently branched pectic polysaccharides with galactan and arabinan side chains but only very small amounts of the galactans or arabinans previously found (29–31).

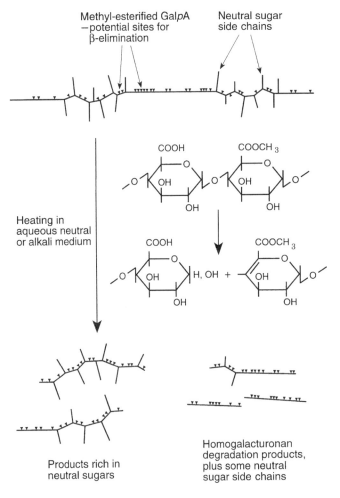

Fig. 3 Diagram showing the mechanism and main products of β-eliminative degradation of pectic polysaccharides.

Table 3 Treatments Used for Sequential Extraction of Purified Cell Wall Material and Major Classes of Polymer Released from Parenchyma Cell Walls at Each Stage

Extraction treatment	Main classes of polysaccharide solubilized
1. CDTA 50 mM	Slightly branched pectic polysaccharides
2. CDTA 50 mM (repeat)	Slightly branched pectic polysaccharides
3. Na_2CO_3 50 mM, 1°C	Branched pectic polysaccharides
4. Na_2CO_3 50 mM	Branched pectic polysaccharides
5. KOH 0.5 M	Branched (and some highly branched) pectic polysaccharides and some highly branched xyloglucans
6. KOH 1 M	Branched xyloglucans
7. KOH 4 M	Branched xyloglucans
8. KOH 4 M + 3% boric acid	Slightly branched xyloglucans

Treatments are carried out at 20°C unless specified.
Material that remains insoluble after step 8 is called α-cellulose residue and invariably contains other polymers including highly branched pectic polysaccharides and some hydroxyproline-rich glycoproteins.
CDTA, cyclohexanediamine tetraacetate, sodium salt.

The extraction of cell wall polymers in an undegraded form is a particular requirement for studies on cooking or processing, where one is studying the degradation caused by these processes. Significant changes could easily be masked by degradative events occurring during cell wall extraction. However, to some extent, the results of work using the earlier methods can be reinterpreted in the light of our understanding of polymer breakdown during extraction. An outline of a method we used for sequential extraction of the purified CWM is given in Table 3, together with the broad categories of polymers released at each stage. This method of extraction has been used on a number of different vegetables and fruits, yielding broadly similar results in the various classes of polymer found. Differences are experienced in the ease of extraction of the polymers depending on the levels of phenolics (as distinct from lignin) in the primary cell wall and on the levels of glycoproteins, as both are agents that appear to reduce the extractability of the polymers in the wall (12,31). One example of the changes that these compounds can cause is red beet, which has a cell wall composition similar to sugar beet. Much work has been done on the composition of the CWM from sugar beet pulp with a view to using it as a DF source (see Chapter 29). The prolonged cooking needed for red beet is a reflection of the extent of phenolic crosslinking throughout the primary wall and across the middle lamella region.

III. POLYMERS FOUND IN THE PLANT CELL WALL

The discussion of the cell wall polymers is divided into three sections: fruits and vegetables, dicotyledonous seeds, and monocotyledonous seeds. Experience of analysis of the cell walls of monocot vegetables (e.g., onion, asparagus) shows that they are very similar to dicots. Monocot vegetables are therefore not discussed separately.

A. Fruits and Vegetables

1. Parenchyma Cell Walls

a. Pectic Polysaccharides. Pectic polysaccharides are chiefly composed of (1,4)-linked α-D-galacturonosyl residues, which are partially methyl esterified. Interspersed with the galacturonosyl residues are rhamnosyl residues, which are joined into the backbone of the pectic polysaccharide by $(1 \to 2)$ linkages and which may also carry side chains composed mainly of galactosyl and arabinosyl residues attached to C-4 (13). The frequency with which the rhamnosyl residues occur in the galacturonan backbone varies, averaging between 1 in 50 and 1 in 15, depending on the tissue and the stage in the sequential extraction at which it is isolated (29–31). The (1,2) linking of rhamnosyl residues alters the conformation of the pectic polysaccharide, because linkage to adjacent carbons on the rhamnose sugar ring puts a bend in the backbone. Evidence for the attachment of side chains mostly to C-4 of (1,2) linked rhamnosyl residues has been obtained for several plant tissues (32). Early estimates of the molecular weight of pectic polysaccharides in the literature give values from 30,000 to 200,000 daltons (28), but milder conditions of extraction give much higher values, and it would appear that these are more reliable. Nevertheless, the estimation of the molecular weight of pectic polysaccharides is not easy because of their tendency to aggregate (28).

At least three classes of pectic polysaccharides can be distinguished, appearing at different stages in the extraction procedure given in Table 3. Cyclohexanediamine tetraacetate, sodium salt (CDTA) solubilizes highly methyl esterified pectic polysaccharides, which have a long backbone containing relatively few rhamnosyl residues and only a few short side chains. In pectic polysaccharides of this type extracted from runner bean and potato, side chains have been estimated from methylation analysis to be two residues long on average (30,31). The fact that the extractant CDTA is a powerful chelating agent suggests that these pectic polysaccharides are bound into the cell wall by calcium bridges (see Sec. IV). The bulk of this class of pectic polysaccharides is believed to be of middle lamella origin, because some tissues show cell separation when they are placed in solutions of CDTA [e.g., tissues from mature unripe tomato and pear, and rhubarb stem (our unpublished observations)]. The molecular weight of the CDTA-extracted pectic polysaccharides from cider apples, determined by light-scattering, is reported to be 600,000–700,000 daltons on average (33).

A second class of pectic polysaccharides is solubilized by dilute Na_2CO_3. Dilute Na_2CO_3 at 1°C deesterifies the pectic polysaccharides without causing significant β-elimination and increases their solubility. These pectic polysaccharides are quite highly branched (Fig. 4) and are generally highly methyl esterified. This can be inferred from the fact that the degree of methyl esterification (DM) of the pectic polysaccharides present in the CDTA-extracted CWM is generally very high. Careful analysis using ^{13}C-NMR (34) and methylation analysis (29,31,34) of pectic polysaccharides extracted with Na_2CO_3 shows that the side chains are from 7–9 residues

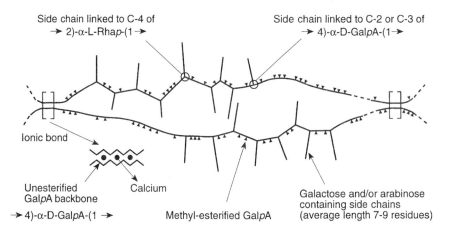

Side chain linked to C-4 of
→ 2)-α-L-Rhap-(1 →

Side chain linked to C-2 or C-3 of
→ 4)-α-D-GalpA-(1 →

Ionic bond

Unesterified
GalpA backbone

Calcium

→ 4)-α-D-GalpA-(1 →

Methyl-esterified GalpA

Galactose and/or arabinose
containing side chains
(average length 7-9 residues)

Fig. 4 Generalized diagram of the structural features of pectic polysaccharides of the primary cell wall.

in length on average. Close analysis of the structure of a similar class of pectic polysaccharides from apples suggests that the molecule is composed of short stretches of polygalacturonic acid interspersed with so-called hairy regions where the rhamnosyl residues are common (28,35), and a significant proportion of the rhamnosyl residues carry side chains composed of a variety of neutral sugars. Removal of the side chains from apple pectin followed by cleavage of the backbone between adjacent rhamnosyl and galacturonosyl residues (with rhamnogalacturonase) has revealed the presence of xylosyl substituents attached to galacturonosyl residues in the backbone of the pectic polysaccharide (36). Pectic polysaccharides extracted with Na_2CO_3 from cider apples and examined with light-scattering techniques behave in a manner consistent with a branched crosslinked microgel structure (33).

The third class of pectic polysaccharides is that associated with the α-cellulose residue, which remains after all the steps in Table 3 have been carried out. From the composition of the residue of a number of plants given in Table 4, it can be seen that pectic polysaccharides account for up to 50% of this residue. In potato this pectic fraction has been shown to be highly branched, containing mainly linear galactose side chains, which have a degree of polymerization (DP) varying between 6 and 10 (P. Ryden, N. M. Rigby, and R. R. Selvendran, unpublished results). The association of pectic polysaccharides with the α-cellulose residue is not found to any significant extent with material from heavily lignified tissues—e.g., runner bean parchment layer (37) and olive seed hull (38). In runner bean parchment layer this residue is approximately 90% cellulose (Table 4). These observations are significant for the structure of the cell wall of soft tissues. They suggest that while the bulk of the pectic polysaccharides (and xyloglucans) can readily be extracted from the CWM, a certain amount of the pectic polysaccharide remains behind because it is enmeshed with the cellulose microfibrils. It is possible that the association of cellulose microfibrils (and associated xyloglucan) with a proportion of the pectic polysaccharides takes place during the extrusion of the cellulose into the cell wall. It is therefore possible to speculate that these highly branched pectic polysaccharides play a role, together with the hydroxyproline-rich glycoproteins, in certain tissues (e.g., runner bean parenchyma) in enmeshing the cellulose microfibrils and associated xyloglucans, helping them to disperse within the wall matrix. The bulk of the pectic polysaccharides in the α-cellulose residue can be released using cellulase digestion to degrade the cellulose of the residue (30). The proportion of the total

Table 4   Composition[a] of α-Cellulose Residue from Different Sources

	Onion (29)	Apple (104)	Potato (31)	Runner bean parenchyma[b] (30) Prechlorite	Runner bean parenchyma[b] (30) Postchlorite	Runner bean parchment layer[c] (81)
Rha	0.7	3	1	1	0.7	0.2
Ara	1	12	5	11	4	0.3
Xyl	0.5	5	0.3	2	0.8	4
Man	2	2	0.8	3	2	0.5
Gal	19	6	35	7	3	0.3
Glc	50	41	42	64	55	86
Uronic acid	10	21	12	10	8	4
Total sugars	83	90	96	98	74	95

[a] Anhydro sugars (g/100 g dry weight).
[b] The runner bean residue was obtained before and after a chlorite/acetic acid extraction, which solubilizes phenolics and glycoproteins.
[c] The parchment layer is as shown in Fig. 1.

pectic polysaccharide of the wall found in each of the classes described above varies from tissue to tissue. The ratio of pectic polysaccharide that is CDTA extractable : Na_2CO_3 + 0.5 M KOH extractable : that in the α-cellulose residue can be estimated from the sum of the galacturonic acid, galactose, and arabinose found in each of the fractions. Typical ratios for parenchyma cell walls are onion (2:6:2), potato (2:3:5), olive pulp (2:3:2), and runner bean (6:3:1).

The recognition of these different classes of pectic polysaccharides in the cell wall has been a direct result of the use of milder nondegradative methods of extraction. As discussed above, previous methods tended to break up the polymer through β-elimination and cause the release of fragments rich in neutral sugars derived from the hairy regions. Careful analysis of the hairy regions of pectic polysaccharides has been carried out by Albersheim and coworkers. Working mainly with suspension culture tissues, they have used polygalacturonase to deliberately degrade the predominantly galacturonic acid containing part of the pectic molecule and release the neutral sugar-rich regions. From this work they have described two polysaccharides, rhamnogalacturonan-I (RG-I) and rhamnogalacturonan-II (RG-II) (15,32). RG-I was first isolated from suspension culture tissues of sycamore. It is a polysaccharide of DP 1000–2000, and it contains alternating rhamnosyl and galacturonosyl residues in a backbone of up to 600 residues. Side chains are attached to half of the rhamnosyl residues, and they average seven residues in length. The side chains have been isolated for further study by cleavage of the backbone with lithium in ethylenediamine to release individual side chains with a rhamnitol residue attached (39). They contain predominantly galactose and arabinose in a wide range of different combinations and may be up to 15 residues long. Pectic polysaccharides containing the RG-I moiety can be inferred to be present in the highly branched pectic polysaccharides of a range of tissues and comprise about 3–4% of the dry weight of the cell walls. RG-II has a DP of about 60 and is notable for the large number of different sugar residues it contains. About 17 different sugars are present, including some very unusual sugars such as aceric acid and ketodeoxyoctulosonic acid. These sugars are believed to be linked as side chains to a rhamnogalacturonan core. Because it has proved possible to isolate pure fractions of specific oligosaccharides, it has been suggested that these sugars appear as side chains of commonly recurring structure (32). The rhamnose linkage pattern within the molecule differs from RG-I in that it can be (1 → 3), (1 → 3, 4), (1 → 2, 3, 4), or terminal, unlike RG-I where the linkage pattern is usually (1 → 2) or (1 → 2, 4). Based on the detection of the unusual sugars found in RG-II, evidence for the presence of this polysaccharide has been found in a wide range of plants (32).

b. Hemicelluloses. Xyloglucans are the predominant hemicellulosic polysaccharides of parenchyma cell walls and make up 7–10% of the wall dry weight. Xyloglucans contain a cellulosic (1 → 4)-β-D-glucan backbone to which short side chains are attached to C-6 of about one half of the glucosyl residues (13). In each side chain xylosyl residues are the first sugar residues attached to the backbone, but these side chains, which are generally one to three residues long, may contain arabinosyl, galactosyl, or fucosyl residues as well. The occurrence of (1, 4)-linked xylosyl residues in highly purified xyloglucans has also been reported (40). The general structural features of xyloglucans are given in Fig. 5. Xyloglucans can be divided into two main classes depending on the frequency with which branch points occur within the molecule. Unlike the different pectic polysaccharides, in all xyloglucans the side chains are only one to three residues long. The (1 → 4)-linked β-D-glucan backbone makes xyloglucans similar in structure to cellulose, and as a result they bind to cellulose in the native cell wall. However, the presence of the side chains has a marked effect on their properties, limiting the extent of binding to cellulose and preventing close intermolecular hydrogen bonding between xyloglucan molecules once solubilized. Thus, unlike cellulose microfibrils, which only swell in alkali, xylog-

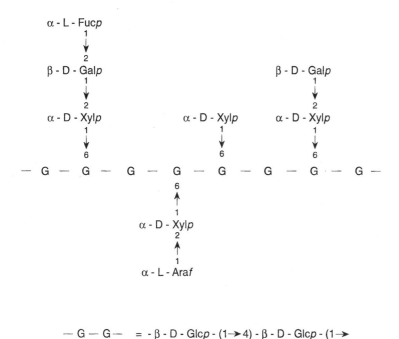

Fig. 5 Structural features of side chains of xyloglucans from parenchyma cell walls.

lucans can be solubilized by alkali from the CDTA- and Na_2CO_3-extracted CWM, the extent of branching determining the ease of extractability. The highly branched xyloglucans are solubilized by 1 M KOH, whereas the less branched xyloglucans require 4 M KOH (Table 3). A small amount of the highly branched xyloglucans can be solubilized with 0.5 M KOH. Estimates of the molecular weight of xyloglucans from runner bean show them to be of the order of 110,000 daltons (41). In general, small but significant amounts of glucomannans are found in the 4 M KOH plus borate extracts, and these polysaccharides are less branched than the xyloglucans (30,31). From the 1 M KOH extracts of a range of products, in addition to xyloglucans, small but significant amounts of hemicellulosic complexes containing xylans, xyloglucans, pectic polysaccharides, proteins, and polyphenolics have been isolated (12,42,43). In runner bean, for instance, about 5% of the total hemicellulose is found in complexes of this type (42). It is possible, however, that some of these complexes are artifacts of the extraction and fractionation procedures.

    c. Cellulose. Cellulose commonly comprises about 20–30% of the dry weight of the parenchyma cell wall (44). Cellulose is a linear polymer of D-glucose linked in a $(1 \rightarrow 4)$-β configuration. The equatorial arrangement of the hydroxyl groups in the cellulose molecule and the alternate inversion of the individual residues caused by the β-linkage allows the cellulose molecules to form strong inter- and intramolecular hydrogen bonds, which render them insoluble. Individual cellulose molecules are 1000–4000 residues long in parenchyma cell walls, but in secondary walls they may be up to 12,000 residues long. Cellulose is laid down in the wall as microfibrils, formed from the association of a large number of individual molecules. An association of 35 cellulose molecules can give rise to a fibril of 3.5 nm diameter. It has been suggested that larger microfibrils may be formed by the association of several of these smaller fibrillar units. Microfibrils from parenchyma cell walls seen under the electron microscope are 8–12 nm in diameter (45). When pectin-depleted sections of the cell wall are prepared by freeze-slamming and viewed by scanning electron microscopy, the relative size and arrangement of the microfibrils gives the wall the appearance of a coarse felt mat (45,46).

X-ray diffraction studies have shown that the cellulose molecules form a crystalline structure in the microfibril. However, a significant proportion of the cellulose in the plant cell wall is present in an amorphous noncrystalline form. Mild acid hydrolysis is capable of releasing about 10% of the cellulose from the cell wall; this treatment increases the degree of crystallinity of the remaining cellulosic material to about 90%, compared with 60% found in the undegraded material (44). Further evidence for the presence of amorphous regions comes from the observation that noncellulosic material remains complexed with the α-cellulose residue after exhaustive extraction—presumably because of interpenetration of the cellulose molecules by other cell wall polymers. In Fig. 6 the amorphous regions are depicted as distinct interruptions in the ordered arrangement of the microfibril. However, other models for the arrangement of the two regions have been proposed, including the suggestion that the less ordered cellulose is present as a loose coating around the microfibril (44). The cellulose microfibrils are believed to be

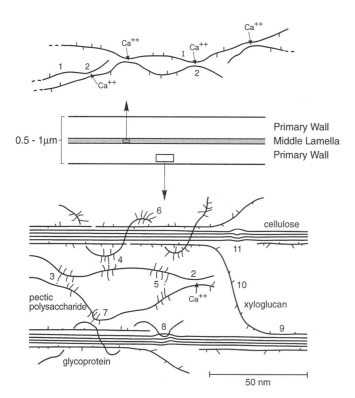

Fig. 6 Diagram of the general arrangement of polymers within the cell wall, together with their possible intermolecular crosslinks: (1) methyl esterified backbone of pectic polysaccharides, (2) calcium bridge ionic crosslink, (3) possible sugar-ester crosslink, (4) phenolic crosslink, (5) boron-mediated crosslink, (6) highly branched pectic polysaccharide twisted around cellulose microfibril, (7) covalent linkage between glycoprotein and pectic polysaccharide, (8) glycoprotein twisted around cellulose microfibril or enmeshed in cellulose amorphous region, (9) xyloglucan hydrogen-bonded to cellulose, (10) xyloglucan molecule associated with more than one cellulose microfibril, (11) amorphous region in cellulose microfibril. Only a few of the cellulose molecules that make up a cellulose microfibril are depicted in the diagram.

coated along their surface with xyloglucan molecules, which serve to disperse the cellulose microfibrils in the wall. As mentioned earlier, it is possible that a proportion of highly branched pectic polysaccharides serve to enmesh and disperse the cellulose microfibrils coated with xyloglucans in the wall matrix.

   d. Proteins. About 2–5% of the dry weight of cell walls purified from free-growing plants is composed of protein. In cell walls purified from suspension culture tissues the protein level is much higher and varies from 5 to 10%. A small proportion of this comes from contamination by intracellular protein; the remainder comes from the enzymes and structural proteins of the cell wall. Almost all of the proteins present in the cell wall are glycoproteins. In work on cell wall structural glycoproteins, the most commonly discussed proteins are the hydroxyproline-rich glycoproteins—also known as extensins (47,48). In these glycoproteins, hydroxyproline is the attachment point for arabinosides of DP 1–4, and galactosyl residues are attached to serine (49,50). The removal of these hydroxyproline-rich glycoproteins from the α-cellulose residue explains the fall in arabinose content of the residue found after treatment with sodium chlorite/acetic acid (Table 4). Similar observations have been made with the α-cellulose from olive pulp (51).

   In culture tissues hydroxyproline-rich glycoproteins are the major cell wall proteins (52), but in free-growing plants the situation is different. In runner beans about half of the cell wall protein can be accounted for by hydroxyproline-poor glycoproteins (42,53,54), and in potato, tomato, asparagus, and onion the figure is nearer 80% (R. R. Selvendran, unpublished results). Studies on the cell walls of runner beans have shown that hydroxyproline-rich glycoproteins are found in a variety of other fractions as well as the α-cellulose residue (30). They appear in the CDTA, Na_2CO_3, 1 M KOH, and 4 M KOH plus borate extracts. Hydroxyproline-poor glycoproteins appear in the CDTA and Na_2CO_3 extracts and are also found in 1 M KOH extracts of depectinated mature runner bean parenchyma (30,42). When assessing the significance of these results it should be borne in mind that the KOH used in the above studies could have caused some hydrolysis of proteins.

   The possible structural role of cell wall glycoproteins depends on the formation of cross-links with other cell wall polymers. Some form of interaction is apparent from the change that can be observed in the ease of extraction of hydroxyproline-rich glycoproteins following wounding (47) and from the difficulties that are experienced in separating different classes of polymers during cell wall fractionation. For instance, pectic polysaccharide-protein complexes have been isolated from leaves of *Vicia faba* using trichloroacetic acid extraction. These complexes have been subject to rigorous separation and purification methods, suggesting that they are not artifacts (55). Work on the glycoproteins in the cell walls of parenchyma tissue of runner beans also confirms that a significant proportion of the hydroxyproline-rich glycoprotein is present in pectic polysaccharide-protein complexes (30). The role of these complexes is not clear.

   One potential mechanism of crosslinking hydroxyproline-rich glycoproteins, which was identified early on, is the formation of phenolic bonds between two tyrosine residues to form isodityrosine (56). Interest in this possibility developed from the observation that treatment with sodium chlorite/acetic acid, which is required to solubilize these proteins from the pectin-depleted cell wall and also from the α-cellulose residue, cleaves phenolic bonds. However, subsequent investigations have not been able to show that this mechanism of crosslinking is of importance. Isodityrosine can be isolated from plant cell cultures (57), but the levels found are low (0.2–1.6 µg/mg), and the linkages that can be detected appear to be intramolecular rather than intermolecular (58). In free-growing plants that have a high content of hydroxyproline-rich glycoproteins (e.g., runner bean parenchyma), attempts to isolate isodityrosine have been unsuccessful (30). More recently evidence has been obtained for the covalent attachment of hydroxyproline-rich glycoproteins to pectic polysaccharides (59). The possibility of ionic interaction between hydroxyproline-rich glycoproteins and pectic polysaccharides has also been a topic of continuing speculation (47,48,58).

In summary, the available evidence suggests that structural glycoproteins are not present in the wall as a single class of molecules linked predominantly by one type of crosslink but exist as a variety of different types closely associated with polysaccharides, phenolics, and other proteins.

   e. Phenolics.   In the parenchyma cell wall, phenolics account for about 5% of the dry weight, and the bulk of the phenolics appear to be closely associated with the hemicellulosic polysaccharides (42). Despite the relatively low proportion of phenolics in the cell wall, they can still play a role in crosslinking (60). As evidence of this, the phenolics isolated generally appear as polysaccharide-protein-phenolic complexes. For instance, in CDTA-extracted runner bean cell wall, 5% of the material is solubilized by 1 M KOH as a complex of this type, made up of approximately 40% carbohydrate, 25% protein, and 20% phenolics (42). In these complexes it is likely that the phenolics are condensed to form small lignin-like domains.

   The cell walls of tissues that are rich in ferulic acid exhibit autofluorescence. This is especially true for sugar beet, red beet, and spinach suspension culture cells. Ferulic acid has been shown to be ester linked to the sugars of the neutral sugar side chains of pectic polysaccharides extracted from sugar beet (61) and spinach suspension culture (62). The presence of additional ether linkages between pectic polysaccharides and ferulic acid is indicated by the failure of alkaline saponification to release all the bound ferulic acid from sugar beet cell walls (B. J. H. Stevens and R. R. Selvendran, unpublished results). Phenolic crosslinking is discussed further below.

   f. Sugar Compositions of Purified Parenchyma Cell Walls.   Table 5 shows the sugar composition of the purified CWM for several tissues. From these data it can be seen that these tissues are rich in cellulose, determined by the difference in glucose values between Saeman hydrolysis and hydrolysis in 1 M H_2SO_4. The latter gives an indication of glucose derived from xyloglucans, but may also hydrolyze a proportion of the noncrystalline cellulose. The xylose in these tissues is derived mostly from the xyloglucans. The abundance of pectic polysaccharides is shown by the high levels of uronic acid (mostly galacturonic acid), arabinose, and galactose; rhamnose is a minor constituent of pectic polysaccharides. In comparing the different tissues it

Table 5   Sugar Composition[a] of Purified Cell Wall Material from Parenchymatous Tissues

	Runner bean (30)	Potato (31)	Onion (29)	Asparagus pith (132)	Apple (104)	Mung bean cotyledon (75)
Rha	2	1	1	0.5	2	1
Ara	16	8	2	3	12	36
Xyl	5	2	2	4	3	4
Man	5	0.7	1	1	4	0.3
Gal	13	29	27	8	6	4
Glc	36	34	24	20	23	16
	(3)[b]	(2)[b]	—	(2)[b]	(3)[b]	(1.3)[b]
Uronic acid	20	24	28	21	33	15
Total sugars	97	98	85	58	83	76

[a] Anhydro sugars (g/100 g dry weight).
[b] From hydrolysis in 1 M H_2SO_4.

can be seen that the pectic polysaccharides of onion and potato are rich in galactose, whereas the pectic polysaccharides of mung bean are rich in arabinose. Apple pectic polysaccharides contain significant amounts of arabinose and galactose.

2. Secondary Thickening

Some specialized tissues undergo secondary thickening of the cell wall. This can lead to a massive increase in wall thickness from 0.5 to 5–10 μm. During secondary thickening cellulose, acidic xylans, lignin, and small amounts of glucomannans are deposited.

The xylans are composed of a $(1 \rightarrow 4)$-linked backbone of β-D-xylosyl residues, a proportion of which are substituted on C-2 with residues of glucuronic acid or 4-O-Me glucuronic acid. The ratio of uronic acid to xylose is normally about 1:10 (63). In the xylans found in dicots 4-O-Me glucuronic acid is the predominant substituent (37), whereas in monocots glucuronic acid is more abundant (64). In dicots, about 7 out of 10 xylosyl residues are acetylated on C-3.

Lignin is a high molecular weight aromatic polymer formed by the enzymatic dehydrogenation and subsequent polymerization of phenylpropanoids. The main monomeric compounds are coniferyl, sinapyl, and p-coumaryl alcohol. The relative proportions of these compounds vary between dicot and monocot plants. About 100 of the monomers make up the polymer of lignin, which is hard and resistant to chemical and biochemical degradation. Lignin stiffens the cell wall and serves to enmesh the various polymers in the wall, and there is good evidence that a proportion of the xylans are linked to lignin.

Secondary thickening appears to begin with the deposition of xylans and lignin in the middle lamella region. As secondary thickening progresses beyond the preexisting primary wall, the wall is thickened by the deposition of cellulose, acidic xylans, and lignin (65–67). The above comments on secondary thickening are deduced from the careful extraction and analysis of cell wall polymers, in addition to histochemical studies on secondary thickening (66) and careful analytical work (68). Detailed analysis from asparagus shoots undergoing lignification has shown that during the initial stage of deposition of xylans and cellulose in the middle lamella, complexes can be isolated that contain pectic polysaccharides, xylans, and phenolic material. The xylans present in these complexes have a relatively low DP. Similar complexes of xylan–pectic polysaccharide–lignin have been isolated from the parchment layers of mature runner bean pods (37), and olive seed hulls (38). The DP of the xylan moieties of the above complexes tends to be low (approximately 30–50) compared with the major alkali-soluble xylans from the same sources, which have a DP of 100–200. During secondary thickening the proportion of the wall composed of pectic polysaccharides drops from 30% to less than 3%, suggesting that additional pectic polysaccharides are not deposited. This has been confirmed in lignified cauliflower stem using monoclonal antibodies for pectic polysaccharides (69). The xylans that are subsequently deposited with cellulose and lignin to thicken the wall appear to have a higher DP of 150–200 (37). The results of these investigations together with those of the histochemical studies are summarized in Figure 7.

Crystallographic studies show that β-$(1 \rightarrow 3)$-linked xylans from algae give a diffraction pattern both in the cell wall and when extracted (70). The diffraction patterns arising from lignified parchment fibers of runner bean, delignified parchment fibers, and delignified parchment fibers that have also been subject to alkali extraction, are all highly comparable with that of crystalline cellulose (M. J. Miles and R. R. Selvendran, unpublished results). This suggests that the high molecular weight β-$(1 \rightarrow 4)$-linked xylans of secondary walls do not exist in crystalline form. It is conceivable that these xylans crystallize without being distinguishable from crystalline cellulose, but this is unlikely.

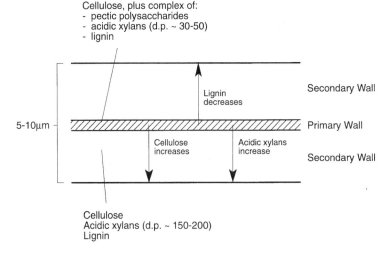

Cellulose, plus complex of:
- pectic polysaccharides
- acidic xylans (d.p. ~ 30-50)
- lignin

Lignin
decreases

Secondary Wall

5-10μm

Primary Wall

Cellulose
increases

Acidic xylans
increase

Secondary Wall

Cellulose
Acidic xylans (d.p. ~ 150-200)
Lignin

Fig. 7 Diagram of secondary thickening of the plant cell wall showing the main polymers deposited. Arrows indicate increasing/decreasing relative abundance of the different polymers.

The deposition of the polysaccharides described above is reflected in the sugar composition of purified CWM from different lignified tissues (Table 6). Runner bean parchment layer and asparagus sclerenchyma sheath are both supporting tissues and have undergone considerable secondary thickening. They are rich in xylose and glucose because of the acidic xylans and cellulose in the secondary wall. About half of the content of uronic acid is due to the glucuronosyl residues of acidic xylans. The CWM derived from the vascular bundles of asparagus and cabbage are from mature tissues, and it was difficult to make these preparations completely free from parenchyma cell walls. Their sugar compositions are comparable with each other and with that from the pea hull. The vascular bundles can be seen to be lignified from their staining reaction to phloroglucinol/HCl. In these tissues, in addition to the cellulose and acidic xylans, which are reflected in the levels of glucose and xylose in the table, there are appreciable levels

Table 6 Sugar Composition[a] of Cell Wall Material from Lignified Vegetable Tissues

	Runner bean parchment[b] (37)	Asparagus sclerenchyma sheath[b] (132)	Asparagus vascular bundles[b] (132)	Cabbage vascular bundles (1)	Pea hull (4)
Rha	0.4	0.3	0.5	2	1
Ara	0.5	0.6	2	4	5
Xyl	29	24	8	6	9
Man	0.4	0.7	1	2	0.2
Gal	0.4	0.9	7	2	1
Glc	38	32	22	23	44
Uronic acid	8	6	10	33	12
Total sugars	77	65	51	72	72

[a] Anhydro sugars (g/100 g dry weight).
[b] The origin of the runner bean and asparagus tissues are shown in Figs. 1 and 2.

of pectic polysaccharides giving rise to arabinose, galactose, and uronic acid (mostly galacturonic acid) on hydrolysis.

3. Epidermal and Cuticular Tissues

Epidermal tissues form the outer protective layer of the plant, providing resistance to desiccation, injury from insects, and attack by pathogens. The cuticular membrane that forms the protective layer on the aerial parts of plants (e.g., for leafy vegetables and fruits) is composed of one or more cuticular layers, which are laid down as incrustations of the cell wall or as adcrustations, together with the cuticle proper, which forms the outermost layer. Outside the cuticular membrane are found waxes. Protection for the underground parts of the plant (e.g., root vegetables) is provided by the suberized epidermal layer. For a full discussion of the structure and chemistry of the cuticular membrane and suberin, the reviews given in the references should be consulted (71–74).

The chemical composition of cutin and suberin are similar in that both are polyesters of fatty acids. Cutin is composed of C-16 and C-18 hydroxy and epoxy fatty acids. Commonly found monomers after acid hydrolysis of cutin include the C-16 fatty acids palmitic acid, 16-hydroxypalmitic acid, and 10,16-dihydroxypalmitic acid (and its isomers) and the C-18 fatty acids stearic acid, oleic acid, linoleic acid, 18-hydroxylinoleic acid, and 9,10,18-trihydroxy-stearic acid, together with the $\delta 12$ unsaturated analogs. While it has proved relatively easy to identify the monomers found in cutin, the intermolecular linkages in the polymer have been difficult to determine. Some of the linkage types have been identified by the use of treatments designed to label the free hydroxyls before depolymerization. Using this type of method in tomato to study the C-16 dihydroxy fatty acids, which are the predominant monomers, about 40% have been shown to be fully esterified and about 50% have the secondary hydroxyl unesterified (73). Phenolic compounds are also found in the cuticular membrane. Both *m*- and *p*-coumaric acids are released from plant cuticles during deesterification, and small amounts of ferulic acid are also released from some tissues. In the case of tomato the level of phenolic acids released increases from 2 to 5% of the cuticle dry weight during maturation of the fruit (71). These acids are believed to be esterified to the rest of the polymer. The analysis of the intermolecular structure of plant cutins has not progressed to a stage where feasible models of its structure can be put forward (72).

The epidermal regions of the underground parts of plants are protected by the deposition of suberin. Suberin contains a higher level of phenolics than cutin, varying from 20 to 60% of the dry weight of the polymer. The phenolics are combined with the aliphatic components, which are mainly hydroxy acids, and the corresponding dicarboxylic acids, varying from C-16 to C-24. The polymer is made up of an aliphatic domain like cutin and a phenolic domain like lignin, which is linked to the cell wall by lignin-like attachments.

B. Seed Tissues of Dicots

In the context of DF the main dicot seed tissues of importance are the legumes. Two very different types of cell walls are found in the storage tissues of legume seeds, depending on whether they are free of an endosperm (i.e., nonendospermic, e.g., pea, mung bean, soybean) or have an endosperm (i.e., endospermic, e.g., guar, locust bean). The former type of seed usually has starch as the main storage polysaccharide, and their cell walls are derived mainly from the tissues of the cotyledons, with some contribution from the testa. The cell wall polysaccharides of the cotyledons are similar to those of parenchymatous tissues and are mainly pectic substances (usually rich in arabinose and/or galactose), cellulose, and hemicelluloses (e.g., xyloglucans). Detailed analysis of CWM from mung bean cotyledons, extracted under nondegradative conditions (175), showed that these cell walls contained cellulose, xyloglucans, and a high content of pectic polysaccharides rich in arabinose. In addition to several ''free'' arabinose-rich pectic polysaccharides, numerous fractions containing arabinose-rich pectic polysaccharides in close association with xyloglucans were isolated (75). However, very few, if any, neutral arabinans were found, and this would suggest that the ''neutral'' arabinans reported in earlier work on legume seed cotyledons (12,76,77) were probably degradation products of more complex pectic polysaccharides.

In endospermic legume seeds there is little or no starch; the cell walls are massively thickened, and the polysaccharides of the cell wall themselves form the reserve food supply (78,79). Examples of polysaccharide food additives derived from seeds of this type are guar gum and locust bean gum. In guar seeds, approximately 80% of the carbohydrate in the cell wall of the endosperm is present as galactomannans. These galactomannans are essentially linear molecules, composed of a backbone of (1,4)-linked mannosyl residues substituted on C-6 with galactosyl residues. Galactosyl substituents are present on about 20–50% of the mannosyl residues. In structure galactomannans are somewhat comparable with xyloglucans, which can also serve as cell wall storage polysaccharides, e.g., in tamarind seeds. Seed storage polysaccharides are partially soluble in water and so can be extracted with hot water and used as food additives. Galactomannans have widespread industrial uses and have nutritional effects: in vitro studies suggest that they slow down the absorption of glucose due to an interaction between the polysaccharide and the intestinal mucosa (80).

The cell walls of the outer covering or ''hull'' of legume seeds are composed mainly of cellulose (about 60%), pectic polysaccharides, acidic xylans, and xyloglucans. Little lignin is found in the hulls of edible legumes (81). The main difference from parenchymatous fruit and vegetable tissues in the context of DF is that the seed tissues are dehydrated. This makes them amenable to grinding for flour production. During cooking starch is gelatinized and rendered soluble and so made amenable to enzymatic degradation. The extent to which gelatinization occurs depends on the type of seed and the extent to which the cell walls permit cell separation and swelling. In general, legume starches are more resistant to enzymatic hydrolysis than tuber starches, because they have a significantly higher content of amylose, which make them susceptible to retrogradation and formation of insoluble complexes upon processing.

C. Monocot Cereal Grains

While commonly referred to as a seed, the cereal grain (or caryopsis) is morphologically a fruit containing a single seed. In wheat, for instance, the outer pericarp (beeswing bran) and inner pericarp (cross cells and tube cells) form the fruit tissue, while the structures inside this, including the aleurone and endosperm, belong to the seed (Fig. 8). The polymers of the grains of monocots differ markedly from those of the dicots, in both unlignified and lignified cells. In addition, they show considerable variation between different species. In monocot grains the flour preparation method has a considerable influence on the DF composition of the resulting flour. In wheat the endosperm tissue accounts for 80% of the whole grain. To obtain refined white flour, 72% of the grain is extracted; this is referred to as 72% extraction flour. In this low-extraction flour, which is virtually pure endosperm, nonstarch polysaccharides account for up to 3% of the dry weight. Higher degrees of extraction yield flours containing significant amounts of bran; in this case the nonstarch polysaccharides increase towards the average for the whole grain of 10%. The level of nonstarch polysaccharides in wheat bran is 42% (5).

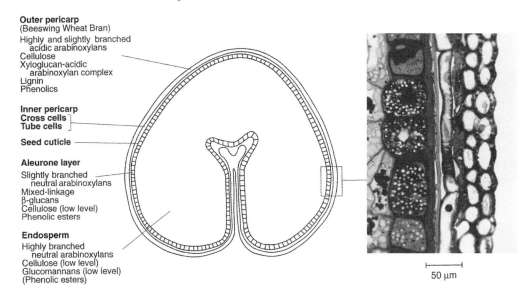

Outer pericarp
(Beeswing Wheat Bran)
Highly and slightly branched
  acidic arabinoxylans
Cellulose
Xyloglucan-acidic
  arabinoxylan complex
Lignin
Phenolics

Inner pericarp
Cross cells
Tube cells

Seed cuticle

Aleurone layer
Slightly branched
  neutral arabinoxylans
Mixed-linkage
β-glucans
Cellulose (low level)
Phenolic esters

Endosperm
Highly branched
  neutral arabinoxylans
Cellulose (low level)
Glucomannans (low level)
(Phenolic esters)

50 μm

Fig. 8 Line diagram of a cross section of a wheat grain showing the main polymers present in the different tissue types. The inset light micrograph, which shows the variation in cell size and cell type, is taken from a grain that is not fully developed. The cells of the inner and outer pericarp, which ultimately collapse, are still visible exterior to the aleurone layer. (Photograph ML Parker.)

1. Endosperm

The endosperm is the main unlignified tissue in the grain. The cell walls of cereal endosperms are generally very different from those of the undifferentiated parenchyma tissue, and it is possible that this is associated with the mode of formation of the cell wall. In most cereals the endosperm develops initially as a multinucleate cell. Cell walls are subsequently laid down in a single phase of wall formation relatively late in endosperm development (82). Rice is the exception among the commonly eaten cereals in having a cell wall composition comparable to that of parenchymatous tissues of dicots. Rice is also distinct in having a low ratio of CWM to starch in the grain, resulting in a low DF content (approximately 1.5% for polished rice). Rice endosperm cell wall contains cellulose, which comprises 40–50% of the cell wall, pectic polysaccharides, which have side chains composed mainly of arabinose and xylose, and xyloglucan hemicelluloses; the cell wall also contains some mixed linkage β-glucans (83,84)

The endosperm of the other common cereals can be grouped into two rather different assemblies with wheat on the one hand, and barley and oats on the other, rye being intermediate between the two. While barley endosperm is discussed together with the other cereals, barley grains are not commonly used as a food product by humans.

Wheat endosperm cell walls account for 80–85% of the DF content of highly refined flours (72% extraction flour). They contain no pectic polysaccharide, little cellulose, and a hemicellulose fraction composed of a mixture of highly branched neutral arabinoxylans, rather than the xyloglucans of parenchyma tissue, together with a small amount of mixed linkage β-glucans (85–87). About 35% of the arabinoxylan is water soluble, and the rest can be solubilized by alkali. It is likely that the alkali-soluble fraction is held in the wall by ester crosslinks. The structure of a similar class of arabinoxylans found in rye has been carefully studied (88). The evidence available suggests that the polysaccharide can be enzymatically degraded into two different fractions. In one the arabinosyl substituents occur as single residues attached to the xylan backbone. In the other the xylosyl residues are doubly substituted. Wheat endosperm arabinoxylan has also been shown to have similar structural features (89).

In barley and oats about 70% of the endosperm cell wall is composed of β-glucans, some of which are associated with proteins, and some with arabinoxylans (90,91). Most but not all of the β-glucan is water soluble. The β-glucans contain a mixture of (1,4)- and (1,3)-linked β-D-glucosyl residues in a ratio of about 7:3 respectively. The use of highly specific enzymes together with methylation analysis and gel chromatography has enabled the following structure to be worked out for mixed linkage β-glucans. They appear to contain β-(1 → 4)-linked residues in groups of three or four separated by single β-(1 → 3) linkages. Groups of two or three contiguous β-(1 → 3) linkages are also found, which cause a marked change in the shape of the molecule. Three β-(1 → 3)-linked residues are sufficient to make the molecule bend back on itself as much as 180 degrees, and their regular occurrence gives rise to a pleated structure. Regions with longer stretches of (1,4)-linked residues also occur regularly throughout the length of the molecule (92–94). The β-glucan chains can form hydrogen bonds in certain regions and thus associate to form viscous solutions when dissolved in water in a manner similar to the galactomannans of guar. The endosperm cell wall of rye is intermediate but closer to barley and oats than wheat. Appreciable amounts of both β-glucans and arabinoxylans are present. Oat bran is distinct from wheat and barley bran in that it is not a true bran and is in fact highly enriched with the thickened outermost cells of the endosperm (subaleurone cells). The walls of these cells are considerably thicker than those of the general endosperm cells and are rich in mixed-linkage β-glucans. Oat bran is used commercially as an enriched form of cereal fiber rich in β-D-glucans.

2. Major Tissues of Wheat Bran

The brans are traditionally a source of added DF. The bran from dehulled wheat is composed mainly of the aleurone layer, seed cuticle, inner pericarp, and the outer pericarp (beeswing bran layer) (Fig. 8).

a. Aleurone Layer. The cell walls of the aleurone layer are much thicker than the endosperm cell walls, and they are autofluorescent due to the presence of covalently linked phenolic acids (e.g., ferulic acid). In wheat the aleurone layer is made up of a single layer of cells, whereas in barley it is three cells thick. While both show autofluorescence, this phenomenon is less pronounced in the barley aleurone layer. The effect of the phenolics is to make the aleurone layer resistant to degradation. It is, however, eventually degraded by colonic bacteria, unlike lignified tissues, which are much more resistant (95,96). The polymers of the aleurone layer contribute a significant proportion to the DF content of the wheat bran. The two main polymers of the aleurone layer cell walls of wheat are slightly branched arabinoxylans (as distinct from endosperm arabinoxylans) and mixed linkage β-glucans. Smaller amounts of cellulose and glucomannans are also present (97,98).

b. Beeswing Wheat Bran. Beeswing wheat bran consists of the outer covering of the grain and is mainly composed of the tissues of the outer pericarp (Fig. 8). Because this material is relatively easy to isolate in large quantity, the CWM from it has been studied in some detail. The cell walls contain 53% hemicelluloses, 30% cellulose, 12% phenolics and lignin, and 5% protein. The hemicelluloses are present as highly branched acidic arabinoxylans, slightly branched acidic arabinoxylans, together with acidic arabinoxylan-xyloglucan complexes (99). The presence of xyloglucans is surprising because xyloglucans are normally only found in soft tissues, but during maturation of the grain the parenchymatous cells of the inner pericarp collapse to leave a layer of cells rich in highly branched arabinoxylans and xyloglucans, which adheres to the outer pericarp.

3.   Nonstarch Polysaccharide Content of Cereal Products

From the data given in Table 7 the following observations can be made. In wheat bran most of the arabinose and xylose is derived from the arabinoxylans of the aleurone layer and the highly branched acidic arabinoxylans of the beeswing bran layer; a small proportion of the xylose is derived from the acidic xylans of the cross cells and tube cells. The latter three tissues also account for the bulk of the glucose from cellulose. Most of the remainder of the glucose is derived from mixed linkage β-glucans of the aleurone layer and is released by hydrolysis in 1 M H_2SO_4. The nonstarch polysaccharides of whole wheat flour are rich in arabinose, xylose, and glucose compared to white flour, and these sugars are largely derived from the polysaccharides of the bran layers. About 70% of the nonstarch polysaccharide content of whole wheat flour is due to the presence of the wheat bran. Xylose and arabinose are the most abundant nonstarch sugars in white flour and come from highly branched arabinoxylans. In this product estimates for cell wall glucose are elevated compared to the values normally found in pure CWM. This suggests some contamination with incompletely removed starch. In the cell walls of wheat endosperm the ratio of arabinose:xylose:glucose is 34:53:3 (86). Using the same ratio, the cell wall glucose level for white flour can be estimated at less than 0.1 g/100 g dry weight, which indicates a very low cellulose level. The values given for rye are for the flour used for making rye biscuits (e.g., Ryvita). The high levels of arabinose and xylose come from the presence of acidic and neutral arabinoxylans. The acidic arabinoxylans are derived from the bran layer. The material is relatively rich in glucose, 40% of which is released by hydrolysis in 1 M H_2SO_4. This is due to the presence of high levels of β-glucans. It can be seen that the DF content of rye flour is significantly higher than that for whole wheat flour and that its overall composition is intermediate between that of wheat and oats. The high DF content is due to higher levels of β-glucans and neutral arabinoxylans in the endosperm of rye. In porridge oats most of the glucose is released by hydrolysis in 1 M H_2SO_4, due to the high levels of β-glucans present. Because the level of glucose derived from cellulose is low, this material can be inferred

Table 7   Nonstarch Polysaccharides[a] in Different Cereal Tissues

	Wheat bran (5)	Whole wheat flour (3)	White flour (3)	Rye flour (3)	Pearl barley (3)	Porridge oats (5)	Brown rice (5)
Ara	9.8	2.7	0.9	3.6	1.2	1.0	0.4
Xyl	18.8	4.3	1.4	5.8	1.6	1.2	0.5
Man	0.2	0.2	0.1	0.3	0.3	0.1	—
Gal	0.7	0.3	0.2	0.3	0.1	0.2	0.1
Glc	11.0	2.6	0.7	3.7	4.5	4.5	0.9
	(3.0)[b]	(1.0)[b]	(0.5)[b]	(2.2)[b]	(4.1)[b]	(4.2)[b]	(0.2)[b]
Uronic acid	1.2	0.3	—	0.2	0.1	0.1	0.2
Nonstarch poly-saccharide	41.7	10.4	3.3	13.9	7.8	7.1	2.1

[a] g/100 g dry weight.
[b] From hydrolysis in 1 M H_2SO_4.

to contain only small amounts of lignified tissue. A significant proportion of the β-glucan is hot water soluble and has beneficial effects similar to guar gum. Pearl barley is very similar in overall composition to oats. The arabinose and xylose in brown rice is mainly derived from arabinoxylans, and most of the glucose is derived from cellulose. However, its overall DF content is even lower than that of white flour.

IV. PLANT CELL WALL ASSEMBLY

Plant primary cell walls exhibit distinct mechanical, physical, and chemical properties. In attempting to understand the molecular basis of these properties it is important to know not only the structure of the component polymers, but also the way the polymers are assembled and organized within the cell wall.

A. Visualizing Cell Wall Structures

The two main techniques that have been used to probe the arrangement of polysaccharides within the wall in recent years are immunocytochemistry and electron microscopy (100). Using gold-labeled antibodies on sections prepared for electron microscopy, the following distributions have been found. In clover leaf and root tissue, antibodies to xyloglucans labeled material only in the cellulose-containing primary wall. Antibodies raised to the pectic fragment RG-I, which recognize RG-I and polygalacturonic acid, labeled material in the middle lamella region and in the areas of middle lamella at the corner junctions of cells (101). In carrot, antibodies for a hydroxyproline-rich glycoprotein extracted from cell walls with $CaCl_2$ were localized in the primary cell wall (102). One of the problems in using antibodies raised to extracted polymers of this type is ensuring their specificity in recognizing a particular polymer. In an approach designed to address this problem, monosaccharides and short lengths of polysaccharide covalently linked to bovine serum albumin have been used (103). In this way antibodies have been raised to a range of specific sugars, including terminal arabinofuranose and D-galactose, and to oligosaccharides containing β-(1,4)-xylose and β-(1,3)-glucose (103). Antibodies to β-(1,4)-xylose (which recognize xylans) were shown to react with the secondary wall of xylem of bean root, the primary wall of isolated cells of *Zinnia elegans*, and bean callus. This latter observation is in agreement with work on cell wall polysaccharides of parenchymatous tissues of runner bean, potato, and apple referred to earlier (30,31,104) where significant amounts of (1,4)-linked xylosyl residues have been found in xylan–pectic polysaccharide–polyphenolic complexes. These "xylan moieties" have relatively low DP, unlike the xylans of secondary walls, which have a DP of 150–200. Antibodies to β-(1,3)-glucose bound to the initial cell plate in dividing cells and to the plasmodesmata, indicating the presence of callose (103). Polysaccharides containing small amounts of (1,3)-linked glucosyl residues have been detected in 0.5 M KOH extracts of runner bean parenchyma, and it is probable that this has arisen from the callose present in the plasmodesmata. Antibodies raised to arabinofuranose detected polymers in the primary wall, but since arabinofuranose substituents are present on all three classes of pectic polysaccharides described above and in the hydroxyproline-rich glycoproteins, it is not possible to infer the distribution of specific polymers from these data alone.

Using monoclonal antibodies it is possible to produce probes that are highly specific, discriminating, for instance, between pectic polysaccharides with different DMs (46,105). In a study on developing root apices it has been shown that there is variation in the distribution of methyl esterified pectic polysaccharides both within the cell wall and between different tissues

(105). Within the primary cell wall, antibodies to unesterified pectic polysaccharides bound to the inner surface of the cell wall adjacent to the plasmamembrane, to the middle lamella, or to the outer surfaces at intercellular spaces. Antibodies to methyl esterified pectic polysaccharides bound evenly throughout the primary cell wall. The structural features of pectic polysaccharides recognized by these antibodies are therefore quite differently distributed within the cell wall. In a similar immunocytochemical labeling study on cauliflower stems it was shown that there is a decrease in the labeling of the primary cell wall by antibodies to methyl esterified pectin with increasing distance from the apical meristem. This change was accompanied by an increase in labeling with antibodies to unesterified pectic polysaccharides (69). In related work using affinity techniques to localize cell wall polymers (106), enzymes have been complexed with colloidal gold and successfully used to show, for instance, the distribution of cellulose in plant-fungal interactions (107) and xylans in the cell walls of hardwood (108).

The approaches described above depend on the use of labeling methods to localize the different components of the cell wall. However, microscopic methods are becoming available that permit molecular features in the cell wall to be visualized directly. One approach has been to improve sample preparation in order to make better use of the resolution available with scanning electron microscopy. Fast freezing combined with methods of chemical extraction has been used to enable the molecular arrangement of cellulose and xyloglucan to be visualized (45). The images produced show parallel cellulose microfibrils apparently cross-linked by the xyloglucan molecules in a regular pattern, rather like the rungs of a ladder. Another approach has been to use atomic force microscopy (AFM) and related techniques, which have a higher level of resolving power. The power of atomic force microscopy is demonstrated by the images produced of individual pectin molecules, which show an unexpected form of branching of the molecular backbone (109).

B. Molecular Cross-Linking

The role of covalent bonds in maintaining the structure of the primary cell wall remains an area of uncertainty. The behavior of different cell wall fractions during isolation suggests that there are covalent cross-links between different components of the cell wall. However, specifically identifying particular covalent cross-links has proved difficult. For instance, problems have been encountered in trying to establish whether or not the mild alkali (Na_2CO_3) that extracts pectic polysaccharides does so by breaking an ester cross-link. Evidence for the existence of other esters, besides methyl esters, between pectic galacturonosyl residues and other cell wall components comes from the discrepancy that has been found between estimates of the total number of esterified galacturonosyl residues and the amount of methanol released by alkali (110). Non-methyl uronyl esters have been detected in the products formed by enzymatic degradation of suspension culture cell walls (111). But attempts to isolate these compounds from free-growing plants in sufficient quantity to characterize them have proved unsuccessful (112). Although the evidence that nonmethyl uronyl esters exist is good, the hypothesis that these esters cross-link cell wall polysaccharides remains unproven. A better case has been made for cross-links between apiose residues (a substituent of RG-II) involving boron (113). In general, for most parenchyma cell walls it appears that assembly is dependent primarily on noncovalent interactions rather than the formation of covalent bonds. However, examples where there are significant levels of covalent cross-linking in the primary wall can be found. For instance, in tissues where autofluorescence of the cell walls is observed (e.g., sugar beet and red beet) the pectic polysaccharides appear to be covalently cross-linked through ferulic acid (27,114). Phenolic dimers, which are presumed to form the cross-link, have been isolated from both beet tissue and Chinese water chestnut (115,116).

Noncovalent interactions occurring between pectic polysaccharides have been the subject of extensive study because of the importance to the food industry of pectins as food additives and gelling agents (28). Within the cell wall the main mechanism for cross-linking pectic polysaccharides appears to be an ionic interaction involving calcium (28,117). Surprisingly, the known ionic behavior of commercially prepared pectic polysaccharides in dilute solution (studied because of its relevance to pectin use in foods) has been of little help in explaining the properties exhibited by pectic polysaccharides in vivo. A minimum number of contiguous unesterified galacturonic acid residues has been found to be necessary for dilute (1% w/w) solutions of pectic polysaccharides to undergo ionic cross-linking with calcium ions (28,117). Randomly esterified pectins need to have a DM below 50% before suitably long blocks of unesterified galacturonic acid occur often enough for gelation to be observed (28). Pectins that contain a nonrandom arrangement of unesterified residues can form gels at higher average DMs. Most pectins extracted under nondegradative conditions do not meet these criteria for the formation of ionic gels in dilute solution. The only native pectin that has been shown to gel at concentrations of 1–2% w/w in the presence of calcium ions is the chelator extracted pectin from unripe tomatoes (20). Although commercial preparations of citrus pectin of relatively high DM (64%) can form gels with calcium, it appears that this is the result of partial degradation by endogenous pectin methylesterase occurring during processing. Examination of more carefully prepared citrus pectin suggests that blocks of unesterified residues occur infrequently (118). Currently the main evidence that ionic interaction between pectic polysaccharides is important for plant cell wall assembly comes from the observations that CDTA can extract pectins and cause cell separation and that addition of calcium increases the stiffness of plant tissues. The level of calcium in the cell wall is therefore of some interest (117). Most of the published estimates of cell wall calcium can be criticized because of the likelihood of redistribution of calcium between the extraction buffer and the cell wall during sample preparation. In view of this we developed a nonaqueous method to obtain accurate estimates of the total level of calcium (and magnesium) in the cell wall (119).

The probable reason for the apparently inconsistent behavior of pectic polysaccharides in the plant cell wall and after extraction is the difference in polymer concentration in the two systems. The concentration of pectic polysaccharide found in the plant cell wall is difficult to determine but is likely to be at least 20% w/w. At this level it is possible that numerous weak ionic interactions provide the crosslinking, whereas in dilute solution a smaller number of highly stable complexes is required. This view is supported by ionic speciation calculations for the major cell wall ions, which predict that pectic polysaccharides in the cell wall will be predominantly complexed with calcium (119). Experimentally it is also possible to show that although commercially prepared apple pectin does not form stable ionic gels at concentrations of 1–2% w/w, nevertheless apple pectin can be stabilized as calcium-containing films at polymer concentrations above 30% w/w (C. W. Tibbits, A. J. MacDougall, and S. G. Ring, unpublished results).

Another noncovalent molecular interaction of importance in the cell wall is the formation of hydrogen bonds between hemicelluloses and cellulose. Binding of xyloglucan and xyloglucan fragments to cellulose has been observed and partially characterized in vitro (120–122). The observation that the nature of the side chains affects the extent of binding is in agreement with the extractability of slightly and highly branched xyloglucans from a range of tissues using alkali of different strengths (30,31). Some success has also been achieved in modeling xyloglucan:cellulose assembly in vitro. By growing a cellulose-extruding bacterium (*Acetobacter xylinum*) in solutions of xyloglucan (123), it has been possible to reproduce the ladder-like physical arrangement of cellulose microfibrils interconnected with xyloglucan molecules seen in pectin-depleted onion cell walls (46).

In contrast to the molecular interactions discussed above, which are all forms of association, it is possible with concentrated mixtures of polymers to observe immiscibility (phase separation). Even quite small structural differences can be sufficient to lead to the incompatibility of different polymers in concentrated solutions. Since there is considerable structural variation in the plant cell wall, immiscibility may be expected to play a role in plant cell wall assembly. This view has been strengthened by the recent demonstration of phase separation of mixtures of isolated cell wall polysaccharides (124). Other interactions that may contribute to self-assembly of the cell wall have been reviewed (125).

C. Physical Properties of the Polymer Network

The physical properties of the plant cell wall polymer network are of direct relevance to its behavior as DF. In attempting to understand the molecular basis of these properties and the extent to which they are affected by the environment surrounding the cell wall, a useful approach has been to consider the extent to which established theories of polymer chemistry can be applied to the plant cell wall.

One example of this is the insight that can be gained into the structural properties of the pectin matrix from examination of the elastic behavior of calcium pectin gels (20). The observation that the stiffness of these materials increases with increasing temperature makes it valid to apply concepts for the elasticity of covalently crosslinked polymer networks to these gels. The main insight gained from this is that the physical behavior of the polymer network can be explained on the basis of a relatively low level of crosslinks.

A second example concerns the swelling behavior of the cell wall. The swelling behavior of calcium pectin gels has been found to be consistent with established theories for the behavior of cross-linked synthetic polyelectrolyte networks (126). The force driving water uptake into the gel or cell wall matrix comes mainly from a difference in the osmotic potential between the bathing solution and the polymer network. This osmotic potential difference arises from an imbalance in the distribution of the mobile counterions, which preferentially congregate in the polymer network to balance the fixed charge carried by the polymer. The extent of this imbalance is much affected by the extent of dissociation of the ionizable groups on the polymer and the salt concentration of the surrounding medium. Consequently it is possible to predict that the porosity and swelling behavior (and hence water-holding capacity) of primary plant cell walls will vary as the pH and ionic environment vary during gut transit.

V. POLYSACCHARIDE FOOD ADDITIVES: GUMS AND STABILIZERS

A. Food Gums

A range of polysaccharides, the majority of which are heteroglycans with branched structures, are used in small amounts in the food industry to give the desired texture to processed products. A significant proportion of these gums are derived from plant cell walls, including pectins, alginates, guar gum, carboxymethyl cellulose, carrageenan, and locust bean gum. Usually the amount of polymer required to produce the desired change in texture in a food product is about 1% of its fresh weight. Therefore, gums are not a major contributor to total DF intake, except in certain special cases (e.g., guar-based breads for diabetics). Several food gums are described in other chapters of this book.

B. Seed Husk (Mucilage)

The husk (epidermal layers) of seeds of a number of species of the plant genus *Plantago*, referred to as ispaghula or psyllium, is obtained from seeds milled and suitably processed to give fiber-enriched pharmaceutical preparations. The mucilage is located in the "thick" mucilage cells, which form the outer epidermis of the spermoderm. A significant amount of the mucilage can be extracted from the husk with water, and the bulk (>90%) can be solubilized with dilute NaOH. The overall structural features of the polysaccharides solubilized by dilute NaOH have been elucidated by fractionation of the methylated mucilage on LH20, and methylation analysis of the separated fractions clearly showed that the constituent polysaccharides are heterogeneous highly substituted xylans (127). However, fractionation of the alkali soluble polysaccharides on Sephadex G-75 failed to resolve the polysaccharides and gave only a single peak, and for convenience this fraction will be referred to as the mucilage polysaccharide (128). The major neutral sugars of the mucilage polysaccharide are D-xylose, L-arabinose, and L-rhamnose, which are present in the molar ratio 10:3.2:1. The polysaccharide has a highly substituted xylan backbone having both (1 → 4) and (1 → 3) linkages in the approximate ratio of 5:2. The majority of the residues in the xylan backbone are variously substituted at C-2 and C-3 with arabinose, xylose, and rhamnose residues, the last of these carrying terminal galacturonic acid residues (128). Presumably these structural features are responsible for the high water-binding capacity of the mucilage. It should be noted that the structural features of these acidic arabinoxylans are quite different from those of the acidic arabinoxylans of beeswing wheat bran and wheat bran (99).

The finely subdivided husk becomes readily dispersible in water, giving apparently viscous, gel-like mucilage, which retains many times its own weight of water. The mucilage has important physiological effects in both the small and the large intestines and, unlike most soluble fibers such as pectins, is only partially degraded by colonic bacteria. Experimental evidence shows continued fermentation of the ispaghula husk in the distal colon (129,130). These properties of the husk are probably some of the factors responsible for its laxative action, and the husk is widely used for treating large bowel disorders such as constipation and diverticular disease (131).

VI. CELL WALL CHANGES DURING GROWTH AND DEVELOPMENT

A. Tissue Toughening

During vegetable maturation, lignin is laid down in certain cell walls leading to secondary thickening and an increase in cell wall strength, which is perceived by the consumer as a toughening of the vegetable. Within a vegetable organ lignification can be seen most obviously in the thickened secondary walls of the xylem elements and structural tissues such as sclerenchyma, but may also occur to a small extent within the primary walls of the parenchyma cells adjacent to tissues which have undergone secondary thickening, for instance those adjacent to the parchment layer of runner bean or between the vascular bundles of asparagus (see Figs 1 and 2) (132). During storage of asparagus, the edible length of the shoot becomes shorter due to lignification of the lower region of the stem (43,133). The other marked change during storage is the decrease in galactose content of all the pectic polysaccharides examined (43,132). Leafy vegetables are often consumed before significant lignification takes place, and some of the toughening found in these vegetables may be attributed to thickening of the cuticle, in addition to lignification of cell walls.

In general toughening of vegetables affects palatability more than DF content. This is because relatively little lignin need be deposited to cause toughening. Where lignin is deposited in massively thickened cell walls, a few cells of this type such as asparagus sclerenchyma sheath or pear stone cells can affect the properties of the overall tissue. Where lignin is thought to be deposited in the parenchyma cell wall, a few crosslinks can have a marked influence on wall strength (134). In a typical vegetable (e.g., runner bean pod) the DF content increases from about 2.5 g/100 g f.wt for tender material to about 4 g/100 g f.wt. for toughened material (135).

B. Fruit Softening

Fruit ripening has been the subject of several reviews (136,137). Changes in the DF quality and content of fruit occur during ripening, but these are not as significant as might at first appear, even in instances where fruit soften markedly. The main cell wall changes that are coincident with ripening and the loss of cell-cell adhesion are an increase in the level of cold-water-soluble pectic polysaccharides and structural modification to the pectic polysaccharides, and possibly the hemicellulosic polymers, which remain in the wall (138–140). There is a significant fall in the level of galactose and or arabinose, depending on the type of fruit (136,137,141–143). In tomato, kiwi fruit, and apple, the loss has been shown to be mainly from pectic polysaccharides (138,142,143). In many fruits there is a fall in the DM of the pectic polysaccharides, but the significance of this is uncertain, since softening is not always accompanied by deesterification of pectic polysaccharides. For instance, in tomatoes both pericarp and locule tissues soften extensively during ripening, but pectin deesterification is only found in the pericarp (144). During the earlier stages of ripening, even in fruit that soften considerably when they become overripe and unfit for consumption, the backbone of the pectic polysaccharides remains relatively undegraded (139). The polymers that can be isolated from cold water extracts of ripening fruit are pectic polysaccharides high in galacturonic acid and low in neutral sugars carrying small side chains typical of middle lamella pectic polysaccharides (described above). Polygalacturonase has been the obvious candidate for a role in middle lamella dissolution and has received much attention (136); however, research in this area has not succeeded in establishing the action of this enzyme as the primary cause of loss of cell-cell adhesion (145). In the DF context it is notable that even in tomatoes where very high levels of endo-polygalacturonase accumulate, the DP of the water soluble pectic polysaccharides is not greatly lower than that of the same fraction from mature green fruit (18). Since the main crosslink found in the middle lamella region is believed to be an ionic calcium bridge, mechanisms that disrupt this linkage could lead to an increase in the cold-water-soluble pectic polysaccharides. One possibility is that intracellular organic acids might leak out into the cell wall space, chelate the calcium and disrupt calcium ionic bonds between the pectic polysaccharides. The role of organic acids in withdrawing calcium from pectic polysaccharide ionic bridges was initially put forward in 1957 (146). Evidence in support of this possibility comes from the observation that citrate increases cell sloughing in potato during cooking (147), and that the permeability of the plasmalemma appears to increase during the ripening process (148). However in a study in which the levels of calcium and organic acids were measured in the cell walls of ripening tomato fruit using a nonaqueous fractionation method, we have found that there is no general withdrawal of calcium from the cell wall, and that the accumulation of organic acids in the apoplast is insufficient to effectively reduce calcium mediated cross-linking of pectic polysaccharides (119). While a variety of different biochemical mechanisms for the solubilization of the pectic polysaccharides can be envisaged, there is currently very little firm evidence supporting any of them.

VII. CELL WALL CHANGES DURING COOKING AND PROCESSING

In the analysis of cell wall changes brought about by cooking, a nondegradative method of extraction is essential. This is highlighted by the difference between the results obtained for pectic polysaccharides when extracted with CDTA and Na_2CO_3 (30,31) compared to hot water and hot oxalate (21,41,104). Using hot water and hot oxalate extractions, extensive degradation of the pectic polysaccharides occurs, and little useful information can be gathered on the effects of the cooking.

Table 8 Comparison of Values Obtained for Soluble and Insoluble DF in Raw Onion Using Standard Methods of DF Analysis with Values Obtained Using Nondegradative Methods of Cell Wall Extraction[a]

| | Raw onion (4) | | Cooked onion (4) | | Raw onion (29) | | Cell wall fractions (29) | | |
	Soluble	Insoluble	Soluble	Insoluble	0.5% SDS (soluble)	Cell wall material (insoluble)	CDTA	Na$_2$CO$_3$ + 0.5 M KOH	α-Cellulose residue
Rha	0.5	tr	0.5	tr	tr	0.3	tr	0.2	0.1
Ara	0.3	0.1	0.3	0.1	0.1	0.4	tr	0.2	0.1
Xyl	0.1	0.5	tr	0.6	tr	0.5	tr	tr	tr
Man	tr	0.2	tr	0.2	tr	0.3	—	—	0.2
Gal	3.6	0.9	3.8	1.0	0.4	5.5	0.4	2.9	1.7
Glc	—	6.6	—	6.2	—	5.0	—	—	4.5
	(tr)[b]	(tr)[b]	(tr)[b]	(0.1)[b]	(tr)[b]	(0.5)[b]	(tr)[b]	(tr)[b]	(tr)[b]
Uronic acid	6.3	0.3	5.9	0.2	0.8	5.7	1.5	2.8	1.0
Nonstarch polysaccharide	10.8	8.6	10.5	8.4	1.4	17.6	2.0	6.0	7.6

Because figures for nonstarch polysaccharides on a dry weight basis from cell wall analysis were unavailable, values given have been made comparable to the figures quoted in columns 1–4 by assuming that the total nonstarch polysaccharide in onion is 19 g/100 g dry weight.

[a] Anhydro sugars (g/100 g dry weight).

[b] Figures in parentheses are for hydrolysis in 1 M H$_2$SO$_4$.

During cooking two main effects are observed. The first is the breakdown of cell membrane compartmentation releasing cell contents and markedly changing the cell wall environment; for instance, in potato the release of citrate from the vacuole leads to increased levels of cell sloughing due to the chelating activity of citrate within the cell wall. The second is the degradation of pectic polysaccharides by β-elimination. Pectic polysaccharides of the primary wall as well as the middle lamella are rendered soluble by β-eliminative degradation. The former are normally not water soluble because of close association with other wall polymers. These effects combine to give a result analogous to fruit ripening and induce cell separation along the middle lamella, but in cooking much more of the nonstarch polysaccharide is rendered soluble than in ripening. The degradation of the pectic polysaccharides within the primary wall has a marked effect on cell wall porosity (149).

Phenolic crosslinks within the wall are not subject to heat-induced degradation. In tissues where these crosslinks are common, cell separation does not occur readily and cooking can be very slow to bring about softening. Examples of such tissues are red beet and Chinese water chestnut, where analysis of the phenolic material released by alkali from the cell wall has shown high levels of ferulic acid dimers (115,116). The same principle applies in the hard-to-cook phenomenon found in legume seeds (150). Under normal circumstances different varieties of legume take different lengths of time to cook. Listed in increasing order of cooking time, the main legume seeds are lentil, mung bean, pinto bean, pea, kidney bean, butter bean, and chick pea. High temperature and humidity during storage can also increase the hard-to-cook phenomenon. Microscopy studies clearly show that poor cooking is associated with failure of cells to separate (134,151). This can also be related to increased permanganate staining in the middle lamella region (134). It would appear that the staining reaction in this study is due to the presence of condensed phenolics in the wall rather than extensive lignin formation.

VIII. CELL WALL SOLUBILITY AND TISSUE STRUCTURE

A. Solubility of Cell Wall Polymers

Careful extraction and analysis of the cell wall polymers under nondegradative conditions is essential if the relative amounts of soluble and insoluble DF in fruit and vegetables are to be assessed accurately. Unfortunately, the methods currently used do not meet these criteria, and as a result values given in the literature for the soluble and insoluble fiber content of a range of foods vary considerably in accuracy. Given the information available from the methods of extraction outlined at the start of this review, it is possible to reevaluate the data and indicate which values are reliable and which are not. The following comments are therefore particularly pertinent to those who are likely to use published data to interpret the results of nutritional and related studies.

The main degradative step in the accepted method for analyzing nonstarch polysaccharides is the heating used to gelatinize starch prior to treatment with amylolytic enzymes. As described above, heat causes degradation of pectic polysaccharides through the β-elimination reaction undergone by methyl esterified galacturonosyl residues in the backbone. This leads to a large release of water-soluble polysaccharide fragments, which come from the largely insoluble crosslinked pectic polysaccharides (Fig. 3). These fragments are rich in galactose and arabinose. This effect is clearly seen in Table 8 in the values for raw onion. Columns 1 and 2 give the values for nonstarch polysaccharides from standard methods of analysis for soluble and insoluble DF (4), whereas columns 5 and 6 give values for comparable fractions prepared using nondegradative methods. During the preparation of purified CWM, less than 10% of the CWM is solubilized as cold-water-soluble polysaccharides, two thirds of this when the cells are separated and the walls teased apart by ball-milling in 0.5% SDS at 2°C (29). During subsequent warming of frozen suspensions of CWM to 20°C a negligible quantity (<0.5%) of the CWM is solubilized. The SDS ball-milled fraction therefore represents the greater part of the soluble DF. The purified CWM is equivalent to cold-water-insoluble DF. It is apparent that while the figures given in columns 1 and 2 show that 55% of the total nonstarch polysaccharide is present as soluble fiber, the true figure is 10% or less. When the individual sugars are examined it can be seen that the results for the nonpectic sugars xylose and mannose are similar in both methods of analysis but that the pectic sugars are at variance, the figure for galactose being particularly striking. This gives strong support to the view that degradation of the pectic polysaccharides is occurring during analysis. This is almost certainly occurring during the gelatinization step; heating for one hour at 100°C, particularly in aqueous buffer, will cause extensive β-eliminative degradation of pectic polysaccharides (9,152), as reflected in the elevated values for soluble DF reported (3,4,153,154). Columns 7–9 give the amounts of sugars solubilized from purified CWM by the sequential extraction method described previously together with the amounts remaining in the α-cellulose residue. It is clear that extraction conditions that deesterify pectins without causing significant β-eliminative degradation are required before appreciable amounts of galactose-rich pectic polysaccharides are solubilized. Even after this series of treatments only 70% of the galactose has been solubilized, whereas in the standard DF analysis of raw onion 80% is solubilized. Comparison of the values for cooked and raw onion provides further evidence that the heat treatment is the cause of degradation. The values for soluble DF for raw and cooked onion are almost identical. From our cell wall work it is clear that the value for soluble DF for onion and a range of other raw vegetables is 10% or less of the total DF (29–31,132), and therefore this figure should be used in preference to values obtained using a gelatinization step. There is thus a need to reassess the solubility of DF polysaccharides at physiological temperature and pH (152). The values are likely to be a little higher than those derived from the nondegradative methods of extraction described here, but nowhere near as high as the values derived from current degradative methods. In ripening fruits where there is an increase in the amounts of pectic polysaccharides that are solubilized as a natural part of ripening, a figure of 15% may be assumed (138,142). Even in the jellified tissues of the locules of kiwi fruit, only 32% of the polysaccharide is cold-water-soluble (142).

Where values are given for cooked vegetables the estimates of nonstarch polysaccharides as a measure of soluble DF are probably more reliable, but even here, from comparative work, it would appear that the effects due to cooking are not as significant as the heat treatment used to gelatinize the starch. In contrast, values for other foods such as cereals, which do not contain pectic polysaccharides with the exception of rice, are likely to be more reliable. It should be kept in mind in these foods that there is likely to be some increase in solubility of the mixed-linkage β-glucans and highly branched neutral arabinoxylans caused by the heat treatment.

B. Tissue Structure and Dietary Fiber

While the analysis of the extracted polymers from purified CWM goes a long way to explaining the composition and some of the properties of DF, in the diet DF is ingested mostly as whole cells rather than as extracted purified polymer. Figure 9 shows the hierarchy of organizational levels found in cell walls above that of the isolated polymers. These higher levels of organization have significant implications for the study of DF but are not generally well appreciated (5,8,135).

Fruit and vegetables before ingestion exist as whole assemblies of cells attached to each other with differing degrees of tenacity. The nature of the food, its preparation, mastication, and to a certain extent the environment of the proximal gastrointestinal tract, determine the

Organizational Level	Example

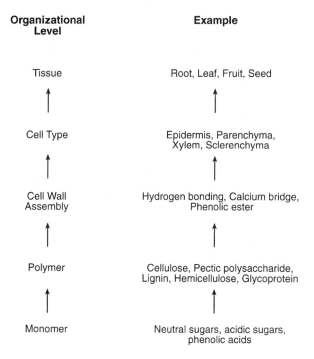

Fig. 9 Organizational levels found in plant organs, illustrated with respect to the cell wall.

structure and properties of the cell aggregates that comprise the food particles of fruit and vegetables during digestion.

When a bite is taken from fresh produce of crisp texture, such as coleslaw, and certain apples, fracture of the cell wall occurs across the primary wall rather than down the middle lamella. Mastication of the food breaks it up into small clusters of cells firmly attached by the middle lamella. In fresh apple, for instance, a wide range of cluster sizes results, varying from 4 to 5 cells to over 200, with the most common size being 20–50 cells, the digesta entering the alimentary canal in this form. In contrast, in cooked vegetables and in some fruit (e.g., apples described as "mealy"), the cells separate more readily along the middle lamella. In cooked apples, although some large clusters remain after mastication, the most common cluster size is in the 1- to 10-cell range, and in general the clusters are more susceptible to disintegration by the physical movement of the intestinal tract. During passage through the alimentary canal, these cell clusters are exposed to the acid environment of the stomach (approximately pH 2.5) and subsequently to the alkaline environment of the small intestine. Both conditions encourage solubilization of the pectic polymers of the middle lamella region and will promote the separation of cells and reduction in particle size. In fresh produce and in cooked material such as legume seeds, or cabbage vascular tissue, where cells are strongly attached to each other, the environment of the upper gut may not be harsh enough to lead to a significant reduction in the size of the cell clusters. In other cooked foods large numbers of single cells may be released. The implications of this for digestion are that starch and protein remains inside the cells and therefore access to these substrates may be restricted. This is particularly true of thick-walled starch-rich foods, such as legume seeds, where large clusters of cells remain. In contrast to this the thin cell walls of rice grain and potato are likely to provide little resistance to starch degradation.

These differences in tissue structure are reflected in the results of simulated digestion studies, where marked variations in rates of starch hydrolysis can be found (155).

Direct measurements of the ability of molecules of differing sizes to move across the cell wall have been made using suspension culture cells, which are likely to be somewhat more porous than free-growing plant cells. In soybean cells a 67,000 dalton globular protein and a 17,900 dalton dextran have been shown to be significantly slower in establishing an equilibrium across the wall than smaller molecules (149). After treatment of the cells with a pectinase, these compounds were able to cross the wall freely. These results underline the importance of cell wall entrapment of starch as a factor in reducing its accessibility to digestion and show that the degree to which the pectic polysaccharides of the primary wall have been degraded during cooking will have a significant influence on digestion rates. In produce made from flour, the cell walls are broken down in the milling process, and so here the starch is not contained within the cell and may be directly acted on by the digestive enzymes. The polysaccharides released from the cell wall are likely to affect the viscosity of the digesta. Cooking, the effect of the pH and ionic environment of the stomach and small intestine, and the effect of proteolytic enzymes in degrading cell wall proteins will all play a role in determining the extent to which solubilization of polysaccharides occurs.

The gross tissue structure of leafy vegetables is also likely to influence the extent to which digestion of food particles is possible. In leaf tissues the cuticular and epidermal layers are resistant to degradation and lie on either side of the thin layer of mesophyll cells. In this way access of bacteria to the more readily degraded material in the internal spaces of the leaf may be restricted. One consequence of this is that leaf tissues retain some of their cellular structure, which serves to trap water.

Passing from the small intestine to the colon, the role of structure and cell organization becomes particularly important because of the effect of this on water retention. Although about 90% of the water is absorbed in the small intestine, a significant amount remains associated with the digesta that passes into the large intestine. The amount of water associated with this digesta depends on the type of fiber consumed. Ispaghula husk retains more water than vegetable or fruit fiber, which in turn retain more water than wheat bran. While vegetable and fruit fiber is readily degraded by colonic bacteria, ispaghula husk and wheat bran are less readily degraded and their fermentation would appear to continue throughout the large intestine (1,129,130). The reason for the slow degradability of isphagula husk is due to its ability to bind water very strongly and thus form a viscous matrix, which appears to restrict bacterial activity, whereas in the case of wheat bran the phenolic ester crosslinks and lignin restrict bacterial activity. The cell walls of the aleurone layer are degraded more readily than the lignified outer layers, but the cellular structure of the bran layers (including the aleurone layer) is retained, which serves to trap water (95,96). Thus the undegraded fiber, associated bacteria, and the water retained by them make a significant contribution to fecal bulking. The importance of tissue structure in water entrapment is demonstrated by the fact that stool weight is significantly higher in subjects fed with coarse bran compared to fine bran (156). Removal of cell wall polysaccharides from wheat bran would expose the associated lignin in the wall matrix, which would serve to bind hydrophobic mutagens effectively and thus remove them with the feces. In this context the in vitro binding studies of mutagens to CWM from beeswing wheat bran and bacterially degraded bran cell wall preparation are highly relevant (157,158).

Digestion of wheat bran in vitro for 24 hours shows that while the aleurone is extensively degraded, the outer lignified layers of bran retain their cellular structure (95,96). Where unlignified tissues show fecal bulking, this is largely due to an increase in bacterial biomass and associated water. The effects of various fiber preparations on fecal bulking have been tested in clinical trials and the results are discussed elsewhere (1,2).

The above considerations clearly show that the nonstarch polysaccharide content alone is inadequate to define the properties of DF during gut transit. The organization of the polysaccharides within the walls and the arrangement of the different tissue types have very significant effects, which need to be taken into account.

ACKNOWLEDGEMENT

We wish to thank the BBSRC for funding the experimental work on dietary fiber and the preparation of this article.

REFERENCES

1. Selvendran RR, Steven BJH, DuPont MS. Dietary fibre: chemistry, analysis, and properties. Adv Food Res 31:117–209, 1987.
2. Selvendran RR. Nutrition, dietary fiber. In: Dulbecco R, ed. Encyclopedia of Human Biology. Vol. 6. 2d ed. San Diego: Academic Press, 1997, pp. 339–349.
3. Englyst HN, Wiggins HS, Cummings JH. Determination of the non-starch polysaccharides in plant foods by gas-liquid chromatography of constituent sugars as alditol acetates. Analyst (London) 107: 307–318, 1982.
4. Englyst HN, Bingham SA, Runswick SA, Collinson E Cummings JH. Dietary fibre (non-starch polysaccharides) in fruit, vegetables and nuts. J Hum Nutr Diet 1:247–286, 1988.
5. Southgate DAT, Englyst H. Dietary fibre: chemistry physical properties and analysis. In: Trowell H, Burkitt D, Heaton K, eds. Dietary Fibre, Fibre-Depleted Foods and Disease. London: Academic Press, 1985, pp. 31–35.
6. Vahouny G, Kritchevsky D. Dietary Fibre—Basic and Clinical Aspects. New York: Plenum Press, 1986.
7. Selvendran RR, Verne AVFV, Faulks RM. Methods for analysis of dietary fibre. In: Linskens HF, Jackson JF, eds. Modern Methods of Plant Analysis, New Series, Vol. 10. Berlin: Springer-Verlag, 1988, pp. 234–259.
8. Selvendran RR, MacDougall AJ. Cell-wall chemistry and architecture in relation to sources of dietary fibre. Eur J Clin Nutr 3(Suppl):S27–S41, 1995.
9. Selvendran RR, O'Neill MA. Isolation and analysis of cell walls from plant material. Methods Biochem Anal 32:25–153, 1987.
10. Selvendran RR, Ryden P. Isolation and analysis of plant cell walls. In: Dey PM, ed. Methods in Plant Biochemistry, Vol. 2, Carbohydrates. London: Academic Press, 1990, pp. 549–579.
11. Selvendran RR. The chemistry of plant cell walls. In: Birch GG, Parker KJ, eds. Dietary Fibre, London: Applied Science Publishers, 1983, pp. 95–147.
12. Selvendran RR. Developments in the chemistry and biochemistry of pectic and hemicellulosic polymers. J Cell Sci 2(suppl):51–88, 1985.
13. Aspinall GO. Chemistry of cell wall polysaccharides. In: Preiss J, ed. The Biochemistry of Plants, Vol. 3, Carbohydrates—Structure and Function. New York: Academic Press, 1980, pp. 473–500.
14. Bacic AC, Harris PJ, Stone BA. Structure and function of plant cell walls. In: J Preiss, ed. The Biochemistry of Plants, Vol. 14. New York: Academic Press, 1988, pp. 297–371.
15. McNeil M, Darvill AG, Fry SC, Albersheim P. Structure and function of the primary cell walls of plants. Annu Rev Biochem 53:625–663, 1984.
16. Fry SC. The Growing Plant Cell Wall: Chemical and Metabolic Analysis. Harlow, UK: Longman, 1988.
17. Carpita NC, Gibeaut DM. Structural models of primary cell walls in flowering plants: consistency of molecular structure with the physical properties of the walls during growth. Plant J 3:1–30, 1993.

18. Seymour GB, Harding SE, Taylor AJ, Hobson GE, Tucker GA. Polyuronide solubilization during ripening of normal and mutant tomato fruit. Phytochemistry 26:1871–1875, 1987.

19. Huber DJ. The inactivation of pectic depolymerase associated with isolated tomato fruit cell-wall—implications for the analysis of pectin solubility and molecular weight. Physiol Plant 86:25–32, 1992.

20. MacDougall AJ, Needs PW, Rigby NM, Ring SG. Calcium gelation of pectic polysaccharides isolated from unripe tomato fruit. Carbohydr Res 923:235–249, 1996.

21. Ring SG, Selvendran RR. An arabinogalactoxyloglucan from the cell wall of *Solanum tuberosum*. Phytochemistry 20:2511–2519, 1981.

22. Wood PJ, Siddiqui IR. Isolation and structural studies of a water soluble galactan from potato (*Solanum tuberosum*). Carbohydr Res 22:212–220, 1972.

23. Stevens BJH, Selvendran RR. Structural investigation of an arabinan from cabbage (*Brassica oleracea* var. Capitata). Phytochemistry 19:559–561, 1980.

24. Darvill AG, NcNeil M, Albersheim P, Delmer DP. The primary cell walls of flowering plants. In: NE Tolbert, ed. The Biochemistry of Plants, Vol. 1, The Plant Cell. New York: Academic Press, 1980, pp. 91–162.

25. Barrett AJ, Northcote DH. Apple fruit pectic substances. Biochem J 96:617–627, 1965.

26. De Vries JA, Den Uijl CH, Voragen AGJ, Rombouts FM, Pilnik W. Structural features of the neutral sugar side chains of apple pectic substances. Carbohydr Polym 3:193–205, 1983.

27. Guillon F, Thibault J-F. Methylation analysis and mild acid hydrolysis of the 'hairy' fragments of sugar-beet pectins. Carbohydr Res 190:85–96, 1989.

28. Voragen AGJ, Pilnik W, Thibault J-F, Axelos MAV, Renard CMGC. Pectins. In: AM Stephen, ed. Food Polysaccharides. New York: Marcel Dekker, 1995, pp. 287–339.

29. Redgwell RJ, Selvendran RR. Structural features of cell-wall polysaccharides of onion *Allium cepa*. Carbohydr Res 157:183–199, 1986.

30. Ryden P, Selvendran RR. Cell-wall polysaccharides and glycoproteins of parenchymatous tissues of runner bean (*Phaseolus coccineus*). Biochem J 269:393–402, 1990.

31. Ryden P, Selvendran RR. Structural features of cell-wall polysaccharides of potato (*Solanum tuberosum*). Carbohydr Res 195:257–272, 1990.

32. O'Neill MA, Albersheim P, Darvill A. The pectic polysaccharides of primary cell walls. In: PM Dey, ed. Methods in Plant Biochemistry, Vol. 2, Carbohydrates. London: Academic Press, 1990, pp. 415–441.

33. Chapman HD, Morris VJ, Selvendran RR, O'Neill MA. Static and dynamic light scattering studies of pectic polysaccharides from the middle lamellae and primary cell walls of cider apples. Carbohydr Res 165:53–68, 1987.

34. Ryden P, Colquhoun IJ, Selvendran RR. Investigation of structural features of the pectic polysaccharides of onion by ^{13}C-N.M.R. spectroscopy. Carbohydr Res 185:233–237, 1989.

35. De Vries JA, Rombouts FM, Voragen AGJ, Pilnik W. Comparison of the structural features of apple and citrus pectic substances. Carbohydr Polym 4:89–101, 1984.

36. Schols HA, Voragen AGJ, Colquhoun IJ. Isolation and characterization of rhamnogalacturonan oligomers, liberated during degradation of pectic hairy regions by rhamnogalacturonase. Carbohydr Res 256:97–111, 1994.

37. Selvendran RR, King SE. Structural features of the cell-wall polysaccharides of the parchment layers of the pods of mature runner beans. Carbohydr Res 195:87–99, 1989.

38. Coimbra MA, Waldron KW, Selvendran RR. Isolation and characterisation of cell wall polymers from the heavily lignified tissues of olive (*Olea europaea*) seed hull. Carbohydr Polym 27:285–294, 1995.

39. Lau JM, McNeil M, Darvill AG, Albersheim P. Treatment of rhamnogalacturonan I with lithium in ethylenediamine. Carbohydr Res 168:245–274, 1987.

40. Karacsonyi S, Kovacik V. Studies of the polysaccharides of *Populus alba* L: isolation and characterisation of xyloglucans. Carbohydr Res 185:199–210, 1989.

41. O'Neill MA, Selvendran RR. Isolation and partial characterisation of a xyloglucan from the cell walls of *Phaseolus coccineus*. Carbohydr Res 111:239–255, 1983.

42. O'Neill MA, Selvendran RR. Hemicellulosic complexes from the cell walls of runner bean (*Phaseolus coccineus*). Biochem J 227:475–481, 1985.

43. Everson HP, Waldron KW, Geeson JD, Browne KM. Effects of modified atmospheres on textural and cell-wall changes of asparagus during shelf-life. Int J Food Sci Technol 27:187–199, 1992.

44. Franz G, Blaschek W. Cellulose. In: PM Dey, ed. Methods in Plant Biochemistry, Vol. 2, Carbohydrates. London: Academic Press, 1990, pp. 291–322.

45. McCann MC, Wells B, Roberts K. Direct visualisation of cross-links in the primary plant cell wall. J Cell Sci 96:323–334, 1990.

46. McCann MC, Roberts K. Architecture of the primary cell wall. In: CW Lloyd, ed. The Cytoskeletal Basis of Plant Growth and Form. London: Academic Press, 1991, pp. 109–129.

47. Showalter AM. Structure and function of plant cell wall proteins. Plant Cell 5:9–23, 1993.

48. Sommer-Knudsen J, Bacic A, Clarke AE. Hydroxyproline-rich plant glycoproteins. Phytochemistry 47:483–467, 1998.

49. Lamport DTA, Catt JW. Glycoproteins and enzymes of the cell wall. In: W Tanner, FA Loewus, eds. Plant Carbohydrates II. New York: Springer-Verlag, 1981, pp. 131–165.

50. O'Neill MA, Selvendran RR. Glycoproteins from the cell wall of *Phaseolus coccineus*. Biochem J 187:53–63, 1980.

51. Coimbra MA, Waldron KW, Selvendran RR. Isolation and characterisation of cell wall polymers from olive pulp (*Olea europaea* L.). Carbohydr Res 252:245–262, 1994.

52. Lamport DTA. The protein component of primary cell walls. Adv Bot Res 2:151–218, 1965.

53. O'Neill MA, Selvendran RR. Glycoproteins from the cell wall of *Phaseolus coccineus*. Biochem J 187:53–63, 1980.

54. Selvendran RR. Cell wall glycoproteins and polysaccharides of parenchyma of *Phaseolus coccineus*. Phytochemistry 14:2175–2180, 1975.

55. Pusztai A, Begbie R, Duncan I. Fractionation and characterisation of water soluble polysaccharide-protein complexes containing hydroxyproline from the leaves of *Vicia faba*. J Sci Food Agric 22: 514–519, 1971.

56. Lamport DTA. The primary cell wall: a new model. In: RA Young, RM Rowell, eds. Cellulose: Structure, Modification and Hydrolysis. New York: John Wiley, 1986, pp. 77–90.

57. Fry SC. Isodityrosine, a new cross-linking amino acid from plant cell-wall glycoprotein. Biochem J 204:449–455, 1982.

58. Kieliszewski MJ, Lamport DTA. Extensin: repetitive motifs, functional sites, post-translational codes, and phylogeny. Plant J 5:157–172, 1994.

59. Qi X, Behrens BX, West PR, Mort AJ. Solubilization and partial characterization of extensin fragments from cell walls of cotton suspension cultures. Plant Physiol 108:1691–1701, 1995.

60. Wallace G, Fry SC. Phenolic components of the plant-cell wall. Int Rev Cytol 151:229–267, 1994.

61. Colquhoun IJ, Ralet M-C, Thibault J-F, Faulds CB, Williamson G. Structure identification of feruloylated oligosaccharides from sugar-beet pulp by NMR spectroscopy. Carbohydr Res 263: 243–256, 1994.

62. Fry SC. Phenolic components of the primary cell wall: feruloylated disaccharides of D-galactose and L-arabinose from spinach polysaccharide. Biochem J 203:493–504, 1982.

63. Timmell TE. Wood hemicelluloses: Part I. In: ML Wolfrom, RS Tipson, eds. Advances in Carbohydrate Chemistry and Biochemistry, Vol. 19. New York: Academic Press, 1964, pp. 247–302.

64. Ring SG, Selvendran RR. Isolation and analysis of cell wall material from beeswing wheat bran (*Triticum aestivum*). Phytochemistry 19:1723–1730, 1980.

65. Northcote DH. The cell walls of higher plants: their composition, structure and growth. Biol Rev Cambridge Philos Soc 33:53–102, 1958.

66. Northcote DH. Changes in the cell walls of plants during differentiation. Symp Soc Exp Biol XVII: 157–174, 1963.

67. Northcote DH. Synthesis and metabolic control of polysaccharides and lignin during the differentiation of plant cells. Essays Biochem 5:89–137, 1969.

68. Meier H. General chemistry of cell walls and distribution of the chemical constituents across the walls. In: Zimmerman MH, ed. The Formation of Wood in Forest Trees. New York: Academic Press, 1964, pp. 137–151.

69. Femenia A, Garosi P, Roberts K, Waldron KW, Selvendran RR, Robertson JA. Tissue-related changes in methyl-esterification of pectic polysaccharides in cauliflower (*Brassica oleracea* L. var. *botrytis*) stems. Planta 205:438–444, 1998.

70. Preston RD. The Physical Biology of Plant Cell Walls. London: Chapman Hall, 1974.

71. Baker EA, Bukovac MJ, Hunt GM. Composition of tomato fruit cuticle as related to fruit growth and development. In: DE Cutter, KL Alvin, CE Price, eds. The Plant Cuticle. London: Academic Press, 1982, pp. 33–44.

72. Holloway PJ. Structure and histochemistry of plant cuticular membranes: an overview. In: DE Cutter, KL Alvin, CE Price, eds. The Plant Cuticle. London: Academic Press, 1982, pp. 1–32.

73. Holloway PJ. The chemical constitution of plant cutins. In: DE Cutter, KL Alvin, CE Price, eds. The Plant Cuticle. London: Academic Press, 1982, pp. 45–85.

74. Kolattukudy PE, Espelie KE, Soliday CL. Hydrophobic layers attached to cell walls. Cutin, suberin and associated waxes. In: W Tanner, FA Loewus, eds. Encyclopedia of Plant Physiology, Vol. 13B, Plant Carbohydrates II: Extracellular Carbohydrates. Berlin: Springer-Verlag, 1981, pp. 225–254.

75. Gooneratne J, Needs PW, Ryden P, Selvendran RR. Structural features of polysaccharides from the cotyledons of mung bean *Vigna radiata*. Carbohydr Res 265:61–77, 1994.

76. Brillouet JM. Non-starchy polysaccharides of legume seeds from the *Papilionoidae* subfamily. Sci Aliment 2:135–162, 1982.

77. Brillouet JM, Carré B. Composition of cell walls of cotyledons of *Pisum sativum, Vicia faba* and *Glycine max*. Phytochemistry 22:841–847, 1983.

78. Meier H, Reid JSG. Reserve polysaccharides other than starch in higher plants. Encycl Plant Physiol New Ser 13A:418–471, 1982.

79. Reid JSG. Cell wall storage carbohydrate in seeds—biochemistry of the seed 'gums' and 'hemicelluloses'. Adv Bot Res 11:125–155, 1985.

80. Johnson IT. Fibre—How and why it works. In: TDR Hockaday, H Keen, eds. Dietary Fibre in the Management of the Diabetic. Oxford: Medical Education Services, 1984, pp. 21–25.

81. Selvendran RR. The plant cell wall as a source of dietary fiber: chemistry and structure. Am J Clin Nutr 39:320–337, 1984.

82. Brink RA, Cooper DC. The endosperm in seed development. Bot Rev 13:423–541, 1947.

83. Shibuya N, Iwasaki T. Polysaccharides and glycoproteins in the rice endosperm cell wall. Agric Biol Chem 42:2259–2266, 1978.

84. Shibuya N, Misaki A. Structure of hemicellulose isolated from rice endosperm cell wall: mode of linkages and sequences in xyloglucan, β-glucan and arabinoxylan. Agric Biol Chem 42:2267–2274, 1978.

85. Ewald CM, Perlin AS. The arrangement of branching in an arabinoxylan from wheat flour. Can J Chem 37:1254–1259, 1959.

86. Mares DJ, Stone BA. Studies on wheat endosperm. I. Chemical composition and ultrastructure of the cell walls. Aust J Biol Sci 26:793–812, 1973.

87. Mares DJ, Stone BA. Studies on wheat endosperm. II. Properties of the wall components and studies of their organisation within the wall. Aust J Biol Sci 26:813–830, 1973.

88. Bengtsson S, Aman P, Andersson RE. Structural studies on water-soluble arabinoxylans in rye grain using enzymatic hydrolysis. Carbohydr Polym 17:277–284, 1992.

89. Hoffman RA, Geijtenbeek T, Kamerling JP, Vliegenthardt JFG. [1]H-N.m.r. study of enzymically generated wheat-endosperm arabinoxylan oligosaccharides: structures of hepta- to tetradeca-saccharides containing two or three branched xylose residues. Carbohydr Res 223:19–44, 1992.

90. Ballance GM, Manners DJ. Structural analysis and enzymic solubilization of barley endosperm cell walls. Carbohydr Res 61:107–118, 1978.

91. Forrest IS, Wainwright T. The mode of binding of β-glucans and pentosans in barley endosperm cell walls. J Inst Brew London 83:279–286, 1977.

92. Carpita NC. The chemical structure of the cell walls of higher plants. In: D Kritchevshy, C Bonfield, JW Anderson, eds. Dietary Fiber: Chemistry, Physiology, and Health Effects. New York: Plenum Press, 1990, pp. 15–30.

93. Kato Y, Nevins DJ. Fine structure of (1-3), (1-4) glucan from *Zea* shoot cell walls. Carbohydr Res 147:69–85, 1986.

94. Woodward JR, Fincher BG, Stone BA. Water-soluble $(1 \to 3)$, $(1 \to 4)$ β-D-glucans from barley (*Hordeum vulgare*) endosperm II. Fine structure. Carbohydr Polym 3:207–225, 1983.

95. Stevens BJH, Selvendran RR. Structural studies on cell wall fractions from wheat bran degraded by human faecal bacteria in vitro. Carbohydr Res 183:311–319, 1988.

96. Stevens BJH, Selvendran RR, Bayliss CE, Turner R. The degradation of cell wall material of apple and wheat bran by human faecal bacteria in vitro. J Sci Food Agric 44:151–166, 1988.

97. Bacic A, Stone BA. Isolation and ultrastructure of aleurone cell walls from wheat and barley. Aust J Plant Physiol 8:453–474, 1981.

98. Bacic A, Stone BA. Chemistry and organisation of aleurone cell wall components from wheat and barley. Aust J Plant Physiol 8:475–495, 1981.

99. DuPont MS, Selvendran RR. Hemicellulosic polymers from the cell walls of beeswing wheat bran: Part 1, polymers solubilised by alkali at 2°. Carbohydr Res 163:99–113, 1987.

100. Moore PJ. Immunogold localization of specific components of plant cell walls. In: HF Linskens, JF Jackson, eds. Modern Methods of Plant Analysis, Vol. 1, Plant Fibres. Berlin: Springer-Verlag, 1989, pp. 70–88.

101. Moore PJ, Staehelin A. Immunogold localization of the cell-wall matrix polysaccharides rhamnogalacturonan I and xyloglucan during cell expansion and cytokinesis in *Trifolium pratense* L.; implication for secretory pathways. Planta 174:433–445, 1988.

102. Stafstrom JP, Staehelin LA. Antibody localisation of extensin in cell walls of carrot storage roots. Planta 174:321–332, 1988.

103. Northcote DH, Davey R, Lay J. Use of antisera to localize callose, xylan and arabinogalactan in the cell-plate, primary and secondary walls of plant cells. Planta 178:353–366, 1989.

104. Stevens BJH, Selvendran RR. Structural features of cell-wall polymers of the apple. Carbohydr Res 135:155–166, 1984.

105. Knox JP, Linstead PJ, King J, Cooper C, Roberts K. Pectin esterification is spatially regulated both within cell walls and between developing tissues of root apices. Planta 181:512–521, 1990.

106. Vian B. Ultrastructural localization of carbohydrates. Recent developments in cytochemistry and affinity methods. In: JA Bailey, ed. Biology and Molecular Biology of Plant-Pathogen Interactions. Berlin: Springer-Verlag, 1985, pp. 49–57.

107. Bonfante-Fasolo P, Vian B, Perotto S, Faccio S, Knox JP. Cellulose and pectin localisation in roots of mycorrhizal *Allium porum*: labelling continuity between host cell wall and interfacial material. Planta 180:537–547, 1990.

108. Vian B, Brillouet JM, Satiat-Jeunemaitre B. Ultrastructural visualisation of xylans in cell walls of hardwood by means of xylanase-gold complex (Lime, *Tilia platyphyllos*). Biol Cell 49:179–182, 1983.

109. Round AN, MacDougall AJ, Ring SG, Morris VJ. Unexpected branching in pectin observed by atomic force microscopy. Carbohydr Res 303:251–253, 1997.

110. Kim J-B, Carpita N. Changes in esterification of the uronic acid groups of cell wall polysaccharides during elongation of maize coleoptiles. Plant Physiol 98:646–653, 1992.

111. Brown JA, Fry SC. Novel *O*-D-galacturonyl esters in the pectic polysaccharides of suspension-cultured plant-cells. Plant Physiol 103:993–999, 1993.

112. Needs PW, Rigby NM, Colquhoun IJ, Ring SG. Conflicting evidence for non-methyl galacturonyl esters in *Daucus carota*. Phytochemistry 48:71–77, 1998.

113. O'Neill MA, Warrenfeltz D, Kates K, Pellerin P, Doco T, Darvill AG, Albersheim P. Rhamnogalacturonan-II, a pectic polysaccharide in the walls of growing plant cell, forms a dimer that is covalently cross-linked by a borate ester—in-vitro conditions for the formation and hydrolysis of the dimer. J Biol Chem 271:22923–22930, 1996.

114. Rombouts FM, Thibault J-F. Feruloylated pectic substances from sugar-beet pulp. Carbohydr Res 154:177–187, 1986.

115. Waldron KW, Ng A, Parker ML, Parr AJ. Ferulic acid dehydrodimers in the cell walls of *Beta vulgaris* and their possible role in texture. J Sci Food Agric 74:221–228, 1997.

116. Parr AJ, Waldron KW, Ng A, Parker ML. The wall-bound phenolics of chinese water chestnut (*Eleocharis dulcis*). J Sci Food Agric 71:501–507, 1996.

117. Jarvis MC. Structure and properties of pectin gels in plant cell walls. Plant Cell Environ 7:153–164, 1984.

118. de Vries JA, Hansen M, Søderberg J, Glahn P-E, Pedersen JK. Distribution of methoxyl groups in pectins. Carbohydr Polym 6:165–176, 1984.

119. MacDougall AJ, Parker R, Selvendran RR. Nonaqueous fractionation to assess the ionic composition of the apoplast during fruit ripening. Plant Physiol 108:1679–1689, 1995.

120. Bauer WD, Talmadge KW, Keegstra K, Albersheim P. The structure of plant cell walls. II. The hemicellulose of the walls of suspension cultured sycamore cells. Plant Physiol 51:174–187, 1973.

121. Hayashi T, Machlachlan G. Pea xyloglucan and cellulose. I. Macromolecular organisation. Plant Physiol 75:596–604, 1984.

122. Levy S, Maclachlan G, Staehelin LA. Xyloglucan side-chains modulate binding to cellulose during in vitro binding assays as predicted by conformational dynamics simulations. Plant J 11:373–386, 1997.

123. Whitney SEC, Brigham JE, Darke AH, Reid JSG, Gidley MJ. In vitro assembly of cellulose/xyloglucan networks. Plant J 8:491–504, 1995.

124. MacDougall AJ, Rigby NM, Ring SG. Phase separation of plant cell wall polysaccharides and its implications for cell wall assembly. Plant Physiol 114:353–362, 1997.

125. Jarvis MC. Self-assembly of plant cell walls. Plant Cell Environ 15:1–5, 1992.

126. Tibbits CW, MacDougall AJ, Ring SG. Calcium binding and swelling behaviour of a high methoxyl pectin gel. Carbohydr Res 310:101–107, 1998.

127. Sandhu JS, Hudson GJ, Kennedy JF. The gel nature and structure of the carbohydrate of Ispaghula husk ex *Plantago ovata* Forsk. Carbohydr Res 93:247–259, 1981.

128. Kennedy JF, Sandhu JS, Southgate DAT. Structural data for the carbohydrate of ispaghula husk ex *Plantago ovata* Forsk. Carbohydr Res 75:265–274, 1979.

129. Marteau P, Flourié B, Cherbut C, Corrèze J-L, Pellier P, Seylaz J, Rambaud J-C. Digestibility and bulking effect of ispaghula husks in healthy humans. Gut 35:1747–1752, 1994.

130. Edwards CA, Bowen J, Brydon WG, Eastwood MA. The effects of ispaghula on rat caecal fermentation and stool output. Br J Nutr 68:473–482, 1992.

131. Godding EW. Therapeutic agents. In: AV Jones, EW Godding, eds. Management of Constipation. London: Blackwell, 1972, pp. 38–76.

132. Waldron KW, Selvendran RR. Composition of the cell walls of different asparagus (*Asparagus officinalis*) tissues. Physiol Plant 80:568–575, 1990.

133. Waldron KW, Selvendran RR. Effect of maturation and storage on asparagus (*Asparagus officinalis*) cell-wall composition. Physiol Plant 80:576–583, 1990.

134. Bhatty RS. Cooking quality of lentils: The role of structure and composition of cell walls. J Agric Food Chem 38:376–383, 1990.

135. Selvendran RR, Robertson JA. The chemistry of dietary fibre—an holistic view of the cell wall matrix. In: DAT Southgate, K Waldron, IT Johnson, GR Fenwick, eds. Dietary Fibre: Chemical and Biological Aspects. Cambridge: The Royal Society of Chemistry, 1990, pp. 27–43.

136. Brady C. Fruit ripening. Annu Rev Plant Physiol 38:155–178, 1987.

137. Knee M, Bartley IM. Composition and metabolism of cell wall polysaccharides in ripening fruit. In: J Friend, MJC Rhodes, eds. Recent Advances in the Biochemistry of Fruits and Vegetables. London: Academic Press, 1981, pp. 133–148.

138. Seymour GB, Colquhoun IJ, DuPont SM, Parsley KR, Selvendran RR. Composition and structural features of cell wall polysaccharides from tomato fruits. Phytochemistry 29:725–731, 1990.

139. Rose JKC, Hadfield KA, Labavitch JM, Bennett AB. Temporal sequence of cell wall disassembly in rapidly ripening melon fruit. Plant Physiol 117:345–361, 1998.

140. Huber DJ. Strawberry fruit softening: the potential roles of polyuronides and hemicelluloses. J Food Sci 49:1310–1315, 1984.

141. Gross KC, Sams CE. Changes in cell wall neutral sugar composition during fruit ripening: a species survey. Phytochemistry 23:2457–2462, 1984.

142. Redgwell RJ, Melton LD, Brasch DJ. Cell-wall polysaccharides of kiwi fruit (*Actinidia deliciosa*):

chemical features in different tissue zones of the fruit at harvest. Carbohydr Res 182:241–258, 1988.

143. Redgwell RJ, Melton LD, Brasch DJ. Cell wall changes in kiwi fruit following post harvest ethylene treatment. Phytochemistry 29:399–408, 1990.

144. Cheng GW, Huber DJ. Alteration in structural polysaccharides during liquefaction of tomato locule tissue. Plant Physiol 111:447–457.

145. Hadfield KA, Bennett AB. Polygalacturonases: many genes in search of a function. Plant Physiol 117:337–343, 1998.

146. Doesburg JJ. Relation between the solubilization of pectin and the fate of organic acids during maturation of apples. J Sci Food Agric 8:206–216, 1957.

147. Selvendran RR, Bushell AR, Ryden P. Pectic polysaccharides in relation to cell sloughing of potatoes. Proceedings of the 11th Triennial Conference of the European Association for Potato Research, Edinburgh, 1990, p. 141.

148. Legge RL, Cheng K-H, Lepock JR, Thompson JE. Differential effects of senescence on the molecular organisation of membranes in ripening tomato fruit. Plant Physiol 81:954–959, 1986.

149. Baron-Epel O, Gharayal PK, Schindler M. Pectins as mediators of wall porosity in soybean cells. Planta 175:389–395, 1988.

150. Stanley DW, Aguilera JM. A review of textural defects in cooked reconstituted legumes—the influence of structure and composition. J Food Biochem 9:277–323, 1985.

151. Shomer I, Paster N, Lindner P, Vasiliver R. The role of cell wall structure in the hard-to-cook phenomenon in beans (*Phaseolus vulgaris* L.). Food Structure 9:139–149, 1990.

152. Monro JA. A nutritionally valid procedure for measuring soluble dietary fibre. Food Chem 47:187–193, 1993.

153. Englyst H. Determination of carbohydrate and its composition in plant materials. In: WPT James, O Theander, eds. Basic and Clinical Nutrition, Vol. 3, The Analysis of Dietary Fiber in Food. New York: Marcel Dekker, 1981, pp. 71–93.

154. Englyst HN, Cummings JH. Simplified method for the measurement of total nonstarch polysaccharides by gas-liquid chromatrgraphy of constituent sugars as alditol acetates. Analyst (London) 109: 937–942, 1984.

155. Gee JM, Johnson IT. Rates of starch hydrolysis and changes in viscosity in a range of common foods subjected to simulated digestion in vitro. J Sci Food Agric 36:614–620, 1985.

156. Brodribb AJM, Groves C. Effect of bran particulate size on stool weight. Gut 19:60–63, 1978.

157. Ryden P. The effects of fermentation on the binding properties of dietary fibre for the hydrophobic mutagen MeIQx (2-amino-3,8-dimethylimidazo[4,5-*f*]quinoxaline). Ph.D. thesis, University of East Anglia, UK, 1995.

158. Ryden P, Robertson JA. The effect of fibre source and fermentation on the apparent hydrophobic binding properties of wheat bran preparations for the mutagen 2-amino-3,8-dimethylimidazo [4,5-*f*]quinoxaline (MeIQx). Carcinogenesis 16:209–216, 1995.

20
Chemistry and Analysis of Lignin

Roger Mongeau
Nutritional Consultant, Ottawa, Ontario, Canada

Stephen P. J. Brooks
Health Canada, Ottawa, Ontario, Canada

I. INTRODUCTION

Historically, lignin has been regarded as an integral component of dietary fiber. Trowell (1974) originally defined dietary fiber as ''that portion of food which is derived from the cell walls of plants and is digested very poorly by human beings.'' Lignin is clearly included in this definition since it is recovered virtually unaltered from fecal material. Later definitions sought to characterize fiber components and human digestive actions more precisely (Trowell et al., 1976) because other plant polymers exist that are not cell wall associated but are also poorly digested by the upper digestive tract. Although there have been several different interpretations of the original dietary fiber hypothesis, one should remember that they all refer to fiber sources from edible plant sources: definitions of dietary fiber have never referred to nonedible plant material because the human digestive tract is not equipped to handle them. More recently, newer definitions of dietary fiber have been proposed that seek to include both historical dietary habits and human physiological responses (Mongeau et al., 1999). The emphasis from Mongeau et al. (1999) is to consume foods in their natural state, avoiding overpeeling and overprocessing foods, to maintain dietary fiber and its associated nutrients.

   In all instances, dietary fiber definitions have included lignin because of its chemical association with cell wall polysaccharides and because of its poor digestibility in the small intestine. Thus lignin is an integral component of dietary fiber. Although lignin is commonly referred to as a single component, it should be noted that lignin is not a single species but has a complex and variable structure. Thus, one should refer to lignins rather than lignin. In the present chapter we shall use the singular term to emphasize the fact that none of the analytical methods can measure pure lignin without losing or destroying part of it (Giger, 1985).

A. General Structure

Unlike the other (primarily polysaccharide-based) components of dietary fiber, lignin is a phenyl-propanoid polymer composed of the monomeric units shown in Table 1. A complete structure for lignin is not well defined in part because the lignin structure itself differs between plant species (i.e., no single structure exists) and because each lignin polymer is formed of a complex pattern of monomeric units attached to protein and to structural carbohydrates. The complexity of the chemical structure of lignin can be explained by random polymerizations involving one of four main phenoxyl radicals formed upon the action of peroxidase (Monties, 1989). These

Table 1   Chemical Structure of Lignin Monomeric Units

Basic carbon skeletal structure of the lignin monomeric unit:

$$HO-\underset{R_2}{\overset{R_1}{\bigcirc}}-{}_\alpha CH={}_\beta CH-X$$

X	R_1	R_2	Common name	Chemical name of substituent
—CH$_2$OH	H	H	Hydroxyphenyl	4-Hydroxyphenyl-
	H	OCH$_3$	Guaiacyl	3-Methoxy-4-hydroxyphenyl-
	OH	OCH$_3$	5-Hydroxyguaiacyl	3-Methoxy-4,5-dihydroxyphenyl-
	OCH$_3$	OCH$_3$	Syringyl	3,5-Dimethoxy-4-hydroxyphenyl-
—COOH	H	H	p-Coumaric	4-Hydroxyphenyl-
	H	OCH$_3$	Ferulic	3-Methoxy-4-hydroxyphenyl-
	OCH$_3$	OCH$_3$	Sinapic	3-Methoxy-4,5-dihydroxyphenyl-

Source: Adapted from Monties, 1989, 1991.

radicals are stabilized by delocalizing the lone electron of the oxygen attached to the C-4 of the phenyl ring, the C-3 and C-1 positions of the phenyl ring itself, or the β-carbon of the 2-propen-1-ol chain (see Table 1). The four positions can, theoretically, be combined in any fashion giving rise to a random mixture of 16 different bonds. This has been demonstrated through studies of peroxidase-catalyzed dehydrogenative polymerization of coniferyl alcohol (3-(4-hydroxy-3-methoxyphenyl)-2-propen-1-ol) (Freudenberg, 1968; Sarkanen, 1971; see Sjöström, 1993, for a review) giving rise to patterns of polymerization that have been observed in purified lignins. The probability of bond formation is not strictly random, however, and depends on steric, solvation, and electronic effects (Sarkanen, 1971; Tanahashi et al., 1976; Glasser, 1980). In accordance with this, different proportions of bonds have been found in different species of wood (Adler, 1977).

    Although a precise structure for "intact" lignin has not been determined, general models have been proposed for softwoods (Fig. 1) (Adler, 1977) and hardwoods (Fig. 2) (Nimz, 1974). These models are not meant to convey a complete picture of lignin but rather illustrate the nature of the interchain bonding as well as give an idea of the branching within the polymer; lignin is a highly branched structure with a complex interunit bonding pattern. Branching patterns different from those of Figs. 1 and 2 are also possible and have been observed in different plant species. For example, evidence for polymers containing repeating syringyl units has been presented for angiosperm woods in syringyl-enriched fractions (Yamazake et al., 1978). These types of studies show that micro-environmental differences may exist within the lignin polymer. Figures 1 and 2 also illustrate that basic interunit bonding patterns may differ between softwood and hardwood lignin.

    Differences between plant lignins are not confined to differences in bonding patterns. Monties (1991) has demonstrated differences in the ratio of syringyl to guaiacyl residues in Klason lignin isolated from hearthwood and stems of various annual plants (Table 2). One can also observe large differences in the total lignin content of plants both between species and between organs within a plant (leaf vs. stem vs. seed). Species differences in monomeric lignin composition and in total lignin content have been related to plant evolution (Higuchi, 1985; Monties, 1991).

    In addition to the phenylpropanoid alcohol units of Table 1, bound phenolic acid residues can also be found in many Gramineae plants (including wheat, corn, and rice). These residues

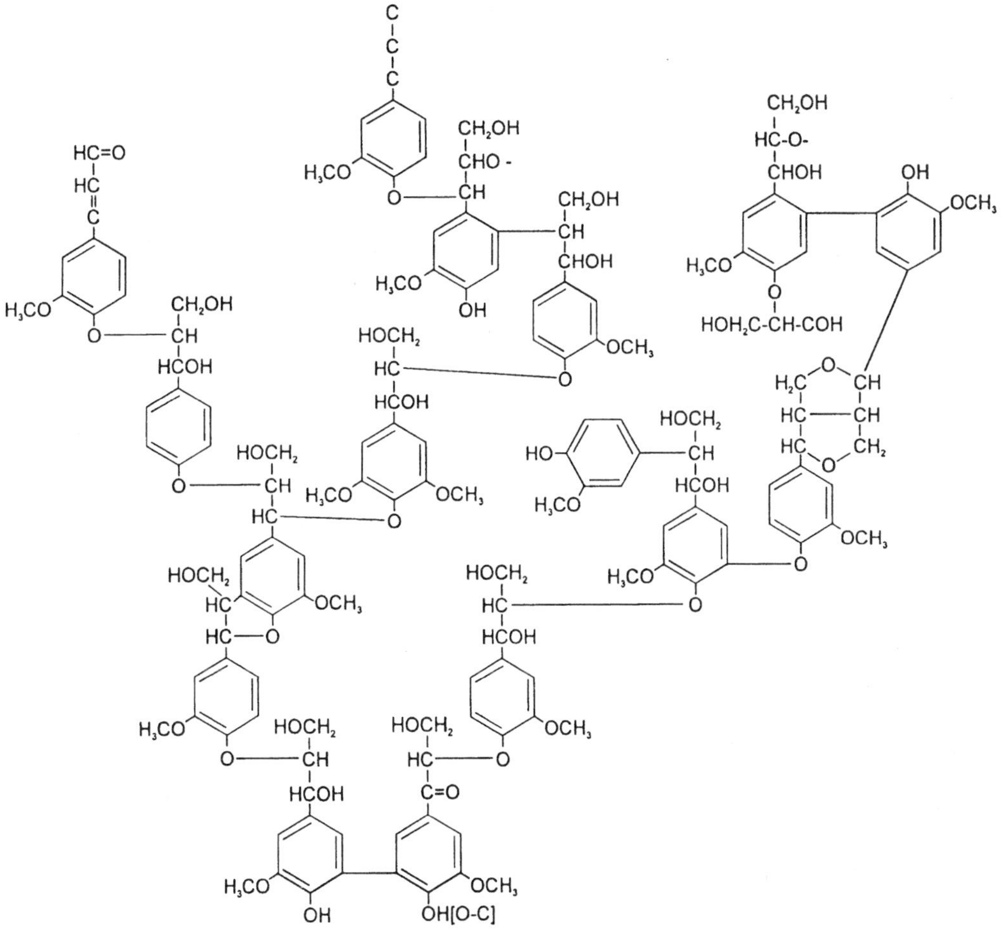

Fig. 1 Partial structural model of spruce wood lignin. The model shows various types of interphenol bonding patterns that are observed in lignin and gives an idea of their relative abundance. (Adapted from Adler, 1977.)

are similar to the phenyl, syringyl, and guaiacyl residues of Table 1 but have a —COOH functional group instead of an —CH$_2$OH functional group on the γ-carbon of the propylene chain. They have been found mostly in the super-order Comelinifloreae (which includes the Gramineae types of Table 2). The carboxylic acid units have been found in association with polysaccharide fractions, suggesting that they are chemically bound to carbohydrate residues. They have also been found as single units after alkaline hydrolysis of lignin at room temperature. Originally it was assumed that they formed part of the basic lignin structure (Higuchi et al., 1967). Yamamoto et al. (1989) later suggested that lignin-associated carboxylic acids may act as lignin cross-linking agents by virtue of their bifunctionality. The cross-bridges could be formed by an ether bond involving the oxygen of the phenol ring on the one end and an ester bond involving the γ-carboxyl group of the propanoid chain on the other end. The exact role of these carboxylic acid units in lignin structure has only recently been discovered; a definitive role for ferulic acid in lignin-carbohydrate bonding has been determined (see Sec. I.B) and the position of p-coumaric acid in the lignin structure has also been discovered. In 1990, Iiyama et al. explained the

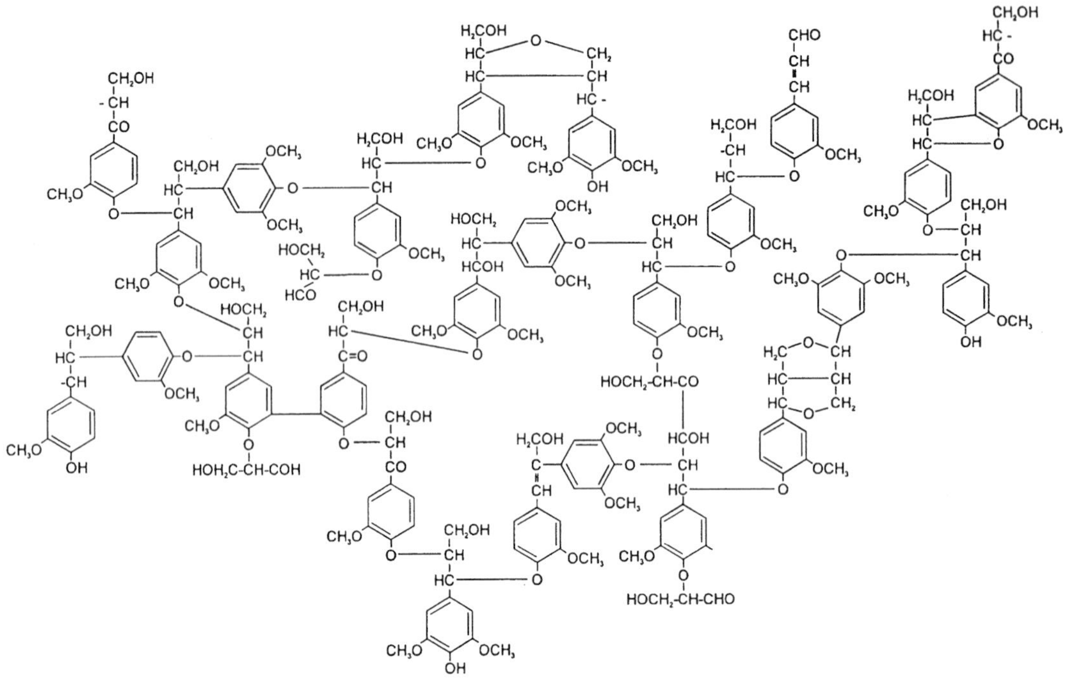

Fig. 2 Partial structural model of beech wood lignin. The model shows various types of interphenol bonding patterns that are observed in lignin and gives an idea of their relative abundance. (Adapted from Nimz, 1974.)

Table 2 Ratio of Guaiacyl to Syringyl Units in Klason Lignin from Various Nonfood and Food Plant Sources

Genus	Common name/Group	Total monomer units (μmol/g Klason lignin)	H/G/S
Notofagus	Evergreen wood	2355	??/12/88
Cratageus	Thorny shrubs	2741	??/21/79
Malus	Apple tree wood	1298	??/26/74
Trifolium	Some fodder plants	1311	??/56/44
Laurelia	Laurel wood (some spices: nutmeg)	1860	??/53/47
Linum	Textile flax	1260	??/80/20
Triticum	Wheat straw	1477	4/43/53
Zea	Corn	606	4/35/61
Oriza	Rice	633	15/40/40

H = Hydroxyphenyl unit; G = guaiacyl unit; S = syringyl unit.
Source: Adapted from Monties, 1989, 1994.

relatively alkaline-labile bonding between phenolic acid and lignin and carbohydrate residues in a proposed structure for wheat internode lignin (Fig. 3). In this model, the ferulic acid units form ester linkages bridging carbohydrate and lignin and the *p*-coumaric acid residues are also found attached to lignin at the end of polymers. It is these ester bonds that are alkali sensitive and yield carboxylic acid monomers after mild alkaline hydrolysis (see also Monties, 1994). Ralph et al. (1994) have also found this arrangement in corn forage fiber. Evidence for the participation of ferulic and *p*-coumaric acids in human dietary fiber has been indirectly obtained. Ferulic acid has been found in wheat flour pentosans (Geissman and Neukom, 1973), and Ring and Selvendran (1980) have found appreciable amounts of ferulic and *p*-coumaric acids in the cell walls of wheat bran. The chemical bond between these compounds and arabinoxylans was sensitive to alkali, suggesting that they were ester linkages.

Ralph et al. (1994) have suggested that the predominance of ester-bonded *p*-coumaric acids (involving the γ-carboxyl group) as well as the lack of ether linkages to the oxygen of the phenol ring argues for a late incorporation of *p*-coumaric acid into the lignin structure. This idea was originally put forward by Iiyama et al. (1990), who observed that concentrations of esterified *p*-coumaric acid increase with physiological maturation in forage plants. Maturation in forage plants involves deposition of a secondary cell wall containing mostly cellulose (Jung, 1977) coupled with extensive lignification to give structural rigidity now that elastic growth has ceased. Thus, Iiyama et al. (1990) postulated that *p*-coumaric acid bound to the core lignin polymer (see below for a discussion of core and noncore terminology) is deposited in the wall during cell maturation and in conjunction with lignification of the secondary plant cell wall (Jung and Deetz, 1993). In rye grass, ferulic acid has been found to participate in cross-bridging of lignin ''strands'' in association with carbohydrate residues (Ralph et al., 1995). These results explain earlier observations that a substantial amount of *p*-coumaric (17%) and ferulic acids (4%) were found associated with the lignin structure after cellulase hydrolysis of wheat straw (Monties, 1991) (see Fig. 4). Wood lignin structures appear to be substantially different from grasses in the type of acid units. Monties (1991) reported that 39% of *p*-hydroxybenzoic and 2% of vanillic acids were associated with the water-insoluble (lignin) fraction after alkaline hydrolysis of poplar wood but *p*-coumaric and ferulic acids are not common in nongrass species.

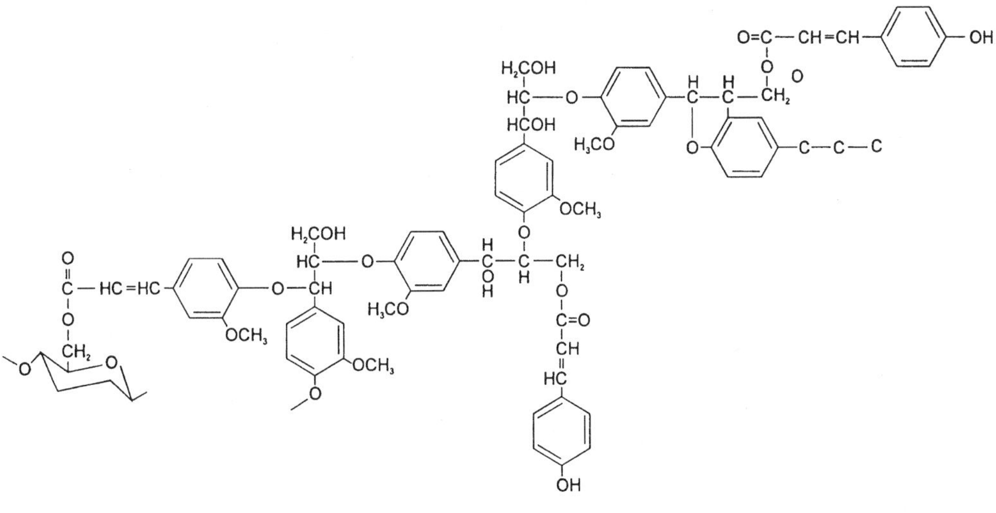

Fig. 3 Proposed chemical structure of lignin in wheat internode cell walls. (Adapted from Iiyama et al., 1990.)

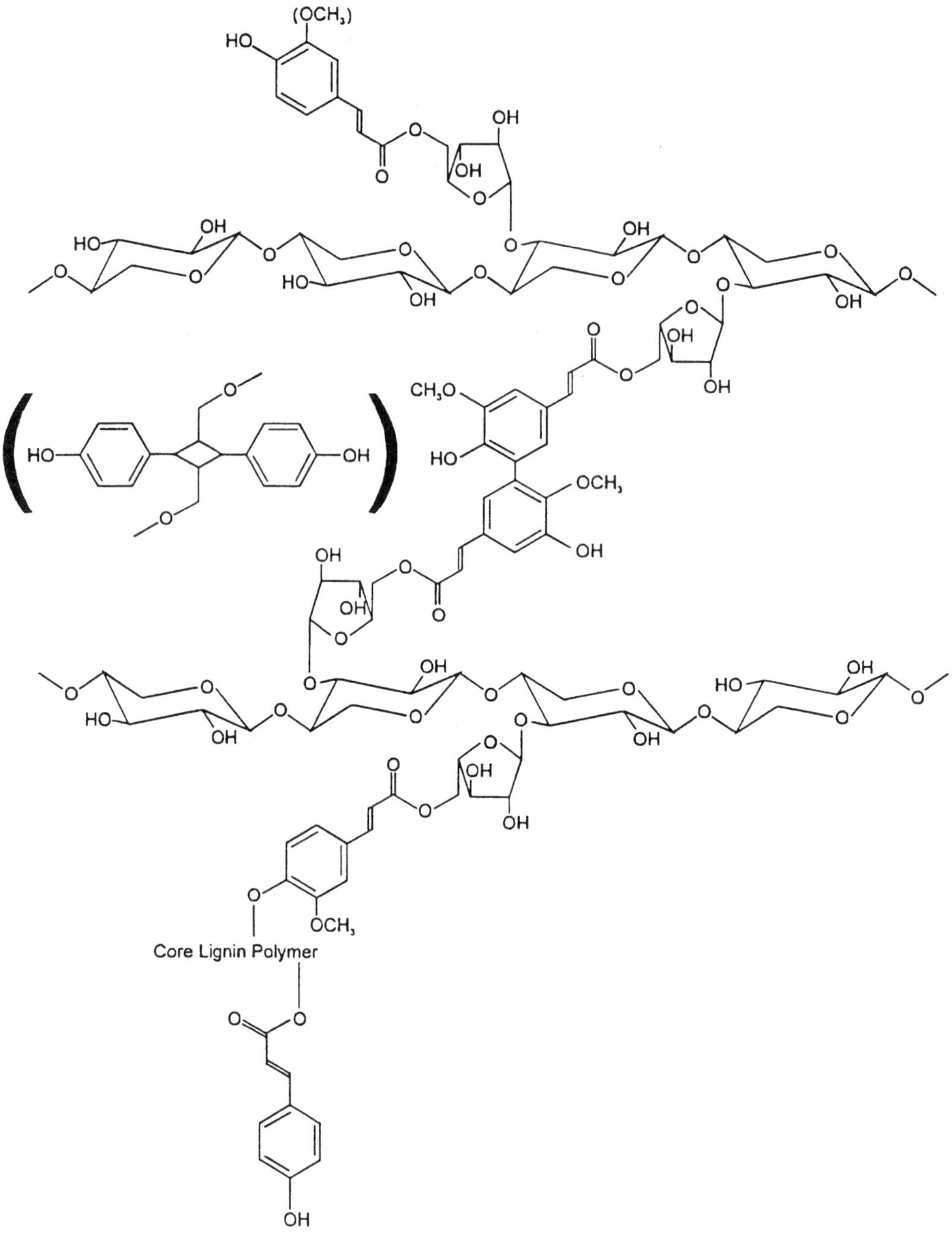

Fig. 4 Model of lignin–ferulic acid–polysaccharide bonding including interhain bridging. Both ferulic and p-coumaric acid participation is noted. Ferulic acids can form intercarbohydrate chain bridges via dehydrodiferulic acid residues ester lined to arabinofuranose residues. The *p*-coumaric acids bridge the chains via truxillic acid esters (shown in parentheses) linked to arabinofuranose units. (Adapted from Jung and Deetz, 1993.)

These results show that a substantial amount of carboxylic acids are intimately associated with lignin structure and not simply bound to carbohydrates.

In addition to the above structural elements, lignin itself has been separated into "core" and "noncore" fractions. This terminology is somewhat confusing, but a paper by Jung and Deetz (1993) clearly illuminates the differences between core and noncore lignin. They point out that the terms core and noncore originated from the use of nonspecific terminology in studies of the "lignin core." The lignin core was first defined by Sarkanen and Ludwig (1971) as "polymeric natural products arising from an enzyme-initiated dehydrogenative polymerization of three primary precursors" (i.e., hydroxyphenyl, guaiacyl, and syringyl units; Table 1). Jung and Deetz (1993) use the following definition provided by Sarkanen and Ludwig (1971) for core lignin: "the phenylpropanoid polymer deposited in the cell wall from polymerization of cinnamyl alcohols during secondary wall thickening." This definition does not physically exclude core lignin to the secondary wall but recognizes the temporal association between lignification and secondary wall thickening (see below). Figure 4 helps clarify the distinction. Ferulic acid and dehydrodiferulic acid residues bridge carbohydrate polymers and are susceptible to alkaline hydrolysis under mild conditions by virtue of their ester bonds. These phenyl compounds are noncore lignins.

Lignin secondary structure also differs depending on the stage of development and the physical location of the lignin. For example, the lignin polymer of the primary wall is more branched and in closer physical association with the polysaccharide portion of the cell wall than is the secondary wall lignin, which is more linear and open in structure. Both primary and secondary wall lignins are thought of as core lignin. Noncore lignin phenolics may participate in chain crosslinking, as discussed above.

B. Lignin-Carbohydrate Bonds

It was not until the early to mid-1800s that researchers began to investigate the chemical nature of wood. These early studies determined that wood was composed of cellulose (the residue left after chemical treatment) and "incrusting material" or lignin (see Merewether, 1951). The resistance of wood to cellulose solvents and the difficulty of separating wood into its various components later (around the mid-1860s) led researchers to conclude that cellulose must be chemically combined with lignin. In the 100 years following these experiments, little more was discovered about the interaction between lignin and carbohydrate. It was clear that extensive chemical treatment was necessary to separate lignin from the carbohydrate fraction of wood, but some researchers believed that the difficulty in extracting lignin from wood was due to a close physical association (Merewether, 1951).

Only recently has a more complete picture of the interaction between lignin and carbohydrate been obtained through studies with chromatography, nuclear magnetic resonance (NMR), and mass spectrometry. Lignin-carbohydrate complexes have been routinely isolated and fractionated and the sugar composition determined. These studies have demonstrated the presence of several different carbohydrate residues (Azuma and Tetsuo, 1988). In order to understand the nature of the carbohydrate-lignin interaction, it is important to understand the cell wall lignification process. Cell wall lignification occurs in stages as plants mature. In immature forage plants, for example, cell walls must be elastic to allow for growth, and primary cell walls are elastic because they lack extensive crosslinking between cell wall polymers. The primary cell wall is made up of several polysaccharides: cellulose, β-glucans, heteroglucans, glucuronarabinoxylans, and heteroxylans (Moore and Hatfield, 1994), but differences in the xylans and pectic substances can be observed between legumes and grasses. In legumes, the pectic substances are substituted with relatively small amounts of ferulic and *p*-coumaric acids, whereas grasses contain high concentrations of ferulic acid esterified to arabinoxylans and small concentrations of p-coumaric acid esters (Jung, 1997). In addition to polysaccharides, proteins are also deposited in primary cell walls.

Lignification is not normally associated with early cell growth because it is thought to impart rigidity to cell structures and young cells must be elastic. However, data from Müsel et al. (1997) show that lignification occurs even in the primary walls of growing maize coleoptyles, long before the deposition of the secondary cell wall during early development when the cells are rapidly extending. The authors showed that lignin was an integral constituent of the primary walls and was associated with proline-rich proteins. After cell extension has stopped, different species deposit different minor sugars in the secondary wall. Lignin polymerization then proceeds through the primary and secondary cell walls, although, as discussed in Section I.A, the branching of lignin is more extensive in the primary wall.

Bonding to carbohydrate may occur through several different interactions. As previously noted (Fig. 3), ferulic acid residues may be directly coupled to carbohydrate residues. Although Iiyama et al. (1990) postulated a direct coupling between lignin polymers and a glucose residue (presumably cellulose), no direct evidence for this type of interaction was presented. It is probable that the bonding pattern more closely resembles that of Fig. 4 (see Jung and Deetz, 1993) with ferulic acid-arabinose (a C-5 sugar) bonding. Direct bonding between ferulic acid and glucose residues (hemicellulose polymers) can be observed, but this represents noncore lignin interactions in forage lignin. For example, hemicellulose–ferulic acid–p-hydroxyphenyl–guaiacyl–syringyl "polymers" can be observed in cell walls of forage plants, but these are not associated with the core lignin polymer (Terashima et al., 1993). In legumes, the cross-linking structure has not yet been identified. However, it is unlikely that ferulic acids are involved because of their known low concentration. Jung (1997) has postulated that tyrosine residues in wall proteins could serve as crosslinking agents since legumes have large amounts of primary wall protein (Jung, 1993).

In woody plants, chemical bonding to almost all the hemicellulose components and even to cellulose has been observed. Sjöström (1993) has reported that 4-O-methyl glucuronic acid can bridge the α-carbon of the propanoid chain and xylan chains via an ester bond. Arabinofuranose and galactopyranose units have also been observed bridging lignin to xylan or mannan chains, respectively, via ether bonds in soft woods.

II. TRADITIONAL METHODS OF LIGNIN ANALYSIS IN NONHUMAN FOODS

Several methods exist for the isolation of lignin from plant material including: ball milling, strong acid and base treatments, periodate treatment, enzymatic treatments, alcohol-HCl isolation, thioglycolic acid treatment, acetic acid treatment, dioxane-HCl solubilization, phenol solubilization, and hydrogenolysis (see Obst and Kirk, 1988). In addition, several chemical processes exist to produce lignin preparations from wood: the Kraft process (hot alkaline sodium sulfide) and soda lignin (hot sodium hydroxide) are the most common examples of these methods. Of all these procedures, ball-milling gives a lignin preparation that most closely resembles native lignin (or protolignin; Obst and Kirk, 1988). Other methods produce various degrees of chemically altered lignin. When considered from a quantitative viewpoint, the major drawback to these methods is that most give a poor yield of lignin (8–30%), and no method efficiently extracts all the lignin from the wood. In addition, chemical analysis of the lignin preparations has shown that differences in the isolation procedure (either a change in the isolation conditions of a particular procedure or utilization of a different procedure) produce lignins of different chemical composition (Browning, 1967; Ben-Ghedalia and Yosef, 1994; Wallace et al., 1995; Terrón et al., 1996). Consequently, these methods have not been used to estimate the concentration of lignin in wood but, rather, to study the structural arrangement of the lignin polymer or to produce lignin on an industrial scale.

In choosing a quantitative method to measure lignin in foods, reproducibility and lack of reaction with interfering substances are important characteristics. No change in the lignin concentration should be noted after heating or processing of the original food unless part of the process involves a refining step. In addition, the method should perform adequately under various conditions using different starting materials. Meeting these criteria does not guarantee that the chosen method is fully adequate but ensures only that it is reproducible from laboratory to laboratory (consistency of results). In many cases lignin is quantified gravimetrically with no subsequent analysis for purity. This means that many methods operate essentially "blind" with respect to verification of the final isolate. This problem is difficult to overcome since lignin itself is difficult to analyze by virtue of its chemical nature and poor solubility in water.

A. Klason Lignin

The most common method for analyzing lignin in nonhuman diets is the Klason procedure. Several variants of the Klason lignin procedure exist, but all are based on the original method described by Ellis et al. (1946). Giger (1985) has reviewed and described the different methodologies. In the Klason method, polysaccharides are removed from wood preextracted using an organic solvent by hydrolysis with strong acids to leave a residue of lignin. Originally, Klason applied 64–72% sulfuric acid to a sample of benzene-extracted wood and let the mixture stand at 15°C for 2 hours with occasional stirring. The sulfuric acid was then diluted to 3% with water, washed with 3% sulfuric acid and refluxed for 4 hours. The residue was measured after filtering. Current modifications allow for the sample to be heated to 30°C for 1 hour in 72% H_2SO_4 followed by dilution (1:25) with water and autoclaving at 120°C for 1 hour. Although this method can be used as a general guide, several authors indicate that the procedure must be optimized for each type of wood. The yield of methoxyl functional groups is used as a monitor of performance. The H_2SO_4 concentration of 72% was chosen because cellulose is not completely hydrolyzed at concentrations below 65% and concentrations ≥80% cause the formation of insoluble polysaccharide complexes (Lai and Sarkanen, 1971).

Problems with the Klason procedure exist despite the fact that it is recognized as a standard method by TAPPI. For example, the final preparation may retain considerable sulfuric acid leading to overestimation of the lignin content (Browning, 1967). When measuring the lignin content of forages, a correction for the content of ash and protein appears necessary. Depending on temperature (van Soest, 1963), moisture content, nitrogen content, and particle size, feed drying may induce high Klason lignin values (Giger, 1985). Lai and Sarkanen (1971) suggested that this may be due to protein condensing with lignin under acidic conditions leading to a (falsely) higher yield of lignin. In support of this conclusion, Klason lignins from trypsin-treated vegetable materials have been found to contain 2.5–15% co-condensed protein (Armitage et al., 1948). Studies on Klason lignin from lucerne, cocksfoot, and switchgrass stem material have also shown appreciable nitrogen content of 1–2% (g/g lignin) (Hatfield et al., 1994). This represents 10–20% of the initial nitrogen content. If one assumes a conversion factor of 6.25 g protein/g nitrogen, one can estimate that 6–12% (g/g) of the Klason lignin was protein. Hatfield et al. (1994) demonstrated that this protein was probably not due to co-precipitation of plant protein as a contaminant since the Klason lignin nitrogen content negatively correlated with the nitrogen content of the original forage sample. In addition, they showed that addition of bovine serum albumin or lysine had no effect on Klason lignin yield. Hatfield et al. (1994) point out that the protein may be chemically bound to the lignin but also note that chemical proof has not been obtained for a protein-lignin bond. One can also add a prehydrolysis step (4 h reflux, 5% H_2SO_4) to remove humin-like degradation products of polysaccharides, but this is known to solubilize some of the lignin and gives lower lignin values (Sharma et al., 1986).

In addition to the potential problem of protein contamination, Klason lignin can be divided into acid-soluble lignin and acid-insoluble lignin portions (Monties, 1984). In woody plants, the amount of acid-soluble lignin has been estimated at around 16% for *Eucalyptus*, birch, and aspen wood (see Lai and Sarkanen, 1971). In addition to the acid pretreatments, wood samples have been preextracted with hot water to remove interfering compounds. This procedure is not recommended since it can reduce the lignin content by 4–10%, depending on the wood sample (see Lai and Sarkanen, 1971). Alkaline pretreatments have also been used to remove some of the tannins and other nonlignin phenolics. These, too, are known to solubilize some of the lignin depending on the temperature and time of pretreatment. As discussed above (Sec. I.A), many of the ferulic and *p*-coumaric acid residues bound to lignin are easily solubilized by mild alkaline treatment. These residues form part of the lignin polymer, although they are found predominantly at the end of chains and are only deposited later during plant maturation. Alkaline treatment (5% NaOH) at high temperatures (200°C) has been shown to solubilize guaiacol and even methoxyl groups (Sarkanen et al., 1963).

Several empirical procedures have been developed to overcome the problems outlined above. Many of these involve the determination of lignin losses during the pre-treatments and during the acid treatment itself. Monties (1989) cautions that these should be extrapolated with care since differences in the monomeric composition have been related to differences in solubility and spectroscopic properties and an unambiguous characterization of acid/base soluble lignin is not possible.

B. Spectrophotometric Methods

The major problem with spectrophotometric procedures is the insolubility of the lignin preparations. In order for the procedure to quantitatively assess total lignin concentrations, the sample must be completely solubilized so that an accurate measurement can be made. The most common method for measuring lignins spectrophotometrically is the acetyl bromide procedure. The original procedure has been modified both by Iiyama and Wallis (1988) and by Morrison (1972a,b). Iiyama recommended addition of perchloric acid to accelerate dissolution of the material permitting coarser samples to be analyzed. In addition they improved the reproducibility by adding twice the conventional concentration of NaOH and omitting the hydroxylamine hydrochloride addition. Dence (1992) gives a summary of the current method. The wording of the original method (Iiyama and Wallis, 1988) is a little ambiguous, and we have been using the following method. Samples are placed in 15 mL glass tubes containing 4.8 mL of 25% (v/v) acetyl bromide in acetic acid plus 0.2 mL of 70% perchloric acid (5 mL total volume). Tubes are sealed with Teflon caps and incubated for 30 minutes at 70°C in an oven. Swirl the samples every 10 minute. The solution is transferred to a 100 mL volumetric flask containing 10 mL of 2 M NaOH and 25 mL of acetic acid. The glass tubes are rinsed with acetic acid, and the solution is made up to 100 mL with acetic acid. The UV absorption is measured against a blank solution. Lignin is calculated from the absorbance at 280 nm as:

$$\%\text{Lignin} = \frac{100 \times (A_S - A_B)}{W \times \varepsilon_{280}} \tag{1}$$

where A_S and A_B are the absorbances of the sample and blank, respectively. W is the weight of the sample (g) and ε_{280} is the absorptivity at 280 nm (L $\cdot$ g^{-1} $\cdot$ cm^{-1}). Equation 1 applies to nonpulped samples. Iiyama and Wallis (1988) used an ε_{280} value of 20 L $\cdot$ g^{-1} $\cdot$ cm^{-1} that could be applied to both softwood and hardwood lignin preparations. No general molar extinction coefficient exists for lignin in human foods. It is important to calibrate the method with lignin isolated from the sample in question because the absorption spectrum can very even within woods and forages (see Monties, 1989, for a review). Fukushima et al. (1991) used purified lignin extracted from alfalfa to follow lignin degradation in alfalfa during digestion. They observed that 48.5% of the lignin disappeared from the solid digesta during in vitro digestion, suggesting that the acetyl bromide procedure measures both core and noncore lignin units.

Problems with interlaboratory standardization can occur with the acetyl bromide method. Standardization with compounds such as vanillin (Bagby et al., 1973) and ferulic acid (Monties, 1989) has been suggested as a remedy. In addition, it is often difficult to obtain a purified lignin preparation from the plant material under study. In this case, practical solutions may provide an answer. For example, Morrison (1972a, b) determined the relationship between the absorptivity of a hot water/ethanol/acetone/diethyl ether extract of forage plants and the Klason lignin content (as measured by the method of Ellis et al., 1946) of these same plants as an estimate of the absorption coefficient of the lignin. The resulting regression equation allowed the calibration of Morrison's extraction method and provided plant Klason lignin contents of grasses (1972a) and legumes (1972b). Even though this method does not provide an absolute measure of the lignin concentration for differently prepared samples, it may point the way to establishing a standard method for measuring lignin in the human diet. To date, no determination of the ε_{280} value for human dietary fiber has been published.

A final problem involves the nature of the derivatized lignin spectrum itself. Figure 5 shows the spectrum of acetyl bromide–derivatized lignin from hard red spring wheat bran after neutral detergent and acid detergent extractions (Goering and van Soest, 1970). It is apparent that the peak at 280 nm, representing the six-membered ring aromatic absorbance maximum, is not the dominant peak even after substraction of the blank. The dominant peak at approximately 254 nm represents conjugated double bonds but cannot be used to measure lignin concentration because of its variability (Iiyama and Wallis, 1988). The spectrum of Fig. 5 shows several anomalies, especially below 245 nm, where absorbance appears constant and finite and the value differs depending on the method of preparation (contrast ADF vs. AF preparations). The loss of absorbency below 245 nm must reflect the action of acetyl bromide on the lignin polymer since purified hard red spring wheat bran has an absorbance maximum below 248 nm (Schwarz et al., 1989). The acetylation process must be incomplete, however, since this absorbance is constant but differs from preparation to preparation. In addition, some of the absorbance must come from the acetyl bromide derivatization method since the blank also shows constant and finite absorbance in this region. This contribution is difficult to estimate because it is not uniform across the range of wavelengths measured. For example, all the sample absorbances approach zero at 400 nm. These considerations mean that the nature of the original sample and the method of sample preparation may greatly influence the final absorbance at 280 nm. In accordance with this conclusion, Reeves and Galletti (1991) have demonstrated that the acetyl bromide method overestimates the lignin concentration because carbohydrates interfere with the spectrophotometric determination. Many of these problems may be avoided by selection of another wavelength to allow calculation of a difference spectrum (acting as an internal control). Several different samples will have to be examined before a definite relationship between the absolute concentration of dietary lignin (human) and the absorbance (as measured by the acetyl bromide method) can be established.

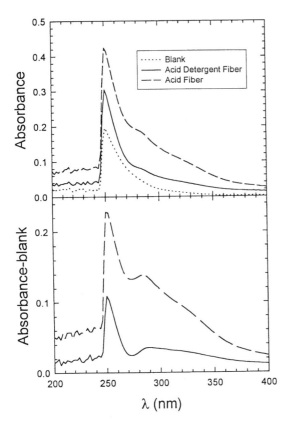

Fig. 5 Spectrum of acetyl bromide–derivatized hard red spring wheat bran. Approximately 15 mg of hard red spring wheat bran was derivatized as outlined in the text. ADF (Goering and van Soest, 1970) or acid fiber (similar to ADF but without the presence of detergent) was prepared and dried. Samples were derivatized with acetyl bromide and their spectra recorded. (Data from S. P. J. Brooks and B. J. Lampi, unpublished.)

C. Other Methods

Several different methods for lignin determination have been published. Most of these are modifications of standard determinations such as the Klason (or acid) lignin method or the spectrophotometric method. For analysis of forage fiber, van Soest (van Soest, 1963; van Soest and Wine, 1967; Goering and van Soest, 1970; van Soest and Robertson, 1980) proposed a milder version of the Klason lignin method that eliminates the acid reflux step present in the original Klason procedure. In this procedure, called the acid detergent lignin (ADL) procedure, the sample is first treated to produce a neutral detergent fiber (NDF) extract and then to produce an acid detergent fiber (ADF) extract. The ADF extract is then incubated in 72% H_2SO_4 at 15°C for 3 hours with stirring to break up the lumps. Lignin is measured as the difference in weight after ashing. Goering and van Soest (1970) indicated that this procedure may be preferable with certain materials since the milder conditions will not produce Maillard products, will help to reduce the amount of acid soluble lignin lost during refluxing, and may reduce protein coprecipitation. Maillard products occur when a reducing sugar and an amino acid such as lysine undergo condensation and polymerization. The new "Maillard polymers" may participate if further polymerization reactions to give a variety of products. These nitrogen-containing polymers may be retained in the final lignin residue giving falsely high values. In accordance with these arguments, the ADL method usually gives lower values when compared with Klason lignin (Hatfield et al., 1994). Some of the improvement in the specificity of the method may result from the detergent treatment. This removes a substantial amount of the protein as shown by a lower nitrogen content in the ADL residue as compared to Klason lignin (Hatfield et al., 1994). Note that part of the lowered ADL yield may also be due to detergent solubilization of the lignin polymer (see Sec. I). In addition, the earlier method of Goering and van Soest (1970) included sodium sulfite in the NDF procedure. It was later found that sulfite has many effects on NDF: it apparently inhibits formation of Maillard products while attacking the lignin polymer (Marlett and Johnson, 1985). Consequently, more modern versions of the NDF method exclude sodium sulfite.

Permanganate has also been used to estimate lignin concentrations. In theory, permanganate oxidizes the lignin components leaving only the sugar residues behind. Permanganate oxidation has been combined with peroxide oxidation to give a complex pattern of digestion products that can be analyzed by GC to give structural information (Tanahashi and Higuchi, 1988; Gellersteat, 1992). The amount of permanganate consumed during the oxidation reaction (the K number) has also been related to the lignin concentration of wood (Browning, 1967). Goering and van Soest (1970), who developed a complete method for analysis of forage fiber after neutral and acid detergent extractions, indicated that the choice between the permanganate and Klason procedures depended on the material and on the final purpose for which the values would be used. However, they favored the permanganate method because it was quicker, the reagents were milder than those used for the Klason procedure, the method did not involve heating the sample (to reduce potential Maillard products and protein-carbohydrate linkages), and it seemed less subject to interference by nonlignin components. In their method, a mixture of saturated $KMnO_4$ is added to an ADF preparation that is contained in Gooch crucibles (placed in a pan containing about 1 cm of water to reduce the flow of permanganate solution out of the bottom). The sample is allowed to sit, covered with $KMnO_4$ solution for 90 minutes at room temperature. It is then washed (with a decolorizing reagent) and dried. The lignin is measured by the change in weight before and after treatment (see also Kirk and Obst, 1988). Compared to the 72% sulfuric acid method after ADF treatment, the permanganate residue includes true lignin and tannins and excludes cutin, damaged protein, and tannin-protein condensation products (van Soest, 1969). In a comparison of methodologies, Nordkvist et al. (1989) found that permanganate lignin values were only one half (wheat straw) or one third (red clover stems) those of the corresponding Klason lignin values. This was also observed when an organic layer of spruce litter was measured by both procedures (Rowland and Roberts, 1994). Giger (1985) and Reeves and Galletti (1991) have also found that sulfuric acid lignin and permanganate lignin values were not strongly correlated ($r = 0.43, p < 0.05, N = 25; r = 0.51, p < 0.07, N =$ not indicated, respectively). This phenomenon has also observed by Rowland and Roberts (1994). Reeves and Galletti (1991) investigated the reasons for these differences. They found that the permanganate procedure may extract some of the carbohydrate in addition to some crude protein (measured as nitrogen).

Many other oxidizing agents have been applied to lignin investigation, including periodate, nitrobenzene, and chlorite. These methods appear to completely solubilize lignin, but it is uncertain how much of the carbohydrate portion is liberated by these methods.

Lignin has also been determined by derivitization with thioglycolic acid. This method has gained popularity since the formation of lignothioglycolic acid was a reported characteristic of lignin (Freudenberg, 1968). In addition, lignothioglycolic acids are apparently free of interfering polymers, such as proteins, in forage material. The method is rather involved: the sample is reacted with thioglycolic acid and BF_3 in 2 N HCl for 4 hours at 100°C. The lignothioglycolic acid is then extracted with 0.5 N NaOH or dimethylformamide. When dimethylformamide is used, the lignin is quantified spectrophotometrically (Kimmins and Wuddah, 1954; Aulin-Erdtman and Hegbom, 1957). Kirk and Obst (1988) indicate that interference by nonlignin components is apparently minimal, but they suggest that methoxyl and other analyses should be performed to verify purity. The residue after NaOH extraction can be weighed to give lignin gravimetrically (Venverloo, 1969; Whitmore, 1978). The gravimetric determination may be confounded by the presence of protein (Whitmore, 1978; Monties, 1988).

It is possible to solubilize lignin from samples using triethylene glycol. Edwards (1973) described a simple procedure where samples were autoclaved for 1 hour at 121°C in triethylene glycol containing 0.2% HCl. The lignin content is obtained from the weight of sample before and after treatment. The method compared favorably to permanganate lignin determinations in pods and stems of lupins. However the triethylene glycol method gave lignin values approximately twofold higher than Klason lignin values. The source of the variability was not investigated, but Edwards (1973) noted that the residue left after the triethylene glycol treatment was almost completely soluble in 72% H_2SO_4. These results are different from those observed by Reeves and Galletti (1991), where triethylene glycol apparently underestimated lignin concentrations because of the inefficiency in extracting the lignin. Obviously, the efficiency and specificity of the methods differ greatly, depending on the nature of the plant material. Lapierre (1993) has extensively reviewed several other methods based on mass spectrometry and gas chromatography.

III. METHODS OF LIGNIN ANALYSIS IN HUMAN FOODS

Although lignin has traditionally been thought of as part of dietary fiber (see Sec. I), not all methods of dietary fiber analysis include lignin in the final analysis. Table 3 shows some common methods for analyzing dietary fiber and indicates whether they include lignin as part of the analysis. Englyst cites two major reasons for not including Klason lignin in his method: ''no important physiological effect of lignin in the human diet has been demonstrated'' and ''no accurate method is available for routine measurement of true lignin'' (Englyst et al., 1995). It is difficult to argue with the second point, as pointed out in Section II. However, lignin appears

Table 3 Comparison of Lignin Determination in Different Methods for Dietary Fiber or Nonstarch Polysaccharide Determination

Method	Includes lignin?	Methodology	Ref.
Prosky enzymatic-gravimetric	Yes	No separate determination; lignin included in insoluble dietary fiber	Prosky et al., 1988
Lee enzymatic-gravimetric	Yes	No separate determination; lignin included in insoluble dietary fiber	Lee et al., 1992
HPB enzymatic-gravimetric	Yes	No separate determination; lignin included in insoluble dietary fiber	Mongeau and Brassard, 1993
Englyst GLC and colorimetric	No	Method determines nonstarch polysaccharides only	Englyst et al., 1994
Uppsala	Yes	Lignin determined as Klason lignin and added to nonstarch polysaccharides	Theander et al., 1995

Source: Adapted from Asp, 1995.

to play an important role in determining overall plant matter fermentability and may play a more specific role in mediating certain biochemical responses (Sec. V).

A. Klason and Acid Detergent Lignins

The method of Klason lignin analysis for human foods can be found in Theander et al. (1995). This method is similar to that used for wood lignin and forage fiber lignin determinations (see Sec. II). In the method of Theander et al. (1995) the sample has been extracted and treated with α-amylase and amyloglucosidase prior to ethanol precipitation. The final pellet is subjected to Klason hydrolysis. Alternately, an acid detergent sample can be prepared prior to analysis. The sample is placed in a glass tube and dispersed with a glass rod. Three mL of 12 M H_2SO_4 is added and the samples are incubated at 30°C in a water bath for 1 hour (capped) with occasional stirring. The tube contents are then quantitatively transferred into a 250 mL beaker with 74.0 mL water. The beakers are covered with aluminum foil and autoclaved at 125°C for 1 hour. The solution is filtered (still warm) through a (preweighed, W_1) glass-fritted crucible and washed with 50 mL of water. Samples are dried for 16 hours in a 105°C oven. The samples plus crucible are weighed accurately (W_2), ashed, and reweighed (W_3). Klason lignin is calculated as the difference: $W_2 - W_3$. The ash is calculated as $W_3 - W_1$.

The ADL method most commonly followed is that of Goering and van Soest (1970), which was originally described for forage fiber. In this method, as mentioned above, ADF residues are treated with cool (15°C) 72% sulfuric acid for 3 hours with mixing in glass filter-bottom crucibles. The sample is filtered, washed, and weighed. ADL is measured as the difference in weight after ashing the material.

When either the Klason or ADL method is applied to human foods, the lignin preparations may contain lignin as well as tannins, cutins, some proteinaceous materials, and nondigestible Maillard reaction products in heat-treated foods (Theander et al., 1995). This has been directly demonstrated in Klason lignin prepared from forage fibers (Reeves and Galletti, 1991). The inclusion of these substances means that the same foods may have differing lignin values depending on the type of processing (raw vs. cooked) (Table 4), and the absolute difference may be a function of carbohydrate or protein content of the specific food. In addition to these concerns, Lowry et al. (1994) have shown that acid treatment solubilizes some lignin. This occurs even in the ADL procedure during the preparation of ADF: the ADF eluate contains the fraction of lignin sensitive to mild alkaline treatment (Lowry et al., 1994). The loss of some fraction of the lignin may partly offset the increased weight that results from incomplete cellulose hydrolysis, sulfuric acid precipitation, and inclusion of Maillard products, but the effect on the final yield is unknown.

Table 4 Klason Lignin Values in Untreated and Heat-Treated Samples

Sample	Klason lignin (g/100 g wet weight)	% of total protein associated with Klason lignin
White wheat flour, untreated	0.2	0.3
White wheat flour, extruded at 168°C	0.4	2.3
Whole wheat flour, untreated	1.4	4.7
Whole wheat flour, extruded at 180°C	2.8	11.0
Potato, raw	0.4	ND
Potato, boiled	1.2	ND
Potato, pressure cooked	2.6	ND

Source: Adapted from Theander and Westerlund, 1993.

Table 5 Dietary Fiber and Lignin Content of Various Human Foods

Food	g/100 g wet weight[a]			Lignin as	Method	Ref.
	Moisture	Fiber[b]	Lignin	% of fiber		
Fruits						
Apple	85.9	1.8	0.1	6	KMnO$_4$	R. Mongeau and R. Brassard, unpublished
Apple	88.3	0.9	0.01	1	Klason	van Soest, 1978b
Apple	84.3	2	0.4	18	Klason	Anderson and Bridges, 1988
Apple, flesh only	??	1.4	0.01	1	Klason	Southgate, 1986
Apple, Granny Smith	83.8	2.7	0.1	4	Klason	Marlett, 1992
Apple, Red Delicious	83.6	2	0.2	10	Klason	Marlett, 1992
Apple, flesh only, Red Delicious	84.6	1.5	0.1	7	Klason	Marlett, 1992
Apple, flesh only, Golden	81.0	1.6	0.11	7	Klason	Vidal-Valverde et al., 1982
Apple, flesh only, Reineta	83.8	2.1	0.28	13	Klason	Vidal-Valverde et al., 1982
Apple, flesh only, Starking	86.6	1.1	0.14	13	Klason	Vidal-Valverde et al., 1982
Apple, peel only	??	3.7	0.49	13	Klason	Southgate, 1986
Applesauce, canned	87.9	1.6	0.1	7	Klason	Anderson and Bridges, 1988
Apricots	85.3	1.7	0.12	7	Klason	Vidal-Valverde et al., 1982
Apricots, canned in syrup	73.4	1.8	0.1	6	Klason	Marlett, 1992
Avocado (CA)	77.3	3.9	0.1	3	Klason	Marlett, 1992
Banana	75.7	1.7	0.6	35	Klason	Marlett, 1992
Banana	73.9	1.9	0.8	44	Klason	Anderson and Bridges, 1988
Banana	??	1.8	0.26	15	Klason	Southgate, 1986
Banana	75.3	1.9	0.1	7	KMnO$_4$	R. Mongeau and R. Brassard, unpublished
Blueberries	85.6	2.5	0.5	19	KMnO$_4$	R. Mongeau and R. Brassard, unpublished
Blueberries	84.8	3.0	0.79	26	KMnO$_4$	Foy et al., 1981
Blueberries	85.4	2.7	0.9	33	Klason	Marlett, 1992
Cantaloupe	88.7	0.7	tr	—	Klason	Marlett, 1992
Carambola	90.2	1.2	0.32	28	KMnO$_4$	Lund and Smoot, 1982
Cherimoya, flesh only	75.8	2.4	0.15	6	Klason	Vidal-Valverde et al., 1982
Cherries	76.3	0.9	0.12	13	Klason	Vidal-Valverde et al., 1982
Cherries	??	1.2	0.07	6	Klason	Southgate, 1986
Cherries, tart, canned	90.9	0.9	0.2	22	Klason	Marlett, 1992

Fig, flesh only	78.4	2.4	0.25	10	Klason	Vidal-Valverde et al., 1982
Fig, flesh only, early	94.9	1.7	0.18	11	Klason	Vidal-Valverde et al., 1982
Grapefruit	85.3	1.2	0.20	16	Klason	Vidal-Valverde et al., 1982
Grapefruit	90.2	0.2	0.03	15	KMnO$_4$	Lund and Smoot, 1982
Grapefruit (FL), yellow	89.5	1.2	0	4	Klason	Anderson and Bridges, 1988
Grapefruit (FL), pink, with membrane	86.9	1.4	tr	—	Klason	Marlett, 1992
Grapefruit (FL), pink, without membrane	88.4	0.5	tr	—	Klason	Marlett, 1992
Grapefruit (TX), pink without membrane	87.9	0.4	tr	—	Klason	Marlett, 1992
Grapefruit (TX), white, without membrane	88.2	0.4	tr	—	Klason	Marlett, 1992
Grapefruit, canned	??	0.4	0.06	14	Klason	Southgate, 1986
Grapes, purple	80.6	1.9	0.2	11	KMnO$_4$	R. Mongeau and R. Brassard, unpublished
Grapes, Rosetti	80.9	0.5	0.16	32	Klason	Vidal-Valverde et al., 1982
Grapes, Thompson, green	80	1	0.2	20	Klason	Marlett, 1992
Grapes, Villanueva	80.2	0.6	0.17	31	Klason	Vidal-Valverde et al., 1982
Greengage, flesh only	74.7	1.7	0.44	26	Klason	Vidal-Valverde et al., 1982
Guavas, canned	??	3.6	0.8	22	Klason	Southgate, 1986
Lemon, flesh only	87.2	2.1	0.22	11	Klason	Vidal-Valverde et al., 1982
Mangoes	84.5	1.1	0.04	4	KMnO$_4$	Lund and Smoot, 1982
Mangoes, canned	??	1	0.03	3	Klason	Southgate, 1986
Medlar, flesh only	85.0	1.6	0.23	14	Klason	Vidal-Valverde et al., 1982
Melon, cantaloupe	90.1	0.9	0.2	19	KMnO$_4$	Mongeau and Brassard, unpublished
Melon, flesh only	88.2	0.6	0.06	11	Klason	Vidal-Valverde et al., 1982
Nectarine	89.7	1.2	0.1	8	Klason	Marlett, 1992
Orange	86	1.8	0.2	11	KMnO$_4$	R. Mongeau and R. Brassard, unpublished
Orange (CA), seedless	87.9	1.4	0	3	Klason	Anderson and Bridges, 1988
Orange (FL)	86.8	1.9	tr	—	Klason	Marlett, 1992
Orange, flesh only	87.1	1.1	0.19	18	Klason	Vidal-Valverde et al., 1982
Orange, flesh only	86.4	0.5	0.24	49	Klason	van Soest, 1978b
Orange, navel	85.5	1.7	tr	—	Klason	Marlett, 1992
Orange, mandarin, flesh only	87.0	0.9	0.11	13	Klason	Vidal-Valverde et al., 1982
Orange, mandarin, canned	??	0.3	0.03	10	Klason	Southgate, 1986
Papaya	86.7	0.9	0.09	9	KMnO$_4$	Lund and Smoot, 1982
Peach	??	2.3	0.62	27	Klason	Southgate, 1986
Peach	87.1	2.1	0.2	7	KMnO$_4$	R. Mongeau and R. Brassard, unpublished
Peach, flesh only	87.7	1.2	0.09	7	Klason	Vidal-Valverde et al., 1982
Peach, canned	91.6	1.6	0.1	9	Klason	Anderson and Bridges, 1988

Table 5 Continued

Food	g/100 g wet weight[a]			Lignin as % of fiber	Method	Ref.
	Moisture	Fiber[b]	Lignin			
Pear	84.5	2.1	0.3	14	KMnO$_4$	R. Mongeau and R. Brassard, unpublished
Pear	83.0	1.9	0.24	13	KMnO$_4$	Flint and Camire, 1992
Pear	83.0	1.9	0.22	12	Klason	Flint and Camire, 1992
Pear, Bartlett	85	2.8	0.4	14	Klason	Marlett, 1992
Pear, flesh only	??	2.4	0.45	18	Klason	Southgate, 1986
Pear, "lemon-like," flesh only	85.5	2.2	0.30	14	Klason	Vidal-Valverde et al., 1982
Pear, "watery," flesh only	82.6	2.5	0.24	10	Klason	Vidal-Valverde et al., 1982
Pear, peel only	??	8.6	2.67	31	Klason	Southgate, 1986
Pear, canned	86.7	1.8	0.25	14	KMnO$_4$	Flint and Camire, 1992
Pear, canned	86.7	1.8	0.24	13	Klason	Flint and Camire, 1992
Pear, canned	90.6	3	0.5	15	Klason	Anderson and Bridges, 1988
Pear, canned in extra light syrup	89.7	1.7	0.2	12	Klason	Marlett, 1992
Pineapple, flesh only	82.4	1.5	0.05	3	Klason	Vidal-Valverde et al., 1982
Pineapple, flesh only	85.1	0.9	0.05	5	KMnO$_4$	Lund and Smoot, 1982
Pineapple, canned	84.2	1	0.1	9	KMnO$_4$	R. Mongeau and R. Brassard, unpublished
Pineapple, canned	82.7	1.7	0	2	Klason	Anderson and Bridges, 1988
Pineapple, canned	83.5	0.9	0.03	3	KMnO$_4$	Lund and Smoot, 1982
Pineapple, canned in unsweetened juice	83.4	0.7	tr	—	Klason	Marlett, 1992
Plantain, flesh only, February	73.3	1.6	0.50	31	Klason	Vidal-Valverde et al., 1982
Plantain, flesh only, July	67.9	2.8	0.20	7	Klason	Vidal-Valverde et al., 1982
Plum	??	1.5	0.3	20	Klason	Southgate, 1986
Plums	85.4	1.5	0.2	14	KMnO$_4$	R. Mongeau and R. Brassard, unpublished
Plum, Friar	87.1	1.2	0.2	17	Klason	Marlett, 1992
Plum, red, flesh only	77.6	1.6	0.47	30	Klason	Vidal-Valverde et al., 1982
Plum, white, flesh only	88.8	1.1	0.07	7	Klason	Vidal-Valverde et al., 1982
Plum, purple, canned	90.4	2.2	0.3	14	Klason	Anderson and Bridges, 1988
Raisins	9.9	4.2	1.8	43	Klason	Marlett, 1992
Raisins, sultanas	??	4.4	1.17	27	Klason	Southgate, 1986
Raspberries	81.0	3.9	0.53	14	KMnO$_4$	Foy et al., 1981
Rhubarb, raw	??	1.8	0.15	8	Klason	Southgate, 1986

Sapodilla	77.9	5.3	2.28	43	KMnO₄	Lund and Smoot, 1982
Strawberries	90.5	1.7	0.3	19	KMnO₄	R. Mongeau and R. Brassard, unpublished
Strawberries	90.2	1.8	0.5	28	Klason	Marlett, 1992
Strawberries	??	2.1	0.81	38	Klason	Southgate, 1986
Strawberries	88.2	1.6	0.19	12	Klason	Vidal-Valverde et al., 1982
Strawberries, canned	??	1	0.33	33	Klason	Southgate, 1986
Tangerine	85.1	1.8	0.1	6	Klason	Marlett, 1992
Watermelon	90.1	0.4	tr	—	Klason	Marlett, 1992
Watermelon	91.1	0.3	0.09	33	Klason	Vidal-Valverde et al., 1982
Vegetables						
Amaranth, green	92.5	3.2	0.46	14	Klason	Chang et al., 1994
Amaranth, red	92.1	3.1	0.21	7	Klason	Chang et al., 1994
Artichoke hearts	87.9	1.5	0.18	12	Klason	van Soest, 1978b
Artichokes, raw	87.5	3.5	0.50	14	ADL	Herranz et al., 1981
Artichokes, raw, frozen	86.4	2.2	0.15	7	ADL	Herranz et al., 1983
Artichokes, boiled	87.5	3.3	0.53	16	ADL	Herranz et al., 1981
Artichokes, frozen, boiled	89.5	1.5	0.16	11	ADL	Herranz et al., 1983
Artichokes, canned	87.7	1.4	0.17	12	ADL	Herranz et al., 1983
Asparagus	91.5	1.1	0.09	9	Klason	van Soest, 1978b
Asparagus	91.8	1.1	0.16	14	ADL	Herranz et al., 1981
Asparagus	87.8	1.8	0.2	9	KMnO₄	R. Mongeau and R. Brassard, unpublished
Asparagus, green	92.8	2.0	0.16	8	Klason	Chang et al., 1994
Asparagus, green	93.9	1.0	0.04	4	ADL	Chen et al., 1982
Asparagus, boiled	91.3	1.3	0.15	12	ADL	Herranz et al., 1981
Asparagus, cooked	91.4	1.9	0.1	5	Klason	Marlett, 1992
Asparagus, canned	93.2	0.9	0.07	7	ADL	Herranz et al., 1983
Asparagus, whole spears, canned	92.7	2.4	0.4	15	Klason	Anderson and Bridges, 1988
Asparagus, whole spears, canned	93.3	1.6	0.2	13	Klason	Marlett, 1992
Balsam-pear	95.1	1.2	0.03	2	ADL	Chen et al., 1982
Bamboo shoots	91.2	2.6	0.00	0	ADL	Chen et al., 1982
Bamboo shoots, green	93.0	1.9	0.09	5	Klason	Chang et al., 1994
Bamboo shoots, canned	97.4	1.5	0.1	7	Klason	Marlett, 1992
Bamboo, water	92.5	2.1	0.03	1	ADL	Chen et al., 1982
Bean sprouts, canned	96.2	1.2	0.1	8	Klason	Marlett, 1992

Table 5 Continued

Food	g/100 g wet weight[a] Moisture	Fiber[b]	Lignin	Lignin as % of fiber	Method	Ref.
Beans, green	91.6	2.6	0.25	10	KMnO$_4$	Foy et al., 1981
Beans, green	88.9	2.3	0.44	19	ADL	Herranz et al., 1981
Beans, green	91.8	2	0.1	7	KMnO$_4$	R. Mongeau and R. Brassard, unpublished
Beans, green	91.3	2.9	0.24	8	Klason	Chang et al., 1994
Beans, green, early	8.0	26.4	6.35	24	KMnO$_4$	Foy et al., 1981
Beans, green, inter	6.7	26.4	4.66	18	KMnO$_4$	Foy et al., 1981
Beans, green, late	6.9	27.0	2.70	10	KMnO$_4$	Foy et al., 1981
Beans, green, cut	92.3	1.4	0.24	18	Klason	van Soest, 1978b
Beans, green, raw, frozen	91.0	1.3	0.15	12	ADL	Herranz et al., 1983
Beans, green, boiled	91.6	2.5	0.28	11	ADL	Herranz et al., 1981
Beans, green, frozen, boiled	93.4	1.3	0.16	13	ADL	Herranz et al., 1983
Beans, green, canned	91.2	3	0.2	8	Klason	Anderson and Bridges, 1988
Beans, green, canned	82.2	3.8	0.2	4	Klason	Anderson and Bridges, 1988
Beans, green, canned	92.1	1.3	0.21	16	ADL	Herranz et al., 1983
Beans, green, whole cut, canned	94.2	1.9	0.2	11	Klason	Marlett, 1992
Beans, green, French cut, canned	93.2	2.1	0.1	5	Klason	Marlett, 1992
Beans, wax	93.7	1.6	0.22	14	KMnO$_4$	Foy et al., 1981
Beans, wax	91.5	1.6	0.18	11	Klason	van Soest, 1978b
Beans, wax, cut	87.5	1.5	0.01	1	Klason	van Soest, 1978b
Beets	88.6	2.7	tr	—	KMnO$_4$	Mongeau and Brassard, unpublished
Beets	89.3	2.6	0.1	2	Klason	Anderson and Bridges, 1988
Beets, canned	92.4	1.7	tr	—	Klason	Marlett, 1992
Beets, canned	91.1	2.6	0.36	14	Klason	Chang et al., 1994
Borecole	90.8	2.2	0.2	8	KMnO$_4$	R. Mongeau and R. Brassard, unpublished
Broccoli	92.7	1.3	0.20	15	Klason	van Soest, 1978b
Broccoli	92.0	1.5	0.22	14	KMnO$_4$	Foy et al., 1981
Broccoli	88.5	3.3	0.3	9	Klason	Marlett, 1992
Broccoli	91.8	1.5	0.14	9	??[d]	Mattheé and Appledorf, 1978
Broccoli	89.8	3.1	0.23	7	Klason	Chang et al., 1994
Broccoli	86.8	2.6	0.28	11	KMnO$_4$	Flint and Camire, 1992

Broccoli	86.8	2.6	0.29	11	Klason	Flint and Camire, 1992
Broccoli, frozen	90.8	2.8	0.1	5	Klason	Anderson and Bridges, 1988
Broccoli, cooked	90.2	3.5	0.3	9	Klason	Marlett, 1992
Broccoli, short cooked	93.9	1.3	0.14	10	??[d]	Mattheé and Appledorf, 1978
Broccoli, long cooked	93.6	1.5	0.19	13	??[d]	Mattheé and Appledorf, 1978
Broccoli, tops, boiled	??	4.1	0.03	1	Klason	Southgate, 1986
Brussels sprouts	89.8	2.2	0.18	8	Klason	van Soest, 1978b
Brussels sprouts	89.0	2.0	0.40	20	KMnO$_4$	Foy et al., 1981
Brussels sprouts	84.6	2.0	0.26	13	ADL	Herranz et al., 1981
Brussels sprouts, boiled	??	2.9	0.07	2	Klason	Southgate, 1986
Brussels sprouts, boiled	88.4	1.7	0.07	4	ADL	Herranz et al., 1981
Brussels sprouts, frozen	83.2	4.5	0.1	2	Klason	Anderson and Bridges, 1988
Brussels sprouts, frozen, cooked	87.2	4.1	0.1	2	Klason	Marlett, 1992
Burdock	74.1	7.6	0.34	4	Klason	Chang et al., 1994
Cabbage	90.9	1.6	0.1	7	KMnO$_4$	R. Mongeau and R. Brassard, unpublished
Cabbage	92.2	1.1	0.05	5	KMnO$_4$	van Soest, 1978b
Cabbage	94.3	1.2	0.21	17	KMnO$_4$	Foy et al., 1981
Cabbage	92.2	1.5	0.10	7	??[d]	Mattheé and Appledorf, 1978
Cabbage	91	2.1	0.1	4	Klason	Anderson and Bridges, 1988
Cabbage	92.7	1.7	tr	—	Klason	Marlett, 1992
Cabbage	92.6	1.7	0.16	9	Klason	Chang et al., 1994
Cabbage, white, spring	89.4	1.2	0.21	17	ADL	Herranz et al., 1981
Cabbage, white, summer	92.7	1.1	0.22	21	ADL	Herranz et al., 1981
Cabbage, boiled	??	2.8	0.38	14	Klason	Southgate, 1986
Cabbage, white, spring, boiled	89.2	1.3	0.17	13	ADL	Herranz et al., 1981
Cabbage, white, summer, boiled	94.5	1.3	0.22	17	ADL	Herranz et al., 1981
Cabbage, short cooked	93.4	1.4	0.08	6	??[d]	Mattheé and Appledorf, 1978
Cabbage, long cooked	93.9	1.3	0.09	7	??[d]	Mattheé and Appledorf, 1978
Cabbage, red	90.0	1.1	0.15	14	ADL	Herranz et al., 1981
Cabbage, red, boiled	90.6	1.5	0.04	3	ADL	Herranz et al., 1981
Cabbage, Chinese	95.7	1.1	0.16	15	Klason	Chang et al., 1994
Carrots	87.8	1.3	0.22	17	ADL	Herranz et al., 1981
Carrots	89.6	1.0	0.15	15	Klason	van Soest, 1978b
Carrots	89.4	2.1	0.47	23	KMnO$_4$	Foy et al., 1981
Carrots	86.5	3.2	0.1	4	Klason	Anderson and Bridges, 1988

Table 5 Continued

Food	g/100 g wet weight[a]			Lignin as % of fiber	Method	Ref.
	Moisture	Fiber[b]	Lignin			
Carrots	87.2	2.5	0.1	4	Klason	Marlett, 1992
Carrots	88.4	1.4	0.15	11	??[d]	Mattheé and Appledorf, 1978
Carrots	88.5	2.7	0.2	8	KMnO$_4$	R. Mongeau and R. Brassard, unpublished
Carrots	88.2	3.3	0.20	6	Klason	Chang et al., 1994
Carrots, boiled	89.1	1.0	0.18	18	ADL	Herranz et al., 1981
Carrots, short cooked	91.6	1.2	0.13	11	??[d]	Mattheé and Appledorf, 1978
Carrots, long cooked	92.5	1.2	0.10	9	??[d]	Mattheé and Appledorf, 1978
Carrots, young, boiled	??	3.7	tr	—	Klason	Southgate, 1986
Cauliflower	92.5	2.3	0.1	4	Klason	Marlett, 1992
Cauliflower	93.8	1.0	0.09	9	Klason	van Soest, 1978b
Cauliflower	88.9	1.4	0.11	8	ADL	Herranz et al., 1981
Cauliflower	91.5	2.5	0.24	9	Klason	Chang et al., 1994
Cauliflower, boiled	??	1.8	tr	—	Klason	Southgate, 1986
Cauliflower, boiled	90.8	1.2	0.10	8	ADL	Herranz et al., 1981
Cauliflower, cooked	94.1	2.1	tr	—	Klason	Marlett, 1992
Cauliflower, frozen	90.4	2.6	0.1	2	Klason	Anderson and Bridges, 1988
Celery	94.6	1.5	0.1	8	KMnO$_4$	R. Mongeau and R. Brassard, unpublished
Celery	95.0	0.7	0.10	14	Klason	van Soest, 1978b
Celery	94.5	1.8	tr	—	Klason	Marlett, 1992
Celery, cooked	95.2	1.8	tr	—	Klason	Marlett, 1992
Celery, Chinese	94.4	2.5	0.42	17	Klason	Chang et al., 1994
Chard, boiled	90.7	2.1	0.22	11	ADL	Herranz et al., 1981
Chard, raw	91.4	1.6	0.26	16	ADL	Herranz et al., 1981
Coba shoot	91.1	3.0	0.26	9	Klason	Chang et al., 1994
Collard greens	90.4	1.8	0.30	17	Klason	van Soest, 1978b
Convolvulus, water	93.2	3.2	0.45	14	Klason	Chang et al., 1994
Corn, kernel	75	2.1	0.3	13	KMnO$_4$	R. Mongeau and R. Brassard, unpublished
Corn, kernel, sweet	79.6	1.6	0.39	24	Klason	van Soest, 1978b
Corn, kernel, sweet, cooked	??	4.7	0.12	3	Klason	Southgate, 1986
Corn, kernel, frozen	75.8	2.1	0.3	14	Klason	Marlett, 1992
Corn, kernel, canned	80.3	1.9	0.1	6	Klason	Anderson and Bridges, 1988

Corn, kernel, canned	76.7	1.9	0.5	25	Klason	Marlett, 1992
Corn, kernel, canned	??	5.7	0.08	1	Klason	Southgate, 1986
Cucumber	96.8	0.9	0.16	17	KMnO$_4$	Foy et al., 1981
Cucumber	95.8	0.9	0.1	11	Klason	Marlett, 1992
Cucumber, small	95.5	0.5	0.01	2	ADL	Chen et al., 1982
Cucumber, small	95.3	1.0	0.01	1	Klason	Chang et al., 1994
Cucumber, large	96.4	0.4	0.01	4	ADL	Chen et al., 1982
Cucumber, large, peeled	96.0	0.7	0.03	5	Klason	Chang et al., 1994
Cucumber, peeled	96.2	0.6	tr	—	Klason	Marlett, 1992
Cucumber, peeled	96.8	0.4	0.05	13	Klason	van Soest, 1978b
Cucumber, skin only	91.5	3.0	0.48	16	Klason	van Soest, 1978b
Daylily flower	88.3	3.2	0.11	3	Klason	Chang et al., 1994
Eggplant	92.7	1.5	0.06	4	ADL	Chen et al., 1982
Eggplant	94.3	1.1	0.26	23	ADL	Herranz et al., 1981
Eggplant	93.1	2.2	0.32	14	Klason	Chang et al., 1994
Eggplant, fried	54.7	2.8	0.24	9	ADL	Herranz et al., 1981
Eggplant, peeled	93.1	1.5	0.23	16	Klason	van Soest, 1978b
Garland chrysanthemum	94.7	1.9	0.22	12	Klason	Chang et al., 1994
Gourd, bottle	93.9	1.1	0.03	3	ADL	Chen et al., 1982
Gourd, bottle	95.8	1.0	0.08	8	Klason	Chang et al., 1994
Gourd, bitter	94.2	2.0	0.32	16	Klason	Chang et al., 1994
Gourd, rag	95.3	0.4	0.02	5	ADL	Chen et al., 1982
Gourd, sponge	94.5	1.0	0.08	8	Klason	Chang et al., 1994
Gourd, wax	95.9	1.1	0.10	9	Klason	Chang et al., 1994
Gourd, wax	97.1	0.6	0.01	1	ADL	Chen et al., 1982
Jerusalem artichokes	81.7	1.3	0.18	14	KMnO$_4$	Foy et al., 1981
Kale	91.6	1.4	0.19	14	Klason	van Soest, 1978b
Kale	90.1	1.6	0.30	19	KMnO$_4$	Foy et al., 1981
Kale, frozen	88.6	3.8	0.4	10	Klason	Anderson and Bridges, 1988
Kohlrabi	91.9	1.1	0.03	2	ADL	Chen et al., 1982
Kohlrabi	92.1	1.7	0.09	5	Klason	Chang et al., 1994
Leek	93.7	1.2	0.13	11	ADL	Chen et al., 1982
Leek	82.8	1.8	0.41	23	ADL	Herranz et al., 1981
Leek, boiled	87.9	2.0	0.27	14	ADL	Herranz et al., 1981

Table 5 Continued

Food	g/100 g wet weight[a]			Lignin as % of fiber	Method	Ref.
	Moisture	Fiber[b]	Lignin			
Leek, Chinese	91.8	3.5	0.48	14	Klason	Chang et al., 1994
Leek, etiolated	94.3	1.8	0.19	11	Klason	Chang et al., 1994
Leek, shoots, yellow	95.8	0.9	0.06	7	ADL	Chen et al., 1982
Leek flower	93.2	1.5	0.14	9	ADL	Chen et al., 1982
Leek flower	91.8	2.5	0.11	5	Klason	Chang et al., 1994
Lettuce	95.9	0.7	0.14	20	KMnO$_4$	Foy et al., 1981
Lettuce	95.8	0.9	0.1	10	Klason	Anderson and Bridges, 1988
Lettuce	??	1.5	tr	—	Klason	Southgate, 1986
Lettuce	93.7	1.1	0.15	14	ADL	Herranz et al., 1981
Lettuce	95.9	1.3	0.19	14	Klason	Chang et al., 1994
Lettuce, leaf, Chinese	94.8	1.6	0.46	29	Klason	Chang et al., 1994
Lettuce, leaf, Chinese	95.4	1.2	0.10	8	ADL	Chen et al., 1982
Lettuce, Romaine	95.1	0.8	0.14	16	Klason	van Soest, 1978b
Lotus root	80.9	2.3	0.21	9	Klason	Chang et al., 1994
Mustard, leaf	93.0	2.4	0.10	4	Klason	Chang et al., 1994
Mushrooms	92.3	1.7	0.15	9	ADL	Herranz et al., 1981
Mushrooms (*Pleurotus ostreatus*)[c]	??	47.5[c]	6.10[c]	13	Klason	Kurasawa et al., 1982
Mushrooms, common (*Agaricus bisporus*)	89.8	3.6	0.17	5	Klason	Chang et al., 1994
Mushrooms, common (*Agaricus bisporus*)[c]	??	29.9[c]	3.60[c]	12	Klason	Kurasawa et al., 1982
Mushrooms, enokitake (*Flammulina velutipes*)[c]	??	38.5[c]	1.00[c]	3	Klason	Kurasawa et al., 1982
Mushrooms, nameko (*Pholiota nameko*)[c]	??	47.6[c]	8.30[c]	17	Klason	Kurasawa et al., 1982
Mushrooms, shiitake (*Lentinus edodes*)[c]	??	41.8[c]	2.00[c]	5	Klason	Kurasawa et al., 1982
Mushrooms, shiitake (*Lentinus edodes*)	90.2	4.0	0.11	3	Klason	Chang et al., 1994
Mushrooms, straw (*Volvariella volvacea*)	91.2	2.4	0.23	10	Klason	Chang et al., 1994
Mushrooms, wood ear (*Auricularia auricula-jude*)[c]	??	55.5[c]	5.00[c]	9	Klason	Kurasawa et al., 1982
Mushrooms, winter (*Flammulina velutipes*)	88.9	3.8	0.06	1	Klason	Chang et al., 1994
Mushrooms, canned	90.9	2.7	0.2	6	KMnO$_4$	Mongeau and Brassard, unpublished
Mushrooms, canned	91.1	2.5	0.1	4	Klason	Marlett, 1992
Mustard greens	92.0	1.9	0.56	30	KMnO$_4$	Foy et al., 1981
Mustard greens	92.4	1.6	0.24	14	Klason	van Soest, 1978b

Food					Method	Reference
Mustard stem	95.3	0.6	0.01	1	ADL	Chen et al., 1982
Okra	92.5	1.1	0.12	11	Klason	van Soest, 1978b
Okra	90.3	1.4	0.14	10	??[d]	Mattheé and Appledorf, 1978
Okra, long cooked	93.4	1.2	0.13	10	??[d]	Mattheé and Appledorf, 1978
Okra, short cooked	92.1	1.3	0.19	15	??[d]	Mattheé and Appledorf, 1978
Olives, black	80.5	2.2	0.6	27	Klason	Marlett, 1992
Olives, green, with pimento	76.5	2	0.4	20	Klason	Marlett, 1992
Onion	92.6	0.6	0.01	3	ADL	Chen et al., 1982
Onion	93.4	0.5	0.04	8	Klason	van Soest, 1978b
Onion, yellow	92.6	1.0	0.05	5	Klason	Chang et al., 1994
Onion, yellow	90.3	1.7	tr	—	Klason	Marlett, 1992
Onion, yellow	??	2.1	tr	—	Klason	Southgate, 1986
Onion, green	92.7	2.2	0.2	9	Klason	Marlett, 1992
Parsnips	??	4.9	tr	—	Klason	Southgate, 1986
Peppers	93.0	1.9	0.41	22	KMnO$_4$	Foy et al., 1981
Peppers, green	93.9	1.7	0.3	18	Klason	Marlett, 1992
Peppers, green	94.5	1.1	0.11	10	ADL	Chen et al., 1982
Peppers, green	93.5	1.9	0.2	8	KMnO$_4$	R. Mongeau and R. Brassard, unpublished
Pepper, green, bell	94.5	1.4	0.14	10	Klason	Chang et al., 1994
Peppers, seedless	90.1	1.7	0.22	13	Klason	van Soest, 1978b
Peppers, cooked	??	0.9	tr	—	Klason	Southgate, 1986
Pe-tsai, Chin-chian	93.5	2.3	0.38	16	Klason	Chang et al., 1994
Pe-tsai	95.5	1.5	0.33	22	Klason	Chang et al., 1994
Pickle	??	1.5	0.12	8	Klason	Southgate, 1986
Pickle, dill	94.9	1.1	0.1	9	Klason	Marlett, 1992
Potato, main crop, raw	??	3.5	tr	—	Klason	Southgate, 1986
Potato, white, raw	80.1	1.2	0.29	24	ADL	Herranz et al., 1981
Potato, white, raw	79	2	0.2	9	Klason	Anderson and Bridges, 1988
Potato, flesh only	80.9	4.2	0.17	4	KMnO$_4$	Foy et al., 1981
Potato, flesh only	77.8	0.6	0.09	16	Klason	van Soest, 1978b
Potato, skin only	80.6	7.0	0.35	5	KMnO$_4$	Foy et al., 1981
Potato, skin only	81.9	2.3	1.18	50	Klason	van Soest, 1978b
Potato, baked	78.9	2.1	0.3	15	KMnO$_4$	R. Mongeau and R. Brassard, unpublished
Potato, baked, with skin	73.3	2.5	0.3	12	Klason	Marlett, 1992
Potato, boiled	79.3	1.1	0.07	6	ADL	Herranz et al., 1981
Potato, boiled, without skin	79.5	1.3	tr	—	Klason	Marlett, 1992

Table 5 Continued

Food	g/100 g wet weight[a]			Lignin as % of fiber	Method	Ref.
	Moisture	Fiber[b]	Lignin			
Potato, canned	??	2.5	tr	—	Klason	Southgate, 1986
Potato, french fries	??	3.2	0.03	1	Klason	Southgate, 1986
Potato, french fries	68.3	2.3	0.1	4	Klason	Marlett, 1992
Potato, fried	56.9	1.5	0.17	11	ADL	Herranz et al., 1981
Potato leaves, sweet	89.7	3.9	0.69	17	Klason	Chang et al., 1994
Pumpkin, canned	90.2	2.9	0.2	7	Klason	Marlett, 1992
Radish	94.2	1.4	tr	—	Klason	Marlett, 1992
Radish	88.1	1.7	0.14	8	Klason	van Soest, 1978b
Radish, Chinese	94.2	1.4	0.11	8	Klason	Chang et al., 1994
Rape	94.5	0.9	0.07	8	ADL	Chen et al., 1982
Rape	93.1	2.2	0.26	12	Klason	Chang et al., 1994
Rutabaga	89	2.2	0.1	6	$KMnO_4$	R. Mongeau and R. Brassard, unpublished
Rutabaga	??	2.4	tr	—	Klason	Southgate, 1986
Rutabaga, peeled	90.0	1.0	0.16	16	Klason	van Soest, 1978b
Spinach	92.4	1.3	0.17	13	Klason	van Soest, 1978b
Spinach	92.3	1.3	0.28	22	$KMnO_4$	Foy et al., 1981
Spinach	86.8	2.3	0.41	18	ADL	Herranz et al., 1981
Spinach	93.3	2.5	0.21	9	Klason	Chang et al., 1994
Spinach	92.4	2.2	0.3	14	Klason	Anderson and Bridges, 1988
Spinach, frozen	88.5	3.3	0.31	9	ADL	Herranz et al., 1983
Spinach, frozen	91.0	3.7	0.28	8	ADL	Herranz et al., 1983
Spinach, frozen, boiled	91.8	1.8	0.22	12	ADL	Herranz et al., 1981
Spinach, boiled	97.5	0.5	0.04	9	ADL	Herranz et al., 1981
Squash	95.0	0.6	0.09	15	Klason	van Soest, 1978b
Squash, summer	94.7	1	0.1	10	Klason	Anderson and Bridges, 1988
Squash, frozen	90.2	1.3	0.07	5	Klason	van Soest, 1978b
Squash, cooked	78.2	1.2	0.05	4	ADL	Herranz et al., 1981
Squash, fried	79.0	1.2	0.07	6	$KMnO_4$	Lund and Smoot, 1982
Sweet potato, flesh only (local market)	77.6	1.1	0.11	10	$KMnO_4$	Lund and Smoot, 1982
Sweet potato, flesh only (Puerto Rico)	86.0	2.1	0.36	17	$KMnO_4$	Lund and Smoot, 1982
Sweet potato, skin (local market)	83.5	3.3	0.41	13	$KMnO_4$	Lund and Smoot, 1982
Sweet potato, skin (Puerto Rico)						

					Method	Reference
Sweet potato, canned	82.7	1.2	0	4	Klason	Anderson and Bridges, 1988
Sweet potato, cut, canned in light syrup	75.6	1.7	0.1	6	Klason	Marlett, 1992
Tomato	94.1	0.7	0.11	16	ADL	Chen et al., 1982
Tomato	93.7	0.8	0.1	13	Klason	Anderson and Bridges, 1988
Tomato	??	1.4	0.3	21	Klason	Southgate, 1986
Tomato	93.7	1.0	0.26	27	ADL	Herranz et al., 1981
Tomato, green, raw	92.2	1.7	0.50	30	ADL	Herranz et al., 1981
Tomato, fried	68.6	1.6	0.36	22	ADL	Herranz et al., 1981
Tomato, canned	93.4	0.7	0.1	14	Klason	Marlett, 1992
Tomato, canned	??	0.85	0.03	4	Klason	Southgate, 1986
Tomato, canned	92.9	0.8	0.12	16	ADL	Herranz et al., 1983
Tomato, canned, fried	77.0	1.2	0.18	16	ADL	Herranz et al., 1983
Turnip	89.2	1.6	0.18	11	KMnO$_4$	Foy et al., 1981
Turnip	??	2.2	tr	—	Klason	Southgate, 1986
Turnip greens	93.4	1.3	0.18	14	Klason	van Soest, 1978b
Turnip greens	87.8	2.2	0.46	21	ADL	Herranz et al., 1981
Turnip greens, frozen	92.9	2.5	0.1	4	Klason	Marlett, 1992
Turnip greens, boiled	89.6	1.9	0.30	16	ADL	Herranz et al., 1981
Yam, D. alata	77.5	1.1	0.15	13	KMnO$_4$	Lund and Smoot, 1982
Yam, D. esculenta	66.7	0.9	0.07	8	KMnO$_4$	Lund and Smoot, 1982
Water chestnut	79.5	1.9	0.04	2	Klason	Chang et al., 1994
Zucchini	95.4	0.6	0.07	13	Klason	van Soest, 1978b
Zucchini	94.5	0.9	tr	—	Klason	Marlett, 1992
Refined grain products						
Biscuits, baking powder	16.7	2.1	0.1	5	Klason	Marlett, 1992
Bran, AACC Certified	8.2	37.5	3.40	9	KMnO$_4$	R. Mongeau and R. Brassard, 1982
Bran, hard red, AACC Certified	8.5	39.8	3.7	9	KMnO$_4$	R. Mongeau et al., unpublished
Bran, white, AACC Certified	8.5	43.5	3.4	8	KMnO$_4$	R. Mongeau et al., unpublished
Bran, bakers	8.4	34.1	2.66	8	Klason	van Soest, 1978b
Bran, cereal	9.6	41.0	4.07	10	Klason	van Soest, 1978b
Bran, rice	7.1	23.5	4.18	18	KMnO$_4$	Flint and Camire, 1992
Bran, rice	7.1	23.5	4.92	21	Klason	Flint and Camire, 1992
Bran, tablets	9.1	7.0	0.73	10	KMnO$_4$	Foy et al., 1981
Bran, unprocessed	8.0	44.6	4.39	10	KMnO$_4$	Mongeau and Brassard, 1982

Table 5 Continued

Food	g/100 g wet weight[a]			Lignin as % of fiber	Method	Ref.
	Moisture	Fiber[b]	Lignin			
Bran, wheat	15.7	42.5	3.12	7	KMnO$_4$	Foy et al., 1981
Bran, wheat (average of 3 grinds)	7.0	29.0	5.52	19	Klason	Flint and Camire, 1992
Bran, wheat (average of 3 grinds)	7.0	29.0	4.16	14	KMnO$_4$	Flint and Camire, 1992
Bran, wheat, Oleoble	6.2	47.1	3.86	8	ADL	Herranz et al., 1981
Bread, cracked wheat	35.6	5.8	0.26	4	KMnO$_4$	Foy et al., 1981
Bread, fiber	46.2	24.6	0.97	4	KMnO$_4$	Foy et al., 1981
Bread, French	29.2	2.7	0.1	4	Klason	Marlett, 1992
Bread, Hovis	??	4.5	0.3	7	Klason	Southgate, 1986
Bread, Italian	26.9	3.8	0.7	18	Klason	Marlett, 1992
Bread, Italian with sesame seeds	34.6	3.4	1	29	Klason	Marlett, 1992
Bread, white, wheat	38.5	4.0	0.12	3	KMnO$_4$	Foy et al., 1981
Bread, white, wheat	36.9	2	0.1	5	Klason	Anderson and Bridges, 1988
Bread, white, wheat	33.1	2.6	0.5	19	Klason	Marlett, 1992
Bread, white, wheat	??	2.7	tr	—	Klason	Southgate, 1986
Bread, white, wheat (10 brands)	37.9	0.5	tr	—	KMnO$_4$	Mongeau and Brassard, 1979
Bread, white, wheat	38.4	1.8	0.4	21	KMnO$_4$	R. Mongeau and R. Brassard, unpublished
Bread, white, wheat, crusted (4 brands)	36.3	0.6	tr	—	KMnO$_4$	Mongeau and Brassard, 1979
Bread, white, enriched	35.8	1.5	0.19	13	Klason	van Soest, 1978b
Bread, whole wheat	35.6	6.8	1.03	15	Klason	van Soest, 1978b
Bread, whole wheat	40.6	9.2	0.42	5	KMnO$_4$	Foy et al., 1981
Bread, whole wheat	40.8	5.5	0.7	12	Klason	Anderson and Bridges, 1988
Bread, whole wheat	??	5.1	0.15	3	Klason	Southgate, 1986
Bread, whole wheat	30.7	9.4	1.32	14	KMnO$_4$	Flint and Camire, 1992
Bread, whole wheat	30.7	9.4	2.43	26	Klason	Flint and Camire, 1992
Bread, 100% whole wheat (10 brands)	37.5	4.5	0.5	11	KMnO$_4$	Mongeau and Brassard, 1979
Bread, 100% whole wheat	39.2	5.4	0.47	9	KMnO$_4$	Mongeau and Brassard, 1989
Bread, 60% whole wheat (6 brands)	38	2.9	0.3	10	KMnO$_4$	Mongeau and Brassard, 1979
Bread, light toasted	17.8	10.9	2.55	23	Klason	Flint and Camire, 1992
Bread, light toasted	17.8	10.9	0.82	8	KMnO$_4$	Flint and Camire, 1992
Bread, dark toasted	14.2	11.3	2.66	23	Klason	Flint and Camire, 1992
Bread, dark toasted	14.2	11.3	1.12	10	KMnO$_4$	Flint and Camire, 1992

Bread, raisin (3 brands)	37.7	0.6	0.2	33	KMnO$_4$	Mongeau and Brassard, 1979
Bread, wholemeal	??	8.5	1.2	14	Klason	Southgate, 1986
Bread, other (10 brands)	36.8	1.0	0.1	10	KMnO$_4$	Mongeau and Brassard, 1979
Bun, hamburger	31.4	2.5	0.2	8	Klason	Marlett, 1992
Cake, yellow	26.9	1.4	0.1	7	Klason	Marlett, 1992
Cookies, chocolate digestive (half-coated)	??	3.5	0.78	22.2	Klason	Southgate, 1986
Cookies, chocolate, (fully coated)	??	3.09	1.31	42.2	Klason	Southgate, 1986
Cookies, ginger snaps	4.8	1.8	0.4	22	Klason	Marlett, 1992
Cookies, ginger snaps	??	2	0.24	12	Klason	Southgate, 1986
Cookies, plain sugar	3.3	1.1	tr	—	Klason	Marlett, 1992
Cookies, semi-sweet	??	2.3	0.22	10	Klason	Southgate, 1986
Cookies, short-sweet	??	1.7	0.13	8	Klason	Southgate, 1986
Cookies, wafers (filled)	??	1.6	0.07	4	Klason	Southgate, 1986
Corn bread	36.1	3	0.4	13	Klason	Marlett, 1992
Crackers, graham	4.4	2.7	0.4	15	Klason	Marlett, 1992
Crackers, graham	3.3	2.4	0.2	8	Klason	Anderson and Bridges, 1988
Crackers, saltine	4.3	3.1	0.5	16	Klason	Marlett, 1992
Crackers, saltine	3.4	3	0.4	15	Klason	Anderson and Bridges, 1988
Crackers, snack	5.2	12.3	1.2	10	Klason	Anderson and Bridges, 1988
Crispbread, rye	??	11.7	1.74	5	Klason	Southgate, 1986
Crispbread, wheat	??	4.8	0.55	11	Klason	Southgate, 1986
English muffin	38	3	0.7	23	Klason	Marlett, 1992
Flour, white, wheat	8	3.7	0.2	7	Klason	Anderson and Bridges, 1988
Flour, white, wheat	??	3.15	0.03	1	Klason	Southgate, 1986
Flour, white, wheat	9.2	2.9	0.2	7	Klason	Marlett, 1992
Flour, whole wheat	11.8	10.9	1.1	10	Klason	Anderson and Bridges, 1988
Flour, whole wheat	??	7.87	0.75	10	Klason	Southgate, 1986
Flour, whole wheat	7.6	10.4	0.83	8	KMnO$_4$	Flint and Camire, 1992
Flour, whole wheat	7.6	10.4	0.92	9	Klason	Flint and Camire, 1992
Flour, wholemeal	??	9.51	0.8	8	Klason	Southgate, 1986
Grits	8.8	2.2	0.3	15	Klason	Anderson and Bridges, 1988
Hominy, white, cooked	85	0.6	tr	—	Klason	Marlett, 1992
Ice cream cone, Comet cup	4.7	3.1	0.5	16	Klason	Marlett, 1992
Macaroni, cooked	69.6	2	0.7	35	Klason	Marlett, 1992
Macaroni, uncooked	10.4	3	0.3	9	Klason	Anderson and Bridges, 1988

Table 5 Continued

Food	g/100 g wet weight[a]			Lignin as % of fiber	Method	Ref.
	Moisture	Fiber[b]	Lignin			
Matzo	??	3.9	0.43	11	Klason	Southgate, 1986
Muffin, plain	27.1	1.5	0.4	27	Klason	Marlett, 1992
Muffin, bran	26.7	5.5	0.53	10	$KMnO_4$	Mongeau and Brassard, 1989
Noodles, Creamette, cooked	67.2	1.7	0.4	24	Klason	Marlett, 1992
Oatbran	8.4	14.4	1.4	10	Klason	Anderson and Bridges, 1988
Oatbran, uncooked	7.4	17	3.5	21	Klason	Marlett, 1992
Oatbran, uncooked	9.2	9.5	0.9	10	Klason	Anderson and Bridges, 1988
Oatcakes	??	4	0.44	11	Klason	Southgate, 1986
Pancake mix	8.3	4.5	0.6	13	Klason	Marlett, 1992
Pie crust	14.9	2.3	0.6	26	Klason	Marlett, 1992
Rice, medium grain, regular, cooked	70.6	0.4	0.1	25	Klason	Marlett, 1992
Rice, white	9.4	0.9	0.6	68	$KMnO_4$	R. Mongeau and R. Brassard, unpublished
Roll, cinnamon	26.4	2.2	0.4	18	Klason	Marlett, 1992
Spaghetti, cooked	60.7	1.5	tr	—	Klason	Marlett, 1992
Spaghetti, whole wheat, uncooked	8.5	9.5	0.8	8	Klason	Anderson and Bridges, 1988
Taco shell	7.7	6.8	0.9	13	Klason	Marlett, 1992
Tortilla, flour	33	1.5	0.3	20	Klason	Marlett, 1992
Wheat germ	4.2	14	1.2	9	Klason	Marlett, 1992
Cereal products						
100% Bran	1.3	28.4	2.62	9	$KMnO_4$	Mongeau and Brassard, 1982
40% Branflakes	3.5	15.3	1.6	10	Klason	Anderson and Bridges, 1988
40% Branflakes	3.2	19.5	1.5	8	Klason	Marlett, 1992
All Bran	2.7	34.2	3.21	9	$KMnO_4$	Flint and Camire, 1992
All Bran	2.7	34.2	2.72	8	Klason	Flint and Camire, 1992
All Bran	2.7	33.0	2.63	8	Klason	van Soest, 1978b
All Bran	1.3	29.4	2.56	9	$KMnO_4$	Mongeau and Brassard, 1982
All Bran	2.7	30.7	3.1	10	Klason	Anderson and Bridges, 1988
All Bran	5.7	30.1	4.3	14	Klason	Marlett, 1992
All Bran	??	26.7	2.88	11	Klason	Southgate, 1986

Alpen	4.3	4.1	0.57	14	KMnO$_4$	Mongeau and Brassard, 1982
Alpha Bits	1.7	1.7	0.39	24	KMnO$_4$	Mongeau and Brassard, 1982
Apple Jacks	1.7	0.9	tr	—	KMnO$_4$	Mongeau and Brassard, 1982
Boo Berry	2.2	1.7	0.29	18	KMnO$_4$	Mongeau and Brassard, 1982
Bran Buds	1.2	24.4	2.07	9	KMnO$_4$	Mongeau and Brassard, 1982
Bran Crunchies	1.5	10.5	0.89	8	KMnO$_4$	Mongeau and Brassard, 1982
Bran flakes, brand 1	2.0	9.5	0.88	9	KMnO$_4$	Mongeau and Brassard, 1982
Bran flakes, brand 2	2.6	10.7	0.73	7	KMnO$_4$	Mongeau and Brassard, 1982
Bran flakes	3.3	12.5	2.2	18	KMnO$_4$	Mongeau and Brassard, 1989
Buckwheat Maple Flavored Wheat Cereal	1.0	6.3	0.89	14	KMnO$_4$	Mongeau and Brassard, 1982
Cap'n Crunch	0.5	1.3	0.20	15	KMnO$_4$	Mongeau and Brassard, 1982
Cheerios	6.0	6.1	1.69	28	Klason	van Soest, 1978b
Cheerios	4.1	3.2	0.77	24	KMnO$_4$	Mongeau and Brassard, 1982
Cocoa Puffs	2.9	1.2	0.29	25	KMnO$_4$	Mongeau and Brassard, 1982
Corn Bran	4.3	81.5	2.2	3	Klason	Anderson and Bridges, 1988
Corn Flakes	3.7	4.2	1.44	34	Klason	van Soest, 1978b
Corn Flakes	10.9	4.3	0.7	16	Klason	Marlett, 1992
Corn Flakes	4.4	1.6	0.6	35	Klason	Anderson and Bridges, 1988
Corn Flakes	??	11	1.32	12	Klason	Southgate, 1986
Corn Flakes	2.2	1.1	0.6	54	KMnO$_4$	R. Mongeau and R. Brassard, unpublished
Corn Pops	1.4	0.5	tr	—	KMnO$_4$	Mongeau and Brassard, 1982
Count Chocula	9.3	0.5	tr	—	KMnO$_4$	Mongeau and Brassard, 1982
Crackling Bran	3.6	1.3	0.58	46	KMnO$_4$	Mongeau and Brassard, 1982
Cream of Wheat, quick	0.8	13.8	1.49	11	KMnO$_4$	Mongeau and Brassard, 1982
Cream of Wheat, mix & eat	8.2	2.2	0.28	13	KMnO$_4$	Mongeau and Brassard, 1982
Cream of Wheat, quick, cooked	9.3	1.4	tr	—	KMnO$_4$	Mongeau and Brassard, 1982
Cream of Wheat, quick, cooked	87.9	0.7	0.1	14	Klason	Marlett, 1992
Cream of Wheat, regular	6.7	2.2	0.09	4	KMnO$_4$	Mongeau and Brassard, 1982
Crunchy Granola, fruits & nuts	2.6	5.1	0.78	15	KMnO$_4$	Mongeau and Brassard, 1982
Crunchy Granola, honey & almonds	2.6	5.1	0.68	13	KMnO$_4$	Mongeau and Brassard, 1982
Crunchy Granola & wheat bran	2.7	4.8	0.68	14	KMnO$_4$	Mongeau and Brassard, 1982
Fiber 1	3.7	42.4	2.9	7	Klason	Anderson and Bridges, 1988
Franken Berry	2.1	1.4	0.20	14	KMnO$_4$	Mongeau and Brassard, 1982
Froot Loops	0.6	0.9	tr	—	KMnO$_4$	Mongeau and Brassard, 1982
Frosted Flakes	0.6	0.3	tr	—	KMnO$_4$	Mongeau and Brassard, 1982

Table 5 Continued

Food	Moisture	Fiber[b]	Lignin	Lignin as % of fiber	Method	Ref.
	g/100 g wet weight[a]					
Frosted Mini Wheats	15	8.2	1	12	Klason	Marlett, 1992
Frosted Rice	0.6	0.3	tr	—	$KMnO_4$	Mongeau and Brassard, 1982
Golden Honey	1.0	1.7	0.20	12	$KMnO_4$	Mongeau and Brassard, 1982
Grain Team	2.1	0.9	tr	—	$KMnO_4$	Mongeau and Brassard, 1982
Granola Vita Crunch, apple & cinnamon	2.8	2.9	0.39	13	$KMnO_4$	Mongeau and Brassard, 1982
Granola Vita Crunch, honey & almonds	1.7	4.7	0.49	10	$KMnO_4$	Mongeau and Brassard, 1982
Granola Vita Crunch, raisins	2.0	5.3	0.59	11	$KMnO_4$	Mongeau and Brassard, 1982
Grape Nuts Flakes	2.9	6.6	0.68	10	$KMnO_4$	Mongeau and Brassard, 1982
Grape-nuts	5.1	7.8	0.95	12	Klason	van Soest, 1978b
Grape-nuts	1.5	8.4	0.89	11	$KMnO_4$	Mongeau and Brassard, 1982
Grape-nuts	3.1	10.1	0.6	6	Klason	Anderson and Bridges, 1988
Grape-nuts	??	7	0.58	9	Klason	Southgate, 1986
Harvest Crunch	0.8	3.5	0.50	14	$KMnO_4$	Mongeau and Brassard, 1982
Harvest Crunch, apple & cinnamon	0.3	4.5	0.40	9	$KMnO_4$	Mongeau and Brassard, 1982
Harvest Crunch, raisin & dates	1.5	3.8	0.59	15	$KMnO_4$	Mongeau and Brassard, 1982
Heartland	2.6	7.2	1.17	16	Klason	van Soest, 1978b
Honey Comb	1.3	0.9	tr	—	$KMnO_4$	Mongeau and Brassard, 1982
Honey Smacks	25.5	2.3	0.1	4	Klason	Marlett, 1992
Lucky Charms	3.1	1.9	0.39	20	$KMnO_4$	Mongeau and Brassard, 1982
Mini Wheats, brown sugar	3.3	6.3	0.58	9	$KMnO_4$	Mongeau and Brassard, 1982
Mini Wheats, Frosted	3.9	7.4	0.58	8	$KMnO_4$	Mongeau and Brassard, 1982
Muffets	2.8	10.4	0.78	7	$KMnO_4$	Mongeau and Brassard, 1982
Muffets, Malt Flavored	3.3	9.7	0.92	10	$KMnO_4$	Mongeau and Brassard, 1982
Naturist Cereal	6.7	6.0	0.75	13	$KMnO_4$	Mongeau and Brassard, 1982
Naturist Cereal, fruits	6.0	5.9	0.85	14	$KMnO_4$	Mongeau and Brassard, 1982
Oats, Oatmeal	7.9	6.7	1.29	19	$KMnO_4$	Mongeau and Brassard, 1982
Oats, Oatmeal	10.6	9.8	0.83	8	$KMnO_4$	Mongeau and Brassard, 1989
Oats, old fashioned, rolled, brand 1	9.2	4.9	0.91	19	$KMnO_4$	Mongeau and Brassard, 1982
Oats, old fashioned, rolled, brand 2	9.5	5.1	0.72	14	$KMnO_4$	Mongeau and Brassard, 1982
Oats, old fashion, cooked	84.2	1.9	0.5	26	Klason	Marlett, 1992

Oats, regular	8.9	6.3	1.00	16	Klason	van Soest, 1978b
Oats, regular, presweetened	7.8	4.3	0.92	21	$KMnO_4$	Mongeau and Brassard, 1982
Oats, Scotch Oatmeal	7.4	5.2	1.02	20	$KMnO_4$	Mongeau and Brassard, 1982
Oats, regular, ready to serve	8.7	4.8	0.91	19	$KMnO_4$	Mongeau and Brassard, 1982
Oats, precooked	8.2	4.5	0.64	14	$KMnO_4$	Mongeau and Brassard, 1982
Oats, cook in 1 min.	9.1	4.9	1.00	20	$KMnO_4$	Mongeau and Brassard, 1982
Oats, instant, cook in 1 min.	9.5	4.7	0.91	19	$KMnO_4$	Mongeau and Brassard, 1982
Oats, quick, brand 1	9.1	4.9	0.82	17	$KMnO_4$	Mongeau and Brassard, 1982
Oats, quick, brand 2	9.2	5.0	0.91	18	$KMnO_4$	Mongeau and Brassard, 1982
Oats, apple & cinnamon, brand 1	7.7	4.2	0.65	16	$KMnO_4$	Mongeau and Brassard, 1982
Oats, apple & cinnamon, brand 2	6.7	4.4	0.75	17	$KMnO_4$	Mongeau and Brassard, 1982
Oats, cinnamon & spices	7.4	4.0	0.93	23	$KMnO_4$	Mongeau and Brassard, 1982
Oats, maple & brown sugar, brand 1	5.9	4.4	0.75	17	$KMnO_4$	Mongeau and Brassard, 1982
Oats, maple & brown sugar, brand 2	7.8	3.7	0.65	18	$KMnO_4$	Mongeau and Brassard, 1982
Oats, raisin & spices	7.3	2.9	0.46	16	$KMnO_4$	Mongeau and Brassard, 1982
Oats, sugar & spices	8.2	4.7	0.83	18	$KMnO_4$	Mongeau and Brassard, 1982
Pep	1.6	5.7	0.59	10	$KMnO_4$	Mongeau and Brassard, 1982
Product 19	1.1	2.6	0.49	19	$KMnO_4$	Mongeau and Brassard, 1982
Product 19	3.4	5.5	1.5	27	Klason	Marlett, 1992
Product 19	2.3	4.4	0.6	13	Klason	Anderson and Bridges, 1988
Puffed rice	6.5	1.3	0.2	15	Klason	Anderson and Bridges, 1988
Puffed rice-1	7.3	0.1	tr	—	$KMnO_4$	Mongeau and Brassard, 1982
Puffed rice-2	3.1	0.2	tr	—	$KMnO_4$	Mongeau and Brassard, 1982
Puffed wheat, brand 1	3.2	4.3	0.77	18	$KMnO_4$	Mongeau and Brassard, 1982
Puffed wheat, brand 2	6.1	3.9	0.56	14	$KMnO_4$	Mongeau and Brassard, 1982
Puffed wheat	5.7	7.2	2.17	30	Klason	van Soest, 1978b
Puffed wheat	0	7.2	0.5	7	Klason	Anderson and Bridges, 1988
Puffed wheat	??	15.4	2.47	16	Klason	Southgate, 1986
Puffed Wheat, Fluffs, roasted	6.7	3.9	0.56	14	$KMnO_4$	Mongeau and Brassard, 1982
Raisin Bran	6.0	8.6	0.80	9	$KMnO_4$	Mongeau and Brassard, 1982
Readibreak	??	7.6	1.22	16	Klason	Southgate, 1986
Red River Cereal	6.3	10.1	1.12	11	$KMnO_4$	Mongeau and Brassard, 1982
Rice Flakes	1.0	tr	tr	—	$KMnO_4$	Mongeau and Brassard, 1982
Rice Krispies	7.8	1.9	0.6	32	Klason	Marlett, 1992
Rice Krispies	1.2	1.2	0.4	33	Klason	Anderson and Bridges, 1988

Table 5 Continued

Food	Moisture	Fiber[b]	Lignin	Lignin as % of fiber	Method	Ref.
		g/100 g wet weight[a]				
Rice Krispies	??	4.5	0.22	4	Klason	Southgate, 1986
Rice Krispies	1.6	0.3	tr	—	$KMnO_4$	Mongeau and Brassard, 1982
Rice Flakes	1	tr	tr	—	$KMnO_4$	Mongeau and Brassard, 1982
Shredded Wheat	6.5	12.5	2.52	20	Klason	van Soest, 1978b
Shredded Wheat	3.7	9.8	0.77	8	$KMnO_4$	Mongeau and Brassard, 1982
Shredded Wheat	7.6	11.3	0.9	8	Klason	Marlett, 1992
Shredded Wheat	??	12.3	0.84	7	Klason	Southgate, 1986
Shredded Wheat	5.3	10.5	0.87	8	$KMnO_4$	Mongeau and Brassard, 1989
Shreddies	1.1	7.3	0.49	7	$KMnO_4$	Mongeau and Brassard, 1982
Special K	1.0	0.6	tr	—	$KMnO_4$	Mongeau and Brassard, 1982
Special K	1.9	3.1	1	31	Klason	Anderson and Bridges, 1988
Special K	12.7	2.7	0.9	33	Klason	Marlett, 1992
Special K	??	5.5	1.05	19	Klason	Southgate, 1986
Spoon Size Shredded Wheat	2.1	10.2	0.73	7	$KMnO_4$	Mongeau and Brassard, 1982
Sugar Crisps	2.7	2.0	0.29	14	$KMnO_4$	Mongeau and Brassard, 1982
Sugar Puffs	??	6.1	1.09	18	Klason	Southgate, 1986
Sugar Smacks	1.1	1.6	0.20	13	$KMnO_4$	Mongeau and Brassard, 1982
Swiss breakfast (mixed brands)	??	7.4	0.74	10	Klason	Southgate, 1986
Total	4	3.1	1.6	52	Klason	Marlett, 1992
Trix	13.1	0.8	tr	—	$KMnO_4$	Mongeau and Brassard, 1982
Vita-B	8.1	7.7	0.69	9	$KMnO_4$	Mongeau and Brassard, 1982
Wheat cereal, uncooked	11.4	5.8	0.3	6	$KMnO_4$	R. Mongeau and R. Brassard, unpublished
Wheat Chex	3.6	9.3	4.24	46	Klason	van Soest, 1978b
Wheat Flakes	13.3	11.0	1.04	9	$KMnO_4$	Mongeau and Brassard, 1982
Wheat germ, brand 1	5.3	13.9	1.28	9	$KMnO_4$	Mongeau and Brassard, 1982
Wheat germ, brand 2	11.3	15.7	1.55	10	$KMnO_4$	Mongeau and Brassard, 1982
Wheat germ	14.9	9.7	0.77	8	$KMnO_4$	Foy et al., 1981
Wheat germ, crude	10.5	7.7	0.36	5	$KMnO_4$	Mongeau and Brassard, 1982
Wheat germ, regular	3.5	11.7	0.77	7	$KMnO_4$	Mongeau and Brassard, 1982
Weetabix	??	12.7	1.19	9	Klason	Southgate, 1986
Weetabix	4.8	7.6	0.81	11	$KMnO_4$	Mongeau and Brassard, 1982
Wheaties	4.7	10.6	2.38	23	Klason	van Soest, 1978b
Wheaties	2.1	7.2	0.69	9	$KMnO_4$	Mongeau and Brassard, 1982

					Method	Reference
Wheaties	2.4	11.4	1.4	12	Klason	Marlett, 1992
Wheaties	0.3	8.3	1.0	12	Klason	Anderson and Bridges, 1988
Wheatlets	10.4	1.4	tr	—	KMnO$_4$	Mongeau and Brassard, 1982
Legumes						
Beans, broad	73.6	5.2	0.39	8	ADL	Herranz et al., 1981
Beans, broad, boiled	76.1	4.9	0.28	6	ADL	Herranz et al., 1981
Beans, broad, frozen, raw	74.8	4.6	0.50	11	ADL	Herranz et al., 1983
Beans, broad, frozen, boiled	80.4	4.6	0.38	8	ADL	Herranz et al., 1983
Beans, French	93.1	1.5	0.20	13	KMnO$_4$	Foy et al., 1981
Beans, kidney	92.3	1.5	0.12	8	ADL	Chen et al., 1982
Beans, kidney, canned	70.4	6.2	1	16	Klason	Anderson and Bridges, 1988
Beans, kidney, canned	77.1	5.2	0.3	6	Klason	Marlett, 1992
Beans, lima	70.2	13.2	0.24	2	Klason	Chang et al., 1994
Beans, lima, baby	66.8	4.0	0.27	7	Klason	van Soest, 1978b
Beans, lima, green, canned	75.3	3.6	0.2	6	Klason	Anderson and Bridges, 1988
Beans, lima, green, canned	74.5	4.2	0.1	2	Klason	Marlett, 1992
Beans, mung, sprouts	94.1	0.9	0.03	3	ADL	Chen et al., 1982
Beans, mung, sprout	94.7	1.4	0.12	8	Klason	Chang et al., 1994
Beans, pinto, dried, raw	8.2	19.4	1.5	7	Klason	Anderson and Bridges, 1988
Beans, pinto, dried, cooked	71.2	6.9	0.8	11	Klason	Anderson and Bridges, 1988
Beans, pinto, canned	73.3	5.1	0.9	17	Klason	Anderson and Bridges, 1988
Beans, red	72.7	13.0	0.66	5	KMnO$_4$	Foy et al., 1981
Beans, runner, boiled	??	3.4	0.21	6	KMnO$_4$	Southgate, 1986
Beans, sprouts	95.5	1.6	0.24	15	KMnO$_4$	Foy et al., 1981
Beans, white	16.9	34.4	0.91	3	KMnO$_4$	Foy et al., 1981
Beans, white, dried, raw	3.6	17.7	1	6	Klason	Anderson and Bridges, 1988
Beans, white, baked	69	5.4	0.49	9	KMnO$_4$	Mongeau and Brassard, 1989
Beans, white, canned	73.6	5.5	0.4	7	Klason	Anderson and Bridges, 1988
Bean, yard long	89.6	3.9	0.49	13	Klason	Chang et al., 1994
Cowpea pods, green	89.8	2.4	0.09	4	ADL	Chen et al., 1982
Garbanzo beans, canned	65.6	3.5	0.4	10	Klason	Anderson and Bridges, 1988
Lentils, dried, cooked	66.5	5.3	1	20	Klason	Anderson and Bridges, 1988
Lentils, dried, raw	9.9	11.5	1.9	17	Klason	Anderson and Bridges, 1988
Peanut butter	1.7	6.3	0.8	13	Klason	Marlett, 1992
Peanut butter	??	7.6	tr	—	Klason	Southgate, 1986
Peanuts	1.6	6.8	0.7	10	Klason	Marlett, 1992

Table 5 Continued

Food	g/100 g wet weight[a]			Lignin as % of fiber	Method	Ref.
	Moisture	Fiber[b]	Lignin			
Peanuts	??	9.3	1.21	13	Klason	Southgate, 1986
Peanuts	1.3	7.5	0.87	12	$KMnO_4$	Mongeau and Brassard, 1989
Peas, green	82.4	4.5	0.37	8	$KMnO_4$	Foy et al., 1981
Peas, green	79.3	2.8	0.10	4	Klason	van Soest, 1978b
Pea, green	88.8	2.5	0.24	9	Klason	Chang et al., 1994
Peas, green, frozen	77.2	3.2	0.31	10	ADL	Herranz et al., 1983
Peas, green, frozen	82.3	3.5	tr	—	Klason	Marlett, 1992
Peas, green, frozen	??	7.8	0.18	2	Klason	Southgate, 1986
Peas, green, frozen, boiled	82.9	3.8	0.39	10	ADL	Herranz et al., 1983
Peas, green, canned	82.0	3.2	0.24	8	ADL	Herranz et al., 1983
Peas, green, canned	??	7.8	0.35	4	Klason	Southgate, 1986
Peas, green, canned	??	6.3	0.01	0.2	Klason	Southgate, 1986
Peas, green, canned, Del Monte	81.5	4.3	0.1	2	Klason	Marlett, 1992
Peas, green, canned, Freshlike	84.7	3.3	0.1	3	Klason	Marlett, 1992
Peas, green, canned, fried	51.8	3.6	0.14	4	ADL	Herranz et al., 1983
Peas, green, with pods	88.0	1.9	0.08	4	ADL	Chen et al., 1982
Peas, black-eyed	65.0	3.2	0.63	20	Klason	van Soest, 1978b
Peas, black-eyed, canned	78.6	3.1	0.5	16	Klason	Marlett, 1992
Peas, black-eyed, canned	65	3.9	0.8	20	Klason	Anderson and Bridges, 1988
Pea leaves	93.8	2.8	0.15	5	Klason	Chang et al., 1994
Pea sprouts	91.0	2.8	0.27	10	Klason	Chang et al., 1994
Pork and beans, canned	75	4.4	0.2	5	Klason	Marlett, 1992
Pork and beans, canned	??	7.3	0.19	3	Klason	Southgate, 1986
Pork and beans, canned	73.5	4.2	0.2	5	Klason	Anderson and Bridges, 1988
Soybean, immature	68.2	11.9	0.61	5	Klason	Chang et al., 1994
Soybean sprouts	91.4	3.0	0.10	3	Klason	Chang et al., 1994
Nuts						
Almonds, with skin	4.7	8.8	1.9	22	Klason	Marlett, 1992
Brazil nuts	??	4.4	1.17	27	Klason	Southgate, 1986
Coconut, shredded	18.5	6.6	0	0	Klason	Marlett, 1992
Walnuts, English	3.5	3.8	0.9	24	Klason	Marlett, 1992

Other foods

Food						
Beef extract, Bovril	??	0.9	0.03	3	Klason	Southgate, 1986
Ketchup	66.7	1.2	0.2	17	Klason	Marlett, 1992
Cocoa	??	43.3	27.9	64	Klason	Southgate, 1986
Chocolate beverage	??	8.2	4.43	54	Klason	Southgate, 1986
Coffee and chicory essence	??	0.8	0.04	5	Klason	Southgate, 1986
Coffee, instant	??	16.4	0.33	2	Klason	Southgate, 1986
Dulse	5.4	28.5	1.04	4	KMnO$_4$	Flint and Camire, 1992
Dulse	5.4	28.5	0.57	2	Klason	Flint and Camire, 1992
Fruit mincemeat	??	3.2	0.5	16	Klason	Southgate, 1986
Lemon curd	??	0.2	tr	—	Klason	Southgate, 1986
Marmalade	??	0.7	0.01	1	Klason	Southgate, 1986
Potato chips (crisps)	??	11.9	0.32	3	Klason	Southgate, 1986
Preserve, jam	??	7.7	1.96	25	Klason	Southgate, 1986
Preserve, plum	??	1	0.03	3	Klason	Southgate, 1986
Preserve, strawberry	??	1.1	0.15	13	Klason	Southgate, 1986
Soup, cream of mushroom, canned	84.1	0.4	0	0	Klason	Marlett, 1992
Soup, minestrone, dried	??	6.6	0.1	2	Klason	Southgate, 1986
Soup, oxtail, dried	??	3.8	0.01	0	Klason	Southgate, 1986
Soup, tomato, dried	??	3.3	0.04	1	Klason	Southgate, 1986
Soup, vegetarian vegetable, canned	82.3	1.8	0.1	6	Klason	Marlett, 1992
Sunchips	3.0	6.2	0.68	11	KMnO$_4$	Flint and Camire, 1992
Sunchips	3.0	6.2	1.75	28	Klason	Flint and Camire, 1992
Yeast extract, Marmite	??	2.7	0.06	2	Klason	Southgate, 1986

[a] Values are reported in grams per 100 g fresh weight with the exception of some mushrooms as noted.
[b] Fiber was measured by various methodologies as reported in the individual papers: Anderson and Bridges, 1988 (modified Prosky method; Prosky et al., 1988); Chen et al., 1982 (NDF; van Soest and Wine, 1967); Foy et al., 1981 (NDF; Flint and Camire, 1992) (nonstarch polysaccharides; Englyst and Cummings, 1988; Goering and van Soest, 1970); Herranz et al., 1981, 1983 (NDF; van Soest and Wine, 1967); Kurasawa et al., 1982 (NDF; van Soest, 1963); Lund and Smoot, 1982 (modified van Soest procedure; Robertson, 1978); Marlett, 1992 (nonstarch polysaccharides + lignin; Marlett, 1992); Matthée and Appledorf, 1978 (NDF; Goering and van Soest, 1970; Mongeau and Brassard, 1979 (NDF, Goering and van Soest, 1970), Mongeau and Brassard, 1982 (unpurified pancreatic amylase/NDF procedure; Goering and van Soest, 1970), Mongeau and Brassard, 1989; R. Mongeau and R. Brassard, unpublished (HPB method; AOAC 992.16; Mongeau and Brassard, 1993); Southgate, 1986 (Southgate method; Southgate, 1969); van Soest, 1978b (NDF; van Soest and Wine, 1967); Vidal-Valverde, 1982 (NDF plus pectic substances; van Soest and Wine, 1967; Vidal-Valverde, 1982).
[c] Values are reported as g/100 g dry weight as no moisture measurements were reported.
[d] Methodology was not specified.

Table 6 Comparison of Lignin Measured by the Permanganate and Klason Methods

	Lignin content (g/100 g fresh weight)			
		Klason		
Product	$KMnO_4$	Method A	Method B	Method C
Apples	0.1	0.1	0.4	>0.01
Bananas	0.1	0.6	0.8	0.3
Blueberries	0.5	0.9	—	—
Pears	0.3	0.4	—	>0.5
Strawberries	0.3	0.5	—	0.8
Celery	0.1	tr	—	0.1
Peanuts	0.9	0.7	—	1.2
Bread, white, wheat	tr	0.5	0.1	tr
Bread, whole wheat	0.5	—	0.7	0.2
All Bran cereal	2.6	4.3	3.1	2.9
Corn Flakes cereal	tr–0.6	0.7	0.6	1.3
Grape-Nuts cereal	0.9	—	0.6	0.6
Product 19 cereal	0.5	1.5	0.6	—
Puffed wheat cereal	0.6–0.8	—	0.5	2.5
Puffed rice	tr	—	0.2	—
Rice Krispies	tr	0.6	0.4	0.2
Shredded Wheat	0.8	0.9	—	0.8
Wheaties	0.7	1.4	1.0	—

Source: Permanganate values from Mongeau and Brassard (1979, 1982, 1989, and unpublished). Klason values from Method A (Marlett, 1992), Method B (Anderson and Bridges, 1988), Method C (Southgate, 1986). See Table 5 for details.

B. Permanganate Lignin

Mongeau and Brassard (1979) directly compared permanganate lignin and ADL values in breads. Both methods included the preparation of ADF prior to analysis so their comparison focused solely on the acid versus permanganate treatments. In general, the permanganate lignin values were about 15% lower than the corresponding ADL values. Flint and Camire (1992) compared permanganate lignin (van Soest and Wine, 1967) and Klason lignin in a selection of foods including vegetables, fruit, breakfast cereals, bread, and toast. They also found that the permanganate values were generally lower, but this was food specific. In 1982, Mongeau and Brassard measured permanganate lignin in 101 breakfast cereals (Table 5). The procedure was similar to that of Goering and van Soest (1970) but used milder conditions for human foods and a specific source of mammalian enzymes (Mongeau and Brassard, 1982, 1989). Unfortunately, no comparison was made to Klason lignin or ADL.

As indicated in the previous section, Klason lignin and ADL may contain varying amounts of Maillard products, precipitated protein and other nonlignin materials depending on the nature of the material being analyzed (Theander and James, 1979; Reeves and Galletti, 1991; Vollendorf and Marlett, 1994; Theander et al., 1995). The permanganate lignin method, on the other hand, is generally less sensitive to the effects of food processing. Nevertheless, the lignin values may be slightly increased in foods containing Maillard products if care is not taken during sample preparation prior to analysis (van Soest, 1978a; Mongeau and Brassard, 1980). Mongeau and Brassard (1980) provided an excellent example of Maillard product interference and proper sample preparation by measuring lignin in toasted whole wheat bread. They measured a permanganate lignin value of 0.4 g/100 g (dry weight basis) in an NDF extract (see Goering and van Soest, 1970) of untoasted whole wheat bread treated with a bacterial α-amylase. After toasting the bread, the lignin value increased to 2.2 g/100 g. When the same toasted bread was treated with an unpurified preparation of porcine pancreatic α-amylase (Sigma Chemical Co., A3176) and an NDF extract prepared, the permanganate lignin was again 0.4 g/100 g. Analysis of the ''lignin'' residues of the toasted breads showed that the 2.2 g residue (obtained after bacterial amylase treatment) contained 10 times more lysine than the 0.4 g residue (obtained after unpurified pancreatic amylase treatment). These results show that NDF permanganate lignin values can be artificially increased under certain heating conditions that are likely to occur with specific foods, but proper treatment of the sample and appropriate choice of the amylase source can avoid this. Mongeau and Brassard (1980) showed that the unpurified pancreatic enzyme improved both the ADL and permanganate lignin values. The NDF extraction is important as well since this step removes much of the digestible and nonfiber protein. In addition, the combined NDF/pancreatic amylase treatment removed the slowly digestible starch fraction, which may have also interfered with the lignin determination. The effect required pretreatment with unpurified α-amylase (5 min) prior to the NDF extraction followed by a second 60-minute α-amylase incubation.

Nonfiber reducing sugars and fiber components such as arabinose may also participate in the Maillard reaction. This may globally increase (or possibly decrease) the apparent fiber and lignin values depending on the food. The data in Table 6 show that the permanganate lignin values obtained using after treatment with pancreatic amylase (Mongeau and Brassard, 1979, 1982, 1991) can be similar to (pears, peanuts, shredded wheat, Grape-Nuts cereal, All Bran cereal) or lower than (bananas, blueberries, strawberries, white bread, Rice Krispies cereal, Wheaties cereal) Klason lignin values. On average, one finds that permanganate lignin values are generally lower than Klason lignin values and ADL values. When human dietary ADL and permanganate lignin values were directly compared, no correlation was observed for wheat bran, black beans, soybean, celery, or oat bran using the pancreatic amylase treatment described above (R. Mongeau and R. Brassard, unpublished data). Similar results were observed when Klason and permanganate lignin values were compared for fruits, breakfast cereals, breads, and toast (Flint and Camire, 1992).

IV. ESTIMATES OF LIGNIN INTAKE

A. Sources of Lignin

In many human foods, lignin is only found associated with spiral and annular bands in xylem-conducting vessels. Thus, lignin is a small component of the human diet since the more heavily woody tissues are not frequently consumed (Southgate, 1993). In human diets, lignins are most commonly found in ''whole'' preparations of cereal grains because of its presence in the cell wall of the seed coat. It can also be found in clumps in the flesh of some fruits (especially the pear) and in fruits that contain edible seeds (such as strawberries). Lignin is also present in mature vegetables such as carrots and other root vegetables (Slavin, 1987). In general, lignin values increase with increasing amounts of nonstarch polysaccharide (Flint and Camire, 1992).

Table 5 presents ADL, Klason lignin, and permanganate lignin values as well as dietary fiber values in various human foods. The table is limited by the fact that lignin is not normally measured in gravimetric procedures but is included in the insoluble dietary fiber isolate along with hemicelluloses, cellulose, and ash. Thus, a separate determination for lignin must be per-

Table 7 Estimate of Daily Lignin Intake in Canadian Populations

Survey food category	Daily intake (g/person/d)		Food category from Table 5	g lignin/100 g food	Total lignin from each food (g/person/d)	
	NS survey[b]	Québec survey[c]			NS survey	Québec survey
Pasta	33.38	63.71	Spaghetti and macaroni, cooked (exclude whole wheat)	0.35	0.1168	0.2230
Rice	13.81	27.06	Rice, medium grain, regular, cooked + white rice	0.35	0.0483	0.0947
Cereal grains	32.03	31.06	Flour, wheat (0.8*white + 0.2*whole)	0.29	0.0929	0.0901
White breads	43.89	43.45	Bread, white wheat	0.16	0.0702	0.0695
Whole wheat breads	17.92	22.23	Bread, whole wheat	0.55	0.0986	0.1223
Other whole grain breads	0.22	0.08	Use ''bread, other'' category	0.10	0.0002	0.0001
Rolls, bagels	17.42	13.86	Bread, French and Italian + hamburger bun	0.33	0.0575	0.0457
Crackers and crisps	4.12	2.95	Average of all types	0.54	0.0222	0.0159
Muffins and English muffins	0	0	Muffin, English and plain (50:50)	0.55	0.0000	0.0000
Pancakes and waffles	0.4	0.59	Pancake mix	0.60	0.0024	0.0035
Croissants	0	0.05	Estimate from flour	0.29	0.0000	0.0001
Dry mixes (cakes)	2.41	3.56	Estimate from Pancakes	0.60	0.0145	0.0214
Whole grain, oats and high fiber cereals	11.74	11.53	Mix of 100% Branflakes, 40% Branflakes, All Bran, Alpen, Bran Buds, Bran Flakes, Fiber 1, Oats, Product 19, Total, Corn bran, Wheaties, Shredded Wheat	1.69	0.1984	0.1949
Other breakfast cereal	9.06	7.18	Mix of Corn Flakes, Cream of Wheat, Frosted Mini Wheats, Grape-nuts, Honey Smacks, Rice Krispies, Special K, Puffed Rice	0.48	0.0435	0.0345
Cookies	6.23	7.38	Cookies, ginger snaps and plain	0.20	0.0125	0.0148
Biscuits	0	0	Biscuits, baking powder	0.10	0.0000	0.0000
Pies, commercial	0.02	0.09	Pie crust	0.60	0.0001	0.0005
Cakes, commercial	0.25	0.67	Cake, yellow	0.10	0.0003	0.0007
Danishes, doughnuts	0	0	Roll, cinnamon	0.40	0.0000	0.0000
Ice creams	8.36	6.16	Ice cream cone, Comet cup	0.50	0.0418	0.0308
Ice milk	1.04	0.24	Ice cream cone, Comet cup	0.50	0.0052	0.0012

Food						
Frozen yogurts	0.96	0.47	Estimate with some fruit	0.10	0.0010	0.0005
Milk, whole	82.63	68.72	No data	0.00	0.0000	0.0000
Milk, 2%	29.82	27.01	No data	0.00	0.0000	0.0000
Milk, 1%	20.16	16.2	No data	0.00	0.0000	0.0000
Milk, skim	44.87	16.58	No data	0.00	0.0000	0.0000
Milk, evaporated whole	6.66	0.86	No data	0.00	0.0000	0.0000
Milk, evaporated 2%	1.18	0.38	No data	0.00	0.0000	0.0000
Milk, evaporated skim	0	0	No data	0.00	0.0000	0.0000
Milk, condensed	0.06	0.19	No data	0.00	0.0000	0.0000
Other types milk	1.72	0.93	No data	0.00	0.0000	0.0000
Whipping cream	0.47	1.39	No data	0.00	0.0000	0.0000
Table cream	2.99	1.35	No data	0.00	0.0000	0.0000
Half & half	5.8	5.15	No data	0.00	0.0000	0.0000
Sour cream	0.66	0.24	No data	0.00	0.0000	0.0000
Cottage cheeses	2.79	0.84	No data	0.00	0.0000	0.0000
Cheeses, <10% BF	0.6	1.89	No data	0.00	0.0000	0.0000
Cheeses, 10–25% BF	7.35	10.16	No data	0.00	0.0000	0.0000
Cheeses, >25% BF	12.97	18.77	No data	0.00	0.0000	0.0000
Yogurts, <2% BF	2.94	8.81	Estimate with some fruit	0.10	0.0029	0.0088
Yogurts, >2% BF	3.28	4.09	Estimate with some fruit	0.10	0.0033	0.0041
Eggs	22.82	24.37	No data	0.00	0.0000	0.0000
Butter	2.57	6.32	No data	0.00	0.0000	0.0000
Regular tub margarine	7.06	9.11	No data	0.00	0.0000	0.0000
Calorie-reduced margarine	0.98	0.2	No data	0.00	0.0000	0.0000
Block margarine	4.84	0.1	No data	0.00	0.0000	0.0000
Vegetable oils	2.43	4.12	No data	0.00	0.0000	0.0000
Animal fats	1.37	2.34	No data	0.00	0.0000	0.0000
Shortening	6.21	5.57	No data	0.00	0.0000	0.0000
Beef, lean only	19	20.05	No data	0.00	0.0000	0.0000
Beef, lean + fat	7.22	10.13	No data	0.00	0.0000	0.0000
Beef, ground	27.06	33.61	No data	0.00	0.0000	0.0000
Veal, lean only	0.2	0.92	No data	0.00	0.0000	0.0000
Veal, lean + fat	0.25	3	No data	0.00	0.0000	0.0000
Lamb, lean only	0.35	0.13	No data	0.00	0.0000	0.0000
Lamb, lean + fat	0.22	0.94	No data	0.00	0.0000	0.0000

Table 7 Continued

Survey food category	Daily intake (g/person/d) NS survey[b]	Daily intake (g/person/d) Québec survey[c]	Food category from Table 5	g lignin/100 g food	Total lignin from each food (g/person/d) NS survey	Total lignin from each food (g/person/d) Québec survey
Pork, fresh, lean	10.3	9.01	No data	0.00	0.0000	0.0000
Pork, fresh, lean + fat	5.66	7.2	No data	0.00	0.0000	0.0000
Bacon	2	1.54	No data	0.00	0.0000	0.0000
Ham, cured, lean	7.19	8.82	No data	0.00	0.0000	0.0000
Ham, cured, lean + fat	3.49	5.47	No data	0.00	0.0000	0.0000
Chicken, meat on	16.44	22.06	No data	0.00	0.0000	0.0000
Chicken, meat + skin	11.94	8.74	No data	0.00	0.0000	0.0000
Turkey, meat only	6.37	3.88	No data	0.00	0.0000	0.0000
Turkey, meat + skin	0.32	0.83	No data	0.00	0.0000	0.0000
Other birds	0.04	0.12	No data	0.00	0.0000	0.0000
Birds, skin only	0.25	0.24	No data	0.00	0.0000	0.0000
Livers	1.19	1.63	No data	0.00	0.0000	0.0000
Liver pates	0.05	0.42	No data	0.00	0.0000	0.0000
Offals	0.14	0.51	No data	0.00	0.0000	0.0000
Sausages	8.74	6.17	No data	0.00	0.0000	0.0000
Game meat	1.28	1.92	No data	0.00	0.0000	0.0000
Luncheon meats	10.74	8.96	No data	0.00	0.0000	0.0000
Nuts	2.14	2.77	Mix of almonds, with skin, Brazil nuts, English walnuts	1.32	0.0282	0.0366
Seeds	0.07	0.34	Estimate from nuts	1.32	0.0009	0.0045
Peanut butter	3.42	3.49	Peanut butter	0.40	0.0137	0.0140
Fish, <6% fat	15.73	6.4	No data	0.00	0.0000	0.0000
Fish, >=6% fat	6.66	4.7	No data	0.00	0.0000	0.0000
Shellfish	14.29	4.31	No data	0.00	0.0000	0.0000
Beans	3.7	4.2	Green and wax	0.21	0.0078	0.0088
Broccoli	4.05	6.88	Broccoli, cooked	0.17	0.0069	0.0117
Cabbage and kale	5.25	5.95	Cabbage, red and white	0.14	0.0074	0.0083
Cauliflower	2.51	3.14	Cauliflower	0.07	0.0018	0.0022
Carrots	14.93	20.68	Carrots	0.16	0.0239	0.0331
Celery	3.61	9.45	Celery	0.07	0.0025	0.0066

Food			Description			
Corn	4.44	5.19	Corn, whole kernel, canned and frozen	0.26	0.0135	0.0115
Lettuces and vegetables leafy	15.75	11.03	Lettuce	0.11	0.0121	0.0173
Mushrooms	4.84	3.39	Mushrooms, canned	0.15	0.0051	0.0073
Onion, green onion	20.48	13.45	Onions	0.05	0.0067	0.0102
Peas and snow peas	3.88	8.21	Peas, green	0.18	0.0148	0.0070
Peppers, red and green	5.92	3.26	Mix of all peppers	0.14	0.0046	0.0083
Squashes	1.24	4.08	Mix of all squash	0.07	0.0029	0.0009
Tomatoes	51.2	36.92	Mix of all tomatoes	0.21	0.0775	0.1075
Juices, tomato and vegetable	16.08	4.94	Estimate from tomatoes	0.21	0.0104	0.0338
Other vegetables	24.48	21.29	Average of vegetables	0.14	0.0298	0.0343
Legumes	5.16	7.15	Average of all legumes	0.47	0.0336	0.0243
Foods made with vegetable protein	0.32	0.47	Estimate as vegetables	0.14	0.0007	0.0004
Potato chips	4.09	5.14	Potato chips (crisps)	0.32	0.0164	0.0131
Fried or roasted potatoes	12.2	15.13	Potato, french fries + fried + baked	0.18	0.0272	0.0220
Potatoes	71.84	83.14	Rest of potatoes	0.12	0.0998	0.0862
Citrus fruits	25.53	24.14	Average of oranges and grapefruit and lemon	0.33	0.0797	0.0842
Apple	54.02	33.01	Mix of all apples	0.15	0.0495	0.0810
Banana	15.63	14.43	Banana	0.44	0.0635	0.0688
Cherries	0.89	0.68	Cherries	0.13	0.0009	0.0012
Grapes and raisin	8.01	2.75	Mix of grapes and raisins	1.00	0.0275	0.0801
Melons	3.1	3.11	Watermelon, + melon	0.09	0.0028	0.0028
Peaches, nectarines	4.92	3.3	Peaches	0.30	0.0099	0.0148
Pears	11.09	4.24	Pear, Bartlett, fresh, unpeeled, canned	0.63	0.0267	0.0699
Pineapple	1.89	2.46	Mix of all pineapples	0.05	0.0012	0.0009
Plums and prunes	2.45	1.59	Mix of all plums	0.26	0.0041	0.0064
Strawberries	1.07	1.75	Strawberries	0.43	0.0075	0.0046
Other fruits	8.77	7.59	Blueberries	0.73	0.0554	0.0640
White and brown sugar	16.49	15.79	No data	0.00	0.0000	0.0000
Jams, jellies and marmalades	4.22	3.73	Estimate fruit	0.10	0.0037	0.0042
Other sugars	9.33	5.61	No data	0.00	0.0000	0.0000
Sugar substitute	0.13	0.11	No data	0.00	0.0000	0.0000
Popcorn, plain & pretzels	0.83	1.36	Guess from corn	0.30	0.0041	0.0025
Salty and high fat snacks	0.49	1.29	No data	0.00	0.0000	0.0000
Candies, gums	1.93	2.18	No data	0.00	0.0000	0.0000
Popsicle, sherbet	0.3	1.02	No data	0.00	0.0000	0.0000
Jello, dessert, commercial pudding	3.66	1.96	No data	0.00	0.0000	0.0000
Chocolate bars	4.04	6.29	No data	0.00	0.0000	0.0000

Table 7 Continued

Survey food category	Daily intake (g/person/d)		Food category from Table 5	g lignin/100 g food	Total lignin from each food (g/person/d)	
	NS survey[b]	Québec survey[c]			NS survey	Québec survey
Fruit juices	64.98	74.22	No data	0.00	0.0000	0.0000
Soft drinks-regular	32.63	22.06	No data	0.00	0.0000	0.0000
Soft drinks with aspartame	56.55	32.17	No data	0.00	0.0000	0.0000
Fruit drinks	33.75	25.2	No data	0.00	0.0000	0.0000
Other beverages	1.05	6	No data	0.00	0.0000	0.0000
Spirits	5.02	2.71	No data	0.00	0.0000	0.0000
Liquors	0.08	0.77	No data	0.00	0.0000	0.0000
Wines	6.6	30.1	No data	0.00	0.0000	0.0000
Beers	0.63	5.58	No data	0.00	0.0000	0.0000
Coolers	1.25	0.08	No data	0.00	0.0000	0.0000
Soups with vegetables	30.32	20.44	Soup, vegetarian vegetable, canned	0.05	0.0158	0.0106
Soups without vegetables	18.24	41.28	No data	0.00	0.0000	0.0000
Gravies	3.84	4.31	No data	0.00	0.0000	0.0000
Sauces	5.17	6.12	No data	0.00	0.0000	0.0000
Salad dressings	7.35	4.31	No data	0.00	0.0000	0.0000
Seasonings	3.25	3.27	No data	0.10	0.0033	0.0033
Meal replacement	0.22	0.61	No data	0.00	0.0000	0.0000
Tea including iced	12.18	21.68	No data	0.00	0.0000	0.0000
Coffee	24.09	61.73	No data	0.00	0.0000	0.0000
Water	6.4	24.64	No data	0.00	0.0000	0.0000
Baby food products	0.06	0.05	Estimate from fiber content and cereal data	0.20	0.0001	0.0001
Infant formula	0	0	No data	0.00	0.0000	0.0000
Spices	0.15	0.15	No data	0.00	0.0000	0.0000
Other food ingredients	0.65	0.79	No data	0.00	0.0000	0.0000
Total					1.6363	1.9861

[a] Data reported as average grams per person per day on a "fresh weight" basis.
[b] Data represent total per capita intake of males and females aged 18–74 years from Nova Scotia survey of food intake (MacLean, 1993).
[c] Data represent total per capita intake of males and females aged 18–74 years from Québec survey of food intake (Santé Québec, 1995).

formed. Many of the procedures that measure nonstarch polysaccharide content by gas chromatography include a separate determination for lignin. The Uppsala and Marlett (1992) methods, for example, measure lignin separately by the Klason procedure.

Table 5 illustrates some of the problems with the various methodologies, and these are highlighted in Table 6. As discussed above, Klason lignin may overestimate lignin and total dietary fiber depending on the sample and the solubility of the lignin in acid solutions (see Sec. II). Thus, the lignin content of some foods in Table 5 is sometimes greater than the "rule of thumb" value of 20% of total dietary fiber (TDF). This predominates in dried/cooked foods that are high in starch (dried noodles, breads) or high in cellulose (breakfast cereals), suggesting that Maillard product formation as well as incomplete cellulose removal by the Klason process may contribute to higher lignin values in some samples.

The permanganate lignin values of Table 5 reported by Mongeau and Brassard (1979, 1982, 1989) were obtained after treatment with unpurified pancreatic amylase (see Sec. III), preparation of a NDF extract, a further treatment with unpurified pancreatic amylase, preparation of an acid detergent extract, and lignin measurement using the permanganate method. For human diets, the results are more reproducible and often lower than those obtained after ADF extraction followed by permanganate treatment (see Sec. III) or after Klason lignin treatment. Table 6 compares lignin values determined by the pancreatic amylase/permanganate method with those determined by the Klason method as reported by Marlett (1992), Anderson and Bridges (1988), and Southgate (1986).

B. Estimates of Population Intake

Table 7 presents an estimate of the average daily intake of lignin per person in grams. Lignin values between 1.6–2 g/d were calculated based on the lignin determinations reported in Table 5. This estimate may be somewhat high because it relies mostly on the use of Klason lignin values, which may overestimate lignin in certain cases (see above). Average TDF intakes for these two populations were 13.5 and 15.2 g/day for Nova Scotia and Québec, respectively. These data show that lignin intake is approximately 13% of TDF intake.

The data of Table 7 give some indication of lignin sources in the Canadian diet. As expected, the major sources of dietary lignin are pasta, wheat flour, bread, and breakfast cereals. This is due to both a higher lignin content in these products as well as a higher per capita intake. Table 7 demonstrates that vegetable and fruit products contribute little to the total lignin intake. This is because vegetables and fruits, themselves, contain very little lignin and because they form a relatively minor portion of total food intake.

V. IMPORTANCE OF LIGNIN IN HUMAN NUTRITION

Dietary fiber represents a diverse group of components with clearly different physiological effects. As Eastwood (1986) pointed out, stating the total dietary fiber content of a diet is about as useful as stating the total vitamin content. It should be noted that Eastwood (1986) was challenging the contemporary view that the physiological effects of dietary fiber could be reasonably predicted by knowing its composition. Several later papers showed that this is not the case. For example, two bran sources (wheat and corn) have similar carbohydrate compositions but exhibit different physiological effects. The less fermentable fiber (corn bran fiber) contains significantly less lignin (Mongeau et al., 1991). In accordance with the present view, and taking into consideration the technical difficulty in separating the various dietary fiber components and

Table 8 Plant Tissue Morphology and Relative Fermentability

Tissue	Fermentability	Notes
Mesophyll	High	Thin wall, no lignin
Parenchyma	Moderate to high	Found in midrib of grass and main vein of legume leaves, leaf sheath and stem of grasses and petiole and stem of legumes
Collenchyma	Moderate to high	Structural cells in legume leaves and stems; thick wall, not lignified
Parenchyma bundle sheath	Moderate	Wall moderately thick and weakly lignified
Phloem fiber	Moderate	Often not lignified; in legume petioles and stems
Epidermis	Low to high	Thickened, lignified outer wall covered with cuticle and waxy layer
Vascular tissue	None to moderate	Phloem and xylem cells; highly lignified
Sclerenchyma	None to low	Thick, lignified wall

Source: Adapted from Buxton and Redfearn, 1997.

determining their contribution to digestive events and physiological responses, researchers have examined comparative trends between fiber sources to extrapolate individual effects.

It is difficult to assess the importance of lignin in human diets because all the studies examining the influence of lignin on fiber fermentation have been performed with ruminants and ruminant fiber. Consequently, we will try to assess the relative importance of lignin in human diets by examining the influence of lignin on forage fermentation while recognizing the fact that human dietary fiber and gastrointestinal tract physiology are very different from ruminant fiber and physiology. In ruminants, Jung and Deetz (1993) stated that lignin is the most important factor in fermentation, limiting microbial digestion of carbohydrate polymers by presenting a physical barrier to access. Buxton et al. (1996) showed that lignin concentration is related to the proportion of indigestible dry matter. Akin and Burdick (1975) showed that plant anatomy influences cell digestibility at least partly through lignin content (Table 8). It is thought that the leaf blades of C_3 plants are more digestible than those of C_4 grasses because they contain more (poorly lignified) mesophyll cells (Buxton and Redfearn, 1997). Lignin is thought to act as a physical barrier to microbes, limiting their capacity for fermentation. This is a result of the high degree of association between lignin and cell wall carbohydrates as well as the degree of crosslinking between carbohydrate polymers caused by noncore lignin bridges in grasses (Fig. 4) (Jung and Allen, 1995). The extent of lignification has been used to explain the high degree of nondigestibility of some legume forages (Buxton and Redfearn, 1997). Direct confirmation of the indigestibility of fiber during fermentation was obtained by feeding oat and cottonseed hulls to cannulated wethers and following acid detergent lignin disappearance. Garleb et al. (1991) observed that only 15% of the lignin disappeared during either in situ or in vivo fermentation. In addition, much of the p-coumaric and ferulic acids were recovered in the fermented fractions, suggesting that noncore lignin losses were responsible for decreases in lignin recovery. Feeding of cabbage and alfalfa fiber derivatives to guinea pigs depressed anaerobic bacterial growth in the cecum. The active agent appeared to be alkali sensitive (see Sec. I), suggesting that it was noncore lignin (Johanning and O'Dell, 1981). It even appears that soluble phenolics inhibit in vitro fermentation of cellulose and protein by rumen microorganisms (Jung and Farley, 1981). Despite these results with cannulated wethers, others, have shown that lignin can be degraded by ruminant microbes when the incubation proceeds for an extended period of time. Specifically, Nordkvist et al. (1989) observed up to 46% of wheat straw lignin and 33–65%

(depending on the methodology) of red clover stem lignin had disappeared after 130 hours in an in vitro system using rumen liquor. These results were similar to alfalfa plant lignin fermentability in an in vitro system where 48.5% of the initial lignin was not detectable using the acetyl bromide procedure after 48 hours (Fukushima et al., 1991). Purified lignin has also been shown to reduce protein digestibility in rats (Shah et al., 1982) and in mice (Keim and Kies, 1979), although the effect was small. Although human dietary fiber and gastrointestinal tract physiology are different from ruminant fiber and physiology, the effects of lignin on limiting fiber fermentation may also be important in human nutrition.

In addition to its effect on fiber fermentation, lignin itself has been associated with various physiological and biochemical responses. In some instances the association is favorable, and in others disease states have been implicated with lignin intake. For example, consumption of harissa (a home-made spice mixture) in Tunisia has been associated with an increased risk for nasopharyngeal carcinoma. To investigate this phenomenon, Bouvier et al. (1995) fractionated harissa and discovered that lignin-containing fractions enhanced an Epstein-Barr virus promotor. This suggested a link between lignin and upregulation of cancer promoters. One must be cautious in interpreting these results because (a) no lignin isolates from other plants were included in the present study, (b) the amount of lignin was not estimated in harissa, (c) there was no comparison to other, highly lignified foods, and (d) phenolics can be cancer promoters at high levels but can serve as potential chemopreventers at levels found in foods (Newmark, 1986; Shahidi and Naczk, 1995).

On the positive side, lignin has been shown to induce apoptosis via production of an ascorbyl radical in the presence of vitamin C (Sakagami and Satoh, 1996), suggesting a possible role in anticancer treatment. This interaction may be especially important in the digestive tract. Lignin may also have a positive effect on lipid balance. Pigs fed purified lignin supplements had significantly reduced plasma triglyceride levels (Valencia and Chavez, 1997), suggesting that the polyphenol chains may bind hydrophobic polymers in the lumen. This has also been suggested for humans where lignin may act to bind bile salts in addition to fatty acids and metals (Jung and Fahey, 1983; Fly et al., 1998). The affinity of lignin polymers for phenolics has been suggested as the mechanisms for the colon-cancer reducing effect of wheat bran (Ferguson and Harris, 1996).

VI. CONCLUSIONS

It is apparent that lignin is a difficult compound to measure. At present, the permanganate method of Mongeau and Brassard (1979, 1982, 1989) appears superior because of its ability to exclude protein and Maillard products from the final pellet, although no measure of the amount of carbohydrate lost during the oxidation product has been provided. In a comparison of methods with forage fiber, Reeves and Galletti (1991) showed that the triethylene glycol and the acetyl bromide procedures excluded protein contamination in addition to the permanganate procedure, but these had problems of carbohydrate interference (acetyl bromide) or incomplete extraction (triethylene glycol). It, therefore, appears that the permanganate procedure is the most preferable current method for measuring dietary lignin values.

Lignin appears to play an important role in ruminant fiber fermentation, limiting fermentation by presenting a physical barrier to bacterial access. This effect may also be expected of human dietary foods, but the extent of ligninification is much lower (see Table 8), which may lower the influence of lignin on colonic (human) fermentation. Lignin may also have other, metabolism-specific, effects that benefit the host. Much work remains to be done to determine the role of lignin in fermentation and colonic metabolism.

ACKNOWLEDGMENTS

The authors wish to thank Dr. Danielle Brulé of the Nutrition Surveys Section of the Nutrition Research Division for providing food intake data and Dr. Mary L'Abbé, Dr. Kevin Cockell, and Ms. Josie Deeks for helpful editorial criticisms.

REFERENCES

Adler, E. (1977). Lignin chemistry—past, present and future. Wood Sci. Technol. 11:169–218.

Armitage, E. R., Ashworth, R. B., and Ferguson, W. S. (1948). The determination of lignin in plant material of high protein content. J. Soc. Chem. Ind. 67:241–264.

Asp, N.-G. (1995). Dietary fiber analysis—an overview. Eur. J. Clin. Nutr. 49(suppl.):S42–S47.

Aulin-Erdtman, G., and Hegbom, L. (1957). Spectrographic contributions to lignin chemistry VII. The ultraviolet absorption and ionization $\Delta\varepsilon$ curves of some phenols. Svensk Papperstidn. 60:671–681.

Azuma, J.-I., and Tetsuo, K. (1988). Lignin-carbohydrate complexes from various sources. In: Methods in Enzymology, Part B. Lignin, Pectin, and Chitin, W. A. Wood and S. T. Kellogg (Eds.), Vol. 161, pp. 12–18. New York: Academic Press.

Bagby, M. O., Cunningham, R. L., and Maloney, R. L. (1973). Ultraviolet spectral determination of lignin. Tappi 56:162–163.

Ben-Ghedalia, D., and Yosef, E. (1994). Effect of isolation procedure on molecular weight distribution of wheat straw lignins. J. Agric. Food Chem. 42:649–652.

Bouvier, G., Hergenhahn, M., Polack, A., Bornkamm, G. W., de Thé, G., and Bartsch, H. (1995). Characterization of macromolecular lignins as Epstein-Barr virus inducer in foodstuff associated with nasopharyngeal carcinoma risk. Carcinogenesis 16:1879–1885.

Browning, B. L. (1967). Methods of Wood Chemistry, pp. 717–746, 785–823. New York: John Wiley & Sons.

Buxton, D. R., and Redfearn, D. D. (1997). Plant limitations to fiber digestion and utilization. J. Nutr. 127:814S–818S.

Buxton, D. R., Mertens, D. R., and Fisher, D. S. (1996). Forage quality and ruminant utilization. In: Cool-Season Forage Grasses, L. E. Moser, D. R. Buxton, and M. D. Casler (Eds.), pp. 229–266. Madison, WI: American Society of Agronomy.

Chen, M. L., Chang, S. C., and Guoo, J. Y. (1982). Fiber contents of some Chinese vegetables and their in vitro binding capacity of bile acids. Nutr. Rep. Int. 26:1053–1059.

Dence, C. W. (1992). The determination of lignin. In: Methods in Lignin Chemistry, S. Y. Lin and C. W. Dence (Eds.), pp. 33–61. Berlin: Springer-Verlag.

Eastwood, M. A. (1986). What does measurement of dietary fiber mean? Lancet 1(8496):1487–1488.

Edwards, C. S. (1973). Determination of lignin and cellulose in forages by extraction with triethylene glycol. J. Sci. Food Agric. 24:381–388.

Ellis, G. H., Matrone, G., and Maynard, L. A. (1946). A seventy-two percent sulfuric acid method for the determination of lignin and its use in animal nutrition studies. J. Anim. Sci. 5:285–297.

Englyst, H. N., and Cummings, J. H. (1988). Improved method for measurement of dietary fiber as non-starch polysaccharides in plant foods. J. Assoc. Off. Anal. Chem. 71:808–816.

Englyst, H. N., Quigley, M. E., and Hudson, G. J. (1994). Determination of dietary fiber as non-starch polysaccharides with gas-liquid chromatographic, high-performance liquid chromatographic or spectrophotometric measurement of constituent sugars. Analyst 119:1497–1509.

Englyst, H. N., Quigley, M. E., Englyst K. N., Bravo, L., and Hudson, G. J. (1995). 'Dietary fiber' measurement by the Englyst NSP procedure. Measurement by the AOAC procedure. Explanation of differences. Report of a Study Commissioned by MAFF, Medical Research Council & University of Cambridge, UK.

Ferguson, L. R., and Harris, P. J. (1996). Studies on the role of specific dietary fibers in protection against colorectal cancer. Mutat. Res. 350:173–184.

Flint, S. I., and Camire, M. E. (1992). Recovery of lignin during nonstarch polysaccharide analysis. Cereal Chem. 69:444–447.

Fly, A. D., Fahey, G. C., and Czarnecki-Maulden, G. L. (1998). Iron bioavailability from diets containing isolated or intact sources of lignin. Biol. Trace Element Res. 62:83–100.

Foy, W. L., Evans, J. L., and Wohlt, J. E. (1981). Detergent fiber analyses on thirty foodstuffs ingested by man. Nutr. Rep. Int. 24:575–580.

Freudenberg, K. (1964). A schematic constitutional formulation for spruce lignin. Holzforschung 18:3–9.

Freudenberg, K. (1968). The constitution and biosynthesis of lignin. In: Constitution and Biosynthesis of Lignin, K. Freudenberg, and A. C. Neish (Eds.), pp. 46–122. Berlin: Springer.

Fukushima, R. S., Behority, B. A., and Loerch, S. C. (1991). Modification of a colorimetric analysis for lignin and its use in studying the inhibitory effects of lignin on forage digestion by ruminal microorganisms. J. Anim. Sci. 69:295–304.

Garleb, K. A., Bourquin, L. D., Hsu, J. T., Wagner, G. W., Schmidt, S. J., and Fahey, G. C., Jr. (1991). Isolation and chemical analyses of nonfermented fiber fractions of oat hulls and cottonseed hulls. J. Anim. Sci. 69:1255–1271.

Geissman, T., and Neukom, H. (1973). Ferulic acid as a constituent of the water-soluble pentosans of wheat flour. Cereal Chem. 50:414–416.

Gellerstedt, G. (1992). Chemical degradation methods: permanganate oxidation. In: Methods in Lignin Chemistry, S. Y. Lin and C. W. Dence (Eds.), pp. 323–333. Berlin: Springer-Verlag.

Giger, S. (1985). Revue des méthodes de dosage de la lignine utilisées en alimentation animale. Ann. Zootech. 34:85–122.

Glasser, W. G. (1980). Lignification: formation of lignin in wood. In: Pulp and Paper, J. P. Casey (Ed.), 3rd ed. Vol. 1., pp. 44–51. New York: John Wiley and Sons.

Goering, H. K., and van Soest, P. J. (1970). Forage fiber analyses. USDA Agric. Handbook 379. Washington, DC: U.S. Gov. Print. Office.

Hatfield, R. D., Jung, H.-G., Ralph, J., Buxton, D. R., and Weimer, P. J. (1994). A comparison of the insoluble residues produced by the Klason lignin and acid detergent lignin procedures. J. Sci. Food Agric. 65:51–58.

Herranz, J., Vidal-Valverde, C., and Rojas-Hidalgo, E. (1981). Cellulose, hemicellulose and lignin content of raw and cooked Spanish vegetables. J. Food Sci. 46:1927–1933.

Herranz, J., Vidal-Valverde, C., and Rojas-Hidalgo, E. (1983). Cellulose, hemicellulose and lignin content of raw and cooked processed vegetables. J. Food Sci. 48:274–275.

Higuchi, T. (1985). Biosynthesis of Lignin in Biosynthesis and Biodegradation of Wood Components, pp. 141–162. London: Academic Press.

Higuchi, T., Ito, Y., Shimada, M., and Kawamura, I. (1967). Chemical properties of milled wood lignin. Phytochemistry 6:1551–1556.

Iiyama, K., and Wallis, A. F. A. (1988). An improved acetyl bromide procedure for determining lignin in woods and wood pulps. Wood Sci. Technol. 22:271–288.

Iiyama, K., Lam, T. B. T., and Stone, B. A. (1990). Phenolic acid bridges between polysaccharides and lignin in wheat internodes. Phytochemistry 29:733–737.

Johanning, G. L., and O'Dell, B. L. (1981). Inhibition of a cecal anaerobe by a dietary fiber component (abstr). Fed. Proc. 40:854.

Jung, H.-J. G. (1997). Analysis of forage fiber and cell walls in ruminant nutrition. J. Nutr. 127:810S–813S.

Jung, H. G., and Allen, M. S. (1995). Characteristics of plant cell walls affecting intake and digestibility of forages by ruminants. J. Animal Sci. 57:1626–1636.

Jung, H. G., and Deetz, D. A. (1993). Cell wall lignification and degradability. In: Forage Cell Wall Structure and Digestibility, H. G. Jung, D. R. Buxton, R. D. Hatfield, and J. Ralph (Eds.), pp. 315–346. Madison, WI: ASA-CSSA-SSSA.

Jung, H. G., and Fahey, G. C. (1981). Effect of phenolic compound removal on in vitro forage digestibility. J. Agr. Food Chem. 29:817–824.

Jung, H. G., and Fahey, G. C. (1983). Nutritional implications of phenolic monomers and lignin: a review. J. Anim. Sci. 57:206–219.

Keim, K., and Kies, C. (1979). Effects of dietary fiber on nutritional status of weanling mice. Cereal Chem. 56:73–78.

Kurasawa, S.-I., Sugahara, T., and Hayashi, J. (1982). Studies on dietary fiber of mushrooms and edible wild plants. Nutr. Rep. Int. 26:167–173.

Lee, S. C., Prosky, L., and DeVries, J. W. (1992). Determination of total, soluble and insoluble dietary fiber in foods: collaborative study. J. Assoc. Off. Anal. Chem. 75:395–416.

Lai, Y. Z., and Sarkanen, K. V. (1971). Isolation and structural studies. In: Lignins. Occurrence, Formation, Structure and Reactions, K. V. Sarkanen and C. H. Ludwig (Eds.), pp. 165–240. New York: Wiley-Interscience, John Wiley & Sons.

Lapierre, C. (1993). Application of new methods for the investigation of lignin structure. In: Forage Cell Wall Structure and Digestibility, H. G. Jung, D. R. Buxton, R. D. Hatfield, and J. Ralph (Eds.), pp. 133–166. Madison, WI: ASA-CSSA-SSSA.

Lowry, J. B., Conlan, L. L., Schlink, A. C., and McSweeney, C. S. (1994) Acid detergent dispersible lignin in tropical grasses. J. Sci. Food Agric. 65:41–50.

Lund, E. D., and Smoot, J. M. (1982). Dietary fiber content of some tropical fruits and vegetables. J. Agric. Food Chem. 30:1123–1127.

Kimmins, W. C., and Wuddah, D. (1977). Hypersensitive resistance determination of lignin in leaves with a localized virus infection. Phytopathology 67:1012–1016.

MacLean, D. (principal investigator) (1993). Nova Scotia Heart Health Program, Health and Welfare Canada, Nova Scotia Department of Health. The Report of the Nova Scotia Nutrition Survey. Halifax, Nova Scotia, 1993.

Matthee´, V., and Appledorf, H. (1978). Effect of cooking on vegetable fiber. J. Food Sci. 43:1344–1345.

Marlett, J. A. (1992). Content and composition of dietary fiber in 117 frequently consumed foods. J. Am. Diet. Ass. 92:175–186.

Marlett, J. A., and Johnson, E. J. (1985). Composition of fecal fiber from human subjects. J. Nutr. 115:650–660.

Merewether, J. W. T. (1951). The existence of a lignin-carbohydrate bond and the isolation of lignin. APPITA 5:226–266.

Mongeau, R., and Brassard, R. (1979). Determination of neutral detergent fiber, hemicellulose, cellulose, and lignin in breads. Cereal Chem. 56:437–441.

Mongeau, R., and Brassard, R. (1980). Rapid digestion of starch and artifact fiber in the measurement of neutral detergent fiber of cereal products. Getreide Mehl Brot 34:125–127.

Mongeau, R., and Brassard, R. (1982). Determination of neutral detergent fiber in breakfast cereals: pentose, hemicellulose, cellulose and lignin content. J. Food Sci. 47:550–555.

Mongeau, R., and Brassard, R. (1986). A rapid method for the determination of soluble and insoluble dietary fiber: Comparison with AOAC total dietary fiber procedure and Englyst's method. J. Food Sci. 51:1333–1336.

Mongeau, R. and Brassard, R. (1989). A comparison of three methods for analyzing dietary fiber in 38 foods. J. Food Compos. Anal. 2:189–199.

Mongeau, R., and Brassard, R. (1993). Enzymatic-gravimetric determination in foods of dietary fiber as sum of insoluble and soluble fiber fractions: summary of collaborative study. J. Assoc. Off. Anal. Chem. 76:923–925.

Mongeau, R., Yiu, S. H., and Brassard, R. (1991). Chemical and fluorescence microscopic analysis of fiber degradation of oat, hard red spring wheat, and corn bran in rats. J. Agr. Food Chem. 39:1966–1971.

Mongeau, R., Scott, F. R., and Brassard, R. (1999). Definition and analysis of dietary fiber. In: Definition and Analysis of Complex Carbohydrates/Dietary Fiber. S. Cho (Ed.). AOAC (in press).

Monties, B. (1984). Lignin biodegradation: experimental evidence, molecular, biochemical and physiological mechanisms. Agronomie 4:387–392.

Monties, B. (1989). Lignins. In: Methods in Plant Biochemistry, Vol. 1, Plant Phenolics, P. M. Dey and J. B. Harborne (Eds.), pp. 113–157. New York: Academic Press.

Monties, B. (1991). Recent advances in structural and biosynthetic variability of lignins. In: Proc. 6th International Symposium on Wood Pulping Chemistry, A. Wallis (Ed.), Vol. 1, pp. 113–123. Carlton, Vic., Australia: APPITA Publishing.

Monties, B. (1994). Chemical assessment of lignin biodegradation some qualitative and quantitative aspects. FEMS Microb. Rev. 13:277–284.

Moore, K. J., and Hatfield, R. D. (1994). Carbohydrates and forage quality. In: Forage Quality, Evolution, and Utilization, G. C. Fahey Jr., M. C. Collins, D. R. Mertens, and L. E. Moser (Eds.), pp. 229–280. Madison, WI: ASA-CSSA-SSSA.

Morrison, I. M. (1972a). A semi-micro method for the determination of lignin and its use in predicting the digestibility of forage crops. J. Sci. Food. Agric. 23:455–463.

Morrison, I. M. (1972b). Improvements in the acetyl bromide technique to determine lignin and digestibility and its application to legumes. J. Sci. Food. Agric. 23:1463–1469.

Müsel, G., Schindler, T., Bergfeld, R., Ruel, K., Jacquet, G., Lapierre, C., Speth, V., and Schopfer, P. (1997). Structure and distribution of lignin in primary and secondary cell walls of maize coleoptiles analyzed by chemical and immunological probes. Planta 210:146–159.

Newmark, H. L. (1986). Plant phenolics as inhibitors of mutational and precarcinogenic events. Can. J. Physiol. Pharmacol. 65:461–466.

Nimz, H. H. (1974). Beech lignin—proposal of a constitutional scheme. Angew. Chem. Int. Ed. 13:313–321.

Nordkvist, E., Graham, P., Aoman, P. (1989). Soluble lignin complexes isolated from wheat straw (*Triticum arvense*) and red clover (*Trifolium pratense*) stems by an in-vitro method. J. Sci. Food Agric. 48:311–321.

Obst, J. R., and Kirk, T. K. (1988). Isolation of lignin. In: Methods in Enzymology. Part B. Lignin, Pectin, and Chitin, W. A. Wood and S. T. Kellogg (Eds.), Vol. 161, pp. 3–12. New York: Academic Press.

Prosky, L., Asp, N.-G., Schweizer, T. F., DeVries, J. W., and Furda, I. (1988). Determination of insoluble, soluble, and total dietary fiber in foods and food products: interlaboratory study. J. Assoc. Off. Anal. Chem. 71:1017–1023.

Ralph, J., Hatfield, R. D., Quideau, S., Helm, R. F., Grabber, J. H., and Jung. H.-J. G. (1994). Pathway of ρ-coumaric acid incorporation into maize lignin as revealed by NMR. J. Am. Chem. Soc. 116:9448–9456.

Ralph, J., Grabber, J. H., and Hatfield, R. D. (1995). Lignin-ferulate cross-links in grasses: active incorporation of ferulate polysaccharide esters into ryegrass lignins. Carbohydr. Res. 275:167–178.

Reeves, J. B., and Galletti, G. C. (1991). Observations on lignin assays: what do they really determine? In: Production and Utilization of Lignocellulosics, G. C. Galletti (Ed.), pp. 183–198. London: Elsevier Applied Science Publishing.

Ring, S. G., and Selvendran, R. R. (1980). Isolation and analysis of cell wall material from beeswing wheat bran (*Triticum aestivum*). Phytochemistry 19:1723–1730.

Robertson, J. B. (1978). The detergent system of fiber analysis. In: Topics in Dietary Fiber Research, G. A. Spiller and D. A. T. Southgate (Eds.), pp. 1–34. New York: Plenum Press.

Rowland, A. P., and Roberts, J. D. (1994). Lignin and cellulose fractionation in decomposition studies using acid-detergent fiber methods. Comm. Soil Sci. Plant Anal. 25:269–277.

Sakagami, H., and Satoh, K. (1996). Stimulation of two step degradation of sodium ascorbate by lignins. Anticancer Res. 16:2849–2852.

Santé Québec, Bertrand, L. (sous la direction de) (1995). Les Québécoises et les Québécois mangent-ils mieux? Rapport de l'Enquête québécoise sur la nutrition, 1990. Montréal: Ministère de la Santé et des Services sociaux, gouvernement du Québec.

Sarkanen, K. V. (1971). Precursors and their polymerization. In: Lignins: Occurrence, Formation, Structure and Reactions, K. V. Sarkanen and C. H. Ludwig (Eds.), pp. 95–164. New York: Wiley Interscience.

Sarkanen, K. V., and Ludwig, C. H. (1971). Definition and nomenclature. In: Lignins: Occurrence, Formation, Structure and Reactions, K. V. Sarkanen and C. H. Ludwig (Eds.), pp. 1–18. New York: Wiley Interscience.

Sarkanen, K. B., Hirkin, G., and Hrutfiord, B. F. (1963). Base-catalyzed hydrolysis of aromatic ether linkages in lignin. 1. The rate of hydrolysis of methoxyl groups by sodium hydroxide. Tappi 46:375–379.

Schwarz, P. B., Youngs, V. L., and Shelton, D. R. (1989). Isolation and characterization of lignin from hard red spring wheat bran. Cereal Chem. 66:289–295.

Shahidi, F., and Naczk, M. (1995). Food phenolics: sources, chemistry, effects, and applications. Lancaster: Technomic Publishing Co. Inc.

Shah, N., Attallah, M. T., Mahoney, R. R., and Pellett, P. J. (1982). Effect of dietary fiber components on fecal nitrogen excretion and protein utilization in growing rats. J. Nutr. 112:658–666.

Sharma, U., Brillouet, J.-M., Scalbert, A., and Monties, B. (1986). Studies on a brittle stem mutant of rice, Oryza sativa L.; characterization of lignin fractions, associated phenolic acids and polysaccharides from rice stem. Agronomie 6:265–271.

Sjöström, E. (1993). Wood Chemistry. Fundamentals and Applications, 2nd ed., pp. 71–89. New York: Academic Press.

Slavin, J. L. (1987). Dietary fiber: classification, chemical analyses, and food sources. J. Am. Diet. Assoc. 87:1164–1171.

Southgate, D. A. T. (1969). Determination of carbohydrates in foods. II. Unavailable carbohydrate. J. Sci. Food Agric. 20:331–338.

Southgate, D. A. T. (1986). Dietary fiber content of selected foods by the Southgate methods (grams per 100 g edible part). In: CRC Handbook of Dietary Fiber in Human Nutrition, G. A. Spiller (Ed.), pp. 447–449. Boca Raton, FL: CRC Press, Inc.

Southgate, D. A. T. (1993). Food components associated with dietary fiber. In: CRC Handbook of Dietary Fiber in Human Nutrition, G. A. Spiller (Ed.), 2nd ed., pp. 23–25. Boca Raton, FL: CRC Press, Inc.

Tanahashi, M., and Higuchi, T. (1988). Chemical degradation methods for characterization of lignins. In: Methods in Enzymology, Part B. Lignin, Pectin, and Chitin, W. A. Wood and S. T. Kellogg (Eds.), Vol. 161, pp. 101–109. New York: Academic Press.

Tanahashi, M., Takeuchi, H., and Higuchi, T. (1976). Dehydrogenative polymerization of 3,5-disubstituted p-coumaryl. Wood Res. 61:44–53.

Terashima, N., Fukushima, K., He, L. F., and Takabe, K. (1993). Comprehensive model of the lignified plant cell wall. In: Forage Cell Wall Structure and Digestibility, H. G. Jung, D. R. Buxton, R. D. Hatfield, and J. Ralph (Eds.), pp. 247–270. Madison, WI: ASA-CSSA-SSSA.

Terrón, M. C., Fidalgo, M. L., Almendros, G., and González, A. E. (1996). Molecular characterization of alkalilignin-1M30C: a valid alternative preparation to the Björkman lignin in the analytical study of wheat straw lignin. Rapid Comm. Mass Spec. 10:413–418.

Theander, O., and James, P. (1979). European efforts in dietary fiber characterization. In: Dietary Fibers: Chemistry and Nutrition, G. E. Inglett, and I. Falkehag (Eds.), pp. 245–249. New York: Academic Press.

Theander, O., and Westerlund, E. (1993). Determination of individual components of dietary fiber. In: CRC Handbook of Dietary Fiber in Human Nutrition, G. A. Spiller (Ed.), pp. 77–98. Boca Raton, FL: CRC Press.

Theander, O., Åman, P., Westerlund, E., Andersson, R., and Pettersson, D. (1995). Total dietary fiber determined as neutral sugar residues, uronic acid residues, and Klason lignin (the Uppsala method): collaborative study. J. Assoc. Off. Anal. Chem. 78:1030–1044.

Trowell, H. (1974). Definitions of fiber. Lancet 1:503.

Trowell, H., Southgate, D. A. T., Wolever, T. M. S., Leeds, A. R., Gassull, M. A., and Jenkins, D. J. A. (1976). Dietary fiber redefined. Lancet 1:967.

Valencia, Z., and Chavez, E. R. (1997). Lignin as a purified dietary fiber supplement for piglets. Nutr. Res. 17:1517–1527.

van Soest, P. J. (1963). Use of detergents in analysis of fibrous feeds. II. Study of effects of heating and drying on yield of fiber and lignin in forages. J. Assoc. Off. Anal. Chem. 48:785–790.

van Soest, P. J. (1969). Chemical properties of fiber in concentrate feedstuffs. Proc. Cornell Nutr. Conf., pp. 17–21.

van Soest, P. J. (1978a). Dietary fibers: their definition and nutritional properties. Am. J. Clin. Nutr. 31(10 suppl):S12–S20.

van Soest, P. J. (1978b). Fiber analysis tables, Table 7. Am. J. Clin. Nutr. 31(suppl):S284.

van Soest, P. J., and Robertson, J. B. (1980). Systems of analysis for evaluating fibrous feeds. In: Standardization of Analytical Methodology for Feeds, W. J. Pigden, C. C. Blach, and M. Graham (Eds.), pp. 49–60. Ottawa: International Development Research Centre (Publ IDRC-134e).

van Soest, P. J., and Wine, R. H. (1967). Use of detergents in the analysis of fibrous feeds. IV. Determination of plant cell-wall constituents. JAOAC 50:50–55.

Venverloo, C. J. (1969). Lignin of *Populus nigra* L. cv. *italica* a comparative study of lignified structures in tissue culture and tissues of tree. Acta Bot. Neerl. 18:241–314.

Vidal-Valverde, C., Herranz, J., Blanco, I., and Rojas-Hidalgo, E. (1982). Dietary fiber in Spanish foods. J. Food Sci. 47:1840–1845.

Vollendorf, N. W., and Marlett, J. A. (1994). Dietary content and composition in home-prepared and commercially baked products: analysis and prediction. Cereal Chem. 71:99–105.

Wallace, G., Russell, W. R., Lomax, J. A., Jarvis, M. C., Lapierre, C., and Chesson, A. (1995). Extraction of phenolic-carbohydrate complexes from graminaceous cell walls. Carbohydr. Res. 272:41–53.

Whitmore, F. W. (1978). Lignin-carbohydrate complex formed in isolated cell walls of callus. Phytochemistry 17:421–425.

Yamamoto, E., Bokelman, G. H., and Lewis, N. (1989). Phenylpropanoid metabolism in cell-walls. In: Plant Cell Wall Polymers: Biogenesis and Biodegradation. ACS Symposium Series, Vol. 399, pp. 68–88. New York: Am. Chem. Soc.

Yamazaki, T., Hata, K., and Higuchi, T. (1978). Isolation and characterization of syringyl component rich lignin. Holzforschung 32:44–45.

21

High-Performance Liquid Chromatography Techniques Used in Dietary Fiber and Complex Carbohydrates Analysis

Alan Henshall
Dionex Corporation, Sunnyvale, California

I. INTRODUCTION

This chapter covers the application of high-performance liquid chromatography (HPLC) to analysis and research on dietary fiber and related complex carbohydrates. It includes applications to both dietary fiber as originally defined by Trowell in 1974 (1), i.e., "that part of plant material in our diet which is resistant to digestion by secretions of the human digestive tract," and to complex carbohydrate food components, such as gums and pectins used as functional food additives, that are included in Trowell's later extended definition (2), i.e., "all the polysaccharides and lignin that are undigested by endogenous secretions of the human digestive tract."

The application of chromatographic techniques to the analysis and characterization of dietary fiber dates back to 1979 when Theander and Åman first published what is now referred to as the Uppsala method (3). In this method, the nonlignin portion of dietary fiber is quantified by gas-liquid chromatography (GLC) of the alditol acetate derivatives of neutral sugars resulting from hydrolysis of nonstarch polysaccharides (NSP).

Subsequent to the publication on the Uppsala method, conventional HPLC techniques for sugar determination using separations on either amino-bonded silica or metal-loaded cation exchange columns coupled with refractive index detection (RI) were applied to dietary fiber determinations (4–6). Although useful for some purposes, these techniques have proved inadequate for separating the mixtures of all the carbohydrates present in NSP hydrolysates (7). They are also limited by the nonspecific nature and relatively low sensitivity of RI compared with the flame ionization detector (FID) used in GLC (8). Consequently, GLC has most often been the chromatographic technique of choice for determination of neutral sugars from NSP since it provides the required resolution and detection sensitivity (9). More recently, an improved HPLC technique has emerged based on high performance anion exchange chromatography coupled with pulsed amperometric detection (HPAEC-PAD) (7,10). This technique offers an attractive alternative to GLC (7,10), since it provides high-resolution separation capability coupled with sensitive and specific detection of NSP-derived neutral sugars and uronic acid residues without requiring derivatization. In addition, the compatibility of HPAEC-PAD with gradient elution is proving to be a valuable tool in fundamental research on dietary fiber characterization for the separation of complex mixtures of oligo- and polysaccharides derived from plant cell-wall carbohydrates (11).

This chapter describes various direct HPLC techniques that can be applied to dietary fiber analysis and reviews their application in the following areas: (a) determination of neutral sugars from enzymatic or chemical hydrolysis of dietary fiber and complex carbohydrates and from in vitro fermentation studies, (b) research on dietary fiber composition, and (c) identification and quantification of complex carbohydrate food ingredients. HPLC techniques involving derivatization of carbohydrates prior to separation are not included since they introduce additional complexity and offer no advantage over direct methods or established GLC derivatization methods for dietary fiber analysis.

II. HPLC INSTRUMENTATION

A detailed review of basic HPLC principles and the design and theory of operation of HPLC instrumentation is beyond the scope of this review. The reader is referred to several excellent texts for this information (12–15). This section will be limited to a brief overview of the types of HPLC components that are applicable to the determination and characterization of the carbohydrate components of dietary fiber.

A schematic of the main components of an HPLC system are shown in Fig. 1. Most commonly, the eluent flowpath is stainless steel; however a metal-free flowpath is highly desirable for ion exchange separations because of the corrosive nature of the eluents. A trap column is optional, depending on the application and eluent, but the use of a guard column is advisable to prevent deterioration of performance of the analytical column due to irreversible adsorption of sample matrix components. The guard column is usually packed with the same stationary phase as the analytical column.

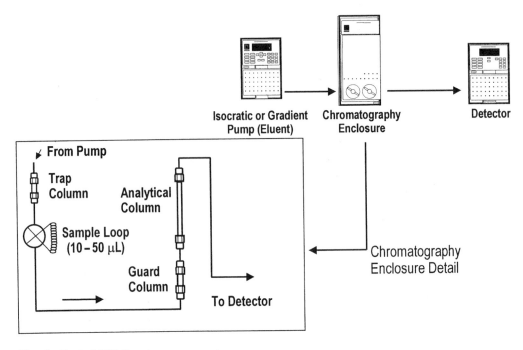

Fig. 1 Typical HPLC system components.

A. Eluent Delivery

HPLC pumping systems are designed to operate at pressures up to 5000 psi (35 MPa) or higher and deliver a constant flow of eluent with minimal pulsation. This is important because most HPLC detectors are sensitive to flow fluctuations. Flow pulsation causes baseline ripple or other disturbances, which limit the usable sensitivity. Good long-term flow accuracy and precision are also essential, since flow variations will affect both peak areas and retention times. Most advanced HPLC pumps are reciprocating-piston pumps with built-in microprocessor-based electronic feedback systems, which control the piston motion to produce virtually constant, pulseless flow. Simpler designs such as single piston pumps without built-in pulsation control require a pulse damper device to be connected between the pump outlet and the injector. Eluent degassing, either by helium sparging or by vacuum degassing (either in-line or off-line), is necessary to prevent bubble formation from dissolved air in the eluent. Bubbles in the eluent will interfere with detection since they will degas in the detector cell and can also become trapped in check valve seats causing flowrate fluctuations. Pumps are available in isocratic (single eluent composition) and gradient versions. Gradient elution provides added capability since it allows the eluent strength to be continuously varied so that analytes with widely differing retention characteristics can be determined in the same run (e.g., mono- and disaccharides along with oligo- and polysaccharides). Gradient pumping systems also greatly facilitate isocratic methods development since they provide on-line mixing of the isocratic eluent components in any proportion. When under the control of a chromatography workstation, optimization of the isocratic conditions can be automated.

B. Injection

All sample and calibration standard solutions should be prefiltered through a 0.2 μm filter. Injection can be performed manually with a syringe or automatically via an electronically or pneumatically activated 6-port valve, as illustrated in Fig. 2, or by variable volume injection systems. Full loop injection generally provides the best precision. The precision of partial loop injection (use <70% of total loop volume) is usually lower than full-loop injection but is more than adequate for most purposes. Partial loop injection is particularly advantageous when sample quantities are limited since no sample is wasted. Automated injection systems are an integral

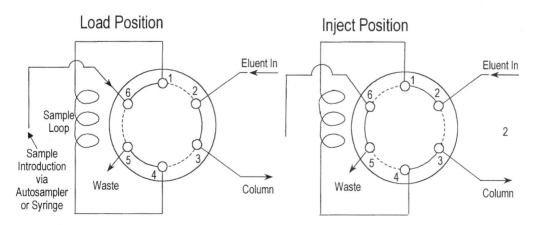

Fig. 2 HPLC sample loading and injection.

part of commercial autosamplers, allowing multiple samples to be analyzed sequentially without requiring operator involvement.

C. Columns

The column is the most critical component of an HPLC system since it effects the separation of the analytes allowing them to be individually detected and quantitated. To achieve high efficiency, commercial columns are packed with small particle size (typically 3–10 μm diameter) stationary phases. All else being equal, the smaller the particle size, the higher the efficiency (and column back pressure at a given flowrate). An important practical consideration when using high-efficiency columns is to minimize extra-column dead volume in the HPLC flowpath since this will cause a loss in efficiency resulting in wider, tailing peaks. Connections between the injector and the column and the exit from the column and the detector should be made with the shortest length possible of small internal diameter tubing. High efficiency results in sharp narrow peaks, but column selectivity is the most important parameter affecting resolution of the analytes. A short guard column is usually installed ahead of the analytical column as shown in Fig. 1 to prevent loss of performance due to irreversible adsorption of sample matrix components. In some cases, a trap column (Fig. 1) may also be necessary to remove trace impurities in the eluent. This is positioned before the injector. Since dietary fiber is largely composed of carbohydrates, the main applications for HPLC in dietary fiber analysis and research involve carbohydrate separations.

There is a wide variety of commercially available HPLC column types with various selectivities and new types under investigation, but only a limited number have so far been used routinely for carbohydrate separations. These are

> Amino-bonded silica columns
> Metal-loaded sulfonated polystyrene divinylbenzene (PSDVB)–based cation exchange
> > resins
> Pellicular anion exchange resins.
> Silica and polymer-based size exclusion columns

The characteristics and applicability of these column types to dietary fiber analysis and research will be discussed in more detail in Sec.III.

D. Detection

HPLC detectors are flow-through devices designed to continuously monitor the eluent exiting from the analytical column and generate an output signal proportional to the concentration or mass of each of the analytes as they pass through the detector cell. Detector cell volumes are usually 5–10 μL or less to minimize peak dispersion. There are many different types of HPLC detectors, but only the refractive index and pulsed electrochemical detectors are routinely used for detection of carbohydrates. Detection of carbohydrates is possible at 190 nm using a variable wavelength UV detector, but this approach has not been widely used because of interference from other types of organic compounds present in the sample or eluent. Carbohydrates only absorb at wavelengths below 200 nm, whereas most other classes of organic compounds exhibit significant end UV absorption in this region. Consequently, the likelihood of interference from sample matrix components is greatly increased, necessitating more extensive sample clean-up. Mass spectrometric detection has been used in research on the characterization of cell-wall carbohydrates. The detection principles and utility of refractive index, pulsed amperometric detection, and mass spectrometry and other detection methods for carbohydrates are discussed in Sec. IV.

III. HPLC COLUMNS FOR CARBOHYDRATE SEPARATIONS

A. Amino-Bonded Silica Columns

The stationary phase in this type of column consists of silica particles with chemically bonded aminopropyl groups, i.e., $Si-O-Si-(CH_2)_3-NH_2$. Depending on the manufacturer, particles range in size from 3 to 10 μM and may be irregular or spherical. Aminopropyl silica columns using an aqueous acetonitrile (65–85% acetonitrile) eluent have been widely used for separation of carbohydrates since becoming commercially available in 1975. The separation mechanism is not fully understood but is classified as hydrophilic interaction (normal phase with an aqueous eluent) since the retention characteristics conform with this definition, i.e., decreasing retention time with increasing eluent polarity (decreasing acetonitrile). The acetonitrile concentration is critical for carbohydrate separations. A concentration in the range of 80–85% (v/v) is required for separation of mono- and disaccharides and 65–75% is required for oligosaccharides to DP 5 (16). In spite of their widespread use, amino-bonded phases have an inherent shortcoming when used for carbohydrate separations in that the amino groups on the stationary phase react with reducing sugars, resulting in loss of analyte and column performance over time (12,16–20). Glucose and galactose are not well resolved on these columns, and chloride interferes with glucose if present in the sample extract (17–19). Other problem separations include glucose/mannitol, glucose/sorbitol, and fructose/xylitol (20). The low solubility of some di- and oligosaccharides in the high concentration of acetonitrile required in the eluent is a limitation for some applications, and environmental and cost considerations associated with the use of large quantities of acetonitrile are also a concern.

B. Metal-Loaded Cation Exchange Resin Columns

These columns are packed with sulfonated PSDVB (4–8% crosslinked) spherical resin particles, which are loaded with a cationic counterion, e.g., Ca^{2+}, Ag^{2+}, Pb^{2+}, or H^+. Particle diameters are in the 7–20 μM range. The predominant separation mode is ligand exchange in which the OH groups on the carbohydrate molecule interact with the metal counterion on the resin by displacing water molecules in the hydration sphere of the metal ion. Column selectivity is determined by the extent of the ligand-metal ion interaction, which in turn depends on the type of counterion and the conformation of the hydroxyl groups in the carbohydrate (Fig. 3). The mobile phase used is usually water at 80–90°C. Elevated temperature is necessary in order to provide

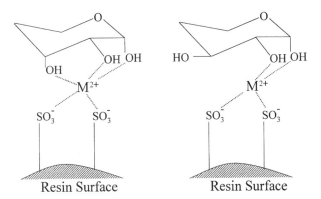

Fig. 3 Retention mechanism in ligand exchange chromatography of carbohydrates. Retention is governed by the ligand-metal ion interaction, which in turn depends on the type of counterion and the conformation of the hydroxyl groups in the carbohydrate.

acceptable resolution and efficiency and to reduce peak tailing and splitting due to the anomeric forms of the carbohydrates (19–21). This type of column has been widely used for simple determinations of the major mono- and disaccharides present in foods and beverages, but coelution of sugars, sugar alcohols, and organic acids can be problematic (17–20). It is possible to resolve some but not all neutral sugars present in dietary fiber hydrolysates, e.g., galactose and rhamnose coelute (20). Individual uronic acids can be chromatographed on these columns at lower temperatures (35°C) than are normally used for cation exchange resin to minimize lactone formation, but only partial resolution of glucuronic, galacturonic and mannuronic is possible (22).

C. Pellicular Anion Exchange Resin Columns

High-performance anion exchange chromatography (also referred to as high pH anion exchange chromatography), is a relatively new separation technique for carbohydrates. Carbohydrates are often thought of as neutral compounds, but in actuality they are weak acids with pK_as in the range of 12–14 (Table 1). At a pH of 12–14, oxyanion formation occurs (Fig. 4), allowing separation by ion exchange. Ion exchange separations are based on the relative affinity of the analyte ion in competition with the eluent ion for the same exchange sites (Fig. 5). The greater the affinity of the ion, the longer the retention time. For carbohydrates, subtle structural differences and small differences in pK_a can cause significant differences in retention characteristics. Pellicular anion exchange columns are commercially available that are specifically designed for carbohydrate separations at high pH. The basic structure of these column packings is shown in Fig. 6. The core of each particle is a sulfonated, highly crosslinked, and impermeable polystyrene divinylbenzene resin bead with a diameter of ~10 μm. This core is covered with a pellicular layer of quaternary amine functionalized porous latex beads with a diameter of ~0.1 μm. Only the pellicular layer is involved in the chromatographic process. This structure allows ion exchange chromatography to be carried out on a stationary phase with extremely small particle diameter (0.1 μm) yet still retaining the flow and backpressure characteristics of a conventional column packing with 10-μm-diameter particles. The extremely small diameter of the pellicular beads results in excellent mass transfer characteristics and highly efficient separations. Sodium or potassium hydroxide solutions with concentrations in the range of 18–100 mM are typically used for separation of mixtures of mono- and disaccharides (Fig. 7), but for separation of all the monosaccharides that are important in dietary fiber analysis, an isocratic water eluent combined with a "reverse" gradient is necessary. This requires a step gradient at the end of each

Table 1 Dissociation Constants of Some Common Carbohydrates (in water at 25°C)

Sugar	pK_a
Fructose	12.03
Mannose	12.08
Xylose	12.15
Glucose	12.28
Galactose	12.39
Dulcitol	13.48
Sorbitol	13.60

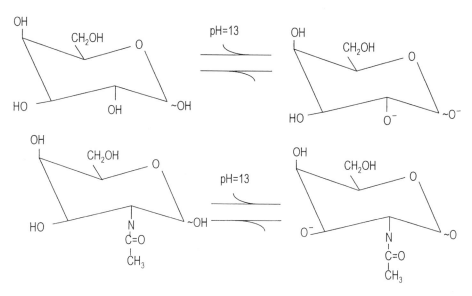

Fig. 4 Carbohydrate oxyanion formation at high pH.

run with 300 mM hydroxide to elute more strongly retained sample matrix components and regenerate the column. Postcolumn addition of 300 mM [OH] is also necessary for detection when using water or hydroxide eluent concentration of less than 18 mM. A typical chromatogram is shown in Fig. 8. To separate uronic acids requires increased eluent strength because they are more strongly retained by the anion exchange stationary phase. Usually a higher [OH] is used in conjunction with a high [acetate] is employed since acetate is a stronger eluting ion than hydroxide. To separate oligo- and polysaccharide mixtures requires gradient elution with hydroxide/acetate eluents. Typically, a sodium hydroxide gradient is used in the first part of the run to elute mono-, di-, and trisaccharides followed by a sodium hydroxide/acetate mixture in which the acetate concentration is gradually increased to elute the more strongly retained

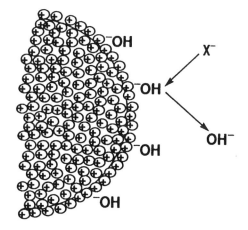

Fig. 5 Ion exchange separations are based on the relative affinity of the analyte ion in competition with the eluent ion for the same exchange sites.

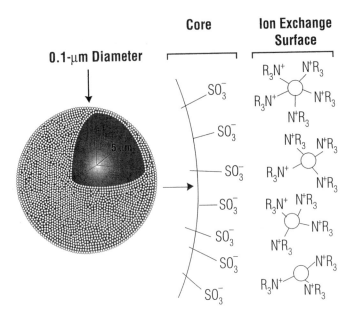

Fig. 6 Structure of pellicular anion exchange column packings used in HPAEC.

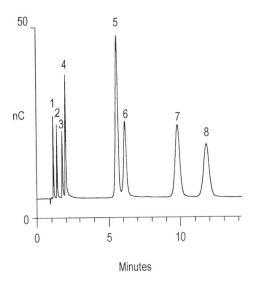

Fig. 7 Isocratic separation of common sugars and sugar alcohols by HPAE-PAD. Column: CarboPac PA10 (10 μM, 250 × 4 mm i.d.) with guard and borate trap. Eluent: 52 mM NaOH. Flowrate: 1.5 mL/min. Detection: pulsed amperometry, Au electrode. Peaks: 1 = glycerol, 2 = xylitol, 3 = sorbitol, 4 = mannitol, 5 = glucose, 6 = fructose, 7 = sucrose, 8 = lactose.

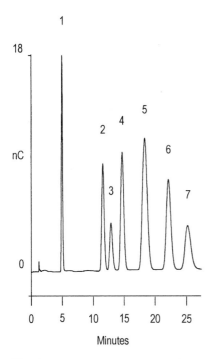

Fig. 8 Isocratic HPAEC separation of monosaccharides important in dietary fiber analysis. Peaks: 1 = glycerol, 2 = xylitol, 3 = sorbitol, 4 = mannitol, 5 = glucose, 6 = fructose, 7 = sucrose.

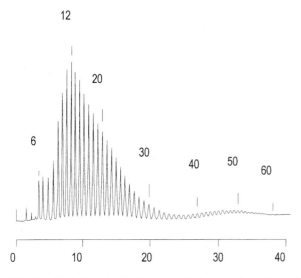

Fig. 9 Chain length distribution of debranched amylopectin from edible canna determined by HPAE-PAD. Column: CarboPac PA1 (10 μM, 250 × 4 mm i.d.) with guard. Eluent A: 150 mM NaOH; Eluent B: 150 mM NaOH/500 mM sodium acetate. Gradient program: 40% B at 0 min, 50% at 2 min, 60% at 10 min, 80% at 40 min. Temp: ambient. Flowrate: 1.0 mL/min. Detector: pulsed amperometric, Au electrode, range 10 μA. (Adapted from Ref. 23.)

oligo- and polysaccharides. In this way resolution of individual polysaccharide chains to DPs in the 60–80 range is possible (11,23) (see Fig. 9).

D. Size Exclusion Chromatography

In size exclusion chromatography (SEC), the sample components elute in order of decreasing molecular size. Stationary phases are ideally noninteractive and have a porous structure. The dimensions of the pores determine the degree to which a particular polymer molecule is retained or excluded. Thus, fractionation occurs based on molecular size. High-efficiency columns are available with plate numbers in the range of 10,000–50,000 per meter. Two or more columns with the same or different pore sizes are usually connected in series either to provide optimal resolution or to extend the molecular weight fractionation range. There are two main types of SEC stationary phases: silica-based with covalently bonded inert phases, such as glycerylpropyl, and polymeric, (such as methacrylate, vinyl, and agarose). For detailed information on the application of SEC to carbohydrate separations and a tabulation of commercially available columns and fractionation ranges, the reader is referred to a recent comprehensive review by Churms (24).

IV. DIRECT HPLC DETECTION TECHNIQUES FOR CARBOHYDRATES

A. Refractive Index Detection

RI is the most widely used detection technique for the major carbohydrates in foods where high sensitivity and specificity is not a prime requirement. There are several designs available, but by far the most commonly used are the deflection and reflection types. The sensitivity of these detectors depends on the difference in RI between the pure eluent and the analyte. As a result the RI sensitivity varies for different eluents. For example, RI sensitivity for carbohydrates in a water eluent is approximately 10 times greater than in a 80:20 acetonitrile:water eluent as used with amino-bonded silica columns (25). The main advantage of the RI detector is that it offers universal detection, since, in principle, any type of analyte will have a different RI than the eluent. In practice, RI detection often lacks the sensitivity needed for quantitation of minor components, e.g., in the determination of total carbohydrate content for nutritional labeling purposes (19). The other major limitation of RI detection is that it is not compatible with gradient elution. Consequently, the main utility of RI is for isocratic separations of samples with a simple or cleaned-up sample matrix. Another fundamental characteristic of RI detection is that the response is extremely temperature sensitive. This problem is addressed in the design of RI detectors by incorporating heated cells or other active temperature-control devices, but these devices sometimes introduce additional dead volume causing increased band broadening and a corresponding decrease in sensitivity and resolution. Improved design of modern RI detectors has increased sensitivity substantially over older detectors so that the lower limits of detection for sugars of the order of 25 ng are possible when using a water eluent. For a 10 μL injection this corresponds to a concentration of 2.5 μg/L in the sample solution.

RI has also been widely used as a detection technique in HPSEC, but increasingly light scattering and more sensitive and specific detectors are being employed (24). RI is particularly useful when used in series with a second detector such as UV or conductivity to provide information on the molecular structure, e.g., the degree of esterification of pectin (26).

B. Pulsed Amperometric Detection

The limitations of traditional HPLC detection methods such as RI and UV for detection of carbohydrates and other nonchromophoric analytes provided the impetus to develop a better detection method and resulted in the development and commercialization of pulsed ampero-metric detection (PAD) (27–30). This detection technique is direct (no derivatization required), highly sensitive and specific, and compatible with gradient elution techniques. When used in conjunction with high-performance anion exchange chromatography (HPAEC-PAD or HPAE-PAD), sugars, sugar alcohols, and oligo- and polysaccharides can be separated with high resolution in a single run and quantitated at the picomole level if necessary. HPAEC-PAD has been successfully applied to food, dietary fiber, and complex carbohydrate analysis (31) and is also widely used for glycoprotein research (32,33). Increasingly, it is being applied to a variety of routine monitoring and research applications (31) and has been approved for use in several official methods (33–35). Dual detection using PAD in series with other detectors is also finding application in fundamental studies of plant cell-wall structure. For example, PAD and UV in conjunction with SEC has been used in the study of plant cell-wall lignin-carbohydrate complexes to monitor lignin and carbohydrate components present in alkaline extracts (36).

Amperometric detection is based on the measurement of a change in current due to oxidation, reduction, or complex formation of an analyte at the surface of an electrode (Fig. 10). In DC amperometry, the electrode is maintained at a constant potential during the determination. This technique has been applied to the determination of a number of compounds and ions, e.g., catecholamines, thiols, phenols, sulfite, iodide, and cyanide (37). Carbohydrates are easily oxidized on gold or platinum electrodes at high pH and are therefore good candidates for electrochemical detection. However, DC amperometry is not useful for carbohydrates since the carbohydrate oxidation products foul the electrode causing a rapidly decreasing response on subsequent determinations (Fig. 11). This problem is solved by pulsed amperometry, which utilizes a triple (38) or more recently a quadruple pulse sequence (39) rather than a constant potential on the working electrode (Fig. 12). By using a rapidly repeating sequence of large positive (E2) and negative potentials (E3) following each measurement, a clean electrode surface is maintained, which ensures consistency in response. The detector signal (E1) is measured at a potential appropriate for the particular analyte by integrating the current for a fixed length of time (typi-

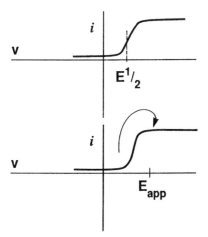

Fig. 10 Amperometric detection is contingent on a change in current due to oxidation, reduction, or complex formation at the applied potential on a specific electrode material.

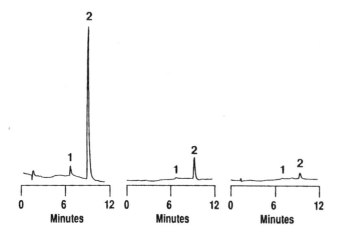

Fig. 11 Decrease in detector response for repeat injections of a carbohydrate and an amino acid (concentration 10 µg/L in both cases) using DC amperometric detection. Peaks: 1, leucine; 2, lactose. Column: CarboPac PA1 (10 µM, 250 × 4 mm i.d.) with guard. Eluent: gradient, 15–150 mM NaOH in 5 min. Detection: DC amperometry, Au electrode, range 1 µA, applied potential 0.15 V vs. Ag/AgCl.

cally 200 ms) and storing the resulting charge in a sample-and-hold amplifier until the next measurement.

An appropriate gold (Au) electrode potential (vs. Ag/AgCl) for oxidation of carbohydrates can be deduced from current vs. potential plots obtained by pulsed voltammetry, as shown in Fig. 13. Since the optimum potential is similar even for different classes of carbohydrates, a single measuring potential setting (E1) can be used for all carbohydrate analytes. In practice, an E1 setting of +0.05V (vs. Ag/AgCl) is typically used since this not only provides good signal to noise ratio (40) but also high specificity since very few classes of organic compounds other than carbohydrates can be oxidized at this low potential. The possibility of interference is thus minimized. In addition, any neutral or cationic components present in the sample matrix are not retained to any degree and elute in or close to the void volume of the column. Potential interference with the analysis of the carbohydrate components from these sources is thus eliminated.

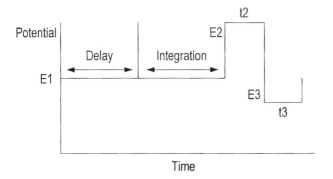

Fig. 12 Triple potential sequence used in pulsed amperometry. A clean electrode surface is maintained by using a repeating sequence of a high positive followed by a negative potential after each measurement

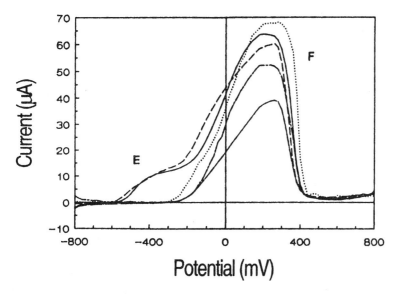

Fig. 13 Pulsed voltammetry response for five carbohydrates in 0.1 M NaOH. Concentrations 0.1 mM: (---) sorbitol; (——) glucose; (— —) fructose; (—·—) sucrose; (···) maltose. (From Ref. 41.)

Pulsed amperometric detection has been commonly used at ambient temperatures in air-conditioned laboratories without temperature thermostatting. For many purposes this is adequate, but PAD response does show some temperature dependence (41), therefore, the column and detector cell should be thermostatted for highest accuracy and reproducibility. The use of an internal standard is also advisable. Detection of carbohydrates is linear over at least three orders of magnitude allowing both minor and major components to be determined in the same run. Limits of detection are in the 1 pmol range (42), i.e., a sample concentration of <20 ng/mL for a 10 μL injection, which is ~100× more sensitive than RI.

C. Light Scattering

Light-scattering detectors, when used in conjunction with HPSEC, facilitate the determination of the molecular weight distribution of carbohydrate polymer fractions. The development of low-angle light scattering (LALLS) and multiple-angle laser light scattering (MALLS) detectors have greatly extended the usefulness of this technique. LALLS and MALLS now makes on-line measurement of molecular weight possible without requiring calibration with a series of standards (in most cases not available for a particular polymer type). Dual detection technique, in which LALLS is used in series with RI, allows the molecular weight distribution and molecular weight average to be determined directly (24). MALLS provides even more capability since information on molecular characteristics such as polymer conformation can be obtained along with molecular weights.

D. Mass Spectrometry

Prior to 1990, very little had been published on the use of on-line HPLC-MS in research on dietary fiber components such as plant cell-wall carbohydrates and their hydrolysis products. More recently, an increasing number of reports have appeared in which on-line HPLC-MS has

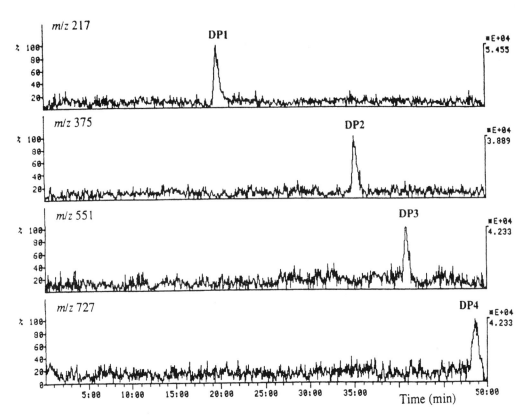

Fig. 14 HPAEC-MS of unsaturated galacturonic acid oligomers (each 10 μg/mL) up to DP 4. The ions indicated are sodiated molecules. (Adapted from Ref. 46.)

been used (43–46). These include studies on the characterization of oligosaccharides derived from cell-wall polysaccharides from soybeans and other sources and the structural analysis of pectic oligosaccharides. The key development that has made this possible has been on-line de-salting of the sodium hydroxide/sodium acetate eluents used in HPAEC-PAD. This has been achieved with suppressor devices that are normally used in conjunction with conductivity detection for ion chromatography (47,48). The suppressor device is positioned either after the PAD detector or directly after the HPAEC column and effectively provides on-line desalting of the sodium hydroxide or sodium hydroxide/sodium acetate eluent by removal of sodium ion. An in-line booster pump is used to deliver the desalted eluent to the inlet of the MS (49) when the MS interface (e.g. thermospray) operates with a back pressure of >0.875 Mpa (125 psi), since this is the upper operating pressure of the suppressor. In recent work using an ionspray interface (46), the booster pump was eliminated, since virtually no back pressure is generated by the MS interface. The HPAEC-MS technique is still evolving but shows great promise. Figure 14 shows HPAEC-MS traces for unsaturated galacturonic acids oligomer standards up to DP4.

V. APPLICATIONS IN DIETARY FIBER ANALYSIS

The increasing utilization of HPLC techniques in dietary fiber and complex carbohydrate analysis can be measured by the growing number of publications during the last few years. These applications, for the most part, fall into four main categories:

1. Determination of neutral sugars
2. Determination of uronic acids
3. Separation of oligo- and polysaccharides
4. Determination of molecular size distribution profiles of complex carbohydrates

The following sections will address each of these types of applications and illustrate the various techniques with examples from published literature.

A. HPLC Techniques for the Determination of Neutral Sugars

Table 2 summarizes the three main HPLC methods that have been used for neutral monosaccharide analysis. Tables 3–5 provide typical retention time data for neutral sugars of interest in dietary fiber analysis for the three main types of columns used for determination of monosaccharides by HPLC. Retention time data are given, rather than k′ data, since these are of more direct practical value. From these tables it is clear that only HPAEC-PAD using a water (or <3 mM [OH]) eluent (Table 4) is capable of resolving the entire set of analytes and also has sufficient sensitivity and dynamic range to detect both major and minor sugar components in the same determination. A number of studies illustrate the use of the HPAEC-PAD technique to determine neutral sugars derived from dietary fiber. Fahey et al. (10,50–52) used HPAEC-PAD extensively to determine the neutral monosaccharide composition of dietary fiber from various vegetables, fruits, gums, animal forage, and other fibrous substances. They also compared dietary fiber methodologies (NDF, TDF, NSP, and Uppsala TDF) using the HPAEC-PAD method to determine the monosaccharide constituents (10,52). Figure 15a shows a chromatogram of standard monosaccharides compared with the neutral monosaccharide profile of a neutral detergent dietary fiber (NDF) residue from apple (Fig. 15b). An estimate of the method precision for monosaccharides was determined for five repeat injections of the same standard solution. Percent relative standard deviations were fucose (0.75), rhamnose (1.60), arabinose (0.43), galactose (0.59), glucose (0.86), xylose (1.98), and mannose (2.10).

Similarly, Englyst et al. (9) used the HPAEC PAD technique to determine dietary fiber. In the Englyst method cell-wall and chemically related nonstarch polysaccharides (NSP) are used as an index of dietary fiber content. NSP is composed of neutral and amino sugars and uronic acids, which are quantified using either GLC or HPLC. In the HPLC method, neutral sugars, hexosamines, and uronic acids from nonstarch polysaccharides are determined by HPAEC-PAD with a CarboPac PA1 column following enzymatic removal of starch and hydrolysis of the NSP residue with sulfuric acid. The treatment of acid hydrolysates for HPLC analysis is minimal. For neutral sugar determinations, the addition of an internal standard is the only step required. Sulfate, which is present in the hydrolysates, is removed during chromatography by a guard column installed ahead of the analytical column. The guard column is automatically switched out of line after 60 seconds to prevent sulfate ions from reaching the analytical column. More recently, Li (53) published details of a simpler procedure that allows sugar, starch, and dietary fiber polysaccharide content to be determined for food products from the same 0.5 g subsample. The procedure involves a simple fractionation scheme in which sugars are extracted into 80% methanol, starches are hydrolyzed to glucose by amylglucosidase, and dietary fiber residues are hydrolyzed with sulfuric acid. HPAEC-PAD (CarboPac PA1) was used for the quantification of the different mixtures of sugars resulting from the various fractionation steps. Results for reduced-calorie bread, cooked instant oatmeal, canned beans with pork and tomato sauce, steamed snap green beans, and microwaved frozen peas correlated well with results obtained previously on the same samples using GLC.

Although HPAEC-PAD is presently the most commonly used HPLC technique for dietary fiber determinations, other HPLC techniques are used in some cases. Redondo et al. (54), in a

Table 2 HPLC Techniques for Neutral Sugar Analysis

Type of column packing	Examples of commercially available columns	Operating temperature range and pH stability	Typical eluent and detection technique	Comments/limitations
Metal-loaded, and H$^+$ form cation exchange PSDVB resin	Aminex series (BioRad) Benson Shodex	65–90°C neutral pH	Water Refractive index	Elevated temperature is necessary to obtain satisfactory column efficiency Resolves some but not all neutral sugars present in dietary fiber hydrolysates Galactose and rhamnose coelute.
Propylamino-bonded silica and amine-modified silica		Ambient to 70°C pH 2–8	80:20 acetonitrile:water for monosaccharides Refractive index	Gradual loss of resolution with use due to column deactivation by reaction of reducing sugars with amino groups Chloride, if present, interferes with glucose Resolves some but not all neutral sugars present in dietary fiber hydrolysates Low solubility of some sugars in the mobile phase is a limitation in some cases Cost and disposal of acetonitrile is increasingly an issue
Pellicular anion exchange resin		Subambient to 30°C pH 1–14	Water, NaOH, or KOH Pulsed amperometric	Resolution of all neutral sugars from dietary fiber hydrolysates requires water or weak hydroxide (1–3 mM [OH]) eluents, hence postcolumn addition of 0.3 M hydroxide is required for detection by PAD Requires fixed postrun column wash with 300 mM [OH] and reequilibration with eluent prior to each run to maintain resolution Gradient elution allows uronic acids and neutral sugars to be determined in the same analysis

Table 3 Typical Retention Times for Neutral Monosaccharides of Importance in Dietary Fiber Analysis on Some Commercially Available Metal-Loaded Cation Exchange Columns

	Retention time (min)						
	Calcium form			Lead form		Hydrogen form	
	BioRad[a] HPX-87C	Supelco[b] SupelcoGel Ca	Waters[c] SugarPak	BioRad[a] HPX-87P	Supelco[b] SupelcoGel Pb	BioRad[a] HPX-87H	Supelco[b] SupelcoGel C-610H
Monosaccharide							
Glucose	10.87	12.0	8.5	12.72	14.9	10.16	12.1
Xylose	12.00	13.2	9.3	13.86	16.1	12.00	12.8
Galactose	12.25	13.4	9.4	14.70	17.6	10.49	12.9
Mannose	12.47	13.8	9.6	16.44	19.8	10.82	12.8
Rhamnose	12.58	—	9.5	14.88	—	11.20	—
(Fructose)	13.58	14.8	10.1	17.04	20.8	10.39	13.1
Arabinose	13.75	15.1	10.4	15.48	19.2	11.34	13.9
Fucose	13.78	14.9	10.4	15.84	—	12.05	—
Conditions							
Col. dimensions	300 × 7.8 mm	300 × 7.8 mm	300 × 6.5 mm	300 × 7.8 mm	300 × 7.8 mm	300 × 7.8 mm	300 × 7.8 mm
Mobile Phase	Water	Water	Water	Water	Water	Water	0.1% H_3PO_4
Flow (mL/min)	0.6	0.5	0.5	0.6	0.5	0.6	0.5
Temperature	85°C	80°C	90°C	85°C	85°C	85°C	30°C
Detection	RI	RI	RI	RI	RI	RI	RI

[a] From HPLC columns methods and applications, Bio-Rad Laboratories, 1993, p. 58.
[b] From Retention Time of Carbohydrates and Sugar Alcohols, Carbohydrate Update 3-2, Supelco Corporation, Jan. 1996.
[c] From Waters Chromatography Handbook, Waters Corporation, 1994, p. 26.

Table 4 Typical Retention Times for Neutral Monosaccharides of Importance
in Dietary Fiber Analysis on Amino-Bonded Silica Columns

	Retention time (min)	
	Waters: μBondapak® carbohydrate[a]	Supelco: Supelcosil LC-NH$_2$[b]
Monosaccharide		
Fucose	4.2	—
Xylose	4.3	6.8
Arabinose	4.8	7.5
(Fructose)	5.7	8.3
Mannose	6.4	9.1
Glucose	7.3	9.8
Galactose	7.7	10.3
Rhamnose	—	—
Conditions:		
Col. dimensions	300 × 3.9 mm	300 × 7.8 mm
Mobile Phase	80:20 acetonitrile:water	75:25 acetonitrile:water
Flow (mL/min)	2.0 mL/min	1.0 mL/min
Temperature	Ambient	Ambient
Detection	RI	RI

[a] From Waters Chromatography Handbook, Waters Corporation, 1994, p. 26.
[b] From Retention Time of Carbohydrates and Sugar Alcohols, Carbohydrate Update 3-2, Supelco Corporation, Jan. 1996.

comparative study of HPLC and GC methods for the determination of nonstarch polysaccharides in raw and processed vegetables, used the Englyst method (55) for isolation of dietary fiber followed by HPLC on a metal (lead)-loaded cation exchange column (Aminex HPX-87P at 85°C, water eluent, and RI detection) to determine neutral sugars and galacturonate. Glucose was the major monosaccharide followed by galactose/rhamnose (coelute), arabinose, cellobiose, xylose, and mannose. In an earlier study (1983), Neilson and Marlett (6) also determined neutral sugar composition using the Aminex HPX-87P. There are very few published articles on the use of amino-bonded silica phases for direct determination of neutral sugars in dietary fiber residues. A μ-Bondapak NH$_2$ column with a 75% acetonitrile mobile phase and RI detection was used to determine free sugars in whole grain foods in a 1987 study by Brighenti et al. (56), but dietary fiber was determined gravimetrically. Similarly, in a 1996 study (57) of sugar, starch, pectin, and insoluble fiber content of frozen green beans and peppers, a Spherisorb NH$_2$ column with 90% acetonitrile mobile phase was used to determine free sugars, glucose from hydrolyzed starch, and galacturonic acid from pectin, but not to determine dietary fiber.

B. HPLC Techniques for the Determination of Uronic Acids

There are a number of methods for determination of the uronic acid constituents of dietary fiber, which usually involve a lengthy digestion with mineral acid(s) and/or enzymes to hydrolyze the uronic acid–containing carbohydrate polymer. Free uronic acids in the hydrolysates are quantified by either spectrophotometry, GLC, or HPLC. Various HPLC techniques have been investigated for determination of uronic acids following hydrolysis.

Table 5 Typical Retention Times for Neutral Monosaccharides of Importance in Dietary Fiber
Analysis on High Performance Pellicular Anion Exchange Columns

	Retention time (min)				
	Dionex CarboPac PA1 with guard column			Dionex CarboPac PA10 with guard column	
Monosaccharide	A H$_2$O	B H$_2$O	C 3 mM NaOH	D 1 mM KOH	E 6 mM KOH
Fucose	6.6	5.9	—	6.4	5.2
Rhamnose	15.2	13.0	—	17.2[a]	11.6
Arabinose	16.1	14.3	15.7	16.0[a]	11.6
Galactose	21.2	20.0	20.8	20.8	14.4
Glucose	24.3	23.6	24.6	25.6	18.0
Xylose	29.3	28.6	29.2	31.2	21.2
Mannose	32.1	31.1	31.6	35.2	22.0

A. Prodolliet et al., J AOAC Int 78(3):749–761 (1995). Water eluent following column wash with 300 mM sodium
  hydroxide. Flowrate = 1.0 mL/min.
B. From Ref. 39. Column wash with 200 mM NaOH. Eluent 10 mM NaOH for 5 min, then water. Flowrate = 1.0
  mL/min.
C. Sullivan J, Douek M. J Chromatogr A. 671:339–350 (1994). Column wash with 350 mM NaOH. 3 mM NaOH
  eluent.
D. Jandik P, Rohrer JS, Henshall A. Poster no. C-901 presented at the 111th AOAC meeting, Montreal, Canada, 1988.
  No column wash. Isocratic 1 mM KOH. Flowrate = 1 mL/min.
E. Jandik P, Rohrer JS, Henshall A. Poster no. C-901 presented at the 111th AOAC meeting, Montreal, Canada, 1988.
  No column wash. Isocratic 6 mM KOH. Flowrate = 1 mL/min.
[a] Note that the elution order for rhamnose and arabinose is reversed under these conditions for the CarboPac PA10 vs.
  the CarboPac PA1 column.

1. Cation Exchange Resin Columns with UV Detection

HPLC methods have been developed (1985) for the determination of uronic acids using a cation
exchange resin column (Aminex HPX-87-H) with UV detection (22). Separations are performed
at lower temperatures (35°C) than are normally used for cation exchange resin to minimize
lactone formation. At 65°C D-glucuronic acid and, to a lesser extent, D-mannuronic acid gave
broad peaks, indicating partial lactonization. Only partial resolution of glucuronic, galacturonic,
and mannuronic acids was achieved. Figure 16 shows the separation of D-glucuronic (RT 7.88
min) and D-mannuronic acids (RT 8.30 min) at 35°C using a 0.0009 N sulfuric acid mobile phase
and UV detection at 220 nm. Based on the reported relative retention time data, galacturonic acid
(RRT 1.09 vs. RRT 1.01 for glucuronic acid) would elute at 8.50 minutes. Under these conditions, accurate quantification of mannuronic and galacturonic acids would not be possible if
both were present.

2. Silica-Based Strong Anion Exchange Columns with RI Detection

In the early 1980s Voragen et al. investigated the use of silica-based strong anion exchange
columns with RI detection (58) for the determination of uronic acids. They were successful in
separating galacturonic, glucuronic, and mannuronic acids using either a Nucleosil 10 SB or
Zorbax SAX column with a 0.7 N acetic acid eluent. A gradual decrease in retention was found
to occur with time using the 0.7 N acetic acid eluent due to deterioration of the column. Column

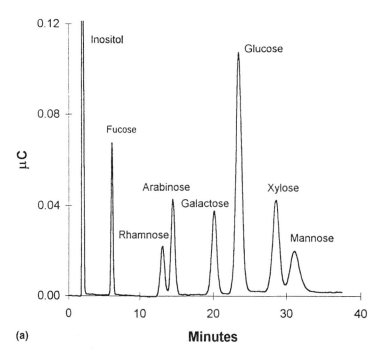

(a)

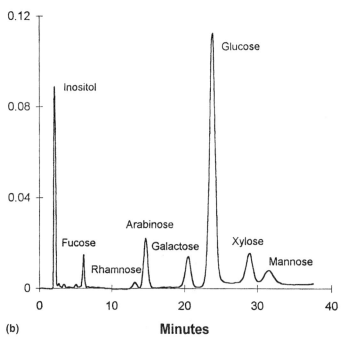

(b)

Fig. 15 (a) HAEC-PAD chromatogram of standard monosaccharides; (b) neutral monosaccharide profile of a Neutral Detergent Dietary Fiber (NDF) residue from apple. Column: Dionex CarboPac ™ PA1 (10 μM, 250 × 4 mm i.d.) with PA1 guard (250 mm × 4 mm i.d.). Eluent: gradient, 10 mM NaOH for 5 minutes to elute inositol and fucose. From 5–7 minutes [NaOH] decreased linearly to zero. Remaining oligosaccharides eluted with 100% water, 35–44 minutes, column wash with 200 mM NaOH. Reequilibrate with 10 mM NaOH for 10 minutes. Detection: Pulsed amperometry, Au electrode. Applied potentials, E1, E2, E3 + 0.05, +0.75, −0.15V vs. Ag/AgCl. (Note: μC = microcoulombs). (Adapted from Ref. 52.)

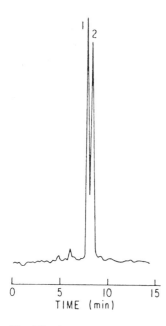

Fig. 16 Separation of D-glucuronic and D-mannuronic acids by HPLC on a cation exchange resin column. Column: Bio-Rad HP-87H. Eluent: Water at 35°C. Flowrate: 0.6 mL/min. UV detection at 220 nm. Peaks: 1, D-mannuronic acid (7.88 min); 2, D-glucuronic acid (8.30 min). (Adapted from Ref. 22.)

lifetime under these conditions was limited to ~6 months, but this might be extended by lowering the acetic acid concentration to 0.3 N since the separation is not affected.

3. Amino-Bonded Silica Columns with RI Detection

Galacturonic acid resulting from NaOH hydrolysis and enzyme treatment of pectin from green beans has been successfully determined using an amino-bonded silica phase using a pH 4.6 acetate buffer eluent and RI detection (59). A second method using a Spherisorb ODS2 alkyl-bonded phase column and a pH2.2 sulfuric acid eluent with UV detection at 215 nm gave similar results.

The possibility of using amino-bonded phase columns for simultaneous separation and determination of several uronic acids has been studied but showed discouraging results (60). Under typical conditions for sugars (80:20 acetonitrile:water) uronic acids did not elute from the Lichrosorb-NH₂ column. Elution of glucuronic and galacturonic acid were achieved using an eluent containing NaH₂PO₄ to lower the pH and increasing the water content. However, separations are very dependent on the water content and pH of the eluent, and peaks are somewhat broad and non-Gaussian.

4. HPAEC-PAD

More recently, Quigley and Englyst (61) have developed methods for the direct determination of neutral sugars and uronic acids using HPAEC-PAD. These methods show good agreement with GC and colorimetric methods but also offer the advantage of an expanded linear range vs. colorimetric methods and quantification of the individual uronic acids (61). Uronic acids by virtue of their carboxyl group are much more strongly retained on CarboPac anion exchange columns than the neutral sugars and therefore require a stronger eluent. In the Englyst HPAEC-

PAD method, uronic acids are determined separately from neutral sugars under isocratic conditions. Baseline separation of galacturonic, glucuronic, and mannuronic acids is achieved with a runtime of less than 13 minutes. Figure 17 shows chromatograms obtained for (a) a standard uronic acid mixture, (b) a citrus pectin hydrolysate, and (c) a sugar beet hydrolysate. The large peak labeled N is due to neutral sugars which coelute under these conditions. It is also possible to determine neutral sugars and uronic acids in a single run by using continuous or step gradient elution. The determination of neutral sugars and uronic acid constituents by HPAE-PAD is now accepted as an alternative method for nutritional labeling purposes in the United Kingdom.

HPAEC-PAD is proving to be valuable not only for the determination of neutral sugars and uronic acids to meet nutritional labeling requirements, but also in development of the methodology. The accuracy of dietary fiber determinations depends on the efficacy of the hydrolysis procedures used, whether they be enzymatic or chemical. HPAE-PAD has been used for determination of monosaccharide constituents in comparing the relative merits of hydrolysis procedures (10,61). The results of a 2 M sulfuric acid hydrolysis of a pectin are shown in Fig. 18. In addition to neutral sugars and galacturonic acid, significant peaks corresponding to uronic acid oligomers are also present, indicating incomplete conversion to the free acid under these conditions.

HPAEC-PAD has also been compared with the standard colorimetric procedure for the determination of galacturonate in pectic substances from fruit and vegetables (50). No significant differences in results were found between the colorimetric and HPLC methods. The direct HPLC procedure was also considered to be superior to GLC derivatization procedures, because sample preparation is much less tedious and the possibility of low values due to incomplete conversion in the derivatization step is eliminated. HPAEC-PAD (CarboPac PA1 column with a hydroxide/acetate gradient) was also used as the method for quantification of uronic acids in comparing four methods for hydrolysis of water-soluble, uronic acid–containing polysaccharides (62). Based on the HPLC data, the best results were obtained using a methanolysis–trifluoroacetic acid (TFA) hydrolysis procedure.

C. HPLC Techniques for the Determination and Characterization of Oligo- and Polysaccharides

HPLC techniques provide powerful tools for characterizing intact NSP and for the determination of the oligo- and polysaccharide residues obtained from partial hydrolysis.

1. Characterization of Carbohydrate Polymers by HPSEC

HPSE-LALLS coupled to RI has been widely used for fractionation and the determination of the molecular weight distribution of soluble dietary fiber components such as carrageenan, alginates, inulin, and pectin (24); however, to prevent aggregation of the polysaccharide chains during chromatography, it is necessary to incorporate electrolytes in the eluent to adjust the ionic strength and operate at elevated temperatures (24). The use of two detectors in series can also provide structural information, as illustrated by the use of a conductivity detector in series with a RI detector to monitor pectins fractionated by HPSEC (26). Peak area ratios for each detector can be correlated with the degree of pectin esterification since the conductivity response is due only to the unesterified galacturonic acid residues.

2. Determination of Chain-Length Distribution

Although limited structural information on NSP can be obtained using HPSEC techniques, further elucidation of the structure requires that these high molecular weight carbohydrate polymers first be broken down by either an enzymatic or a chemical treatment to provide lower molecular

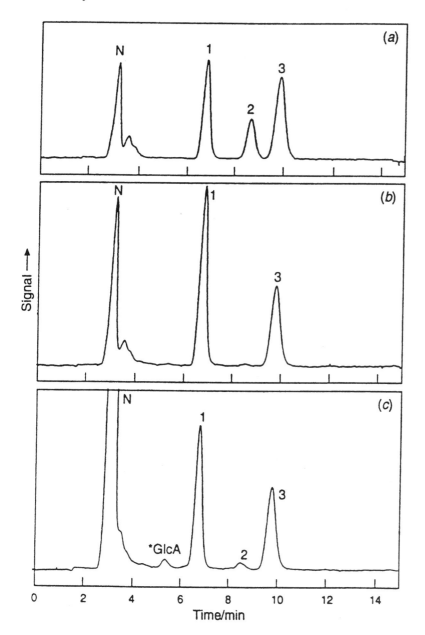

Fig. 17 Chromatogram of (a) a standard uronic acid mixture, (b) a pectin (citrus) hydrolysate, and (c) a sugar beet hydrolysate. Column: CarboPac PA1 (10 μM, 250 × 4 mm i.d.) with guard. Eluent: 25 mM NaOH/150 mM sodium acetate. Flowrate: 1.0 mL/min. Detection: pulsed amperometry, Au electrode, range 300 nA. Peaks: 1, galacturonic acid; 2, glucuronic acid; 3, mannuronic acid (internal standard). The largest peak N represents the neutral sugars; *GlcA is an unidentified peak, which appears to convert to glucuronic acid on further hydrolysis. (Adapted from Ref. 61.)

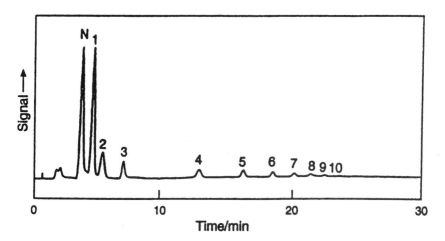

Fig. 18 HPAEC-PAD chromatogram of a pectin hydrolysate showing incomplete conversion to free uronic acids by the 2 M sulfuric acid hydrolysis treatment. Column: CarboPac PA1 (10 μM, 250 × 4 mm i.d.) with guard. Eluent: gradient, 100 mM NaOH/240 mM sodium acetate to 100 mM NaOH/480 mM sodium acetate in 15 minutes. Temp.: ambient. Detection: pulsed amperometric, Au electrode, range 300 nA. (Adapted from Ref. 61.)

weight residues, which are amenable to chromatographic analysis. Traditional HPLC techniques have proved inadequate for separating these complex mixtures of oligo- and polysaccharides resulting from the hydrolysis of starch and other carbohydrates such as inulin and pectin (7,11). A major limitation is the incompatibility of RI with gradient elution, but equally important is the requirement for a column to resolve carbohydrate polymers of DP >20 differing only by a single sugar unit. The problem is illustrated in Fig. 19a, which shows the separation of a hydrolyzed corn syrup using a conventional metal-loaded cation exchange column with RI detection. The limitation of this approach is apparent since the oligosaccharides with DP >2 are only weakly retained and the elution order is from high to low DP. Only the monosaccharide is baseline resolved from the oligosaccharides, which elute as a poorly resolved envelope of peaks with the larger DP oligosaccharide chains crowding to the front of the chromatogram and virtually no resolution at DP >5.

An alternative approach is to use pulsed amperometric detection in conjunction with hydrophilic interaction chromatography on amino-bonded silica columns to study glucooligosaccharides derived from hydrolysates of Polycose, starch, and amylopectin (63). Separations of oligosaccharides up to a DP of ~30 were achieved using gradient elution with acetonitrile:water in the range 67:33 to 50:50 over 70 minutes and also postcolumn addition of sodium hydroxide to the eluent prior to the detector. Good resolution was achieved for DP <15, but the insolubility of higher polysaccharides in the acetonitrile:water eluent is a limiting factor.

The advent of the HPAEC-PAD technique using gradient elution has in many cases provided a general solution to the problem of separating polysaccharide mixtures (64). Figure 19b shows a separation using HPAEC-PAD with sodium hydroxide gradient elution of the same hydrolyzed corn syrup run on the cation exchange column shown in Fig. 19a. For HPAEC-PAD, the elution order is reversed as compared with the cation exchange separation, i.e., retention time increases with increase in DP. Resolution is achieved up to a DP of >20.

3. Structural Studies on Amylopectins

HPAEC-PAD with gradient elution has been used for structural studies on starch-derived materials such as amylopectins since the chain length distribution is an important parameter for charac-

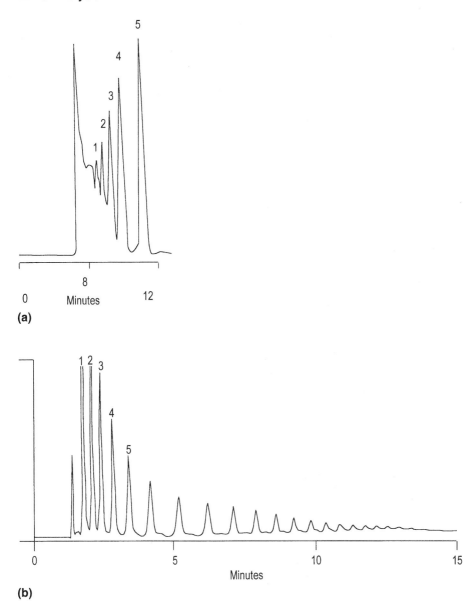

Fig. 19 (a) Separation of a hydrolyzed corn syrup by ion moderated partition chromatography on a cation exchange resin (calcium form). Eluent: water. Flowrate: 0.6 mL/min. Temp.: 80°C. Detector: refractive index. Peaks: 1, DP 5; 2, DP 4; 3, DP 3; 4, DP 2; 5, glucose. (b) Separation of a hydrolyzed corn syrup by HPAE-PAD using gradient elution. Column: CarboPac PA1 (10 μM, 250 × 4 mm i.d.) with guard. Eluent: 150 mM sodium hydroxide with sodium acetate gradient from 250 to 500 mM from 1 to 9 minutes, then hold at 150 mM NaOH : 500 mM NaOH. Flowrate: 1.0 mL/min. Temp: ambient. Detector: pulsed amperometric, Au electrode. Peaks: 1, glucose; 2, DP 2; 3, DP 3; 4, DP 4; 5, DP 5.

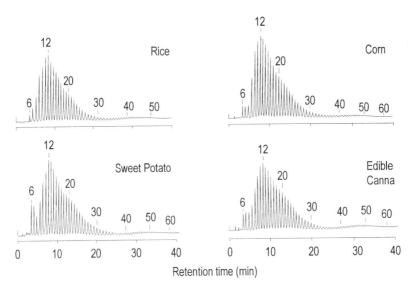

Fig. 20 Chain length distribution of debranched amylopectins from various sources determined by HPAE-PAD. Column: CarboPac PA1 (10 µM, 250 × 4 mm i.d.) with guard. Eluent: A, 150 mM NaOH; B, 150 mM NaOH/500 mM sodium acetate. Gradient program: 40% B at 0 min, 50% at 2 min, 60% at 10 min, 80% at 40 min. Temp: ambient. Flowrate: 1.0 mL/min. Detector: pulsed amperometric, Au electrode, range 10 µA. (From Ref. 23.)

terizing the molecular structure (65–67). Figure 20 shows the chain length distribution up to a DP of 55 for debranched amylopectins from various sources (67). These distributions can be used as fingerprints for the amylopectin source.

4. Quantitation of Polysaccharides

For exact quantitation by HPLC, the detector response for each polysaccharide over the DP range of interest is required. Relative PAD detector response for maltose oligomers in the DP range of 2–7 determined by Koizumi et al. are shown in Table 6 (68). For the maltooligomers in the DP range of 6–17, the relative response factors were determined after first isolating quantities of the individual maltosaccharides (56). The data in Table 7 show that the relative response on a molar basis increases linearly for chain lengths from DP 6 to DP 15 and more

Table 6 Relative PAD Responses of Maltosaccharides (DP 2–6)

DP	Relative response (molar basis)	Relative response (mass basis)
2	1.00	1.00
3	1.39	0.94
4	1.72	0.88
5	2.06	0.85
6	2.33	0.80
7	2.59	0.77

Table 7 Relative PAD Responses of
Maltosaccharides (DP 6–17)

DP	Relative response (molar basis)	Relative response (mass basis)
6	0.74	1.10
7	0.82	1.05
8	0.89	1.00
9	1.00	1.00
10	1.10	0.99
11	1.20	0.98
12	1.31	0.99
13	1.38	0.94
14	1.46	0.94
15	1.55	0.94
16	1.59	0.90
17	1.65	0.88

slowly for the DP 16 and DP 17 maltosaccharides. This suggests that the difference in relative response for higher oligomers becomes smaller with increasing chain length. With the availability of semi-preparative scale (9 and 22 mm i.d.) CarboPac columns, isolation of milligram quantities of individual polysaccharides in a single injection becomes feasible for any polysaccharide mixture, allowing pure standards to be prepared and the relationship between DP and response factor to be accurately determined. An alternative approach is to use an in-line postcolumn enzyme (amyloglucosidase) reactor to convert each oligo- and polysaccharide to glucose, which is quantified using the PAD. This technique has been successfully applied to the study of debranched amylopectin from tapioca (65). Figure 21 shows chromatograms for debranched tapioca amylopectin with and without passage through the enzyme reactor. As would be predicted, the PAD response is enhanced by the reactor. Detection of amylodextrin up to a DP of 77 was achieved.

D. Determination of Inulins and Other Fructans

Inulin and fructooligosaccharides (FOS) are increasingly being used as functional food ingredients. FOS products are typically mixtures of small oligosaccharides such as the FOS shown in Figure 22. Analysis of these types of products is straightforward using either HPAEC-PAD (69), as shown in Fig. 23, or hydrophilic interaction chromatography on amino-bonded silica with RI detection (70,71). Chain-length distribution profiles of commercial products such as those derived from inulin can be determined by using HPAEC-PAD with gradient elution (Fig. 24a). By adjusting the initial gradient profile (Fig. 24b), smaller oligofructose (F_n) chains can be distinguished from the inulin (GF_n) chains and separations up to DP 80 are possible (72). Quantitation of individual inulin oligomers requires a knowledge of the PAD response factors. These have been determined for the F_n and GF_n oligomers from DP 2 to 8 and from DP 11 to 17 by isolation of 5–20 mg quantities of the pure oligomers using preparative scale RP-18 HPLC (73). Unfortunately, pure fractions of the oligomers in the DP range of 6–10 could not be obtained using the RP-18 technique due to coelution problems. The response factors for the DP 6–10 region are obtained by linear regression of the DP 2–5 and DP 11–17 series followed by interpolation. For DP >17 the response factor appears to change very slowly with increasing

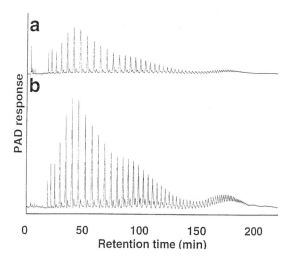

Fig. 21 HPAEC chromatograms of debranched amylopectin (0.5 mg/mL) (a) without and (b) with passage through a postcolumn amyloglucosidase reactor. Column: CarboPac PA1 (10 µM, 250 × 4 mm i.d.) with guard. Eluent: A, 100 mM NaOH; B, 100 mM NaOH/300 mM sodium nitrate. Gradient program: 0–5 minutes 94% A and 6% B; 5–10 minutes, linear gradient to 10% B; 10–150 minutes, linear gradient to 30%; 150–200 minutes, linear gradient to 40% C; 200–220 minutes, linear gradient to 45% B. Temp.: ambient. Flowrate: 0.5 mL/min. Detector: pulsed amperometric, Au electrode (Adapted from Ref. 65.)

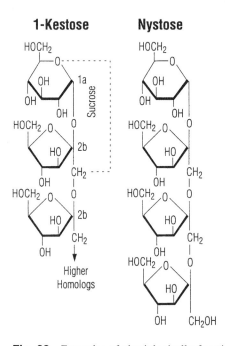

Fig. 22 Examples of physiologically functional fructooligosaccharides.

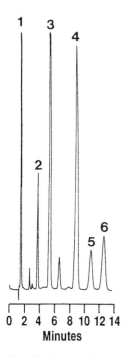

Fig. 23   Determination of kestoses and related sugars by HPAE-PAD. Column: CarboPac PA1 (10 μM, 250 × 4 mm i.d.) with guard. Eluent 100 mM NaOH/20 mM sodium acetate. Flowrate: 1.0 mL/min. Temp.: ambient. Detector: pulsed amperometric, Au electrode, range 1 μA. Peaks: 1, galactinose; 2, sucrose; 3, 1-kestose; 4, 6-kestose; 5, neo-kestose; 6, nystose.

DP, and relative response factors can be obtained by interpolation. As noted previously, semi-preparative scale (9 and 22 mm i.d.) CarboPac PA1 columns are available commercially and could be used for isolation of mg quantities of all the inulin oligomers. This would allow accurate PAD response factors to be obtained directly over the entire DP range.

For regulatory and labeling purposes, methods are also needed both to quantify and iden-tify these types of products since they are not determined by AOAC or other official methods for dietary fiber (74,75). Methodology has been developed for the determination of inulin and oligofructose in food products (74), which subsequently received first action approval by AOAC International in 1997 as AOAC method 997.08 (75) following an interlaboratory validation study. The method involves three steps: (a) an initial water extraction at 85°C for 15 minutes to determine free fructose and glucose, (b) treatment of the residue with amyloglucosidase to convert starch and maltodextrins to glucose, and (c) treatment of the residue from (b) with inulinase (commercially available as Fructozym from Novo Nordisk and Megazyme) to convert the fructan to fructose and glucose. Released sugars are determined at each stage and the concen-tration of glucose and fructose released from the fructan calculated by difference from the three determinations. Commercial food ingredient products derived from the lower molecular weight fractions of inulin (DP 3–20), referred to as fructooligosaccharides or oligofructose are also determined by AOAC Method 997.08. However, the method does not give any information regarding the concentration of each FOS in the food product. This has spurred the development of a method that both identifies and quantifies FOS products directly (76). The method uses HPAEC-PAD and hinges on a finely tuned gradient elution profile, which allows commercially available FOS and inulin products to be identified and quantified in a variety of foods. Identifica-

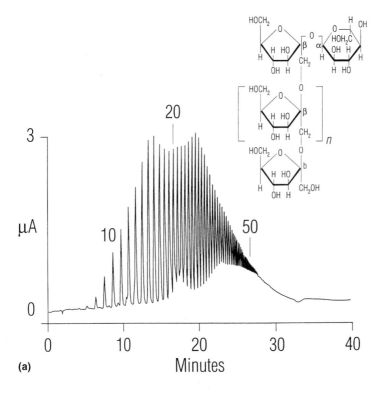

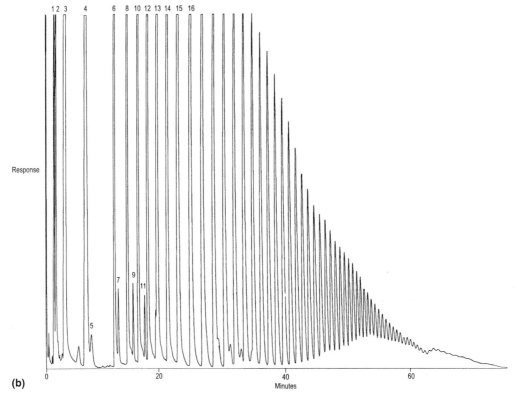

(a)

(b)

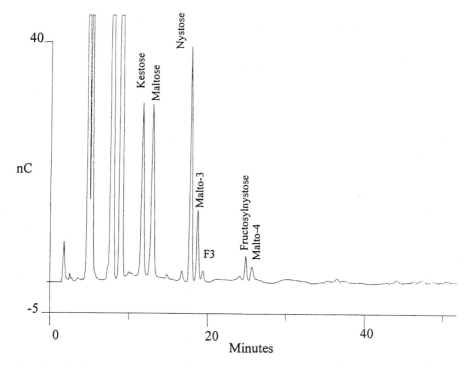

Fig. 25 HPAEC-PAD chromatogram of a strawberry yogurt containing Actilight-95®. (Adapted from Ref. 76.)

tion is based on the unique "fingerprint" pattern of fructooligosaccharides for each FOS product. For example, Figure 25 shows the HPAEC-PAD chromatogram for a strawberry yogurt containing the FOS product Actilight-95®. The kestose, nystose, and fructosylnystose peaks and their relative amounts are characteristic of Actilight-95®.

E. Determination of Pectin

Pectin is routinely quantified as galacturonic acid following hydrolysis with NaOH and an enzymatic treatment, as described previously in the section on uronic acids. The structure of pectin, however, has yet to be fully characterized (11). Structural studies aimed at characterizing the complex mixture of acidic and neutral polysaccharides following partial hydrolysis of pectin have been hampered in the past due to the limitations of the chromatographic techniques (11). Prior to the development of HPAEC-PAD, the largest underivatized oligogalacturonic acid that

---

Fig. 24 Determination of chain length distribution profiles of inulins. (a) HPAEC-PAD analysis of purified inulin. Column: CarboPac PA1 (10 μM, 250 × 4 mm i.d.) with guard. Eluent A, 0.1 M NaOH, eluent B 0.1 M NaOH/1.0 M sodium acetate. Gradient 20–60% B in 40 minutes. Flow rate: 1.0 mL/min. Detection: pulsed amperometry, Au electrode, range 3 μA. (Sample courtesy of Dr. C. Mitchell, California Natural Products, Manteca, CA.) (b) HPAEC-PAD analysis of Raftiline, a commercial inulin-based product using HPAEC-PAD. Peaks: 1, glucose; 2, fructose; 3, sucrose; 4, GF_2; 5, F_3; 6, GF_3; 7, F_4; 8, GF_4; 9, F_5; 10, GF_5; 11, F_6; 12, GF_6. (Chromatogram and peak assignments kindly provided by H. Hoebregs, Raffinerie Tirlmontoise S.A., Tienen, Belgium.)

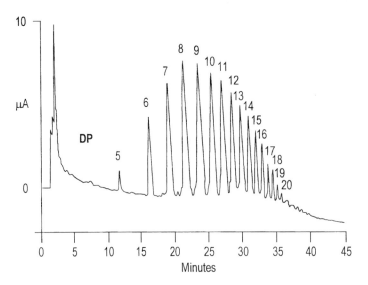

Fig. 26 Chromatogram of a pectin hydrolysate showing incomplete conversion to free uronic acids by the hydrolysis treatment. Column: CarboPac PA1 (10 μM, 250 × 4 mm i.d.) with guard. Eluent: gradient, 100 mM NaOH/240 mM sodium acetate to 100 mM NaOH/480 mM sodium acetate in 15 minutes. Temp.: ambient. Detection: pulsed amperometric, Au electrode, range 300 nA.

could be separated was DP 11 (11). Separation of oligogalacturonic acids in the DP range of 2–50 have been reported by Hotchkiss et al. (11). Figure 26 shows a typical chromatogram of underivatized oligogalacturonic acids from a pectin hydrolysate using HPAEC-PAD. HPLC has also been used in the determination of the methyl esterification pattern in pectin (77). In this case HPAEC-PAD was used to separate and quantitate unesterified galacturonic acid–containing oligomers.

F. Determination of Hydrocolloids

Hydrocolloids such as guar and locust bean gum are widely used food ingredients that also fall under Trowell's extended definition of dietary fiber. The high molecular weight of these materials has made them difficult to identify and quantitate. A method has been developed for isolation, identification, and determination of these materials in food products (78). The method utilizes standard techniques for starch removal and hydrolysis in conjunction with gradient HPAEC-PAD to generate chromatograms, including both monosaccharides and uronic acid components. These monosaccharide/uronic acid "fingerprints" allow gums and pectin from various sources to be distinguished and quantified. Figure 27 shows (a) a reference chromatogram for guar gum and (b) a chromatogram for a fruit preparation that contains guar gum. The galacturonic acid peak is due to pectin from the fruit.

G. Determination of Polydextrose

Polydextrose is a synthetic carbohydrate polymer that is produced from dextrose, sorbitol, and citric acid by a vacuum polycondensation process, which is marketed commercially as a functional food ingredient. A recent article (79) and Chapter 3 of this handbook provide detailed information on the properties and analysis of polydextrose. Methodology for the determination of polydextrose in low-calorie foodstuffs has been developed that utilizes HPAEC-PAD (80).

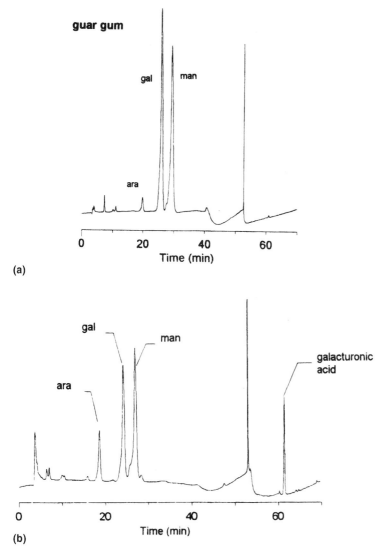

guar gum

gal

man

ara

0   20   40   60
Time (min)

(a)

gal

man

galacturonic
acid

ara

0   20   40   60
Time (min)

(b)

Fig. 27 HPAEC-PAD analysis of hydrocolloid food ingredients: (a) reference chromatogram for guar gum and (b) a chromatogram for a fruit preparation containing guar gum. The galacturonic acid peak is due to pectin from the fruit. Columns: 2 Dionex CarboPac PA1 (10 μM, 250 × 4 mm i.d.) in series, with CarboPac PA1 guard (50 × 4 mm i.d.). (Adapted from Ref. 76.)

Sample clean-up involves extraction of polydextrose with water and enzymatic degradation of interfering polysaccharides such as starch and inulin. Recoveries ranged from 94 to 106% for unbaked goods and from 100 to 115% for baked goods. An improved version of this method has been developed (79) and has been approved for an AOAC interlaboratory validation study.

H. Determination of β-Glucan

β-Glucans are naturally occuring glucose polymers that qualify as dietary fiber since they are nondigestable due to the absence in humans of an enzyme capable of hydrolyzing β-glucosidic linkages (81). They are important as functional food additives (81). HPLC has been utilized in structural studies on β-glucans (82) to separate and quantify the water-soluble and water-insoluble oligosaccharides released by the action of lichenase on oat and barley β-glucans. HPAEC-PAD of the major products 3-O-β-cellobiosyl-D-glucose and 3-O-β-cellotriosyl-D-glucose allowed rapid definition of the major structural features of different β-glucans without prior purification (82). Figure 28 shows chromatograms of oligosaccharides released following lichenase digestion of oat and barley β-glucans.

I. Determination of Pentosans

The pentosans are the major nonstarch polysaccharides of wheat and rye endosperm and consist mainly of arabinoxylans (83,84). They are important because they markedly influence the functional properties of wheat and rye flour in spite of the fact that they are present at relatively low levels (<5%) (83). Determination of the pentosan content is therefore necessary both for

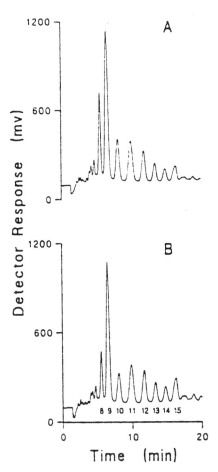

Fig. 28 HPAEC-PAD chromatograms of oligosaccharides in water-insoluble material released during lichenase digestion from (A) oat and (B) barley β-glucans. Column: CarboPac PA1 (10 μM, 250 × 4 mm i.d.) with guard. Eluent: 150 mM sodium hydroxide/105 mM sodium acetate for 1 minute, 1–9 minutes linear gradient to 150 mM sodium hydroxide/150 mM sodium acetate, then hold at 150 mM sodium hydroxide/150 mM sodium acetate for 2 minutes. Flowrate: 1.0 mL/min. Temp.: ambient. Detector: pulsed amperometric, Au electrode. (Adapted from Ref. 82.)

research and for routine analysis of commercial food constituents and products, e.g., flours, doughs, and baked products. GLC and colorimetric methods have been developed but require a time-consuming sample pretreatment to remove interferences from starch-derived glucose (84). A fast and simple HPLC method has been developed (84). Wheat flour is first hydrolyzed with 2 M HCl (9 minutes at 100°C), then neutralized and treated with glucose oxidase to remove excess glucose by conversion to gluconic acid. Arabinose, galactose, glucose, and xylose are determined isocratically (2-deoxy-D-glucose internal standard) on a CarboPac PA1 column with PAD. Gluconic acid does not interfere since it elutes much later than the monosaccharides. RSDs for pentosan content determinations were in the range of 0.03–1.84%.

VI. CONCLUSIONS

The use of HPLC in research and analysis of dietary fiber has expanded rapidly in the last decade. Methods for the determination of dietary fiber have been developed that offer attractive alternatives to previous wet chemical and gravimetric techniques, in that they provide information on composition as well as total amount. Accurate determination of each of the neutral sugars present in hydrolysates of complex carbohydrates and dietary fiber can be made directly without requiring derivatization. Similarly, uronic acids and oligouronic acids derived from complete or partial hydrolysis of pectin can be determined either separately or concurrently with the neutral sugars by using gradient elution. HPLC techniques also lend themselves to the analysis and identification of natural and synthetic carbohydrate food ingredients for which methods have previously been lacking. In dietary fiber research, the compatibility of the HPAEC-PAD technique with gradient elution is proving to be a powerful tool for fundamental studies on cell-wall carbohydrates since it makes possible the high-resolution separation of oligo- and polysaccharide chains. As a result, the determination of chain length distribution profiles of starch and nonstarch oligo- and polysaccharide mixtures can be achieved up to degrees of polymerization as high as 80 in a single run. The technique can also be scaled up to the semi-preparative scale for purification and isolation of milligram quantities of each oligo- or polysaccharide. High-performance size exclusion chromatography with light scattering detection is extremely valuable for on-line determination of the molecular weight of cell-wall carbohydrate fractions, and HPSEC with multiple detection such as conductivity in combination with RI can provide structural information (e.g., the degree of pectin esterification). Future developments in column and detector technology should result in even wider use of HPLC both for automated routine dietary fiber determinations and in research applications.

ACKNOWLEDGMENTS

The author wishes to acknowledge the contribution of the applications and research staff of Dionex Corporation, who performed the chromatographic separations shown in Figs. 6, 7, 11, 18, 22, 23, and 26.

REFERENCES

1. Trowell H. Definition of dietary fibre. Lancet i:503 (1974).
2. Trowell H, Southgate DAT, Wolever TMS, Leeds AR, Sassull MA, Jenkins DJA. Dietary fiber redefined. Lancet i:976 (1976).

3. Theander O, Åman P. Studies on dietary fibres. I. Analysis and chemical characteristics of water-soluble and water insoluble dietary fibres. Swedish J Agric Res 9(3):97–106 (1979).

4. Slavin JL, Marlett JA. Evaluation of high-performance liquid chromatography for measurement of the neutral saccharides in neutral detergent fibre. J Agric Food Chem 31(3):467–471 (1983).

5. Windham WR, Barton FF, II, Himmelsbach DS. High-pressure liquid chromatographic analysis of component sugars in neutral detergent fiber for representative warm- and cool-season grasses. J Agric Food Chem 31:471–475 (1983).

6. Neilson MJ, Marlett JA. Comparison between detergent and non-detergent analyses of dietary fibre in human foodstuffs using high-performance liquid chromatography to measure neutral sugar composition. J Agric Food Chem 31(6):1342–1347 (1983).

7. Quigley ME, Englyst HN. Determination of neutral sugars and hexosamines by high performance liquid chromatography with pulsed amperometric detection. Analyst 117:1715–17181 (1992).

8. Harris PJ, Blakeney AB, Henry RJ, Stome BA. Gas chromatographic determination of the monosaccharide composition of plant cell wall preparations. J AOAC 71(2):272–275 (1988).

9. Englyst HN, Quigley ME, Hudson GJ, Cummings JH. Determination of dietary fibre as non-starch polysaccharides by gas-liquid chromatography. Analyst 117:1207–1717 (1992).

10. Garleb KA, Bourquin LD, Fahey Jr GC. Neutral monosaccharide composition of various fibrous substances: a comparison of hydrolytic procedures and use of anion-exchange high-performance liquid chromatography with pulsed amperometric detection. J Agric Food Chem 37:1287 (1989).

11. Hotchkiss Jr AT, Hicks KB. Analysis of oligogalacturonic acids with 50 or fewer residues by high performance anion-exchange chromatography and pulsed amperometric detection. Anal Biochem 184:200–206 (1990).

12. Nollet LML, ed. Food Analysis by HPLC. New York: Marcel Dekker, Inc., 1992.

13. Robards K, Haddad PR, Jackson PE. Principles and Practice of Modern Chromatographic Methods. London: Academic Press, Harcourt Brace and Company, 1994.

14. Scott RPW. Techniques and Practices of Chromatography. New York: Marcel Dekker, 1995.

15. Meyer VR. Practical High-Performance Liquid Chromatography, 2nd ed. New York: Wiley, 1994.

16. Churms SC. Recent progress in carbohydrate separation by high performance liquid chromatography based on hydrophilic interaction. J Chromatogr A 720(1–2):75–91 (1996).

17. DeVries JW, Nelson AL. Meeting analytical needs for nutritional labeling, Food Technol. 48(7):77 (1994).

18. Lee SC, DeVries JW, Sullivan DM. Carbohydrate/dietary fiber analysis for nutrition labeling. Methods of Analysis for Nutrition Labeling, p. 74. Gaithersburg, MD: AOAC International, 1993.

19. Shaw PE. Handbook of Sugar Separations in Foods by HPLC., p. 29. Boca Raton, FL: CRC Press Inc., 1988.

20. Scott FW. In: Food Analysis by HPLC, Nollet LML, ed., pp. 262, 268, 271. New York, Marcel Dekker, 1992.

21. Nishikawa T, Suzuki S, Kubo H, Ohtani H. On-column isomerization of sugars during high-performance liquid chromatography: analysis of the elution profiles. J Chromatogr A 720:167–172 (1996).

22. Hicks KB, Lim PC, Haas J. Analysis of uronic and aldonic acids, their lactones and related compounds by high performance liquid chromatography on cation-exchange resins. J Chromatogr 319:159–171 (1985).

23. Koizumi K, Fukuda M, Hizukuri S. High performance anion exchange chromatography of homogeneous D-gluco-oligosaccharides and polysaccharides (polymerization degree $\geq$ 50) with pulsed amperometric detection. J Chromatogr 585:233–238 (1991).

24. Churms SC. Recent progress in carbohydrate separation by high performance liquid chromatography based on size exclusion. J Chromatogr A 720:151–166 (1996).

25. Shaw PE. Handbook of Sugar Separations in Foods by HPLC, p. 31. Boca Raton, FL: CRC Press, Inc., 1988.

26. Plöger A. Conductivity detection of pectin: a rapid HPLC method to analyze degree of esterification. J Food Sci 57(5):1185–1186 (1992).

27. Johnson DC, Polta JA. Amperometric detection in liquid chromatography with pulsed cleaning and reaction of noble metal; electrodes. Chromatogr Forum 1:37 (1986).

28. Rocklin RD, Pohl CA. Determination of carbohydrates by anion exchange chromatography with pulsed amperometric detection. J Liquid Chromatogr 6:1577 (1983).
29. Johnson DC, LaCourse WR. Liquid chromatography with pulsed electrochemical detection at gold and platinum electrodes. Anal Chem 62(10):589A–596A (1990).
30. Rocklin RD, Henshall A, Rubin RB. A multimode electrochemical detector for non-UV-absorbing molecules. Am Lab 22(3):34–49 (1990).
31. HPAEC-PAD in food and beverage analysis. Semin Food Anal 2(1/2):1–127 (1997).
32. Lee YC. Carbohydrate analysis with high performance anion exchange chromatography. J Chromatogr A 720(1/2):137–149 (1996).
33. Method for the analysis of sucrose, glucose, and fructose in cane molasses, officially adopted at the 21st session of the International Commission for Uniform Methods of Sugar Analysis, Havana, 1994 (1st action approval AOAC Method 996.04).
34. ISO Method 11292:1995. Instant coffee: determination of free and total carbohydrates—method by high performance anion-exchange chromatography (1st action approval AOAC Method 995.13).
35. 1st action approval AOAC Method 997.08, Determination of fructans in food products.
36. Wong KKY, de Jong E. Size exclusion chromatography of lignin- and carbohydrate-containing samples using alkaline eluents. J Chromatogr A 737:192–203 (1996).
37. Rocklin RD. In: A Practical Guide to HPLC Detection. New York: Academic Press, Inc., 1993, p. 149.
38. LaCourse WR, Dasenbrock CO, Zook CM. Fundamentals and applications of pulsed electrochemical detection in food analysis. Semin Food Anal 2(1/2):5–41 (1997).
39. Rocklin RD, Clarke AP, Weitzhandler M. Improved long-term reproducibility for pulsed amperometric detection of carbohydrates via a new quadrupole-potential waveform. Anal Chem 70:1496–1501 (1998).
40. Technical Note 21, Dionex Corporation, 1228 Titan Way, Sunnyvale, CA 94088.
41. LaCourse WR, Johnson DC. Optimization of waveforms for pulsed amperometric detection (PAD) of carbohydrates following separation by liquid chromatography. Anal Chem 65:55 (1993).
42. Technical Note 40, Dionex Corporation, 1228 Titan Way, Sunnyvale, CA 94088.
43. Niessen WMA, Schols HA, van der Hoeven RAN, Voragen AGJ, van der Grief J. Characterization of oligosaccharides derived from plant cell wall polysaccharides by on-line high performance anion-exchange chromatography thermospray mass spectrometry. In: Modern Methods of Plant Analysis, Vol. 87, Plant Cell Wall Analysis, H. F. Liebern and J. W. Jackson (Eds.), pp. 147–163. Berlin: Springer, 1996.
44. Schols HA, Mutter M, Voragen AGJ, Niessen WMA, van der Hoeven RAM, van der Greef J, Bruggink C. The use of combined high-performance anion-exchange chromatography-thermospray mass spectrometry in the structural analysis of pectic oligosaccharides. Carbohydr Res 261:335–342 (1994).
45. Schols HA, Luca-Lockhorst G, Voragen AGJ. Isolation and characterization of cell wall polysaccharides from soybeans. Carbohydr Netherlands:7–10 (1993).
46. van der Hoeven RAM, Hofte AJP, Tjaden UR, van der Greeg J, Torto N, Gorton L, Marko-Varga G, Bruggink C. Sensitivity improvements in the analysis of oligosaccharides by on-line high-performance anion exchange chromatography/ion spray mass spectrometry. Rapid Comm Mass Spec 12:69–74 (1998).
47. Rabin S, Stillian J, Barreto V, Friedman K, Toofan M. New membrane-based electrolytic suppressor device for suppressed conductivity detection in ion chromatography. J Chromatogr 640:97–109 (1993).
48. Henshall A, Rabin S, Statler J, Stillian J. A recent development in ion chromatography detection. Am Lab 330:20R (1992).
49. van der Hoeven RAM, Niessen WMA. Characterization of sugar oligomers by on-line high performance anion exchange chromatography-thermospray mass spectrometry. J Chromatogr 627:63–73 (1992).
50. Garleb KA, Bourquin LD, Fahey Jr GC. Galacturonate in pectic substances from fruits and vegetables: comparison of anion exchange HPLC with pulsed amperometric detection to standard colorimetric procedure. J Food Sci 56(2):423–426 (1991).

51. Bourquin LD, Garleb KA, Merchen NR, Fahey Jr GC. Effect of intake of forage levels on site and extent of digestion of plant cell wall monomeric components of sheep. J Anim Sci 68:2479–2495 (1990).

52. Cambell JM, Flickinger EA, Fahey Jr GC. A comparative study of dietary fiber methodologies using pulsed electrochemical detection of monosaccharide constituents. Semin Food Anal 2:43–53 (1997).

53. Li EW. Analysis of food carbohydrates: sugars, starches, and dietary fiber polysaccharides. In: New Techniques in the Analysis of Food. New York: Plenum Publishing Corp., pp. 193–200.

54. Redondo A, Villaneuva MJ, Rodriguez MD. High performance liquid chromatographic determination of dietary fiber in raw and processed carrots. J Chromatogr A 677(2):273–278 (1994).

55. Englyst MN, Cummings JH. Improved method for the determination of dietary fiber in plant foods. J AOAC 71(4):808–814 (1988).

56. Brighenti F, Testolini G, Ciappellano S, Porrini M, Simonetti P. Total fiber and qualitative and quantitative composition of available carbohydrates in commercial whole grain foods: an analysis procedure combining enzymatic and chromatographic steps. Riv Soc Ital Aliment 16(3):199–204 (1987).

57. Rodriguez MD, Redondo A, Villaneuva MJ, Wolters M, Bos KD. Comparative study of two chromatographic methods: HPLC and GC, for the determination of non-starch polysaccharides in vegetables. Alimentaria 34(276):79–83 (1996).

58. Voragen AG, Schols HA, De Vries JA, Pilnik W. High-performance liquid chromatographic analysis of uronic acids and oligogalacturonic acids. J Chromatogr 244:327–336 (1982).

59. Vazquez-Blanco ME, Lopez-Hernandez J, Vazquez-Oderiz ML, Simal-Lozano J, Gonzalez-Castro MJ. Determination of pectins by HPLC. A comparison of two methods applied to green beans. J Chromatogr Sci 33(10):551–553 (1995).

60. Wei Y-A, Fang J-N. Studies on the chromatographic behavior of some uronic acids on an aminobonded phase column. J Chromatogr 513:227–235 (1990).

61. Quigley ME, Englyst HN. Determination of the uronic acid constituents of non-starch polysaccharides by high-performance liquid chromatography with pulsed amperometric detection. Analyst 119:1511–1518 (1994).

62. De Ruiter GA, Schols HA, Voragen AGJ, Rombouts FM. Carbohydrate analysis of water-soluble uronic acid-containing polysaccharides with high performance anion exchange chromatography using methanolysis combined with TFA [trifluoroacetic acid] hydrolysis is superior to four other methods. Anal Biochem 207(1):176–185 (1992).

63. Feste AS, Khan I. Separation of gluco-oligosaccharides and polysaccharide hydrolysates by gradient-elution hydrophilic interaction chromatography with pulsed amperometric detection. J Chromatogr 630:129–139 (1993).

64. Churms SC. Recent progress in carbohydrate separation by high performance liquid chromatography based on size exclusion. J Chromatogr A 720:156 (1996).

65. Wong KS, Jane J. Quantitative analysis of debranched amylopectin by HPAEC-PAD with a post-column reactor. J Liq Chromatogr Rel Technol 20(2):297–310 (1997).

66. Wong KS, Jane J. Effects of pushing agents in the separation and detection of debranched amylopectin by high performance anion-exchange chromatography with pulsed amperometric detection. J Chromatogr 18(1):63–80 (1995).

67. Koizumi K, Fukuda M, Hizukuri S. High performance anion exchange chromatography of homogeneous D-gluco-oligosaccharides and polysaccharides (polymerization degree $\geq$ 50) with pulsed amperometric detection. J Chromatogr 585:233–238 (1991).

68. Koizumi K, Kubota Y, Tanomoto T, Okada Y. High-performance anion-exchange chromatography of homogeneous D-gluco-oligosaccharides and -polysaccharides (polymerization degree greater than or equal to 50) with pulsed amperometric detection. J Chromatogr 464:365–373 (1989).

69. Chatterton J, Harrison PA, Thornley WR, Bennett JH. Purification and quantification of kestoses (fructosylsucroses) by gel permeation and anion exchange chromatography. Plant Physiol Biochem 27(2):289–295 (1989).

70. Supri JL. Analysis of 1-kestose, nystose, 1-f-fructofuranosyl nystose in a lactose powder matrix. Poster #89D-20, IFT Annual Meeting, New Orleans, LA, June 22–26, 1996.

71. Ling S-C, Lee W-C. Separation of a fructo-oligosaccharide mixture by hydrophilic interaction chromatography using silica-based micropellicular sorbents. J Chromatogr A 803:302–306 (1998).

72. Hubert Hoebregs, Tiense Suikerraffinaderij NV, Raffinerie Tirlemontoise SA. Private communication, Tienen, Belgium.
73. Timmermans JW, van Leeuwen MB, Tournois H, deWit D, Vliegenthart J. Quantitative analysis of the molecular weight distribution of inulin by means of anion exchange HPLC with pulsed amperometric detection. J Carbohydr Chem 13(6):881–888 (1994).
74. Quemener B, Thibault JF, Coussement P. Determination of inulin and oligofructose in food products and integration in the AOAC method for measurement of total dietary fiber. Lebensm-Wiss Technol 27:125–132 (1994).
75. Hoebregs H. Fructans in foods and food products, ion exchange-chromatographic method: collaborative study J AOAC Int 80(5):1029–1037 (1997).
76. Durgnat J-M, Martinez C. Determination of fructooligosaccharides in raw materials and finished products by HPAE-PAD. Semin Food Anal 2:85–97 (1997).
77. Mort AJ, Qiu F, Maness NO. Determination of the pattern of methyl esterification in pectin. Distribution of contiguous nonesterified residues. Carbohydr Res 247:321–335 (1993).
78. Koswig S, Fuchs G, Hofsommer HJ. Semin Food Anal 2:71–83 (1997).
79. Craig SA, Holden JP, Auerbach MH, Frier HI. Polydextrose as soluble fiber: physiological and analytical aspects. Cereal Foods World 43(5):370–376 (1998).
80. Stumm I, Baltes W. Determination of polydextrose in food by means of ion chromatography and pulsed amperometric detection. Zeitschrift Unters Forsch 195:246–249 (1992).
81. Jezequel V. Curdlan: a new functional β-glucan. Cereal Foods World 45(5):361–364 (1988).
82. Wood PJ, Weisz J, Blackwell BA. Structural studies of (1 → 3), (1 → 4)-β-D-glucans by 13C-nuclear magnetic resonance spectroscopy and by rapid analysis of cellulose-like regions using high-performance anion-exchange chromatography of oligosaccharides released by lichenase. Cereal Chem 70(3):301–307 (1994).
83. Rouau X, Surget A. A rapid semi-automated method for the determination of total and water-extractable pentosans in wheat flours. Carbohydr Polym 24:123–132 (1994).
84. Houben R, de-Ruijter CF, Brunt K. Determination of the pentosan content of wheat products by hydrolysis, glucose oxidase treatment and analysis by HPAEC-PAD. J Cereal Sci 26(1):37–46 (1997).

22

Dietary Fiber–Associated Compounds: Chemistry, Analysis, and Nutritional Effects of Polyphenols

Fulgencio D. Saura-Calixto and Laura Bravo
Instituto del Frío, Consejo Superior de Investigaciones Científicas, Madrid, Spain

I. INTRODUCTION

Phenolic compounds or polyphenols (PP) constitute one of the most numerous and widely distributed group of substances in the plant kingdom. They are present in all plant organs, having important significance in plant physiology. Thus, PP are involved in the resistance of plants to pathogens, parasites, and predators, protecting crops from preharvest seed germination and plague. On the other hand, some phenolic compounds such as flavonoids have therapeutical applications as antibiotics, antidiarrheic, or anti-inflammatory agents or in the treatment of hypertension, vascular fragility, radiation damage, allergies, hypercholesterolemia, and other diseases (1). Besides their pharmacological uses, PP have a range of industrial applications such as in the manufacture of paints, in cosmetics, as tanning agents, or in the food industry as additives. Moreover, being ubiquitous in all plant organs, polyphenols inevitably constitute an integral part of both human and animal diets.

Considering all these factors, polyphenols clearly stand out as a most important group of plant substances. Consequently, in spite of their great chemical complexity, efforts have been made to study PP in a number of plant products with different approaches: chemical, biochemical, pharmacological, nutritional, agronomic, etc. Within the scope of the present book, we intend to approach polyphenolic compounds from a nutritional point of view, specifically addressing the importance of PP in the analysis of dietary fiber. A brief description of the chemistry of polyphenolic compounds and their occurrence in plant foods will also be included.

A. Chemistry of Polyphenolic Compounds

Polyphenols are products of the secondary metabolism of plants, biogenetically arising from two main synthetic pathways: the shikimate pathway and the acetate pathway (2). They range from simple molecules like phenolic acids to highly polymerized substances such as tannins, their basic chemical structures being benzene and flavone. Phenolics are mostly found in plants in conjugated form, principally with one or more sugar residues linked to hydroxyl groups. The associated sugars can be present as mono-, di-, tri-, or tetrasaccharides and include glucose, galactose, arabinose, rhamnose, xylose, mannose, apiose, allose, and glucuronic and galacturonic acids, among others. Association with other compounds such as carboxylic and organic acids, amines, lipids, and also linkages with other phenols are known. For instance, the most commonly occurring flavonoid, quercetin, is known to occur in 135 different associations (*O*-glycosides, *O*-sulfates, and conjugated with sugars acylated with aromatic and aliphatic acids) (2). Therefore, the study of such a large and complex group of compounds, with over 8000 phenolic structures known to date (3), is considerably difficult.

Polyphenols can be divided into at least 10 different classes according to their basic chemical structure. The most important single group, the flavonoids, can be further subdivided into 15 classes, with over 5000 compounds described by 1990 (3). A number of comprehensive reviews on the chemistry of plant phenolics can be found in the literature (2–7).

Table 1 and Fig. 1 show the main classes of PP found in plant foods according to Harborne (2). Simple phenols, phenolic acids and derivatives, and phenylpropanoids are among the most common low molecular weight phenolic compounds. Phenylpropanoid derivatives such as the cinnamyl alcohols are the basic constituents of lignin and thus form one of the major groups of plant phenolics, present in the cell walls of all vascular plants. On the other hand, flavonoids are the most ubiquitous group of polyphenols, occurring in all plant organs (roots, tubers, stems, flowers, fruits, etc.) and even in plant exudates. All of these compounds conform the vast majority of plant phenolics. They can be found free, although their corresponding methyl and ethyl esters and glycosides occur very commonly. Most of these compounds, of relatively low molecular weights, are soluble according to their polarity and chemical structure (degree of hydroxyla-

Table 1 Main Classes of Food Polyphenols

Class (basic chemical structure)	Examples
Simple phenols (C_6)	Resorcinol, orcinol, thymol, cresol, phenol
Phenolic acids and aldehyes (C_6-C_1)	Gallic acid, vanillin, *p*-hydroxybenzoic acid, syringaldehyde
Phenylpropanoids (C_6-C_3)	Hydroxycinnamic acids (*p*-coumaric, caffeic, ferulic, sinapic)
	Cinnamyl alcohols (guaiacyl, *p*-coumaryl alcohol, syringyl)
	Coumarins (umbilliferone, aesculetin, scopoletin)
Stilbenes (C_6-C_2-C_6)	Resveratrol
Flavonoids (C_6-C_3-C_6)	
Flavones	Apigenin, luteolin
Flavonols	Quercetin, myricetin, kaempferol
Flavanones	Naringenin, hesperidin
Flavanols	Catechin, epicatechin
Flavandiols	Leucoanthocyanidins
Anthocyanidins	Pelargonidin, malvidin, cyanidin
Isoflavonoids	Daidzein, genistein
Tannins	
Hydrolyzable tannins	
Condensed tannins or proanthocyanidins (C_6-C_3-C_6)$_n$	
Lignin (C_6-C_3)$_n$	
Other less common polyphenols	
Benzoquinones, naftoquinones, anthraquinones, acetophenones, phenylacetic acids, benzophenones, xanthones, chromones, phenanthrenes, chalcones, aurones, flavans, biflavonoids, etc.	

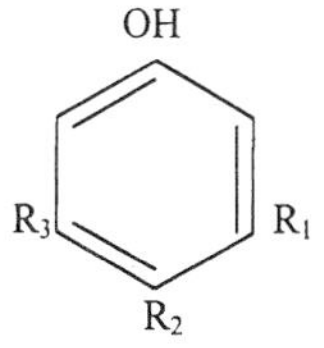

1. $R_1 = R_2 = R_3 = H$: phenol
2. $R_1 = R_3 = H; R_2 = CH_3$: *p*-cresol
3. $R_1 = OH; R_2 = R_3 = H$: resorcinol
4. $R_1 = R_3 = OH; R_2 = H$: phloroglucinol

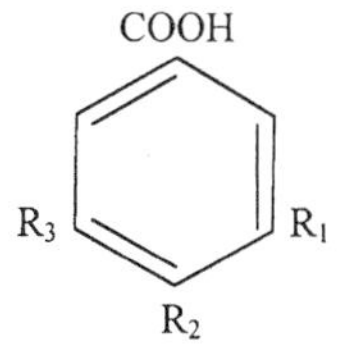

5. $R_1 = OCH_3; R_2 = OH$: vanillic acid
6. $R_1 = R_2 = R_3 = OH$: gallic acid
7. $R_1 = R_3 = OCH_3; R_2 = OH$: syringic

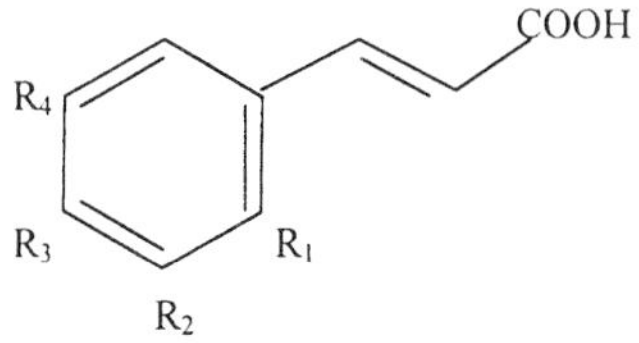

8. $R_1 = R_2 = R_4 = H; R_3 = OH$; *p*-coumaric
9. $R_1 = R_2 = H; R_3 = R_4 = OH$; caffeic
10. $R_1 = R_4 = H; R_2 = OMe; R_3 = OH$: ferulic

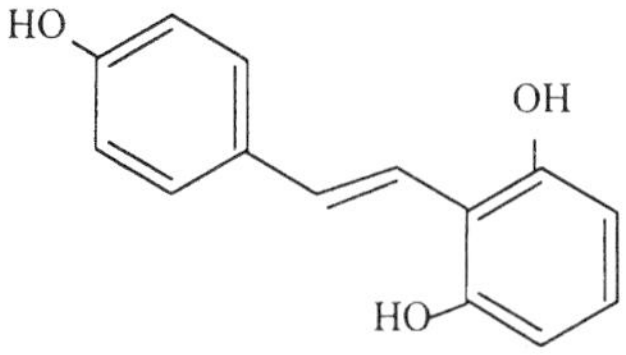

11. Resveratrol

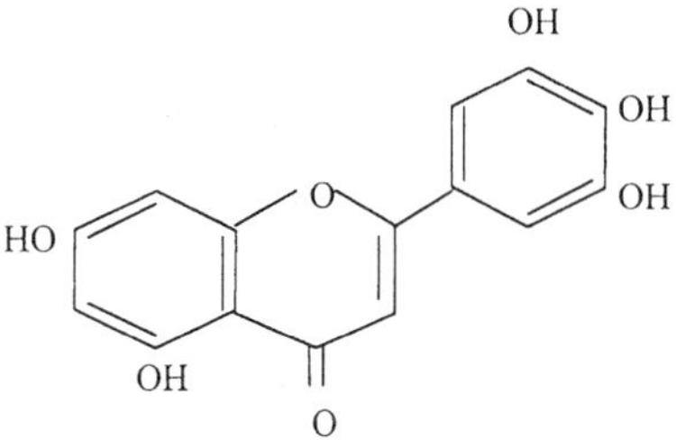

12. Quercetin

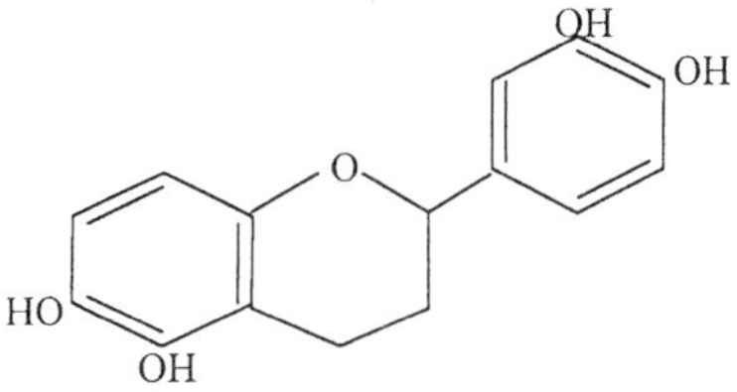

13. Catechin

Fig. 1 Examples of some common food polyphenols

tion, glycosylation, acylation, etc.). Some of them, however, can be linked to cell wall components (polysaccharides, lignin). Due to the nature of the ester linkages, they can be solubilized in alkaline conditions, otherwise being retained in the fiber matrix. When ingested, intestinal pH or degradation of fiber constituents during fermentation would release some of these polyphenols.

Another group of polymeric polyphenols widely distributed in plant foods are the tannins. Tannins are compounds of intermediate to high molecular mass. Average molecular weights of around 5000 daltons are common, although they can occur as polymers of molecular mass up to 32,000 (8). Tannins are characterized by their high degree of hydroxylation, which confers upon them the ability to form insoluble complexes with carbohydrates and protein.

Plant tannins are classified in two major groups: hydrolyzable and condensed (9). Another group, the phlorotannins, is only found in marine brown algae and is not commonly consumed by humans (10).

Hydrolyzable tannins consist of gallic acid and derivatives esterified to a polyol, mainly glucose (9). These compounds are easily hydrolyzed with acid, alkali, or hot water or by enzymatic action. They can be further subdivided into gallotannins or ellagitannins, according to the nature of the monomeric phenolic constituent. The best-known hydrolyzable tannin is tannic acid, a gallotannin consisting of a pentagalloyl glucose molecule that can further esterify with another five gallic acid units.

Condensed tannins (CT) or proanthocyanidins are polymers of high molecular weight. The monomeric unit is a flavan-3-ol (catechin, epicatechin, etc.), the precursor of which is a flavan-3,4-diol or leukoanthocyanidin molecule. The proanthocyanidins most commonly referred in the literature are oligomers (dimers, trimers, tetramers) due to the difficulty in the analysis of highly polymerized molecules. However, they can occur as polymers with degrees of polymerization of 50 and greater, and condensed tannins of molecular weights over 30,000 have been described (8). Interflavanoid linkages are acid labile, rendering monomeric anthocyanidins upon acid hydrolysis in alcoholic solutions. This reaction is used for determination of proanthocyanidin molecules.

Oligomeric proanthocyanidins and lower molecular weight hydrolyzable tannins are soluble in the usual solvents (aqueous acetone and methanol, water, etc.). However, high molecular weight condensed and hydrolyzable tannins are insoluble. Also, when tannins are forming complexes with protein or cell wall polysaccharides, they remain insoluble, resisting enzymatic hydrolysis and modifying protein and carbohydrate digestibility.

B. Food Polyphenols

As constituents of plant foods, PP are partly responsible for their sensory and nutritional quality. At low concentrations PP protect plants from oxidation, being involved in the disease resistance of plants. The browning reaction of phenolic compounds via enzymatic (catalyzed by the polyphenol oxidase) or nonenzymatic reactions is responsible for the formation of undesirable color and flavor in fruits and vegetables (11,12). On the other hand, oxidative changes of PP during processing result in the development of distinctive and desirable organoleptic characteristics of certain foods, such as the browning of cocoa or the oxidative polymerization of tea polyphenols during the manufacture of black tea. Also, the astringency and bitterness of foods and beverages depends on their polyphenolic compound content.

Dietary PP are almost ubiquitous in plant foods (fruits, vegetables, cereals, legumes, nuts, etc.) and beverages (tea, wine, cider, beer, cocoa, etc.). Their levels in plants vary greatly even between cultivars of the same species and are largely influenced by genetic factors and environmental conditions, as well as by factors such as germination, ripening, processing, or storage (13). Nevertheless, due to the complexity of this group of substances, there is no total agreement as to the nomenclature of phenolic compounds or in the adoption of an appropriate methodology to analyze the different types of families of polyphenolic compounds. As a consequence of this, information in the literature on the content and composition of PP in plant foods is not only incomplete but also sometimes contradictory and difficult to compare.

The range of polyphenolic content of different foods and beverages is shown in Table 2. For extensive data, readers are referred to the monograph recently published by Shahidi and Naczk (12) and to Kühnau's comprehensive review on food flavonoids (1). Most polyphenols analyzed in foods are phenolic acids and flavonoids (including anthocyanins, flavanones, flavanols, etc.), while the tannin contents referred to in the literature are usually very low. Nonethe-

Table 2 Polyphenolic Content of Different Foods and Beverages

Food	Polyphenolic content[a]	Beverage	Polyphenolic content
Legumes	0.1–1.5 (% d.m.)	Tea	15–30 (% dry leaves)
			150–210 (mg/200 mL)
Cereals	0.1–10 (% d.m.)	Coffee	6–9 (% dry beans)
			200–550 (mg/150 mL)
Vegetables	0.3–10 (% d.m.)	Cocoa	12–18 (% dry beans)
Fruits	2–225 (mg/100 g f.m.)	Wine	250–4000 (mg/L)
Berries	20–400 (mg/100 g f.m.)	Fruit juices	2–7000 (mg/L)
Nuts	0.1–34 (% d.m.)	Beer	60–100 (mg/L)
Olive oil	0.5–8%		

[a] d.m.: dry matter; f.m.: fresh matter.

less, most analyses are performed in extracts obtained from plant foods. In this case, insoluble tannins (highly polymerized molecules or tannins bound to cell wall constituents and protein) are not determined following the usual quantitative methodologies, and the actual content of tannins is usually underestimated. Foods like legumes, grapes, cocoa, nuts, etc. are likely to contain appreciable amounts of insoluble tannins.

Concerning the intake of dietary polyphenols, there is no accurate information. Kühnau (1) estimated an average daily flavonoid intake in the United States of 1 g in winter and spring increasing to up to 1.1 g in summer and autumn, at which time consumption of fruits is also increased. Nevertheless, these data were restricted to the intake of flavonoids in 1971, when only about 800 different flavonoids were known. Considering that the number of flavonoid structures known by 1990 increased to over 5000 (3), these figures would be expected to be considerably higher. However, recent investigations report on much lower intakes of two types of flavonoids (flavonols and flavones, 23 mg/d in the Dutch diet) (14) than those reported by Kühnau (115 mg/d of these two flavonoids in the U.S. diet) (1). Nevertheless, none of these studies considered the intake of other phenolic compounds. Moreover, as mentioned before, the actual polyphenolic content of plant foods is often underestimated since analysis of many PP, mainly insoluble compounds that can be quantitatively more important than flavonoids, is neglected, and therefore their actual content in foods not considered in the estimation of PP intake. Thus, accurate estimations of total polyphenolic intakes are not available. On the other hand, information on the bioavailability of food phenolics is rather limited, and this is a most determinant factor when evaluating the nutritional significance of these compounds.

II. POLYPHENOL-RICH DIETARY FIBER—ANALYTICAL IMPLICATIONS

A. Problems Derived from the Presence of Polyphenolic-Associated Compounds in the AOAC Method for Dietary Fiber Determination

The most widely used method for the determination of dietary fiber (DF) in foods is the AOAC enzymatic-gravimetric method (15), official in most European countries and the United States. Briefly, it consists of the enzymatic removal of most starch and protein from the food sample and the gravimetric quantification of the remaining residues after correction for their ash and protein content. Separate values for soluble and insoluble DF fractions can be obtained, or alternatively the total DF content can be directly quantified after precipitation of soluble fiber components. This method quantifies dietary fiber as nonstarch polysaccharides plus lignin, according to the official definition (16). However, the presence of high amounts of polyphenolic compounds in certain plant foods can lead to errors in the quantification of their DF content, resulting in many cases in the overestimation of their real DF content.

Insoluble polyphenols, both highly polymerized condensed tannins or proanthocyanidins and PP that are covalently linked to protein and polysaccharides from cell walls, are highly indigestible compounds that resist enzymatic hydrolysis with the amylolytic and proteolytic enzymes used in the analysis of DF (17–20). Therefore, these compounds would be recovered in the residues gravimetrically quantified as insoluble dietary fiber (IDF). Moreover, PP have a wide range of solubilities. During precipitation of soluble dietary fiber (SDF) in 80% ethanol, low and intermediate molecular weight phenolics can also co-precipitate. This, along with the presence of PP associated to the SDF matrix, would result in the quantification of these polyphenolic compounds as DF constituents. Therefore, even in foods with low polyphenolic content, the presence of these associated substances can result in overestimation of their actual DF content.

Data confirm these facts. Thus, the analysis of a variety of food samples with CT concentrations ranging from <1% to >30% of the dry matter showed the presence of significant amounts of CT in the IDF residues (Table 3) (17–23). Up to 97% of the CT present in the original material can be recovered after the enzymatic treatments. Even lower molecular weight CT such as the oligomeric proanthocyanidins analyzed in acetone:water (70:30 v/v) extracts in lentils and cocoa were significantly resistant to enzymatic hydrolysis, although to a lesser extent than the highly polymerized molecules. When polyphenols are not minor constituents of the food sample, no correction for their content in fiber residues can involve important quantitative errors as shown in Table 4. Moreover, qualitative errors may also occur since polyphenolic compounds exhibit some physiological properties that can be wrongly attributed to DF (26,27)

The amount of CT present in the IDF residues would depend on the complexity of these compounds: the higher the degree of polymerization, the higher the resistance to enzymatic hydrolysis. Also the capacity of CT to bind to protein and cell wall polysaccharides will determine the amount of tannins present in the fiber residues.

Table 3 Condensed Tannins (CT) and Protein Content in Fractions of Different Plant Materials (g/100 g dry matter)

	Sample		IDF		KL	
	CT	Protein	CT[a]	Protein[a]	Protein[a]	Ref.
Carob pod[b]	17.9	2.7	17.1 (95.5)	1.8 (66.7)	0.8 (29.6)	17
Carob pod concentrate[b]	27.6	5.1	12.7 (46.0)	3.3 (64.7)	—	21
Mesquite pod[b]	0.41	8.1	0.33 (80.5)	2.2 (27.2)	—	22
Spanish sainfoin[b]	7.0	8.2	5.6 (80.0)	2.1 (25.6)	ND	18
Apple pulp[b]	1.6	5.0	1.0 (62.5)	2.7 (54.0)	—	21
Cider wastes[b]	3.1	5.4	3.0 (96.8)	3.0 (55.6)	1.9 (35.2)	19
White grape pomace[b]	14.5	10.7	—	7.5 (70.1)	2.6 (24.3)	20
Red grape pomace[b]	36.4	13.8	—	12.2 (88.4)	2.8 (20.3)	20
Lentils[c]	0.19	21.0	0.05 (26.3)	3.3 (15.6)	—	23
Cocoa[c]	1.15	11.9	0.44 (38.3)	6.8 (56.9)	—	23

ND: Not detected.
[a] Values in parentheses expressed as percentage of condensed tannins (CT) or protein in the original sample.
[b] CT directly analyzed in solid material after boiling in 5% HCl/butanol and reading absorbances at 550 nm (24).
[c] CT analyzed in acetone:water (70:30 v/v) extracts (proanthocyanidins oligomers) after boiling in HCl/butanol and reading absorbances at 550 nm (25).

Table 4 Total Dietary Fiber and Polyphenolic Content of Plant Materials (g/100 g dry matter)

	TDF[a]	PP in DF residue	Corrected TDF[b]	Ref.
Carob pod	36.9	18.0	18.9	17
Spanish sainfoin	68.4	5.9	59.1	18
Cider wastes	65.5	3.1	62.4	19
White grape pomace	59.0	14.5	45.5	20
Red grape pomace	60.8	36.4	24.8	20

[a] Total dietary fiber determined by the AOAC method (15).
[b] Corrected TDF = TDF (AOAC) − PP.

CT have a great affinity for protein, forming insoluble tannin-protein complexes that are not hydrolyzed by digestive enzymes (28–30). Moreover, CT can also inhibit proteolytic enzymes (31–34). Both factors result in reduced digestibility of dietary protein, with increased amounts of resistant protein in the IDF residues, as shown in Table 3. Between 15 and 90% of the initial protein can be present as resistant protein in the IDF fractions. Correction for protein content in the fiber residue would eliminate this interference caused by CT in the official AOAC quantification of DF. Nevertheless, in many cases a modification of the AOAC enzymatic-gravimetric method is used, mostly for research purposes. In this modification, constituent neutral sugars and uronic acids are chemically analyzed in both soluble and insoluble DF fractions after acid hydrolysis (35–39). The residue remaining after acid hydrolysis of IDF (dispersion in 12 M sulfuric acid, 1 h, 30°C, followed by hydrolysis with 1 M sulfuric acid, 90 min, 100°C) is gravimetrically quantified as Klason lignin (KL) without further corrections. However, tannin-protein linkages are strong enough to resist acid hydrolysis, and significant amounts of resistant protein remain in these KL residues, as can be seen in Table 3. Moreover, CT also remain in the KL residues after acid hydrolysis in the form of phlobaphene-like substances (20,40).

In summary, the presence of insoluble polyphenols in plant foods, even in low quantities, would result in the overestimation of the DF content of these foods due to the presence of these tannins in the DF residues (including the KL ones) and to an increased amount of resistant protein being erroneously quantified as KL.

Resistance to enzymatic hydrolysis and presence in DF fractions, however, is not restricted to CT. Soluble phenolic compounds can also be detected in both soluble and insoluble DF fractions, as shown in Table 5. Table 6 shows the presence of total soluble polyphenols (SPP) and

Table 5 Presence of Soluble Polyphenols in Original Samples and Dietary Fiber Fractions of Different Plant Materials (g/100 g dry matter)

	SPP sample	SPP in IDF residue[a]	SPP in SDF[a]	Ref.
Carob pod[b]	1.3	—	0.72 (55.4)	17
Spanish sainfoin[b]	1.1	—	0.30 (27.3)	18
Pear[c]	0.34	0.15 (44.1)	0.19 (55.9)	23
Lentils[c]	0.78	0.27 (34.6)	0.34 (43.6)	23
Cocoa[c]	5.88	1.91 (32.5)	0.20 (3.4)	23

SPP: Soluble polyphenols; IDF: insoluble dietary fiber; SDF: soluble dietary fiber.
[a] Values in parentheses expressed as percentage of SPP in the original sample.
[b] Analyzed in water extracts using the Folin Denis reagent (41). Expressed as catechin equivalents.
[c] Analyzed in acetone:water (70:30 v/v) extracts following the Prussian blue method (42). Expressed as tannic acid equivalents.

Table 6 Presence of Soluble Polyphenols in Fractions from Different Plant Materials (g/100 g dry matter)[a]

		Apple pulp[f]	Carob pod concentrate[f]	Red grape skins[g]	White grape skins[g]	White grape seeds[g]
Extract[b]	SPP[d]	0.34	1.36	3.27	4.02	4.79
	Flavan-3-ol[e]	0.20	0.53	3.29	4.05	5.56
Residue[c]	SPP	0.28	2.18	0.49	0.46	0.42
	Flavan-3-ol	0.12	1.08	0.42	0.33	0.32
IDF gravimetric	SPP	—	—	1.44	1.70	2.27
	Flavan-3-ol	—	—	1.47	1.44	1.98
IDF hydrolysate	SPP	—	—	—	0.34	0.31
	Flavan-3-ol	—	—	—	0.43	0.47
SDF gravimetric	SPP	0.11	0.59	—	—	—
	Flavan-3-ol	0.06	0.17	—	—	—
SDF dialysate	SPP	0.21	2.02	0.68	1.14	1.08
	Flavan-3-ol	0.05	0.60	0.24	0.19	0.20

[a] Soluble polyphenols (SPP) extracted in methanol:water (50:50 v/v) and acetone:water (70:30 v/v). Analysis performed in the combined supernatants. IDF: Insoluble dietary fiber; SDF: soluble dietary fiber.
[b] Methanol:water plus acetone:water extracts except for apple pulp and carob pod (ethanolic extraction only in these samples).
[c] Residue from extraction of SPP subject to a second extraction with methanol:water plus acetone:water.
[d] SPP analyzed using the Folin-Cioclateau reagent (44). Expressed as gallic acid equivalents.
[e] Flavan-3-ol polyphenols analyzed using the HCl/vanillin reagent (41). Expressed as catechin equivalents.
[f] From Ref. 43.
[g] From Ref. 44.

flavan-3-ol phenolics in fractions from different plant materials. Even after extraction, significant amounts of PP remain in the residues obtained after a second extraction treatment. What is most noteworthy is the fact that SPP remain in both insoluble and soluble dietary fiber fractions, their concentration exceeding that analyzed in the residue after the second extraction with methanol: water and acetone:water (for details of the extraction procedure, see Sec. II.B). It is feasible that enzymatic treatments of samples render some phenolic compounds soluble, either by partial depolymerization of condensed polyphenols or by liberation of polyphenols bound to other food components or included within cell structures such as vacuoles. Even after acid hydrolysis of the IDF residue, important amounts of SPP can be detected. Also, after dialysis high amounts of PP remain in the soluble dietary fiber (SDF) fraction, partly co-polymerized to cell wall polysaccharides. Therefore, polyphenolic compounds bring about errors in the gravimetric quantification not only of IDF fractions, but also of SDF either after precipitation or in methods where this fraction is quantified after dialysis and lyophilization (36,46).

To avoid such errors, correction for the PP content of food samples should be introduced in the analytical methods for DF determination. CT should be analyzed in the IDF residue and their content subtracted from the corresponding gravimetric value of IDF or KL. Also protein should be analyzed and corrected in the KL residues. Likewise, correction for SPP present in the SDF fraction should also be introduced when this fiber fraction is quantified gravimetrically (43). Analysis and correction of SPP in IDF is also advisable, although they are a minor component of this fraction and will not greatly affect the gravimetric value, their protein-precipitating capacity being negligible in comparison with CT. However, SPP have important physiological properties that can be wrongly attributed to DF. Therefore, although the quantitative errors derived from the presence of SPP associated to DF residues would be less significant, much more important qualitative errors would derive from these associated bioactive compounds when their occurrence in DF is ignored.

Alternatively, in view of the persistence of this fraction of plant foods in the indigestible residues quantified as DF and considering the physiological properties of polyphenolic compounds, which will be described later in this chapter, it could be reasonable to consider polyphenols as dietary fiber constituents (20,43).

B. Analysis of Polyphenolic Compounds Associated with Dietary Fiber

Whether PP are considered as DF constituents or not, appropriate analysis of these compounds is required either for correction of DF gravimetric values or for estimation of their actual content in plant foods. As mentioned above, however, accurate determination of polyphenols is not a straightforward matter.

The first difficulty in the analysis of plant phenolics relates to the complete extraction of these compounds from the plant material. Polyphenols are polar compounds and moderately soluble in polar solvents such as ethanol, methanol, acetone, diethyl ether, and dimethyl sulfoxide. PP often appear as glycosides attached to one or more sugar molecules, rendering the compound more water soluble, and thus combinations of organic solvents with water are usually employed.

Most analytical procedures measure PP after extraction with one or more solvents. Nonetheless, as shown in Table 6, even combination of several solvent mixtures in a sequential extraction does not attain the total extraction of soluble polyphenols. Moreover, polymeric polyphenols or PP bound to protein or cell wall polysaccharides are not extracted with the usual solvents. These compounds remain in the insoluble residues and usually their quantification is omitted. This results in quantitative and qualitative errors, including an underestimation of the polyphenolic content of certain plant foods, and ignoring or wrongly attributing some of their physiological effects to other food constituents.

Most methods for the analysis of PP employs spectrophotometric techniques, although chromatographic analysis using reversed-phase HPLC has gained great popularity in recent years. Excellent monographs on the analysis of plant phenolics (2) or specifically on flavonoid identification (6) are available. Due to the enormous number of polyphenolic compounds, further problems in the analysis of these substances arise from the lack of appropriate standards.

Terrill et al. (47) developed a method for the separate determination of condensed tannins bound to protein and dietary fiber. This method was based on the extraction with sodium dodecyl sulfate of protein-bound CT from residues obtained after previous removal of extractable CT with acetone:water (70:30 v/v). Soluble and protein-bound CT are determined in the corresponding extracts, whereas fiber-bound CT are analyzed directly in the residue remaining after the extraction of protein-bound tannins.

C. Methodology for the Extraction and Analysis of Polyphenolic Compounds

1. Extraction of Soluble Polyphenols

Aiming at the correction of the PP content of DF fractions, SPP in SDF can be analyzed in this fiber fraction after precipitation or in the dialysates prior to lyophilization. In the case of precipitated SDF fractions, as in food samples, a sequential extraction with aqueous methanol and acetone can be carried out. Samples (SDF residues or 1 g of food sample) are extracted with 40 mL of methanol:water (50:50 v/v) for 1 hour at room temperature with constant agitation. Samples are then centrifuged (15 min, 3000 g) and supernatants transferred into volumetric flasks. The pellets are resuspended in 40 mL acetone:water (70:30 v/v) and the extraction procedure repeated. The supernatants are combined and made up to 100 mL (44). Analysis of soluble polyphenols is performed in the combined supernatants. If chromatographic determinations are carried out for identification of individual phenolics, concentration under vacuum should be performed.

2. Analysis of Soluble Polyphenols

Total soluble polyphenols can be determined in the extracts or in dialysates. A rapid colorimetric method using the Folin-Ciocalteau's reagent is suitable to measure the content of total soluble polyphenols in DF residues or whole sample foods. Aliquots (0.5 mL) are pipetted into 25 mL volumetric flasks and 0.5 mL of Folin-Ciocalteau's reagent is added. After 3 minutes at room temperature, 10 mL of sodium carbonate solution (75 g/L) are added and the volume made up to 25 mL with water. After 1 hour at room temperature with occasional shaking, absorbances are read at 750 nm against a blank prepared in parallel with water instead of sample (45). Tannic acid or gallic acid can be used as standards. This is a nonselective method useful for the determination of the total content of polyphenolic compounds. However, protein interferes with this method. Alternatively, the Prussian blue method can be used (42), which has been reported to interfere less with protein (48).

Additionally, flavan-3-ol derivatives can be quantified in the extracts and dialysates by assaying with the vanillin-HCl reagent using catechin as standard (41). Aliquots (2 mL) are pipetted into 10 mL volumetric flasks and mixed with 2 mL of freshly prepared vanillin-HCl solution (1 g/100 mL 24.5% HCl). Final volume is made up to 10 mL with 24.5% HCl (prepared diluting 700 mL of 35% HCl with 300 mL water). After 25 minutes at room temperature with occasional shaking, absorbances are read at 500 nm against a reagent blank.

3. Analysis of Condensed Tannins

Concerning insoluble PP, proanthocyanidins should be analyzed in the IDF residues. Since these polymeric tannins resist acid hydrolysis, the value analyzed in the IDF can also be used for correction of the KL residue when separate values for constituent neutral sugars, uronic acids, and Klason lignin are required. For quantitative estimation of the CT content of IDF residues or foodstuffs, 10 mL of butanol-HCl (95:5 v/v) are added to samples (50 mg of IDF residues or the plant fraction insoluble in aqueous acetone and methanol) and incubated for 3 hours at 100°C. Absorbances of the anthocyanidin solutions obtained are read at 550 nm against a reagent's blank (24). Purified quebracho, carob pod or grape tannins, or commercial cyanidin could be used as standard. Due to the ability of CT to react with different dietary constituents, they can partly lose their capacity to form anthocyanidins after treatment with butanol-HCl, failing to produce the red solutions quantified spectrophotometrically. This is the case when CT are analyzed in fecal samples. To avoid this problem, an alternative gravimetric method can be used (49). Since CT remain quantitatively in the KL residue after acid hydrolysis (12 M H_2SO_4, 30°C, 30 min plus 1 M H_2SO_4, 100°C, 90 min) (20), gravimetric quantification of this residue corrected for the resistant protein content (determined by the Kjeldahl method as N $\times$ 6.25) would render the CT value.

III. NUTRITIONAL SIGNIFICANCE OF DIETARY FIBER–ASSOCIATED POLYPHENOLS

The nutritional significance of food phenolics will be greatly influenced by the behavior of polyphenols within the gastrointestinal tract. Systemic effects of polyphenolic compounds, either beneficial as in antioxidant polyphenols or deleterious as in some toxic phenols considered as antinutrients, depends on their capacity to interact with macronutrients, digestive enzymes, and the colonic microflora, thus determining the digestibility of food components and/or on their absorption through the intestinal mucosa and metabolism in target organs. Conversely, the digestive fate of polyphenols will depend on their chemical structure, molecular size, and solubility, since not all phenolic compounds seem to be equally susceptible to intestinal digestion and absorption. However, the study of polyphenol bioavailability and physiological implications is greatly hindered by the enormous variability of chemical structures and conjugates found in nature.

Most works in the literature dealing with either the nutritional effects of PP or their intestinal digestibility use extracts of different plant materials made up of a complex mixture of soluble phenolic compounds, which hinders the interpretation of the specific effects and metabolism of individual PP. Also, the metabolism of a specific group of food phenolics, the flavonoids, has been studied either with pure standards or with complex foods in laboratory animals and in humans. Differences in the absorption and metabolism of these compounds when administered as part of a complex foodstuff or as a supplement cannot be ruled out. Besides, the significance of results obtained in animal models into humans is unclear. Moreover, partly due to the difficulty in the analysis and characterization of insoluble PP—highly polymerized or bound tannins—very few data on the intestinal fate of these compounds and their nutritional and physiological importance are reported in the literature, and usually this insoluble fraction is simply ignored.

In order to better understand the nutritional implications of dietary phenols and taking into account their different behavior, PP can be classified according to their solubility in extractable and nonextractable polyphenols (27,50). Extractable polyphenols (EPP) are low and intermediate molecular weight phenolics that can be extracted using different solvents (water, aqueous methanol, acetone), including some hydrolyzable tannins and oligomeric proanthocyanidins.

On the other hand, nonextractable polyphenols (NEPP) are high molecular weight compounds and phenols bound to other food components (protein or cell wall polysaccharides) that remain insoluble in the usual solvents. The main characteristics and physiological properties of these compounds are summarized in Table 7.

One of the best known properties of food phenolics is their capacity to bind and precipitate dietary protein. Insoluble polyphenol-protein complexes pass unaltered through the gastrointestinal tract, being excreted in feces and thus resulting in a reduced protein digestibility (51–53). This protein-binding capacity affects other endogenous proteins, such as salivary proteins (53,54) or digestive enzymes, causing their inhibition (31–34,55). However, although this prop-

Table 7 Nutritional Classification and Main Physiological Properties of Food Polyphenols

Property/Effect	Nonextractable polyphenols (NEPP)	Extractable polyphenols (EPP)
Type of compounds	High MW and/or bound to other food components (protein and cell wall)	Low and intermediate MW (<5000)
	Insoluble[a]	Soluble[a]
Fate in the gastrointestinal tract		
Mouth, complexation with salivary proteins	Minor	Yes
Stomach, hydrolysis	Not affected	Partly (acid pH)
Small intestine		
Endogenous protein complexation	Minor	Yes
Mineral complexation	No	Yes
Enzymatic inhibition	Minor	Yes
Hydrolysis	Minor (some bound phenolics released; alkaline pH)	Partial (bacterial hydrolysis of glycosides; terminal ileum)
Absorption	No	Partial
Large intestine		
Fermentation	Minor; only some fiber-bound NEPP released after fiber fermentation	Bacterial hydrolysis of glycosides and aglycones
Absorption	Only released PP; highly polymerized and bound PP not absorbed	Yes
Effect on colonic microflora	None	Partial interference (by phenolic acids, not flavonoids)
Fecal excretion	Major	Minor
Main physiological effects		
	Decreased protein digestibility	Antioxidants
	Bulking effect	Astringency
	Reduced postprandial glycemia	Reduced postprandial glycemia
	Increased fat excretion	Increased fat excretion
		Mineral malabsorption
Overall behavior (digestibility/physiological effects)	Comparable to IDF	Comparable to SDF

PP, Polyphenols; MW, molecular weight; IDF, insoluble dietary fiber; SDF, soluble dietary fiber.
[a] Solubility in water, aqueous methanol, and acetone as described in Sec. II.B.

erty is common to most polyphenols thanks to their high degree of hydroxylation, the ability of NEPP to form protein-polyphenol complexes would be limited to those molecules physically accessible to soluble proteins. Insoluble NEPP often form part of a complex matrix with cell wall polysaccharides (56), or they can also form insoluble tannin granules (8), which reduce their ability to precipitate salivary proteins or to inhibit digestive enzymes. Therefore, these effects are more pronounced with EPP, mainly with those soluble compounds of higher molecular weight (oligomeric proanthocyanidins and hydrolyzable tannins) (34), the simple phenols having no protein-precipitating capacity (30).

Likewise, PP can also form complexes with polysaccharides other than those conforming the plant cell wall (i.e., starch) (57,58), resulting in a reduced postprandial glycemic response (59), although this property has been poorly investigated and can be partly due to inhibition of amylolytic enzymes (55). Another property of food phenolics scarcely studied is their effect on lipid metabolism. Increased levels of fat excretion with both NEPP (49,60–62) and EPP (62–64) have been reported. Also, hypocholesterolemic effects have been attributed to polyphenolic compounds, mainly EPP (grape proanthocyanidins, tannic acid) (64–66), their action probably being mediated by a reduced intestinal cholesterol absorption, yet the exact mechanism is not known.

Another important effect of polyphenolic compounds on nutrient bioavailability in the small intestine is their influence on mineral absorption. EPP have been reported to form complexes with nonheme iron, reducing Fe absorption in animals and humans (67,68). This effect has been attributed to galloyl and catechol groups (69). The influence of flavonoids on Fe absorption has not been clearly established, and contradictory results are reported in the literature (68,69). EPP have also been found to interfere in the absorption of copper and zinc, with inhibitory or enhancing effects depending on the animal model used (70,71). These compounds have no apparent effect on calcium, magnesium, or manganese absorption (70,72).

Concerning the metabolism of polyphenolic compounds in the upper intestine, only EPP may be affected by the acid pH of the stomach fluids, causing the partial hydrolysis of some hydrolyzable tannins. Through their passage along the small intestine, only a minor number of polyphenols bound to cell wall polysaccharides or protein (NEPP) can be released upon hydrolysis of their alkali-labile linkages (73). Also, some flavonoid glycosides can be hydrolyzed, rendering the free aglycones thanks to the action of bacteria colonizing the terminal ileum (73,74). Some EPP (aglycones and free simple phenolic compounds) can be absorbed through the small intestinal mucosa. The major part of the polyphenolic compounds, namely NEPP and a significant amount of unabsorbed EPP (flavonoid glycosides and oligomeric tannins), would resist the pH and the action of digestive enzymes, passing unaltered into the large intestine. These facts are confirmed by in vitro data showing the presence of both EPP and NEPP in dietary fiber residues, as previously discussed (Tables 3–6) (17–22,44).

Once in the large intestine, only a minor portion of NEPP is metabolized by the colonic microflora, corresponding to those PP bound to cell wall polysaccharides that are released after dietary fiber fermentation. Most NEPP (highly polymerized tannins, tannin-protein complexes, and a significant fraction of fiber-bound phenolics) are not absorbed or metabolized in the colon, being extensively excreted in feces. Between 70 and over 95% of the ingested NEPP can be excreted, depending on their complexity and the degree of polymerization to other cell components (49,75). NEPP would pass inert through the colon, not affecting the intestinal microflora or its fermentative capacity towards other substrates, and normal levels of short-chain fatty acids (SCFA)—acetic, propionic, and butyric acids—the main end-products of colonic fermentation, are produced (27,76,77).

In contrast, EPP are extensively hydrolyzed by the intestinal bacteria, and some EPP (phenolic acids) can slow down colonic metabolism, resulting in reduced SCFA levels due to a decreased capacity of the colonic microflora towards fermentation of carbohydrates and protein (63,77–79). EPP are mostly fermented and/or absorbed in the large intestine, and only minor amounts are excreted in feces (50,80–82). Metabolism of EPP requires an initial hydrolysis of glycosides to their corresponding aglycones by bacterial enzymes in the small intestine and colon, since mammals lack the appropriate intestinal β-glycosidases. Aglycones are absorbed by the gut epithelium and methylated and/or conjugated with glucuronic acid or sulfate in the liver. These metabolites are excreted in the bile and can enter an enterohepatic cycle when deconjugated by the action of the colonic microflora and reabsorbed, thus ensuring significant plasmatic levels of circulating phenols. Alternatively, they can be fully metabolized and converted into simple phenolic acids after hydrolysis of their flavone structure (cleavage of the heterocyclic ring) mediated by bacterial enzymes. These phenolic acids, like free, soluble phenolics, are absorbed through the intestinal mucosa and excreted in the urine (82–86).

Only minor amounts of ingested flavonoids can be detected in plasma [less than 1% of catechins (86)], which suggests predominant fermentation of EPP. This is a crucial subject, since the extent to which EPP are absorbed and metabolized in the organism will determine their effects as bioactive compounds. Most of the physiological properties that can be ascribed to dietary polyphenols are derived from their interaction with endogenous and exogenous compounds along the digestive tract. Thus, EPP are markedly astringent due to their capacity to precipitate proline-rich salivary proteins, an ability that is thought to be a protective strategy of plants against predators (54). Also, PP can modify the digestibility of certain macro- and micronutrients, the NEPP having a strong bulking capacity due to their nondigestible compound content (Table 7). However, systemic effects of EPP related to their potential health effects depend on the amount of absorbed compound.

Recent interest in food phenolics has increased enormously due to their role as antioxidants, antimutagens, and scavengers of free radicals (87–90). Many studies on the antioxidant capacity of PP are based on in vitro methods (90–92), and phenolic compounds are classified according to their potential antioxidant capacity or antiradical power (93,94). However, this efficiency will greatly depend on the extent of metabolization and absorption of the polyphenol within the gut. As mentioned before, very low levels of tea catechin could be detected in plasma 1 hour after tea ingestion (86), although these levels seem to be enough to exert a potent antioxidant action in vivo as reported in studies with human volunteers (95,96). Moreover, epidemiological studies suggest that increased consumption of phenolic antioxidants is correlated with a reduced risk of cardiovascular disease and certain types of cancer (97–99) Similarly, moderate consumption of red wine—rich in polyphenols—has been associated with a low risk of coronary heart disease (100), suggesting that a reduced absorption does not prevent the biological effects of food phenolics.

IV. CONCLUSIONS

Polyphenolic compounds are closely associated to dietary fiber constituents and very often interfere with the analysis of this fraction of foods. The association between DF and PP hinders the complete removal of polyphenolic compounds, and consequently they are usually present in dietary fiber–rich foods. This not only results in significant errors in the quantitative determination of the DF content of such products, but, more importantly, qualitative mistakes can also occur due to the parallelism existing in the physiological effects caused by DF and PP.

Indeed, when considering together all the effects of dietary polyphenols and their behavior within the digestive tract (Table 7), certain similarities between dietary fiber constituents and polyphenols can be drawn. NEPP, like the insoluble dietary fiber constituents, are also insoluble, nondigestible compounds that are scarcely affected by the fermentative microflora and can reduce the digestibility of other dietary constituents, resulting in increased fecal bulk and protein and fat excretion. On the other hand, EPP are soluble compounds that are mostly metabolized by the colonic bacteria, also affecting mineral absorption, reducing postprandial glycemia, and increasing fat excretion, similar to soluble dietary fiber.

All these facts, along with the permanence of PP associated to DF, constitute the rationale for the suggested inclusion of polyphenolic compounds as DF constituents (20,43). A new type of DF, namely antioxidant dietary fiber (ADF), has recently been defined as a dietary fiber–rich material containing high amounts of antioxidant polyphenols associated to the fiber matrix (101). This ADF would combine the beneficial health effects of dietary fiber and polyphenols.

REFERENCES

1. Kühnau J. The flavonoids. A class of semi-essential food components: their role in human nutrition. World Rev Nutr Diet 24:117–191 (1976).
2. Harborne JB. Methods in Plant Biochemistry. I. Plant Phenolics. London: Academic Press, 1989.
3. Harborne JB. The Flavonoids: Advances in Research Since 1986. London: Chapman and Hall, 1993.
4. Harborne JB. The Flavonoids: Advances in Research Since 1980. London: Chapman and Hall, 1988.
5. Hemingway RW, Karchesy JJ. Chemistry and Significance of Condensed Tannins. New York: Plenum Press, 1989.
6. Markham KR. Techniques of Flavonoid Identification. London: Academic Press, 1982.
7. Scalbert A. Polyphenolic Phenomena. Paris: INRA Editions, 1993.
8. Würsch P, del Vedovo S, Rosset J, Smiley M. The tannin granules from ripe carob pod. Lebensm Wiss Technol 17:351–354 (1984).
9. Porter LW. Tannins. In: Harborne JB. ed. Methods in Plant Biochemistry. I. Plant Phenolics. London: Academic Press, 1989, pp. 389–419.
10. Ragan MA, Glombitza K. Phlorotannins, brown algal polyphenols. Prog Phycol Res 4:177–241 (1986).
11. Ho C-T, Lee CY, Huang M-T. Phenolic Compounds in Food and Their Effects on Health I. Analysis, Occurrence, and Chemistry. Washington, DC: American Chemical Society, 1992.
12. Shahidi F, Naczk M. Food Phenolics. Sources, Chemistry, Effects, Applications. Lancaster, PA: Technomic Publishing Co., 1995.
13. Peleg H, Naim M, Rouseff RL, Zehavi U. Distribution of bound and free phenolic acid in oranges (*Citrus sinensis*) and grapefruits (*Citrus paradisi*). J Sci Food Agric 57:417–426 (1991).
14. Hertog MGL, Hollman PCH, Katan MB, Kromhout D. Intake of potentially anticarcinogenic flavonoids and their determinants in adults in the Netherlands. Nutr Cancer 20:21–29 (1993).
15. Prosky L, Asp N-G, Schweizer TF, Devries JW, Furda I. Determination of insoluble, soluble and total dietary fiber in foods and food products: interlaboratory study. J Assoc Off Anal Chem 71: 1017–1023 (1988).
16. Trowell H. Definition of dietary fiber and hypothesis that it is a protective factor in certain diseases. Am J Clin Nutr 29:417–427 (1976).
17. Saura-Calixto F. Effect of condensed tannins in the analysis of dietary fiber in carob pods. J Food Sci 53:1769–1771 (1988).
18. Saura-Calixto F. Dietary fibre complex in a sample rich in condensed tannins and uronic acid. Food Chem 23:95–103 (1987).
19. Goñi I, Torre M, Saura-Calixto F. Determination of dietary fibre in cider wastes. Comparison of methods. Food Chem 33:151–159 (1989).
20. Saura-Calixto F, Goñi I, Mañas E, Abia R. Klason lignin, condensed tannins and resistant protein as dietary fibre constituents: determination in grape pomaces. Food Chem 39:299–309 (1991).

21. Bravo L. Propiedades de los Compuestos Polifenólicos como Constituyentes de la Dieta. Comparación con Componentes de la Fibra Dietética. PhD dissertation, Universidad Autónoma de Madrid, 1993.

22. Bravo L, Grados N, Saura-Calixto F. Composition and potential uses of mesquite pods (*Prosopis pallida* L): comparison with carob pods (*Ceratonia siliqua* L). J Sci Food Agric 65:303–306 (1994).

23. Bartolomé B, Jiménez-Ramsey LM, Butler LG. Nature of the condensed tannins present in the dietary fibre fractions in foods. Food Chem 53:357–362 (1995).

24. Reed JD, McDowell RE, Van Soest PJ, Horvart PJ. Condensed tannins: a factor limiting the use of cassava forage. J Sci Food Agric 33:213–220 (1982).

25. Porter LJ, Hrstich LN, Chan BC. The conversion of procyanidins and prodelphinidins to cyanidin and delphinidin. Phytochemistry 25:223–230 (1986).

26. Bravo L, Abia R, Goñi I, Saura-Calixto F. Possible common properties of dietary fibre constituents and polyphenols. Eur J Clin Nutr 49 (suppl 3):S211–S214 (1995).

27. Bravo L, Abia R, Saura-Calixto F. Polyphenols as dietary fiber associated compounds. Comparative study on in vivo and in vitro properties. J Agric Food Chem 42:1481–1487 (1994).

28. Hagerman AE, Butler L. Condensed tannin purification and characterization of tannin-associated proteins. J Agric Food Chem 28:947–952 (1980).

29. Hagerman AE. Tannin-protein interaction. In: Ho CT, Lee CY, Huang MT, eds. Phenolic Compounds in Food and Their Effects on Health. I. Analysis, Occurrence, and Chemistry. Washington, DC: American Chemical Society, 1992, pp. 236–247.

30. Hagerman AE. Chemistry of tannin-protein complexation. In: Hemingway RW, Karchesy JJ, eds. Chemistry and Significance of Condensed Tannins. New York: Plenum Press, 1989, pp. 323–333.

31. Oh HI, Hoff JE. Effect of condensed grape tannins on the in vitro activity of digestive proteases and activation of their zymogens. J Food Sci 51:577–580 (1986).

32. Ahmed AE, Smithard R, Ellis M. Activity of enzymes of the pancreas, and the lumen and mucosa of the small intestine in growing broiler cockelers fed on tannin-containing diets. Br J Nutr 65: 189–197 (1991).

33. Longstaff MA, McNab JM. The effect of concentration of tannin-rich bean hulls (*Vicia faba* L.) on activities of lipase (EC 3.1.1.3) and α-amylase (EC 3.2.1.1) in digesta and pancreas and on the digestion of lipid and starch by young chicks. Br J Nutr 66:139–147 (1991).

34. Quesada C, Bartolomé B, Nieto O, Gómez-Cordovés C, Hernández T, Estrella I. Phenolic inhibitors of α-amylase and trypsin enzymes by extracts from pears, lentils, and cocoa. J Food Prot 59:185–192 (1996).

35. Theander O, Åman P. Studies on dietary fibre. A method for the analysis and chemical characterisation of total dietary fibre. J Sci Food Agric 33:340–344 (1982).

36. Asp N-G, Johansson CG, Hallman H, Siljeström M. Rapid enzymatic assay of insoluble and soluble dietary fiber. J Agric Food Chem 31:476–482 (1983).

37. Brillouet J-M, Rouau X, Hoebler C, Barry J-L, Carré B, Lorta E. A new method for determination of insoluble cell walls and soluble nonstarchy polysaccharides from plant materials. J Agric Food Chem 36:969–979 (1988).

38. Marlett JA, Chesters JG, Longacre MJ, Bogdanske JJ. Recovery of soluble dietary fiber is dependent on the method of analysis. Am J Clin Nutr 50:479–485 (1989).

39. Theander O, Åman P, Westerlund E, Graham H. Enzymatic/chemical analysis of dietary fiber. J Assoc Off Anal Chem 77:703–709 (1994).

40. Saura-Calixto F, Bravo L. Determination of polyphenolic compounds associated with dietary fibre. In: Sørensen AM, Bach Knudsen KE, Englyst HN, Gudman-Høyer E, Nyman M, eds. Recent Progress in the Analysis of Dietary Fibre. Luxembourg: Office for Official Publications of the European Communities, 1995, pp. 87–92.

41. Swain T, Hillis WE. The phenolic constituents of *Prunus domestica*. 1. The quantitative analysis of phenolic constituents. J Sci Food Agric 10:63–68 (1959).

42. Price ML, Butler LG. Rapid visual estimation and spectrophotometric determination of tannin content of sorghum grain. J Agric Food Chem 25:1268–1273 (1977).

43. Mañas E. Análisis de Fibra Alimentaria. Fuentes de Error en los Métodos Actuales y Propuesta de Nueva Metodología. PhD dissertation, Universidad Autónoma de Madrid, 1992.

44. Bravo L, Saura-Calixto F. Characterization of dietary fiber and the in vitro indigestible fraction of grape pomace. Am J Enol Vitic 49:135–141 (1998).

45. Montreau FR. Sur le dosage des composés phénoliques totaux dans les vins par la méthode Folin-Ciocalteau. Conn Vigne Vin 24:397–404 (1972).

46. Arrigoni E, Caprez A, Amadò R, Neukom H. Gravimetric method for the determination of insoluble and soluble dietary fibres. Z Lebensm Unters Forsch 178:195–198 (1984).

47. Terrill TH, Rowan AM, Douglas GB, Barry TN. Determination of extractable and bound condensed tannin concentrations in forage plants, protein concentrate meals and cereal grains. J Sci Food Agric 58:321–329 (1992).

48. Carmona A, Seidl DS, Jaffé WG. Comparison of extraction methods and assay procedures for the determination of the apparent tannin content of common beans. J Sci Food Agric 56:291–301 (1991).

49. Bravo L, Mañas E, Saura-Calixto F. Dietary non-extractable condensed tannins as indigestible compounds: effects on faecal weight, and protein and fat excretion. J Sci Food Agric 63:63–68 (1993).

50. Saura-Calixto F, Bravo L. Intestinal degradation of polyphenols. In Mälkki Y, Cummings JH, eds. COST Action 92. Dietary Fibre and Fermentation in the Colon. Luxembourg: Office for Official Publications of the European Communities, 1996, pp. 174–180.

51. Shahkhalili Y, Finot PA, Hurrell R, Fern E. Effects of foods rich in polyphenols on nitrogen excretion in rats. J Nutr 120:346–352 (1990).

52. Alzueta C, Treviño J, Ortiz L. Effect of tannin from faba beans on protein utilization in rats. J Sci Food Agric 59:551–553 (1992).

53. Butler LG. Effects of condensed tannins on animal nutrition. In: Hemingway RW, Karchesy JJ, eds. Chemistry and Significance of Condensed Tannins. New York: Plenum Press, 1989, pp. 391–402.

54. Charlton AJ, Baxter NJ, Haslam E, Williamson MP. Salivary proteins as a defence against dietary tannins. In: Amadò R, Andersson H, Bardócz S, Serra F, eds. Polyphenols in Food. Luxembourg: Office for Official Publications of the European Communities, 1998, pp. 179–185.

55. Carmona A, Borgudd L, Borges G, Levy-Benshimol A. Effect of black bean tannins on in vitro carbohydrate digestion and absorption. Nutr Biochem 7:445–450 (1996).

56. Andary C, Mondolot-Cosson L. Histolocalization of plant polyphenols in tissues and cell walls. Some applications. In: Amadò R, Andersson H, Bardócz S, Serra F, eds. Polyphenols in Food. Luxembourg: Office for Official Publications of the European Communities, 1998, pp. 41–47.

57. Ya C, Gaffney SH, Lilley TH, Haslam E. Carbohydrate-polyphenol complexation. In: Hemingway RW, Karchesy JJ, eds. Chemistry and Significance of Condensed Tannins. New York: Plenum Press, 1989, pp. 307–322.

58. Desphande SS, Shalunke DK. Interactions of tannic acid and catechin with legume starches. J Food Sci 47:2080–2081, 2083 (1982).

59. Thompson LU, Yoon JH, Jenkins DJA, Wolever TMS, Jenkins AL. Relationship between polyphenol intake and blood glucose response of normal and diabetic individuals. Am J Clin Nutr 39:745–751 (1984).

60. Würsch P. Influence of tannin-rich carob pod fiber on the cholesterol metabolism in the rat. J Nutr 109:685–692 (1979).

61. Martín-Carrón N, García-Alonso A, Goñi I, Saura-Calixto F. Nutritional and physiological properties of grape pomace as a potential food ingredient. Am J Enol Vitic 48:328–332 (1997).

62. Bravo L, Saura-Calixto F. Soluble polyphenols and non-extractable condensed tannins as dietary constituents: effect on fat excretion. In: Brouillard R, Jay M, Scalbert A, eds. Polyphenols 94. Paris: INRA, 1995, pp. 409–410.

63. Bravo L, Abia R, Eastwood MA, Saura-Calixto F. Degradation of polyphenols (catechin and tannic acid) in the rat intestinal tract. Effect on colonic fermentation and faecal output. Br J Nutr 71:933–946 (1994).

64. Tebib K, Bitri L, Besançon P, Rouanet J-M. Polymeric grape seed tannins prevent plasma cholesterol changes in high-cholesterol-fed rats. Food Chem 49:403–406 (1994).

65. Tebib K, Besançon P, Rouanet J-M. Dietary grape seed tannins affect lipoproteins, lipoprotein lipases and tissue lipids in rats fed hypercholesterolemic diets. J Nutr 124:2451–2457 (1994).

66. Yugarani T, Tan BKH, Das NP. The effects of tannic acid on serum and liver lipids of RAIF and RICO rats fed on high fat diet. Comp Biochem Physiol 104A:339–343 (1993).
67. Reddy MB, Cook JD. Assessment of dietary determinants of nonheme-iron absorption in humans and rats. Am J Clin Nutr 54:723–728 (1991).
68. Hurrell RF, Reddy M, Cook JD. Influence of polyphenol-containing beverages on iron absorption. In: Amadò R, Andersson H, Bardócz S, Serra F, eds. Polyphenols in Food. Luxembourg: Office for Official Publications of the European Communities, 1998, pp. 169–172.
69. Brune M, Rossander L, Hallberg L. Iron absorption and phenolic compounds: importance of different phenolic structures. Eur J Clin Nutr 43:547–558 (1989).
70. Jansman AJM, Houdijk JGM, Verstegen MWA. Effects of condensed tannins in faba beans (*Vicia faba* L.) on the availability of minerals in pigs. In: Schlemmer U, ed. Bioavailability 93. Nutritional, Chemical and Food Processing Implications of Nutrient Availability. Karlsruhe: Federation of European Chemical Societies, 1993.
71. Vaquero MP, Veldhuizen M, Van Dokkum W, van den Hamer CJA, Schaafsma G. Copper bioavailability from breakfasts containing tea. Influence of the addition of milk. J Sci Food Agric 64:475–481 (1994).
72. Fraile AL, Flynn A. The absorption of manganese from polyphenol-containing beverages in suckling rats. Int J Food Sci Nutr 43:163–168 (1992).
73. Buchanan CJ, Wallace G, Fy SC, Eastwood MA. In vivo release of ^{14}C-labelled phenolic groups from intact dietary spinach cell walls during passage through the rat intestine. J Sci Food Agric 71:459–469 (1996).
74. Hollman PCH, de Vries JHM, van Leeuwen SD, Mengelers MJB, Katan MB. Absorption of dietary quercetin glycosides and quercetin in healthy ileostomy volunteers. Am J Clin Nutr 62:1276–1282 (1995).
75. Bravo L, Saura-Calixto F, Goñi I. Effects of dietary fibre and tannins from apple pulp on the composition of faeces in rats. Br J Nutr 67:463–473 (1992).
76. Martín-Carrón N, Goñi I. Prior exposure of cecal microflora to grape pomaces does not inhibit in vitro fermentation of pectin. J Agric Food Chem 46:1064–1070 (1998).
77. Arrigoni E, Balzer P, Amadò R. Influence of polyphenols on the fermentability of polysaccharides. In: Amadò R, Andersson H, Bardócz S, Serra F, eds. Polyphenols in Food. Luxembourg: Office for Official Publications of the European Communities, 1998, pp. 187–192.
78. Mañas E, Lebet V, Arrigoni E, Amadò R. In vitro studies of polyphenol fermentability. In: Mälkki Y, Cummings JH, eds. COST Action 92. Dietary Fibre and Fermentation in the Colon. Luxembourg: Office for Official Publications of the European Communities, 1996, pp. 186–190.
79. Levrat M-A, Texier O, Régerat F, Demigné C, Rémésy C. Comparison of the effects of condensed tannin and pectin on cecal fermentations and lipid metabolism in the rat. Nutr Res 13:427–433 (1993).
80. Degen AA, Becker K, Makkar HPS, Borowy N. *Acacia saligna* as a fodder tree for desert livestock and the interaction of its tannins with fibre fractions. J Sci Food Agric 68:65–71 (1995).
81. Jimenez-Ramsey LM, Rogler JC, Housley TL, Butler LG, Elkin RG. Absorption and distribution of ^{14}C-labeled condensed tannins and related sorghum phenolics in chickens. J Agric Food Chem 42:963–967 (1994).
82. Manach C, Morand C, Texier O, Favier ML, Agullo G, Demigné C, Régérat F, Rémésy C. Quercetin metabolites in plasma of rats fed diets containing rutin or quercetin. J Nutr 125:1911–1922 (1995).
83. Williams RT. Metabolism of phenolics in animals. In: Harborne JB, ed. Biochemistry of Phenolic Compounds. London: Academic Press, 1964, pp. 205–248.
84. Griffiths LA. Mammalian metabolism of flavonoids. In: Harborne JB, Mabry TJ, eds. The Flavonoids: Advances in Research. London: Chapman and Hall, 1982, pp. 681–718.
85. Hackett AM. The metabolism of flavonoid compounds in mammals. In: Cody V, Middleton E, Harborne JB, eds. Plant Flavonoids in Biology and Medicine: Biochemical, Pharmacological, Structure-Activity Relationships. New York: Alan R. Liss, Inc., 1986, pp. 177–197.
86. Hollman PCH. Bioavailability of flavonoids. Eur J Clin Nutr 51(suppl 1):S66–S69 (1997).
87. Shahidi F, Wanasundara PKJPD. Phenolic antioxidants. Crit Rev Food Sci Nutr 32:67–103 (1992).

88. Jacob RA. The integrated antioxidant system. Nutr Res 15:755–766 (1995).
89. Larson RA. Naturally Occurring Antioxidants. Boca Raton, FL: Lewis Publishers, 1997.
90. Yen G-C, Chen H-Y. Antioxidant activity of various tea extracts in relation to their antimutagenicity. J Agric Food Chem 43:27–32 (1995).
91. Kanner J, Frankel E, Granit R, German B, Kinsella JE. Natural antioxidants in grapes and wines. J Agric Food Chem 42:64–69 (1994).
92. Teissedre PL, Frankel EN, Waterhouse AL, Peleg H, German JB. Inhibition of in vitro human LDL oxidation by phenolic antioxidants from grapes and wines. J Sci Food Agric 70:55–61 (1996).
93. Brand-Williams W, Cuvelier ME, Berset C. Use of a free radical method to evaluate antioxidant activity. Lebensm Wiss Technol 28:25–30 (1995).
94. Sánchez-Moreno C, Larrauri JA, Saura-Calixto F. A procedure to measure the antiradical efficiency of polyphenols. J Sci Food Agric 76:270–276 (1998).
95. Serafini M, Ghiselli A, Ferro-Luzzi A. Red wine, tea and antioxidants. Lancet 344:626 (1994).
96. Serafini M, Ghiselli A, Ferro-Luzzi A. In vivo antioxidant effect of green and black tea in man. Eur J Clin Nutr 50:28–32 (1996).
97. Hertog MGL, Feskens EJM, Hollman PCH, Katan MB, Kromhout D. Dietary antioxidant flavonoids and risk of coronary heart disease. The Zutphen Elderly Study. Lancet 342:1007–1011 (1993).
98. Hertog MGL, Feskens EJM, Hollman PCH, Katan MB, Kromhout D. Dietary flavonoids and cancer risk in the Zutphen Elderly Study. Nutr Cancer 22:175–184 (1994).
99. Hertog MGL, Sweetnam PM, Fehily AM, Elwood PC, Kromhout D. Antioxidant flavonols and ischemic heart disease in a Welsh population of men: the Caerphilly Study. Am J Clin Nutr 65:1489–1494 (1997).
100. Renaud S, De Lorgeril M. Wine, alcohol, platelets and the French paradox for coronary heart disease. Lancet 339:1523–1526 (1992).
101. Saura-Calixto F. Antioxidant dietary fiber product: a new concept and a potential food ingredient. J Agric Food Chem 46:4303–4306 (1998).

23
Food Uses of Fiber

Janette Gelroth and Gur S. Ranhotra
American Institute of Baking, Manhattan, Kansas

I. INTRODUCTION

Epidemiological and clinical studies, especially those reported by British researchers a few decades ago, have linked the inadequacy of fiber in the Western diet with the higher incidence of chronic diseases among us. Numerous aspects of this relationship have been investigated and expanded, including the definition of dietary fiber and its constituents and the correct methods by which to measure them.

As a result of these investigations, fiber's health benefits have become increasingly recognized. This has led to the marketing of a plethora of new fiber-containing food products. Many of these are highly successful, but others have failed. New laws have been enacted to regulate the labeling of fiber in fiber sources and fiber-containing foods, and restrictions have also been placed regarding health claims that can and cannot be made on food labels and in advertising.

Over the years, various fiber sources have fallen into and out of acceptance by the food industry and consumers alike. However, the use of fiber in foods has continued to grow and expand, with an ever-increasing number of fiber sources becoming available for food applications. In addition, functional characteristics of fiber sources have also been recognized and developed. This chapter discusses various aspects of fiber ingredients and their use in foods.

II. SOURCES OF FIBER

Fiber is found only in foods of plant origin—cereal grains, legumes, fruits, vegetables, nuts, and seeds. In many Western countries, including the United States, fiber has traditionally been obtained by consumption of plant-based foods. Over the years, however, food-consumption patterns, which increasingly included more animal-based than plant-based foods, have shown a significant decline in fiber intake; currently, fiber intake in the United States averages only 10–15 g per day.

Increasing awareness of the health benefits of fiber has led to various dietary recommendations, which suggest that we increase our fiber intake substantially (1). A daily intake of 25 g is now widely suggested—i.e., a doubling of the current intake. Toward this goal, an increasing number of fiber ingredients for food use have been developed from a variety of different sources. Table 1 lists many of these sources and an approximate range of fiber contents in ingredients

Table 1 Selected Sources of Fiber for Use in Food Applications

Source	Total dietary fiber[a] (%)
Grains	
Amaranth	NA
Barley	35–70
Corn	50–95
Oats	15–95
Rice	30–80
Rye	NA
Wheat	10–65
Legumes	
Soy	45–75
Peas	50–95
Peanuts	50–55
Sweet lupin	60–95
Vegetables	
Carob	45–50
Cocoa	55–75
Potato pectin	50–55
Sugar beet	60–80
Sugar cane	72–86
Tomato	45–65
Tapioca	70
Fruits	
Apple	43–60
Black currant	43
Citrus[b]	25–70
Cranberry	6–8
Date	44–52
Fig	12–64
Peach	10
Pear	13–14
Prune	16–57
Raisin	6–8
Raspberry	2–5
Nuts and seeds	
Almond	2–12
Cottonseed	NA
Flaxseed	30–40
Hazelnut	3
Mustard	NA
Pecan	2–3
Psyllium	NA
Sunflower	NA
Cellulose and cellulose derivatives[c]	75–100
Gums	
Agar	75–85
Carrageenan	85–90
Guar	85–90
Gum arabic	80–90
Locust bean	90
Pectin	100
Tragacanth	80
Xanthan	75
Others	
Oligosaccharides	NA
Polydextrose	NA
Resistant starch	30–40

NA = Not available

[a] Range values of processed sources (not of raw materials).

[b] e.g., grapefruit, lemon, lime, and orange.

[c] e.g., cellulose, methylcellulose, carboxymethylcellulose, and hydroxypropyl-methylcellulose.

Source: Refs. 2–6.

derived from them (2–6). As is evident from Table 1, different sources of fiber can yield products that differ greatly in fiber content.

For all practical purposes, fiber is viewed as total dietary fiber (TDF) and not as crude fiber—a term now rarely used, primarily because the method involved grossly underestimates fiber in most foods. For health and nutrition labeling purposes, TDF is broadly classified into insoluble fiber (IF) and soluble fiber (SF).

III. PROCESSING AND CONCENTRATING FIBER

A variety of processing techniques are employed in the production of fiber ingredients for use in food. These techniques include such things as various milling processes, simple extraction and drying procedures, and enzyme and additive treatments, to name a few. Using these techniques, fiber ingredients can be isolated from raw materials and concentrated or otherwise modified to serve a particular function within a food system. Fiber ingredients can even be produced from sources that might otherwise be considered waste products. For example, wheat straw, soy hulls, oat hulls, peanut and almond skins, corn stalks and cobs, spent brewer's grains, and waste portions of fruits and vegetables processed in large quantities (7–10) can be converted into fiber ingredients, which may be highly functional in certain food applications.

The extent or degree of processing used in the manufacture of fiber ingredients can have a substantial impact on characteristics of the finished products. Often this accounts for the wide range of TDF contents observed for fiber ingredients from various sources (Table 1). For cereal grains, TDF content would also differ greatly based on the portion of the grain (e.g., whole grain, bran, or hull) utilized as the starting material. For example, oat groats, which are produced by removal of the outer layer (hulls) of whole oats, contain about 10% TDF. Additional milling and fractionating of the groats produce oat bran. Cleaning, bleaching, and grinding of the hulls removed in the initial step result in an additional fiber product (Table 2) (11).

Modified fiber ingredients are products that are subjected to additional processing to yield an altered product, which may have a higher fiber content, different functional characteristics, or other attributes useful when incorporating the ingredients into food products. In one study, for example, fine grinding followed by air classification of a wheat bran formed a fraction containing 10% more fiber (51% vs. 61% TDF) (12). In another study, an alcoholic extraction process followed by heat drying of oat bran produced an oat bran concentrate in which the TDF content increased from 15.4% to 37.1% (13).

Cellulose is another example of a fiber source which, based on additional processing techniques utilized, can result in different types of fiber ingredients. Cellulose is the principal structural component of plants and can be obtained in highly purified form (virtually 100% IF) from

Table 2 Comparison of the Fiber Content from Various Oat Fractions

	Content (%)	
Product	Total dietary fiber	Soluble fiber
Oat groats	8–12	3–5
Oat bran	15–18	4–8
Oat hulls	79–96	0–4

Source: Ref. 11.

various sources, mainly wood pulp but also products such as sugar beets, sugar cane, and linters (the fuzz retained on cottonseed after the ginning process) (14). Modification of cellulose, through changes such as in the length of the fibers or in chemical substitutions at the molecular level, forms products (Table 1) which are adapted to suit particular performance needs (15–17).

Modification of fiber length was used in the production of two types (B-Trim™ and Z-Trim™) of fiber ingredients developed by the U.S. Department of Agriculture (USDA). Processing techniques used in their manufacture include shearing conditions, which result in a reduction of the cellular structure length (18,19).

Blending of fiber sources is another technique used to tailor-make ingredients suited to particular food applications. Incorporation of these blends into food products can maximize dietary fiber levels as well as meet the necessary functionality requirements. One example of blending of fiber sources is to combine grain products with other grains or with fruit fibers. This may result in products with different proportions of IF and SF than were present in the original ingredients or with different functional characteristics. Another example of blending grain products is in the production of Z-Trim ™. This USDA-developed product can be manufactured from a variety of sources such as oat, pea, corn, rice, soybean, and wheat. Blending of Z-Trim products from different sources can have a synergistic effect on the viscosity of gels made from the final blend (19). Another blending example is that of gums with IF sources. Because IF frequently settles out in liquids, some applications require the addition of a colloid, such as xanthan gum or carrageenan, to keep the insoluble particles in suspension (20).

Some fiber sources require certain pretreatments before they are suitable for use in food products. Rice bran, for example, contains the enzyme lipase, which, if left intact, will break down fat leading to rancidity and a substantial reduction in shelf life. Thus, this enzyme must be deactivated before rice bran can successfully be used as a food ingredient. Traditionally, lipase has been destroyed by a dry heat extrusion process, which has the disadvantage of adversely affecting native proteins, vitamins, flavor, and color. However, a nonheat inactivation method that can be used to stabilize the rice bran involves treatment with a proteolytic enzyme, which destroys the lipase (9,21).

Enzyme treatments are also involved in the preparation or modification of other fibers. For example, α-amylase is used in the production of Oatrim™, a food ingredient developed from oats and high in SF (22), and a fructooligosaccharide can be prepared from sucrose by an enzyme treatment (8). Modification of the textural characteristics of pectins can also be performed by utilizing enzymes.

Hydrogen peroxide modification is another example of a pretreatment of fiber sources. By using hydrogen peroxide to break down lignin (a structural fiber component in plant cells), a variety of what might otherwise be considered waste products—wheat straw, cornstalks and cobs, and soy and oat hulls, to name a few—can be converted into low-calorie, high-fiber "flours" (7).

Another processing technique used to impart a particular flavor to fiber ingredients is malting. Grains that have undergone the controlled sprouting process of malting are dried and ground into flour or further processed to form flakes or kibble. Because of its role in brewing, barley has traditionally been the most commonly malted grain. Now, however, wheat, rye, and oats are being used, with each grain type imparting its own distinctive flavor and color to food products (23).

Heating and cooling of starch is a processing technique that results in the formation of resistant starch (24,25). Although technically not a fiber, resistant starch, like other fibers, escapes digestion in the small intestine. Analytically, it is measured as fiber, and because of its characteristics it is considered to be a "functional fiber" (26).

Obviously, processing techniques will have a dramatic effect on the content and functionality characteristics of fiber in the source intended for food use. These techniques must be taken into consideration when choosing a particular fiber ingredient for use in foods.

IV. FUNCTIONAL CHARACTERISTICS OF FIBER

Fiber sources can provide a multitude of functionalities when added to food products. Specific requirements of particular food systems can often be targeted by using certain fiber sources or combinations of sources, with combinations often providing synergistic effects. Fiber ingredients can vary substantially in the functionalities, and the degree thereof, that they possess. Thus, when incorporating fiber into foods, these functionalities must be considered. A summary of various functionality characteristics of fiber is given below:

1. Health benefits: Because of its reported protective effect against certain forms of cancers and cardiovascular disease, fiber fortification of foods can have a wide consumer appeal. Listing fiber content on the nutrition label and/or making health claims about fiber can be a valuable marketing tool for food companies.

2. Calorie reduction: Because fiber is generally considered as noncaloric, foods containing added fiber could show, depending on the use level, a substantial reduction in caloric value compared to a reference product. The nutrition labeling regulations currently in place in the United States allow subtracting IF, but not SF, from the total carbohydrate content prior to calculation of caloric content of foods (27). SF, because of its extensive degradation by intestinal microflora, may provide some caloric value, but this value is likely to be much less than 4 kcal/g, the value traditionally assigned to available carbohydrates—starches and sugars (28). Because of its noncaloric characteristic, fiber can be used as a ''bulking agent'' in combination with high-intensity sweeteners to replace large quantities of caloric sweeteners (e.g., sugar) in reduced-calorie food products.

3. Water-holding capacity: Fiber, in general, has a high water-holding capacity. This, in addition to fiber's noncaloric characteristic, enables reducing the caloric content of the finished foods. A high water-holding capacity also helps to retard staling, control moisture migration and ice crystal formation, increase freeze/thaw stability, and reduce syneresis or weeping.

4. Fat mimetic: Fat contributes several functional properties to a food system. As a result, it is often difficult or impossible to find a single ingredient that can effectively replace fat. In a ''systems-based'' approach (combination of two or more ingredients) to replacing fat, fiber sources can fulfill vital functions associated with fat (29). Utilization of fiber ingredients that exhibit lubricity, thickening, emulsion, opacity, and gel texture simulation characteristics can enable development of a fiber system that may successfully replace at least a good portion, if not all, of the fat in many food products.

5. Anticaking agent: This attribute helps to prevent caking and clumping and improves flowability. Thus, performance of packaging equipment can be improved and, as a result, efficiency is increased.

6. Antisticking agent: In extrusion processing, resistance of the dough, through sticking to the walls and screw element of the extruder, can adversely affect the rate of extrusion. Fiber added to the dough can decrease this stickiness and, thus, facilitate the extrusion process.

7. Dimensional stabilizer: Because of the ''fibrous'' nature of a number of fiber sources,

addition of fiber ingredients to certain food systems may stabilize or modify the physical structure of the food. This may help to minimize shrinkage or improve product density.

8. Texturizing agent: The particulate nature of many fiber ingredients can contribute to the mouthfeel of the product. In addition, varying particle sizes can result in differences in water-holding capabilities. This factor also contributes to mouthfeel.

9. Thickening/viscosity/gelling agent: The water-holding and gel-forming capabilities of fiber ingredients can contribute to an increase in the thickness or viscosity of a food product. The composition and chemical nature of the various fibers can have a significant impact on the ability of the fiber to function as a thickener or gelling agent. Variations in the drying processes of the fiber sources can even affect their viscosity characteristics (19). Blending of different sources can also be performed to develop a product specifically suited to the needs of a particular food system.

Incorporation of fiber into foods requires consideration of the functionalities provided by the fiber sources. Since different fibers have different functionalities, careful selection of the source or sources most appropriate for the particular food system is necessary.

V. LABELING FIBER-CONTAINING FOODS

In the mid-1970s, a number of high-fiber breads were introduced to the American market. Among these was Fresh Horizons bread, marketed by Continental Baking Company (now part of the Interstate Brands Corporation). It was advertised as a reduced-calorie/high-fiber product, and claims were made regarding its potential in a weight loss regimen and its other health benefits. Within a few months after its introduction, U.S. Food and Drug Administration (FDA) issued warnings to the company that, unless changes were made, Fresh Horizons bread would be considered a drug. Specifically, FDA objected to the statement ''and now there is increasing scientific and medical opinion that fiber may even help prevent serious diseases'' (30). Restrictions were imposed on the product's labeling to eliminate the ''therapeutic claims,'' and orders were issued to destroy point-of-sale pamphlets. These actions led to investigation of certain breakfast cereals, which also carried packaging statements suggesting a relationship between insufficient fiber intake and serious digestive disorders.

In the ensuing years, FDA's stance regarding labeling and health claims has changed substantially. Reports by the Surgeon General and the National Research Council, as well as a growing body of scientific evidence, have emphasized the need to provide consumers with information that may assist them in choosing a healthful diet. FDA has responded to this need by passing regulations regarding nutrition labeling and by allowing for the use of certain health claims, with the requirement that specific rules are followed (27). Two of these health claims relate to health benefits (protection against colon cancer and cardiovascular disease) associated with fiber-containing foods.

A. Nutrition Labeling

The Nutrition Labeling and Education Act of 1990 (NLEA), which became effective in May 1994, made nutrition labeling of most FDA-regulated foods mandatory, and specific rules for this labeling were enacted (27). Under the NLEA, declaration in the nutrition label (Nutrition Facts Panel) of the total carbohydrates (in g per serving and rounded to the nearest g) in a food is mandatory, and the definition is such that TDF is included as part of the total carbohydrates. Separate declaration of dietary fiber (in g per serving) is also mandatory unless the food contains less than 1 g of fiber. In this case, declaration is not required (the statement "not a significant source of dietary fiber" must then be placed at the bottom of the table of nutrient values) or the declaration "contains less than 1 g" or "less than 1 g" is made. If a serving contains less than 0.5 g of dietary fiber, it may be declared as zero. Declarations of IF and SF (in g per serving and rounded to the nearest g) are voluntary, unless claims are made regarding their content, which then makes the declarations mandatory. Amounts less than 1 g are declared as "contains less than 1 g" or "less than 1 g," and amounts less than 0.5 g may be declared as zero. Calculation of the caloric value of the food (frequently determined using conversion factors 4, 9, and 4 kcal per g for protein, fat, and carbohydrates, respectively) allows, as mentioned earlier, for the subtraction of IF (but not SF) from the total carbohydrates.

B. Nutrient Content Claims

FDA regulations allow for the use of particular descriptors in food labels and in labeling. For example, a serving of a food containing 10–19% of the recommended daily intake of fiber (25 g) can be labeled as a "good source of" or "contains" fiber; a contribution of 20% or more allows labeling the food as "high in" or "rich in" fiber. These descriptors apply to other nutrients, also.

C. Health Claims

FDA initially approved the use of eight specific health claims. Two of these apply, as mentioned earlier, to fiber. Because of insufficient scientific evidence, health claims for fiber pertain to fiber-containing foods and not to fiber per se. In other words, claims can only be made regarding the relationship between "fiber-containing grain products, fruits, and vegetables" and cancer or cardiovascular diseases, and specific requirements for wording of the claims must be met (27). Since the regulations state that the food "shall be or shall contain" a grain product, fruit, or vegetable, formulated or processed foods may also use the claim. Such a food must also qualify as "low saturated fat" (≤1 g saturated fat per serving), "low cholesterol" (≤20 mg cholesterol per serving), and "low fat" (≤3 g fat per serving) (31).

Another requirement regarding fiber-related health claims pertains to foods containing a certain level of fiber "without fortification." Interpretation of this requirement is such that a grain-based product, e.g., a bakery food or breakfast cereal, may contain added wheat bran or other concentrated fiber from wheat and not be considered fortified. As such, that product would be allowed to make a "fiber food" health claim. A grain-based product with added fiber from a nongrain source would be considered to be fortified and would, thus, not be allowed to make the claim (27).

At the time of this writing, four more health claims have been approved, two of which pertain to fiber. In one of these, FDA allowed food specific claims for two foods—oats and psyllium—rich in SF that reduce the risk of coronary heart disease. Food products must contain at least 0.75 g of SF from eligible oat products (oat bran, rolled oats, or whole oat flour) or 1.7 g of SF from psyllium husk per serving. In another approved health claim, the connection between whole grain foods and a reduction in the risk of heart disease and certain cancers is addressed. Products must contain ≥ 51% whole grain ingredients as well as meet other requirements.

VI. FOOD USES OF FIBER

Fiber fortification of food products began in the 1970s with the introduction of several different brands of white and wheat (brown) breads containing added fiber. Initially, this was done for the health benefits associated with weight loss, as these breads contained fewer calories than regular products. Since that time, other functional aspects of fiber have been determined and developed, and a wide array of foods now utilize these advances. Listed below are a number of food categories in which fiber has become a valuable ingredient. Examples are given for each category to illustrate some of the fibers that might be used in those food products.

A. Bakery Products

A number of factors must be considered when adding fiber to foods, and bakery products are no exception. A main consideration in bakery products is the effect fiber has on the rheological properties of the dough or batter. Because of the high water-holding capacity of most fibers, the formula absorption generally needs to be increased with increasing levels of fiber used. In addition, incorporation of fiber results in a reduced tolerance to overmixing, reduced extensibility, and, depending on the fiber used, may either increase or decrease the resistance to extension. Viscosity and stickiness may also be affected. These factors influence such things as loaf volumes, need for additional ingredients such as vital wheat gluten, and production schedules and interruptions (32). These may sound intimidating, but incorporation of fiber into bakery products has been accomplished quite successfully over the years. Many different fibers, such as stabilized flax (6), oat fibers (33), psyllium (34), powdered cellulose (35), barley fractions (36,37), resistant starch (26), and numerous others (4,14,38–41), can be used. These fibers are effectively added to products such as breads, buns, cakes, cookies, crackers, muffins, biscuits, bagels, pizza, tortillas, pie crusts, pancakes, waffles, and doughnuts. In these products, fiber fulfills a number of functions, including inhibiting ice crystal formation in frozen foods and decreasing fat uptake in fried foods such as doughnuts.

Gums are also used in baked goods. For some applications, the level of gum (e.g., agar, guar, xanthan, cellulose gum) used is high enough to be considered a source of fiber enhancement. Other applications, however, are based on functionality (e.g., emulsifier, stabilizer, thickening agent, etc.) and use low levels of gums. In baked goods, gums are used not only in doughs and batters but are also important ingredients in icings, glazes, toppings, fillings, pipings, and meringues (42–45).

Development of yeast-leavened and chemically leavened bakery products containing added fiber has been extensively discussed by Stauffer (46,47). As mentioned earlier, a variety of processing and formula changes may be necessary to successfully incorporate fiber ingredients into bakery products. Representative formulas for reduced-calorie (one-fourth fewer calories than the standard product) bread and fiber cookies are provided in Tables 3 and 4, respectively.

B. Breakfast Cereals

The fiber content of ready-to-eat (RTE) breakfast cereals varies greatly depending on the ingredients used in the formula. Unless the cereal is an all bran or whole grain type, the fiber content is probably only 1–2 g per serving. The potential for including a health claim on the front panel (Principal Display Panel) of the packaged food has prompted many manufacturers to increase the dietary fiber content of their cereals.

Many different fiber ingredients can be used to increase the fiber content of RTE cereals. Because of the relationship between SF and cardiovascular disease, a number of breakfast cereal

Table 3 Formula for Reduced-Calorie Bread

Ingredient	Baker's percent[a]
Sponge	
Flour	60
Bleached oat fiber or alpha cellulose	40
Vital wheat gluten	5
Compressed yeast	3
Mineral yeast food	0.6
Ethoxylated monoglycerides (emulsifier)	1
Stearoyl-2-lactylates (emulsifiers)	0.5
Water	110
Dough	
Flour	40
High-fructose corn syrup	7
Vital wheat gluten	5
Salt	3
Compressed yeast	2
Calcium propionate	0.5
Water	20
Ascorbic acid	0.01

[a] Flour equal to 100%
Source: Refs. 14, 33.

Table 4 Formulas for Reduced-Calorie Cookies

Ingredient	Peanut butter cookies[a]	Chocolate chip cookies[a]
First stage		
Oat fiber	29	19
Sugar beet fiber	2	—
Cocoa fiber	—	12
Unemulsified shortening	—	15
Crunchy peanut butter	30	—
High-fructose corn syrup	70	70
Soy lecithin	—	2
Second stage		
Flour	69	69
Dry whole eggs	1.4	1.4
Salt	0.9	0.9
Sodium bicarbonate	0.4	0.4
Barley malt	0.15	0.15
Natural peanut flavor	0.3	—
Water	40	50
Chocolate chips	—	20

[a] Based on fibers (oat, sugar beet, cocoa) and flour equal to 100%.
Source: Refs. 14, 33.

manufacturers incorporate oat or psyllium fiber to qualify for using the relevant health claim as discussed earlier. Use of other sources, such as wheat bran, whole wheat, oat hulls, sugar beet or pea, if incorporated in sufficient levels, would allow for the use of the "good source of" or "high in" nutrient content descriptors. Fruit fibers may also be used and would impart a distinct flavor or color to the cereal. Soy- and barley-based fibers have also been used (48,49).

Addition of fiber may affect the structure and texture of the cereal product. A coarsely ground fiber might provide more fiber appearance in the product, but it may also result in a gritty mouthfeel; a finer granulation has less grittiness and may lead to a more shelf-stable cereal. Too much fiber, however, can act as an avenue of breakage, and loss of cereal piece integrity may occur (50).

In a recently reported study, incorporation of resistant starch into extruded cereals resulted in greater crispness and an improvement in texture due to better expansion (26). Most conventional fibers tend to hamper extruded cereal expansion, so the observed improvement resulting from the resistant starch is advantageous. In general, though, modification of formulas or processing conditions can overcome any problems associated with the addition of fiber to extruded breakfast cereal products.

C. Pastas and Noodles

As part of the foundation of the Food Guide Pyramid (51), pasta and noodle products are low in fat and are good sources of complex carbohydrates. In general, though, they are not good sources of fiber. However, a variety of fiber ingredients, such as cellulose (14), oats (33), barley (36), soy (39,52), rice bran (38), and others (4,39), can be incorporated into these products to increase their fiber content as well as provide functional attributes. For pastas, the antisticking characteristic of certain fibers helps to facilitate the extrusion process. Other fibers may also contribute to dough strength or improve steam table life of the cooked pasta. Addition of gums to certain Asian noodle products makes the noodles firmer and easier to rehydrate upon cooking or soaking (53).

D. Beverages

Beverages are common products to which fiber is often added. Reasons for this addition include the potential for fiber enrichment as well as utilization of numerous fiber functionalities. The emerging trend in development of nutraceuticals (functional foods), designed to positively impact health, physical performance, or state of mind above and beyond normal nutritive value, is a driving force in fiber enrichment of beverages. Currently, Japan has shown the greatest interest in "functional foods," and many fiber-rich soft drink products such as FibeMini™ and Fibi™ are available in that country (54). Growing awareness of these types of products will lead to a greater demand for fiber-enriched beverages in the United States and elsewhere. Because of their soluble nature as well as their cholesterol-lowering abilities and low viscosity levels, oat fibers such as Oatrim™ are often used in this type of application. Some of the beverages in which oats have been incorporated include milk, milk shakes, hot chocolate, instant-type breakfast drinks, fruit and vegetable juices, ice tea, sports drinks, cappuccino, and wine (18,22,39,55). Other beverages that can benefit from the addition of fiber include liquid diet beverages—both those created for people with special dietary needs as well as weight loss or meal-replacement beverages (56).

From a functionality perspective, fiber ingredients have a lot to offer in terms of use in beverages. In these applications, the main functional purpose of fiber is as a thickening agent, and fiber ingredients such as alginates, carrageenan, cellulose gums, pectins, xanthan, guar gum, gum arabic, and other gums are frequently used (45,54–57). Viscosities of these fibers vary, but some modification of the thickening effect may be possible through processing techniques, changes in particle size, or by combining two or more fiber sources. Added viscosity from fiber is a valuable asset in modification of the texture and mouthfeel of reduced-calorie or reduced-fat beverages such as skim milk. In addition to affecting the beverage's flow rate and mouthfeel, viscosity of added fiber ingredients can also influence flavor. A more viscous liquid remains in the mouth longer and can increase perception of flavor. Additionally, other fibers may mask tart or bitter flavors that are often intensified in reduced-fat or reduced-sugar beverage applications (56).

Another functionality of fiber in beverages is that of stabilization of dispersions. Incorporation into liquids of some fibers, such as corn or soy, which have limited solubility, often results in gravitational settling of the particles. Addition of a hydrocolloid stabilizer (e.g., xanthan gum, carrageenan, or microcrystalline cellulose) stabilizes these beverages to keep the particles in suspension (56). Other fibers may act as foam or emulsion stabilizers when incorporated into beverages.

Another application for fiber is in texturally modified beverages (TMBs). In these products, various hydrocolloid materials such as alginates, xanthan, gellan, or carrageenan gums are used to suspend pulp, gel balls, or other components in beverages. With just a slight increase in viscosity, opportunities such as incorporation of different and distinct flavor phases (e.g., spicy floating balls in a fruit-flavored drink) or striking visual effects (e.g., colored floating material suspended in a clear solution) are possible (54).

E. Meat Products

Fiber incorporation into meat products would appeal to many health-conscious consumers looking for low- and reduced-fat products. A variety of red meat and pork products can benefit from the lubrication, slipperiness, body, and mouthfeel resulting from the utilization of fiber as a fat replacer. Carrageenan, particularly the iota form, is highly recommended for use in meat products due to its cold solubility, freeze/thaw stability, gelling and water-binding properties (49). Gel-like pieces can also be formed and added to low-fat meats such as breakfast sausages to provide the visual appearance of fat.

Other fiber sources, such as oat, soy, pea, psyllium, vegetable fibers, and cellulose, are also suitable for use in meats (4,34,39,49,52). Cellulon™, a bacteria-formed cellulose, has been used in the production of surimi, a minced fish product popular in Japan. The Cellulon serves as a low-cost extender of the expensive surimi protein as well as improving the texture and adding whiteness to the color of the surimi (58). In the production of synthetic meats (meat analogs from plant protein), addition of psyllium mucilloid aids in modifying the texture to impart a meat-like chewiness (34).

Thus, fiber, because of numerous functional characteristics including water-holding capacity, lubricity, freeze/thaw stability and texture modification, to name a few, is a valuable extender, binder, and fat-replacement ingredient in the manufacture of various meat products.

F. Dairy Products

There is currently a great deal of interest in reducing the fat and calorie content of dairy products, and fiber ingredients are valuable tools in this endeavor. As indicated previously, fiber (often Oatrim™ or a cellulose gel) can be used to modify the texture and mouthfeel of skim milk products (16,55). Furthermore, this modification improves the visual appearance of the product. Other types of milk products, such as reduced-fat, evaporated, condensed and chocolate milks, also benefit from the addition of hydrocolloid gums, which suspend solids as well as provide body.

Table 5 Suppliers of Dietary Fiber Ingredients

Supplier	Fiber source(s)	Address	Telephone #	Fax #	Online address
ADM Milling Co.	Corn bran, oat bran	Box 7007, Shawnee Mission, KS 66207	913/491-9400	913/491-0035	admworld.com
California Natural Products	Soy bran	P.O. Box 1219, Lathrop, CA 95330	209/858-2525	209/858-4076	californianatural.com
Can-Oat Milling	Oat bran	Portage La Prairie, MB Canada R1N 3W1	204/857-9700	204/857-9500	can-oat.com
Canadian Harvest	Corn bran, multigrain, oat bran, oat fiber	1001 S. Cleveland St., Cambridge, MN 55008	612/689-5800	612/689-5949	chusa.com
ConAgra Grain Processing	Barley, corn bran, multigrain, oat bran	9 ConAgra Drive, Omaha, NE 68102-5002	402/595-4370	402/595-4111	
Durey-Libby Edible Nuts, Inc.	Apple, fruit (low moisture), pear, prune, sunflower	100 Industrial Road, Carlstadt, NJ 07072	201/939-2775	201/939-0386	
Farmers' Rice Cooperative	Rice bran	P.O. Box 15223, Sacramento, CA 95851	916/923-5100	916/920-3321	
Freeman Industries, LLC	Apple, citrus, corn bran, fruit (low moisture), oat bran, oat fiber, rice bran, tomato, vegetable	100 Marbledale Road, Tuckahoe, NY 10707	914/961-2100	914/961-5793	
Fruitrim Fat Replacers & Sweeteners, Adept Solutions, Inc.	Apple, barley, fruit (low moisture), oat bran, oat fiber, pear, prune, rice bran, sugarbeet	331 Capitola Ave, Suite L, Capitola, CA 95010	888/477-6644 408/477-1344	408/477-1348	
Functional Foods	Cellulose, psyllium	470 Route 9, Englishtown, NJ 07726	800/442-9524 908/972-2232	908/536-9179	
International Grain Products Co.	Barley, corn bran, multigrain, pea bran, wheat bran	P.O. Box 677, Wayzata, MN 55391	800/845-5750 612/474-6573	612/397-7232	
Kellogg	Wheat bran	1 Kellogg Square, Battle Creek, MI 49016-3599	616/961-2336	616/961-6764	kelloggs.com
Lauhoff Grain Co., Bunge Corp.	Corn bran, wheat bran	Box 571, Danville, IL 61834	217/442-1800	217/443-9849	

Company	Fiber	Address	Phone	Fax	Website
Mid-America Food Sales, Ltd.	Amaranth bran, apple, barley, citrus, corn bran, fruit (low moisture), multigrain, mustard, oat bran, oat fiber, pea bran, prune, psyllium, rice bran, soy bran, sugarbeet, vegetable	P.O. Box 904, Northbrook, IL 60065-0904	847/945-0104	847/945-0424	
Miller Brewing Co.	Barley	3939 W. Highland Blvd., Milwaukee, WI 53208	414/931-3739	414/931-4285	
Minn Dak Growers Ltd,	Mustard	Hwy 81 N P.O. Box 13276, Grand Forks, ND 58208	701/746-7453	701/780-9050	minndak.com
National Oats Co. Inc.	Oat bran, oat fiber	701 16th St. NE, Cedar Rapids, IA 52402	800/364-0585	319/364-1695	
Quaker Oats Co., Food Ingredients Dept.	Corn bran, oat bran	321 N. Clark St., #19-14, Chicago, IL 60610	312/222-7107	312/222-8407	
Red River Commodities Inc.	Sunflower	P.O. Box 3022 501 42nd St., NW (58102), Fargo, ND 58108	800/437-5539 701/282-2600	701/282-5325	
Roman Meal Milling Co.	Oat bran, wheat bran	4014 15th Ave, NW P.O. Box 46, Fargo, ND 58102	701/282-9656	701/282-9743	
J.M. Swank Co.	Cellulose, corn bran, oat bran, oat fiber, soy bran, wheat bran	P.O. Box 365, North Liberty, IA 52317	800/593-6375	319/626-3662	jmswank.com
TIC Gums Inc.	Cellulose	4609 Richlynn Drive, P.O. Box 369, Belcamp, MD 21017-0369	800/221-3953 410/273-7300	410/273-6469	ticgums.com
Tree Top Inc.	Apple	P.O. Box 248, Selah, WA 98942	509/697-7251	509/697-0409	
United Soybean Board	Soy bran	190 Queen Anne Ave. N., Seattle, WA 98109	800/TALK-SOY	206/285-2551	talksoy.com
Vacu-Dry Co.	Apple, fruit (low moisture), prune	7765 Healdsburg Ave. P.O. Box 2418, Sebastopol, CA 95473	888/822-8379 707/829-4646	707/829-4643	vacu-dry.com
Watson Foods Co. Inc.	Cellulose, wheat bran	301 Heffernan Drive, West Haven, CT 06516	203/932-3000	203/932-8266	

Source: Ref. 59.

As for milk, reduction of fat in cultured dairy products such as sour cream, cottage cheese, and yogurt raises concerns regarding viscosity, texture, and mouthfeel. In these products, one or more gums, often blended with other ingredients (e.g., starch, emulsifiers, or corn syrup solids), can supply the necessary emulsification, stabilization, and water-retention characteristics as well as the proper texture and mouthfeel of the product (16). Some of the gums that can be used include carrageenan, guar gum, locust bean gum, and xanthan gum (16,49). When incorporating fiber into these types of dairy products, care must be taken to utilize fiber sources that will not interfere with the fermentation rate or overall product quality resulting from the active cultures essential to the manufacture of the products.

Fat reduction in milk and cultured dairy products is fairly easy due to their relatively low fat content. Ice creams and frozen yogurts, on the other hand, have higher fat levels, and as a result fat reduction becomes more complicated. By their nature, these frozen products also place greater demands on the functionalities of fat-replacing ingredients. Here again, fiber ingredients, particularly hydrocolloid gums, fulfill many of the requirements for these applications. Some of the gums that are particularly useful include alginates, carrageenan, locust bean and guar gums, and cellulose gels. They serve to provide viscosity, improve emulsion, foam, and freeze/thaw stability, control melting properties, prevent casein precipitation, reduce syneresis, promote formation of smaller ice crystals, and facilitate extrusion (16).

Cheese products, having an even higher fat content, present a greater challenge for fat reduction than ice creams and frozen yogurts. Additionally, their higher solids levels, use of cultures, and dependence on protein structures contribute to the difficulties. As a result, fat reduction is more easily accomplished in products such as processed cheeses, dips, and spreads. In these applications, combinations of microcrystalline cellulose and various hydrocolloid gums (e.g., carrageenan or guar gum) contribute successfully to the fat reduction. These fibers assist in achieving the proper deformability and melting properties and reduce stickiness and rubbery texture in the products (16).

G. Miscellaneous Products

As is evident from the previous sections, fiber ingredients can be utilized in a number of different food categories. Beyond these, many other foods can benefit substantially from fiber enrichment or the functional characteristics of fibers. Food items such as soups, sauces, gravies, salad dressings, puddings, whipped toppings, tofu, peanut butter, mayonnaise, margarine, granola bars, extruded snacks, fried snacks, jams, confectionery items, microwave reheatable foods, dry mixes, and pet foods all have specific requirements for their particular applications. Fiber ingredients may be suited to addressing some of these requirements.

VII. PRODUCT QUALITY

The ultimate emphasis in production of a food must be placed on taste and quality, since these are main factors involved in successful marketing of the product. Food product designers and technologists should be aware of the multitude of fiber ingredients, and the modifications and variations thereof, that are available for use. Inability of one fiber source to fulfill a particular requirement for a food application may indicate a need to try another fiber source or to use a systems-based approach in blending two or more fibers or combining fiber sources with other functional ingredients. Fiber ingredients may contribute a variety of functional characteristics to the development or manufacture of many different foods. Also, as consumers become more aware of the health benefits of fiber, there will be an increased demand for more numerous and varied food products enriched with fiber.

VIII. INGREDIENT SUPPLIERS

Many different companies serve as suppliers of fiber ingredients. These suppliers can provide guidance to food developers regarding functional characteristics and application suitability of their fiber products. A partial listing of fiber suppliers is given in Table 5 (59). For a more complete or updated listing, consult buyers' guides and directories.

IX. SUMMARY

For health and functional reasons, fiber is finding increasingly greater application in both plant-derived and animal-derived food products. Highly concentrated forms of fiber, prepared from a variety of sources, can be used for these applications. Many different companies serve as suppliers of processed fibers. These suppliers can provide guidance to research and development operations on functional characteristics and application suitability of their fiber products. A partial list of fiber suppliers is presented (Table 5). Additional information can be obtained by consulting buyers' guides and other relevant resource materials.

REFERENCES

1. Lee SC, Prosky L. Perspectives on complex carbohydrate definition. Cereal Foods World 41:88–89, 1996.
2. Vetter JL. Commercially available fiber ingredients and bulking agents. Manhattan, KS: American Institute of Baking, Technical Bulletin, Vol. X, issue 5, 1988.
3. Dietary fiber guide. Cereal Foods World 32:555–570, 1987.
4. Przybyla AE. Formulating fiber into foods. Food Eng 60(10):77–88, 1988.
5. Ranhotra GS, Gelroth JA, Glaser BK. Energy value of resistant starch. J Food Sci 61:453–455, 1996.
6. Duxbury DD. Stabilized flax: high-fiber protein source. Food Proc 54(4):93, 1993.
7. McNeillie A, Bieser J. Hydrogen peroxide uses for the year 2000. Food Proc 54:59–65, 1993.
8. Katz F. Putting the function in functional foods. Food Proc 57(2):56–58, 1996.
9. Hammond N. Functional and nutritional characteristics of rice bran extracts. Cereal Foods World 39:752–754, 1994.
10. Weber FE, Chaudhary VK. Recovery and nutritional evaluation of dietary fiber ingredients from a barley by-product. Cereal Foods World 32:548–550, 1987.
11. Vollendorf NW, Marlett JA. Dietary fiber methodology and composition of oat groats, bran, and hulls. Cereal Foods World 36:565–570, 1991.
12. Posner ES. Mechanical separation of a high dietary fiber fraction from wheat bran. Cereal Foods World 36:553–556, 1991.
13. Ranhotra GS, Gelroth JA, Astroth K, Rao CS. Relative lipidemic responses in rats fed oat bran or oat bran concentrate. Cereal Chem. 67:509–511, 1990.
14. Matz SA. Formulating and Processing Dietetic Foods. McAllen, TX: Pan-Tech International, Inc., 1996.
15. Ang J. Use of powdered cellulose in grain-based foods. Manhattan, KS: American Institute of Baking, Technical Bulletin, Vol. XVI, issue 7, 1994.
16. Alexander RJ. Moo-ving toward low-calorie dairy products. Food Product Design 7(1):74–98, 1997.
17. Kevin K. Carbohydrates: the next generation. Food Proc 57(2):52–54, 1996.

18. Modified Oatrim finds use in healthy beverages. Food Eng 65(1):22, 1993.

19. Inglett GE. Development of a dietary fiber gel for calorie-reduced foods. Cereal Foods World 42: 382–385, 1997.

20. Penichter KA, McGinley EJ. Cellulose gel for fat-free food applications. Food Technol 45(6):105, 1991.

21. Deis RC. Functional ingredients from rice. Food Product Design 6(10):45–56, 1997.

22. Inglett GE, Grisamore SB. Maltodextrin fat substitute lowers cholesterol. Food Technol 45(6):104, 1991.

23. Kevin K. A marriage of fiber and flavor. Food Proc 56(9):83–84, 1995.

24. Kevin K. Starch de resistance, Food Proc 56(1):65–67, 1995.

25. Ranhotra GS, Gelroth JA, Eisenbraun GJ. High-fiber white flour and its use in cookie products. Cereal Chem 68:432–434, 1991.

26. Yue P, Waring S. Resistant starch in food applications. Cereal Foods World 43:690–695, 1998.

27. Vetter JL. Food Labeling—Requirements for FDA Regulated Product. Manhattan, KS: American Institute of Baking, 1993.

28. Ranhotra GS, Gelroth JA, Glaser BK. Usable energy value of selected bulking agents. J Food Sci 58:1176–1178, 1993.

29. Abboud A. Systems approach to reducing fat in baked goods. Manhattan, KS: American Institute of Baking, Technical Bulletin, Vol. XVII, issue 12, 1995.

30. FDA forces change in Fresh Horizons' 'therapeutic claims.' Advertising Age, Oct. 18, 1976.

31. CFR. Code of Federal Regulations 21 (Parts 100 to 169). Washington, DC: U.S. Government Printing Office, 1998.

32. Lang CE, Walker CE. Effect of fiber on dough rheology. Manhattan, KS: American Institute of Baking, Technical Bulletin, Vol. XII, issue 11, 1990.

33. Dougherty M, Sombke R, Irvine J, Rao CS. Oat fibers in low calorie breads, soft-type cookies, and pasta. Cereal Foods World 33:424–427, 1988.

34. Chan JK, Wypyszyk V. A forgotten natural dietary fiber: psyllium mucilloid. Cereal Foods World 33:919–922, 1988.

35. Ang JF, Miller WB. Multiple functions of powdered cellulose as a food ingredient. Cereal Foods World 36:558–564, 1991.

36. Knuckles BE, Hudson CA, Chiu MM, Sayre RN. Effect of β-glucan barley fractions in high-fiber bread and pasta. Cereal Foods World 42:94–99, 1997.

37. Newman RK, Ore KC, Abbott J, Newman CW. Fiber enrichment of baked products with a barley milling fraction. Cereal Foods World 43:23–25, 1998.

38. Duxbury D. Dietary fiber: many sources, multi-functional. Food Proc 52(5):136–140, 1991.

39. Duxbury DD. Fiber: form follows function. Food Proc 54(3):44–54, 1993.

40. Bahr PS. New ways to apply fiber. Food Product Design 6(7):77–94, 1996.

41. Matz SA. Ingredients for Bakers. McAllen, TX: Pan-Tech International, Inc., 1996.

42. Ward F, Andon S. The use of gums in bakery foods. Manhattan, KS: American Institute of Baking, Technical Bulletin, Vol. XV, issue 4, 1993.

43. Ward FM. Hydrocolloid systems as fat mimetics in bakery products: icings, glazes and fillings. Cereal Foods World 42:386–390, 1997.

44. Penichter KA, McGinley EJ. Cellulose gel for fat-free food applications. Food Technol 45(6):105, 1991.

45. Greenberg NA, Sellman D. Partially hydrolyzed guar gum as a source of fiber. Cereal Foods World 43:703–706, 1998.

46. Stauffer CE. Fiber and Baking. Kansas City, MO: Sosland Publishing Co., 1991.

47. Stauffer CE. Fiber: choosing the right one. Baking Snack 14(6):28–32, 1992.

48. Ready-to-eat breakfast cereal processing gets a big boost from extrusion and impingement technology. Baking Snack 14(7):34–38, 1992.

49. Mauro DJ, Wang Y-J. Breakfast food ingredients. Cereal Foods World 42:440–443, 1997.

50. Knehr E. Bowl 'em over: Adding value to breakfast cereal. Food Product Design 7(3):103–124, 1997.

51. The Food Guide Pyramid. Home and Garden Bulletin No. 252. Hyattsville, MD: USDA, Human Nutrition Information Service, 1992.
52. Andres C. Multi-functional fiber provides nutrition, texture, and increased functionality. Food Proc 47(13):39–40, 1986.
53. Hou G, Kruk M. Asian Noodle Technology. Manhattan, KS: American Institute of Baking, Technical Bulletin, Vol. XX, issue 12, 1998.
54. Giese J. Developments in beverage additives. Food Technol 49(9):64–72, 1995.
55. Pszczola DE. Oatrim finds application in fat-free, cholesterol-free milk. Food Technol 50(9):80–81, 1996.
56. Hegenbart S. Using fiber in beverages. Food Product Design 5(3):68–78, 1995.
57. Andon S. Applications of soluble dietary fiber. Food Technol 41(1):74–75, 1987.
58. Kent RA, Stephens RS, Westland JA. Bacterial cellulose fiber provides an alternative for thickening and coating. Food Technol 45(6):108, 1991.
59. Food Processing 1999 Guide & Directory Issue. Food Proc 59(9):100–103, 261–311, 1998.

24
Wheat Bran: Physiological Effects

Susan Sungsoo Cho and Celeste Clark
Kellogg Company, Battle Creek, Michigan

Wheat bran is a component of whole wheat, a food used by humans for millennia. Wheat bran itself has been in use as a food for over a century in the United States.

Wheat bran consists of the outer coats of the wheat grain, which can be separated from the germ and various grades of flour during the milling process. The commercial product usually contains some of the wheat embryo and a small amount of endosperm because of the difficulty of making a sharp separation. The bran amounts to approximately 12–15% of the grain. It has come into prominence since the development of modern methods of milling, which date back to about 1870. At first it was used almost exclusively for feeding farm animals, but subsequently it was introduced as an item of the human diet. From the standpoint of human nutrition, it should be mentioned that there are two principal varieties of bran on the market. Untreated bran is the mill product widely used for feeding animals and also, after cleaning, to some extent for incorporation into dough mixtures for making certain bakery products such as bran muffins. The prepared type of bran has been subjected to processes designed to improve its palatability, and it is distributed primarily as a so-called breakfast cereal food. The processing may vary somewhat. The general procedure consists of washing the crude bran (sometimes with dilute acid, then with water) and mixing with malt syrup, sugar, salt, and water. The mixture is cooked and finally dried and packaged. Frequently it is shredded or toasted before being packed in cartons. In connection with the use of wheat bran or whole wheat in ready-to-eat (RTE) breakfast cereals, the basic patent for shredded wheat was issued in 1895, and various manufacturers (including Kellogg) have produced shredded wheat biscuit cereals for decades. A variation on the production process of shredded bran cereal was obtained by John Leonard Kellogg in 1916 (U.S. Patent 67,504). Kellogg also has produced a variety of other wheat bran cereals for similarly lengthy periods.

I. WHEAT BRAN AND COLORECTAL CANCER

It has been recognized by U.S. health authorities that diet can play a role in reducing the risk of some cancers, including colorectal cancers. Diet is considered to be linked to approximately 50% of all cancers (Hunter et al., 1980) and has been called the most important environmental factor associated with colon cancer (Kashtan and Stern, 1992).

Various U.S. health authorities have recognized the role that wheat bran or whole wheat consumption can play in reducing the risk of certain types of cancer. For example, the National

Research Council (1989) noted that there is an inverse relationship between insoluble fiber and cancer, noting specifically that wheat bran, a source of water-insoluble fiber, was more consistently associated with lower risk of colon cancer than other fiber sources. As a consequence, the Surgeon General recommended a higher intake of whole-grain cereal fibers based on evidence that foods high in fiber might decrease the risk for colon cancer.

Colorectal cancer is an especially significant form of cancer with respect to morbidity/mortality statistics. This form of cancer is the third most common malignant neoplasm worldwide (Shike et al., 1990) and the second leading cause of cancer deaths (irrespective of gender) in the United States (Boring et al., 1993). Between 1973 and 1989, mortality from colorectal cancer declined by 12.8%, but incidence increased by 2.5% in the United States. The overall 5-year mortality rate is approximately 50% (National Cancer Institute, 1995). The National Cancer Institute (NCI) has estimated that in 1994, 56,000 people died from colorectal cancer, and another 149,000 contracted the disease (NCI, 1996). Incidence rates for the period 1987–91 based on statistics from NCI indicate that, for every 100,000 white persons, 47.8 develop colorectal cancer; the corresponding figure among blacks is 52.4. NCI (1996) has further estimated that the average number of years of life lost due to colorectal cancer was estimated to be 13.3. The risk of colorectal cancer begins to increase after the age of 40 and rises sharply at age 50–55; the risk doubles with each succeeding decade, reaching a peak by age 75. Despite advances in surgical technique and adjuvant therapy, there has been only a modest impact on patients who present with advanced neoplasms. (Moertel, et al., 1990). Hence, effective primary and secondary preventive approaches must be developed to reduce the morbidity and mortality from this disease.

The Life Sciences Research Office (LSRO) (Kritchevsky, 1991) of the Federation of American Societies for Experimental Biology (FASEB) (Pilch, 1987) found particular types of fiber (especially fiber from wheat bran) to have protective effects in animals. Specifically, LSRO noted that both human epidemiological and animal studies suggest that certain kinds of dietary fiber play a role in the etiology of colon cancer, strengthening the hypothesis regarding insoluble fiber and cancer. LSRO stated that human studies demonstrate whole wheat/wheat's implication in colon carcinogenesis, independently of fat intake. As it explained, dietary fiber, particularly whole-grain cereals and bread, may reduce the production and/or excretion of fecal mutagens and decrease the concentrations of secondary bile acids that play a role in colon carcinogenesis. LSRO also noted that animal studies suggest that certain kinds of dietary fiber play a role in the etiology of colon cancer. It noted in this connection that 13 of 17 studies demonstrated evidence of protection by dietary wheat bran against colon tumor development, whereas three studies showed no effect and one study showed an enhancing effect. International correlational studies, considered together, were also found to indicate that the inverse relationship between fiber and fiber-containing foods and colon cancer risk is strong, consistent, and not likely due to artifacts of the analyses from particular studies. LSRO therefore recommended a daily fiber intake of 25–30 g, including fiber from whole-grain cereal sources. In 1991, LSRO, as part of a request by the U.S. Food and Drug Administration (FDA) to FASEB in connection with the investigation of science regarding a dietary fiber/cancer health claim, also analyzed two case-control studies demonstrating that insoluble fiber is associated with decreased risk of colon cancer, and the magnitude of association increased after controlling for fat intake (Kritchevsky, 1991). At that time, LSRO discussed additional studies that confirmed the consistently protective effect of wheat bran in animals.

The National Research Council's 1989 volume on diet and health also discusses wheat bran consumption and cancer risk. It noted animal studies that indicate a protective effect of dietary fiber against colon cancer. While this effect varied depending upon the source of the fiber, wheat bran has the most consistent inhibiting effect. (Animal studies suggest that wheat bran in particular is an effective inhibitor of experimentally induced carcinogenesis.) Likewise, the 1986 Recommended Dietary Allowances discussed plausible mechanisms for the anticarcinogenic effect of fiber, including decreased intestinal transit time or contact time between carcinogens and the intestine and dilution of fecal contents (along with dilution of any carcinogens) (NRC, 1989). Decreased intestinal transit time and increased fecal output are associated with reduction in incidence and number of colonic tumors. Because insoluble fibers (such as those in whole wheat or wheat bran) are most strongly implicated in these mechanisms, there is support for a health claim about insoluble fiber from wheat bran and cancer, particularly regarding colorectal cancers (NRC, 1996).

In sum, U.S. health authorities uniformly recognize the importance of increased fiber consumption in reducing the risk of colon cancer. Yet, 25% of men and women consume less than 6–8 g of fiber per day, and perhaps 90% of American men and women consumed less than 20 and 15 g of fiber, respectively, per day (Block and Subar, 1992).

There is extensive evidence from comparative and case-control studies that consumption of dietary fiber, including dietary fiber from cereal sources, is associated inversely with the incidence of colorectal cancer. Greenwald et al. (1987) examined 40 epidemiological studies in 55 reports published between 1970 and 1986 and concluded that a large fraction of the diverse studies of different populations consuming a variety of foods reported a common and consistent trend. Those groups consuming high-fiber diets generally had lower colon cancer rates than comparable populations consuming a low-fiber diet. While other dietary factors potentially interacted, dietary fiber and its interaction with fat remains the single most comprehensive explanation of the available evidence.

Likewise, Trock et al. (1990) conducted a meta-analysis of the data from 37 observational studies and 16 of 23 case-control studies conducted between 1970 and 1988 and concluded that critical evaluation of epidemiological studies of fiber and colon cancer provides considerable evidence that a diet rich in fiber and vegetables is associated with a reduced risk of colon cancer. At least 25 studies showed a strong to moderate protective effect for fiber; the data from case-control studies suggest a reduction in risk of approximately 40% for persons consuming diets high in fiber and vegetables. Shankar and Lanza (1991) offered a similar observation, noting that since 1980 a protective effect has been found in six out of seven within-country or national correlation studies, 12 out of 17 case-control studies, and four out of five metabolic studies. Their conclusion was that a large body of literature suggests that eating a variety of high-fiber foods has a protective effect against colon cancer.

Similarly, Howe et al. (1992) did a combined analysis of the data from 13 case-control studies involving 5,287 colon cancer cases and 10,470 controls. Their conclusion was that the present analysis has provided strong evidence of monotonically decreasing risk with increasing intake of fiber, an association that, in essence, could not be due to chance. It was estimated that if the United States and Canadian populations increased their fiber intake to 39 g/day, the reduction in colon cancer risk would be 31%, or 50,000 fewer cases per year in the United States alone. Most recently, Friedenreich et al. (1994) undertook a pooled analysis of the data from 13 case-control studies on diet and colorectal cancer published between 1983 and 1992 and found an odds ratio for dietary fiber, scaled by interquintile range of intake (27 g/d), of 0.46 (95% confidence interval = 0.34–0.64). If seven additional studies measuring dietary fiber intake were included, the ratio was 0.53 (95% CI = 0.37–0.65) (Dwyer 1993). As one group of scientists has noted, the inverse relationship between fiber consumption and colon cancer incidence is generally recognized (Jacobs, 1987).

There are four general types of studies presenting scientific evidence relating to consumption of insoluble fiber from wheat bran or whole wheat and the risk of colorectal cancer: (1) correlational (or ecological) studies; (2) case-control (or retrospective) studies; (3) cohort (or prospective) studies; and (4) experimental studies (or clinical trials) (Byers, 1988). With respect to correlation studies, the analyses by Englyst et al. (1982), McKeown-Eyssen and Bright-See (1984, 1985), Maisto and Bremner (1981), and Powles and Williams (1984) all found protective effects for wheat bran or whole wheat. Two other studies involving correlational analyses of case-control pairs found reduced risk of colon or rectal cancer among those who consumed whole wheat or wheat bran, but not at levels that reached statistical significance (Pickle et al., 1984; Randall et al., 1992). No prospective cohort study deals specifically with wheat bran or whole wheat.

With respect to case-control studies, the most significant recent dietary intervention analyses are (a) the Arizona Prevention Trial involving 52 patients with a history of colon adenoma resection fed 2.0 or 13.5 g/d of wheat bran for 9 months (Alberts et al., 1996); (b) the New York study of 58 patients with familial adenomatous polyposis treated with up to 22.5 g/d of wheat bran over 4 years (DeCosse et al., 1989); (c) the Canadian Intervention Trial involving 201 polypectomy patients fed varying amounts of dietary fiber (up to 35 g/d), most of which came from wheat bran, during 2 years of dietary counseling (McKeown-Eyssen et al., 1994); and (d) the Australian Polyp Prevention Trial, involving 424 patients with a history of adenomatous polyps, portions of whom received 25 g/d of wheat bran over 4 years (MacLennan et al., 1995). These four key studies found that wheat bran as part of a total diet exhibited some degree of protective effect against colon cancer. In a randomized, double-blind, placebo-controlled study on humans (Alberts et al., 1996), 9 months of high daily intakes of wheat bran fiber supplements were associated with a statistically significant reduction in fecal bile acid concentrations and excretion rates. As the authors summarized, epidemiological and nutritional studies demonstrate that complex interactions among dietary factors, genetic susceptibility, and environmental factors affect colorectal carcinogenesis. Their measurement of fecal bile acids among test subjects suggested a potential mechanism for reduction of colorectal cancer risk by dietary interventions. The results were that all mean fecal bile acid concentrations and excretion rates were lower at 9 months than at zero months or 3 months for those in the high-dose fiber treatment group, and the high-dose fiber effect at 9 months of supplementation was statistically significant with respect to virtually all geometric mean fecal bile acid concentrations and excretion rates. Pointing to the association with statistically significant reductions in both total and secondary fecal bile acid concentrations and excretion rates in patients with resected colon adenomas, the authors indicated that their study suggests that reductions in fecal bile acid concentrations may represent the major mechanism through which wheat bran fiber exerts its preventive effects on colon carcinogenesis (Wargovich and Levin, 1996). The results obtained in the Arizona Prevention Trial undertaken by Alberts and colleagues were prefigured in a randomized, double-blind, placebo-controlled study conducted in the late 1980s by DeCosse and colleagues in New York. There, 58 patients with familiar adenomatous polyposis were given 4 g of vitamin C and 400 mg of vitamin E daily, either alone or in conjunction with 22.5 g/d of fiber from wheat bran. Over the 4 years of the trial, patients underwent proctosigmoidoscopy every 3 months. The results showed that those on a high-fiber diet had a lower median polyp number ratio than controls or those on vitamins alone; while this analysis could not be statistically demonstrated among those for whom there was an intent to treat, when adjustments were made for dietary compliance over the course of the 4 years, significant and consistent results showed that polyp number decreased as the amount of ingested, prescribed fiber increased. The authors noted that benefit from the prescribed fiber appeared to be concentrated among those study patients who consumed more than 11 g of fiber daily, suggesting a threshold level of ingested grain fiber for a treatment effect. Total energy (caloric) intake and consumption of polyunsaturated fat did not alter results.

More equivocal results were obtained in the Canadian Intervention Trial, reported by McKeown-Eyssen et al. (1994). This was a randomized dietary intervention trial involving 201 patients who had undergone polypectomy for adenomatous colorectal polyps. The patients were assigned to either a group on a normal diet high in fat and low in fiber or a diet low in fat (the lesser of 50 g/d or 20% of energy) and high in fiber (50 g/d, principally from a wheat bran snack product). After 12 months of counseling, fat consumption was 25% of energy in the high-fiber group and 33% of energy in the normal diet group; respective fiber consumption was 35 and 16 g/d. Biochemical indicators were obtained on a blinded basis over 2 years of follow-up through annual 24-hour stool collections and quarterly blood samples; 165 of the patients had follow-up colonoscopic examinations. Among those in the high-fiber group, 21.8% had at least one pathologically confirmed neoplastic polyp, while the corresponding incidence rate was only 18.4% among those on the regular diet. However, noticeably higher incidence rates were observed among men than among women (relative risk of 1.6 vs. 0.7).

The Australian Polyp Prevention Trial yielded no significant gender-based differences. It was a randomized, partially double-blind, placebo-controlled factorial trial involving 424 patients with a history of colorectal adenomas. Patients were divided into eight intervention groups, consisting of controls and persons eating a diet low in fat (25–30% of energy), high in fiber (25 g of finely milled raw wheat bran in All-Bran cereal), and containing 20 mg of β-carotene, alone or in combination. The study lasted 4 years and 306 patients completed it; blinded colonoscopies were conducted at 24 and 48 months. No single intervention had a protective effect against adenomas of any size. However, the combination of low fat and high fiber yielded zero large adenomas at 24 and 48 months, a finding that was statistically significant. The authors concluded that the bran supplement had no effect on the incidence of total adenomas, but our data suggest that bran may interact with low fat to reduce the incidence of large adenomas. They found that their trial supports current guidelines for cancer prevention, particularly with regard to reducing fat intake and at the same time eating more fiber-rich foods (specifically, wheat bran). Case-control studies other than these four large clinical trials have typically involved significantly fewer numbers of subjects and have examined the effect of wheat bran or whole wheat intake on recognized physiological factors associated with colorectal cancer risk, particularly fecal bile acid concentrations, enzyme activity, fecal weights, intestinal transit time, and epithelial cell proliferation in rectal mucosa.

As a last category, there is the subgroup of case-control studies involving experiments on rats or mice. The typical structure of many of these studies involves determination of the effect of wheat bran or whole wheat intake on tumor incidence among animals in whom cancer is chemically induced. Several authors have pointed out that research involving 1,2-dimethylhydrazine (DMH) and male Sprague-Dawley rats is particularly useful in identifying dietary influences of colorectal cancer that may have significance for humans (McIntosh et al., 1993; McIntyre et al., 1993). Thirteen animal studies involving administration of DMH (and usually involving male Sprague-Dawley rats, unless otherwise indicated) found a protective effect for wheat bran [Abraham et al., 1980; Barbolt and Abraham, 1978; Barnes et al., 1983 (Fischer-344 rats); Calvert et al., 1987 (Fischer-344 rats); Chen et al., 1978 (CF female mice); Clapp et al., 1980 (Fischer-344 rats); Fleiszer et al., 1978 (male Chester Beatty hooded weanling rats); McIntosh 1993; McIntyre et al., 1993; Scheutte and Rose, 1986; Wilson et al., 1977; Young et al., 1996]. Two found no effect (Bauer et al., 1979; Cruse et al., 1978), and three found a possible promoting effect with respect to tumor incidence, at least under certain conditions [Clapp et al., 1980 (male Balb-c/mice); Jacobs, 1983, 1984]. A number of other studies involved carcinogenesis in animals induced through other chemicals, principally azoxymethane (AOM), methylnitrosurea (MNU), 3,2′-dimethyl-4-aminobiphenyl (DMAB), or N-methyl-N′-nitro-N-nitroso-guanidine. In

8 of these 10 studies (which involved either Wistar or Fischer-344 rats), a protective effect for wheat bran or whole wheat was found. Various researchers (Alabaster et al., 1993 (in conjunction with psyllium), 1995; Reddy et al., 1980, 1981; Shivapurkar et al., 1995; Sinkeldam et al., 1990; Tatsuta et al., 1988; Watanabe et al., 1979) found protective effects against AOM-induced tumors but not against MNU-induced tumors. Only Nigro et al. (1979) and Shivapurkar et al. (1995) found no statistically significant difference in AOM-induced tumors among controls and subjects fed wheat bran in some circumstances.

Finally, a group of animal studies involved analysis of the effect of wheat bran ingestion on a variety of biomarkers associated with the incidence of colorectal cancer, such as fecal weight, epithelial cell proliferation, gastrointestinal transit time, short-chain fatty acid (SCFA) production, crypt cell formation, fecal bile acid concentration, and thymidine kinase activity, where no chemically induced carcinogenesis was part of the study design. Of the 27 studies falling in this category, all found some protective effect associated with wheat bran ingestion (Barbolt and Abraham, 1978, 1980; Boffa et al., 1992; Calvert and Reicks, 1988; Calvert et al., 1990; Edwards and Eastwood, 1992; Folino et al., 1995; Furukawa et al., 1995; Gallaher and Franz, 1990; Gestel et al., 1994; Gibson et al., 1995; Glauert and Bennink, 1983; Jacobs and White, 1983; Jacobs and Schneeman, 1981; Jacobs and Lupton, 1982; Kawata et al., 1992; Lupton and Jacobs, 1983; McIntyre et al., 1991; Malville-Shipan and Fleming, 1992; Mathers and Fotso Tagny, 1994; Munakata et al., 1995; Otsuka et al., 1988; Reddy et al., 1980; Robblee et al., 1989 (effect on mitotic activity); Roland et al., 1994, 1995; Topping et al., 1993). Schneeman and Richter (1993) also reported the effects of psyllium, wheat bran, and oat bran on mucosal weight and DNA contents.

The animal studies overwhelmingly support the proposition that wheat bran has a protective effect against colorectal carcinogenesis. The few studies that yielded a contrary conclusion usually involved administration of DMH or, in one instance, AOM. Reddy pointed out cogently that the few differing results—contained principally in the 1983 study by Jacobs, the 1979 study by Bauer and colleagues, the 1978 study by Cruse and colleagues, and the 1979 study by Nigro and colleagues—are all anomalous.

Dietary inhibitory effects with respect to colorectal cancer have been attributed to the following physiological effects: increase in fecal weight, frequency of defecation, and microbial growth; decrease in gastrointestinal transit time and bile acid hydroxylation; dilution of colonic contents and adsorption of organic and inorganic substances; and production of hydrogen, methane, carbon dioxide, and SCFAs (Mendeloff, 1977; Calvert et al., 1987; Kritchevsky, 1991, 1995). In an overview article, Ausman (1993) noted at least 17 potential mechanisms by which dietary fiber may prevent colon cancer, including alteration of aqueous phase bile acids, fecal pH, mucosal enzyme activity, intestinal microflora, colonic mucin, colonic cell proliferation, or fecal bulk; dilution of fecal bile acids, reduction in fecal mutagenicity or fecal transit time, neurogenic effects caused by changes in fecal bulk or SFCAs, factors related to gut hormones of other peptide growth or enterohepatic circulation of hormones; and decreased availability of total dietary energy. In recent articles, some authors have distinguished between direct and indirect protective mechanisms. Harris and Ferguson (1993) differentiate between direct effects of fiber in the colon and indirect effects after fiber is degraded by bacterial enzymes and fermented; they further note that these classifications can be subdivided into mechanisms affecting the carcinogen before DNA lesions (e.g., binding of carcinogens or increasing the bulk of colon contents among the direct effects, changes in intestinal microflora among the indirect effects) and mechanisms that affect any stages in the progression from epithelial cells with DNA lesions to fully developed tumors (e.g., binding of bile acids among the direct effects, lowering of pH and butyrate action among the indirect effects).

Of course, all dietary fibers are not identical, and each can have different effects on colon carcinogenesis. Wheat bran is a source of cellulose, hemicellulose, and lignin (Ausman, 1993). Huang et al. (1978) estimated that bran is 35–40% dietary fiber and only 8–10% crude fiber; the dietary fiber fraction in turn is typically 67% hemicellulose, 23% lignin, and 10% cellulose. These fibers are insoluble or relatively less soluble and are poorly fermented. Other constituents of wheat bran also may have a protective effect. Moreover, it has been suggested that wheat bran may suppress colon cancer in part because it contains phytic acid (inositol hexaphosphate), which forms chelates with various metals and inhibits damaging ion-catalyzed redox reactions (Graf and Eaton, 1993). As a result, phytic acid can suppress oxidant damage to intestinal epithelium and neighboring cells by colonic bacteria that produce oxygen radicals.

A number of recent studies have sought to quantify and measure changes in bile acid concentrations brought about by wheat bran intake. One recent analysis of the topic was provided in the Arizona Prevention Trial discussed earlier and reported in Alberts et al. (1996). The authors pointed out that fecal bile acids are well recognized as colon cancer promoters; the major mechanism through which wheat bran fiber may exert its preventive effects is in connection with fecal bile acid concentration reduction. The increase in fecal bile acid excretion accompanying a significant decrease in fecal bile acid concentrations has been explained as due to increased stool bulk from wheat bran fiber. The conflicting results of epidemiological studies investigating the relationship between fecal bile acid concentrations and colorectal neoplasia may be attributed in part to differences in methods of fecal sampling, pH, transit time, and water content or differences in colonic function among the various case groups.

Another recent study of significance is that of Reddy et al. (1994), which demonstrated how different bran sources affect fecal bile acid concentration. They used a randomized dietary intervention study to examine the effects of certain fiber sources (wheat, oat, and corn brans) on fecal bile acids, fecal neutral sterols, and fecal bacterial enzymes, all of which have been implicated in tumorigenesis and carcinogenesis. These fiber sources were chosen due both to their differences in solubility, composition, and fermentability and to their importance as sources of grain fiber in the U.S. diet. Subjects comprised 74 premenopausal women who were not following any special diets (including fat-modified diets) and who had no gastrointestinal disease. After a 4-week dietary baseline/control period, subjects were randomly assigned to one of the fiber regimens for 8 weeks. Fiber supplementation was accomplished by adding three to four muffins per day (approximately 15 g/d dietary fiber) to the subjects' normal diets, bringing their total fiber intake to 30 g/d. Nutrient intakes were measured, which revealed slightly but significantly higher caloric and fat intakes (versus the control period) on wheat bran. Beyond that and the twofold increase in fiber intake versus the control period for all three diets, there were no other significant differences in nutrient intakes. After 8 weeks, total fecal secondary bile acid concentrations were significantly ($p < 0.0001$) reduced on the wheat bran diet. In contrast, the corn bran diet did not significantly reduce total bile acid concentrations. Oat bran had no significant effect on bile acids. With respect to neutral sterols, wheat bran decreased and oat bran increased concentrations significantly ($p < 0.05$). The authors concluded from this and earlier human metabolic studies, in addition to animal studies, that the type of fiber is important in affecting positive mechanisms of colon carcinogenesis, including excretion of secondary bile acids, and that insoluble fiber, particularly from wheat bran, appears to decrease these factors most strongly.

In addition to mechanisms involving bile acids, dietary fiber may modulate carcinogenesis via fermentation to SCFAs in the colon with butyrate (one of the SCFAs), which is reported to be the preferred substrate for colonic epithelial cells (Klurfeld, 1992). Starch fermentation increases butyrate production, and butyrate is a well-recognized and antiproliferative agent, acting as an inhibitor of DNA synthesis and cell growth (Bingham, 1993).

Clausen et al. (1991) have shown that wheat bran doubles the production of SCFAs and, in in vitro fermentation, resulted in reduced production of butyrate in subjects with colonic adenomas or suffering from colon cancer. Lupton and Kurtz (1993) showed that the concentration of SCFAs in the cecum and proximal colon was much higher among rats fed wheat bran; indeed, wheat bran produced butyrate-rich fermentations in those sites and in the distal colon. The authors concluded that the effect of SCFA on colonocytes is different in normal cells versus transformed cells. Butyrate seems to inhibit growth in transferred cells while enhancing proliferation in normal human and rat mucosa. Topping et al. (1993) also found that wheat bran increased butyrate levels in the distal colons of pigs. McIntyre et al. (1991), in another animal study, found that wheat bran intake resulted in high SCFA concentrations in both the feces and the cecum and in high butyrate excretion rates. They pointed out that wheat bran may be particularly important since, because of its lesser degree of fermentability, it can have an effect in the distal colon. Mathers and Fotso Tagny (1994) noted similarly that, in addition to reducing cecal transit time, wheat bran increased butyrate production by a factor of 1.62 in the distal colon. Boffa et al. (1992) did a comparative analysis in rats, considering colonic luminal butyrate levels among rats fed 0, 5, 10, and 20% fiber from wheat bran. The authors found that total SCFA concentration increased by a factor of 1.8 between the 0 and 5% levels, remained stable between the 5 and 10% levels, and increased 3.4 times over controls between the 10 and 20% levels. There was an inverse correlation between luminal butyrate levels and colonic cell proliferation and a positive linear correlation between those levels and colon epithelial cell histone acetylation. The authors did warn that while diets with moderate levels of fiber may have a protective effect, ingestion of too much fiber could promote carcinogenesis, citing the fact that wheat bran at the 20% level increased hyperplasia and colonic cell hyperproliferation. However, this concern is belied by human studies where subjects were fed large daily amounts of wheat bran over time without any promoting effects being discerned. Butyrate production may be important for another, related reason as well, in that there may be a mechanism by which butyrate may protect against tumor progression through regulation of extracellular proteolysis (Antalis and Reeder, 1995). The authors therefore concluded that investigation of key factors in the regulation of gene expression by butyrate may provide potential targets for intervention (noting that gene expression may be a biomarker for colon cancer and that dietary fiber may affect molecular factors through SCFA production that modulate inherited risk). Butyrate appears to affect epithelial cell growth, which may be a significant factor in colorectal carcinogenesis. This proposed mechanism is closely related to SCFA and butyrate levels and the fermentability of the dietary fiber in question. The scientific evidence as to whether wheat bran intake can inhibit cellular proliferation is mixed. In a study involving patients with a history of colon cancer fed 13.5 g/d of wheat bran fiber for 2 months, Alberts et al. (1990) concluded that a wheat bran fiber supplement can inhibit DNA synthesis and epithelial cell proliferation within rectal mucosa crypts of patients at high risk for colon cancer. On the other hand, in other human studies, Gregoire and colleagues (1992) noted no effect of a wheat bran–supplemented diet on fecal pH or epithelial cell proliferation. Among the animal studies, Malville-Shipan and Fleming (1992) and Otsuka et al. (1988) (looking at thymidine kinase activity) also found no such effect. On the other hand, Folino et al. (1995) found that coarse wheat bran intake resulted in high epithelial proliferative rates in the distal colon along with high crypt depths.

There have been disparities in the published evidence about wheat bran's effects on colonic microflora, but many of the studies have demonstrated some lowering of colonic enzyme activity among those fed wheat bran. Gestel et al. (1994) found lower fecal α-glucuronidase, mucinase, and nitroreductase activity in a study of rats fed 10% fiber from wheat bran. Goldin et al. (1980) found reduced 7-α-dehydroxylase activity, but no changes in α-glucuronidase, nitroreductase, or azoreductase levels among subjects fed 30 g/d of wheat bran for one month. An earlier human trial by Goldin et al. (1978) also found no significant changes in the levels of these latter three enzymes. Jenkins et al. (1975) found that 46 g/d of wheat bran fiber (including All-Bran) for 3 weeks significantly decreased fecal neutral steroid concentrations. On the other hand, Bauer et al. (1979) found no significant changes in bacterial α-glucuronidase activity in feces from the distal colon between rats on the control diet and those fed wheat bran. Then again, Kawata et al. (1992), in a study involving rats fed 5% wheat bran and injected with 3-methylchloranthene, found much lower 7-ethoxycoumarin 0-deethylase activity in the colonic microsomes of animals on the bran diet, as opposed to controls. Reddy et al. (1992), in a study of premenopausal women fed 13–15 g/d of wheat bran for 8 weeks, found that wheat bran led to highly significant reductions in the activities of fecal bacterial α-glucuronidase, dehydroxylase, nitroreductase, and azoreductase. In sum, while the key studies do not present a unanimous picture by any means (possibly due to their respective durations, at least in the human trials), they do suggest that wheat bran intake can lead to reductions in the activity of certain colonic microflora associated with colon cancer risk.

In sum, much remains to be learned and studied about the physiological mechanisms by which wheat bran supplementation of the diet exerts a protective effect against colorectal cancer. Nonetheless, numerous plausible mechanisms have been posited to explain that effect.

II. WHEAT BRAN AND CONSTIPATION

There is general agreement among U.S. health authorities that dietary fiber is an important part of a healthful diet. As discussed above, U.S. health authorities uniformly advise Americans to increase their consumption of fiber-rich foods, including wheat and other whole-grain cereals. Moreover, the inclusion of fiber in the human diet is necessary in order to maintain normal functioning of the gastrointestinal tract and promotes regularity. Dietary fiber has many health-promoting effects on the gastrointestinal tract (Anderson et al., 1994; Gorman and Bowman, 1993). As noted earlier, foods rich in insoluble fiber decrease intestinal transit time and increase fecal bulk and stool number (Anderson et al. 1994). In general, cereal grains are more effective than fruits and vegetables in increasing the bulk of stools and preventing constipation. Wheat bran, in a variety of forms and doses, has been found to significantly increase stool weight and volume (Balasubramanian et al., 1987; Jenkins, 1987; Müller-Lissner, 1988; Lampe et al., 1993; Munakata et al., 1995). Wheat bran is able to increase fecal bulk because it traps water, increases the amount of undigested material, and increases the bacterial cell mass in the stool (National Research Council, 1989). Increase in stool weight and volume due to increased fiber consumption results in the dilution of fecal contents (Munakata et al., 1995). Wheat bran has also been shown to increase stool frequency and decreases transit time (Balasubramanian et al., 1987).

Many clinical studies have shown that dietary fiber, particularly wheat fiber, is useful in the prevention and treatment of constipation. Constipation becomes increasingly prevalent with increasing age; it has been estimated that constipation afflicts 20–25% of the elderly in Western populations (Read et al., 1995). The benefits shown in these studies include reducing transit time, increasing the number of bowel movements, and reducing or eliminating the need for laxatives.

III. WHEAT BRAN AND DIVERTICULAR DISEASE

Diverticulosis of the colon is an acquired pathological defect characterized by small, saccular herniations of the mucosa through the muscular wall of the colon, most often the sigmoid colon.

The disease appears almost exclusively in patients over 40 years of age and increases in incidence and severity with age (Cheskin and Lamport, 1995). It has been estimated that in the United States, most people over 60 years of age have diverticulosis.

A great deal of evidence supports the proposition that diverticulosis is caused by insufficient fiber content in the diet (Cheskin and Lamport, 1995). Diverticulosis was almost unknown before this century. It appeared with increasing frequency in industrialized countries in the 1900s, concomitant with the decrease in fiber intake and increase in consumption of refined carbohydrates (Burkitt, 1969; Trowell, 1976; Heller and Hackler 1978; Ohi et al., 1983). In addition, the modern prevalence of diverticulosis is much lower in nonindustrialized populations, where fiber consumption is relatively high, than it is in industrialized populations (Fatayer et al., 1983; Ihekwaba, 1992). Also, vegetarians have a lower incidence of diverticular disease and consume more fiber than nonvegetarians (Gear et al., 1979).

Although the mechanism by which reduced fiber intake promotes diverticulosis is not clear, it is believed that prolonged transit time and decreased stool volume result in increased intraluminal pressure, which may contribute to development of the disease (Cheskin and Lamport, 1995). LSRO concluded that epidemiological data showed an etiological relationship between low fiber intake and the development of diverticular disease and that clinical evidence suggests that a diet high in wheat fiber may relieve the symptoms of uncomplicated diverticular disease. The NRC noted that several studies have demonstrated a beneficial effect of fiber-rich diets in treating uncomplicated diverticular disease. A recent article reviewing the literature Cheskin and Lamport (1995) reiterated that dietary fiber in the form of wheat bran has been shown to be an effective therapy for diverticulosis. In both constipated geriatric patients and patients with symptomatic diverticular disease, wheat bran decreases colonic transit time. Wheat bran also has been shown to decrease intraluminal pressures (Cheskin and Lamport, 1995).

Most importantly, bran has been shown by most studies, but not all, to decrease symptoms in patients with confirmed diverticular disease (Cheskin and Lamport, 1995). In a review article, Freeman (1993) noted that a number of uncontrolled trials have suggested that bran supplements may be therapeutically beneficial. In one study of the effects of a high-fiber diet, 90% of patients reporting compliance with a high-fiber diet remained symptom-free at 5 years. A high-fiber diet can be particularly useful for the elderly (Cheskin and Lamport, 1995).

IV. WHEAT BRAN AND IRRITABLE BOWEL SYNDROME

Irritable bowel syndrome is a chronic disorder considered to be functional because no specific structural or biochemical cause has been found. The common symptoms of irritable bowel syndrome are abdominal pain associated with altered bowel habits, including constipation and diarrhea. Symptoms compatible with irritable bowel syndrome are reported in 10–22% of adults.

Wheat bran has been widely used therapeutically in treating irritable bowel syndrome (Pilch, 1987). Two studies cited by LSRO (Manning et al., 1977; Hillman et al., 1984) reported improvement in irritable bowel symptoms following the use of a high-fiber diet (Pilch, 1987). Two other studies cited by LSRO (Soltoft et al., 1976; Cann et al., 1984) found that irritable bowel syndrome symptoms were improved for patients consuming a high-fiber diet, but also found similar improvement for patients consuming a placebo. LSRO concluded that the available evidence showed that the patients with irritable bowel syndrome most likely to benefit from an increased intake of dietary fiber such as wheat bran are those whose chief complaint is constipation. In a recent study, Lambert et al. (1991) assessed 72 irritable bowel syndrome patients before and up to 6 months after being advised to eat a high-fiber diet. A significant inverse relationship was found between fiber intake and incidence of symptoms, including incomplete defecation, urgency, and hard stools. All patients with constipation, mucus, urgency, or water stools at the beginning of the study who were consuming more than 30 g/d of fiber by the end of the study reported improvement. Some studies have suggested that the benefits of bran supplementation may be due in part to placebo effect. Snook and Shepherd (1994), in a block-randomized, placebo-controlled crossover study, found that symptomatic improvement was reported in approximately equal percentages of the bran and placebo patients. Francis and Whorwell (1994) questioned 100 irritable bowel patients who had received wheat bran and found that 55% of the patients reported worsening of symptoms, while 10% reported improvement. A recent review article noted that wheat bran supplementation is emphasized for treatment of irritable bowel syndrome (Lynn and Friedman, 1993).

V. WHEAT BRAN AND WEIGHT CONTROL

The routine use of high-fiber foods has been found to reduce the risk for obesity and assist in weight maintenance (Anderson, 1990; Anderson and Akanji, 1993; Seim and Holtmeier, 1992; Kaul and Nidiry, 1993). Obesity is a critical factor in the development and progression of cardiovascular disease, hypertension, and diabetes (Gorman and Bowman, 1993). High-fiber foods may help reduce the risk of obesity because of the following mechanisms: high-fiber foods are lower in energy; they take longer to eat, which increases the feeling of satiety; they slow gastric emptying, thereby increasing the feeling of fullness; they decrease serum insulin concentration, thereby decreasing food intake because insulin stimulates appetite; and they decrease energy absorption (Anderson, 1990; Anderson and Akanji, 1993; Gorman and Bowman, 1993).

Epidemiological evidence suggests that higher-fiber diets are lower in energy and are less likely to contribute to the development of obesity (Gorman and Bowman, 1993). Although further research may be needed to fully document the effect of fiber on obesity, several clinical studies have found that fiber supplements have a relatively small but significant impact as part of a weight-reducing diet (Anderson and Akanji, 1993). Thus, the Position Statement of the American Dietetic Association states that dietary fiber is known to be beneficial in the management of obesity (Gorman and Bowman, 1993). LSRO concluded similarly that dietary fiber may have a beneficial, although limited, role in the treatment of obesity (Pilch, 1987). The AMA's Council on Scientific Affairs observed that high-fiber diets may reduce energy intake, even when more food is eaten, and that, although fiber has no magical effects in promoting weight loss, it can be an important part of a balanced diet with restricted energy intake (Council on Scientific Affairs, 1989).

VI. WHEAT BRAN AND HYPERTENSION

Epidemiological studies have demonstrated lower mean blood pressures in vegetarians and other groups consuming diets high in fiber than in nonvegetarians and other groups consuming diets lower in fiber (National Research Council, 1989; Pilch, 1987). Studies of populations worldwide have shown that those groups eating a diet predominantly composed of vegetable products have low average blood pressure levels (Sacks et al., 1995). Within industrialized countries, vegetarians have lower average blood pressure levels than do comparable nonvegetarian populations. Studies of Seventh-Day Adventist vegetarian groups show that they consume high levels of fiber from sources including whole grain cereals and demonstrate comparatively low blood pressure levels (Beilin, 1994).

Similarly, clinical studies indicate a fairly consistent blood pressure–lowering effect of diets with high levels of fiber from various sources in normal as well as hypertensive subjects (Pilch, 1987). Several more recent studies have shown that increased dietary fiber tends to lower blood pressure (Eliasson et al., 1992; Nami et al., 1995). Other studies have failed to show such an effect (Little et al., 1991; Sciarrone et al., 1992). The NRC and LSRO noted that no firm conclusions could be drawn about the effect of high levels of dietary fiber on blood pressure, because the high-fiber diets observed in many studies also differed from average diets in that they were low in fat and refined sugar and high in complex carbohydrates.

VII.   WHEAT BRAN AND GALLSTONES

Epidemiological evidence shows an inverse relationship between dietary fiber level and incidence of gallstones (Pilch, 1987). The incidence of gallstones is markedly higher in urban, Westernized societies than in primitive, rural societies where diets contain a higher proportion of fiber (Heaton and Pomare, 1974). Vegetarians have been found to exhibit a lower incidence of gallstones (Nair and Mayberry, 1994). A possible mechanism by which fiber inhibits the formation of gallstones is that fiber-depleted foods encourage overnutrition and hyperinsulimia, i.e., that fiber-depleted sugar evokes a greater insulin response.

Although some clinical studies have not found a preventive effect of dietary fiber on gallstone disease (Diehl et al., 1989), several studies have confirmed the role of fiber in preventing gallstone disease (Zhang et al., 1992). Studies have shown that humans with gallstones or highly lithogenic bile tend to improve when fed wheat bran, while normal persons are not affected (Hayes et al., 1992). Animal studies have also demonstrated a role of insoluble and soluble fibers in protecting against gallstone formation.

After reviewing the scientific evidence concerning the effect of dietary fiber on gallstone formation, Heaton and Pomare (1974) concluded that a low intake of wheat bran or similar cereal fiber is likely to promote gallstones. Published studies show that increased intake of wheat bran reduces the percentage of deoxycholic acid content and cholesterol content in bile acids. Deoxycholic acid has been shown to be a risk factor for bile supersaturated with cholesterol and hence for gallstones. LSRO and the NRC concluded similarly that supplemental wheat bran can lower both the cholesterol saturation index and the deoxycholic acid content of bile. LSRO concluded, however, that the influence of dietary fiber on gallstone formation is still unresolved.

VIII.   WHEAT BRAN AND DIABETES

Epidemiological evidence shows that diabetes mellitus is more prevalent in populations with low fiber intakes than in populations with high-fiber intakes (Anderson and Akanji, 1993). LSRO observed that much of the available epidemiological data supports the hypothesis that consumption of a low-fiber diet is an important factor in the etiology of diabetes but stopped short of concluding that this evidence provides a proven causal relationship (Pilch, 1987). The prevalence of diabetes is comparatively low in groups in nonindustrialized areas consuming high-fiber diets, such as Africa (Trowell, 1976).

Extensive clinical studies have documented the benefits of high fiber intakes for individuals with diabetes (Anderson et al., 1994; Pilch, 1987). LSRO observed that in both insulin-dependent and non–insulin-dependent diabetics, a majority of studies have shown that high-fiber, high-carbohydrate diets significantly lowered insulin requirements, decreased fasting plasma glucose concentration, reduced the urinary excretion of glucose, and substantially reduced plasma cholesterol concentration. Such diets have also been reported to provide other beneficial effects for diabetic patients, such as lowering blood pressure and promoting weight loss in some instances. Likewise, the American Diabetes Association (1979) advises the consumption of a diet rich in high-fiber carbohydrate foods.

In a recent review article, Anderson and Akanji (1993) examined the results of 53 studies that investigated the effects of fiber supplements on diabetic individuals and another 53 studies that investigated the effects of high-fiber diets on diabetics. The authors concluded that both types of study offered persuasive evidence that fiber supplements and high-fiber diets improve glycemic control, increase sensitivity to insulin, lower serum lipids, decrease blood pressure, and assist in weight management. Many of the high-fiber diets tested provided high carbohydrate content as well as high fiber content, but high-fiber diets with carbohydrate contents similar to control diets also benefited diabetic subjects. In addition, high-fiber diets may have special advantages for obese diabetics. Weight-reducing high-fiber diets promptly decrease the need for insulin or oral hypoglycemic agents and quickly decrease serum glucose and lipids. Special groups such as children, pregnant women, and geriatric subjects benefit from fiber supplementation (Anderson and Akanji, 1993). While soluble fibers appear to be the most beneficial in the treatment of diabetes, insoluble fibers, such as those found in wheat bran, also afford significant benefits to diabetics (Vinik and Jenkias, 1988). Thus, Anderson and Akanji (1993) concluded that wheat bran supplements improve glycemic control and reduce the requirements for insulin and/or oral hypoglycemic agents.

REFERENCES

R Abraham, TA Barbolt, JB Rodgers. Inhibition by bran of the colonic cocarcinogenicity of bile salts in rats given dimethylhydrazine. Exp Mol Pathol 33:133–143, 1980.

O Alabaster, ZC Tang, A Frost, N Shivapurkar. Potential synergism between wheat bran and psyllium: Enhanced inhibition of colon cancer. Cancer Lett 75(1):53–58, 1993.

O Alabaster, Z Tang, A Frost, N Shivapurkar. Effect of beta-carotene and wheat bran fiber on colonic aberrant crypt and tumor formation in rats exposed to azoxymethane and high dietary fat. Carcinogenesis 16(1):127–132, 1995.

DS Alberts, J Einspahr, S Rees-McGee, P Ramanujam, MK Buller, L Clark, C Ritenbaugh, J Atwood, P Pethigal, D Earnest, H Villar, J Phelps, M Lipkin, M Wargovich, FL Meyskens, Jr. Effects of dietary wheat bran fiber on rectal epithelial cell proliferation in patients with resection for colorectal cancers. J Natl Cancer Inst 82(15):1280–1285, 1990.

DS Alberts, C Ritenbaugh, JA Story, M Aickin, S Rees-McGee, MK Buller, J Atwood, J Phelps, PS Ramanujam, S Bellapravalu, J Patel, L Bettinger, L Clark. Randomized, double-blinded, placebo-controlled study of effect of wheat bran fiber and calcium on fecal bile acids in patients with resected adenomatous colon polyps. J Natl Cancer Inst 88(2):81–92, 1996.

American Diabetes Association, Committee on Food and Nutrition. Principles of nutrition and dietary recommendations for individuals with diabetes mellitus. Diabetes 28:1027–1030, 1979.

JA Anderson. Food allergy or sensitivity terminology, physiologic bases, and scope of clinical problem. In: JE Perkin, ed. Food Allergies and Adverse Reactions. Aspen Publication, 1990, pp 1–13.

JW Anderson, AO Akanji. Treatment of diabetes with high fiber diets. In: GA Spiller, ed. Dietary Fiber in Human Nutrition. 2nd ed. Boca Raton, FL: CRC Press, 1993, pp 443–470.

JW Anderson, BM Smith, NJ Gustafson. Health benefits and practical aspects of high-fiber diets. Am J Clin Nutr 59(5 suppl):1242S–1247S, 1994.

TM Antalis, JA Reeder. Butyrate regulates gene expression of the plasminogen activating system in colon cancer cells. Int J Cancer 62(5):619–626, 1995.

LM Ausman. Fiber and colon cancer: Does the current evidence justify a preventive policy? Nutr Rev 51(2):57–63, 1993.

R Balasubramanian, EJ Johnson, JA Marlett. Effect of wheat bran on bowel function and fecal calcium in older adults. J Am Coll Nutr 6(3):199–208, 1987.

TA Barbolt, R Abraham. The effect of bran on dimethylhydrazine-induced colon carcinogenesis in the rat. Proc Soc Exp Biol 157:656–659, 1978.

TA Barbolt, R Abraham. Dose-response, sex difference, and the effect of bran in dimethylhydrazine-induced intestinal tumorigenesis in rats. Toxicol Appl Pharmacol 55:417–422, 1980.

DS Barnes, NK Clapp, DA Scott, DL Oberst, SG Berry. Effects of wheat, rice, corn, and soybean bran on 1,2-dimethylhydrazine-induced large bowel tumorigenesis in F344 rats. Nutr Cancer 5(1):1–9, 1983.

HG Bauer, NG Asp, R Oste, Dahlqvist, PE Fredlund. Effect of dietary fiber on the induction of colorectal tumors and fecal beta-glucuronidase activity in the rat. Cancer Res 39(9):3752–3756, 1979.

LJ Beilin. Vegetarian and other complex diets, fats, fiber, and hypertension. Am J Clin Nutr 59(5 suppl):1130S–1135S, 1994.

S Bingham. Food components and mechanisms of interest in cancer and diet in relation to their measurement. Eur J Clin Nutr 47(suppl. 2):S73–S77, 1993.

G Block, AF Subar. Estimates of nutrient intake from a food frequency questionnaire: the 1987 National Health Interview Survey. J Am Diet Assoc 92(8):969–977, 1992.

LC Boffa, JR Lupton, MR Mariani, M Ceppi, HL Newmark, A Scalmati, M Lipkin. Modulation of colonic epithelial cell proliferation, histone acetylation, and luminal short chain fatty acids by variation of dietary fiber (wheat bran) in rats. Cancer Res 52:5906–5912, 1992.

C Boring, TS Squires, T Tong. Cancer statistics. Ca Cancer J Clin 43(1):7–26, 1993.

DP Burkitt. Related disease-related/cause? Lancet 2:1229–1231, 1969.

T Byers. Diet and cancer: Any progress in the interim? Cancer 62(8):1713–1724, 1988.

RJ Calvert, M Reicks. Alterations in colonic thymidine kinase enzyme activity induced by consumption of various dietary fibers. Proc Soc Exp Biol Med 189(1):45–51, 1988.

RJ Calvert, DM Klurfeld, S Subramaniam, GV Vahouny, D Kritchevsky. Reduction of colonic carcinogenesis by wheat bran independent of fecal bile acid concentration. J Natl Cancer Inst 79(4):875–880, 1987.

RJ Calvert, S Satchithanandam, RP Schaudies. Dietary wheat bran reduces colonic mucosal immunoreactive epidermal growth factor (EGF) levels in rats. (abstr) FASEB: A782, 1990.

PA Cann, NW Read, CD Holdsworth. What is the benefit of coarse wheat bran in patients with irritable bowel syndrome? Gut 25:168–173, 1984.

W-F Chen, AS Patchefsky, HS Goldsmith. Colonic protection from dimethylhydrazine by a high fiber diet. Surg Gynecol Obstet 147:503–506, 1978.

LJ Cheskin, RD Lamport. Diverticular disease. Epidemiology and pharmacological treatment. Drugs Aging 6(1):55–63, 1995.

NK Clapp, DS Barnes, DA Scott, DL Oberst, SG Berry. Effect of dietary bran on 1,2-dimethylhydrazine (DMH) tumorigenesis in rats. AACR Abstracts, March:121 [Abstract 483], 1980.

MR Clausen, H Bonnén, PB Mortensen. Colonic fermentation of dietary fibre to short chain fatty acids in patients with adenomatous polyps and colonic cancer. Gut 32(8):923–928, 1991.

Council on Scientific Affairs, American Medical Association. Dietary fiber and health. JAMA 262(4):542–546, 1989.

JP Cruse, MR Lewin, CG Clark. Failure of bran to protect against experimental colon cancer in rats. Lancet 2:1278–1280, 1978.

JJ DeCosse, HH Miller, ML Lesser. Effect of wheat fiber and vitamins C and E on rectal polyps in patients with familial adenomatous polyposis. J Natl Cancer Inst 81(17):1290–1297, 1989.

AK Diehl, SM Haffner, JA Knapp, HP Hayuda, MP Stern. Dietary intake and the prevalence of gallbladder disease in Mexican-Americans. Gastroenterology 97:1527–1533, 1989.

J Dwyer. Dietary fiber and colorectal cancer risk. Nutr Rev 51(5):147–148, 1993.

CA Edwards, MA Eastwood. Comparison of the effects of ispaghula and wheat bran on rat caecal and colonic fermentation. Gut 33(9):1229–1233, 1992.

K Eliasson, KR Ryttig, B Hylander, S Rössner. A dietary fibre supplement in the treatment of mild hypertension. A randomized, double-blind, placebo-controlled trial. J Hypertens 10(2):195–199, 1992.

HN Englyst, SA Bingham, HS Wiggins, DAT Southgate, R Seppänen, P Helms, V Anderson, KC Day, R

Choolun, E Collinson, JH Cummings. Nonstarch polysaccharide consumption in four Scandinavian populations. Nutr Can 4(1):50–60, 1982.

WT Fatayer, MM A-Khalaf, KA Shalan, AV Toukon, MR Daker, MA Arnaout. Diverticular disease of the colon in Jordan. Dis Colon Rectum 26(4):247–249, 1983.

D Fleiszer, D Murray, J MacFarlane, RA Brown. Protective effect of dietary fibre against chemically induced bowel tumours in rats. Lancet 2:552–553, 1978.

M Folino, A McIntyre, GP Young. Dietary fibers differ in their effects on large bowel epithelial proliferation and fecal fermentation-dependent events in rats. J Nutr 125:1521–1528, 1995.

CY Francis, PJ Whorwell. Bran and irritable bowel syndrome: time for reappraisal. Lancet 344:39–40, 1994.

HJ Freeman. Human epidemiological studies on dietary fiber and colon cancer. In: GA Spiller, ed. Dietary Fiber in Human Nutrition. 2nd ed. Boca Raton, FL: CRC Press, 1993, pp 477–486.

CM Friedenreich, RF Brant, E Riboli. Influence of methologic factors in a pooled analysis of 13 case-control studies of colorectal cancer and dietary fiber. Epidemiology 5(1):66–79, 1994.

K Furukawa, I Yamamoto, N Tanida, T Tsujiai, M Nishikawa, T Narisawa, T Shimoyama. The effects of dietary fiber from lagenaria, scineraria (yugao-melon) on colonic carcinogenisis in mice. Cancer 75(6 suppl):1508–1515, 1995.

DD Gallaher, PM Franz. Effects of corn oil and wheat brans on bile acid metabolism in rats. J Nutr 120(11): 1320–1330, 1990.

JSS Gear, P Fursdon, DJ Nolan, A Ware, JI Mann, AJM Brodribb, MP Vessey. Symptomless diverticular disease and intake of dietary fibre. Lancet 1:511–514, 1979.

G Gestel, P Besancon, JM Rouanet. Comparative evaluation of the effects of two different forms of dietary fibre (rice bran vs. wheat bran) on rat colonic mucosa and faecal microflora. Ann Nutr Metab 38(5): 249–256, 1994.

P Gibson, M Folino, A McIntyre, O Rosella, C Finch, G Young. Dietary modulation of colonic mucosal urokinase activity in rats. J Gastroenterol Hepatol 10:324–330, 1995.

HP Glauert, MR Bennink. Influence of diet or intrarectal bile acid injections on colon epithelial cell proliferation in rats previously injected with 1,2-dimethylhydrazine. J Nutr 113(3):475–482, 1983.

B Goldin, J Dwyer, SL Gorbach, W Gordon, L Swenson. Influence of diet and age on fecal bacterial enzymes. Am J Clin Nutr 31(10 suppl):S136–S140, 1978.

BR Goldin, L Swenson, J Dwyer, M Sexton, SL Gorbach. Effect of diet and Lactobacillus acidophilus supplements on human fecal bacterial enzymes. J Natl Cancer Inst 64(2):255–261, 1980.

MA Gorman, C Bowman. Position of The American Dietetic Association: health implications of dietary fiber. J Am Diet Assoc 93(12):1446–1447, 1993.

E Graf, JW Eaton. Suppression of colonic cancer by dietary phytic acid. Nutr Can 19(1):11–19, 1993.

P Greenwald, E Lanza, GA Eddy. Dietary fiber in the reduction of colon cancer risk. J Am Diet Assoc 87(9):1178–1188, 1987.

RC Gregoire, H Kashtan, HS Stern, KS Yeung, J Stadler, GA Neil, R Furrer, S Langley, WR Bruce. The effect of lowering faecal pH on the rate of proliferation of the normal colonic mucosa. Surg Oncol 1(1):43–47, 1992.

PJ Harris, LR Ferguson. Dietary fibre: its composition and role in protection against colorectal cancer. Mutat Res 290(1):97–110, 1993.

KC Hayes, A Livingston, EA Trautwein. Dietary impact on biliary lipids and gallstones. Ann Rev Nutr 12:299–326, 1992.

KW Heaton, EW Pomare. Effect of bran on blood lipids and calcium. Lancet 1:49–50, 1974.

SN Heller, LR Hackler. Changes in the crude fiber content of the American diet. Am J Clin Nutr 31: 1510–1514, 1978.

LC Hillman, NH Stace, EW Pomare. Irritable bowel patients and their long-term response to a high fiber diet. Am J Gastroenterol 79(1):1–7, 1984.

GR Howe, E Benito, R Castelleto, J Cornée, J Estève, RP Gallagher, JM Isovich, J Dengao, R Kaaks, GA Kune, S Kune, KA L-Abbé, HP Lee, M Lee, AB Miller, RK Peters, JD Potter, E Riboli, ML Slattery, D Trichopoulos, A Tuyns, A Tzonov, AS Whittemore, AH Wu-Williams, Z Shu. Dietary intake of fiber and decreased risk of cancers of the colon and rectum: Evidence from the combined analysis of 13 case-control studies. J Natl Cancer Inst 84(24):1887–1896, 1992.

CTL Huang, GS Gopala Krishna, BL Nichols. Fiber intestinal sterols and colon cancer. Am J Clin Nutr 31:516–526, 1978.

K Hunter, MW Linn, R Harris. Dietary patterns and cancer of the digestive tract in older patients. J Am Ger Soc 28(9):405–409, 1980.

FN Ihekwaba. Diverticular disease of the colon in black Africa. J Roy Coll Surg Edinb 37(1):107–109, 1992.

LR Jacobs. Enhancement of rat colon carcinogenesis by wheat bran consumption during the stage of 1,2-dimethylhydrazine administration. Cancer Res 43(9):4057–4061, 1983.

LR Jacobs. Stimulation of rat colonic crypt cell proliferative activity by wheat bran consumption during the stage of 1,2-dimethylhydrazine administration. Cancer Res 44(6):2458–2563, 1984.

LR Jacobs. Effect of dietary fiber on colonic cell proliferation and its relationship to colon carcinogenesis. Prev Med 16(4):566–571, 1987.

LR Jacobs, JR Lupton. Dietary wheat bran lowers colonic pH in rats. J Nutr 112(3):592–594, 1982.

LR Jacobs, BO Schneeman. Effects of dietary wheat bran on rat colonic structure and mucosal cell growth. J Nutr 111(5):798–803, 1981.

LR Jacobs, FA White. Dietary wheat bran inhibits DNA synthesis and enhances 5-fluorouracil toxicity in rat pancreas. Nutr Cancer 5(3–4):131–136, 1983.

DJA Jenkins, MS Hill, JH Cummings. Effect of wheat fiber on blood lipids, fecal steroid excretion and serum iron. Am J Clin Nutr 28(12):1408–1411, 1975.

DJA Jenkins, RD Peterson, MJ Thorne, PW Ferguson. (1987) Wheat fiber and laxation: Dose response and equilibration time. Am J Gastroenterol 82(12):1259–1263, 1987.

H Kashtan, HS Stern. Colonic proliferation and colon cancer risk. A review of clinical studies. Isr J Med Sci 28(12):904–910, 1992.

L Kaul, J Nidiry. High-fiber diet in the treatment of obesity and hypercholesterolemia. J Natl Med Assoc 85(3):231–232, 1993.

S Kawata, S Tamura, Y Matsuda, N Ito, Y Matsuzawa. Effect of dietary fiber on cytochrome P450IA1 induction in rat colonic mucosa. Carcinogenesis 13(11):2121–2125, 1992.

DM Klurfeld. Dietary fiber-mediated mechanisms in carcinogenesis. Cancer Res 52(7 suppl):2055s–2059s, 1992.

D Kritchevsky. Evaluation of Publicly Available Scientific Evidence Regarding Certain Nutrient-Disease Relationships: 6. Dietary Fiber and Cardiovascular Disease. Prepared by LSRO/FASEB for Center for Food Safety and Applied Nutrition, FDA, DHHS, under FDA Contract No. 223-88-2124, Task Order #9, 1991.

D Kritchevsky. Epidemiology of fibre, resistant starch and colorectal cancer. Eur J Cancer Prev 4(5):345–352, 1995.

JP Lambert, PW Brunt, NAG Mowat, CC Khin, CKW Lai, V Morrison, JWT Dickerson, MA Eastwood. The value of prescribed ''high fibre'' diets for the treatment of the irritable bowel syndrome. Eur J Clin Nutr 45(12):601–609, 1991.

JW Lampe, RF Wetsch, WO. Thompson, JL Slavin. Gastrointestinal effects of sugarbeet fiber and wheat bran in healthy men. Eur J Clin Nutr 47(8):543–548, 1993.

P Little, G Girling, A Hasler, A Trafford. A controlled trial of a low sodium, low fat, high fibre diet in treated hypertensive patients: effect on antihypertensive drug requirement in clinical practice. J Hum Hypertens 5(3):175–181, 1991.

JR Lupton, LR Jacobs. Differential response of rat gastric mucosa to dietary oat bran, wheat bran, pectin and guar (abstr). Fed Proc 42(4):1063, 1983.

JR Lupton, PP Kurtz. Relationship of colonic luminal short-chain fatty acids and pH to in vivo cell proliferation in rats. J Nutr 123(9):1522–1530, 1993.

RB Lynn, LS Friedman. Irritable bowel syndrome. N Engl J Med 329(26):1940–1945, 1993.

R MacLennan, F Macrea, C Bain, D Battistutta, P Chapuis, H Gratten, J Lambert, RC Newland, M Ngu, A Russell, M Ward, ML Wahlqvist, and the Australian Polyp Prevention Project. Randomized trial of intake fat, fiber, and beta carotene to prevent colorectal adenomas. J Natl Cancer Inst 87:1760–1766, 1995.

OE Maisto, CG Bremner. Cancer and the colon and rectum in the coloured population of Johannesburg: relationship to diet and bowel habits. S Afr Med J 60:571–573, 1981.

K Malville-Shipan, SE Fleming. Wheat bran and corn oil do not influence proliferation in the colon of healthy rats when energy intakes are equivalent. J Nutr 122(1):37–45, 1992.

AP Manning, KW Heaton, RF Harvey, P Uglow. Wheat fibre and irritable bowel syndrome: a controlled trial. Lancet:417–418, 1977.

JC Mathers, J-M Fotso Tagny. Diurnal changes in large-bowel metabolism: short-chain fatty acids and transit time in rats fed on wheat bran. Br J Nutr 71(2):209–222, 1994.

GH McIntosh, L Jorgensen, P Royle. The potential of an insoluble dietary fiber-rich source from barley to protect from DMH-induced intestinal tumors in rats. Nutr Cancer 19(2):213–221, 1993.

A McIntyre, GP Young, T Taranto, PR Gibson, PB Ward. Different fibers have different regional effects on luminal contents of rat colon. Gastroenterology 101(5):1274–1281, 1991.

A McIntyre, PR Gibson, GP Young. Butyrate production from dietary fibre and protection against large bowel cancer in a rat model. Gut 34(3):386–391, 1993.

GE McKeown-Eyssen, E Bright-See. Dietary factors in colon cancer: international relationships. Nutr Cancer 6(3):160–170, 1984.

GE McKeown-Eyssen, E Bright-See. Dietary factors in colon cancer: international relationships. An update. Nutr Cancer 7(4):251–253, 1985.

GE McKeown-Eyssen, E Bright-See, WR Bruce, V Jazmaji, and the Toronto Polyp Prevention Group. A randomized trial of a low fat high fiber diet in the recurrence of colorectal polyps. J Clin Epidemiol 47:525–536, 1994.

AI Mendeloff. Dietary fiber and human health. N Engl J Med 297(15):811–814, 1977.

CG Moertel, TR Fleming, JS MacDonald, DG Haller, JA Laurie, PJ Goodman, JS Ungerleider, WA Emerson, DC Tormey, JH Glick, MH Veeder, JA Mailliard. Levamisole and fluorouracil for adjuvant therapy of resected colon carcinoma. N Engl J Med 322(6):352–358, 1990.

SA Müller-Lissner. Effect of wheat bran on weight of stool and gastrointestinal transit time: a meta analysis. Br Med J 296:615–617, 1988.

A Munakata, S Iwane, M Todate, S Nakaji, K Sugawara. Effects of dietary fiber on gastrointestinal transit time, fecal properties and fat absorption in rats. Tohoku J Exp Med 176:227–238, 1995.

P Nair, JF Mayberry. Vegetarianism, dietary fibre and gastro-intestinal disease. Dig Dis 12(3):177–185, 1994.

R Nami, V Gallo, G Pavese, F Panza, C Gennari. Antihypertensive activity of a vegetable fibre preparation: a preliminary, double-blind, placebo-controlled study. Eur J Clin Nutr 49 (suppl. 1):S201–206, 1995.

National Cancer Institute. PDQ Supportive Care/Screening/Prevention Information, Screening for colorectal cancer (208/04726) (obtained from Cancer Net), 1995.

National Cancer Institute. Cancer statistics (from the SEER Program) (obtained from Cancer Net), 1996.

National Cholesterol Education Program. Bethesda, MD: DHHS, Public Health Service, National Institutes of Health. Eating to Lower Your High Blood Cholesterol. NIH Publication No. 89-2920, 1989.

National Research Council. (1989) Evidence of dietary components and chronic diseases: dietary fiber: implications for reducing chronic disease risk. Diet and Health 291–309, 696, 1989.

National Research Council. Carcinogens and Anticarcinogens in the Human Diet. Washington, DC: National Academy Press, 1996, pp 82–83.

ND Nigro, AW Bull, BA Klopfer, MS Pak, RL Campbell. Effect of dietary fiber on azoxymethane-induced intestinal carcinogenesis in rats. J Natl Cancer Inst 62(4):1097–1102, 1979.

G Ohi, K Minowa, T Oyama, M Nagahashi, N Yamazaki, S Yamamoto, K Nagasako, K Hayakawa, K Kimura, B Mori. Changes in dietary fiber intake among Japanese in the 20th century: a relationship to the prevalence of diverticular disease. Am J Clin Nutr 38(1):115–121, 1983.

M Otsuka, S Satchithanandam, RJ Calvert. Influence of meal distribution of wheat bran on fecal bulk, gastrointestinal transit time and colonic thymidine kinase activity in the rat. J Nutr 119(4):566–572, 1988.

SM Pilch, ed. Physiological effects and health consequences of dietary fiber. Fed Am Soc for Exp. Biol; Prepared for Center For Food Safety and Applied Nutrition, FDA, DHHS, under Contract No. FDA 223-84-2059, 1987.

JW Powles, DRR Williams. Trends in bowel cancer in selected countries in relation to wartime changes in flour milling. Nutr Cancer 6(1):40–48, 1984.

NW Read, AF Celik, P Katsinelos. Constipation and incontinance in the elderly. J Clin Gastroenterol 20: 61–70, 1995.

BS Reddy, K Watanabe, A Sheinfil. (1980) Effect of dietary wheat bran, alfalfa, pectin and carrageenan on plasma cholesterol and fecal bile acid and neutral sterol excretion in rats. J Nutr 110:1247–1254, 1980.

BS Reddy, A Engle, B Simi, M Goldman. Effect of dietary fiber on colonic bacterial enzymes and bile acids in relation to colon cancer. Gastroenterology 102(5):1475–1482, 1992.

BS Reddy, B Simi, A Engle. Biochemical epidemiology of colon cancer: effect of types of dietary fiber on colonic diacylglycerols in women. Gastroenterology 106(4):883–889, 1994.

NM Robblee, EA McLellan, RP Bird. Measurement of the proliferative status of colonic epithelium as a risk marker for colon carcinogenesis: effect of bile acid and dietary fiber. Nutr Cancer 12(4):301–310, 1989.

N Roland, L Nugon-Baudon, J-P Flinois, P Beaune. Hepatic and intestinal cytochrome P-450, glutathione-S-transferase and UDP-glucuronosyl transferase are affected by six types of dietary fiber in rats inoculated with human whole fecal flora. J Nutr 124(9):1581–1587, 1994.

N Roland, L Nugon-Baudon, C Anderieux, O Szylit. Comparative study of the fermentative characteristics of inulin and different types of fibre in rats inoculated with a human whole faecal flora. Br J Nutr 74(2):239–249, 1995.

FM Sacks, E Obarzanek, MM Windhauser, LP Svetkey, WM Vollmer, M McCullough, N Karanja, P-H Lin, P Steele, MA Proschan, MA Evans, LJ Appel, GA Bray, TM Vogt, TJ Moore. Rationale and design of the Dietary Approaches to Stop Hypertension trial (DASH). A multicenter controlled-feeding study of dietary patterns to lower blood pressure. Ann Epidemiol 5(2):108–118, 1995.

BO Schneeman, D Richter. Changes in plasma and hepatic lipids, small intestinal histology and pancreatic enzyme activity due to aging and dietary fiber in rats. J Nutr 123(7):1328–1337, 1993.

SA Schuette, RC Rose. The effect of diets high in fat and/or fiber on colonic absorption of DMH in the rat. Nutr Cancer 8(4):257–265, 1986.

SEG Sciarrone, LJ Beilin, IL Rouse, PB Rogers. A factorial study of salt restriction and a low-fat/high-fibre diet in hypertensive subjects. J Hypertens 10(3):287–298, 1992.

HC Seim, KB Holtmeier. Effects of a six-week, low-fat diet on serum cholesterol, body weight, and body measurements. Fam Pract Res J 12(4):411–419, 1992.

S Shankar, E Lanza. Dietary fiber and cancer prevention. Hematol Oncol Clin North Am 5(1):25–41, 1991.

M Shike, SJ Winawer, PH Greenwald, A Bloch, MJ Hill, SV Swaroop, the WHO Collaborating Centre for the Prevention of Colorectal Cancer. Primary prevention of colorectal cancer. Bull WHO 68(3): 377–385, 1990.

N Shivapurkar, Z Tang, A Frost, O Alabaster. Inhibition of progression of aberrant crypt foci and colon tumor development by vitamin E and beta-carotene in rats on a high-risk diet. Cancer Lett 91(1): 125–132, 1995.

EJ Sinkeldam, CF Kuper, MC Bosland, VMH Hollanders, DM Vedder. Interactive effects of dietary wheat bran and lard on N-Methyl-N′-nitro-N-nitrosoguanidine-induced colon carcinogenesis in rats. Cancer Res 50(4):1092–1096, 1990.

J Snook, HA Shepherd. Bran supplementation in the treatment of irritable bowel syndrome. Alim Pharmacol Ther 8:511–514, 1994.

J Søtoft, B Krag, E Gudmand-Høyer, E Kristensen, HR Wulff. A double-blind trial of the effect of wheat bran on symptoms of irritable bowel syndrome. Lancet (Feb. 2):270–272, 1976.

M Tatsuta, H Iishi, H Yamamura, H Taniguchi. Inhibition by tetragastrin of experimental carcinogenesis in rat colon: effect of wheat bran consumption. Int J Cancer 41(1):239–242, 1988.

DL Topping, RJ Illman, JM Clarke, RP Trimble, KA Jackson, Y Marsono. Dietary fat and fiber alter large bowel and portal venous volatile fatty acids and plasma cholesterol but not biliary steroids in pigs. J Nutr 123(1):133–143, 1993.

B Trock, E Lanza, P Greenwald. Dietary fiber, vegetables, and colon cancer: critical review and meta-analyses of the epidemiologic evidence. J Natl Cancer Inst 82(8):650–661, 1990.

H Trowell. Definition of dietary fiber and hypotheses that it is a protective factor in certain diseases. Am J Clin Nutr 29:417–427, 1976.

AI Vinik, DJA Jenkins. Dietary fiber in management of diabetes. Diabetes Care 11(2):160–173, 1988.

MJ Wargovich, B Levin. Grist for the mill: role of cereal fiber and calcium in prevention of colon cancer. J Natl Cancer Inst 88(2):67–69, 1996.

K Watanabe, BS Reddy, JH Weisburger, D Kritchevsky. Effect of dietary alfalfa, pectin, and wheat bran on azoxymethane- or methylnitrosourea-induced colon carcinogenesis in F344 rats. J Natl Cancer Inst 63(1):141–145, 1979.

RB Wilson, DP Hutcheson, L Wideman. Dimethylhydrazine-induced colon tumors in rats fed diets containing beef fat or corn oil with and without wheat bran. Am J Clin Nutr 30:176–181, 1977.

GP Young, A McIntyre, V Albert, M Folino, JG Muir, PR Gibson. Wheat bran suppresses potato starch-potentiated colorectal tumorigenesis at the aberrant crypt stage in a rat model. Gastroenterology 110(2):508–514, 1996.

JX Zhang, E Lundin, G Hallmans, F Bergman, E Westerlund, P Petterson. Dietary effects of barley fibre, wheat bran and rye bran on bile composition and gallstone formation in hamsters. APMIS 100(6): 553–557, 1992.

25
Psyllium: Food Applications, Efficacy, and Safety

Susan Sungsoo Cho and Celeste Clark
Kellogg Company, Battle Creek, Michigan

I. FOOD APPLICATIONS OF PSYLLIUM

Psyllium is used as a food or food component and has been so used for centuries. Psyllium is a harvestable grain. It comes from plants of the *Plantago* genus. The genus is widely distributed, with several species being common weeds (buckhorn and plantain). Several types of psyllium are available, depending on growing region. Commercial psyllium is primarily cultivated in France, Spain, and India, with some small quantities also grown in the American Southwest. The French or black psyllium comes from *P. indica* (L.). Spanish psyllium comes from *P. psyllium* (L.) and is also known as zaragatona. Indian or blonde psyllium comes from *P. ovata*, also known as ispaghula (BeMiller, 1973).

Psyllium has been known in India since Ayurvedic times and in China was cited in Shen Nung's Pen T'sao, written 3,000 years before Christ (Montague, 1932). British, American, and Indian authors have noted a wide variety of traditional food uses for the substance. Thus, it has been mixed in water, often with sugar, to create a cooling drink (Fluckinger and Hanburg, 1874; Council for Scientific Information and Research [CSIR], 1969). It has also been mixed with fruit extracts, such as coconut water, orange juice, or prune juice (Figg, 1931). Sometimes it has been mixed in lieu of arrowroot into a conjee, a type of Indian beverage (Nadkarni, 1927). Other traditional uses involve spreading psyllium on bread, mixing it with honey, marmalade, or stewed fruits, using it in soup, or mixing it with wheat flour as a thickener. Psyllium has also traditionally been used as an ingredient in the making of chocolates and in jellies. The substance has additionally been utilized as a confectionery base, with other ingredients such as sugar, aniseed, or cardamom (Nadkarni, 1927; Singh and Virmani, 1982). Nadkarni also reported on its use with curds and rosewater and in sherbet. And, of course, its use as a sizing agent or thickener has consistently been recognized.

A more recent use of the substance in this century has been as an ice cream stabilizer (Kumar, 1973). A current application in this context is manufactured by Meer Corporation of North Bergen, New Jersey, which makes psyllium-based stabilizers marketed as Merecol IC (for ice cream), Merecol SH (for sherbet), and Merecol Y (for yogurt) (Dairy Foods, 1990). There have also been numerous recent food uses of psyllium in the United States. At least three ready-to-eat (RTE) cereals have included psyllium as a component since 1989: Heartwise (now

Table 1   Recent Food Uses of Psyllium

Product	Manufacturer
Super Diet Fast Wafers, in vanilla and chocolate flavors	Advantage Supplements
Louise Tenney's Ultimate Cookie, in peanut butter, pineapple coconut, and oatmeal raisin flavors	Enrich International
Fiberall Wafers, in oatmeal raisin and fruit and nut flavors	Fiberall
Green Mountain Farms Easy Oats, a multifiber, high-soluble fiber drink mix, also used as a thickener for soups, stews, and salad dressings	Futurbiotics
Great Cakes, in seven flavors—apple, peach, raspberry, blueberry, summer fruits, tropical fruits, and carob	Great Cakes, Inc.
Super Diet Cookie, with psyllium and oat bran	Laci Le Beau
Kee-Noa, instant beverage granules, with quinoa and psyllium	Lewis Laboratories, Inc.
Fabulous Fiber, instant beverage granules with psyllium, pectin, and guar gum	Lewis Laboratories, Inc.
Weigh Down, diet beverage in vanilla and chocolate flavors, with psyllium and oat bran	Lewis Laboratories, Inc.
Diet Smart, meal replacement shake, in French vanilla and dutch chocolate flavors	Naturade Products, Inc.
Diet Smart Between Meal Snacks, wafers in strawberry-banana and chocolate malt flavors	Naturade Products, Inc.
Weight Reduction Program, beverage in vanilla flavor, with oat bran, psyllium, and tofu	Naturade Products, Inc.
Psyllium Plus, whole wheat bread with psyllium	Natural Way Bakery
Carrot-Tien, instant beverage granules	Nature's Plus
Spiru-Tein Energy Packed Meal Replacement, chocolate, strawberry, and vanilla flavors	Nature's Plus
Spiru-Tein Wafers, banana and vanilla flavors	Nature's Plus
Smooth Food 3, synergetic herb powder with corn bran and psyllium	New Moon Extracts, Inc.
Daily Fiber Formula beverage	Yerba Prima
Health Chips	Wysong, Inc.
Fiber-Psyll Soup mix	Holistic Products, Inc.
Fantastic Fiber, fruit and grain beverage concentrate	Plus Products
Brewer's Yeast with fiber	GNC
Bran Buds	Kellogg's

discontinued), Bran Buds, and Benefit (now discontinued). It has also been used recently in this country in a variety of other foods including those listed in Table 1.

Psyllium has been used in beverages, cereals, and candy and that one company, Botanicals International, Inc. of Long Beach, California, manufactures products containing psyllium that are used in cake icings and instant fruit fillings (Chan and Wypyszyk, 1988).

II.   PSYLLIUM AND CORONARY HEART DISEASE RISK REDUCTION

The U.S. Food and Drug Administration (FDA) has authorized a health claim for soluble fiber from psyllium husk and the risk of coronary heart disease (CHD) (Anon., 1998b). It is based on the totality of publicly available scientific evidence supporting the relationship between soluble fiber from psyllium husk and CHD. There are 57 human studies between 1965 and 1996 that, taken as a whole, demonstrate that consumption of psyllium (typically 7–15 g daily) leads to decreased levels of serum total cholesterol (TC) and low-density lipoprotein cholesterol (LDL-C) and a concomitant reduction in the risk of CHD. These studies include abundant evidence of beneficial results obtained with respect to test subjects who are mild to moderate hypercholesterolemics and who are therefore subject to a greater risk of contracting the disease. Every 1% reduction in average serum cholesterol level within a population represents a 2–4% reduction in CHD risk. As a result, psyllium consumption can lead to health benefits that will save lives. Soluble fiber from psyllium has been shown to be efficacious in lowering cholesterol levels more consistently and in more studies than soluble fiber from oatmeal or oat bran.

CHD is a disease having a multifactorial etiology that is associated with a number of risk factors (Stampfer et al., 1999). Among those factors, serum levels of TC and LDL-C are considered to be among the most important (Expert Panel, 1993). A number of human trials have reported a significant decline in mortality due to CHD as a result of intervention aimed at reducing serum cholesterol levels in subjects, including those without established clinical evidence of the disease. Based on the results of such studies, it has been estimated that for every 1% decrease in mean TC levels within a population, the risk of a fatal or nonfatal CHD-related incident in that population decreases by 2% (Lipid Research Clinics Program, 1984). After modification of these statistics to take into account differing cholesterol measurements, it has been concluded that a 1% decline in serum TC may actually be associated with a 3–4% decrease in CHD risk. Thus, reductions in mean total cholesterol of as little as 3% can reduce the number of CHD-related incidents in the United States by as much as 6–12%. Reductions in CHD risk of these magnitudes could potentially affect the lives of between 420,000 and 840,000 people annually. Since 1963, the number of deaths associated with CHD in this country has declined by 54% (Johnson et al., 1993). This decline in mortality has been attributed primarily to dietary changes that helped lower serum cholesterol. Between 1968 and 1976 alone, 30% of the decline was the result of reductions in blood cholesterol levels. Data from the National Health and Nutrition Examination Surveys (NHANES) have indicated a consistent decline in serum TC levels from 1960 through 1991, with more than half of the decline occurring within the period from 1976 to 1991 (Johnson et al., 1993). These same data suggest that this decline in total cholesterol was due primarily to a reduction in LDL-C levels.

The foregoing reductions in serum TC and LDL-C levels during the last three decades have been paralleled by dietary changes in consumption of fatty foods. Since the 1960s, consumption of red meat, butter, eggs, and whole fat dairy products has decreased; this has been largely responsible for the observed decrease in total fat intake in adult men and women from approximately 40–42% of calories to about 34–35% of calories (Stephen and Wald, 1990; Alaimo et al., 1994). Consumption of grain products has also increased since the mid-1970s. However, the dietary goal set by public health authorities in the United States of consuming 6–11 grain servings per day is not being met by the population as a whole. Data from NHANES III show that median intakes of fiber are 11–15 g, well below FDA's recommended daily value of 25 g and the National Cancer Institute's (NCI) recommended daily value of 20–30 g (Block and Subar, 1992; Alaimo et al., 1994) (noting daily dietary fiber intake of only 7–14 g). Thirty years of epidemiological, animal-experimental, and clinical studies have documented the hypocholesterolemic effects of soluble fiber (Anderson et al., 1994; Glore et al., 1994; Roberts et al., 1994; Truswell, 1995). The majority of this effect has been attributed to grain sources of soluble fiber such as cereals and legumes (Pilch, 1987; Glore et al., 1994). Indeed, in a recent study in the *Journal of the American Medical Association* analyzing data from the Health Professionals Follow-Up Study, it was indicated that consumption of dietary fiber has an inverse association with the risk of CHD-related incidents independently of fat intake (Rimm et al., 1996). The authors concluded that higher intake of dietary fiber, particularly from cereal and grain sources, can substantially reduce the risk of coronary heart disease. Cold breakfast cereal intake contributed about 9% of the total fiber intake among men in this study. The Nurses' Health Study, a prospective cohort study of U.S. women followed for 10 years from 1984, also indicated that only cereal fiber, among different sources of fiber, was strongly associated with a reduced risk of CHD (Wolk et al., 1999). A 10 g/day increase in total fiber intake (the difference between the lowest and highest quintiles), the multivariate RR of total CHO event was 0.81. NHANES III analysis indicated that breakfast meal pattern affected mean daily fiber intake status: cold breakfast cereals at breakfast showed the highest fiber intake of 20.3 g, followed by fruit/fruit drink consumers, 17.7 g; bread eaters, 16.9 g; egg/bacon eaters, 16.1 g; and breakfast skippers with the lowest fiber intake of 14.2 g daily (Cho et al., 2001).

A. Clinical Trials

The evidence on soluble fiber from psyllium, totaling 60 studies over the last 30 years, is persuasive. Those studies are summarized in Table 2; studies marked with an asterisk indicate human trials involving use of breakfast cereals containing psyllium. Of these latter studies, those by Anderson et al. (1992), Rippe (unpublished), Summerbell et al. (1994), and Wolever et al. (1994a) involved the use of Heartwise, a cereal containing psyllium, marketed by Kellogg Company. The studies by Jenkins et al. (unpublished) and Wolever et al. (1994a, 1994b) involved the use of Bran Buds. Other studies by Stoy et al. (1993) and Rippe et al. (unpublished) involved the use of test cereals by Kellogg that are not currently marketed.

These studies, many of which were controlled, demonstrate the hypocholesterolemic effects of psyllium intake ranging from as little as 2.5 to as much as 30 g/day. The effects are shown among both normocholesterolemics and mild to moderate hypercholesterolemics, among both men and women, among both adults (including elderly adults) and children, and among both free-living subjects and those undergoing clinical test conditions. The studies range from as little as 9–10 days to as long as 29 months. Some of the studies demonstrate that psyllium has a hypocholesterolemic effect even among people on a low-fat diet (Jenkins et al., 1993; Sprecher et al., 1993). The only studies demonstrating no decreases in serum TC and/or LDL-C levels were those of Rippe et al. (1990) and Dennison and Levine (1993). Two other studies comparing psyllium alone with drug intervention are distinguishable because of the focus of the study design (Maciejko et al., 1994; Spence et al., 1995), as is the study by Frape and Jones (1995), which was intended to measure only immediate postprandial plasma cholesterol levels. In a recent study, as little as 1.3 g/day of soluble fiber from psyllium proved to be efficacious in lowering plasma LDL cholesterol in both normal and hypercholesterolemic individuals (Romero et al., 1998).

Animal studies have yielded similar results. Psyllium intake has been found to lower cholesterol levels in studies involving African green monkeys (McCall, 1986, 1992a, 1992b), rabbits (Kritchevsky and Tepper, 1995), guinea pigs (Fernandez et al., 1995; Shen et al., 1998), hamsters (G. Kakis et al., unpubd.), and rats (Hara et al., 1994).

B. Meta-Analysis of Selected Studies

To verify the conclusions drawn from the human trials summarized above, Olson et al. (1997) conducted a meta-analysis of 11 published and unpublished studies utilizing psyllium-enriched RTE cereal in order to determine the hypocholesterolemic effects of soluble fiber from psyllium. Average baseline estimates for TC, LDL-C, and high-density lipoprotein (HDL) cholesterol levels are reported in Table 3. For the study by Roberts et al. (1994), data were broken down between test populations from Sydney and from Newcastle, Australia. No differences between mean baseline lipid values for the two treatment groups were found, given the randomization of subjects into those groups ($p < 0.05$).

Evaluation of the effects of psyllium intake on the difference between baseline and ending TC, HDL-C, and LDL-C was accomplished using a general linear model and PROC GLM in SAS7 software. Least-squares means were used to provide the estimates of the size of the effect of psyllium on lipid values. The ratio of ending to baseline lipid values was first transformed using natural logarithms to more closely approximate normally distributed data before it was analyzed. Estimates of the size of the effect of ratio data were obtained using nontransformed data, with conclusions drawn only about transformed lipid values. Factors in the full model included treatment, study, age category, gender, the interaction of treatment with each of the others, and the three-way interaction of treatment, gender, and age category. Results of the difference between baseline and ending lipid values and the ratio measurement are included in Table 4. Reduction of the full model by elimination of nonsignificant interactions yielded no change in the significance of the treatment factor and had little change on the size of the effect difference, so results from a model including only major effects will be discussed.

As a result of this meta-analysis, it was concluded that (a) psyllium intake had a significant effect ($p < 0.03$) on the lowering of serum TC and LDL-C levels, but no significant effect on serum HDL-C levels and (b) these effects were stable across the studies analyzed, i.e., the effect of psyllium occurred without regard to the study in which they participated. Estimates of the degree to which psyllium reduced TC and LDL-C levels in the studies analyzed are listed in Table 5. Also included are the 95% confidence intervals (CI) for the true values of the average difference and ratio estimates. Using the main effects linear model that pools all of the information across all studies, estimates for the overall average difference were obtained. The conclusion derived from these data is that subjects eating a psyllium-supplemented RTE cereal experienced a significant decrease in TC of approximately 0.31 mmol/L and a significant decrease in LDL-C of approximately 0.35 mmol/L compared with subjects eating control cereal. Similarly, a value in the ratio column of less than 1.0 represents a drop in TC, HDL-C, or LDL-C. Using the same pooled model, a common ratio of -0.05 was estimated for TC. Also, a common ratio for low-density lipoproteins of -0.09 was estimated for LDL-C. Thus, the subjects eating a psyllium-supplemented cereal tended to experience, on average, a 5% greater drop in TC and a 9% greater drop in LDL-C than their counterparts eating control cereal.

C. Suggested Explanations for Psyllium's Hypocholesterolemic Effects

The mechanism by which soluble fiber from psyllium reduces serum TC and LDL-C levels is admittedly not yet completely understood, but several hypotheses have been offered (Bell et al., 1989; Haskell et al., 1992; Everson et al., 1992; Sprecher et al., 1993; Glore et al., 1994; Fernandez et al., 1995;). These include:

1. The hypothesis that soluble fiber from psyllium may physically entrap bile acids, resulting in increased fecal excretion of such acids in a manner similar to that seen with bile acid sequestrants, and thus preventing their normal reabsorption
2. The hypothesis that soluble fiber from psyllium may interfere with micelle formation in the proximate small bowel, resulting in alterations in the quantity of cholesterol or fatty acids absorbed by the intestine
3. The hypothesis that fermentation of soluble fiber from psyllium into short-chain fatty acids by colonic bacteria may secondarily decrease hepatic cholesterol synthesis

Table 2 Leading Human Trials Concerning Psyllium Intake and Cholesterol Levels, 1965–1995

Study (study design)	Subjects	Dose (g/day)	Length of trial	Diet used	% Cholesterol reduction TC	% Cholesterol reduction LDL-C
1. Garvin et al., 1965 (intervention)	15 normal	9.6	5 weeks	Usual or usual + 6–8 eggs	−7 to −9	N/A
2. Forman et al., 1968 (intervention)	Normal males; number N/A	9.6	6 weeks	Usual or egg-supplemented	−17	N/A
3. Lieberthal and Martens, 1975 (intervention)	10 hyper-cholesterolemic (HC), 9 normal	11.5	5 weeks	Usual	−14.4 (HC) −9.8 (normal)	N/A
4. Tarpila and Miettinen, 1977 abstract (comparison after treatment)	9 HC	30	10 days		Mean decrease was significant	N/A
5. Danielsson et al., 1979 (intervention)	13 hyperlipidemics (HL)	7.2–10.8	2–29 months (avg. of 8 months)	Usual	−16.9 among those with cholesterol levels above 300 mg/dl	N/A
6. Capani et al., 1980 (intervention)	9 non–insulin-dependent diabetics (NIDD)	21	9 days	N/A	Significant decrease (approximately −12)	N/A
7. Enzi et al., 1980 (intervention)	22 obese	6	30 days	N/A	Significant decrease (approximately −14)	N/A
8. Fagerberg, 1982 (intervention)	40 NIDD	3.6–7.2 for 2 months, 10.8 for 2 months	4 months	Usual	−5 (approx.)	N/A
9. Burton and Manninen, 1982 (intervention)	12 elderly, recovering from hemiplegia	25–30 or less	16 weeks	Usual	−20	N/A
10. Nakamura et al., 1982 (intervention)	9 normal	6–12	5 weeks	Usual	−14.4	−25.6

	Reference	Subjects	Dose	Duration	Diet	Change 1	Change 2
11.	Frati-Munari et al., 1983 (intervention)	19 obese, 8 NIDD	15	10 days	Usual	−12.6 (tot. grp.) −14.1 (obese) −10.5 (diabetics)	−18.4 (tot. grp.) −19.3 (obese) −17 (diabetics)
12.	Borgia et al., 1983 (intervention)	65	10.5	4 weeks	Usual	−2.6	N/A
13.	Kies, 1983 (pooled analysis)	85	14–20	N/A	Usual	−8	N/A
14.	Abraham and Mehta, 1988 (intervention)	7 normal	21	3 weeks	Usual	−16	−15
15.	Anderson et al., 1988 (randomized, double-blind, placebo-controlled parallel)	26 HC	10.2	8 weeks	Usual	−14.8	−20.2
16.	Reynolds et al., 1988 abstract (randomized, double-blind, placebo-controlled)	75 (mean TC of 229 mg/dl)	10.2	8 weeks	NCEP Step 1	Significant reduction (approx. −4.4)	N/A
17.	Spark et al., 1989 abstract (intervention)	36 HC Children	5–10	6 months	Low-fat diet (10% of cal. from fat)	−18	−23
18.	Sugerman et al., 1989 abstract (intervention)	59 HC	20	3 weeks	Usual	Reduction (exact figure N/A)	−16.3
19.	Bell et al., 1989 (randomized, double-blind, placebo-controlled parallel)	75 HC (40 on psyllium)	10.2	8 weeks	AHA Step 1	−4.2 (from baseline) −4.8 (from controls)	−7.7 (from baseline) −8.2 (from controls)
20.	Taneja et al., 1989 (intervention)	11 normal adolescents	25	3 weeks	Usual	Significant decrease (approx. −7)	N/A

Table 2 Continued

Study (study design).	Subjects	Dose (g/day)	Length of trial	Diet used	% Cholesterol reduction TC	% Cholesterol reduction LDL-C
21. Rippe et al., 1989, unpublished (single-blind, placebo-controlled parallel)	24 HC (12 on psyllium)	9.5	4 weeks	AHA Step 1	−15.7	−24
22. Miettinen and Tarpila, 1989 (lead-in, followed by treatment phase)	9 hyperlipidemics ("HL")	30	11 days	Low cholesterol (110 mg/2400 kcal)	−6 (but inconsistent among subjects)	−9
23. Rippe et al., 1990, unpublished (single-blind, placebo-controlled longitudinal)	66 HC	5.6–16.8	8 weeks	AHA Step 1	No significant reductions	
24. Lerman-Garber et al., 1990 (lead-in, followed by treatment phase)	14 HC	10.2	6 weeks	Isocaloric, 10% of cal from fat	−8	−11
25. Bell et al., 1990 (double-blind, placebo controlled)	58 HC	6	6 weeks	AHA Step 1	−5.9	−5.7
26. Neal and Balm, 1990 (parallel open-label)	54 HC (27 on psyllium)	20.4	13 weeks	AHA Step 1	−7.1	−8.6
27. Levin et al., 1990 (randomized double-blind parallel)	58 HC	10	16 weeks	AHA Step 1	−5.6	−8.6
28. Glassman et al., 1990 (intervention)	36 HC children	2.5–10	8 months	N.Y. Med. Cntr. modified	−18 (from baseline) −14 (from controls)	−23 (from baseline) −19 (from controls)

No.	Study	Subjects	Dose	Duration	Diet	Outcome 1	Outcome 2
29.	Anderson et al., 1991 (randomized, placebo-controlled parallel)	105 HC	10.2	8 weeks	AHA Step 1	−4.3	−8.8
30.	Williams et al., 1995 (parallel)	25 HC children	6.4	12 weeks	AHA Step 1	−9.6	−15.7
31.	Stewart et al., 1991 (intervention)	175 elderly	9–19	1 month–1 year	Usual	−4.1 (for those taking 15–17 g daily)	N/A
32.	Everson et al., 1992 (randomized, double-blind crossover)	20 HC	15.3	40 days	Usual	−6 (from baseline) −3.5 (from controls)	−8 (from baseline) −6 (from controls)
33.	Mueller et al., 1992 abstract (randomized, controlled crossover) (earlier version of study listed below as number 52)	13 HC	6	2 weeks	AHA Step 1	−7.4	−11.1
34.	Haskell et al., 1992 (randomized, double-blind placebo-controlled)	55 HC total on psyllium mixture (3 out of 4 studies)	2.1–6.3 (as part of water soluble fiber mixture)	4–12 weeks	Usual	−3.0 (study 1) −8.3 (study 3) −4.9 to −12.2 (study 4)	−5.7 (study 1) −12.4 (study 3) −6.8 to −14.9 (study 4)
35.	Anderson et al., 1992 (randomized double-blind parallel)	44 HC	114 of psyllium mixture	6 weeks	AHA Step 1	−8.36	−12.9
36.	Huff et al., 1992, unpublished (double-blind, randomized parallel)	104 HC (22 on psyllium, 27 on psyllium + Colestipol)	15 psyllium or 7.5 psyllium + 7.5 Colestipol	10 weeks	Usual	−6.5 (psyllium only) −12 (psuyllium+ Colestipol	−8.8 (psyllium only) −18 (psyllium + Colestipol)

Table 2 Continued

Study (study design)	Subjects	Dose (g/day)	Length of trial	Diet used	% Cholesterol reduction TC	% Cholesterol reduction LDL-C
37. Jenkins et al., 1992, unpublished (randomized crossover)	12 HL	7.4/1000 kcal	1 month	Metabolic diet, 20% or less of calories from fat	−3.4	−5.1
38. Jenkins et al., 1993 (randomized crossover)	43 HL	High soluble fiber additions, including fiber from legumes, psyllium, and oat bran	4 months	NCEP Step 2	−4.9	−4.8
39. Jensen et al., 1993 (double-blind parallel)	29 HC	15 of soluble fiber mixture, including psyllium, pectin, and guar gum	4 weeks	Typical fat-modified	−10	−14
40. Dennison and Levine, 1993 (randomized, double-blind, placebo-controlled crossover)	20 HC children	6	4–5 weeks	Low fat, low saturated fat, low cholesterol	No significant reductions reported	
41. Kies, 1993 abstract (n/a)	130	10–30	7–28 days	Usual	−10.8	−6.3
42. Schechtman et al., 1993 (comparisons of psyllium vs. drug treatment)	297 HL (103 on psyllium)	10.4	46 months	Usual	−2.8	−2.2 (−8 in subjects <60)
43. Sprecher et al., 1993 (double-blind placebo-controlled parallel)	118 HC (59 on psyllium)	10.2	8 weeks	High- and low-fat diets	−4.5	−5.8
44. Stoy et al., 1993 (randomized crossover)	23 HC	15 soluble fiber from psyllium	5–8 weeks	NCEP Step 1	−4.4	−5.6

45.	Stoy et al., 1993 unpublished (randomized crossover)	22 HC	84 g psyllium cereal yielding 30 g of soluble fiber	5–8 weeks	NCEP Step 1	−4.4	−5.6
46.	Summerbell et al., 1994 (randomized double-blind placebo-controlled)	37 HC	9.6	6 weeks	Low-fat diet (30% of cal from fat)	−7.3	−10.6
47.	Gelissen et al., 1994 (controlled with washout period)	6 normal 4 ileostomy patients	9.9 psyllium seed	3 weeks	Usual	−6.4	−10.1
48.	Gupta et al., 1994 (controlled)	24 NIDD with HC	7	90 days	30 cal/kg of body weight	−19.7	−23.7
49.	Roberts et al., 1994 (double-blind crossover)	81 HC	12 mostly from psyllium	6 weeks	Low–saturated fat diet	−3.2	−4.4
50.	Maciejko et al., 1994 (double-blind, placebo-controlled crossover)	18 HC	10.2 in addition to cholestyramine	6 weeks	NCEP Step 1	No significant changes over cholestyramine alone	
51.	Wolever et al., 1994a (randomized, controlled crossover)	42 HL	6.7	2 weeks	AHA Step 2	−6.4	−7.8
52.	Wolever et al., 1994b (randomized three 2-wk. experimental periods separated by 2-week washout periods)	18 HC	7.3	2 weeks	NCEP Step 2	−8.4	−11.3
53.	Anderson et al., 1994 unpublished (multicenter, double-blind, placebo-controlled, randomized clinical trial)	248 HC	10.2	26 weeks	AHA Step 1	−4.7	−6.7

Table 2 Continued

Study (study design).	Subjects	Dose (g/day)	Length of trial	Diet used	% Cholesterol reduction TC	% Cholesterol reduction LDL-C
54. Keane et al., 1994, unpublished (parallel study with placebo control)	79 elderly HC (40 on psyllium)	10.2	12 weeks	AHA Step 1	−2.0	−5.2
55. Frape et al., 1995 (controlled double-blind)	12 HC	2.2 after each of two high fat meals	3 weeks	High-fat breakfasts and lunches	No significant effect on postprandial plasma measurements reported	
56. Spence et al., 1995 (randomized, double-blind parallel)	49 HC	15 of psyllium or 7.5 of psyllium + Colestipol	10 weeks	NCEP Step 2	No significant effects on TC; psyllium + Colestipol most effective in reducing LDL-C	
57. Williams et al., 1995 (randomized, single-blind placebo-controlled parallel)	50 children	3.2–6.4	12 weeks	NCEP Step 1	−9.6	−15.7
58. Davidson et al., 1996a (double-blind, placebo-controlled crossover)	25 HC children	6.4	6 weeks	NCEP Step 1	−5.2	−6.8
59. Davidson et al., 1996b, unpublished (double-blind, placebo-controlled parallel)	227 HC (197 on psyllium)	3.4–10.4	24 weeks	NCEP Step 1	−3.4	−5.3
				People consuming 10.2 g compared to controls; for lower consumption levels, no significant differences at the end of the treatment period		
60. Weingand et al., unpublished	23 HC	10.2	8 weeks	AHA Step 1	−2	−6.5

Table 3 Baseline Lipid Values by Study and Treatment Group and for Pooled Data

Study (n)	TC (mmol/L)		HDL-C (mmol/L)		LDL-C (mmol/L)	
	Control	Psyllium	Control	Psyllium	Control	Psyllium
Stoy et al., 1993	5.99	6.04	1.22	1.09	3.98	4.20
Stoy et al., 1993, unpublished	5.85	6.19	1.36	1.19	3.91	4.19
Jenkins et al., 1993	7.04	7.26	1.41	1.48	4.80	5.07
Jenkins et al., 1992, unpublished	7.07	7.25	1.41	1.57	4.91	5.15
Roberts et al., 1994	6.83	6.69	1.27	1.24	4.72	4.60
Roberts et al., 1994	6.41	6.64	1.12	1.19	4.38	4.55
Summerbell et al., 1994	6.07	6.14	1.37	1.44	4.02	4.15
Anderson et al., 1992	6.73	6.67	1.19	1.20	4.80	4.62
Rippe et al., 1989, unpublished	4.98	5.26	1.13	1.23	3.22	3.42
Rippe et al., 1990, unpublished	5.64	5.41	1.09	1.12	3.68	3.71
Bell et al., 1990	5.50	5.54	1.18	1.21	3.68	3.81
Wolever et al., 1994a	6.56	6.37	1.03	1.25	4.51	4.36
Overall average	6.16	6.39	1.33	1.36	4.14	4.33
Pooled SEM	0.10	0.09	0.05	0.04	0.10	0.09

4. The hypothesis that psyllium increases the activity of HMG CoA reductase secondary to lower insulin levels and reduced postprandial nutrient fluxes, which may have an effect on enterohepatic circulation of bile acids and cholesterol synthesis

With respect to fecal excretion of bile acids, with a few exceptions, increasing the intake of soluble fiber from psyllium has been shown to elevate bile acid fecal excretion in both humans and animals. However, increased sterol or acid excretions would not seem to account fully for the cholesterol reductions typically observed. Everson and colleagues (1992), who found that 15 g per day of psyllium increased total bile acid synthesis by 43% in hypercholesterolemic men, suggested that increased bile acid excretion may be related to its interference with the intestinal absorption of such acids. With respect to micelle formation, decreased micellular formation or interference with micellular solubilization of cholesterol was suggested to be caused by the viscosity of the soluble fiber in psyllium.

Table 4 Linear Model Analysis of Difference and Ratio Measurements

	Observed significance levels for difference = (baseline-ending)			Observed significance levels for log (ratio) = (ending/balance)		
	TC	HDL-C	LDL-C	TC	HDL-C	LDL-C
Study	0.0001	0.0002	0.0001	0.0001	0.0045	0.01
Treatment	0.0002	0.34	0.0001	0.0008	0.86	0.03
Age category	0.68	0.94	0.13	0.66	0.94	0.65
Gender	0.24	0.93	0.25	0.33	0.97	0.84

Table 5 Estimates of the Size of Effect of Psyllium-Supplemented Cereal on Lipid Fractions

	Difference = (baseline-ending)			Difference of ratios: (end/begin)		
	TC	HDL-C	LDL-C	TC	HDL-C	LDL-C
Control	−0.01	0.01	−0.03	1.01	1.00	1.02
95% CI	(−0.11, 0.10)	(−0.02, 0.04)	(−0.13, 0.07)	(0.99, 1.03)	(0.97, 1.03)	(0.99, 1.05)
Psyllium	0.30	0.01	0.32	0.96	1.02	0.93
95% CI	(0.20, 0.40)	(−0.03, 0.04)	(0.22, 0.42)	(0.94, 0.97)	(0.99, 1.04)	(0.90, 0.94)
Overall	0.31	No significant change	0.35	0.05	No significant change	0.09
95% CI	(0.25, 0.37)		(0.29, 0.40)	(0.03, 0.08)		(0.04, 0.13)

The hypothesis of fermentability has been challenged with respect to psyllium because it is not fermented as rapidly as other cholesterol-lowering soluble fibers. Thus, for example, pectin is completely degraded in the human gut, while psyllium is degraded only partially. The final suggested mechanism has numerous aspects, all of which appear to be related to the liver's processing of cholesterol. Psyllium's effect on enzymatic activity in the liver may be critical due to that organ's role in cholesterol synthesis. Psyllium appears to affect the enterohepatic circulation of bile acids. Several studies have shown that psyllium treatment expands the bile acid pool and stimulates the activity of 7α-hydroxylase, the initial and rate-limiting enzyme in the bile acid biosynthetic pathway as well as HMGCoA reductase activity (Turley and Dietschy, 1991; Fernandez et al., 1995; Horton, et al., 1993).

III. PSYLLIUM POSES NO PROBLEMS WITH RESPECT TO VITAMIN AND MINERAL ABSORPTION

Psyllium intake also raises no issues of significance with respect to vitamin or mineral absorption. There are 32 reported human and animal studies in this area, which are summarized in Table 6.

The conclusions in these studies are largely positive. Thus, Lawrence et al. (1990) noted that psyllium had no adverse effect on vitamin and mineral status. Vahouny et al. (1987) came to a similar conclusion. Likewise, Paulini et al. (1988) and Buth and Mehta (1983), in two long-term feeding studies of African green monkeys, reported, respectively, increased iron utilization and no adverse effects on zinc or copper absorption. Jacobs (1989), Bell et al. (1989), Anderson et al. (1988), Burton and Manninen (1982), and Mehta and Poetter (1984) offer similar conclusions as to zinc and/or iron. Jacobs (1987) likewise reports no changes in serum levels of magnesium, calcium, or zinc, a conclusion (with respect to the first two minerals) supported by Spiller et al. (1979) and by Rampton (1984). Solter and Lorenz (1983) and the five Italian studies reported in SCOGS likewise find no changes in biochemical, hematochemical, and/or hematological parameters.

Even the few studies reporting adverse results raise no concerns. While Roe et al. (1988) reported a reduction in the absorption of vitamin B_2 (riboflavin), their findings are of limited value because (a) they studied only the absorption of pharmacological doses of riboflavin, conceding that further research is needed to investigate the effect of psyllium supplements on the absorption of riboflavin from foods, (b) the study lasted only 24 hours and they conceded that further research is needed on the long-term effects on riboflavin nutriture, and (c) the effect on riboflavin absorption found was small, involving only reduction in absorption of about five percentage points. Similarly, while Kies (1983) noted increases in fecal copper and zinc losses after ingestion of psyllium, she pointed out that less copper was excreted than after ingestion of wheat bran.

In its 1989 report on Diet and Health, the National Research Council likewise concluded that there was little evidence that high fiber intake impedes mineral absorption and bioavailability and that any differences caused by fecal or urinary excretion seem too small to pose a major health hazard (NRC, 1989). Pilch (1987) concluded that the results of the animal and human studies on the influence of psyllium on mineral absorption and metabolism suggest that, at psyllium intakes contemplated for its use as a food ingredient, no significant adverse effects would be likely unless dietary intakes of minerals were marginal.

Table 6 Human and Animal Studies on Vitamin and Mineral Status and Psyllium

Author	Dosage	Duration	Subjects	Comments
1. Dennison et al., 1993	6 g/d	4–5 weeks	Humans	Zn, vitamin D, vitamin A, vitamin E, Ca levels unchanged; Fe levels were higher
2. Levin et al., 1990	10.2 g/d of Metamucil	16 weeks	Humans	No significant differences in indicators of vitamin K status
3. Lawrence et al., 1990	1–5% diets	91 days	Fischer 344 rats	No apparent effect on Na and K status; urinary P excretion decreased as psyllium increased; urinary Mg excretion decreased with psyllium; serum and bone Mg and P status unchanged; no apparent adverse effect on other mineral status
4. Ganji and Kies, 1990	Not reported	10 days	Humans	Zn balance not adversely affected by combined intake of psyllium and Fe supplements
5. Jacobs and Domek, 1989	1–5% diets	4 weeks	Sprague-Dawley rats	Hepatic and serum Cu increased; hepatic and serum Zn was unchanged; intestinal absorption of Zn and Cu was unchanged
6. Bell et al., 1989	10.2 g/d of Metamucil	8–16 weeks	Humans	No effect on serum Fe levels.
7. Anderson et al., 1988	10.2 g/d of Metamucil	8 weeks	Humans	No effects on serum levels of Fe and Zn
8. Roe et al., 1988	2.3–5.7 g of soluble fiber/d	1 day	Humans	Reduced absorption of pharmacological doses of vitamin B$_2$
9. Paulini et al., 1988	10% diet	3 years (monkeys) 10 weeks (rats)	African green monkeys, Sprague-Dawley rats	In monkeys, no effect on Zn status; serum Cu decreased, but liver and kidney Cu unchanged. In rats fed marginal Zn, tibia Zn decreased slightly, but no effects were seen on intestinal absorption of Zn or Cu. Conclusion: short- or long-term feeding of psyllium did not affect adversely Zn or Cu status with nonmarginal diets
10. Jacobs et al., 1987	1–5% diets	4 weeks	Sprague-Dawley rats	Fecal concentrations of Cu, Zn, Mg, Mn, Ca, and Fe were diluted dose-responsively; serum Cu levels increased while Mg, Zn, and Ca were unchanged; psyllium modifies intestinal mineral metabolism
11. Vahouny et al., 1987	5% diet	4 weeks	Wistar rats	Positive balances of intake vs. fecal output recorded for Ca, Fe, Mg, and Zn
12. Gillooly et al., 1984	5 g of Mucilose	1 day	Humans	Decrease in Fe status noted

No.	Reference	Dose	Duration	Species	Findings
13.	Rampton, 1984	7 g/d	8 weeks	Humans	Fecal excretion of K, Ca, and Mg increased while that of P decreased; no effects on plasma P, Ca, and K
14.	Mehta and Poetter, 1984	5–10% diets	10 weeks	Weanling rats	With marginal Zn diet, slight effect on tibia Zn, but none on absorption
15.	Solter and Lorenz, 1983	2 tsp of Prodiem/d	7 days–12 weeks	Humans	No significant effect on Na and K levels
16.	Kies, 1983	14–20 g/d	Various	Humans	Increased fecal Cu, Zn, Ca, and Mg
17.	Buth and Mehta, 1983	9.7% diet	16 months	African green monkeys	Fe utilization increased and fecal loss decreased
18.	Kies et al., 1983	5.3 g/d	6–7 days	Humans	Fecal Zn loss increased among both omnivores and vegetarians, but less so among the latter
19.	Burton and Manninen, 1982	maximum daily dose that could be taken comfortably, <25 d/g	16 weeks	Humans	No changes in serum Cu or Fe
20.	Fernandez and Phillips, 1982	not reported	1 day (perfusion)	Dogs	Fe absorption decreased in healthy dogs
21.	Enzi et al., 1980	<6 g/d	30–150 days	Humans	Plasma Fe and Ca levels decreased slightly after 30 days, but stabilized thereafter
22.	Spiller et al., 1979	20 g/d	21 days	Humans	No significant differences in fecal excretion of Ca or Mg; no abnormal changes in plasma chemistry
23.	Mercatelli et al., 1982	250–750 mg/kg/d	6 months	Beagle dogs	Inorganic P concentrations greater in dogs given 250 mg/kg/d, while Na and K levels higher in females given 750 mg/kg/d
24.	McHale et al., 1979	10–20 g/d	18 days total	Humans	No effect on Ca serum level and only a minor effect on Mg serum levels
25.	Drews et al., 1979	14.2 g/d	4 days	Humans	Increased Zn, Fe, and Mg fecal excretions
26.	Kies et al., 1979	4.2–24.2 g/d	50 days (total)	Humans	Urinary and blood serum Zn levels unaffected, but fecal Zn levels increased
27.	Fraschini, 1982	0.5–1.0 g/kg/d	25 weeks	Sprague-Dawley rats	No differences in results of hematological, hematochemical, and urine tests
28.	Giovannini and Careddu, (reported in SCOGS, 1982)	3.6 g/d	10–14 days	Humans	No changes in mean values of hematological or blood chemistry parameters
29.	Davi and Strano, 1982	7 g/d	10 days	Humans	No changes in hematological parameters
30.	Slaerno et al., 1982	800 mg/kg/d	15 days	Beagle dogs	No changes in blood biochemistry
31.	Beshgetoor et al., 1977	4.2–14.2 g/d	14–28 days	Humans	Increased Zn loss noted
32.	Kies and Fox, 1976	4.2–24.2 g/d	42 days total	Humans	Zn balance negatively affected for high dosage level only

IV. PSYLLIUM AND ALLERGENICITY

The surveys of the incidence of reactions among pharmaceutical workers and health care providers sensitized by prior inhalation of psyllium are important in that they suggest that the rate of significant sensitization is, at most, 25%, and probably much less. For example, Goransson and Michaelson (1979) found that only 12 of 64 pharmaceutical workers (19%) had positive reactions to both skin and provocation tests for psyllium. McConnochie et al. (1990) similarly found a prevalence of specific (IgE and/or skin test) positivity to psyllium in only 11 of 92 pharmaceutical workers (12%). Marks et al. (1991) found a similar response in only 7.6% of 125 workers, and Nelson's (1987) epidemiological study of health care providers in chronic care facilities disclosed that only 18% (136 of 743) displayed allergic responses to psyllium. Thus, the subpopulation of exposed individuals at risk appears to be a relatively small one. The more recent research examining the topic uniformly concludes that sensitization to psyllium was mediated through an IgE mechanism (Seggev et al., 1984; Cartier et al., 1987; Schwartz et al., 1989).

REFERENCES

ZD Abraham, T Mehta. Three-week psyllium-husk supplementation: effect on plasma cholesterol concentrations, fecal steroid excretion, and carbohydrate absorption in men. Am J Clin Nutr 47:67–74, 1988.

K Alaimo, MA McDowell, RR Briefel, AM Bischof, CR Caughman, CM Loria, CL Johnson. Dietary intake of vitamins, minerals, and fiber of persons ages 2 months and over in the United States: third national health and nutrition examination survey, phase 1, 1988–91. Advance Data 258:1–26, 1994.

JW Anderson, N Zettwoch, T Feldman, J Tietyen-Clark, P Oeltgen, CW Bishop. Cholesterol-lowering effects of psyllium hydrophilic mucilloid for hypercholesterolemic men. Arch Intern Med 148:292–296, 1988.

JW Anderson, TL Floore, PB Geil, D Spencer, TK Balm. Hypercholesterolemic effects of different bulk forming hydrophilic fibers as adjuncts to dietary therapy in mild to moderate hypercholesterolemia. Arch Intern Med 151:1597–1602, 1991.

JW Anderson, S Riddell-Mason, NJ Gustafson, SF Smith, M Mackey. Cholesterol lowering effects of psyllium enriched cereal as an adjunct to a prudent diet in the treatment of mild to moderate hypercholesterolemia. Am J Clin Nutr 56:93–98, 1992.

JW Anderson, AE Jones, S Riddell-Mason. Ten different dietary fibers have significantly different effects on serum and liver lipids of cholesterol-fed rats. J Nutr 124(1):78–83, 1994.

Anon. Food labeling: Health claims: Soluble fiber from certain food and coronary heart disease. Fed Reg 63:8103–8121, 1998.

LP Bell, K Hectorne, H Reynolds, TK Balm, DB Hunninghake. Cholesterol-lowering effects of psyllium hydrophilic mucilloid—adjunct therapy to a prudent diet for patients with mild to moderate hypocholesterolemia. JAMA 261(23):3419–3423, 1989.

LP Bell, KJ Hectorne, H Reynolds, DB Hunninghake. Cholesterol-lowering effects of soluble-fiber cereals as part of a prudent diet for patients with mild to moderate hypercholesterolemia. Am J Clin Nutr 52:1020–1026, 1990.

JN BeMiller. Industrial gums: polysaccharides and their derivatives. In: RL Whistler, JN BeMiller, eds. Quince Seed, psyllium seed, flax seed, and okra gums. New York: Academic Press, 1973, pp 339–367.

D Beshgetoor, C Kies, HM Fox. Zinc utilization by human adults as affected by dietary pectin, cellulose and hemicellulose (abstr). Fed Proc 36(3):1118, 1977.

G Block, AF Subar. Estimates of nutrient intake from a food frequency questionnaire: the 1987 national health interview survey. J Am Diet Assoc 92:969–977, 1992.

M Borgia, N Sepe, V Brancato, G Costa, P Simone, R Borgia, R Lugli. Treatment of chronic constipation by a bulk-forming laxative (Fibrolax). J Int Med Res 11:124–127, 1983.

M Buth, T Mehta. Effect of psyllium husk on iron bioavailability in monkeys. Nutr Reports Intl 28:743–752, 1983.

R Burton, V Manninen. Influence of a psyllium based fibre preparation on faecal and serum parameters. Acta Med Scand 668(suppl):91–94, 1982.

F Capani, A Consoli, A Del Ponte, G Lalli, S Sensi. A new dietary fibre for use in diabetes. IRCS Med Sci 8:661, 1980.

A Cartier, J-L Malo, J Dolovich. Occupational asthma in nurses handling psyllium. Clin Allergy 17:1–6, 1987.

JKC Chan, V Wypyszyk. A forgotten natural dietary fiber: psyllium mucilloid. Cereal Foods World 33(11): 919–922, 1988.

SS Cho, G Block, S Steinburg, C Clark. Dietary fiber sources of American population. Manuscript in preparation.

Council for Scientific Information and Research (CSIR). Wealth of India: a dictionary of Indian raw materials and industrial products, Vol. VIII. 1969, pp 146–154.

Dairy Foods. Using fiber in ice cream: psyllium stabilizer appeals to label-readers. Dairy Foods 91(10): 120–121, 1990.

A Danielsson, B Ek, H Nyhlin, L Steen. Effect of long-term treatment with hydrophilic colloid on serum lipids. Acta Hepato-Gastroenterol 26:148–153, 1979.

MH Davidson, LD Dugan, JH Burns, D Sugimoto, K Story, K Duncan. A psyllium enriched cereal for the treatment of hypercholesterolemia in children: a controlled, double-blinded, crossover study. Am J Clin Nutr 1996:96–102, 1996.

G Davi, A Strano. Sperimentazione clinica controllata su Metamucil. Report and English translation submitted to SCOGS by G.D. Searle & Company, Chicago, IL. (As reported in SCOGS II-23, 1982.)

BA Dennison, DM Levine. Randomized, double-blind, placebo-controlled, two-period crossover clinical trial of psyllium fiber in children with hypercholesterolemia. J Pediatr 123(1):24–29, 1993.

LM Drews, C Kies, HM Fox. Effect of dietary fiber on copper, zinc, and magnesium utilization by adolescent boys. Am J Clin Nutr 32:1893–1897, 1979.

G Enzi, EM Inebman, G Crepaldi. Effect of a hydrophilic mucilage in the treatment of obese patients. Pharmatherapeutics 2:421–428, 1980.

GT Everson, BP Daggy, C McKinley, JA Story. Effects of psyllium hydrophilic mucilloid on LDL-cholesterol and bile acid synthesis in hypercholesterolemic men. J Lip Res 33:1183–1192, 1992.

Expert Panel on Detection, Evaluation, and Treatment of High Blood Cholesterol in Adults. Summary of the second report of the National Cholesterol Education Program (NCEP) expert panel on detection, evaluation, and treatment of high blood cholesterol in adults (adult treatment panel II). JAMA 269: 3015–3023, 1993.

SE Fagerberg. The effects of a bulk laxative (Metamucil) on fasting blood glucose, serum lipids and other variables in constipated patients with non-insulin dependent adult diabetes. Curr Ther Res 31(2): 166–172, 1982.

ML Fernandez, LR Ruiz, AK Conde, Dong-Ming Sun, SK Erickson, DJ McNamara. Psyllium reduces plasma LDL in guinea pigs by altering hepatic cholesterol homeostasis. J Lip Res 36(5):1128–1138, 1995.

R Fernandez, SF Phillips. Components of fiber impair iron absorption in the dog. Am J Clin Nutr 35:107–112, 1982.

HB Figg. Psyllium seeds. Pharm J Pharmacist 126(4):29, 1931.

FA Fluckinger, D Hanbury. A history of the Principal Drugs of Vegetable Origin, Met with in Great Britain and British India. London: Macmillan and Co., 1874, pp 440–441.

DT Forman, JE Garvin, JE Foresiner, CB Taylor. Increased excretion of fecal bile acids by an oral hydrophilic colloid. Proc Soc Exp Biol Med 127:1060–1063, 1968.

DL Frape, AM Jones. Chronic and postprandial responses of plasma insulin, glucose and lipids in volunteers given dietary fibre supplements. Br J Nutr 73(5):733–751, 1995.

F Fraschini. Toxico-pharmacological tests on Metamucil (in Italian). Report and its English translation submitted to FASB for SCOGS by G.D. Searle & Co., Inc., Chicago, IL. (As reported in SCOGS II-23, 1982.).

A Frati-Munari, J Fernandez-Harp, M Becerril, A Chavez-Negrete, M Banales-Ham. Decrease in serum lipids, glycemia and body weight by plantago psyllium in obese and diabetic patients. Arch Invest Med 14:259–268, 1983.

VK Ganji, C Kies. Psyllium fiber interactions with regular iron and time release iron supplements: effects on zinc bioavailability to humans (abstr). FASEB 4(3):A395, 1990.

J Garvin, D Forman, W Eiseman, C Phillips. Lowering of human serum cholesterol by an oral hydrophilic colloid. Proc Soc Exp Biol Med 120:744–746, 1965.

IC Gelissen, B Brodie, MA Eastwood. Effect of plantago ovata (psyllium) husk and seeds on sterol metabolism: studies in normal and ileostomy subjects. Am J Clin Nutr 59(2):395–400, 1994.

M Gillooly, TH Bothwell, RW Charlton, JD Torrance, WR Bezwoda, AP MacPhail, DP Derman, L Novelli, P Morrall, F Mayet. Factors affecting the absorption of iron from cereals. Br J Nutr 51(1):37–46, 1984.

M Giovannini, P Careddu. Efficacia e tollerabilita di una mucillagine di plantaginis ovatae (Metamucil) nelle turbe della peristalsi intestinale in pediatria. Report and its English translation submitted to SCOGS by G.D. Searle & Company, Chicago. (As reported in SCOGS II-23, 1982.).

M Glassman, A Spark, S Berezin, S Schwarz, M Medow, LJ Newman. Treatment of type IIa hyperlipidemia in childhood by a simplified American Heart Association diet and fiber supplementation. AJDC 144:973–976, 1990.

SR Glore, D Van Treeck, AW Knehans, M Guild. Soluble fiber and serum lipids: a literature review. J Am Diet Assoc 94(4):425–436, 1994.

K Goransson, NG Michaelson. Ispaghula powder: an allergen in the work environment. Scand J Work Environ & Health 5:257–261, 1979.

RR Gupta, CG Agrawal, GP Singh, A Ghatak. Lipid-lowering efficacy of psyllium hydrophilic mucilloid in non insulin dependent diabetes mellitus with hyperlipidaemia. Indian J Med Res 100:237–241, 1994.

H Hara, Y Saito, M Nagata, M Tsuji, K Yamamoto, S Kiriyama. Artificial fiber complexes composed of cellulose and guar gum or psyllium may be better sources of soluble fiber for rats than comparable fiber mixtures. Am Inst Nutr 124(8):1238–1247, 1994.

WL Haskell, GA Spiller, CD Jensen, BK Ellis, JE Gates. Role of water-soluble dietary fiber in the management of elevated plasma cholesterol in healthy subjects. Am J Cardiol 69(5):433–439, 1992.

JD Horton, JA Cuthbert, DK Spady. Regulation of hepatic 7á-hydroxylase expression by dietary psyllium in the hamster. J Clin Inv 93(5):2084–2092, 1993.

MW Huff, P Heidenheim, A Viswanatha, H Burton, D Mills, JD Spence. Psyllium enhances the efficacy of colestipol in hypercholesterolemic subjects (abstr). Circulation 86(suppl 1):I-144, 1992.

LR Jacobs, M Domek. Dose-response reduction of serum cholesterol in rats fed psyllium fiber and its relationship to increased hepatic and serum copper. Gastroenterology 96:A233, 1989.

LR Jacobs, M Domek, B Lonnerdal. Influence of psyllium fiber supplements on rat colonic mucosal cytokinetics and mineral metabolism. Gastroenterology 92:1450, 1987.

DJA Jenkins, TMS Wolever, V Rao, R Hegele, S Mitchell, T Ransom, D Boctor, P Spadafora, A Jenkins, C Mehling, L Katzman Relle, P Connelly, J Story, E Furamoto, P Corey, P Wursch. Effect of blood lipids of very high intakes of fiber in diets low in cholesterol. N Engl J Clin Nutr 329(1):21–26, 1993.

CD Jensen, GA Spiller, JE Gates, AF Miller, JH Whittan. The effect of acacia gum and a water-soluble dietary fiber mixture on blood lipids in humans. J Am Clin Nutr 12:147–154, 1993.

CL Johnson, BM Rifkind, CT Sempos, MD Carroll, PS Bachorik, RR Briefel, DJ Gordon, VL Burt, CD Brown, K Lippel, JI Cleeman. Declining serum total cholesterol levels among U.S. adults. The national health and nutrition examination surveys. JAMA 269:3002–3008, 1993.

C Kies. Purified Psyllium Seed Fiber, Human Gastrointestinal Tract Function, and Nutritional Status of Humans. ACS Symp Ser 214, 1983, pp 61–70.

C Kies. Psyllium fiber supplementation of human diets: impact on blood serum lipid concentrations and intestinal efficacy. XV International Congress of Nutrition 2:659 (abstract), 1993.

C Kies, HM Fox. Zinc nutritional status of human subjects as affected by dietary hemicellulose (abstr). Cereal Foods World 8:453, 1976.

C Kies, HM Fox, D Beshgetoor. Effect of various levels of dietary hemicellulose on zinc nutritional status of men. Cereal Chem 56(3):133–136, 1979.

D Kritchevsky, SA Tepper. Influence of dietary fiber on establishment and progression of atherosclerosis in rabbits. J Nutr Biochem 6:509–512, 1995.

S Kumar. Famous plants isubgol. Botanica (Delhi) 24:39–42, 1973.

AT Lawrence, FE Wood, SJ Stoll. The effect of psyllium husk and cellulose on mineral excretion and status in young male rats (abstr). FASEB 4(3):A530, 1990.

IM Lerman-Garber, M Lagunas, JCS Pereez, MA Ayala, A Saldana, GC Saldana, CP Romero. Effect of psyllium plantago on patients with moderately high hypercholesterolemia. Arch Inst Cardiol Mex 60:535–539, 1990 (in Spanish).

EG Levin, VT Miller, RA Muesing, DB Stoy, TK Balm, JC LaRosa. Comparison of psyllium hydrophilic mucilloid and cellulose as adjuncts to a prudent diet in the treatment of mild to moderate hypercholesterolemia. Arch Intern Med 150(9):1822–1827, 1990.

MM Lieberthal, RA Martens. Lowered serum cholesterol following the ingestion of a hydrophilic colloid. Digest Dis 20(5):469–474, 1975.

Lipid Research Clinics Program. The Lipid Research Clinics Coronary Primary Prevention in Trial Results: I. Reduction in incidence of coronary heart disease. JAMA 251(3):351–364, 1984.

GB Marks, CM Salome, AJ Woolcock. Asthma and allergy associated with occupational exposure to ispaghula and senna products in a pharmaceutical work force. Am Rev Respir Dis 144:1065–1069, 1991.

MR McCall. The effect of psyllium husk on plasma lipoproteins, cholesterol metabolism and atherosclerosis in African green monkeys. Ann Arbor, MI: U.M.I. Dissertation Information Services, 1986.

M McCall, T Mehta, C Leathers, D Foster. Psyllium husk I: Effect on plasma lipoproteins, cholesterol metabolism, and atherosclerosis in African green monkeys. Am J Clin Nutr 56:376–384, 1992a.

M McCall, T Mehta, C Leathers, D Foster. Psyllium husk II: effect on the metabolism of apolipoprotein B in African green monkeys. Am J Clin Nutr 56:385–393, 1992b.

K McConnochie, JH Edwards, R Fifield. Ispaghula sensitization in workers manufacturing a bulk laxative. Clin Exp Allergy 20(2):199–202, 1990.

M McHale, C Kies, HM Fox. Calcium and magnesium nutritional status of adolescent humans fed cellulose or hemicellulose supplements. J Food Sci 44(5):1412–1417, 1979.

JJ Maciejko, R Brazg, A Shah, S Patil, M Rubenfire. Psyllium for the reduction of cholestyramine-associated gastrointestinal symptoms in the treatment of primary hypercholesterolemia. Arch Fam Med 3:955–960, 1994.

T Mehta, C Poetter. Effect of psyllium husk on small intestine morphology and bioavailability of zinc and copper in rats. Fed Proc 43:4480A, 1984.

P Mercatelli, AA Storino, RO Salerno, A Nunziata, GC Perri. CRF Centro Ricerca Farmaceutica S.P.A., Roma. Tossicita cronica nel cane ''beagle'' del prodotto Metamucil; report a 1 mesi. Report and its English translation submitted to SCOGS by G.D. Searle & Company, Chicago. (As reported in SCOGS II-23, 1982.)

T Miettenen, S Tarpila. Serum lipids and cholesterol metabolism during guar gum, plantago ovata and high fibre treatments. Clin Chim Acta 183:253–262, 1989.

JF Montague. Psyllium seed: the latest laxative. New York: Montague Hospital for Intestinal Ailments, 1932.

S Mueller, TMS Wolever, T Ransom, D Boctor, G Buckley, R Patten, DJA Jenkins. Low glycemic index breakfast cereal reduces CHD lipid risk factors (abstr). Am J Clin Nutr 56(4):60, 1992.

KM Nadkarni. The Indian Materia Medica. Bombay: K.M. Nadkarni, 1927, pp 689–693.

H Nakamura, T Ishikawa, N Tada, A Kagami, K Kondo, E Miyazima, S Takeyama. Effect of several kinds of dietary fibres on serum and lipoprotein lipids. Nutr Rpts Int 26(2):215–221, 1982.

National Research Council/National Academy Of Sciences. Diet and Health: Implications for Reducing Chronic Disease Risk. Washington, DC: National Academy Press, 1989.

GW Neal, TK Balm. Synergistic effects of psyllium in the dietary treatment of hypercholesterolemia. South Med J 83:1131–1137, 1990.

WL Nelson. Allergic events among health care workers exposed to psyllium laxatives in the workplace. J Occup Med 29(6):497–499, 1987.

BH Olson, SM Anderson, MP Becker, JW Anderson, DB Hunninghake, DJ Jenkins, JC LaRosa, JM Rippe, DC Roberts, DB Stoy, CD Summerbell, AS Trowell, TM Wolever, DH Morris, VL Fulgoni. Psyllium enriched cereals lower blood total cholesterol and LDL cholesterol, but not HDL cholesterol, in hypercholesterolemic adults: Meta-analysis. J Nutr 127:1973–1980, 1997.

I Paulini, C Poetter, T Mehta, R Kincaid. Zinc and copper bioavailability in monkeys and rats with psyllium consumption. Nutr Res 8:401–412, 1988.

SM Pilch, ed. Physiological effects and health consequences of dietary fiber. Prepared for Center for Food Safety and Applied Nutrition, FDA, DHHS. NTIS Publication No. DB-87-212619, 1987.

DS Rampton, SL Cohen, V deB Crammond, J Gibbons, MF Lilburn, JY Rabet, AJ Vince, JD Wager, OM Wrong. Treatment of chronic renal failure with dietary fiber. Clin Nephrol 21(3):159–163, 1984.

HR Reynolds, LP Bell, K Hectorne, DB Hunninghake. Effect of psyllium mucilloid on serum lipids. Abstracts 1988 Am Diet Assoc Ann Meeting, 1988, p. 167.

EB Rimm, A Ascherio, E Giovannucci, D Spielgeman, MJ Stampfer, WC Willett. Vegetable, fruit, and cereal fiber intake and risk of coronary heart disease among men. JAMA 275(6):447–451, 1996.

JM Rippe, DH Morris, A Ward. Effects of a psyllium-supplemented cereal on blood cholesterol levels in hypercholesterolemic men. Unpubl. 1990.

DC Roberts, AS Truswell, A Bencke, HM Dewar, E Farmakalidis. The cholesterol-lowering effect of a breakfast cereal containing psyllium fibre. Med J Aust 161(11–12):660–664, 1994.

DA Roe, H Kalkwarf, J Stevens. Effect of fiber supplements on the apparent absorption of pharmacological doses of riboflavin. J Am Dietetic Assoc 88(2):211–213, 1988.

A Romero, JE Romero, S Galaviz, ML Fernandez. Cookies enriched with psyllium or oat bran lower plasma LDL cholesterol in normal and hypercholesterolemic men from northern Mexico. J Am Coll Nutr 17:601–608, 1998.

RO Salerno, T Bianco, A Nunziata. Studio farmacologico nel cane Abeagle@del Metamucil. Report and its English translation submitted to SCOGS by G.D. Seale and Company, Chicago, IL (As reported in SCOGS II-23, 1982.).

G Schechtman, J Hiatt, A Hartz. Evaluation of the effectiveness of lipid-lowering therapy for treating hypercholesterolemia in veterans. Am J Cardiol 10:759–765, 1998.

HJ Schwartz, JL Arnold, KP Strohl. Occupational allergic rhinitis reaction to psyllium. J Occup Med 31:624–626, 1989.

JS Seggev, K Ohta, WR Tipton. IgE mediated anaphylaxis due to a psyllium-containing drug. Ann Allergy 53(10):325–326, 1984.

H Shen, L He, RL Price, ML Fernandez. Dietary soluble fiber lowers plasma LDL cholestrol concentrations by altering lipoprotein metabolism in female guinea pigs. J Nutr 128:1434–1441, 1998.

AK Singh, OP Virmani. Cultivation and utilisation of isubgol (plantago ovata Forsk): a review. Curr Res Med Aromatic Plants 4(2):109–120, 1982.

H Solter, D Lorenz. Summary of clinical results with Prodiem Plain, a bowel-regulating agent. Today's Ther Trends 1:45–59, 1983.

A Spark, MS Glassman, LJ Newman. A psyllium-supplemented simplified diet for treatment of primary type II-A hypercholesterolemia in children (abstr). JADA (suppl):A112, 1989.

JD Spence, MW Huff, P Heidenheim, A Viswanatha, C Munoz, R Lindsay, B Wolfe, D Mills. Combination therapy with colestipol and psyllium mucilloid in patients with hyperlipidemia. Ann Intern Med 123:493–499, 1995.

GA Spiller, EA Shipley, MC Chernoff, WC Cooper. Bulk laxative efficacy of a psyllium seed hydrocolloid and a mixture of cellulose and pectin. J Clin Pharmacol 19:313–320, 1979.

DL Sprecher, BV Herris, AC Goldberg, EC Anderson, LM Bayuk, BS Russell, DS Crane, C Quinn, J Bateman, BR Kuzmak. Efficacy of psyllium in reducing serum cholesterol levels in hypercholesterolemic patients on high- or low-fat diets. Ann Intern Med 119(7 Pt. 1):545–554, 1993.

MJ Stampfer, FB Frank, JE Manson, EB Rimm, WC Willett. The primary prevention of coronary heart disease in women through diet and lifestyle. Circulation 110:1868–1869, 1999.

AM Stephen, NJ Wald. Trends in individual consumption of dietary fat in the United States, 1920–1984. Am J Clin Nutr 1990:457–469, 1990.

RB Stewart, WE Hale, MT Moore, FE May, RG Marks. Effect of psyllium hydrophilic mucilloid on serum cholesterol in the elderly. Dig Dis Sci 36(3):329–334, 1991.

DB Stoy, JC LaRosa, BK Brewer, M Mackey, RA Muesing. Lipid lowering effects of ready-to-eat cereal containing psyllium. JADA 93(87):910–912, 1993.

CS Sugerman, et al. Physiological effects of four types of dietary fiber in healthy subjects (abstr). JADA: A112, 1989.

CD Summerbell, P Manley, D Barnes, A Leeds. The effects of psyllium on blood lipids in hypercholesterolemic subjects. J Human Nutr Diet 7:147–151, 1994.

A Taneja, CM Bhat, A Arora, AP Kaur. Effect of incorporation of isabgol husk in a low fibre diet on faecal excretion and serum levels of lipids in adolescent girls. Eur J Clin Nutr 43:197–202, 1989.

S Tarpila, TA Miettinen. Effects of plantago fibre on serum lipids and fecal composition in hypercholesterolemic patients. Scand J Gastro (suppl 45)12:105, 1977.

AS Truswell. Dietary fibre and blood lipids. Curr Opin Lipidol 6:14–19, 1995.

SD Turley, BP Daggy, JM Dietschy. Cholesterol-lowering action of psyllium mucilloid in the hamster: sites and possible mechanisms of action. Metabolism 40(10):1063–1073, 1991.

GV Vahouny, R Khalafi, S Satchithanandam, DW Watkins, JA Story, MM Cassidy, D Kritchevsky. Dietary fiber supplementation and fecal bile acids, neutral steroids and divalent actions in rats. J Nutr 117(12):2009–2015, 1987.

CL Williams, M Bollella, A Spark, D Puder. Soluble fiber enhances the hypercholesterolemic effect of the Step I diet in childhood. J Am Coll Nutr 14(3):251–257, 1995.

TMS Wolever, DJA Jenkins, S Mueller, R Patten, LK Relle, D Boctor, TP Ransom, ES Chao, K McMillan, VK Fulgoni III. Psyllium reduces blood lipids in men and women with hyperlipidemia. Am J Med Sci 4:269–273, 1994a.

TMS Wolever, DJA Jenkins, S Mueller, DL Boctor, TP Ransom, R Patten, ES Chao, K McMillan, VK Fulgoni III. Method of administration influences the serum cholesterol-lowering effect of psyllium. Am J Clin Nutr 59(5):1055–1059, 1994b.

A Wolk, JE Manson, MJ Stampfer, GA Colditz, FB Hu, FE Speizer, CH Hennekens, WC Willett. Long-term intake of dietary fiber and decreased risk of coronary heart disease among women. JAMA 281: 1998–2004, 1999.

26

Oat Fiber

Production, Composition, Physicochemical Properties, Physiological Effects, Safety, and Food Applications

Yrjö Mälkki
Cerefi Ltd., Espoo, Finland

I. INTRODUCTION

By tradition, oats have been used as human food since ancient times and have been a staple food in many countries. It has been regarded as a healthy food without a clear knowledge of its specific health-related effects. However, today we know that its effects on satiety and retarded absorption of nutrients and as a deterrent of various disorders of the gastrointestinal tract account for this reputation. These beneficial effects are a result of oats soluble fiber content. Today oats are one of the richest and most economical sources of soluble dietary fiber; they also contain insoluble fiber.

The present interest in soluble oat fiber originated from animal and human studies of de Groot et al. in 1963 (1), which showed a hypocholesterolemic effect of relatively massive amounts of rolled oats. This launched an extensive series of both animal and clinical studies, the majority of which confirmed this effect. However, not until 1988 was public attention drawn to the possibilities of exploiting this effect therapeutically. An econometric study (2) based on the available clinical studies indicated potentially drastic cost savings using oat bran–based treatments as compared to chemotherapy.

The use of oats as food in the United States increased during 1985–1990 2.5-fold (3). This so-called oat boom was suddenly interrupted as a result of a well-publicized but less well-planned and performed study (4), which did not find a hypocholesterolemic effect of oat fiber. Although serious drawbacks of this study were soon indicated in the scientific journals by several authors, the demand for oat bran decreased somewhat but remained elevated level during the 1990s (5) and is again increasing since the allowance of health claims in the marketing.

In other industrialized countries the interest in the effects of oat soluble fiber has followed the same trend, but changes in the demand have been more modest. In addition to oats' hypocholesterolemic effect, focus on other physiological effects, in particular on hypoglycemic effect, started gradually to grow.

In addition to oat bran fiber, products made from oat hulls are also on the market. Their fiber is nearly entirely insoluble. They are used in the food industry mainly as a water-binding and structure-giving ingredient and have less and different physiological effects than oat bran fiber.

II. PRODUCTION AND CONSUMPTION OF OATS

The principal oat species cultivated and marketed today are *Avena sativa* (white oats) and *Avena byzantina* (red oats). The principal oat-producing areas in 1997, in order of magnitude of production, were Russia, the European Union, Canada, the United States, central Europe, and Australia. The principal oat-exporting countries are Canada, Sweden, Finland, and Australia. Of the total amount produced, 23% is used globally for food. The per capita consumption (kg/year) is highest in Russia (12.0), Canada (8.5), Australia (8.1), the Scandinavian countries (4–6), and the United States (5.2) (5). Dietary fiber obtained from these amounts is 0.6–1.7 g/day, but since individual consumption of oats varies greatly, regular users of oat products can obtain a substantial part of their total and soluble dietary fiber intake from oats.

III. AMOUNT AND LOCATION OF FIBER IN THE OAT KERNEL

Of the total weight of oat kernels of common cultivar varieties, 20–35% consists of hulls, which in an unprocessed state contain approximately 85% insoluble dietary fiber. Exceptions are naked cultivar varieties, where the hull content is less than 5%. Hulls can be further processed to bleached oat hull fiber, which has a dietary fiber content of more than 90%, all of it being insoluble.

In the remaining edible part, the groat, the total content of dietary fiber is usually 6–9%, about half of which is insoluble fiber, located mainly in the tissues outside the aleurone layer (Fig. 1). The principal component of the soluble fiber is a linear polysaccharide $(1 \rightarrow 3),(1 \rightarrow 4)$-$\beta$-D-glucan, usually called β-glucan. It is located in endosperm cell walls, which are thickest adjacent to the aleurone layer, in the subaleurone layer. However, the size of endosperm cells, the thickness of the cell walls throughout the groat, and thus the distribution of β-glucan vary widely among the different cultivar varieties (6).

The total β-glucan content of oat groats is influenced by both genetic and environmental factors, the genetic influence being the greatest (6–10). Reported contents vary from 1.8 to 8.5%, but the varieties having the highest β-glucan content are not commonly cultivated, and in the oat trade the content of β-glucan usually varies from 3.5 to 5.5%. Cultivar varieties that develop large kernels usually also have a high β-glucan content, and there is a negative correlation between the protein and β-glucan contents (9,11).

The effects of environmental conditions are less clear, and some effects observed are valid only for some of the varieties commonly cultivated. This might at least in part be due to the fact, that an effect on the β-glucan level can be indirect and affected by several simultaneously contributing factors. All the published cultivation studies have been made under field conditions, and thus have been subject to the natural variation of weather and soil conditions.

The effect of growing location—often a combined effect of climatic conditions and soil type—is evident. Studies from Germany (12) and Australia (13) show that on average the growing location can cause a difference of 0.3–0.7% units in the β-glucan content. In both German (12) and Finnish studies (14) the influence of the harvest year conditions outweighed the influence of location.

A highly significant correlation ($p < 0.001$) between the mean temperature of growing time and the content of β-glucan has been reported (14). There is a negative correlation between the content of β-glucan and the growing time, as measured from time of sprouting to ripeness (7). The effects of rainfall are complicated. A negative correlation often reported (14) could be caused by the fact that under dry growing conditions the ripening of the kernel starts prematurely

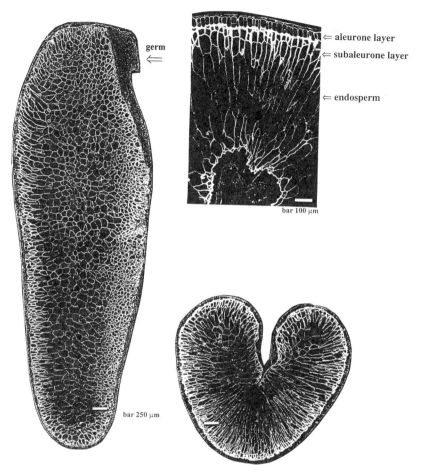

Fig. 1   Structure of oat groat. β-Glucan is located in the white cell walls of the inner endosperm and subaleurone layer. (Micrographs courtesy of Dr. K. Autio, VTT Biotechnology, Espoo, Finland.)

and leads to a small kernel size in which the relative amount of fiber-rich outer layers is higher.

Relatively high values of β-glucan are obtained on soils with low but not excessively low pH value (14). A high phosphorus content limits the β-glucan content (14), possibly by favoring an increase in phytic acid, which has a negative correlation with β-glucan content (15).

IV. PROCESSING

A. Hulling

After pretreatments for cleaning and grading, the first stage of the conventional oat milling process is hulling, where the outer layers of the kernel are removed by impact and aspiration treatments (16,17). Hulls as such do not contain soluble fiber, but any hulling loss exceeding the share of hulls also means losses of soluble fiber into the hull fraction.

B. Heat Treatments

Heat treatments serve several purposes. Dry heat treatments are used for creating a roasted flavor and/or, when performed before hulling, for enhancing the release of hulls. Hydrothermal treatments serve to inactivate enzymes, especially lipase and lipoxygenase, which can cause rancidity and a bitter taste, and β-glucanase and to improve the solubility of β-glucan.

A conventional hydrothermal treatment involves steaming and dry heating at 95–105°C for 0.5–2 hours. The process parameters are chosen based on the known time-temperature dependence of enzyme inactivation (16,18). The process is usually controlled by determining residual tyrosinase activity as an indicator for inactivation of lipase and lipoxygenase. A more effective stabilization and simultaneously hydratation of β-glucan is achieved by mild heat treatments under pressure. For controlling inactivation of β-glucanases, the most relevant method in regard to preserving the physiological activity is to test the absence of a viscosity-reducing effect in suspensions of hydrated β-glucan–containing material.

C. Oatmeal and Rolled Oats

Traditional oat flakes are prepared from hulled and heat-treated groats by rolling between cast-iron rolls that have equal speeds. This is typically performed immediately following steaming, which serves both to enzyme inactivation and for plasticising the groats. More rapidly cooking flakes and instant oat flakes are prepared by steel-cutting the groats in three to five pieces before rolling, by decreasing the flake thickness, and by more intensive steaming.

Traditional whole oat flour is prepared from oat groats by milling. When further treated by removing bran fractions by sieving, the resulting flour is called refined oat flour. For details of the preparation see Ref. 17.

D. Oat Bran

In contrast to many other cereal materials, oat bran does not consist of a sharply limited distinct part of the oat groat. In conventional milling operations, the subaleurone layer, which consists of thick-walled cells (see Fig. 1), follows the coarse outer layers of the groat and is thus included in the bran.

In the United States, the following definition for oat bran is valid (19): "Oat bran is produced by grinding clean oat groats or rolled oats and separating the resulting oat flour by suitable means into fractions, such that the oat bran fraction is not more than 50 percent of the original starting material and provides at least 5.5 percent (dwb) β-glucan soluble fiber and a total dietary fiber content of 16 percent (dwb), and such that at least one-third of the total dietary fiber is soluble fiber."

In conventional oat milling processes, hulled and heat-treated oat groats are subjected to grinding and sieving operations in one or several stages to separate the major part of starchy endosperm from the outer layers of the groat. Bran is separated as the coarse fraction. A practical upper limit for β-glucan in the traditional milling process is 10%; in commercial oat brans the content varies from 5.5 to 9%. The present industrial practice has been reviewed in Refs. 17 and 20.

E. Dry Enrichment of Oat Fiber

To enable physiologically effective amounts of oat soluble fiber to be ingested without simultaneously ingesting excessive amounts of other oat constituents, efforts to concentrate oat fiber further from oat bran or oat flour have been made since that late 1980s. Preparations from an unexplained "nonsolvent fractionation" process containing 10.9–12.3% β-glucan (21,22) have been supplied to animal studies. In published laboratory and pilot-scale dry fractionations (23), brans containing up to 12.8% β-glucan have been obtained. In recent studies (Y. Mälkki and O. Myllymäki, unpublished), the highest contents of β-glucan in enriched full-fat bran in laboratory and pilot-scale experiments were 17.5 and 16.1% of dry weight, respectively.

F. Concentrations After Defatting or in Organic Solvent

To avoid difficulties in clogging and material flow caused by fat content, several groups have used defatting of oat groats or flakes and subsequently performed grinding and sieving or air classification operations in a dry state. After defatting with hexane, pin milling or abrasive milling and air classifications, concentrated brans containing 11.2–30% β-glucan have been achieved (23–25). A disadvantage in the dry sieving operations is the transfer of β-glucan into the fine fraction, which reduces the yields of concentrates obtainable. By sieving in aqueous or organic solvent, sieves with smaller openings can be used and thus losses of β-glucan into the fine fraction reduced. In earlier studies (for review, see Ref. 20) the point was mainly to separate protein, and the most common solvent was hexane. Contents of β-glucan were not analyzed, but as now estimated from the yield of the bran fraction, concentrations of β-glucan have probably been between 8 and 12%. In later studies using ethanol or 2-propanol as a solvent (23,26), β-glucan concentrations in the coarse fraction could be elevated up to 15–18% and even up to 27%. (Y. Mälkki and O. Myllymäki, unpublished).

A concentration of oat fiber based on soaking groats in 50°C water and a subsequent wet milling in ethanol has been presented (27). According to the patent specification, the content of β-glucan in the final bran fraction is 19.4%; in the commercial product it is declared to be more than 16% (28). At the time of the manuscript of this paper, the product is marketed mainly to the cosmetic industries.

A method for concentration of β-glucan to 30% or even 40% level has been developed (29). It is based on a hydrothermal treatment with or without a combination with enzymatic degradation of protein and removal of starch by further sieving. Simultaneously, the solublity of β-glucan is improved.

G. Aqueous Processes

In an aqueous wet milling process (30), use is made of the low and slow solubility of β-glucan in cold water, and starch is removed by a rapid screening of oat flour in cold water. In the patent description the content of β-glucan was said to be 31%; in the commercial product it was 15%. Marketing of this concentrated bran was discontinued in 1996.

Concentration of soluble fiber by removal of insoluble fiber is used in an enzymatic process (31). Oat flour or oat bran is hydrolyzed by thermostable α-amylases to convert the starch into maltodextrins, and β-glucan is dissolved. Insoluble components are separated by centrifugation. Commercial preparations have found a market mainly based on the properties of maltodextrin; the β-glucan content in the different preparations varies from 1 to 20%.

H. Isolation of β-Glucan

Methods presented are based on the well-known solubility of β-glucan in hot water and in alkaline solutions, separation of the dissolved proteins by isoelectric precipitation, and precipitating the β-glucan by ammonium sulfate, 2-propanol, or ethanol (32,33). Preparations usually contain 60–80% β-glucan, the remaining part being mainly protein (7–22%), mineral substances (3%), pentosans, starch, and lipid (0.1–1.0%) (34,35). Since 1996 isolated β-glucan has been produced on a small scale for cosmetic, skin care, and immunological applications. In further purification for research purposes, repeated precipitations and enzymatic hydrolysis of residual starch are used, and a purity of 99% has been reached (35).

I. Oat Hull Fiber

A minimal process is to grind and sieve the material to obtain a particle size of 0.2–0.4 mm. Another type of preparation involves bleaching with alkaline hydrogen peroxide to dissolve partially the lignin (36). The process reduces the original tan color, improves the speed of hydratation and water-holding capacity, and reduces the gritty mouthfeel of the untreated material.

V. CHEMICAL STRUCTURE

A. β-Glucan

The main component of oat soluble fiber, β-glucan, is a linear polysaccharide composed of (1 → 3) and (1 → 4)-β-linked glucosidyl subunits (Fig. 2). (1 → 3) linkages occur singly, linking together (1 → 4)-β-linked oligosaccharidyl subunits. Structurally related mixed-linkage β-D-glucans differ in the ratio of tri-and tetrasaccharidyl residues, which for β-glucan of oats is 2.1–2.4, for barley 2.8–3.3 (37), and for wheat 3.0–3.8 (35). Other frequently occurring sequences have a degree of polymerization (DP) of 5 or 9, but sequences with a DP up to 15 have been found (37).

Isolated and purified β-glucan frequently contains 0.5–1% or even more nitrogen, which usually is interpreted to derive from proteins, peptides, or amino acids. It is still uncertain whether protein or peptide is covalently bound to the β-glucans (38). It may bind β-glucan to the cell wall structure, as has been suggested for barley (39), or it may bind macromolecule chains to each other. An indication for binding is the reduction of viscosity by trypsin (40), which is dissimilar in different cultivar varieties (41).

The highest peak molecular weights, $2.9–3.1 \times 10^6$ daltons, have been reported for β-glucan extracted in sodium carbonate solutions from ground oat groats or oat bran (42). These values are higher than those found for β-glucan from barley ($1.3–2.7 \times 10^6$), waxy barley ($1.3–1.5 \times 10^6$) or rye (1.1×10^6) (42). In commercial oat products, the peak molecular weights have varied from 0.6 to 3.0×10^6 daltons. In commercial oat brans the peak molecular weight in hot water extracts varied from 1.4 to 1.8×10^6 daltons, and in an extract made by simulating physiological conditions from 1.1 to 1.9×10^6 daltons (43).

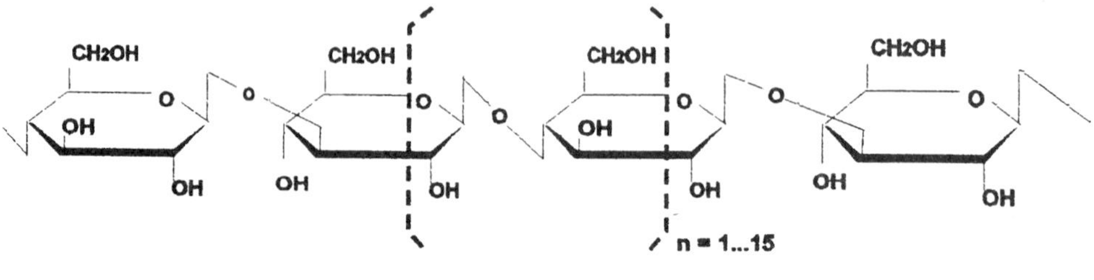

Fig. 2   Structure of oat β-glucan, (1 → 3),(1 → 4)-β-D-glucan.

A drastic decrease in molecular weight can occur in isolation procedures, on both a laboratory and technical scale, and in technical processing (23). Factors affecting a reduction are temperature, alkalinity, acidity, shear forces, and enzymatic breakdown. In isolated β-glucan weight average molecular weights have varied from 0.7 to 1.63×10^6 daltons (42), and in physiological extracts of oat bran muffins peak molecular weights vary from 0.6 to 1.2×10^6 daltons (43). In breads weight average molecular weights from 0.5 to 2.0×10^6 daltons have been found (44; T. Suortti, personal communication). Incubation of unheated oat bran for 0.5 hour at pH 5 and room temperature is sufficient to reduce the molecular weight from 1.5×10^6 to 3.7×10^5 daltons (40) The molecular weight has also been found to decrease during storage of ground oat material in a dry state, even in frozen storage (45).

B. Oat Hull Fiber

Unprocessed oat hull fiber typically contains 70–75% carbohydrates, the remaining part being protein, lignin, and ash. The content of cellulose is reported to be 30.9%, that of other hexosans 2.6% and of pentosans 33.2% (46). In bleached hull fiber, the carbohydrate content is usually above 90%.

VI. PHYSICAL PROPERTIES

A. Water Solubility and Extractability of β-Glucan

The "final rule" for food labeling health claims (19,47) refers to "β-glucan soluble fiber" and to an enzymatic method for the determination of β-glucan (48), which does not differentiate between soluble and insoluble β-glucan. For declaration purposes, valid standard methods for soluble dietary fiber must be applied, although all of these (49) involve an initial heating step and thus do not as such simulate physiological conditions.

Solubility of β-glucan is dependent, on the one hand, on the pretreatment of the preparation and, on the other hand, on the extracting conditions. Dissolving of β-glucan occurs gradually, the principal factors being temperature, moisture content, possible barriers for water penetration and for diffusion of the dissolved material, and the possible presence of endogenous or microbial enzymes degrading the macromolecules.

In studies in which unheated oat grain samples or commercially heated oat bran have been extracted at 38 or 40°C (40,50,51), 79.5–90% of β-glucan has been extractable. Under the same conditions, only 40.4–44.0% of β-glucan was extracted from hot-ethanol wet milled oat bran concentrates (40). The difference is probably due to the solubilization of β-glucan by the endogenous enzymes. At 80°C, the extractability of β-glucan from an ethanol enzyme-inactivated material was 46% (42) and at 90°C in water containing thermostable α-amylase 72–79% (52). As expected, milling treatments and particle size have a great influence on the extractability, not only by increasing the contact surface of the solid particle and water, but also by opening the physical barriers of the plant tissue structure for water penetration.

Extractability of β-glucan under simulated physiological conditions has been found to be from oat brans 12.9–28.7%, from rolled oats 33.2%, and from oat bran muffins 30.3–85.3%, the latter depending on the formulation and starting material (43). The solubility of β-glucan in muffins decreased in frozen storage (−20°C) during 8 weeks to about a half of the starting value: "the decline in solubility . . . possibly reflects changes in molecular organization and crystallinity" (43). These changes might be similar to those leading to the decreased solubility of ethanol enzyme inactivated samples. No studies exist on the reversibility of these changes.

B. Rheological Properties

At low shear rates (<10/s) or frequencies, the apparent viscosity of aqueous solutions of unhydrolyzed oat gum is independent of shear rate, which indicates no macromolecular interactions (53). At higher shear rates and above a concentration of 0.2% the solutions are shear-thinning but do not exhibit a time-dependent behavior. Starting from concentrations of 0.3–0.4%, the viscosity increases very steeply, and the concentration dependency is similar to that of guar gum (53). The viscosity level is sensitive to changes in molecular weight. Thus, e.g., β-glucan concentrations needed to give an apparent viscosity of 200 mPa·s at a shear rate of 30/s were 0.58, 1.39, and 5.5%, when the weight average molecular weights were 1.2, 0.36, or 0.1×10^6 daltons, respectively (53). The viscosity is not affected by sodium chloride but is increased by 25 and 50% sucrose concentrations (54).

Micelle-like aggregations have been observed with low molecular weight oat gum preparations (53,55), and these can lead either to a suspension or to a weak network (53). Aggregations are not found with unhydrolyzed preparations (53). Oat maltodextrin containing 10% of β-glucan exhibited in a 5% suspension a shear thickening behavior at shear rates from 20 to 80/s, returning to the shear thinning behavior again at higher shear rates, whereas cooked oat bran showed constantly a shear thinning behavior (56).

In suspensions of β-glucan–containing oat products, the viscosity is for the main part determined on the amount of β-glucan dissolved from the material and its molecular weight. Less refined and not intensively heat-treated oat products give lower viscosities, which also develop slowly, but the viscosity can be drastically increased by hydrothermal treatments. Losses of viscosity during isolation procedures are most probably mainly due to shear forces involved. Losses in bread baking are mainly due to hydrolysis by β-glucanase enzymes deriving from yeast, contaminating microorganisms, or other cereal ingredients (57) but can also be in part due to thermal degradation (44). Contaminating microorganisms are an important source of endogenous β-glucanases (58).

Diminution of particle size improves water penetration, as stated above, but the rapid water absorption can lead to caking and clogging effects and to the so-called fish-eye formation, in which the outer layers of an agglomerate absorb water, forming a heavily viscous layer that delays diffusion of additional water for hydrating the inner parts of the agglomerate. This effect can be prevented by, for example, mixing the β-glucan–containing preparation with inert materials such as maltodextrin (59) or by precipitating the β-glucan during the preparation on an inert material (29).

Enzymatic degradations of several components of the material often initially elevate the extractability of β-glucan, but they usually lead to reduced viscosities due to the breakdown of β-glucan macromolecules.

Table 1 Water Hydration Capacity of Some Natural and Processed Fibers

Fiber source	Water hydration capacity (g/g dry substance)	Ref.
Cellulose	4.7	Opta Food Ingredients, Bedford, MA
Wheat bran	1.67	20
Oat hull fiber	1.76	20
Oat hull fiber HDF-90	6.0–7.0	National Oats, Cedar Rapids, IA
Oat bran, commercial	4.12	20
Oat bran, experimental	7.76	20, 23
Oat bran, experimental	12.74	20, 27

C. Water Binding

Both soluble and insoluble fiber affect the water-binding capacity of oat fractions. This alters the behavior in the processing as well as properties of the products. Representative data are presented in Table 1. As expected, the hydration capacity increases with increasing content of β-glucan, but it is also greatly improved by hydrothermal treatments (not shown). In preparations with the highest hydration capacities there is a gradual transition to viscous suspensions.

VII. PHYSIOLOGICAL EFFECTS

A. Cholesterol and Lipid Metabolism

1. Occurrence and Magnitude of the Effect

Reduction of blood total and low-density lipoprotein (LDL) cholesterol are the most well-known physiological effects of oat soluble fiber. It is unanimous that the principal causative component is oat β-glucan, although effects of other components are not excluded.

Three recent reviews of the clinical studies on this effect are available. A meta-analysis (60) covering 20 original studies, all of which were randomized and controlled, resulted in the following conclusions:

Initial cholesterol level	Change, β-glucan < 3 g/day	Change, β-glucan ≥ 3 g/day
<5.9 mmol/L	−0.09 ± 0.10 mmol/L	−0.13 ± 0.12 mmol/L
≥5.9 mmol/L	−0.27 ± 0.04 mmol/L	−0.41 ± 0.21 mmol/L

Earlier metabolic studies as well as recent human and animal studies and the mechanism of action are reviewed in Ref. 61. The U.S. Food and Drug Administration (FDA) (62) reviewed 37 clinical studies in view of the significance and dose-response of the effect. On this basis, FDA later (19,47) authorized the use of health claims addressing the association between soluble fiber from whole oats and a reduced risk of coronary heart disease. Preconditions for the claim are that the product should contain at least 0.75 g of β-glucan soluble fiber per serving and that the β-glucan soluble fiber is derived from whole oats.

To determine the dose response based on the total existing experimental material, a litera- ture survey was made without prescreening the studies. Fifty-three original clinical studies were identified, 37 of which reported a significant reduction of cholesterol, 10 others a nonsignificant reduction. The reason for nonsignificance was often the small number of subjects who partici- pated in the study; several of these studies showed a mean reduction of more than 8%. However, the dose response was very scattered (Fig. 3). Below an evident threshold of 3 g β-glucan a day, the reduction of cholesterol was minimal, after which a trend for dose response is evident. As a rule, the reason for a weak response or for no effect has been one or several of the following:

> A too low β-glucan content in the experimental diets
> A low solubility of β-glucan, e.g., use of unheated oat bran
> A weak compliance to the prescribed intake of soluble fiber
> Participation of subjects with initially low blood cholesterol
> Participation of subjects nonresponding for genetic reasons
> Faults in the experimental design

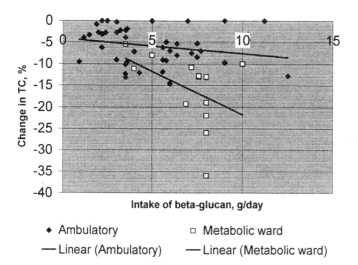

Fig. 3 Dose response of the cholesterol-lowering effect of β-glucan in 53 clinical studies published between 1963 and 1998. In cases where the amount of β-glucan has not been given in the original paper, it has been estimated on the basis of the average content of β-glucan in the components of the experimental diet.

The great difference in the dose response between the ambulatory and metabolic ward studies shown in Fig. 3 is evidently caused partly by the better control of compliance and partly by the route of administration. In most of the metabolic ward studies, oat soluble fiber has been given as porridge or as oat muffins, thus in both cases in a prehydrated state, which has enabled a rapid development of viscosity in the stomach and in the upper small intestine. In many of the ambulatory studies the oat preparation has been given to the subjects in a dry state; its further preparation or intake in a dry state has varied among the test subjects, and control of leftovers has in most cases been lacking or insufficient. The trend of ambulatory studies thus does not give a true picture of the dose response.

Due to the commercial unavailability of preparations, only a few studies have been made using isolated β-glucan. In one of them (63) a dose of 2.9 g of β-glucan twice daily for 4 weeks was used. The test subjects had an average baseline blood total cholesterol of 6.77 mmol/L. A reduction of 9.2% in total cholesterol and 10.0% of LDL cholesterol was observed. Five of the 19 subjects proved to be nonresponders. In another study (64), no reduction of cholesterol was observed despite a daily dose of 9 g of β-glucan. Possible reasons for the lack of effect on total cholesterol are a verified reduction of molecular weight of β-glucan in the isolation (65) and the low initial serum cholesterol content (4.23 mmol/L) of the subjects.

Data on the effect of oat β-glucan obtained from other concentrated sources show varying responses. A ready to eat (RTE) cereal made from a concentrated oat bran prepared by an undisclosed ''nonsolvent process'' gave with a similar dose of β-glucan a reduction of total cholesterol similar to that of oat bran (66), but was in rat studies more effective than oat bran (21,22,67). Oat bran concentrates made by ethanol wet milling, used at a level of 9 g β-glucan a day, gave a reduction of total cholesterol of 13.6% and of LDL cholesterol 23% (68). The same preparation showed in two rat studies (40,69) higher responses than oat bran with a similar dose of β-glucan. Oat fiber extracts prepared by the enzymatic method (31) given at levels corresponding to 0.95 or 6.0 g β-glucan a day caused reductions in total cholesterol of 9.5 or

14.6%, respectively (70). Oat bran concentrates prepared by an aqueous wet milling process were less effective than oat bran. In two clinical studies with daily doses of β-glucan of 10.3 or 11.2 g, a reduction of cholesterol was observed after 4 weeks, but after 8 weeks the cholesterol levels returned to near the initial level (71,72). The weak response has most probably been due to a weak solubility of β-glucan and to the weak viscosity properties of the water-soluble fraction of β-glucan (40).

Individual responses have in at least 12 clinical studies been reported to show nonresponding subjects, reports of the share of such persons varying from 20 to >50%. Different responses have been in a few studies related to apolipoprotein E polymorphism, but the results are controversial (71,73,74; Å. Lia et al., unpublished). The subject has been reviewed briefly (75).

2. Mechanism of Action

The reduction of cholesterol is evidently a sum of several effects. However, it is a commonly accepted concept the main part of the effect is due to the decreased absorption of bile acids, which causes a removal of steroids from the body by fecal excretion. The probable main consequence is an increased catabolism of cholesterol, an increase in the secretion of bile acids (76), a decrease in lipoprotein cholesterol secretion, and a reduction in the total body pool of cholesterol.

Direct indications of this mechanism are an increase in excretion of bile acids via feces: reported increases of bile acid excretion vary from 35 to 65% (77–80). There is no direct proof for a mechanism of the reduced absorption, but it is probably for the main part caused by the increased viscosity in the small intestine. This explanation is supported merely by the physical effect of the viscosity on the diffusion rates and the thickness of the unstirred layer on the site of absorption, but also by a study on cholesterol and galactose absorption in rat small intestine in vitro (81). This is related to the effects of β-glucan and its viscosity on the absorption of glucose (59).

Due to a decrease in bile acid content in the small intestine, emulsification of fats is decreased, which in addition to the viscosity effects mentioned reduces fat absorption. As a result, excretion of fat is increased. In a study with ileostomics (80) this excretion was 5.5 g/day, which does not significantly alter the amount of fat available daily but might have a positive long-term effect. Reduction and retardation of absorption of nutrients can also have effects via hormonal pathways.

Less attention has been paid to a possible role of apolipoprotein B_{100}. This is the major structure protein of LDL cholesterol and the binding site for the LDL receptor. In one study (82) oat bran reduced its content by 25%, while LDL cholesterol was simultaneously reduced by 10.5%. Elevated levels of $apoB_{100}$ are known to be a risk factor for coronary heart disease. Additional experimental data are needed to confirm this effect and to evaluate its relative importance for reducing the risk of coronary heart disease.

A suggested mechanism for cholesterol reduction is the action of short-chain fatty acids. Soluble fiber entering the colon is fermented nearly completely, the main end products being acetic, propionic, and butyric acids. Since propionic acid inhibits cholesterol synthesis in isolated rat hepatocytes at concentrations of 1.0–2.5 mM (83), it has been suggested that it would have an inhibiting effect on liver cholesterol synthesis. However, in rats fed oat bran the concentration of propionate in the hepatic portal vein has been shown to be maximally 0.35 mmol/L (76), and this mechanism seems thus to be unlikely or have a minor effect, if any in humans. This view is also supported by the fact that fructosan- and oligosaccharide-based food ingredients having no viscosity-elevating effect but acting as substrates in colon fermentations have in most studies had no or only minor cholesterol-reducing effects.

B. Hypoglycemic Effects

Diets giving a slow postprandial release of glucose and insulin have been studied and practiced actively since the late 1970s. The importance of viscosity was shown in experiments with guar gum, hydrolyzed guar gum, and other thickeners or fiber sources (84). In one case study from 1980 (36), a daily intake of a coarse oat fraction enabled a diabetic patient to reduce his insulin intake to zero while keeping his serum glucose in a normal range. Compared to many other foods, oats have a low postprandial glycemic response (85). In vitro studies with rat small intestine rings (81) have shown that oat gum retards monosaccharide uptake due to the increased viscosity and its effect on the reduction of diffusion and due to the thickness of the so-called unstirred layer on the absorption site.

In glucose tolerance tests, doses of 1.8, 7.2, and 14.5 g of β-glucan have effected reductions in the peak glucose value of 17, 40, and 60%, respectively (59,86). The relationship of increment in peak plasma glucose and peak plasma insulin to viscosity was the same as for guar gum (59).

Effects of β-glucan from oat gum and from oat bran as ingredients in meals have been studied with both healthy and type 2 diabetic (NIDDM) subjects (87) with doses of 8.8 g of β-glucan per meal. In healthy control subjects, glucose excursions (differences between the highest and lowest glucose levels) were 43 or 38% lower with oat gum or oat bran than with control meal, and the 3-hour areas under the curve above baseline were 28.5 or 27.2% lower, respectively, than with controls. With type 2 diabetic subjects, the levels of excursions were higher and the duration longer than with healthy subjects, and with the oat gum and oat bran meals the glucose excursions were 27.4 or 33.9% lower, respectively, than those of controls. Changes in insulin followed the same pattern.

In a study with NIDDM patients (88), β-glucan deriving from an ethanol wet-milled oat bran concentrate was incorporated in a cooked extruded breakfast cereal. With doses of 4.0, 6.0, or 8.4 g of β-glucan per meal, peak elevations of glucose were reduced by 33, 59, or 62%, respectively, from the control meal values, and 4-hour areas under curve above basal values by 29, 39, and 65%, respectively, from the control. Peak insulin values were reduced by 33, 38, or 41%, respectively. The higher responses compared to those of the previous study (87) might be due to differences in the solubility of β-glucan.

In a long-term study (68), eight men with NIDDM received in bread products for 12 weeks 9 g of β-glucan per day originating from ethanol wet-milled oat bran concentrate. The total carbohydrate level of the diet was 55%. During the oat bran concentrate period, total glucose response area was reduced by 46% ($p \leq 0.05$) and total insulin response area by 19% (not significantly). The glucose peak values after breakfast and lunch decreased by 15 and 25%, respectively.

There has also been interest in applying the hypoglycemic effect of oat soluble fiber to improving performance in sports. In a comparison of the effects of corn, wheat, and oat cereals on the respiratory quotient and on blood glucose, insulin, and amino acids at rest and during exercise (89), oat cereal gave the lowest glucose and insulin values for 90 minutes after the meal. After the first 20 minutes of exercise the glucose level was higher than with corn or wheat, but subsequently the differences were small, and no difference was observed in performance. The amount of β-glucan obtained from the oat cereal was, however, only approximately 1.1 g, and in view of the results of diabetic studies, more favorable effects would have been expected with higher doses.

The above results indicate that an effective dose for reducing postprandial elevations of glucose and insulin is about 6 g per meal provided that it is prehydrated or in an easily hydratable state and that its macromolecules have not been degraded.

C. Gastrointestinal Effects

Both soluble and insoluble oat fiber have gastrointestinal effects—soluble fiber mainly due to its high swelling and water-binding ability and as a substrate of colon fermentations, and insoluble fiber mainly due to its bulking effect.

Data on the effect of oat fiber on stomach emptying are controversial. The high swelling and water-binding properties of oat soluble fiber would lead one to expect delayed stomach emptying. Using radioactivity counting it was found (90) that an amount of 9 g of total dietary fiber per meal from oat bran caused no difference in the emptying rate as compared to semolina porridge control. In studies with pigs, use of relatively larger amounts of oat bran has been possible, and a viscosity-related delaying effect has been observed (91,92). A dose of 16 g of β-glucan from oat flour per kg dry matter of feed, elevating the viscosity of the liquid fraction in the stomach to approximately 15 mPa·s at a shear rate of 45 s^{-1}, caused an increased retention of liquid and solid markers, of digesta and of dry matter.

In the small intestine of humans, β-glucan remains intact, since no mammalian enzymes are capable of hydrolyzing it. In pigs, the molecular weight of β-glucan decreases, especially in the distal end, due to the effect of bacterial enzymes (92). Due to physical barriers to hydration and enzymatic action, intact remnants of the plant tissue are still observed, and the individual variations in viscosity ranged from 2 to 195 mPa·s, with the highest mean value (90 mPa·s) in the distal third of the small intestine 3 hours postprandial (92). In human ileal effluents (93), 88.5% of the β-glucan ingested was recovered.

Published clinical studies (Table 2) and animal studies (96) show that oat soluble fiber increases the fecal wet weight and reduces total transit time. Because β-glucan as such decomposes in the large intestine, the increase in dry weight is caused mainly by an increase in microbial cells, as shown in animal studies (97). The microbial cell material also retains more water than insoluble fiber, which increases the water content of the stool. Like other fiber sources that act as substrates for fermentation in the large intestine, oat soluble fiber can cause evolution of gas, especially when the amount ingested in the diet is changed suddenly. Compared to wheat bran, oat bran is reported to induce less discomfort and less formation of hydrogen and methane (94). Individual variations in the evolution of gas are large, but on average the amount of hydrogen produced from isolated oat gum, uncooked oats, or cooked oats is 58, 91, or 68%, respectively, of the amount produced from lactulose (98). Oat soluble fiber also causes a reduction in stool pH (97).

Insoluble oat fiber from oat hulls also increases the wet and dry weight of feces, but relatively less than oat soluble fiber. Oat hull fiber is not fermented in the large intestine (46).

D. Other Effects

In diets for weight reduction, oat soluble and insoluble fibers can act as water-binding and fat-mimicking ingredients. As stated earlier, oat fiber also increases the excretion of fat through the feces. An important function is its often reported effect on the feeling of satiety, probably caused by several simultaneous mechanisms.

In the large intestine, β-glucan is completely decomposed by bacterial enzymes and acts as a substrate for fermentations similar to other sources of soluble fiber. The physiological effects of these fermentations are described in other chapters of this book. The most important of these are probably the reduction of risk of intestinal and other cancers, effects on satiety, renal nitrogen load reduction, and prebiotic function.

In regard to the reduction of cancer risk, a special advantage of oat fiber is its lignan and

Table 2 Effect of Oat Soluble and Insoluble Fiber on Colon Function[a]

Preparation	Subjects no., sex, age	Insol. fiber (g/d)	Sol. fiber (g/d)	Fecal wet weight (g/d)	Fecal dry weight (g/d)	Transit time (h)	Stool frequency/day	Ref.
Control	6 f 65–73 yr			57.0	13.7		1.4	94
Oat bran		3	3	124.6	31.1		1.8	
Wheat bran		9.1	0.45	205.4	38.3		3.4	
Oat gum			7.5	73.1	22.0		1.8	
Raffinose			7.5	73.9	14.3		3.0	
Control	10 m 39–66 yr			134	27			79
Oat bran		8	8	191	42			
Control	6 m 4 f 24–36 yr			114	29	36		77
Rolled oats		5	5	125	34	30		
Control	8 m 35–62 yr			147	34.9			78
Oat bran		8	8	169	42.6			
Control	9 m 19–27 yr	15.5	2.7	85.3	24.6	73.1	0.68	95
Wheat bran		26.0	2.8	135.6	37.7	62.5	0.9	
Control		10.3	3.3	110.7	29.4	62.6	0.88	
Oat bran		18.8	9.1	156.4	42.4	53.0	0.92	
Control	10 m 20–37 yr			113	22.2	44.3		46
Oat hull fiber		17		155	45	42.0		

[a] Amounts fiber recalculated.

isoflavone content. These phytoestrogens are converted by intestinal bacteria to biologically active substances (for review, see Ref. 99). Over the long term these compounds probably reduce risks of mammary, prostate, and colon cancer. Reported total content of these compounds in oat bran varies from 2 to 7 mg/kg (100,101). The principal lignan components of oat bran are matairesinol and secoisolariciresinol, which are converted during intestinal fermentation to enterolactone and enterodiol. The level of lignans in oat bran is similar or higher than in rye, and in a dry enrichment of β-glucan content it is enriched in the same proportion. (H. Adlercreutz, unpublished).

One effect of oat soluble fiber seldom mentioned but having potential therapeutic value is an increase in the excretion of nitrogen through feces. This is a result of the increase in the microbial cell mass excreted and has been shown in pigs to elevate the amount protein excreted through feces fourfold compared to wheat flour (97,102). Increased fecal nitrogen excretion reduces correspondingly the urinary excretion and renal nitrogen load (103).

E. Effect of Processing and Storage on Physiological Efficiency

As stated above, the main effects of β-glucan depend on its viscosity. Processes that improve extractability of oat β-glucan thus increase its physiological efficiency, provided the macromolecules are not degraded in the process enzymatically or by shear forces, as stated above in connection with physical properties. Processing or storage conditions that lead to diminution of the extractability, such as formation of a glassy state or physical barriers for solubility in drying or semi-dry heat treatments or frozen storage (43), are expected to affect the physiological efficiency correspondingly.

VIII. SAFETY

Both oat meal and oat bran are generally recognized as safe (GRAS) under Sec. 170.30 (d) (21 CFR 170.30 (d)) (62). Oat gum has received GRAS status for specified uses; the applications listed include several types of cheese spreads, vegetables, meats, and frozen desserts, and no information on the possible carcinogenity or mutagenicity of oat gum is known (104). Use of oat hull fiber is permitted in the United States.

Some concern has arisen regarding reduced mineral absorption in connection with high intakes of dietary fiber. This is a problem common to several dietary fiber sources. Some minor components, especially phenolic compounds and phytic acid, accompanying fiber-rich plant tissues can bind divalent metal ions. Physiologically the most noticeable of these is binding of zinc and iron. In a long-term study with rats (105) absorption was affected by the level of the total mineral in the diet and not by the kind of fiber source. Diet did not appreciably affect mineral levels in soft tissues and bone. Nonheated oat bran reduces calcium availability and impairs absorption of mineral calcium (106). Magnesium absorption and retention as percent of intake are reduced, but the reduction is offset by the magnesium output from oat bran (106). Absorption and retention of iron, zinc, and phosphorus are increased (106). Ingestion of baked oat bran results in lower calcium and iron availability but has no effect on zinc, phosphorus, or magnesium absorption (106). Since fiber ingredients form only a minor part of the human diet, it is commonly suggested that these effects are easily compensated for by intakes from other food sources and might only in extreme cases result in low levels of zinc. In contrast, the complexing of iron by phytate and phenolic substances might be beneficial due to reduced fat peroxidation and formation of free radicals.

In animal studies where lipotropic substances—usually cholesterol and cholic acid—are added to feed to induce a hypercholesterolemic condition, infiltration of fat in the liver independent of addition of insoluble or soluble fiber has been reported (21,107). With increasing amounts of β-glucan in the diet, the changes in the liver become more severe, but lipid infiltration into the liver occurs only when lipotropic substances are added to the feed (108).

In some earlier data residues of oat hulls were regarded as a health risk due to sharp silica crystals on their outer surface and their potential to cause internal bleeding. With present hulling technologies the amount of such residues has been reduced to less than one piece per serving (one ounce), and the problem is presently regarded to be nonexistent.

Oat is in general relatively free of agrochemical residues due to the fact that in cultivation the need for such chemicals is smaller than for other crops. Important chemical contaminants include fungal toxins.

A physical risk common to all easily hydratable polysaccharides exists for oat gum as well. If ingested in tablet form, rapid swelling and adhesive action might cause blockage of the upper digestive tract. At least one fatal case of esophagus blockage by a glucomannan preparation is known. The risk can be avoided by incorporating the fiber in food items or administrating it in powder or granular form accompanied by a large amount of water.

IX. FOOD APPLICATIONS

Up to now oat fiber applications have been almost completely limited to traditional cereal products, such as hot and cold breakfast cereals, breads, biscuits, snacks, and pasta products. However, there is no reason for this limitation. Possible other product groups include meat products, ready-to-eat meals, drinks or drink powders, dairy products, and desserts. Persons who want to increase their daily intake of soluble dietary fiber need a variety of choices of palatable food items to continuously maintain a diet rich in soluble fiber. Attention should, however, be paid not only to the minimal amount of β-glucan. To achieve the health effects desired, it is even more important that the β-glucan in the preparation has solubility and viscosity properties adequate for the end use. To maintain good compliance, sensory properties are a key factor. It is a challenge for the food industry to provide consumers of both conventional foods and dietetic foods with such variety.

REFERENCES

1. de Groot AP, Luyken R, Pikaar NA. Cholesterol-lowering effect of rolled oats. Lancet Aug. 10: 303–304, 1963.
2. Kinosian BP, Eisenberg JM. Cutting into cholesterol. Cost-effective alternatives for treating hypercholesterolemia. JAMA 259:2249–2254, 1988.
3. Sparks Commodities Inc. The United States Market for Oats. Washington, DC: Sparks Commodities Inc., 1990.
4. Swain JF, Rouse IL, Curley CB, Sacks FM. Comparison of the effects of oat bran and low-fiber wheat on serum lipoprotein levels and blood pressure. N Engl J Med 322:147–152, 1990.
5. Pullinen T, and Sparks Commodities. Oats: a strategic assessment. Helsinki: Finnish Ministry of Agriculture and Forestry, 1998.
6. Fulcher RG, Miller SS. Structure of oat bran and distribution of dietary fiber components. In: Wood P, ed. Oat Bran. St. Paul, MN: American Association of Cereal Chemists 1993, pp 1–24.
7. Welch RW, Lloyd JD. Kernel $(1 \rightarrow 3),(1 \rightarrow 4)$-β-D-glucan content of oat genotypes. J Cereal Sci 9:35–40, 1989.
8. Lim HS, White PJ, Frey KJ. Genotypic effects on β-glucan content of oat lines grown in two consecutive years. Cereal Chem 69:262–265, 1992.

9. Miller SS Wood PJ, Pietrzak LN, Fulcher RG. Mixed-linkage β-glucan, protein content, and kernel weight in Avena species. Cereal Chem 70:231–235, 1993.

10. Cho KC, White PJ. Enzymatic analysis of β-glucan content in different oat genotypes. Cereal Chem 70:539–542, 1993.

11. Saastamoinen M, Plaami S, Kumpulainen J. Genetic and environmental variation in β-glucan content of oats cultivated in Finland. J Cereal Sci 16:279–290, 1992.

12. Ganssmann W. β-Glucangehalte in deutschen Hafersorten und Laborversuche zur Anreicherung von β-Glucan und Gesamt-Ballaststoffen. Getreide Mehl Brot 48 (6):45–49, 1994.

13. Mugford DC. Oat bran—an Australian "definition." In: Barr AR, ed. Proc. of the IV Int. Oat Conference Vol. 1. The Changing Role of Oats in Human and Animal Nutrition. Adelaide: Amanda Imprint, 1992, pp 96–100.

14. Saastamoinen M. Effects of environmental factors on the β-glucan content of two oat varieties. Acta Agric Scand Sect B Soil Plant Sci 45:181–187, 1995.

15. Saastamoinen M, Plaami S, Kumpulainen J. β-Glucan and phytic acid content of oats cultivated in Finland. Acta Agric Scand Sect B Soil Plant Sci 42:6–11, 1992.

16. Dorn V. New machinery in oat milling. Association of Operative Millers Bulletin, 1989, pp 5493–5502.

17. Caldwell EF, Dahl M, Fast RB, Seibert SE. Hot cereals. In: Fast RB, Caldwell EF, eds. Breakfast Cereals and How They Are Made. St. Paul, MN: American Association of Cereal Chemists, 1990, pp 243–272.

18. Vorwerk K. Hydrothermische Behandlung von Hafer. Getreide Mehl Brot 42:199–202, 1988.

19. Department of Health and Human Services. Food labeling: health claims; oats and coronary heart disease. Final rule. Fed Reg 62: 3584–3601, 1997.

20. Paton D, Lenz MK. Processing: Current practice and novel processes. In: Wood PJ, ed. Oat Bran, St. Paul, MN: American Association of Cereal Chemists, 1993, pp. 25–47.

21. Shinnick FL, Ink SL, Marlett JA. Dose responses to a dietary oat bran fraction in cholesterol-fed rats. J Nutr 120:561–568, 1990.

22. Shinnick FL, Longacre MJ, Ink SL, Marlett JA. Oat fiber: composition versus physiological function in rats. J Nutr 118:144–151, 1988.

23. Wood PJ, Weisz J, Fedec P, Burrows V. Large-scale preparation and properties of oat fractions enriched in $(1 \rightarrow 3)(1 \rightarrow 4)$-β-D-glucan. Cereal Chem 66:97–103, 1989.

24. Knuckles BE, Chiu MM, Betschart AA. β-Glucan-enriched fractions from laboratory-scale dry milling and sieving of barley and oats. Cereal Chem 69:198–202, 1992.

25. Wu YV, Stringfellow AC. Enriched protein- and β-glucan fractions from high-protein oats by air classification. Cereal Chem 72:132–134, 1995.

26. Myllymäki O, Mälkki Y, Autio K. Process for fractionating crop into industrial raw material. Finnish Pat. 84775, U.S. Pat. 5,312,636 (1991, 1994).

27. Collins FW, Paton D. Method of producing stable bran and flour products from cereal grains. U.S. Pat. 5,169,660, (1992).

28. Ceapro Inc., Internet pages *http://www.ceapro.com/canamino.html*, 1998.

29. Mälkki Y, Myllymäki O. A method for enriching soluble dietary fibre. Finnish Pat. 94015, International PCT publication WO 94/28742 (1994).

30. Lehtomäki I, Karinen P, Bergelin R, Myllymäki O. Beta-glucan enriched alimentary fiber and a process for preparing the same. Finnish Pat. 85796, U.S. Pat. 5,106,640 (1992).

31. Inglett GE. Method of making soluble dietary fiber compositions from cereals. U.S. Pat. 5,082,673 (1992).

32. Hohner GA, Hyldon RG. Oat groat fractionation process. U.S. Pat. 4,028,468, (1977).

33. Wood PJ, Siddiqui IJ, Paton D. Extraction of high-viscosity gums from oats. Cereal Chem 55:1038–1049, 1978.

34. Paton D, Breasciani S, Han NF, Hart J. Oats: chemistry, technology and potential uses in the cosmetic industry. Cosmet Toiletries Mag 110 (3):63–70, 1995.

35. Wood PJ, Weisz J, Blackwell BA. Molecular characterization of cereal β-glucans. Structural analysis of oat β-D-glucan and rapid structural evaluation of β-D-glucans from different sources by high-

performance liquid chromatography of oligosaccharides released by lichenase. Cereal Chem 68: 31–39, 1991.

36. Gould JM. Alkaline peroxide treatment of agricultural byproducts. U.S. Pat. 4,806,475 (1989).

37. Wood PJ, Weisz J, Blackwell BA. Structural studies of (1 → 3),(1 → 4)-β-D-glucans by ^{13}C-nuclear magnetic resonance spectroscopy and by rapid analysis of cellulose-like regions using high-performance anion-exchange chromatography of oligosaccharides released by lichenase. Cereal Chem 71: 301–307, 1994.

38. Vårum KM, Smidsrød O. Partial chemical and physical characterization of (1 → 3),(1 → 4)-β-D-glucans from oat (*Avena sativa* L.) aleurone. Carbohydr Polym 9:103–117, 1988.

39. Forrest IS, Wainwright T. The mode of binding of β-glucans and pentosans in barley endosperm cell walls. J Inst Brew 83:279–286, 1977.

40. Mälkki Y, Autio K, Hänninen O, Myllymäki O, Pelkonen K, Suortti T, Törrönen R. Oat bran concentrates: physical properties of β-glucan and hypocholesterolemic effects in rats. Cereal Chem 69: 647–653, 1992.

41. Autio K, Myllymäki O, Suortti T, Saastamoinen M, Poutanen K. Physical properties of β-glucan preparates isolated from Finnish oat varieties. Food Hydrocolloids 5:513–522, 1992.

42. Wood PJ, Weisz J, Mahn W. Molecular characterization of cereal β-glucans. II. Size-exclusion chromatography for comparison of molecular weight. Cereal Chem 68:530–536, 1991.

43. Beer MU, Wood PJ, Weisz J, Fillion N. Effect of cooking and storage on the amount and molecular weight of (1 → 3),(1 → 4)-β-D-glucan. Cereal Chem 74:705–709, 1997.

44. Suortti T, Poutanen K. Analysis of β-glucan in Finnish oat bread. Cereal Foods World 43:511, 1998.

45. Knuckles BE, Chiu MM, Yokoyama W, Sayre R. Changes in physical characteristics of β-glucan. Cereal Foods World 41:569–570, 1996.

46. Stephen AM, Dahl WJ, Johns DM, Englyst HN. Effect of oat hull fiber on human colonic function and serum lipids. Cereal Chem 74:379–383, 1997.

47. Department of Health and Human Services. Food labeling: health claims; oats and coronary heart disease. Amendment. Fed Reg 62:15343–15344, 1997.

48. Association of Official Analytical Chemists International (AOAC). Official Methods of Analysis, 16th ed. Method No. 992.28, 1995

49. Asp N-G, Schweizer TF, Southgate DAT, Theander O. Classification of carbohydrates in foods as related to dietary fibre analysis. In: Schweizer TF, Edwards CA, eds. Dietary Fibre—A Component of Food. Nutritional Function in Health and Disease. London: Springer-Verlag, 1992, pp. 57–101.

50. Åman P, Graham H, Tilley A. Content and solubility of mixed-linked (1 → 3),(1 → 4)-β-D-glucan in barley and oats during kernel development and storage. J Cereal Sci 10:45–50, 1989.

51. Lee CJ, Horsley RD, Manthey FA, Schwarz PB. Comparisons of β-glucan content of barley and oat. Cereal Chem 74:571–575, 1997.

52. Beer MU, Wood PJ, Weisz J. Molecular weight distribution and (1 → 3),(1 → 4)-β-D-glucan content of consecutive extracts of various oat and barley cultivars. Cereal Chem 74:476–480, 1997.

53. Doublier J-L, Wood PJ. Rheological properties of aqueous solutions of (1 → 3)(1 → 4)-β-D-glucan from oats (*Avena sativa* L.). Cereal Chem 72:335–340, 1995.

54. Autio K, Myllymäki O, Mälkki Y. Flow properties of solutions of oat β-glucans. J Food Sci 52: 1364–1366, 1987.

55. Vårum KM, Smidsrød O, Brant DA. Light scattering reveals micelle-like aggregation in the (1 → 3),(1 → 4)-β-D-glucans from oat aleurone. Food Hydrocolloids 5:497–511, 1992.

56. Carriere CJ, Inglett GE. Solution viscoelastic properties of OATRIM-10 and cooked oat bran. Cereal Chem 75:354–359, 1998.

57. Mälkki Y. Effect of oat bran on blood cholesterol—a critical review. In: Aalto-Kaarlehto T, Salovaara H, eds. Proc. 25th Nordic Cereal Congress. Helsinki: Helsinki University Press, 1993, pp 25–33.

58. Zhang D, Doehlert DC, Moore WR. Factors affecting viscosity of slurries of oat groat flours. Cereal Chem 74:722–726, 1997.

59. Wood PJ, Braaten JT, Scott FW, Riedel KD, Wolynetz MS, Collins MW. Effect of dose and modifi-

cation of viscous properties of oat gum on plasma glucose and insulin following an oral glucose load. Br J Nutr 72:731–743, 1994.

60. Ripsin CM, Keenan JM, Jacobs DR, et al. Oat products and lipid lowering. A meta-analysis. JAMA 267:3317–3325, 1992.

61. Anderson JW, Bridges SR. Hypocholesterolemic effects of oat bran in humans. In: Wood PJ, ed. Oat Bran. St. Paul, MN: American Association of Cereal Chemists, 1993, pp 139–157.

62. Department of Health and Human Services. Food labeling: Health claims; oats and coronary heart disease. Fed Reg 61:296–337, 1996.

63. Braaten JT, Wood PJ, Scott FW, Wolynetz MS, Lowe MK, Bradley-White P, Collins MW. Oat β-glucan reduces blood cholesterol concentration in hypercholesterolemic subjects. Eur J Clin Nutr 48:465–474, 1994.

64. Beer M, Arrigoni E, Amadò R. Are the oat β-glucans responsible for serum cholesterol lowering? In: Lairon D, ed. Mechanism and Action of Dietary Fibre on Lipid and Cholesterol Metabolism. Luxembourg: Commission of the European Communities, 1993, pp 145–148.

65. Beer MU, Arrigoni E, Amadò R. Extraction of oat gum from oat bran: effects of process on yield, molecular weight distribution, viscosity and $(1 \rightarrow 3),(1 \rightarrow 4)$-β-D-glucan content of the gum. Cereal Chem 73:58–62, 1996.

66. Demark-Wahnefried W, Bowering J, Cohen PS. Reduced serum cholesterol with dietary change using fat-modified and oat bran supplemented diets. J Am Diet Assoc 90:223–229, 1990.

67. Ney DM, Lasekan JB, Shinnick FL. Soluble oat fiber tends to normalize lipoprotein composition in cholesterol-fed rats. J Nutr 118:1455–1462, 1988.

68. Pick ME, Hawrysh ZJ, Gee MI, Toth E, Carg ML, Hardin RT. Oat bran concentrate bread products improve long-term control of diabetes: a pilot study. J Am Diet Assoc 96:1254–1261, 1996.

69. Ranhotra GS, Gelroth JA, Astroth K, Rao CS. Relative lipidemic responses in rats fed oat bran and oat bran concentrate. Cereal Chem 67:509–511, 1990.

70. Behall KM, Scholfield DJ, Hallfrisch J. Effect of beta-glucan level in oat fiber extracts on blood lipids in men and women. J Am Coll Nutr 16:46–51, 1997.

71. Uusitupa MIJ, Ruuskanen E, Mäkinen E, Laitinen J, Toskala E, Kervinen K, Kesäniemi A. A controlled study on the effect of beta-glucan-rich oat bran on serum lipids in hypercholesterolemic subjects: relation to apolipoprotein E phenotype. J Am Coll Nutr 11:651–659, 1992.

72. Törrönen R, Kansanen L, Uusitupa M, Hänninen O, Myllymäki O, Härkönen H, Mälkki Y. Effects of an oat bran concentrate on serum lipids in free-living men with mild or moderate hypercholesterol-aemia. Eur J Clin Nutr 46:621–627, 1992.

73. Jenkins DJA, Hegele RA, Connelly PW, Hallak K, Bracchi P, Kashtan H, Corey P, Pintila M, Stern H, Bruce R. The apoprotein E gene and the serum low-density lipoprotein cholesterol response to dietary fiber. Metabolism 42:585–593, 1993.

74. Wolever TMS, Hegele RA, Connelly PW, Ransom TPP, Story JA, Furumoto EJ, Jenkins DJA. Long-term effect of soluble-fiber foods on postprandial fat metabolism in dyslipidemic subjects with apo E3 and apo E4 genotypes. Am J Clin Nutr 66:584–590, 1997.

75. Uusitupa M. Hypo-cholesterolaemic effects of dietary fibre in relation to genetic factors. In: Guillon F, et al., eds. Functional Properties of Non-digestible Carbohydrates. Nantes: Institut National de la Recherche Agronomique, 1998, pp 97–100.

76. Illman RJ, Topping DL. Effects of dietary oat bran on faecal steroid excretion, plasma volatile fatty acids and lipid synthesis in rats. Nutr Res 5:839–846, 1985.

77. Judd PA, Truswell AS. The effect of rolled oats on blood lipids and fecal steroid excretion in man. Am J Clin Nutr 34:2061–2067, 1991.

78. Kirby RW, Anderson JW, Sieling B, Rees ED, Chen W-JL, Miller RE, Kay RM. Oat-bran intake selectively lowers serum low-density lipoprotein cholesterol concentrations of hypercholesterolemic men. Am J Clin Nutr 34:824–829, 1981.

79. Anderson JW, Story L, Sieling B, Chen W-JL, Petro MS, Story J. Hypocholesterolemic effects of oat bran or bean intake for hypercholesterolemic men. Am J Clin Nutr 40:1146–1155, 1984.

80. Lia Å, Hallmans G, Sandberg A-S, Sundberg B, Åman P, Andersson H. Oat β-glucan increases bile acid excretion and a fiber-rich barley fraction increases cholesterol excretion in ileostomy subjects. Am J Clin Nutr 62:1245–1251, 1995.

81. Lund EK, Gee JM, Brown JC, Wood PJ, Johnson IT. Effect of oat gum on the physical properties of the gastrointestinal contents and on the uptake of D-galactose and cholesterol by rat small intestine in vitro. Br J Nutr 62:91–101, 1989.

82. Bartram P, Gerlach S, Scheppach W, Keller F, Kasper H. Effect of a single oat bran cereal breakfast on serum cholesterol, lipoproteins, and apolipoproteins in patients with hyperlipoproteinemia type II a. J Parent Ent Nutr 16:533–537, 1992.

83. Wright RS, Anderson JW, Bridges SR. Propionate inhibits hepatic lipid synthesis. Proc Soc Exp Biol Med 190:26–29, 1990.

84. Jenkins DJA, Wolever TMS, Leeds AR, Gasull MA, Haisman P, Dilawari J, Goff DV, Metz GL, Alberti KGMM. Dietary fibers, fiber analogues, and glucose tolerance: Importance of viscosity. Br Med J 1:1392–1394, 1978.

85. Wolever TMS, Katzman-Relle L, Jenkins AL, Vuksan V, Josse RG, Jenkins DJA. Glycaemic index of 102 complex carbohydrate foods in patients with diabetes. Nutr Res 14:651–659, 1994.

86. Braaten JT, Scott FW, Wood PJ, Riedel KD, Poste LM, Collins MW. Oat gum lowers glucose and insulin after oral glucose load. Am J Clin Nutr 53:1425–1430, 1991.

87. Braaten JT, Scott FW, Wood PJ, Riedel KD, Wolynetz MS, Brulé D, Collins MW. High β-glucan oat bran and oat gum reduce postprandial blood glucose and insulin in subjects with and without type 2 diabetes. Diabetic Med 11:312–318, 1994.

88. Tappy L, Gügolz E, Würsch P. Effects of breakfast cereals containing various amounts of β-glucan fibers on plasma glucose and insulin responses in NIDDM subjects. Diabetes Care 19:831–834, 1996.

89. Paul GL, Rokusek JT, Dykstra GL, Boileau RA, Layman DK. Oat, wheat or corn cereal ingestion before exercise alters metabolism in humans. J Nutr 126:1372–1381, 1996.

90. Lia Å, Andersson H. Glycemic response and gastric emptying rate of oat bran and semolina porridge meals in diabetic subjects. Scand J Nutr 38:154–158, 1994.

91. Johansen HN, Bach Knudsen KE, Sandström B, Skjøth F. Effects of varying content of soluble dietary fibre from wheat flour and oat milling fractions on gastric emptying in pigs. Br J Nutr 75: 339–351, 1996.

92. Johansen HN, Bach Knudsen KE, Wood PJ, Fulcher RG. Physicochemical properties and the degradation of oat bran polysaccharides in the gut of pigs. J Sci Food Agric 73:81–92, 1997.

93. Lia Å, Sundberg B, Åman P, Sandberg A-S, Hallmans G, Andersson H. Substrates available for colonic fermentation from oat, barley and wheat diets. A study in ileostomy subjects. Br J Nutr 76: 797–808, 1996.

94. Meyer S, Calloway DH. Gastrointestinal response to oat and wheat milling fractions in older women. Cereal Chem 54:110–119, 1977.

95. Hosig KB, Shinnick FL, Johnson MD, Story JA, Marlett JA. Comparison of large bowel function and calcium balance during soft wheat bran and oat bran consumption. Cereal Chem 73:392–398, 1996.

96. De Schrijver R, Fremaut D, Verheyen A. Cholesterol-lowering effects and utilization of protein, lipid, fiber and energy in rats fed unprocessed and baked oat bran. J Nutr 122:1318–1324, 1992.

97. Bach Knudsen KE, Hansen I, Borg Jensen B, Østergård K. Physiological implications of wheat and oat dietary fiber. In: Furda I, Brine CJ, eds. New Developments in Dietary Fiber. New York: Plenum Press, 1990, pp 135–150.

98. Lund EK, Johnson IT. Fermentable carbohydrate reaching the colon after ingestion of oats in humans. J Nutr 121:311–317, 1990.

99. Adlercreutz H. Lignans and isoflavonoids. In: Mälkki Y, Cummings JH, eds. Dietary Fibre and Fermentation in the Colon. Cost Action 92, Luxembourg: European Commission, 1996, pp 324–332.

100. Axelson M, Sjövall J, Gustafson BE, Setchell KDR. Origin of lignans in mammals and identification of precursors from plants. Nature 298:659, 1982.

101. Thompson LU, Ronn P, Serraino M, Cheung F. Mammalian lignan production from various foods. Nutr Cancer 16:43–52, 1991.

102. Bach Knudsen KE, Borg Jensen B, Andersen JO, Hansen I. Gastrointestinal implications in pigs of wheat and oat fractions. 2. Microbial activity in the gastrointestinal tract. Br J Nutr 65:233–248, 1991.

103. Rémésy C, Younes H, Demigné C. Fermentable carbohydrates may shift nitrogen disposal towards the fecal excretion by enhancing urea transfer into the large intestine. In: Mälkki Y, Cummings JH, eds. Dietary Fibre and Fermentation in the Colon. Cost Action 92, Luxembourg: European Commission, 1996, pp 223–236.

104. Federation of American Societies for Experimental Biology. Evaluation of the health aspects of oat gum, okra gum, quince seed gum, and psyllium seed husk gum as food ingredient. Bethesda, MD: Report No FDA/BF/82/61, 1982.

105. Shah BG, Malcom S, Belonje B, Trick KD, Brassard R, Mongeau R. Effect of dietary cereal brans on the metabolism of calcium, phosphorus and magnesium in a long-term rat study. Nutr Res 10: 1015–1028, 1990.

106. De Schrijver R, Conrad S. Availability of calcium, magnesium, phosphorus, iron and zinc in rats fed oat bran containing diets. J Agric Food Chem 40: 1166–1177, 1992.

107. Lopez-Guisa JM, Harned MC, Dubelzieg R, Rao SC, Marlett JA. Processed oat hulls as potential dietary fiber sources in rats. J Nutr 118:953–962, 1988.

108. Mälkki Y, Törrönen R, Pelkonen K, Myllymäki O, Hänninen O, Syrjänen K. Effects of oat-bran concentrate on rat serum lipids and liver fat infiltration. Br J Nutr 70:767–776, 1993.

27
Barley Fiber

Christine E. Fastnaught
Castle Dome Foods, Inc., Fargo, North Dakota

I. INTRODUCTION

Barley is recognized as a unique substrate in the malting and brewing industry. Barley not used as malt is typically used as feed. However, as one of the first domesticated grains, barley was a major source of fiber and nutrients in the human diet. Barley fiber provides a unique balance of soluble and insoluble fibers distributed throughout the mature seed. Nutritional studies during the past 20 years have focused the medical community and consumer attention on increasing fiber in the diet and renewed the interest in barley as a source of β-glucan–rich balanced fiber.

A definition for barley fiber is complicated by the variation produced by growing environment and plant genetics. There are no major genes to control fiber production in the barley grain, but a number of genes influence the fiber level and change the composition. Cultivated barley varies in number of kernel rows on the spike (2 vs. 6), presence of a cemented hull (hulled vs. hulless), and amylose content of the starch (waxy, normal, high amylose). Breeding programs have introduced or selected variation in starch granule morphology (fractured), protein content (high lysine genes), cell wall thickness, and enzyme concentration. Understanding the major effects and interactions of these genes on fiber production and composition has been a significant research effort for scientists working with barley.

II. COMPOSITION

A barley seed produces fiber in the hull, pericarp, and the cell walls of the aleurone and starchy endosperm. Fiber from these anatomical sources differs in composition (Table 1). Cellulose is a major component of the hull (1), while arabinoxylan and β-glucan are the major components of the aleurone and starchy endosperm cell walls (2), respectively. Scanning microspectrofluorometry of barley seed cross sections confirm high concentrations of β-glucan in the central endosperm (3). Thus, there can be many different barley fibers, first, depending on the anatomical source and, second, determined by the genetic background of the barley cultivar.

Hull and starchy endosperm represent 85% of the seed, thus the composition of whole grain dietary fiber is strongly influenced by these two sources. Oscarsson et al. (4) and Xue et al. (1) have compared the components of dietary fiber in hulled and hulless cultivars (Table 2). On average, hulless cultivars had 19–26% less total dietary fiber than the hulled cultivars. Cellulose was 40–50% lower, lignin was 46–55% lower, and arabinoxylan was 30% lower in the

Table 1 Composition (% of total fiber) of Major Sources of Fiber in Mature Barley Grain

| Type of fiber | Hulls[a] | Cell walls[b] | |
		Aleurone	Starchy endosperm
Arabinoxylan	39	71	20
Cellulose	37	2	2
β-Glucan	3	26	75
Glucomannan	na	2	2
Klason lignin	17	na	na

[a] Values estimated from data presented in Ref. 1.
[b] Taken in part from Ref. 2.
na = Not available.

hulless cultivars. β-Glucan content was 18% higher. The variation between these two studies is a reflection of the cultivar variation, which included waxy and high–amylose starch, high-protein, and low–β-glucan cultivars. While Oscarsson et al. (4) reported that cellulose represented an average of 17.5% of the dietary fiber in a hulless cultivar, individual hulless cultivars ranged from 11.1 (waxy) to 24.8% (high protein) cellulose in the fiber. This suggests that characteristics of the pericarp and cell walls may influence cellulose content as much as hull presence.

Recent focus on the nutritional importance of dietary fiber has influenced the development of methods of analysis that give an accurate total dietary fiber content and distinguish between insoluble and soluble dietary fiber. Total dietary fiber (TDF) in barley is reported to vary from 11.2 to 34.0% and soluble dietary fiber (SDF) from 3.3 to 19.6% (Table 3). Fiber data from 12 studies was compiled to generate the means reported in Table 3. Aalto et al. (5) analyzed 118 malt/feed cultivars grown in Finland and found that 2-row cultivars had slightly less total dietary fiber than 6-row cultivars but slightly higher soluble dietary fiber. Separate studies investigating the influence of hull presence and starch type on dietary fiber conclude that normal starch, hulless genotypes have less total and soluble fiber content than hulled genotypes but a higher SDF/TDF ratio. Soluble dietary fiber is higher in waxy starch, hulled genotypes compared to

Table 2 Total Fiber Composition (%) of Hulled (covered) and Hulless Barley

| Component | Oscarsson et al. (4) | | Xue et al. (1) | |
	Hulled (10)[a]	Hulless (6)	Hulled (4)	Hulless (8)
Total fiber	20.6[b]	16.6	18.6	13.8
Arabinoxylan	7.9 (38.3[c])	5.7 (34.3)	6.5 (35.0)	4.5 (32.3)
A-X ratio[d]	0.44	0.72	na[e]	na
Cellulose	4.8 (23.3)	2.9 (17.5)	4.1 (22.1)	2.0 (14.5)
β-Glucan	4.8 (23.3)	5.7 (34.3)	5.2 (27.9)	5.6 (40.8)
Klason lignin	1.3 (6.3)	0.7 (4.2)	2.0 (10.8)	0.9 (6.5)
Uronic acid	0.8 (3.9)	0.7 (3.6)	na	na
Galactose	0.3 (1.5)	0.3 (1.8)	na	na
Mannose	0.4 (1.9)	0.4 (2.4)	na	na

[a] Number of cultivars.
[b] % of dry matter.
[c] % total fiber calculated from original data.
[d] Ratio of arabinose to xylose.
[e] na = Not available.

Table 3 Mean (range) Total and Soluble Dietary Fiber in Diverse Barley Genotypes

Genotype	N^a	Dietary fiber (% dry wt)		Soluble/ Total ratio	Ref.
		Total	Soluble		
2-row	68	19.9 (15.0–23.9)	4.9 (3.4–5.9)	0.25 (0.19–0.29)	5
6-row	50	20.9 (17.7–24.1)	4.3 (3.3–5.8)	0.21 (0.17–0.26)	5
Hulled	8	20.0 (19.0–22.4)	5.3 (3.8–6.7)	0.27 (0.20–0.32)	6–9
Hulless	19	13.0 (11.0–15.7)	4.5 (3.0–7.0)	0.35 (0.23–0.45)	7–12
Waxy starch, hulled	3	20.7 (20.0–21.0)	6.7 (6.4–7.2)	0.32 (0.31–0.34)	6,7
Waxy starch, hulless	20	15.8 (13.1–20.1)	7.0 (5.2–10.2)	0.44 (0.32–0.55)	7,9–16
Waxy starch, high protein, hulless	2	33.7 (33.4–34.0)	18.9 (18.1–19.6)	0.56 (0.54–0.58)	14,17
High-amylose starch hulless	2	17.6 (17.2–17.9)	7.2 (6.8–7.5)	0.40 (0.40–0.42)	9,15

^{a} Number of cultivars/samples used to calculate mean.

normal starch genotypes even though the total dietary fiber is similar. Genotypes that carry both the waxy starch and hulless traits have lower total dietary fiber but significantly higher soluble fiber. This generally results in a higher SDF/TDF ratio (0.32–0.53). A high-protein, waxy starch, hulless cultivar, Prowashonupana, is listed separately from the other waxy hulless cultivars because it has 2.5 times higher total and soluble fiber and a TDF/SDF ratio of 0.56. The high-protein genes in barley are generally associated with lower kernel weight (18), which may partially explain this significant increase in fiber. A high–amylose starch, hulless genotype is reported to contain levels of total dietary fiber and soluble dietary fiber similar to the waxy hulless genotypes.

β-Glucan and arabinoxylan are the primary components of soluble fiber in barley. High levels of β-glucan have been associated with poor malt quality, thus the emphasis in cultivar development has been for low β-glucan or high β-glucanase enzyme. But β-glucan is also associated with many of the beneficial health effects of barley (19,20), and this has promoted interest in high–β-glucan cultivars. Barley β-glucans are linear chains of β-glucosyl residues joined through both $(1{\rightarrow}3)$ and $(1{\rightarrow}4)$ linkages. MacGregor and Fincher (21) reviewed estimates of β-glucan content worldwide prior to 1993 and reported variation from 2.0 to 10.7% in malt and feed cultivars. More recently, the effect of specific genotypes on β-glucan content has been investigated and the range has increased to include genotypes with 17.5% β-glucan. The mean and range of β-glucan content of data from 28 studies is grouped by genotype in Table 4. Most of the studies reported utilizing an enzymatic procedure (42) to determine total β-glucan [hydrolysis with a purified $(1{\rightarrow}3),(1{\rightarrow}4)$-β-glucan endohydrolase] and the procedure of Aman and Graham (43) to determine soluble β-glucan content (water, 2 hr, 38°C).

Head type (2-vs. 6-row) probably does not have a major effect on β-glucan content. Research concluded that in cultivars grown in Finland (22) 2-row cultivars had higher β-glucan, in cultivars grown in Canada (23) 6-row cultivars had higher β-glucan, and in the United States (9) no difference was observed between 2- and 6-row cultivars. These different results are probably due to interactions with environment and background genotype of the cultivars grown in

Table 4 Mean (range) of β-Glucan Content in Diverse Barley Genotypes

Genotype	N(n)[a]	β-Glucan (% dry wt)		Soluble/ Total ratio	Ref.
		Total	Soluble		
2-row	101	4.2 (3.3–5.2)	na[b]	na	9,22,23
6-row	98	3.9 (3.0–5.6)	na	na	9,22,23
Hulled	44 (20)	4.4 (2.0–5.9)	2.6 (1.7–3.8)	0.56 (0.42–0.79)	4,7,8,9,15,17, 24–32
Hulless	55 (12)	5.1 (4.1–6.4)	3.0 (2.2–3.7)	0.61 (0.47–0.72)	4,7,8,9,12,25, 27,29–31, 33
Waxy starch, hulled	10 (5)	5.8 (4.7–7.3)	3.3 (2.7–4.2)	0.58 (0.50–0.69)	4,7,9,24
Waxy starch, hulless	35 (7)	7.0 (5.1–11.3)	4.0 (3.2–4.8)	0.67 (0.55–0.73)	4,9,12,15,24–26, 28,29,32–38
High protein, hulless	3 (2)	6.9 (5.9–8.0)	3.8 (3.5–4.1)	0.60 (0.51–0.69)	4,26,39
Waxy starch, high protein, hulless	4 (1)	16.6 (14.7–17.5)	6.6	0.40	14,17,28,39
High-amylose starch, hulless	5 (2)	7.2 (6.0–7.9)	2.5 (2.1–2.9)	0.36 (0.35–0.37)	4,9,15,40,41

[a] N = Number of cultivars/samples averaged to calculate mean total β-glucan; n = number of cultivars/samples averaged to calculate mean soluble β-glucan.
[b] na = Data not available.

each of these countries. When all of these observations are averaged, the mean and range (Table 4) of β-glucan content is similar for 2- and 6-row cultivars. Hulless genotypes consistently have a higher β-glucan content than hulled genotypes (1) because removal of the hull decreases cellulose and arabinoxylan more than β-glucan. Data averaged from 11 studies of hulled and hulless cultivars with normal starch confirm a 15% higher mean total and soluble β-glucan content as well as a higher ratio of soluble to total β-glucan in the hulless genotypes. However, the range of β-glucan content was similar in the hulled and hulless cultivars.

Changing the amylose:amylopectin ratio in barley starch or the protein content of the seed has a significant effect on β-glucan content. Hulled genotypes with waxy starch have 32% more β-glucan than normal starch, hulled genotypes and a similar soluble-to-total ratio (Table 4). Hulless genotypes with waxy or high–amylose starch or high protein have 35–41% more β-glucan than normal starch, hulless genotypes. When the waxy starch and high-protein genes are combined into one cultivar, β-glucan increases of 325% are reported. Separate but interacting mechanisms may explain these increases. Amylose production is blocked in the waxy starch genotypes, and it has been suggested that glucose normally shunted to the starch biosynthetic pathways is taken up by the β-glucan biosynthetic pathway. Xue et al. (1) observed that the waxy starch genotypes had lower starch content and higher levels of free sugars. The high-amylose (40) and high-protein (4) genotypes have lower starch content and lower kernel weights. Interaction of these traits may explain the exceptional increase in β-glucan content in the high-protein, waxy hulless genotypes.

Independent of these factors are two characteristics considered part of a cultivar's background genotype, i.e., cell wall volume and β-glucanase activity. It is generally agreed that cell walls vary in thickness, but few data have been collected to quantify this observation. However, breeding programs have developed mutants with thin cell walls (44,45), which have been crossed to waxy genotypes to produce low–β-glucan waxy cultivars. Swanston (45) reported that breeding lines having waxy starch contained 3.5–6.5% β-glucan after crossing to the thin cell wall mutant, Chalky Glenn. This suggests that there are distinct genes controlling cell wall thickness that may be manipulated to achieve lower β-glucan and potentially higher β-glucan.

Cell wall volume may also be increased by increasing cell numbers with decreased size. Swanston et al. (46) observed an extremely compressed endosperm in a breeding line that contains both the waxy and high-amylose genes. Cell wall modification during malt processing occurred at half the rate in this double starch mutant compared to the normal genotypes. The compactness of the endosperm may increase β-glucan content, although this was not measured.

Enzyme activity can also influence β-glucan content, especially during processing. Brennan et al. (47) used calcofluor to investigate cell wall modification after 136 hours of malting. The cell walls of the cultivar Hart showed little degradation at the end of this period, while the cell walls of Chariot were gone. This suggests lower levels of β-glucanase in Hart. β-Glucanase development prior to harvest (environmental factors leading to sprouting) and during storage and processing would decrease β-glucan and fiber content of a potentially high-fiber cultivar.

β-Glucan content is significantly affected by environment (9,29,48,49) as well as interactions between environment and genotype. Swanston et al. (48) compared total and soluble β-glucan content of two cultivars grown in Spain and Scotland. These cultivars had 1.2–1.5 times more total β-glucan and 2.3–5 times more soluble β-glucan when grown in the hot, drier Spanish climate. Fastnaught et al. (9) collected samples of the waxy hulless cultivar Wanubet from 42 commercial fields and reported β-glucan content varied from 4.6 to 9.5%. This helps to explain the variation reported in the literature.

The arabinoxylans found in barley fiber are (1 → 4)-β-xylan chains with arabinose residues attached through β-(1→2) or β-(1→3) linkages or both. Total arabinoxylan content is reported to vary from 1.2 to 11% of the whole grain (Table 5). Levels of this mostly insoluble polysaccharide are also influenced by genotype and environment (51,52). Studies of both Finnish (50) and Canadian (51) cultivars concluded that 6-row cultivars have higher levels of total and water-soluble arabinoxylan than 2-row cultivars. This is likely due to the smaller seed found in the 6-row cultivars and the proportionately higher levels of hull. Data averaged from seven studies (Table 5) indicate that hulled cultivars have 50% more total arabinoxylan than the hulless cultivars. However, the hulless cultivars have a slightly higher water-soluble arabinoxylan content

Table 5 Mean (range) of Arabinoxylan Content in Diverse Barley Genotypes

Genotype	N_1, N_2, N_3[a]	Arabinoxylan (% dry wt)		Arabinose/ Xylose ratio	Ref.
		Total	Soluble		
2-row	75, 18, —	7.9 (5.4–9.8)	0.52 (0.43–0.62)	na[b]	50,51
6-row	58, 20, —	9.3 (5.7–11.0)	0.63 (0.48–0.82)	na	50,51
Hulled	27, 25, 7	6.4 (4.4–8.3)	0.54 (0.40–0.69)	0.39 (0.29–0.48)	4,8,52–54
Hulless	22, 21, 3	4.3 (1.2–5.4)	0.60 (0.50–0.73)	0.41 (0.40–0.42)	4,8,51,54,55

[a] $N_{1,2,3}$ = Number of cultivars/samples averaged to calculate mean total and soluble arabinoxylan and A/X ratio, respectively.

[b] na = Data not available.

and similar ratio of arabinose to xylose. Oscarsson et al. (4) reported cultivars having waxy starch had similar arabinoxylan content as normal starch cultivars. Cultivars having high-amylose starch or high protein had higher levels of arabinoxylan than similar hulled or hulless cultivars.

Type 3 resistant starch, formed from retrograded amylose following heat treatment, resembles dietary fiber in that it passes through the small intestine undigested and is analyzed as dietary fiber using standard procedures of analysis. Szczodrak and Pomeranz (56) found no native resistant starch present in isolated starch from High Amylose Glacier (40% amylose). But recently, using a slightly different isolation and methods of analysis, Vasanthan and Bhatty (165) found 3% resistant starch in the isolated native starch of this same cultivar.

III. PHYSICOCHEMICAL PROPERTIES

The physical and chemical properties of barley fiber are a function of the component polysaccharides, particularly β-glucan and arabinoxylan. Two of these properties, solubility in water and high viscosity in solution, are influenced by the chemical structure. The molecular weight (M_w of β-glucan from whole barley or extracts from whole barley has been reported to range from 0.19 to 3.30 $\times$ 10^6 (Table 6). Knuckles et al. (28) suggested that lower molecular weights may be an artifact of β-glucanase activity or mechanical damage during extraction. β-glucanase activities of 83 U/kg observed in untreated ground flours from sound grain were reduced only 20% by refluxing in 70% hot ethanol for 4 hours. Extraction without degradation was reported using 1 N NaOH + 1% $NaBH_4$ at 65°C for 1 hour and M_w of total β-glucan from two waxy hulless cultivars ranged from 2.9 to 3.3 $\times$ 10^6 (Table 6). Water-extractable β-glucan (23°C) from the same cultivars had M_w 50–75% lower. Beer et al. (58) reported lower M_w β-glucan in water extracts from waxy starch Compana isotypes compared to normal starch isotypes after hot ethanol refluxing for 2 hours. However, a higher concentration of β-glucan was extracted from the waxy starch isotypes. Total extraction of β-glucan from these genotypes with 5% NaOH + 0.5% $NaBH_4$ for 16 hours decreased peak molecular weight, suggesting degradation of the β-glucan molecule under severe extraction procedures.

Digestion studies of β-glucan using lichenase, a (1→3),(1→4)-β-D-glucan-4-glucanohydrolase (E.C.3.2.1.73), have concluded that the (1→3) linkages occur singly and most of the (1→4) linkages occur in groups of two or three (62). Lichenase cleaves the (1→4) linkage of the 3-O-substituted units in β-glucan (Fig. 1). HPLC can separate and quantify the released oligosaccharides, primarily β-(1→3)-linked cellotriosyl and cellotetraosyl units. Edney et al. (63) reported that perchloric acid–extracted β-glucan, representing total β-glucan, contained 88% cellotriosyl and cellotetraosyl residues after lichenase digestion in a 1.8-to-2.4 ratio depending on the cultivar. Alkaline extracted β-glucan from the cultivar Wanubet was reported to have a tri/tetra ratio of 3.2 (60), which was similar to the average ratio (3.0) reported for 16 cultivars by Wood et al. (62). The remaining residues vary from DP 5 to 20 (64). Izawa et al. (65) suggest that longer blocks of contiguous cellotriosyl residues separated by single β-(1→3) linkages were responsible for the insolubility rather than longer blocks of adjacent β-(1→4) linkages. This is consistent with the observation that oat β-glucan has a lower tri/tetra ratio and is more soluble in water at 37°C than barley β-glucan.

Sequential extracts of water-and alkali-extractable nonstarch polysaccharides (NSP) followed by ammonium sulfate fractionation provide evidence of the heterogeneous structure of β-glucan and arabinoxylan along with their influence on solubility and viscosity. Izydorczyk et al. (66) extracted 1.3 and 1.4% of the dry weight from Harrington barley in water at 40 and

Table 6 Summary of Barley β-Glucan Molecular Weight Studies

Barley sample	Average M_W (g/mol)	Method (extraction)	Ref.
Azhul	3.30×10^6	HPSEC, MALLS[a]	28
Waxbar	2.92×10^6	(1N NaOH-1% NaBH$_4$, 1 hr, 65°C)	
Azhul	0.72×10^6	HPSEC, MALLS	28
Waxbar	1.57×10^6	(Water, 1 hr, 23°C)	
Crystal	1.54×10^6		
Prowashonupana	2.34×10^6		
Compana-normal	1.67×10^6	HPSEC, RALLS	58
Compana-waxy	1.39×10^6	(Water/Termamyl, 2 hr, 90°C)	
Sigma Standard	0.25×10^5	HPSEC, MALLS	59
Megazyme Standard	0.23×10^5	(Water, α-amylase, 2 hr, 65°C)	
Spanish cultivar	0.57×10^5		
Azhul bran	2.00×10^6	Gel filtration (Water, sequential 40, 65 and 95°C combined)	35
Wanubet	2.66×10^6	Gel filtration (NaCarbonate, pH 10, 30 min, 45°C)	60
Four cultivars	$1.70–2.66 \times 10^6$	HPSEC, LALLS	61
Four malts	$0.97–1.48 \times 10^6$	(NaCarbonate, pH 10, 2 hr, 60°C)	
Biocon standard	0.19×10^5		

[a] HPSEC = High-pressure size exclusion chromatography; MALLS = multiple-angle laser light-scattering; LALLS = low-angle laser light-scattering.

65°C, respectively. The NSP of the 65°C extract had higher molecular weight, viscosity, glucose content, and ratio of tri-/tetrasaccharide oligomers. Subfractions of both extracts precipitated at increasing saturation levels of ammonium sulfate contained more arabinoxylan and less β-glucan. Subsequent alkali extracts (5.9% of dry weight) had higher intrinsixc viscosity and levels of arabinoxylans as well as higher xylose/arabinose ratios than the water extracts. β-Glucans extracted in these fractions had high ratios of the tri-/tetra units and large amounts of contiguously linked β-(1→4) linkages (66). Saulnier et al. (67) reported that NSP in a 40°C water extract from barley with waxy starch had higher molecular weight and intrinsic viscosity but lower tri/tetra ratio than a normal starch cultivar.

Viscosity of wholemeal or flour extracts from barley has been used as an indicator of β-glucan content. But, as discussed previously, molecular structure may impact viscosity. While many research studies have reported viscosity, the variation in solvent pH, temperature, concentration, and instruments make comparisons between studies difficult. Acid and alkaline extract viscosity avoid the confounding factor of β-glucanase activity, which reduces viscosity very quickly in a water extract. This can be partially overcome by refluxing with hot ethanol for

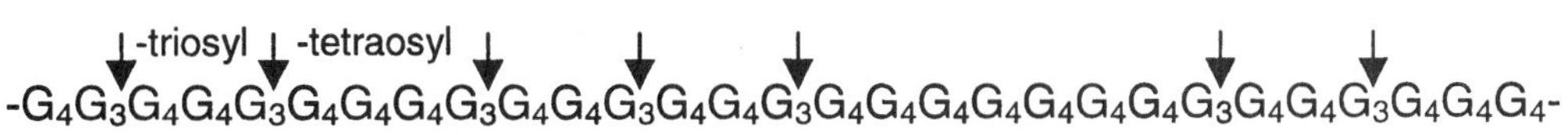

Fig. 1 Schematic representation of barley β-glucan structure. G$_3$ and G$_4$ represent positions at which the glucose residue is linked. Arrows show the β-(1→4) linkage cleaved by lichenase.

extended periods. Extraction temperature generally is kept below 55°C (25–50°C) to avoid the interference of starch gelatinization. Most studies use 4 or 10% w/v, but concentrations as high as 27% can be found (12). Two classes of instruments are generally used to measure viscosity: falling ball viscometers and rotating cone/cylinder viscometers. When using the latter, rotation speed can be varied, which allows observations on the effect of shear rate. Measurement of viscosity has been used extensively in breeding programs to identify potential low–β-glucan cultivars for malting and high–β-glucan cultivars as a functional food ingredient. Genotypic differences in extract viscosity correspond to the differences in β-glucan content. Thus, hulless cultivars with waxy or high-amylose starch generally have higher extract viscosities (regardless of method) than covered normal starch cultivars (1,9,24,25). One exception is the cultivar Wafranubet, which has extract viscosities of only half those of other waxy cultivars with the same β-glucan content (9).

The rheological properties of isolated β-glucan have been compared to other food gums and found to be most similar to methylcellulose. Schwarz and Lee (60) produced a 90% pure β-glucan isolate, which had stable viscosity and exhibited pseudoplastic flow properties. Both viscosity and pseudoplasticity decreased with increasing temperature, suggesting that barley β-glucan could be used in applications requiring fluidity at high temperatures followed by thickening upon cooling. Addition of sodium chloride or adjustment of pH had little effect upon viscosity, while addition of sugar decreased viscosity. Blends of the isolated β-glucan and methylcellulose had a synergistic increase in viscosity. β-Glucan (0.45%) doubled the pasting viscosity of an 8% wheat starch suspension (69) and had higher viscosity than 0.45% carboxymethylcellulose. Temelli (70) tested the whippabilty, foam stability, and emulsion-stabilizing capacity of 57–89% barley β-glucan isolates. Dispersions of 2.5% β-glucan achieved whipping volumes of 60–185% and were 40–85% stable after 2 hours. Emulsions formed using 0.05% β-glucan in water mixed with oil were 45–63% stable following centrifugation. Girhammar and Nair (57) reported water-binding capacity of an extracted barley nonstarch polysaccharide to be 0.49 g/g and emulsifying capacity to be 600 mL oil in water/g polysaccharide. Gamma irradiation (10 Mrad) increased the solubility of β-glucan but significantly altered the rheological characteristics by reducing molecular weight and viscosity (71).

IV. PRODUCTION

Barley fiber can be a byproduct of other processing (malting, brewing, ethanol production) or one of the primary products from dry or wet milling. The byproducts of malting and fermentation processes have been called brewers spent grains (BSG) or spent barley grain (SBG) or dried distillers grains (DDG). They consist of the hull and other water-insoluble components remaining after the grain is malted, macerated, and washed to remove soluble components. These products are a rich source of insoluble (98%) dietary fiber containing 48–59% TDF (72–75). Weber and Chaudhary (72) describe two products, barley bran flour and barley high-protein flour, derived from the BSG by milling and sieving to concentrate fiber and protein, respectively (Table 7). Kanauchi and Agata (76) describe a similar fiber product called germinated barley foodstuff (GBF) prepared from BSG by a combination of pressing with a roller-mill and sieving. GBF is similar to the high-protein flour in total fiber content but has less cellulose and significantly higher protein and glutamine content.

Milling procedures to concentrate barley β-glucan and/or fiber fit into three categories: (a) conventional roller-milling with associated sieving, (b) impact or abrasive milling (pin mill, hammermill, etc.) followed by air classification or sieving, and (c) pearling. Regardless of the type of milling, hulled cultivars are generally dehulled to eliminate the husk. Products derived

Table 7 Nutrient Composition of Brewer's Spent Grains and Derived Fiber Products

Component (% dry wt)	Brewer's spent grain[a]	Barley bran flour[a]	Barley high-protein flour[a]	Brewer's spent grain[b]	Germinated barley foodstuff[b]
Total fiber	53.3	70.0	35.5	59.0	34.0
Insoluble	na	67.0	33.9	na	na
Soluble	na	3.0	1.6	na	na
Cellulose	16.5	23.3	15.0	25.4	8.9
Hemicellulose	33.5	42.9	21.5	21.8	17.0
Lignin	4.1	5.3	3.8	11.9	8.2
Protein	24.5	18.5	35.5	24.0	46.0
Lipid	na	6.8	8.7	10.6	10.2
Ash	na	4.6	4.6	2.4	2.0

[a] From Ref. 72.
[b] From Ref. 76.

from conventional milling are classified as flour, shorts, or bran depending on particle size. Often the bran and shorts are combined because the brittleness of barley bran precludes a clean separation from the shorts (12). Thus, barley bran will contain pericarp, testa, aleurone, and subaleurone and the fiber content will increase as flour yield increases. Flour yields of 26.3–83.1% have been reported for barley (33,36,54,77–79). Bhatty (33) milled a hulless and a waxy hulless barley at six different moisture levels and concluded that the highest flour yield for both cultivars (83.1 and 66.4, respectively) was obtained by milling grain at 5% moisture. Compared to raw grain, β-glucan concentrations were 15 and 29% higher in the bran and 4 and 16% lower in the flour, respectively. Levels of β-glucan and fiber reported in flour and bran are summarized in Table 8. The variability reflects the many types of mills (brands and pilot vs. commercial scale), cultivars, growing environments, and omission of the dehulling step for hulled cultivars. In general, milling hulled cultivars without dehulling produced bran with high total fiber content (up to 58%) but low β-glucan content. Impact and abrasive milling have been used to grind dehulled or hulless barley into whole grain meal with varying particle size. Sieving the meal effectively concentrates fiber and β-glucan in the coarse fractions. The effectiveness of these procedures vary with type of mill and cultivar. Knuckles et al. (26) examined particle size

Table 8 β-Glucan and Fiber Content of Roller-Milled Products from Barley

Fiber	Grain	Flour	Shorts	Bran
Total fiber %[a]	12.6–22.1	3.8–8.5	18.2–30.4	16.3–58.7
Change (%)[b]	—	−59.8 to −65.1	+21.0 to +67.7	+29.4 to +165.0
No. samples	6	8	6	4
Soluble fiber%	5.5–6.5	1.6–3.8	8.8–9.5	6.6
Change (%)	—	−69.1	+35.4 to +72.7	+20.0
No. samples	2	5	2	1
β-Glucan %	3.6–11.3	1.9–6.1	5.0–10.0	1.5–15.4
Change (%)	—	−4.3 to −69.6	+21.7 to +73.9	−56.0 to +46.7
No. samples	15	30	9	14

[a] % dry matter.
[b] % difference from whole grain.
Source: Refs. 33,35,36,54,77–83.

distribution of barley meal produced on five mills and selected an abrasive Udy mill with a 0.25 mm screen for experimental sized samples. Fifty to seventy percent of the particles produced on this mill passed through a 325-mesh screen (45-μm openings) chosen because it would allow starch granules to pass through. The β-glucan content of this material ranged from 1.2 to 2% (71.4–82.4% lower than the raw grain), varying with cultivar. The β-glucan content of the material remaining on top of the screen ranged from 11.4 to 19.5% (67.6–181.1% increase). Regrinding of the meal remaining on top of the screen resulted in 4 to 19% more of the meal passing through the 325-mesh screen. The final coarse fraction (18.7–30.1% yield) contained 16.0–19.9% β-glucan representing a 135.3–245.1% increase. This was further separated into fractions containing up to 22.5% β-glucan, but only in small quantities. These results varied only slightly among the four cultivars examined (Table 9). Pilot scale testing of this process produced similar results (84) and was utilized to produce glucan-enriched barley (GEB) containing 43–46% total fiber and 18–23% β-glucan (86,87).

A single grind with a hammermill followed by sieving with a 140-mesh screen (103 μm) produced coarse fractions in three cultivars containing 38–88% more β-glucan, 25–77% more total fiber, and 45–106% more soluble fiber (88,85). The material passing through the sieve contained 67–75% less β-glucan, similar to material sieved with a 325-mesh screen (26). Dudgeon-Bollinger et al. (37) ground pearled barley with a commercial hammermill and sieved with a 100-mesh screen (150 μm) to produce coarse fractions containing 47% higher β-glucan and 57% higher soluble fiber. However, the material passing through the screen still contained 4.8% β-glucan.

Air classification has also been used to concentrate fiber and β-glucan (89,84). Wu et al. (39) described repeated pinmilling of barley to produce a high proportion (74–86%) of particles smaller than 30 μm. The coarse fractions (>30 μm) separated with air classification had 59.7–153.4% higher β-glucan content than the raw barley. However, this differed between cultivars. β-Glucan enrichment (45.5–93.4% increase) was observed in fractions with particle sizes from

Table 9 Fiber and β-Glucan Content of Enriched Fractions Produced by Impact or Abrasion Milling

Cultivar	Type[a]	Yield	Total fiber %	Total fiber % increase	β-Glucan %	β-Glucan % increase	Particle size (Ref.)
Steptoe	1	20.7	nd	nd	17.6	232.1	>45 μm
Klages	1	18.7	nd	nd	17.6	245.1	(26)
CI 4362	3	30.1	nd	nd	16.0	135.3	
Wanubet	2	25.0	nd	nd	19.9	176.4	
Steptoe	1	24.5	45.1	162.4	18.3	319.7	>45 μm
Crystal	1	19.9	43.1	214.1	17.6	357.8	(84)
Waxbar	2	25.1	36.9	165.5	15.8	262.1	
Apollo	2	59.4	28.6	31.8	11.3	44.9	>103 μm
Wanubet	2	67.8	22.7	22.7	9.5	36.5	(85)
Robust	1	67.0	19.9	25.9	7.0	28.9	
Merlin	2	42.1	17.3	24.5	9.0	40.6	>150 μm (37)
Portage	1	13.2	nd	nd	14.7	153.4	>30 μm
CI 4362	3	27.3	nd	nd	14.6	82.5	(39)
Prowashonupana	4	31.0	nd	nd	31.3	59.7	

[a] 1 = Normal starch, hulled; 2 = waxy starch, hulless; 3 = normal starch, high protein, hulless; 4 = waxy starch, high protein, hulless.
nd = Not determined.

18–30 μm in the cultivar Prowashonupana. This cultivar has very low starch content, 25%, which may explain fiber enrichment occurring in fractions with such small particle size.

Pearling barley grain removes the outer layers, which contain much of the cellulose and arabinoxylan found in barley. Using photomicrographs, Bhatty (33) showed that pearling 30% of the hulless cultivar Condor removed the pericarp, testa, aleurone, and subaleurone, producing true bran. Barley bran produced by pearling has higher ash and phosphorus content and lower starch and β-glucan content (90) than bran produced by roller-milling. Pearling 20% of the waxy hulless cultivar Merlin (37) and the hulless cultivar Condor (33) produced bran having similar composition except β-glucan content (Table 10). β-Glucan content of the Merlin bran was lower than the raw grain (2.8% vs. 6.1%), whereas the Condor bran had higher β-glucan content (6.6% vs. 4.6%). A higher concentration of β-glucan in the starchy endosperm of Merlin may explain this difference. Bhatty (12) observed considerable variation in 45% pearled products from nine hulless and three waxy hulless barley cultivars. Total fiber ranged from 35 to 50% lower in the pearled products compared to the raw grain. Changes in β-glucan and soluble fiber varied, depending on the cultivar. β-Glucan ranged from a 6.3% decrease to a 11.1% increase and soluble fiber ranged from a 34% decrease to a 31.6% increase. The variation among these hulless barley cultivars did not appear to be related to type of starch. Additional studies reported that 40% of pearled products of covered and hulless cultivars had from 5 to 26% increase in β-glucan content (91,92).

Various combinations of solvents, pH, temperature, and enzymes have been utilized in the production of barley β-glucan isolates (93). Initially, procedures to purify β-glucan developed from the research on molecular weight and solubility. Hot water (up to 100°C) with or without enzyme digestion is reported to solubilize up to 86% of the β-glucan in barley producing concentrates having 33.1–89.1% β-glucan (35,67,70,86,94,95). Temelli (70) reported that soluble β-glucan yield and viscosity increased as temperature increased up to 55°C. Extractions at four temperature (40–55°C) and pH (7–10, using sodium carbonate) combinations gave the highest yields at pH 7 and 8 but the highest viscosity at pH 9, indicating the need to balance extraction yield with functionality. Bhatty (35) also observed the highest viscosity when β-glucan was extracted with sodium carbonate but the highest solubility and recovery using 4% NaOH (54% vs. 81%, respectively). Solubility increased to 98% using 1 N NaOH (80), but recovery decreased to 77% lowering overall yield. Knuckles et al. (28) reported 100% β-glucan solubility in 1 N NaOH + NaBH₄ (1%) at 65°C. The extracted β-glucan, which represented the total β-glucan, had a higher molecular weight than β-glucans extracted in water. Burkus and Temelli (96) reported that viscosity stability is improved by refluxing with 70% ethanol prior to purification of β-glucan.

Table 10 Composition (% dry weight) of Raw Grain and Products Derived from 20% Pearling

Cultivar	Product	Fiber			Starch	Lipid	Protein
		Total	Soluble	β-Glucan			
Merlin[a]	Grain	16.0	6.2	6.1	55.9	3.8	14.9
	Bran	31.7	4.4	2.8	11.2	12.8	23.9
	Pearled	13.9	6.6	6.4	63.9	1.8	12.7
Condor[b]	Grain	12.9	4.2	4.6	67.8	—	15.8
	Bran	26.1	3.4	6.6	13.0	—	28.6
	Pearled	9.6	4.4	4.1	81.5	—	12.6

[a] Waxy hulless (37).
[b] Hulless (33).

Extracted β-glucans are typically precipitated with alcohol. However, Morgan and Ofman (97) developed a new method of β-glucan isolation using hot water extraction followed by freeze-thawing of the extract to precipitate the β-glucans. The presence of endogenous enzyme resulted in lower molecular weight β-glucan unless extraction time was kept to a minimum. Inglett (98) developed a process of extracting β-glucan soluble fiber from oat and barley along with gelatinized, soluble starch resulting in a dietary fiber-maltodextrin product containing 7–8% dietary fiber. Patents have been granted for barley β-glucan extraction methods utilizing water alone or combined with an enzyme digestion (98–100), NaOH and enzyme digestion (101), and acid (102).

Resistant starch (RS) can be enhanced in some types of barley through heat and chemical processing. Formation of resistant starch increases with increasing amylose content in barley starch (6,15). Sundberg and Falk (103) found that bread and porridge made from barley having normal starch had higher RS (0.8 and 1.1%) than the same products made from barley with waxy starch (0.2%). Szczodrak and Pomeranz (56) increased RS in isolated starch of High Amylose Glacier from 0 to 26% by repeated cycles of autoclaving and found that lipids and emulsifiers interfered with the formation of RS in barley (104). Vasanthan and Bhatty (165) found that starch gels made with high-amylose barley starch had 7% RS. After three heating and cooling cycles, the RS was increased to 13%. Further processing of the dried retrograded starch gels with pullanase or acid increased RS to 20% and 21.5%, respectively.

V. PHYSIOLOGICAL EFFECTS

The combination of soluble and insoluble fiber in barley creates complex interactions in the direct effect on the digestive and immune systems and the indirect effect of reducing risk for coronary heart disease, diabetes, and cancer.

A. Digestion

The effect of barley insoluble fiber in the digestive system has been clearly documented in both animal and human studies. Ingestion of BSG (brewer's spent grains, 97% insoluble fiber) or derived products is associated with increased fecal weight (76,105–108), accelerated transit time (105), increased cholesterol and fat excretion (109), and a decrease in gallstones (73,108). Rats fed GBF (a high–insoluble fiber, glutamine-rich protein derived from BSG) had higher fecal weights and jejunum mucosal protein than rats fed only fiber or protein isolated from GBF (76,110). The isolated protein had no effect on fecal weight. GBF also prevented diarrhea in rats fed diarrhea-inducing soluble fiber (111).

Barley soluble fiber is also associated with increased fat and cholesterol excretion from the digestive system. Lia et al. (112) reported 55% higher cholesterol excretion in ileostomists consuming 13 g/d β-glucan from barley flour. Increased fecal fat excretion ranging from 70% to 200% has been reported in hamsters (16), chicks (113), and rats (114) consuming significant quantities of β-glucan–containing barley products. Bowles et al. (115), using ^{13}C NMR spectroscopy, found no evidence of specific binding between β-glucan and the bile acid salt glycocholic acid.

Collection of ileal effluents in animals and humans has been a valuable tool in studying the digestion and fermentation of barley fiber. Fardet et al. (116) collected ileal effluents from swine fed barley bran that contained 3.4% β-glucan and 29.3% total fiber. β-Glucan represented 11.6% of the total cell wall sugars in the raw grain but only 2% in the ileal insoluble residue and effluent. During in vitro fermentation of these residues using human fecal bacteria, 42% of the cell wall sugars disappeared including 50% of the arabinose and xylose and 30% of the glucose. These levels of in vitro fermentation are similar to the in vivo fermentation of insoluble barley fiber reported in humans (117) and swine (118). Ileal digestibility of barley NSP varied from 23 to 37% when three hulless cultivars were fed to swine (30). The digested NSP represented 7–12% of the xylose, 2–18% of the arabinose, and 44–60% of the glucose. The higher ileal digestibility of glucose in these cultivars may reflect the higher levels of β-glucan (4.5–5.9%) present. Robertson et al. (119) reported increased solubility and decreased molecular weight of β-glucan collected from ileal effluents indicating substantial degradation prior to reaching the colon. Bach Knudsen et al. (120) reported 60–65% apparent digestibility of NSP from an insoluble barley fiber in humans. Partial digestible energy values (107,121) for this fiber range from 0.4 to 0.8 kcal/g NSP (1.6–8 kJ/g NSP).

B. Cardiovascular Disease

The hypocholesterolemic effect of barley fiber and fiber products has been documented in chick, rat, hamster, and human clinical trials during the past 10 years (Table 11). Cholesterol reduction has been observed in studies involving both insoluble and soluble (β-glucan) fiber, indicating more than one mechanism of cholesterol lowering.

Brewer's spent grains containing insoluble fiber, lipid, and protein reduced cholesterol 30% in hamsters when added at the 15% level but not at the 5 or 10% level (73,128). α-Tocotrienol, a component of the lipids in BSG, was shown to inhibit HMG-CoA reductase activity in the liver and reduce in vivo cholesterol synthesis (123). This mechanism may explain

Table 11 Change in Total Serum Cholesterol of Test Subjects Ingesting Barley Products

Product	Decrease (%) in total cholesterol			
	Chicks	Rats	Hamsters	Humans
Brewer's spent grains				
Average	31	13	15	9.1
Range	23 to 39	—	nc to 30	8.2 to 10
N[a] (Ref.)	2 (20)	1 (124)	2 (73, 128)	2 (109, 129)
Isolated β-glucan (wet extraction)				
Average	—	27.4	—	—
Range	—	16 to 52	—	—
N (Ref.)	—	5 (20, 85, 94, 114, 125)	—	—
Flours and brans				
Average	30.1	21.7	16.8	5.4
Range	13 to 47	10 to 31	12 to 24	3 to 9.9
N (Ref.)	9 (13, 19, 20, 41, 83, 113, 122, 123, 128)	7 (10, 14, 20, 124, 126, 127)	3 (16, 86, 87)	5 (19, 130, 131, 156)
Barley oil				
Average	29.5	—	nc	7
Range	25 to 34	—	—	—
N (Ref.)	2 (20, 123)	—	1 (16)	1 (129)

nc = No change.

[a] N = Number of studies; Refs. 19 and 20 are review articles.

the observation that barley oil isolated from BSG decreased cholesterol in humans almost as effectively as the intact BSG (129) In addition, Oda et al. (125) extracted and separated soluble and insoluble fiber from defatted ground barley and found that the insoluble fiber had no effect on total serum cholesterol when fed to rats. But more recently, barley oil extracted from barley flour did not decrease cholesterol in hamsters (16), even though it contained significant levels of tocotrienols and tocopherols. Thus, while BSG and the oil extracted from it appear to lower cholesterol, the mechanism is not clear because of the contrasting results when the oil and fiber are extracted from flour.

Definitive studies have confirmed the role of β-glucan soluble fiber as one of the cholesterol-reducing components in barley. β-Glucan isolated from barley using wet extraction methods reduced total cholesterol in rats from 16 to 52% (Table 11). The levels of isolated β-glucan fed rats (2–7.8%) were not strongly correlated to the percent decrease in cholesterol, suggesting that the isolation processes may have altered the cholesterol-reducing characteristics of the β-glucan. Treatment of barley flour with β-glucanase reduces or eliminates the cholesterol-lowering effects in hamsters (16) and chicks (83,113,122). Wang et al. (113) observed no reduction in cholesterol and lower intestinal viscosity in chicks fed β-glucanase–treated barley. This supports the hypothesis that viscosity produced by the β-glucan reduces absorption of lipids and cholesterol and reabsorption of bile acids. Peterson and Qureshi (122) reported that hexane extracted barley flour reduced HMG CoA reductase activity and increased cholesterol hydroxylase in chicks as much as unextracted barley and similarly to a tocotrienol-rich fraction of palm oil. The effect of the soluble fiber on these enzymes is most likely a feedback mechanism related to the increased fat, cholesterol, and bile acid excretion brought on by the increased viscosity.

The extrusion process appears to increase the cholesterol-reducing characteristics of barley, possibly by increasing the solubility of the β-glucan. Wang and Klopfenstein (126) reported that raw barley significantly reduced cholesterol in rats by 13% but the same barley extruded reduced cholesterol 38%. Sundberg et al. (83) observed a similar reduction (13%) in chicks fed an unprocessed mill concentrate. After drum drying this barley decreased cholesterol in chicks 27%, and following extrusion the decrease was 38%.

C. Glucose and Insulin Response

Barley has a low glycemic index (GI), with published estimates of 31–48 for pearl barley (132,133). A low GI indicates slower digestion and absorption of food carbohydrates, resulting in a lowering of blood glucose and insulin response. However, GI is a function of structure, starch type, fiber content, and the interaction of these characteristics (15). Foods containing viscous β-glucan soluble fiber from oats and barley can reduce glucose and insulin response in the blood stream by 50% compared to white bread (134).

Livesey et al. (135) found that ileostomists eating finely ground barley had 2% undigested starch compared to 17% when they consumed barley flakes. Light microscopy of the ileal effluent showed starch granules surrounded by intact cell walls. Liljeberg and Bjorck (136) reported breads made with ground wholemeal barley were similar to white bread (GI = 100) while breads containing 80% intact barley kernels were significantly lower (GI = 33). Granfeldt et al. (15) reported GI was lowered to 66 when ground wholemeal barley flour was boiled and eaten as a porridge and suggested that boiling released the soluble fiber more effectively than baking. More recently, Liljeberg et al. (17) reported a lower GI (71–77) for both porridge and bread made from a barley flour containing 18% β-glucan. Pasta containing 7.7% β-glucan from a β-glucan–enriched barley flour produced 63% lower peak glucose and 53% lower insulin response in subjects compared to the control durum pasta (137). A longer-term study involving 11 non–insulin-dependent diabetics (38) eating barley bread products that provided 5.2 g/d β-glucan reported lower glycemic response but, in contrast to studies with healthy test subjects, a higher insulin response. This resulted in four subjects reducing their dosage of hypoglycemics. A 6-month community-based study of non–insulin-dependent diabetes subjects (138) reported lower glycosylated hemoglobin and diastolic blood pressure after consuming barley breads providing 5g/d β-glucan.

D. Cancer

The role of barley fiber in reducing risk of colon cancer has not been studied extensively. McIntosh et al. (74,124) compared barley bran diets that varied in insoluble and soluble fiber content to a wheat bran diet in tumor-induced rats. Some of the barley brans were comparable to wheat bran in decreasing tumor incidence and tumor mass index. One of the most effective barley brans, BB1, was prepared in a manner similar to oat bran and contained 13% total fiber, which was 40% soluble (74). In an earlier study (124), SBG (same as BSG, brewer's spent grains) containing mostly insoluble fiber was comparable to wheat bran. Thus, the mechanism of cancer prevention is not clear. Zhang et al. (73) reported that ingestion of BSG reduced the secondary-to-primary bile acid ratio in hamsters, and preferential adsorption of lithocholic acid by barley fiber has been demonstrated (139). Excessive concentrations of secondary bile acids have been suggested as one cancer-promoting mechanism (75).

E. Immune Response

The cell walls of many bacteria and fungi contain hemicelluloses similar to the β-glucans found in barley and oats but comprised of β-(1→3)-linked glucosyl residues with small numbers of β-(1→6) linkages rather than the β-(1→4) linkages. These glucans have the ability to enhance the immune system (140), resulting in antitumor, antibacterial, antiviral, anticoagulatory, and wound-healing activities. A leukocyte membrane receptor, CR3, has been identified as the binding site (141) that recognizes β-glucans, including barley β-glucan (142,143). While no in vivo studies have utilized barley β-glucan, Yun et al. (144) restored immune function in immunosuppressed mice with both intragastric and subcutaneous treatments of oat β-glucan. They suggested that follicle-associated cells (M cells) in the intestinal epithelium, which specialize in the transport of macrophage from the intestinal lumen to the lymph system, may be involved in the actual uptake of β-glucan molecules. Disappearance of barley β-glucan in the intestine has been reported in balance studies with no explanations provided. Future research in this area may clarify the role of barley fiber in human nutrition and disease.

VI. SAFETY

The mineral-binding capacity of fibers can result in loss of mineral nutrients via excretion. Persson et al. (95) isolated soluble fiber from barley that contained 5.5% phytic acid and examined the in vitro binding capacity of the fiber to copper, cadmium, and zinc with and without phytase. Phytase treatment reduced binding only slightly. A barley fiber that contained 25% acid detergent fiber and 4.4% lignin was reported to contain 2000 µg/g of magnesium, 52 µg/g of zinc, and 2.9 µg/g of copper (145). This barley fiber had a high total binding capacity for copper and zinc at pH 6.8 and a low capacity for magnesium when compared to 15 fibers from other botanical sources. The variation in total binding capacity of these three minerals among the various fibers reflects the confusion that surrounds the relationship between fiber and minerals. Fibers can contain a diverse array of compounds, which must be quantified in order to understand this relationship. Wisker et al. (106) examined the calcium, magnesium, and zinc balances and iron absorption in young women eating a diet containing 15 g/day of barley fiber which was 97% insoluble and low in phytic acid (0.06%). This fiber was derived from the outer layers of the grain and contained no husk. The fiber had no effect on the mineral balances or absorption of iron except when protein intake was decreased. Kalra and Jood (31) reported that barley hull fiber decreased total digestibility and biological value of protein, whereas β-glucan had little effect on protein quality parameters in rats.

VII. FOOD APPLICATIONS

The wide range of fiber products available from barley suggests that food applications would be diverse. At the present time, many more research studies are available on food applications than there are marketed foods containing barley or barley fiber. Similar to other cereal grains, barley can be minimally processed into flakes and grits to be utilized as a hot breakfast cereal or a baking ingredient (146–148). In fact, a commercial barley meal similar to oatmeal has the highest β-glucan content, 5.08%, of all the commercial cereals sold in Finland (149). Flaked barley cereals made from waxy hulless barley sold in the United States contain 7% β-glucan providing 2 g per 1 oz. serving. Minimal processing also produces the pearled barley most often found in soups and can provide 1–2 g of β-glucan per 1 oz. serving depending on the type of barley pearled. In Japan, barley is pearled and split to look similar to rice and can be used to supplement fiber content without changing traditional recipes (12,131).

Extrusion processing of barley for foods has significant benefits over other processing. High temperature and high pressure increases the solubility of β-glucan and can increase resistant starch producing an increase in both soluble and insoluble fiber of the products (11,150). Ostergard et al. (151) extruded whole grain hammermilled barley with a twin screw extruder and reported significantly higher soluble dietary fiber in all of the extruded products and higher insoluble dietary fiber in products extruded at a temperature greater than 120°C and feed moisture greater than 18%. Marlett (34) made a ready-to-eat cereal from a waxy hulless and a waxy covered (dehulled prior to processing) barley variety using a process similar to that used for oven-puffed crisp rice. Processing increased the solubility of the fiber and β-glucan by 23%. Lee and Schwarz (150) examined the physical properties and dietary fiber content of extruded barley and barley/corn blends. Using barley with 12.6% dietary fiber they found that increasing feed moisture and temperature produced products with higher bulk density and breaking strength. The bulk density of 100% barley was 2.5 times greater than corn extrudates. Extrudates containing 50% barley had a similar bulk density to 100% corn but slightly less expansion, higher breaking strength, higher water-holding capacity (8%) and higher oil-absorption capacity (25%). These products had 2.3% soluble and 5.8% total dietary fiber compared to only 0.4% and 2.6%, respectively, in the corn products. Berglund et al. (11) compared extrusion of four barley cultivars, rice, and barley/rice blends in the production of a crisp rice cereal. Cereals made with 100% barley had 165–238% higher bulk density as the rice cereal. But 50% barley cereals were only 30% higher. Cereals containing 2.7% soluble and 8% total dietary fiber were scored similar in hedonic sensory testing to the rice cereal with 1.3% total dietary fiber. Extrusion (37) of barley flours containing variable levels of lipid (1.3–3.8%) and fiber (10–17.3%) into snack products indicated that expansion ratio was negatively correlated to fiber content. However, the product having the best expansion and rated highest by a trained sensory panel still had 5% soluble and 10% total dietary fiber.

Noodles containing small amounts of barley are reported to have acceptable cooking and sensory qualities and increased β-glucan contents. Baik and Czuchajowska (152) found that the texture profile analysis of udon noodles containing 15% ground pearled nonwaxy barley was similar to 100% wheat flour noodles but required a shorter cooking time. Waxy barley reduced hardness and chewiness of this type of noodle. Spaghetti (153) made with 15% barley had similar cooking quality to 100% durum spaghetti and 0.5–1.4% β-glucan (depending on the cultivar). Knuckles et al. (154) used milled fiber enriched barley fractions and an extracted water-soluble barley fiber to make pasta containing 4.1–8.6% β-glucan. A pasta made with 20% of the extracted fiber (7.1% β-glucan) had an overall acceptability rating and color equal to the durum pasta. Spaghetti containing 70% barley bran or flour has been rated acceptable and similar to a whole wheat control (155,156).

Barley β-glucan incorporated at low levels in yeast bread is similar to other gums used as gluten substitutes. Lee et al. (69) reported that 1% of an extracted 85% pure barley β-glucan increased water absorption and dough development time but improved bread grain and texture while maintaining loaf volume. Higher levels (5–26%) of barley β-glucan isolates (154,157) flours (77,82,136,155), and brans (158) have been incorporated into breads to provide consumers with adequate levels of fiber and β-glucan in their diet. All of these studies have reported a decrease in loaf volume as barley β-glucan or fiber is increased in bread. However, sensory tests showed that breads with significant levels of barley β-glucan (1 to 3%) or fiber are rated similar in overall acceptability to the control breads. Bhatty (159) reported that hulless barley flour has twice the water-holding capacity and alkaline water retention capacity as wheat flour but similar oil absorption. Alexander (160) has a patent for making bread products without shortenings or oils by using flour made from waxy barley to increase moisture and as a replacement for fats. Heavier type breads (38,77,136,156), flatbreads (17), and biscuits (155,156) can been made using 30–100% barley flour or bran.

Cookies, muffins, quick breads, and tortillas have been made using various levels of flour, brans, and concentrates. Berglund et al. (155) incorporated 50–100% waxy hulless barley flour (6.6% β-glucan) into cookies, a no-fat muffin, and quick breads, which were rated by consumer panels as having overall acceptability similar to the control products. Muffins made with 100% barley flour (78) having β-glucan content ranging from 3.8 to 4.9% have been described as moister and gummier, but were preferred over the wheat control. These muffins had similar physical characteristics to the control but were darker and more tender. High β-glucan mill fractions used at lower levels (25%) in muffins and cookies (82) produce products comparable to whole wheat products but containing twice as much soluble dietary fiber. Hudson et al. (161) used a similar fraction to develop a muffin that had three times the total dietary fiber (7 g/100 g muffin), four times (3.8 g/100 g muffin) the β-glucan content, and one third of the fat of a commercial oat bran muffin mix. It was necessary to increase leavening by 10% and liquid by 20–25% because of the moisture-absorbing characteristic of the barley fraction. Fastnaught et al. (162) found that muffins containing between 1 to 3% β-glucan had higher volume and were more tender when fat was decreased as much as 66%. An extracted barley fiber concentrate containing 55.6% β-glucan was used to develop tortillas with 12.5% total dietary fiber which were slightly more tender and had similar storage stability as control tortillas (114). Robertson et al. (163) reported that β-glucan extractability in biscuits was increased as a result of cooking.

Hulless barley cultivars can be used to produce malt and malt extract containing higher levels of soluble fiber. Vis and Lorenz (32) malted waxy hulless barley to produce a beer containing 1.5% β-glucan compared to 0.35% in the control. Malted hulless barley or ''food'' malt (164) contains no hulls, thus can be used to make malt extracts with 1.5% β-glucan compared to 0.1% in commercial extracts.

Barley fiber can be utilized in its many forms in a variety of food products. The genotypic, environmental, and processing effects on barley fiber necessitate strict definition and characterization of the individual fiber products by processors. Documentation of the health benefits associated with barley fiber is an ongoing process, which will generate demand by the medical community and consumers. Development of foods containing barley fiber can increase to meet this demand only when manufacturers understand the benefits, unique attributes, and impact on specific products.

REFERENCES

1. Xue Q, Wang L, Newman RK, Newman CW, Graham H. Influence of the hulless, waxy starch and short-awn genes on the composition of barleys. J Cereal Sci 26:251–257, 1997.
2. Fincher GB. Cell wall metabolism in barley. In: Shewry PR, ed. Barley: Genetics, Bioochemistry. Molecular Biology and Biotechnology. Oxford: CAB International, 1992, pp 413–437.
3. Miller SS, Fulcher RG. Distribution of (1-3),(1-4)-β-d-glucan in kernels of oats and barley using microspectrofluorometry. Cereal Chem 71:64–68, 1994.
4. Oscarsson M, Andersson R, Salomonsson AC, Aman P. Chemical composition of barley samples focusing on dietary fibre components. J Cereal Sci 24:161–170, 1996.
5. Aalto T, Lehtonon M, Varo P. Dietary fiber content of barley grown in Finland. Cereal Chem 65: 284–286, 1988.
6. Bjorck I, Eliasson AC, Drews A, Gudmundsson M, Karlsson R. Some nutritional properties of starch and dietary fiber in barley genotypes containing different levels of amylose. Cereal Chem 67:327–333, 1990.
7. Xue Q, Newman RK, Newman CW, McGuire CF. Waxy gene effects on β-glucan, dietary fiber content and viscosity of barleys. Cereal Res Comm 19:399–404, 1991.
8. Boros D, Rek-Cieply B, Cyran M. A note on the composition and nutritional value of hulless barley, J Animal Feed Sci 5:417–424, 1996.
9. Fastnaught CE, Berglund PT, Holm ET, Fox GJ. Genetic and environmental variation in β-glucan content and quality parameters of barley for food. Crop Sci 36:941–946, 1996.
10. Ranhotra GS, Gelroth JA, Astroth K, Bhatty RS. Relative lipidemic responses in rats fed barley and oat meals and their fractions. Cereal Chem 68:548–551, 1991.
11. Berglund PT, Fastnaught CE, Holm ET. Physicochemical and sensory evaluation of extruded high-fiber barley cereals. Cereal Chem 71:91–95, 1994.
12. Bhatty RS, Rossnagel BD. Comparison of pearled and unpearled Canadian and Japanese barleys. Cereal Chem 75:15–21, 1998.
13. Martinez VM, Newman RK, Newman CW. Barley diets with different fat sources have hypocholesterolemic effects in chicks. J Nutr 122:1070–1076, 1992.
14. Newman RK, Klopfenstein CF, Newman CW, Guritno N, Hofer PJ. Comparison of the cholesterol-lowering properties of whole barley, oat bran, and wheat red dog in chicks and rats. Cereal Chem 69:240–244, 1992.
15. Granfeldt Y, Liljeberg H, Anders D, Newman R, Bjorck I. Glucose and insulin responses to barley products: influence of food structure and amylose-amylopectin ratio. Am J Clin Nutr 59:1075–1082, 1994.
16. Wang L, Behr SR, Newman RK, Newman CW. Comparative cholesterol-lowering effects of barley β-glucan and barley oil in golden syrian hamsters. Nutr Res 17:77–88, 1997.
17. Liljeberg HGM, Granfeldt YE, Bjorck IME. Products based on a high fiber barley genotype, but not on common barley or oats, lower postprandial glucose and insulin responses in healthy humans. J Nutr 126:458–466, 1996.
18. Munck L. The case of high-lysine barley breeding. In: Shewry PR, ed. Barley: Genetics, Biochemistry, Molecular Biology and Biotechnology. Oxford: CAB International, 1992, pp 573–601.
19. Kahlon TS, Chow FI. Hypocholesterolemic effects of oat, rice, and barley dietary fibers and fractions. Cereal Foods World 42:86–92, 1997.
20. McIntosh GH, Newman RK, Newman CW. Barley foods and their influence on cholesterol metabolism. World Rev Nutr Diet 77:89–108, 1995.
21. MacGregor AW, Fincher GB. Carbohydrates of the barley grain. In: MacGregor AW, Bhatty RS, eds. Barley: Chemistry and Technology. St Paul, MN: Am Assoc Cereal Chem, 1993, pp 73–130.

22. Lehtonen M, Aikasalo R. β-glucan in two- and six-rowed barley. Cereal Chem 64:191–192, 1987.

23. Narasimhalu P, Kong D, Choo TM, Ferguson T, Therrien MC, Ho KM, May KW, Jui P. Effects of environment and cultivar on total mixed-linkage β-glucan content in eastern and western Canadian barleys (*Hordeum vulgare* L.). Can J Plant Sci 75:371–376, 1995.

24. Ullrich SE, Clancy JA, Eslick RF, Lance RC. β-glucan content and viscosity of extracts from waxy barley. J Cereal Sci 4:279–285, 1986.

25. Rossnagel BG, Bhatty RS. Acid-extract viscosity and % βeta-glucan in barley. Barley Newslett 34: 121–122, 1990.

26. Knuckles BE, Chiu M-CM, Betschart AA. β-Glucan-enriched fractions from laboratory-scale dry milling and sieving of barley and oats. Cereal Chem 69:198–202, 1992.

27. Horsley RD, Schwarz PB, Faue AC, Manthey FA. Survey of β-glucan content of barley cultivars adapted to North Dakota. North Dakota Farm Res 49:24–26, 1992.

28. Knuckles BE, Yokoyama WH, Chiu M-CM. Molecular characterization of barley β-glucans by size-exclusion chromatography with multiple-angle laser light scattering and other detectors. Cereal Chem 74:599–604, 1997.

29. Lee CJ, Horsley RD, Manthey FA, Schwarz PB. Comparisons of β-glucan content of barley and oat. Cereal Chem 74:571–575, 1997.

30. Baidoo SK, Liu YG. Hull-less barley for swine: Ileal and faecal digestibility of proximate nutrients, amino acids and non-starch polysaccharides. J Sci Food Agric 76:397–403, 1998.

31. Kalra S, Jood S. Biological evaluation of protein quality of barley. Food Chem 61:35–39, 1998.

32. Vis RB, Lorenz K. Malting and brewing with a high β-glucan barley, Lebensm Wiss Technol 31: 20–26, 1998.

33. Bhatty RS. Milling of regular and waxy starch hull-less barleys for the production of bran and flour. Cereal Chem 74:693–699, 1997.

34. Marlett JA. Dietary fiber content and effect of processing on two barley varieties. Cereal Foods World 36:576–578, 1991.

35. Bhatty RS. Extraction and enrichment of (1-3),(1-4)-β-D-glucan from barley and oat brans. Cereal Chem 70:73–77, 1993.

36. Danielson AD, Newman RK, Newman CW. Proximate analyses, β-glucan, fiber and viscosity of select barley milling fractions. Cereal Res Comm 24:461–468, 1996.

37. Dudgeon-Bollinger AL, Fastnaught CE, Berglund PT. Extruded snack products from waxy hull-less barley. Cereal Foods World 42:762–766, 1997.

38. Pick ME, Hawrysh ZJ, Gee MI, Toth E. Barley bread products improve glycemic control of type 2 subjects. Int J Food Sci Nutr 49:71–78, 1998.

39. Wu YV, Stringfellow AC, Inglet GE. Protein-and β-glucan enriched fractions from high-protein, high β-glucan barleys by sieving and air classification. Cereal Chem 71:220–223, 1991.

40. Oscarsson M, Parkkonen T, Autio K, Aman P. Composition and microstructure of waxy, normal and high amylose barley samples. J Cereal Sci 26:259–264, 1997.

41. Sundberg B, Xue Q, Newman RK, Newman CW. Glycaemic responses and hypocholesterolaemic effects of high-amylose barley diets on broiler chicks. J Sci Food Agric 76:457–463, 1998.

42. McCleary BV, Glennie-Holmes M. Enzymic quantification of (1-3),(1-4)-β-D-glucan in barley and malt. J Inst Brew 91:285–295, 1985.

43. Aman P, Graham H. Analysis of total and insoluble mixed-linked (1-3),(1-4)-β-D-glucans in barley and oats. J Agric Food Chem 35:704–709, 1987.

44. Ellis RP, Swanston JS, Rubio A, Perez-Vendrell AM, Romagosa I, Molina-Cano JL. The development of β-glucanase and degradation of β-glucan in barley grown in Scotland and Spain. J Cereal Sci 26:75–82, 1997.

45. Swanston JS. Waxy starch barley genotypes with reduced β-glucan contents, Cereal Chem 74:452–455, 1997.

46. Swanston JS, Ellis RP, Stark JR. Effects on grain and malting quality of genes altering barley starch composition. J Cereal Sci 22:265–273, 1995.

47. Brennan CS, Amor MA, Harris N, Smith D, Cantrell I, Griggs D, Shewryll RR. Cultivar differences in modification patterns of protein and carbohydrate reserves during malting of barley. J Cereal Sci 26:83–93, 1997.

48. Swanston JS, Ellis RP, Perez-Vendrell A, Voltas J, Molina-Cano JL. Patterns of barley grain development in Spain and Scotland and their implications for malting quality. Cereal Chem 74:456–461, 1997.

49. Perez-Vendrell AM, Brufau J, Molina-Cano JL, Francesch M, Guasch J. Effects of cultivar and environment on β-(1,3)-(1,4)-D-glucan content and acid extract viscosity of spanish barleys. J Cereal Sci 23:285–292, 1996.

50. Lehtonen M, Aikasalo R. Pentosans in barley varieties. Cereal Chem 64:133–134, 1986.

51. Fleury MD, Edney MJ, Campbell LD, Crow GH. Total, water-soluble and acid-soluble arabinoxylans in western Canadian barleys. Can J Plant Sci 77:191–196, 1997.

52. Henry RJ. Genetic and environmental variation in the pentosan and β-glucan contents of barley, and their relation to malting quality. J Cereal Sci 4:269–277, 1986.

53. Henry RJ. Pentosan and (1-3),(1-4)-β-glucan concentrations in endosperm and wholegrain of wheat, barley, oats and rye. J Cereal Sci 6:253–258, 1987.

54. Sundberg B, Aman P. Fractionation of different types of barley by roller milling and sieving. J Cereal Sci 19:179–184, 1994.

55. Bhatty RS, MacGregor AW, Rossnagel BG. Total and acid-soluble β-glucan content of hulless barley and its relationship to acid-extract viscosity. Cereal Chem 68:221–227, 1991.

56. Szczodrak J, Pomeranz Y. Starch and enzyme-resistant starch from high-amylose barley. Cereal Chem 68(6):589–596, 1991.

57. Girhammar U, Nair BM. Certain physical properties of water soluble non-starch polysaccharides from wheat, rye, triticale, barley and oats. Food Hydrocolloids 6:329–343, 1992.

58. Beer MU, Wood PJ, Weisz J. Molecular weight distribution and (1-3)(1-4)-β-D-glucan content of consecutive extracts of various oat and barley cultivars. Cereal Chem 74:476–480, 1997.

59. Gomez C, Navarro A, Manzanarea P, Horta A, Carbonell JV. Physical and structural properties of barley (1-3)(1-4)-β-D-glucan. Part I. Determination of molecular weight and macromolecular radius by light scattering, Carbohydrate Polym 32:7–15, 1997.

60. Schwarz PB, Lee Y-T. Rheological and chemical characterization of (1,3),(1,4)-β-glucans from hull-less barley. In: Meuser F, Manners DT, Seibel W, eds. Progress in Plant Polymeric Carbohydrate Research. Hamburg: Behr's Verlag, 1995, pp 99–103.

61. Wood PJ, Weisz J, Mahn W. Molecular characterization of cereal β-glucans. II. size-exclusion chromatography for comparison of molecular weight. Cereal Chem 68:530–536, 1991.

62. Wood PJ, Weisz J, Blackwell BA. Structural studies of (1-3),(1-4)-β-D-glucans by c-nuclear magnetic resonance spectroscopy and by rapid analysis of cellulose-like regions using high performance anion-exchange chromatography of oligosaccharides released by lichenase. Cereal Chem 71:301–307, 1994.

63. Edney MJ, Marchylo BA, MacGregor AW. Structure of total barley beta-glucan. J Inst Brew 97:39–44, 1991.

64. Izydorczyk MS, Macri LJ, MacGregor AW. Structure and phsicochemical properties of barley non-starch polysaccharides-I. Water-extractable β-glucans and arabinoxylans. Carbohydrate Polym 35:259–269, 1998.

65. Izawa M, Yukinobu K, Koshino S. Relationship between structure and solubility of (1-3),(1-4)-β-D-glucan from barley. J Am Soc Brew Chem 51:123–127, 1993.

66. Izydorczyk MS, Macri LJ, MacGregor AW. Structure and physicochemical properties of barley non-starch polysaccharides-II. Alkali-extractable β-glucans and arabinoxylans. Carbohydrate Polym 35:249–258, 1998.

67. Saulnier L, Gevaudan S, Thibault J-F. Extraction and partial characterisation of β-glucan from the endosperms of two barley cultivars. J Cereal Sci 19:171–178, 1994.

68. Bengtsson S, Aman P, Graham H, Newman CW, Newman RK. Chemical studies on mixed-linked β-glucans in hulless barley cultivars giving different hypocholesterolaemic responses in chickens. J Sci Food Agric 52:435–445, 1990.

69. Lee Y-T, Schwarz PB, D'Appolonia BL. Effects of beta-(1-3),(1-4)-D-glucans from hull-less barley on the properties of wheat, starch, flour and bread. Barley Newslett 39:60–65, 1995.

70. Temelli F. Extraction and functional properties of barley β-glucan as affected by temperature and pH. J Food Sci 62:1194–1201, 1997.

71. Bhatty RS, MacGregor AW. Gamma irradiation of hulless barley: effect on grain composition, β-glucans and starch. Cereal Chem 65(6):463–470, 1988.
72. Weber FE, Chaudhary VK. Recovery and nutritional evaluation on dietary fiber ingredients from a barley by-product. Cereal Foods World 32:548–550, 1987.
73. Zhang J, Lundin E, Hallmans G, Bergman F, Westerlund E, Petterson P. Dietary effects of barley fibre, wheat bran and rye bran on bile composition and gallstone formation in hamsters. APMIS 100:553–557, 1992.
74. McIntosh GH, Le Leu RK, Royle PJ, Young GP. A comparative study of the influence of differing barley brans on DMH-induced intestinal tumours in male Sprague-Dawley rats. J Gastroenterol Hepatol 11:113–119, 1996.
75. McIntosh GH. Colon cancer: dietary modifications required for a balanced protective diet. Prev Med 22:767–774, 1993.
76. Kanauchi O, Agata K. Protein, and dietary fiber-rich new foodstuff from brewer's spent grain increased excretion of feces and jejunum mucosal protein content in rats. Biosci Biotech Biochem 61:29–33, 1997.
77. Marklinder I, Johansson L, Haglund A, Nagel-Held B, Seibel W. Effects of flour from different barley varieties on barley sourdough bread. Food Qual Pref 7:275–284, 1996.
78. Newman RK, McGuire CF, Newman CW. Composition and muffin baking characteristics of flours from four barley cultivars. Cereal Foods World 35:563–566, 1990.
79. Miller MC, Froseth JA, Wyatt CL, Ullrich SE. Effect of starch type, total β-glucans and acid detergent fiber levels on the energy content of barley (*Hordeum vulgare* L.) for poultry and swine. Can J Animal Sci 49:679–686, 1994.
80. Bhatty RS. Laboratory and pilot plant extraction and purification of β-glucans from hull-less barley and oat brans. J Cereal Sci 22:163–170, 1995.
81. Newman CW, Newman RK. Barley as a food grain. Cereal Foods World 36:800–805, 1991.
82. Newman RK, Ore KC, Abbott KJ, Newman CW. Fiber enrichment of baked products with a barley milling fraction. Cereal Foods World 43:23–25, 1998.
83. Sundberg B, Pettersson D, Aman P. Nutritional properties of fibre-rich barley products fed to broiler chickens. J Sci Food Agric 67:469–476, 1995.
84. Knuckles BE, Chiu M-CM. β-glucan enrichment of barley fractions by air classification and sieving. J Food Sci 60:1070–1074, 1995.
85. Yoon SH. Evaluation of waxy hulless and nonwaxy hulled barley cultivars and their fractions for beta-glucan enrichment, M.S. thesis. North Dakota State University, Fargo, ND, 1993.
86. Kahlon TS, Chow FI, Knuckles BE, Chiu M-CM. Cholesterol-lowering effects in hamsters of β-glucan-enriched barley fraction, dehulled whole barley, rice bran, and oat bran and their combinations. Cereal Chem 70:435–440, 1993.
87. German JB, Xu R, Walzem R, Kinsella JE, Knuckles B, Nakamura M, Yokoyama WH. Effect of dietary fats and barley fiber on total cholesterol and lipoprotein cholesterol distribution in plasma of hamsters. Nutr Res 16:1239–1249, 1996.
88. Yoon SH, Berglund PT, Fastnaught CE. Evaluation of selected barley cultivars and their fractions for β-glucan enrichment and viscosity. Cereal Chem 72:187–190, 1995.
89. Foehse KB. Method of dry milling and preparing high soluble fiber barley fraction. U.S. Pat. 5,063,078 (1991).
90. Bhatty RS. Hull-less barley bran: A potential new product from an old grain. Cereal Foods World 40:819–824, 1995.
91. Czuchajowska Z, Klamczynski A, Paszczynska B, Baik B-K. Structure and functionality of barley starches. Cereal Chem 75:747–754, 1998.
92. Klamczynski A, Baik B-K, Czuchajowska Z. Composition, microstructure, water imbibition, and thermal properties of abraded barley. Cereal Chem 75:677–685, 1998.
93. Jadhav SJ, Lutz SE, Ghorpade VM, Salunkhe DK. Barley: chemistry and value-added processing. Crit Rev Food Sci 38:123–171, 1998.
94. Oda T, Aoe S, Imanishi S, Kanazawa Y, Sanada H, Ayano Y. Effects of dietary oat, barley, and guar gums on serum and liver lipid concentrations in diet-induced hypertriglyceridemic rats. J Nutr Sci Vitaminol 40:213–217, 1994.

95. Persson H. Binding of mineral elements by dietary fibre components in cereals-in vitro(III). Food Chem 40:169–183, 1991.

96. Burkus Z, Temelli F. Effect of extraction conditions on yield, composition, and viscosity stability of barley β-glucan gum. Cereal Chem 75:805–809, 1998.

97. Morgan KR, Ofman DJ. Glucagel, a gelling β-glucan from barley. Cereal Chem 75:879–881, 1998.

98. Inglett GE. Method of making soluble dietary fiber compositions from cereals. U.S. Pat. 5,082,673 (1992).

99. Lehtomaki I. Beta-glucan enriched alimentary fiber. U.S. Pat. 5,183,677 (1993).

100. Wang L. Production of β-glucan and β-glucan product. U.S. Pat. 5,512,287 (1996).

101. Bhatty RS. Methods for extracting cereal β-glucans. U.S. Pat. 5,518,710 (1996).

102. Fox GJ. Food ingredients derived from the viscous barley grain and the process of making. U.S. Pat. 5,614,242 (1997).

103. Sundberg B, Falk H. Composition and properties of bread and porridge prepared from different types of barley flour. Am J Clin Nutr 59:780S, 1994.

104. Szczodrak J, Pomeranz Y. Starch-lipid interactions and formation of resistant starch in high-amylose barley. Cereal Chem 69:626–632, 1992.

105. Lupton J, Morin JL, Robinson MC. Barley bran flour accelerates gastrointestinal transit time. J Am Diet Assoc 93:881–885, 1993.

106. Wisker E, Nagel R, Tanudjaja TK, Feldheim W. Calcium, magnesium, zinc, and iron balances in young women: effects of a low-phytate barley-fiber concentrate. Am J Clin Nutr 54:553–559, 1991.

107. Wisker E, Bach-Knudsen KE, Daniel M, Eggum BO, Feldheim W. Energy values of non-starch polysaccharides: comparative studies in humans and rats. J Nutr 127:108–116, 1997.

108. Gallaher DD, Locket PL, Gallaher CM. Bile acid metabolism in rats fed two levels of corn oil and brans of oat, rye and barley and sugar beet fiber. J Nutr 122:473–481, 1992.

109. Zhang JX, Lundin E, Andersson H, Bosaeus I, Dahlgren S, Hallmans G, Stenling R, Aman P. Brewer's spent grain, serum lipids and fecal sterol excretion in human subjects with ileostomies. J Nutr 121:778–784, 1991.

110. Kanauchi O, Agata K, Fushki T. Mechanism for the increased defecation and jejunum mucosal protein content in rats by feeding germinated barley foodstuff. Biosci Biotech Biochem 61:443–448, 1997.

111. Kanauchi O, Nakamura T, Agata K, Fushiki T. Preventive effect of germinated barley foodstuff on diarrhea induced by water-soluble dietary fiber in rats. Biosci Biotech Biochem 61:449–454, 1997.

112. Lia A, Hallmans G, Sandberg AS, Sundberg B, Aman P, Anderson H. Oat β-glucan increases bile acid excretion and a fiber-rich barley fraction increases cholesterol excretion in ileostomy subjects. Am J Clin Nutr 62:1245–1251, 1995.

113. Wang L, Newman RK, Newman CW, Hofer PJ. Barley β-glucans alter intestinal viscosity and reduce plasma cholesterol concentrations in chicks. J Nutr 122:2292–2297, 1992.

114. Hecker KD, Meier ML, Newman RK, Newman CW. Barley β-glucan is effective as a hypocholesterolaemic ingredient in foods. J Sci Food Agric 77:179–183, 1998.

115. Bowles RK, Morgan KR, Furneaux RH, and Coles GD. ^{13}C CP/MAS NMR study of the interaction of bile acids with barley β-glucan. Carbohydrate Polym 29(1):7–10, 1996.

116. Fardet A, Guillon F, Hoebler C, Barry J-L. In vitro fermentation of beet fibre and barley bran, of their insoluble residues after digestion and of ileal effluents. J Sci Food Agric 75:315–325, 1997.

117. Daniel M, Wisker E, Rave G, Feldheim W. Fermentation in human subjects of nonstarch polysaccharides in mixed diets, but not in a barley fiber concentrate, could be predicted by in vitro fermentation using human fecal inocula. J Nutr 127:1981–1988, 1997.

118. Bell JM, Keith MO. Effect of pig weight and barley hulls on the digestibility of energy, protein and fiber in wheat, corn, and hulless barley diets. Nutr Res 11:1307–1316, 1991.

119. Robertson JA, Majsak-Newman G, Ring SG. Release of mixed linkage (1-3),(1-4)-β-D-glucans from barley by protease activity and effects on ileal effluent, Int J Biol Macromol 21:57–60, 1997.

120. Bach Knudsen KE, Wisker E, Daniel M, Feldheim W, Eggum BO. Digestibility of energy, protein, fat and non-starch polysaccharides in mixed diets: comparative studies between man and the rat. Br J Nutr 71:471–487, 1994.

121. Wisker E, Godau A, Daniel M, Peschutter G, Feldheim W. Contribution of barley fiber to the metabolizable energy of human diets. Nutr Res 12:1315–1323, 1992.

122. Peterson DM, Qureshi AA. Effects of tocols and β-glucan on serum lipid parameters in chickens. J Sci Food Agric 73:417–424, 1997.

123. Wang L, Newman RK, Newman CW, Jackson LL, Hofer PJ. Tocotrienol and fatty acid composition of barley oil and their effects on lipid metabolism. Plant Foods Human Nutr 43:9–17, 1993.

124. McIntosh GH, Jorgensen L, Royle P. The potential of an insoluble dietary fiber-rich source from barley to protect from DMH-induced intestinal tumors in rats. Nutr Cancer 19:213–221, 1993.

125. Oda T, Aoe S, Sanada H, Ayano Y. Effects of soluble and insoluble fiber preparations isolated from oat, barley, and wheat on liver cholesterol accumulation in cholesterol-fed rats. J Nutr Sci Vitaminol 39:73–79, 1993.

126. Wang WM, Klopfenstein CF. Effect of twin-screw extrusion on the nutritional quality of wheat, barley, and oats. Cereal Chem 70:712–715, 1993.

127. Jackson KA, Suter DAI, Topping DL. Oat bran, barley and malted barley lower plasma cholesterol relative to wheat bran but differ in their effects on liver cholesterol in rats fed diets with and without cholesterol. J Nutr 124:1678–1684, 1994.

128. Zhang J-X, Bergman F, Hallmans G, Johansson G, Ludin E, Stenling R, Theander O, Westerlund E. The influence of barley fibre on bile composition, gallstone formation, serum cholesterol and intestinal morphology in hamsters. APMIS 98:568–574, 1990.

129. Lupton J, Robinson MC, Morin JL. Cholesterol-lowering effect of barley bran flour and oil. J Am Diet Assoc 94:65–70, 1994.

130. Narain JP, Shukla K, Bijlani RL, Kochhar KP, Karmarkar MG, Bala S, Srivastava LM, Reddy KS. Metabolic responses to a four week barley supplement. Int J Food Sci Nutr 43:41–46, 1992.

131. Ikegami S, Tomita M, Honda S, Yamaguchi M, Mizukawa R, Suzuki Y, Ishii K, Ohsawa S, Kiyooka N, Higuchi M, Kobayashi S. Effect of boiled barley-rice feeding in hypercholesterolemic and normolipemic subjects. Plant Foods Human Nutr 49:317–328, 1996.

132. Collier GR, Wolever T, Wong GS, Hosse RG. Prediction of glycemic response to mixed meals in noninsulin-dependent diabetic subjects. Am J Clin Nutr 44:349–352, 1986.

133. Wolever TMS, Bolognes C. Source and amount of carbohydrate affect postprandial glucose and insulin in normal subjects. J Nutr 126:2798–2806, 1996.

134. Wursch P, Pi-Sunyer FX. The role of viscous soluble fiber in the metabolic control of diabetes. Diabetes Care 20:1774–1780, 1997.

135. Livesey G, Wilkinson JA, Roe M, Faulks R, Clark S, Brown JC, Kennedy H, Elia M. Influence of the physical form of barley grain on the digestion of its starch in the human small intestine and implications for health. Am J Clin Nutr 61:75–81, 1995.

136. Liljeberg H, Bjorck I. Bioavailability of starch in bread products. Postprandial glucose and insulin responses in healthy subjects and in vitro resistant starch content. Eur J Clin Nutr 48:151–163, 1994.

137. Yokoyama WH, Hudson CA, Knuckles BE, Chiu M-CM, Sayre RN, Turnlund JR, Schneeman BO. Effect of barley β-glucan in durum wheat pasta on human glycemic response. Cereal Chem 74:293–296, 1997.

138. Hawrysh ZJ, Gee MI, Pick ME, Toth E, Hardin RT. Barley bread products in the diet: community study with diabetic subject. Cereal Foods World 42:620, 1997.

139. Huang CM, Dural NH. Absorption of bile acids on cereal type food fibers. J Food Proc Eng 18:243–266, 1995.

140. Bohn JA, BeMiller JN. (1-3)-β-D-Glucans as biological response modifiers: a review of structure-functional activity relationships. Carbohydrate Polym 28:3–14, 1995.

141. Vetvicka V, Thornton BP, Ross GD. Soluble β-glucan polysaccharide binding to the lectin site of neutrophil or natural killer cell complement receptor type 3 (CD11b/CD18) generates a primed state of the receptor capable of mediating cytotoxicity of iC3b-opsonized target cells. J Clin Invest 98:50–61, 1996.

142. Czop JK, Austen FK. Properties of glycans that activate the human alternative complement pathway and interact with the human monocyte β-glucan receptor. J Immunol 135:3388–3393, 1985.

143. Thornton BP, Vetvicka V, Pitman M, Goldman RC, Ross GD. Analysis of the sugar specificity and

molecular location of the β-glucan-binding lectin site of complement receptor type 3 (CD11b/ CD18). J Immunol 156:1235–1246, 1996.

144.   Yun CH, Estrada A, Van Kessel A, Gajadhar AA, Redmond MJ, Laarveld B. β-(1-3,1-4) Oat glucan enhances resistance to *Eimeria vermiformis* infection in immunosuppressed mice. Int J Parasitol 27:329–337, 1997.

145.   Idouraine A, Hassani BZ, Claye SS, Weber CW. In vitro binding capacity of various fiber sources for magnesium, zinc, and copper. J Agric Food Chem 43:1580–1584, 1995.

146.   Alexander DJ. Cereal food ingredients from waxy barley. U.S. Pat. 5,360,619 (1994).

147.   Sundberg B, Abrahamsson L, Aman P. Quality of rolled barley flakes as affected by batch of grain and processing technique. Plant Foods Human Nutr 45:145–154, 1994.

148.   Lewis VM, Lewis DA. Cereal food product for hot and cold usages. U.S. Pat. 5,391,388 (1995).

149.   Plaami SP, Kumpulainen JT. Soluble and insoluable dietary fiber and β-glucan contents in domestic and imported breakfast cereals consumed in Finland. J Food Composition Analysis 6:307–315, 1993.

150.   Lee WJ, Schwarz PB. Effect of twin-screw extrusion on physical properties and dietary fiber content of extrudates from barley/corn blends. Foods Biotechnol 3:169–174, 1994.

151.   Ostergard K, Bjorck I, Vainionpaa J. Effects of extrusion cooking on starch and dietary fibre in barley. Food Chem 34:215–227, 1989.

152.   Baik BK, Czuchajowska Z. Barley in udon noodles. Food Sci Technol Int 3:423–435, 1997.

153.   Faccini N, Vale G, Grossi M, Reggiani F, Baravelli M, Giorni E, Stanca AM. Use of barley beta-glucan for the qualitative improvement of spaghetti. Informatore-Agrario 52:55–56, 1996.

154.   Knuckles BE, Hudson CA, Chiu MM, Sayre RN. Effect of β-glucan barley fractions in high-fiber bread and pasta. Cereal Foods World 42:94–99, 1997.

155.   Berglund PT, Fastnaught CE, Holm ET. Food uses of waxy hull-less barley. Cereal Foods World 37:707–714, 1992.

156.   McIntosh GH, Whyte J, McArthur R, Nestel PJ. Barley and wheat foods: influence on plasma cholesterol concentrations in hypercholesterolemic men. Am J Clin Nutr 53:1205–1209, 1991.

157.   Klopfenstein CF, Hoseney RC. Cholesterol-lowering effect of beta-glucan-enriched bread. Nutr Rep Int 36:1091–1098 (1987).

158.   Rasco BA, Rubenthaler G, Borhan M, Dong FM. Baking properties of bread and cookies incorporating distillers' or brewer's grain from wheat or barley. J Food Sci 55:424–429, 1990.

159.   Bhatty RS. Physiochemical and functional (breadmaking) properties of hulless barley fractions. Cereal Chem 63:31–35, 1986.

160.   Alexander DJ. Method of making bread products without shortenings and/or oils. U.S. Pat. 5,510,136 (1996).

161.   Hudson CA, Chiu MM, Knuckles BE. Development and characteristics of high-fiber muffins with oat bran, rice bran, or barley fiber fractions. Cereal Foods World 37:373–376, 1992.

162.   Fastnaught CE, Bond JM, Berglund PT. Oil reduction in muffins using waxy hulless barley β-glucan. Cereal Foods World 42:666, 1997.

163.   Robertson JA, Majsak-Newman G, Ring SG, Selvendran RR. Solubilisation of mixed linkage (1-3),(1-4)β-D-glucans from barley: effects of cooking and digestion. J Cereal Sci 25:275–283, 1997.

164.   Bhatty RS. Production of food malt from hull-less barley. Cereal Chem 73:75–80, 1996.

165.   Vasanthan T, Bhatty RS. Enhancement of resistant starch (RS3) in amylomaize, barley, field pea and lentil starches. Starch/Starke 50:286–291, 1998.

28

Rice Bran
Production, Composition, Availability, Healthful Properties, Safety, and Food Applications

Talwinder S. Kahlon and Faye I. Chow
U.S. Department of Agriculture, Albany, California

I. PRODUCTION

The world production of rice paddy from 1993 to 1997 was 527–571 million metric tons. The five top rice-growing countries are China, India, Indonesia, Bangladesh, and Thailand, producing 34.8, 21.5, 8.6, 4.9, and 3.7% of the world rice crop, respectively. The United States contributes 1.4% (8 million metric tons) to the annual world rice production. One hundred pounds of paddy yields 18–20 lb husk, 10–12 lb rice bran, 10–12 lb broken rice, and 56–58 lb milled white rice. Rice is a major cereal food providing nourishment to over half the world's population and is usually consumed as milled white, polished rice. Rice bran, a by-product obtained from the milling process, contains lipase, which rapidly degrades the oil in rice bran to free fatty acids and glycerol, making the bran unpalatable. Research at the Western Regional Research Center, USDA-ARS (Albany, CA) resulted in successfully stabilizing rice bran by subjecting it to 125–135°C for 1–3 seconds at 11–15% moisture and holding the extruded bran at an elevated temperature for 3 minutes prior to cooling, thereby deactivating the lipase (1). Stabilized rice bran (SRB) has an estimated shelf life of about 6 months and potential use as a food ingredient as well as a source of edible oil. In the United States, more than 90% of the rice bran which results from the milling process is used as animal feed. The remainder is stabilized and could be used as food; however, the largest current market for SRB is as horse-feed supplement. Parboiling, which is a steam treatment of paddy rice, results in gelatinization of the starch beneath the bran layer of the rice kernel and results in a higher yield of white rice, less broken rice, and higher-fiber bran. The parboiling process also stabilizes rice bran by deactivating lipase, but it also destroys many of the antioxidants in rice bran.

II. COMPOSITION

The composition of stabilized and parboiled rice bran is given in Table 1 and that of rice bran oil in Table 2. Most studies testing the healthful properties of rice bran have focused on its dietary fiber, oil, and protein components. The total dietary fiber (TDF) content of rice bran ranges from 20 to 27%, with less than 2% as soluble dietary fiber (Table 1). Rice bran contains

Table 1 Composition of Rice Bran (%)

	Stabilized rice bran	Parboiled rice bran
Total dietary fiber	20.9	27.0
Soluble dietary fiber	1.9	1.9
Nitrogen	2.4	3.0
Fat	22.4	29.6

Source: Ref. 10.

22–29% crude fat, which includes approximately 1.8% gum and 0.4% wax (2). The fatty acid composition of rice bran oil consists of 19% saturates, 40% monounsaturates, and 35% polyunsaturates (Table 2). Rice bran oil (RBO) is unusually high in unsaponifiable matter (U), containing over 4% compared with 0.3–1% in peanut oil (3). Rice bran unsaponifiable matter is a mixture of 43% plant sterols (campesterol, stigmasterol, β-sitosterol, and others), 28% triterpene alcohols (24-methylene cycloartanol and cycloartenol), 10% 4-methyl sterols, and 19% less polar compounds such as aliphatic alcohols and other hydrocarbons (4). Oryzanol, a mixture of ferulic acid esters of triterpenoid alcohols and reported to have hypocholesterolemic activity, is present at about 20–30% of the unsaponifiable matter or 1.1–2.6% of the oil (5). The protein content of stabilized rice bran ranges from 12 to 16% and in parboiled rice bran from 14 to 20%. Rice bran protein is of relatively high digestibility and nutritional value, with a protein efficiency ratio of 1.6 for rice bran and 2.0–2.2 for protein concentrates isolated from rice bran, compared to 2.5 for casein (6).

III. HEALTHFUL PROPERTIES: CHOLESTEROL-LOWERING BY RICE BRAN

A. Hamster Studies

The hamster has come to be the preferred rodent model for cholesterol studies, since it has a gall bladder, which is absent in the rat, and the lipoprotein profile of hamster plasma by density

Table 2 Composition of Rice Bran Oil

Component	%
Unsaponifiable matter	4.1
Saturated fatty acids	
Palmitic	17.0
Stearic	1.7
Arachidic	0.6
Monounsaturated fatty acids	
Oleic	39.4
Vaccenic	0.9
Gadoleic	0.6
Polyunsaturated fatty acids	
Linoleic	34.3
Linolenic	1.3

Source: Ref. 11.

gradient ultracentrifugation contains distinct very low-density (20%), low-density (25%), and high-density (55%) lipoprotein fractions. Furthermore, hamsters and humans are reported to be similar in having significant levels of circulating plasma cholesterol and an intrinsically low rate of hepatic cholesterol synthesis and in their response to diet modification and drugs (7).

Cholesterol lowering in hamsters by stabilized or parboiled rice bran in the United States was first reported by USDA-ARS (Albany, CA) scientists (8) and was acknowledged by a feature article in the *Journal of the American Oil Chemists' Society* (9) in which the need was expressed for funding a human study to validate the findings in hamsters. Diets containing 10% TDF from intact full-fat rice bran (stabilized or parboiled) resulted in significantly lower plasma and liver cholesterol elevations compared with the 10% cellulose control diet in hamsters fed 0.5% cholesterol (10). Replacing one third of the stabilized rice bran fiber with wheat bran fiber also resulted in significantly lower plasma and liver cholesterol elevations. In a subsequent study (11), diets containing 10% TDF from stabilized rice bran significantly reduced plasma cholesterol compared to those fed a cellulose control diet, both in the presence and absence of 0.3% cholesterol in the diet (Table 3). In the cholesterol-fed hamsters, diets containing 11, 22, 33, and 44% rice bran resulted in plasma cholesterol reductions of 8, 11, 15, and 21%, respectively, compared with control values. Although plasma cholesterol reductions were significantly correlated with the level of rice bran in the diet ($r = 0.38$), the low correlation coefficient suggested that the rice bran level alone was a poor predictor of plasma cholesterol lowering.

Several fractions of rice bran were evaluated for cholesterol-lowering properties. Defatted rice bran resulted in a loss of cholesterol-lowering ability (10,11), suggesting that the lipid fraction was necessary for maximum cholesterol-lowering potential (Table 3). A combination of defatted rice bran plus RBO or degummed, dewaxed RBO resulted in significant liver cholesterol reductions (2,11). However, RBO extracted at 4 or 54°C and wax and gum fractions of RBO had no significant influence on cholesterol status compared with their respective corn oil controls (2). When recombined, it appeared that defatted rice bran and RBO were less effective in lowering cholesterol compared with intact full-fat rice bran, suggesting that there was a loss or inactivation of cholesterol-lowering activity in the rice oil fractionation process.

Since the liver is the principal organ responsible for the regulation of plasma cholesterol levels, liver cholesterol levels also provide a measure of the influence of diet on cholesterol metabolism. Liver cholesterol was significantly lowered in hamsters by diet containing 10% TDF from rice bran or a 5:5 TDF combination of rice bran and a β-glucan–enriched (19% total β-glucans) barley fraction in diets containing 0.25% cholesterol (12). In the same study, a diet containing a combination of rice bran and oat bran (5:5, TDF) with 2.6% total β-glucans (0.3% from rice bran, 2.3% from oat bran) resulted in significant plasma and liver cholesterol reduc-

Table 3 Hamster Studies: Plasma and Liver Cholesterol Lowering by Rice Bran

	Control	Rice bran	Effect	Ref.
Plasma cholesterol, mg/dL	402	274	Significant	10
	327	255	Significant	11
	322	237	Significant	2
	302	276	Not significant	12
	281	266	Not significant	13
Liver cholesterol, mg/g	57	31	Significant	10
	37	28	Significant	11
	36	23	Significant	2
	54	43	Significant	12
	46	32	Significant	13

tions, suggesting that the contribution of rice bran in lowering cholesterol in hamsters is likely due to components other than β-glucans or soluble fiber. Measurement of diet slurry viscosities revealed rice bran diet viscosity to be similar to that of the cellulose (insoluble fiber) control diet (<10 cP over a 3-hour period), rather than to oat bran diet viscosity (104 cP), indicating that cholesterol lowering by rice bran is related to a mechanism other than sequestering or entrapment of lipid, bile acids, or their metabolites.

In the earlier studies (2,10,11) in which either 0.3 or 0.5% cholesterol was fed, rice bran resulted in significant plasma cholesterol reductions, but when dietary cholesterol was lowered to 0.25% (12) plasma cholesterol was not significantly reduced by the rice bran diet, suggesting that the plasma cholesterol response is dependent on the level of hypercholesterolemia induced in the animals (Table 3).

The source of dietary protein is an additional influence on plasma cholesterol elevations. It is common knowledge that vegetarians have lower plasma cholesterol levels than persons consuming animal protein. In each of the aforementioned hamster studies, the control diets contained casein as the sole source of protein, while treatment diets contained some plant protein. Therefore, a study was designed in which the contribution of plant protein was made equal in all treatments (13). Diets contained 0.3% cholesterol, 10% TDF, 10.1% fat, and 3% nitrogen with the same plant-to-animal N ratio (44:56), using soy protein and casein in the control diet. Plasma cholesterol was elevated in the control animals to 281 mg/dL, 13% lower than that (322–325 mg/dL) observed in previous studies (2,11) in which hamsters were fed 0.3% cholesterol with casein as the sole source of protein in the control diet (Table 3). In this study, the unsaponifiable matter was isolated from rice bran oil and added to cellulose or rice bran diets to provide a total of 0.4 or 0.8% U in the diets. Probably as a result of the lower level of hypercholesterolemia in the control animals, plasma cholesterol was not significantly lower in animals fed rice bran without added U but was significantly lower in animals fed stabilized or raw rice bran with 0.4% additional U from RBO, compared to the control group. Liver cholesterol was significantly lowered by stabilized or raw rice bran with or without added U (0.8% or 0.4% U, respectively), and by cellulose diets with added U (0.8%). A dose response to U was observed for both plasma and liver cholesterol reductions. Rice bran diets lowered cholesterol up to twice as much as cellulose diets with equivalent levels of U. Fecal fat excretion was significantly negatively correlated to liver ($r = -0.97$) and plasma ($r = -0.83$) cholesterol values. The results of these hamster studies suggest that unsaponifiable matter and other components of rice bran have cholesterol-lowering activity, possibly through increased fecal excretion of lipids.

B. Rat Studies

Although the current preference among researchers is to use the hamster model for the evaluation of diet ingredient effects on cholesterol metabolism, earlier work was conducted primarily with the laboratory rat. In cholesterol-fed rats, Ayano et al. (14) reported that the neutral detergent fiber fraction (high in hemicellulose) of rice bran had serum cholesterol-lowering effects, while the acid detergent fiber fraction was ineffective. The hemicellulose fraction was isolated from defatted rice bran and fed to rats at 2% of the diet, resulting in significantly reduced plasma cholesterol levels (15); however, liver cholesterol was not significantly influenced in either study. Data from the latter investigation suggested that the hypocholesterolemic effect of rice bran hemicellulose involved increased excretion of bile acid, but not liver accumulation of cholesterol or suppression of cholesterol absorption. Others reported no significant plasma cholesterol reductions with diet containing 10% stabilized rice bran from parboiled rice compared to 10% cellulose or fiber-free control diets fed to rats for 4 weeks (16); however, none of the diets contained added cholesterol and the level of rice bran in the diet was low. When diets containing 1% cholesterol, 0.2% cholic acid, 10% TDF from raw or parboiled rice bran, and 17–19% fat were fed to rats for 21 days, both plasma and liver cholesterol levels were significantly reduced by the rice bran diets compared with the fiber-free control diet (17). Topping et al. (18) found significantly lower plasma and liver cholesterol in rats fed cholesterol-free diets containing 7% TDF from heat-stabilized rice bran compared to 7% TDF from unprocessed wheat bran. The cholesterol reductions were related to increased hepatic low-density lipoprotein (LDL) receptor activity.

Cholesterol-lowering effects of rice bran oil and rice bran oil U were reported in rats fed 1% cholesterol and 0.5% cholic acid diets for 8 weeks (19). Results showed that either 10% RBO or 0.4% rice bran oil U significantly lowered total plasma cholesterol (TC) and liver cholesterol compared to peanut oil. In another study with cholesterol-fed rats, significantly lower TC, LDL cholesterol, and very low-density lipoprotein (VLDL) cholesterol were observed with 10% RBO compared with those fed peanut oil (20). Addition of 0.5% oryzanol to RBO diet showed a further significant decrease in TC. Rice bran oil also lowered liver cholesterol and triglycerides significantly. Evidence of a possible mechanism for the hypocholesterolemic activity of oryzanol was reported in a subsequent study in which a significant increase in fecal cholesterol and bile acid excretion and a 20% reduction in cholesterol absorption in vitro were observed after rats were fed 0.5% oryzanol and 1% cholesterol diet (21). An additional mechanism for reducing atherosclerotic risk with oryzanol was suggested by significantly lower ADP-induced platelet aggregation and total inhibition of aggregation by collagen when 0.5% oryzanol was added to 1% cholesterol rat diet (22).

Other components of rice bran reported to have cholesterol-lowering activity in rats include wax isolated from RBO, which significantly lowered plasma and liver cholesterol and increased fecal fat excretion when fed at 10% of the diet (23), and rice bran protein, which significantly lowered serum cholesterol compared to casein or fish protein in rats fed cholesterol-free diet (24). The hypocholesterolemic effect of rice protein was attributed to the higher arginine/lysine ratio in rice protein relative to animal protein.

C. Other Species

Rabbits fed 20% rice protein diet had significantly lower TC, VLDL cholesterol, and LDL cholesterol compared to those fed casein (25). In addition to the higher arginine/lysine ratio of rice protein compared to that of casein (1.13 vs. 0.44), the authors also suggested that the lower percentage of acetate-generating amino acids (valine, leucine, isoleucine, phenylalanine, tryptophan, and lysine) in rice protein versus casein (33.49 vs. 38.17%, respectively) may have been partly responsible for the cholesterol-lowering effects.

In male cynomolgus monkeys, rice bran oil significantly lowered TC and LDLc without affecting high density lipoprotein (HDL) cholesterol compared with a diet containing a mixture of butter oil, corn oil, and olive oil in an 8-week feeding study (26). In contrast, feeding a 50% rice bran diet to female cynomolgus monkeys fed increasing amounts of cholesterol for 9 months resulted in no plasma cholesterol reductions (27).

A stabilized rice bran diet with 7% TDF significantly lowered plasma cholesterol but not liver cholesterol in C57BL/6 mice compared to a fiber-free control diet when diets contained 0.06% cholesterol from ground beef (28).

In chicks fed a diet containing 0.5% cholesterol, 60% full-fat rice bran, and 24% fat, TC and LDL cholesterol were significantly lowered while HDL cholesterol was significantly increased, compared with the 7% fat control diet; however, when diets were made isocaloric (10.8% fat), LDL cholesterol significantly decreased and HDL cholesterol increased with no effect on TC (29). Defatted rice bran appeared to be devoid of any effect, suggesting that TC-lowering properties of rice bran in chicks may be associated with rice bran oil.

D. Human Studies

Unpolished rice showed a repressive effect on serum cholesterol and triglyceride elevations in adult males compared with those fed polished rice; the beneficial effect was attributed to the dietary fiber of the unpolished rice (30). Five healthy young men consumed brown rice with 27.9 g of neutral detergent fiber (NDF) per day for 14 days, resulting in significant increases in fecal wet weight, dry weight, water and fat excretion compared with those fed white rice with 13.7 g of NDF per day (31). Total plasma and HDL cholesterol levels were not significantly different from those with a polished rice diet, possibly due to the fact that total cholesterol concentrations in the subjects were in the lower part of the normal range. In a 4-week study, 24 mildly hypercholesterolemic men consuming 60 g/d of rice bran had 4% (nonsignificant) reductions in plasma LDL cholesterol and apo-B, significant increases in their HDL cholesterol/total cholesterol ratio, and no change in TC compared to those consuming wheat bran (32) (Table 4). It was concluded that a consumption of realistic amounts of a single food source of dietary fiber could provide a modest benefit to the antiatherogenic profile of plasma lipoproteins. In a 3-week crossover design study, significant reductions in plasma total and LDL cholesterol were observed in 11 subjects with moderately elevated blood cholesterol after consuming 100 g/d of rice bran or oat bran (33). Reductions were 10% (significant) during the first 3 weeks and 5% (nonsignificant) during the second 3-week period, with an overall reduction of 7% (Table 4). Cholesterol reductions with rice bran and oat bran were similar. In a recent 6-week noncrossover design study (34), moderately hypercholesterolemic adults achieved significant reductions in serum total and LDL cholesterol by consuming 84 g/d of a heat-stabilized, full-fat medium grain rice bran product or oat bran. The bran supplements were added to the subjects' usual daily intake of a low-fat, low-cholesterol diet and did not replace any dietary components. There were no significant differences between the serum cholesterol reductions with the rice bran product (8.3%) versus those with the oat bran (13.0%).

Addition of a mixture of 30 g each of rice bran and oat bran to the daily diets of 17 moderately hypercholesterolemic and hypertriglyceridemic individuals for 6 weeks resulted in no significant reductions in TC or HDL cholesterol (35). The authors suggested that the level of dietary fiber tested may have been inadequate or that increasing soluble fiber intake may not be the sole answer to reduce hyperlipidemia. Consuming 15 or 30 g/d of rice bran by 18 normocholesterolemic subjects for 3 weeks resulted in no significant changes in TC, LDL cholesterol, or HDL cholesterol, although triglycerides were significantly reduced with 15 g/d rice bran consumption compared with 15 g/d wheat bran (36). Again, the normocholesterolemic state of the subjects may have been partly responsible for the lack of effect.

Table 4 Plasma Cholesterol Lowering by Rice Bran in Human Studies

| | Plasma cholesterol, mg/dL | | | |
	Control	Treatment	Effect	Study
Phase I	235	211	Significant	33
Phase II	217	208	Not significant	33
15 days	247	204	Significant	38
30 days	247	183	Significant	38
4 weeks	245	242	Not significant	32

A 60-g mixture of rice bran oil and safflower oil (70:30) given for 7 days to 10 females per group was more effective in lowering TC than either of the oils alone (37,38); most of the subjects had normocholesterolemic basal levels at the start of each treatment. Other investigators also reported a beneficial effect when customary cooking oil was replaced with rice bran oil for 15 and 30 days, resulting in significant reductions in TC and triglycerides in 12 hypercholesterolemic and hypertriglyceridemic subjects (39) (Table 4). Significant cholesterol-lowering effects of γ-oryzanol were reported in hyperlipidemic patients who were given 300 mg/d γ-oryzanol for 3 months (40). Consuming a diet supplemented with 35.5 g/d of full-fat rice bran for 18 days significantly lowered serum cholesterol in 10 subjects, compared to a fiber-free control period, whereas 30 g/d of defatted rice bran was not effective (41), suggesting that cholesterol reductions were due to the lipid component of rice bran.

IV. SUMMARY

Animal and human studies show cholesterol-lowering from a hypercholesterolemic status with rice bran, with reductions occurring usually in the LDL (atherogenic) fraction. Specific rice bran fractions showing hypocholesterolemic activity include rice bran oil, unsaponifiable matter, and protein. There is a dose response to the level of rice bran and rice bran oil unsaponifiable matter for cholesterol reductions, but intact full-fat rice bran appears to be the most effective. This suggests that incorporation of intact stabilized rice bran into food products would be more effective than the fortification of food with isolated individual concentrated fractions of rice bran.

Possible mechanisms for cholesterol-lowering with rice bran include interference with absorption/reabsorption of dietary and/or endogenous lipid in the gastrointestinal tract and increased excretion of bile acids, which results in utilization of more cholesterol for bile acid synthesis. In addition, changes in hepatic LDL receptor activity have been reported with rice bran feeding (18), and the inhibition of cholesterol synthesis by tocols and tocotrienols (42) present in rice bran oil may also contribute to cholesterol reduction. The evidence to date suggests that several mechanisms may be simultaneously involved in the cholesterol-lowering effects of rice bran.

Atherosclerosis is a disease that apparently takes from 40 to 50 years to develop. The concept of a 2% reduction in risk with each 1% reduction in cholesterol in high-risk individuals is well accepted. With reported plasma total and LDL cholesterol reductions of 4–10% in subjects with moderate hypercholesterolemia, the available information suggests that inclusion of rice bran in the diet, along with a reduction of fat calories to 30% and saturated fat to less than one third of total fat, could prove to be healthful for the general population. Commercial interest generated by the health effects of rice bran has contributed to the introduction of numerous value-added rice bran–containing foods and food products such as breads, breakfast cereals, cakes, cookies, extruded snacks, muffins, pies, and snack bars. The popularity of the new rice bran products is encouraging and expected to continue with health-conscious consumers. Incentives are needed for the rice industry to increase the production and availability of stabilized rice bran for its incorporation into more healthful, value-added foods for human consumption.

REFERENCES

1. Randall JM, Sayre RN, Schultz WG, Fong RY, Mossman AP, Tribelhorn RE, Saunders RM. Rice bran stabilization by extrusion cooking for extraction of edible oil. J Food Sci 50:361, 1985.
2. Kahlon TS, Saunders RM, Sayre RN, Chow FI, Chiu MM, Betschart AA. Cholesterol-lowering ef-

fects of rice bran and rice bran oil fractions in hypercholesterolemic hamsters. Cereal Chem 69:485, 1992.

3. Sharma RD, Rukmini C. Rice bran oil and hypocholesterolemia in rats. Lipids 21:715, 1986.

4. Itoh T, Tamura T, Matsumoto T. Sterol composition of 19 vegetable oils. J Am Oil Chemists Soc 50:122, 1973.

5. Seetharamaiah GS, Prabhakar JV. Oryzanol content of Indian rice bran oil and its extraction from soap stock. J Food Sci Technol 23:270, 1986.

6. Connor MA, Saunders RM, Kohler GO. Rice bran protein concentrates obtained by wet alkaline extraction. Cereal Chem 53:488, 1976.

7. Spady DK, Dietschy JM. Rates of cholesterol synthesis and low-density lipoprotein uptake in the adrenal glands of the rat, hamster and rabbit in vivo. Biochim Biophys Acta 836:167, 1985.

8. Kahlon TS, Saunders RM, Chow FI, Chiu MM, Betschart AA. Effect of rice bran and oat bran on plasma cholesterol in hamsters. Cereal Foods World 34:768, 1989.

9. Haumann BF. Rice bran linked to lower cholesterol. J Am Oil Chemists Soc 66:615, 1989.

10. Kahlon TS, Saunders RM, Chow FI, Chiu MM, Betschart AA. Influence of rice bran, oat bran, and wheat bran on cholesterol and triglycerides in hamsters. Cereal Chem 67:439, 1990.

11. Kahlon TS, Chow FI, Sayre RN, Betschart AA. Cholesterol-lowering in hamsters fed rice bran at various levels, defatted rice bran and rice bran oil. J Nutr 122:513, 1992.

12. Kahlon TS, Chow FI, Knuckles BE, Chiu MM. Cholesterol-lowering effects in hamsters of β-glucan-enriched barley fraction, dehulled whole barley, rice bran, and oat bran and their combinations. Cereal Chem 70:435, 1993.

13. Kahlon TS, Chow FI, Chiu MM, Hudson CA, Sayre RN. Cholesterol-lowering by rice bran and rice bran oil unsaponifiable matter in hamsters. Cereal Chem 73:69, 1996.

14. Ayano Y, Ohta F, Watanabe Y, Mita K. Dietary fiber fractions in defatted rice bran and their hypocholesterolemic effect in cholesterol-fed rats. J Nutr Food (Japan) 33:283, 1980.

15. Aoe S, Ohta F, Ayano Y. Effect of rice bran hemicellulose on the cholesterol metabolism in rats. Nippon Eiyoshokuryo Gakkaishi 42:55, 1989.

16. Johnson IT, Gee JM, Brown JC. A comparison of rice bran, wheat bran and cellulose as sources of dietary fibre in the rat. Food Sci Nutr 42F:153, 1989.

17. Rouanet J-M, Laurent C, Besancon P. Rice bran and wheat bran: selective effect on plasma and liver cholesterol in high-cholesterol fed rats. Food Chem 47:67, 1993.

18. Topping DL, Illman RJ, Roach PD, Trimble RP, Kambouris A, Nestel PJ. Modulation of the hypolipidemic effect of fish oils by dietary fiber in rats: studies with rice and wheat bran. J Nutr 120:325, 1990.

19. Sharma RD, Rukmini C. Hypocholesterolemic activity of unsaponifiable matter of rice bran oil. Indian J Med Res 85:278, 1987.

20. Seetharamaiah GS, Chandrasekhara N. Studies on hypocholesterolemic activity of rice bran oil. Atherosclerosis 78:219, 1989.

21. Seetharamaiah GS, Chandrasekhara N. Effect of oryzanol on cholesterol absorption & biliary & fecal bile acids in rats. Indian J Med Res [B] 92:471, 1990.

22. Seetharamaiah GS, Krishnakantha TP, Chandrasekhara N. Influence of oryzanol on platelet aggregation in rats. J Nutr Sci Vitaminol 36:291, 1990.

23. Ishibashi G, Yamamoto M. Effect of rice wax, garlic, and gingko seed component on plasma and liver cholesterol levels in rats. Kyushi Women's Univ 16:115, 1980.

24. Sugano M, Ishiwaki N, Nakashima K. Dietary protein-dependent modification of serum cholesterol level in rats. Ann Nutr Metab 28:192, 1984.

25. Alladi S, Gilbert R, Shanmugasundaram KR. Lipids, lipoproteins and lipolytic activity in plasma with dietary protein changes. Nutr Rep Int 40:653, 1989.

26. Nicolosi RJ, Ausman LM, Hegsted DM. Rice bran oil lowers serum total and low density lipoprotein cholesterol and apo B levels in nonhuman primates. Atherosclerosis 88:133, 1991.

27. Malinow MR, McLaughlin P, Papworth L, Naito HK, Lewis LA. Effect of bran and cholestyramine on plasma lipids in monkeys. Am J Clin Nutr 29:905, 1976.

28. Hundemer JK, Nabar SP, Shriver BJ, Forman LP. Dietary fiber sources lower blood cholesterol in C57BL/6 mice. J Nutr 121:1360, 1991.

29. Newman RK, Betschart AA, Newman CW, Hofer PJ. Effect of full-fat or defatted rice bran on serum cholesterol. Plant Foods Hum Nutr 42:37, 1992.

30. Suzuki M. Repressive effect of dietary fiber fractions in unpolished rice on the increase in cholesterol and triglyceride. J Nutr Food (Japan) 35:155, 1982.

31. Miyoshi H, Okuda T, Oi Y, Koishi H. Effects of rice fiber on fecal weight, apparent digestibility of energy, nitrogen and fat, and degradation of neutral detergent fiber in young men. J Nutr Sci Vitaminol 32:581, 1986.

32. Kestin M, Moss R, Clifton PM, Nestel PJ. Comparative effects of three cereal brans on plasma lipids, blood pressure, and glucose metabolism in mildly hypercholesterolemic men. Am J Clin Nutr 52: 661, 1990.

33. Hegsted M, Windhauser MM, Morris SK, Lester SB. Stabilized rice bran and oat bran lower cholesterol in humans. Nutr Res 13:387, 1993.

34. Gerhardt AL Gallo NB. Full-fat rice bran and oat bran similarly reduce hypercholesterolemia in humans. J Nutr 128:865, 1998.

35. Ranhotra GS, Gelroth JA, Reeves RD, Rudd MK, Durkee WR, Gardner JD. Short-term lipidemic responses in otherwise healthy hypercholesterolemic men consuming foods high in soluble fiber. Cereal Chem 66:94, 1989.

36. Sanders TAB, Reddy S. The influence of rice bran on plasma lipids and lipoproteins in human volunteers. Eur J Clin Nutr 46:167, 1992.

37. Suzuki S, Oshima S. Influence of blending of edible fats and oils on human serum cholesterol level (Part 1). Blending of rice bran oil and safflower oil. J Nutr (Japan) 28:3, 1970.

38. Suzuki S, Oshima S. Influence of blending oils on human serum cholesterol (Part 2). Rice bran oil, safflower oil, sunflower oil. J Nutr (Japan) 28:194, 1970.

39. Raghuram TC, Rao UB, Rukmini C. Studies on hypolipidemic effects of dietary rice bran oil in human subjects. Nutr Rep Int 39:889, 1989.

40. Yoshino G, Kazumi T, Amano M, Tateiwa M, Yamasaki T, Takashima S, Iwai M, Hatanaka H, Baba S. Effects of gamma-oryzanol and probucol on hyperlipidemia. Curr Therap Res 45:975, 1989.

41. Tsai CE, Ting H, Wang L-J, Lin T. The effect of rice bran on blood lipids in man. J Chinese Agric Chem Soc 30:484, 1992.

42. Qureshi AA, Burger WC, Peterson DM, Elson CE. The structure of an inhibitor of cholesterol biosynthesis isolated from barley. J Biol Chem 261:10544, 1986.

29

Sugar Beet Fiber
Production, Composition, Physicochemical Properties, Physiological Effects, Safety, and Food Applications

Jean-François Thibault, C. M. G. C. Renard, and F. Guillon
Institut National de la Recherche Agronomique, Nantes, France

I. INTRODUCTION

Sugar beet fiber is primarily derived from the sugar beet industry, where it is obtained from the co-product (sugar beet pulp) after extraction of sucrose. Sugar beet roots contain about 15% sucrose and about 5% cell wall polysaccharides on a wet weight basis. For sugar production, the roots are first washed to eliminate sand and other inorganic materials and then are sliced. Heat treatments aiming at facilitating diffusion and increasing sugar recovery are then applied to the slices. These treatments typically consist of heating at 85°C for approximatively 15 minutes followed by diffusion by water, typically 2 hours at ~65°C and pH ~ 6.5. The resultant products are a sucrose-containing juice (which is treated to produce crystallised sugar) and pulp. The pulp (dry matter ~ 8%) may be pressed (dry matter ~ 20%) or dried (dry matter ~ 90%). It is a very abundant and cheap by-product—production in France is equivalent to 1.5 million tons (dry matter) of beet pulp per year.

The pulp is primarily used as animal feed. However, alternative uses are currently proposed in order to increase the value of the pulp. The extraction of polysaccharides (pectins, arabinans, cellulose) or monomeric components (arabinose, galacturonic acid, rhamnose, ferulic acid) may be one method to increase its value (Vogel, 1991; Broughton et al., 1995; Micard et al., 1996). For example, arabinan extracted from the pulp has been investigated as a fat replacement (Cooper et al., 1992).

Another possibility is to find direct uses for the pulp. Because this residue consists mainly of cell wall polysaccharides, several if not all sugar companies have studied the use of sugar beet pulp as a high-fiber food ingredient or dietary fiber.

II. PRODUCTION OF THE FIBER

A. Sugar Beet Pulp Processing

Beet pulp must be processed before it can be used in food systems because it has an unpleasant flavor, may be too brightly colored, and also may contain large amounts of soil or sand (Tjebbes, 1988). The way of drying (Miranda Bernardo et al., 1990), the removal of most of the taste, color, and odor are especially important for beet fiber, as is the removal of all traces of soil. Physical treatments including cleaning, extraction, sieving, and heating have been mainly described, although some chemical treatments have been also proposed. With special processing it is possible to produce a dietary fiber with an off-white color and unobstrusive flavor, suitable for human food. The fiber may be milled to a given particle size from coarse to fine, depending on the intended use, or treated with steam in a flaking process.

Another method is to use not the beet pulp but the beet root as a starting material and to mimic the sugar extraction while minimizing or avoiding color/odor formation as well as the presence of soil or sand by special washing of the roots.

Several processes have been patented and trade names have been given for such fibers as DuoFiber by American Crystal Sugar Company (Lee, 1988), Fibrex by Fibrex S.A., Danisco Sugar AB (Tjebbes, 1988), and Betafiber/Atlantis by British Sugar (Williams et al., 1994). Fibers have also been developed in the United States by General Foods (Beale et al., 1984) and in France by SRD (Michel et al., 1985a, 1988). Fibrex and Atlantis are the main commercial products today.

Steam drying for Fibrex uses superheated steam to extract moisture from the fiber, preventing overdrying and reducing energy costs. The process optimizes temperature, pressure, and time, as well as removing sand from the end product.

British Sugar developed Betafiber in the late 1980s (Harland, 1993) and patented the process to obtain, directly from beet roots, palatable products with partial or complete sugar extraction (Williams et al., 1994). The products are sold by a Atlantis Food Ingredients, founded in 1994 by British Sugar.

The commercial fibers are generally claimed to consist of one third water-soluble and two thirds water-insoluble fibers; however, the values may be obtained by methods that overestimate the water-soluble dietary fibers because of some extraction of pectic material (Thibault et al., 1994).

B. Modification of Beet Fiber

In order to increase the ratio of soluble to insoluble dietary fiber in sugar beet as well as to change its hydration properties, some modifications have been proposed. Physical treatments such as extrusion cooking (Thibault et al., 1988; Ralet et al., 1991) or enzyme treatment combined with extrusion cooking (Jezek et al., 1996), autoclaving (Guillon et al., 1992), or chemical means (Bertin et al., 1988) have been applied to the fibers, mainly at a laboratory scale, in order to modulate the nutritional effects and/or to improve their functional properties.

III. COMPOSITION AND STRUCTURE

Dietary fiber in the sugar beet comes exclusively from its cell walls and is devoid of resistant starch or other reserve polysaccharides. The structure and composition of the dietary fiber from sugar beet is different of that of fiber from cereals for two reasons: (a) botanical origin—the cell walls of the Poaceae (formerly Gramineae) are actually an exception among land plants, and (b) tissue type—the part of beet that is used is a reserve parenchyma, with thin, nonsecondarized cell walls, in contrast to brans. This leads to very different physicochemical properties, with high hydration capacities and a high proportion of soluble dietary fiber. As such, beet fiber can be considered as an intermediate between the insoluble dietary fibers from cereals and the soluble dietary fibers.

Table 1 Dietary Fiber Composition of Sugar Beet Fiber Preparations

	TDF	SDF	IDF	ADF	NDF
Sugar beet fiber (1)					
native	871 ± 40	154 ± 2	717 ± 38		
autoclaving 122°C	784 ± 19	259 ± 11	525 ± 80		
autoclaving 136°C	786 ± 19	297 ± 11	489 ± 8		
Sugar beet fiber (2)	723	202	521		
	723	125	603		
Sugar beet fiber (3)	722	161	561		
Sugar beet fiber (4)	740	245	⌐ 495	267	556
(pepsin/pancreatin)	874	205	669	304	748
Sugar beet fiber (5)				291	569
Sugar beet fiber (6)				245	560
Apple AIS	859	225	634		
Apple fiber	597	134	463		

Source: (1) Guillon et al., 1992; (2) Thibault et al., 1994; (3) Dongowski et al., 1998; (5) Ozboy et al., 1998; (4) Schweizer and Wursch, 1979; (6) Michel et al., 1988; (7) Renard and Thibault, 1991.

A. Composition

Sugar beet pulp has a high dietary fiber content, typically >750 mg/g, and is known for its high soluble fiber content (10–20%) (Table 1). The AOAC method, because of its lengthy enzyme incubations at pH close to neutral, may overestimate the amount of fiber actually solubilized in the upper parts of the digestive tract. Extraction of beet pulp with water at low pH only leads to solubilization of approximately 20 mg of polymeric material per g of beet pulp (Rombouts and Thibault, 1986a; Thibault et al., 1994) (Table 2). The lignin content of beet fiber is low (Table 1 and 3). The remainder of the fiber preparations (Table 1 and 3) consist of proteins, in amounts varying according to the mode of preparation, ash, and lipids (<20 mg/g) (Harland, 1993). Some sugar beet pulp fractions may be high in ash (Michel et al., 1988) arising from contamination by soil particles.

Global characterization of beet fiber often refers to a high "hemicellulose" content (Table 1), (Harland 1993; Clarke and Edye, 1996), but the methods used, developed for grasses or forage crops, do not adapt very well to this type of material. Whether measured by difference between "neutral detergent soluble fraction" and "acid detergent soluble fraction," by difference between total carbohydrates and the sum of cellulose and galacturonic acid, or as pentosans (by analogy with cereals in which pentose sugars are present as hemicellulosic heteroxylans), in beet cell walls this mainly refers to arabinose, by far the main pentose present (>90%). This

Table 2 Global Composition of Beet Fibers

	Cellulose	Hemicellulose[a]	Pectin[b]	Lignin	Proteins	Ash
Sugar beet fibre (1)	230–270	260–290	240–290	30–50		
Sugar beet pulp (2)	220	320	270	20	70	80
Sugar beet fiber (3)	272	221		19	87	32
Beta fibre (4)	184	294	220		95	35

Source: (1) Clarke & Edye, 1994; (2) Dinand et al., 1997; (3) Ozboy et al., 1998; (4) Harland, 1993.
[a] Pentosans or difference between cellulose and galacturonic acid; here mainly as arabinan components of beet pectin.
[b] Galacturonic acid.

Table 3 Composition of Sugar Beet Cell Walls and Fiber Preparations (mg/g)

	Rha	Ara	Xyl	Man	Gal	Glc	GalA	MeOH	AcOH	Phenolic acids (FeA)	Protein	Lignin	Ash
Sugar beet AIS (1)	18	189	15	11	58	263	194	25	44	15	86		41
Sugar beet fiber (2)	10	201	14	12	49	216	221	26	38	(8)	36		44
Sugar beet fiber (3)	11	173	15	15	43	217	189	23	36	13 (9)	80	18	84
Sugar beet pulp (4)	24	209	17	11	51	211	211	18	39	8	113		36
Sugar beet NSP (5)	12	190	14	14	40	243	153						
Apple AIS (6)	15	81	51	18	64	277	345	36	21	0	69		22
Apple fiber (6)	7	62	33	23	35	266	142	17	12		67		29

AIS = Ethanol insoluble solids (from fresh beets or apples); NSP = nonstarchy polysaccharides.
Source: (1) Renard and Thibault, 1993; (2) Guillon et al., 1992; (3) Bertin et al., 1988; (4) Micard et al., 1996; (5) Spagnuolo et al., 1997; (6) Renard and Thibault, 1991.

arabinose forms arabinan and the arabinogalactan side chains of the sugar beet pectins and is a small part of hemicellulose.

In more detailed studies of their composition, beet cell walls, and therefore sugar beet fiber, are characterized by a very high pectin content (Table 3), with about 200 mg/g each of galacturonic acid and arabinose. This amount of pectin and more specifically of arabinose is exceptionally high even in comparison to cell walls from other dicotyledons (Table 3). Sugar beet fiber also contains approximatively 200 mg/g of glucose, mainly of cellulosic origin; in total, sugars add up to about 80% of the dry weight, with remarkably low amounts of xylose and mannose, again also in comparison with other dicotyledons. The pectin in sugar beets is methylated (DM 50–70), although with a lower DM than apple or citrus, and is also acetylated (DAc ~ 60 on the whole cell wall). Sugar beet cell walls also contain phenolic acids (<10 mg/g), mainly ferulic acid. Although quantitatively minor, these phenolic acids are thought to be of major importance in the structure of the beet cell wall.

There are few differences in global sugar composition between cell wall material isolated from raw beets and sugar beet pulp (Table 3). Le Quéré et al. (1981) found 45 mg of water-soluble pectin per g of alcohol-insoluble solids (AIS) for beet slices and, surprisingly, still 33 mg/g for beet pulp after diffusion. This low extraction of pectins could be due to physical limitations to diffusion of the pectic polymers from the cell wall network or to the structure of beet cell walls. Little material is extracted from beet cell walls in mild, nondegradative conditions. Dea and Madden (1986) only extracted a total of 50 mg/g dry matter from whole beets by successive cold and hot water treatments at pH 3.7, and Renard and Thibault (1993) only extracted 56 mg/g from whole beet AIS by buffer at pH 4.5 and room temperature, in contrast to 289 mg/g at pH 6.5 and 80°C. This material as well as the soluble dietary fiber in sugar beet are of pectic nature, rich in galacturonic acid and arabinose; soluble dietary fiber of beet probably has a relatively low viscosity, as might be inferred from low intrinsic viscosities obtained for pectin extracts, whatever the method (Table 4).

B. Structure

Sugar beets are mainly composed of parenchymal tissue with thin, supple and hydrophilic cell walls. Typical primary cell walls of dicotyledonous plants are composed of almost equal amounts of three types of polysaccharides: (a) pectin, rich in galacturonic acid and containing the main neutral sugars galactose, arabinose, and rhamnose, (b) hemicelluloses, typically xyloglucans with minor amounts of (gluco)mannans, and (c) cellulose. The structure of these cell walls has

Table 4 Composition (mg/g) of Beet IDF and SDF According to the AOAC Method and of Water-Insoluble and Soluble Material

	Yield[a]	Rha	Ara	Xyl	Man	Gal	Glc	GalA	MeOH	AcOH	Protein	Ash
AOAC method:												
IDF	603	16	246	16	14	61	296	196	14	35	—	—
SDF	125	9	79	tr.	42	31	6	434	44	43	—	—
Water at 20–22°C												
Residue	815	12	192	14	10	49	222	217	20	38	95	54
Soluble polymers	18	12	161	tr.	tr.	61	12	316	—	—	—	—

[a] In mg/g beet pulp.

—: Not determined; tr.: traces.

Source: Thibault et al., 1994.

given rise to a number of models (Carpita and Gibeaut, 1993) and can be summarized as three interlocking networks, namely cellulose/xyloglucans, pectin, and cell wall glycoproteins. Sugarbeet cell walls differ from this blueprint in a number of key points which will be unterlined in the next paragraphs.

1. Pectins

Most data on the structure of the constitutive polysaccharides of sugar beet cell walls and fiber deal with the pectic fraction (Table 5). Sugar beet pectins have distinctive features, notably high acetic acid contents and presence of phenolic esters on their side chains. They also contain a high proportion of "hairy regions," with very high arabinose and lesser rhamnose contents.

The pectins from sugar beet do not form gels in the usual conditions, i.e., either with calcium or with high sugar concentrations and acidic conditions (Michel et al., 1985b; Williamson et al., 1990). This inability has been ascribed variously to the presence of acetyl groups (Pippen et al., 1950), which indeed hinders binding of ions (Kohn and Malovikova, 1978), to low molecular weight (Roboz and Van Hook, 1946; Michel et al., 1985b), or to excessive amounts of side chains (Keenan et al., 1985). Acetyl groups are the most likely candidates for this inhibition of gelification. The presence of phenolic acids (mostly ferulic acid) (Rombouts and Thibault, 1986a) as esters on the side chains can, however, be used for chemical crosslinking of pectins, which can lead to gel formation in vitro (Thibault and Rombouts, 1986).

a. Backbone. The backbone of pectins is composed of α-(1 → 4)-linked D-galacturonic acid units interrupted by the insertion of α-(1 → 2)-rhamnose. Controlled acid hydrolysis of beet pectins (Thibault et al., 1993) led to isolation of homogalacturonans of DP 70–100, comprising less than one rhamnose unit per polymer. The rhamnose residues are concentrated in rhamnogalacturonans, where they alternate with the galacturonic acid residues (Sakamoto and Sakai, 1994; Renard et al., 1998). Beet pectins, with a rhamnose: galacturonic acid ratio of >1: 10 in the cell wall, are rich in rhamnose (Table 3). In the pectins, about 40% of the rhamnose residues are further substituted at position 4 by neutral sugar side chains (Table 6).

Rhamnogalacturonan II, a small complex pectic polysaccharide, and its boron-crosslinked dimer can be isolated from beet after enzymic digestion (Ishii and Matsunaga, 1996).

b. Side Chains. Other constituent sugars are attached in side chains. In beet pectins, the side chains are composed of arabinose and galactose; other sugars (xylose, glucose, mannose) are present in negligible amounts (Rombouts and Thibault, 1986a; Guillon and Thibault, 1989). The xylogalacturonan subunit of pectins is thus very low if not absent in beet pectins.

Methylation analysis (Table 6) shows presence of arabinans with a backbone of α-(1→5)-linked arabinofuranosyl residues carrying ramifications predominantly on O-3. With similar amounts of chain and ramified residues, beet arabinans are highly branched.

The galactose residues are mostly present as type I galactans, i.e., linear chains of β-(1→4)-linked galactose residues, but the partially methylated derivatives also indicate presence of type II galactans (Table 6) (Guillon and Thibault, 1989; Oosterveld et al., 1996).

NMR analysis of sugar beet pectin supports the evidence of methylation analysis with presence of 1→5-linked α-L-arabinose and 1→4-linked β-D-galactose residues (Keenan et al., 1985).

c. Nonsugar Substituents. In sugar beet, the pectin backbone carries both methyl esters (on the carboxylic group) and acetyl esters on the secondary alcools. Sugar beet pectins are not highly methylated, having a degree of methylation of about 50–60 (Table 5). The degree of acetylation of extracted beet pectins is generally 20–30, slightly lower in acidic extraction conditions (Table 5). The precise location of the acetyl groups is not known, but they are present both on the homogalacturonans of the "smooth regions" and on the rhamnogalacturonans of

Table 5 Extraction Conditions and Characteristics of Beet Pectins

	Yield	GalA	Rha	Ara	Gal	MeOH (DM)	AcOH (DAc)	FeA	[η] (mL/g)
HCl pH 1.5, 80°C, 4 h (1)	177	682				122 (75)	47 (25)		110
Oxalate NH₄ 0.25%, pH 3.5, 75°C, 1 h (1)	218	641				110 (67)	53 (29)		158
EDTA 0.5% + HCl 0.01 M 90°C 1 h (1)	189	532				97 (59)	49 (27)		208
EDTA 2% 85°C 1 h (2)	136	552	19	337	73				
HNO₃ pH 1 85°C 1 h (3)	129	623				(53)	(25)		
Cold water (pH 3.7)(4)[a]	23	600				57 (54)	74 (55)		200
Hot water (pH 3.7, 70°C)(4)[a]	28	520				39 (40)	90 (71)		140
Water 3 × 30 min, 20–22°C (5)[a]	22	544	9	84	65	72 (76)	57 (31)	1.0	259
Oxalate NH₄ 1%, 3 × 30 min, 20–22°C (5)[a]	5	779	9	19	24	81 (60)	40 (15)	0.4	57
HCl 0.05 M, 3 × 30 min, 85°C (5)[a]	199	651	23	100	59	71 (62)	75 (35)	4.8	225
NaOH 0.05M, 3 × 30 min, 4°C (5)[a]	111	549	32	125	81	7 (8)	7 (4)	5.7	181
Buffer pH 4.5 20–22°C (6)	56	513	13	101	51	28 (63)	56 (32)		187
CDTA pH 4.5 20–22°C (6)	71	484	11	82	46	46 (52)	44 (27)		257
Buffer pH 6.5 80°C (6)	289	456	19	164	55	43 (52)	53 (34)		70
CDTA pH 6.5 80°C (6)	275	484	16	143	48	48 (55)	57 (35)		100
Water 20–22°C (7)[a]	64	76	3	73	40	6 (41)	11 (41)	0	
NaOH 0.15 M + EDTA 0,05 M, 20–22° (7)[a]	151	388	30	293	46	—	—	1.5	
Autoclave pH 5.2 121°C (7)[a]	178	399	21	267	39	51 (70)	65 (48)	6.1	

[a] As part of a fractionated extraction scheme.

Source: (1) Arslan, 1995; (2) Wen et al., 1988; (3) Michel et al., 1985b; (4) Dea and Madden, 1986; (5) Rombouts and Thibault, 1986; (6) Renard and Thibault (1993); (7) Oosterveld et al., 1996.

Table 6 Glycosidic Linkage Analysis of Beet Cell Walls and Some Fractions Thereof (linkage types in mol%)

Derivatives	Linkage	Total fiber (1)	Pectin (HCl)(2)	Pectin (Autoclave) Total (3)	Pectin (Autoclave) DEAE (4)	4 M NaOH Total (3)	4 M NaOH DEAE (4)
Rhamnose		2.6 (2.1)[a]	9.3 (10.5)	1.3	5.7	2.6	0.4
2,3,4-Me3 Rha	Rhap-(1→			0.5	0.9	0.5	0.4
3,4-Me2 Rha	→2)-Rhap-(1→		5.6	0.4	2.8	1.1	
3-Me Rha	→2,4)-Rhap-(1→	2.6	3.7	0.4	2.1	1.0	
Arabinose		37.7 (40.6)	67.9 (67.5)	47.0	73.3	71.0	44.2
2,3,5-Me3 Ara	Araf-(1→	11.8	22.5	17.4	27.2	25.3	19.4
2,3,4-Me3 Ara	Arap-(1→		tr.				
3,5-Me2 Ara	→2)-Araf-(1→	0.6	0.7	0.5	0.7	0.8	
2,5-Me2 Ara	→3)-Araf-(1→		1.5				
2,3-Me2 Ara	→5)-Araf-(1→	14.0	20.6	14.2	21.4	23.1	13.3
2-Me Ara	→3,5)-Araf-(1→	11.7	18.7	11.8	17.5	16.9	10.2
3-Me Ara	→2,5)-Araf-(1→		2.3	0.9	1.2	1.5	
Ara	→2,3,5)-Araf-(1→	tr.	1.6	2.2	5.3	3.4	1.4
Galactose		7.6 (9.6)	22.8 (22.0)	3.7	13.9	7.9	4.0
2,3,4,6-Me4 Gal	Galp-(1→	0.7	5.2	1.8	4.1	2.7	2.2
2,4,6-Me3 Gal	→3)-Galp-(1→	1.2	3.8				
2,3,6-Me3 Gal	→4)-Galp-(1→	4.6	8.0	0.9	2.7	2.6	1.8
2,3,4-Me3 Gal	→6)-Galp-(1→	0.9	1.1	0.4	1.8	1.5	0.1
2,6-Me2 Gal	→3,4)-Galp-(1→	0.9	1.9				
2,4-Me2 Gal	→3,6)-Galp-(1→		2.8	0.3		0.3	
2,3-Me2 Gal	→4,6)-Galp-(1→			0.3	5.4	0.8	

Residue	Linkage					
Xylose		4.1 (3.2)	1.9	5.7	6.9	12.9
2,3,4-Me$_3$ Xyl	Xyl$p$-(1→	0.8	0.8	1.9	1.2	6.7
2,3-Me$_2$ Xyl[b]	→4)-Xyl$p$-(1→	3.3	0.3	2.5	5.3	6.1[c]
3-Me Xyl	→2,4)-Xyl$p$-(1→		0.4	1.7	0.2	
2-Me Xyl	→3,4)-Xyl$p$-(1→		0.4	0.6	0.2	
Mannose		2.4 (2.1)	0.8	0	2.2	7.3
2,3,6-Me$_3$ Man	→4)-Man$p$-(1→	2.4	0.8	0	2.2	7.3
Glucose		45.3 (42.2)	1.0	1.3	3.2	31.1
2,3,4,6-Me$_4$ Glc	Glc$p$-(1→	0.3				
2,3,6-Me$_3$ Glc	→4)-Glc$p$-(1→	40.9	0.9	0.5	2.8	21.1
2,6-Me$_2$ Glc	→3,4)-Glc$p$-(1→	0.5	0.1		0.4	
3,6-Me$_2$ Glc	→2,4)-Glc$p$-(1→	1.5				
2,3-Me$_2$ Glc	→4,6)-Glc$p$-(1→	2.1		0.8		10.1
Galacturonic acid[d]			44.2		6.1	
2,3,4,6-Me$_4$ Gal	GalAp-(1→		2.3		0.6	
2,3,6-Me$_3$ Gal	→4)-GalAp-(1→		39.4		4.2	
2,6-Me$_3$ Gal	→3,4)-GalAp-(1→		2.5		1.3	

[a] Total (based on analysis of alditol acetates).
[b] Not distinguished from 3,4 Me$_2$ Xyl.
[c] 3,4 Me$_2$ Xyl exclusively.
[d] Determined as galactose residues after carboxyl reduction.

Source: (1) Thibault and Rouau, 1990; (2) Guillon and Thibault, 1989; (3) Oosterveld et al., 1996.

the "hairy regions" (Rombouts and Thibault, 1986b). The rhamnogalacturonan fraction could have a higher degree of acetylation and lower degree of methylation than the homogalacturonans (Oosterveld et al., 1996). Location of the acetyl groups at position 2 or 3 of galacturonic acid is still uncertain; Keenan et al. (1985) by ^{13}C-NMR and Dea and Madden (1986) by ^{1}H-NMR identified three signals for acetyl groups, which would imply location at one position or both positions at once. In other plant materials, acetylation occurs mainly at O-2 in rhamnogalacturonans (Ishii, 1995) and at O-3 in homogalacturonans (Ishii, 1997a).

Among the dicotyledons, Chenopodiaceae in particular contain cell wall–bound phenolic acids (Table 3) (Ishii, 1997b). These include mainly ferulic acid, which represents about 0.8% of beet cell walls, and to a lesser extent p-coumaric acid (Rombouts and Thibault, 1986a). These phenolic acids are carried by the neutral sugar side chains of pectins (Rombouts and Thibault, 1986a, b). More precisely, they are esterified about 50–60% to the O-2 position of arabinose moieties and 40–50% to the O-6 position of galactose residues (Ishii, 1994; Ralet et al., 1994). Structural analysis of longer oligosaccharides (up to DP 8) showed that the feruloyl groups are linked to arabinose residues of the core chain of arabinans and to galactose residues of the core chain of type I galactans and not to extremities of the side chains (Colquhoun et al., 1994).

Phenolic acids are bifunctional and thus a potential crosslink of the beet cell wall (Fry, 1986). Indications in favor of that role are the presence of dehydrodimers of ferulic acid in sugar beet pulp (Table 7) and the possibility of crosslinking extracted beet pectins in vitro by oxidation of their feruloyl groups (Thibault and Rombouts, 1986; Oosterveld, 1997).

   d.   Distribution of Structural Elements.   After degradation of extracted pectins either by chemical β-elimination or using enzymes, two fractions are obtained, with the neutral sugars concentrated in a high molecular weight fraction and the galacturonic acid in a low molecular weight population (Rombouts and Thibault, 1986b; Guillon and Thibault, 1988). These results are in conformity with the perception of pectins as composed of "smooth," homogalacturonic regions and "hairy regions" where the rhamnogalacturonic backbone carries neutral sugar side chains (Voragen et al., 1995). The highest degradation occurred with polygalacturonase or pectatelyase after saponification (Rombouts and Thibault, 1986b). After degradation with polygalacturonase (Guillon and Thibault, 1988), most of the galacturonic acid is obtained as oligomer, with less than 20% of the galacturonic acid initially present being recovered in the high molecular weight fraction. This fraction ("hairy region") is composed mostly of neutral sugars, notably arabinose, galactose, and rhamnose.

The distribution of arabinans and galactans in the "hairy regions" has been studied by degradation with dilute acids (Guillon and Thibault, 1989) or specific enzymes (Guillon et al., 1989; Sakamoto et al., 1993; Sakamoto and Sakai, 1994). Digestion by a mixture of endoarabinase and arabinofuranosidase can lead to complete separation of the arabinose while the galactose is retained with the rhamnogalacturonan. These results indicate that galactan chains are directly linked to the backbone, while arabinans might be connected through an interposed

Table 7   Contents (mg/g) of Ferulic Acid and Its Dehydrodimers in the Cell Walls of Sugar Beet and in Extracted Pectins

	FeA	Total diFeA	Repartition of the types of dimers				
			8-8′	8-5′	5-5′	8-O-4′	4-O-5′
Sugar beet pulp (1)	8	1.40	12	48	9	31	nd
Sugar beet pectin (2)	15	1.43	27	21	16	37	nd
Sugar beet cell walls (3)	4	1.30	3.5	40.3	10.6	45.6	nd

nd: Not detected.
Source: (1) Micard et al., 1997; (2) Oosterveld et al., 1997; (3) Waldron et al., 1997.

galactan (Sakamoto et al., 1993; Sakamoto and Sakai, 1994). This is confirmed by the isolation of a small polymer composed exclusively of galactose, rhamnose, and galacturonic acid (molar ratio 1:1:2) after autoclaving and acid hydrolysis (C.M.G.C. Renard, unpublished results).

  e. Extraction and Molecular Weight. Sugar beet cell walls contain a very low amount of readily extractable pectin (by water or chelating agents at room temperature) even prior to the diffusion step (Table 5). Although calcium is present in sugar beet in amounts sufficient to neutralize most nonmethylated uronic acid (K. Farès et al., unpublished results), calcium cross-links do not seem to be the main mechanism holding the pectins in the beet cell wall.

  Efficient extraction can be obtained either by heating or by alkaline treatments (i.e., demands degradation of pectin). Autoclaving as well as heating at pH $\sim$ 6.5 (either with buffer, EDTA, or CDTA) leads to degradation of the pectic backbone through β-elimination and therefore to extraction. This results in the presence in the extract of two populations, namely a high molecular weight, neutral sugar–rich fraction (analogous to the "hairy regions" obtained after enzymic degradation) and a lower molecular weight fraction almost exclusively composed of galacturonic acid (Guillon et al., 1992; Renard and Thibault, 1993, Oosterveld et al., 1996).

  Hot acid treatments, comparable to those used for industrial extraction of pectins, lead to degradation first of the arabinan side chains. Acid-extracted sugar beet pectins can thus be characterized by a low neutral sugar content and conversely high galacturonic acid (Table 5). These acid-extracted sugar beet pectins have relatively low intrinsic viscosities and molecular weight (Rombouts and Thibault, 1986; Michel et al., 1985b; Arslan, 1995), compared in particular to pectin extracted in similar conditions from citrus or apple.

  Some pectins can be extracted from beet cell walls by alkali at room temperature (Oosterveld et al., 1996) and are therefore thought to be held in the wall by ester bonds, i.e., in beet cell walls to be crosslinked by dehydrodiferulates.

2. Hemicelluloses

Hemicelluloses can be defined as cell wall polysaccharides that have the capacity to bind strongly to cellulose microfibrils by hydrogen bonds (Roland et al., 1989). The common structural features of hemicelluloses are a main chain with a structural resemblance to cellulose and either short side chains that result in a pipe cleaner–shaped molecule or a different sugar interpolated in the main chain, both modifications preventing further aggregation (Carpita and Gibeaut, 1993). In the cell walls of land plants, three classes of polymers correspond to that definition, namely xyloglucans, heteroxylans, and mannans. In the primary cell wall of dicotyledons, the main hemicellulose is usually xyloglucan, which accounts for 15–20% of the dry weight of the wall.

  Beet cell walls have very low concentrations of the sugars that denote hemicelluloses, i.e., xylose, mannose, noncellulosic glucose, and fucose (Table 3), and their hemicelluloses have been very little studied. One of the problems encountered is prevalence of arabinans in all steps of fractionnated extraction schemes, as can be seen in Table 8. Oosterveld (1997) isolated from a 4 M NaOH beet extract a fraction enriched in hemicelluloses (Table 8), and methylation analysis of this material indicated presence of xyloglucans and mannans (Table 5). Degradation by a purified endo-glucanase of this fraction allowed identification of xyloglucan oligomers, which confirmed the presence, though in very low amounts, of a standard fucogalactoxyloglucan in beet cell walls.

3. Cellulose

Cellulose is the second most abundant polymer in beet fiber ($>$200 mg/g). Cellulose is a linear chain of β-(1→4)-linked glucopyranose. In cell walls, these chains form microfibrils with a

Table 8 Concentrated Alkali Extracts of Sugar Beet Pulp

	Yield	GalA	Rha	Fuc	Ara	Xyl	Man	Gal	Glc
NaOH 4 M, 20–22°C (after autoclave)(1)	263	123	29		296	30	17	71	36
NaOH 4 M, 20–22°C (after NaOH 0.15 M)(1)	208	106	47		389	43	20	91	42
KOH 1 M, 20–22°C (after oxalate 100°C)(2)	150	370	52	4	432	0	6	126	10
KOH 4 M, 20–22°C (after oxalate 100°C)(2)	95	231	46	12	379	123	4	138	66
NaOH 2.5 M, 20–22°C (after EDTA 85°C and pectinase) pH 5 precipitate (3)	168	5	108		140	232	220	130	214
NaOH 2.5 M, 20–22°C (after EDTA 85°C and pectinase) pH 5 supernatant (3)	88	41	105		217	125	144	169	260

Source: (1) Osterveld et al., 1996; (2) Kobayashi et al., 1993; (3) Wen et al., 1988.

parallel arrangement of the polymer chains. Beet cell walls contain typical primary cell wall microfibrils, 2–4 nm in diamater (Dinand et al., 1996). X-ray diffraction patterns indicate presence of cellulose IVI, i.e., of a type I cellulose with limited lateral order, probably due to limited size of the microfibrils (Dinand, 1997). Solid-state NMR of beet cell walls (C. M. G. C. Renard and M. C. Jarvis, unpublished results) indicates presence of 42% of crystal-surface chains, in good agreement with the diameter observed by microscopy (Dinand et al., 1996).

IV. PHYSICOCHEMICAL PROPERTIES

A. Cation-Exchange Capacity

Fibers from sugar beet behave as weak monofunctional cation-exchange resins with a CEC of about 0.5 mEq/g (Table 9). This ion-binding capacity is due to the presence of nonmethylesterified galacturonic residues, and the CEC is equal to the concentration of nonmethylated galacturonic acid residues calculated from independent galacturonic and methyl groups measurements (Bertin et al., 1988; Dronnet et al., 1997). Beet fibers are devoid of phytic acid, the main ion-binding species in cereal fibers. Beet pulp itself contains enough calcium to neutralize most of the free galacturonic acid (K. Farès et al., unpublished results). This calcium may be endogenous but may also arise from the pressing aids used during the sugar recovery process.

In spite of the presence of acetyl groups (Dronnet et al., 1996), pectin in sugar beet pulp is able to bind divalent cations, with higher affinities than in solution (Dronnet et al., 1997) but with the same selectivity scale: $Cu \sim Pb \gg Zn \sim Cd > Ni > Ca$.

B. Hydration Capacities

Basically, three different parameters can be measured: (a) swelling, (b) water retention capacity (WRC), i.e., the amount of water retained by a known weight of fiber measured by methods such as centrifugation, and (c) water absorption capacity (WAC), i.e., the ability of the fiber to absorb water measured using a Baumann apparatus or osmotic pressure/dialysis techniques.

Beet fiber has generally high hydration capacities, especially compared to fibers from cereal brans. However, these hydration properties are very variable depending on the fiber preparation and also on the conditions of measurement (Table 9). The main intrinsic factors are particle size and drying condition. High-temperature drying results in a decrease of hydration capacities (Cloutour, 1997), as does a decrease in particle size (Table 9). The effect of particle size on swelling can be due to increased interparticular spaces rather than increased hydration of the particles. Thermal or thermomechanical treatments increase the amount of soluble fiber in beet pulp and modify its hydration properties.

In addition, the measured hydration capacities are sensitive to extrinsic factors, such as ionic strength of the hydrating solution (Table 9) and its ion composition. These effects are mostly visible after conversion to the H^+ or Na^+ form or after saponification. Beet pulp then appears to behave as a polyelectrolyte resin. Presence of divalent cations results in a decrease in observed hydration capacities of deesterified beet pulp (Renard et al., 1994). A number of these effects might be masked in native beet pulp by the presence of a high calcium concentration. The conditions of hydration also play a role: presence of shear forces in the form of intense stirring can lead to a destructuring of the beet fiber and an increase in apparent WRC. This sensitivity to the exact method and conditions of measurement explains the variability of the results.

Table 9 Physicochemical Properties of Beet Fibers

Substrat	CEC (meq/g)	Swelling (mL/g)	WAC	WRC (centrifugation)
Beet pulp (1)	0.62			
Beet fiber (2)	0.47			
Native		11.5[a]		26.5[a]
Na[+] form		32.6[a]		30.8[a]
Beet fiber (3)	0.42	23.0[a]		34.0[a] (18.0[a])
Beet pulp (4)	0.48			
Native		11.0[a] (10.0[d])		26.6[a]
H[+] form		25.0[a]		22.5[a]
Beet pulp (5)	0.55			
H[+] form		17.8[a] (13.4[d])		23.9[a] (16.0[d])
Na[+] form		32.0 (15.3[a])		
Beet fiber (6)	0.60			
Beet fiber (7)	0.64		16.6	
Beet fiber (8)				
φ 540 μm		21.5[a] (19.8[d])	8.5[a] Baumann	24.2[b] 12.6[c] (11.8[d])
φ 385 μm		21.4[a] (19.3[d])	8.8[a]	22.6[b] 12.0[c] (10.9[d])
φ 205 μm		15.9[a] (16.3[d])	7.3[a]	19.2[b] 9.2[c] (9.6[d])
Beet fiber NDF fraction (9)	0.70			
Beet fiber NDF fraction (10)	0.57			
Saponified beet pulp (4)	1.12			
Native		25.0[a] (20.0[b])		24.8[a]
H[+] form		20.0[a]		20.7[a]
Saponified beet pulp (11)	1.13			
H[+] form		21.9[a] (12.6[b])		18.3[a] (8.3[d])
Na[+] form		32.4[a] (19.3[b])		
Extruded beet pulp (12)	0.39	14.4[a]		28.2[a]
Autoclaved beet pulp (3)				
at 122°C	0.35	20.0[a] (21.3[b])		35.0[a] (30.0[d])
at 136°C	0.20	21.0[a] (26.7[b])		38.4[a] (40.0[d])

NDF: neutral detergent fiber.

[a] In water.

[b] Long incubation, heavy stirring (in water).

[c] Short incubation, gentle stirring (in water).

[d] In presence of supporting salts.

Source: (1) Langenhorst et al., 1961; (2) Bertin et al., 1988; (3) Guillon et al., 1992; (4) Renard et al., 1994; (5) Dronnet et al., 1997; (6) Michel et al., 1988; (7) Özboy et al., 1998; (8) Auffret et al., 1994; (9) McBurney et al., 1983; (10) Allen et al., 1985; (11) Dronnet et al., 1998; (12) Ralet et al., 1991.

V. NUTRITIONAL STUDIES

A. Apparent Fermentability or Apparent Digestibility

Apparent fermentability and apparent digestibility were investigated in vitro with fecal inoculate (Guillon et al., 1992, 1998; Auffret et al., 1993; Salvador et al., 1993; Fardet et al., 1997) or in vivo in rats (Nyman et al., 1981; Champ et al., 1989) or in pigs (Graham et al., 1986; Longland et al., 1993). All indicated a high fermentability or apparent digestibility of sugar beet fiber, in the range of 70–90%. Galacturonic acid and arabinose were virtually completely digested; glucose about 85–88%; only xylose, present in small amount, was of low digestibility. It was shown in vitro that all sugars are not fermented at the same rate; glucose disappearance began more slowly than that of uronic acid and arabinose (Guillon et al., 1992, 1998; Auffret et al., 1993; Salvador et al., 1993; Fardet et al., 1998). The tridimensionnal arrangement of the polymers within the cell wall, and thus the access of bacteria or associated enzymes to the polymers, may account for this difference.

In these studies, the chemical composition of the fibers were identical or very close but their physical form and hydration properties varied greatly (Table 10), leading to differences in the rate of fermentation (Table 10). Processing of fiber, such as autoclaving or chemical extraction followed by drying, also influenced its fermentability (Table 10). Porosity, which could be approached by measurement of the swelling and water retention capacity, is an important factor controlling the fiber fermentation (Guillon et al., 1998).

The production of short chain fatty acids (SCFA) was analyzed in vitro (Rumney and Henderson 1990; Guillon et al., 1992, 1998; Auffret et al., 1993; Salvador et al., 1993; Fardet et al., 1997) and in vivo. In the latter case, the production was deduced either from measurement of SCFA in feces or cecal digesta of animals (Champ et al., 1989) or from dynamic analysis of porto arterial differences in the concentration of SCFA and of the portal blood flow rate in pigs (Michel and Rérat, 1998). The data confirmed the high fermentability of sugar beet fiber, especially when compared to other insoluble fibers (from cereal or legumes). Fermentation profiles, expressed as molar percent of each of the major SCFA—acetic (C2), propionic (C3), and butyric (C4)—was characterized by a high ratio of C2 (60–80) followed by C3 (11–23) and then C4 (9–15). In vitro, no alterations in the SCFA profile were observed when modulating the chemical composition and physicochemical properties of sugar beet fiber (Auffret et al., 1993; Guillon et al., 1998). The fact that both uronic acid and cellulose produced high amounts of acetate could be the explanation (McBurney and Thompson, 1989; Vince et al., 1990).

B. Sugar Beet Fiber, Transit Time, and Stool Output

The effect of sugar beet fiber on transit time and stool output was evaluated in healthy subjects (Cherbut et al., 1991), in patients complaining of chronic constipation (Giacosa et al., 1990), and in rats (Nyman and Asp, 1982; Johnson et al., 1990; Gallaher et al., 1992; Harland, 1993). Supplementation with sugar beet fiber increased wet fecal mass and number of daily stools. More diverse were the effects on transit time and dry fecal mass.

Sugar beet fiber (33 g/day) in the diet decreased transit time by 25%, as did the wheat bran supplemented diet (Cherbut et al., 1991). Both increased the number of daily stools and wet fecal mass. Weight of fecal water but not the dry fecal mass changed, while wheat bran increased both dry weight of fecal mass and fecal water. In rats the sugar beet diet increased the fecal output, as did the other fiber diets (Nyman and Asp, 1982; Johnson et al., 1990; Gallaher et al., 1992; Harland, 1993). Nyman and Asp (1981), Johnson et al. (1990), and Harland (1993) reported both wet and dry fecal mass increase. In constipated patients, a marked decrease in severe and moderate constipation at both the 15th and 30th days of treatment with sugar beet fiber was found, with a significant increase in fecal frequency normalization (Giacosa et al., 1990). Moreover, fecal consistency changed from hard and semi-hard stools to soft ones.

The mechanisms by which fiber influences transit time are still not fully understood. Different mechanisms have been suggested, which depend on the physical properties and fermentability of the fiber (Cherbut, 1995, 1998; Cherbut et al., 1998). The fiber may act by increasing the lumen volume, depending on the amount of indigestible residue in the colon, the water retention capacity of the residue, the stimulation of microbial growth, and the production of gas. The fiber can also reduce transit time through modulating colonic motility either by a mechanical stimulation of mechanoreceptors by the edges of the fiber particle (Tomlin and Read,

Table 10 Apparent Total Sugar Disappearance of Sugar Beet Fiber Samples after 6, 12, and 24 Hours of Incubation with Fecal Bacteria

Ref.	Treatment	Particle size (geometric mean particle size)	Water retention capacity (g water/g pellet dry matter)	Apparent total sugar disappearance (%)		
				6 h	12 h	24 h
Guillon et al., 1992	No	570 μm	18	32	64	86
Auffret et al., 1993	No	390 μm	17	43	72	85
Salvado et al., 1993	No	<80 μm	7	45	68	81
Guillon et al., 1998	No	480 μm	12	55	73	84
Guillon et al., 1992	Autoclaving	Not indicated	28	69	80	88
Guillon et al., 1998	Pectin extraction followed by soft drying	430 μm	15	28	48	72
Auffret et al., 1993		120 μm	22	58	81	87
Guillon et al., 1998	by harsh drying	120 μm	6	24	33	41

1988), or by a chemical stimulation by the products of fermentation (Cherbut, 1995), or by the release of compounds trapped by fiber, such as biliary acids or fatty acids (Cherbut, 1998). In the latter case, these products can stimulate not only colon motility but also secretion (Cherbut et al., 1998). Except for stimulation of mechanoreceptors, the different mechanisms mentioned above could contribute to the effect of sugar beet fiber on transit.

The increase in stool output by dietary fiber intake may have several causes (Cherbut, 1998); it could be related to the amount of excreted residue and its water-binding capacity. The increase of the bacterial mass can also contribute, since bacteria contain 80% water. Finally, the excreted water could be water not absorbed in the colon because of the short transit time or changes in colonic motility. Again, these different mechanisms can all participate in the increase in stool output.

C. Sugar Beet Fiber and Minerals

The effect of sugar beet fiber on the absorption of zinc, iron, copper, calcium, and magnesium was investigated in humans (Sandström et al., 1987; Cossack et al., 1992; Coudray et al., 1997) or rats (Fairweather-Tait and Wright, 1990; Harland, 1993) and led to the same conclusions. Sugar beet fiber has no negative effect on any of the minerals studied. These studies stressed the fact that beet fiber generally has a relatively high mineral content and can therefore contribute to mineral intake.

D. Sugar Beet Fiber and Glucose Metabolism

The effects of sugar beet fiber on glucose metabolism were investigated with different objectives. The effects on fasting plasma glucose and insulin values and on glucose tolerance of sugar beet fiber intake over a period of several weeks (from 3 to 8) were studied in normal (Tredger et al., 1991), normal but with high fasting cholesterol value (Frape and Jones, 1995), or non–insulin-dependent diabetes mellitus (NIDDM) subjects (Hagander et al., 1988, 1989). These parameters were regarded together with lipid parameters in order to better understand the mechanisms by which daily intake of dietary fiber can decrease the risks of cardiovascular disease. Experiments were also concerned with glucose tolerance (Tredger et al., 1981; Morgan et al., 1990; Leclère et al., 1993; Thordottir et al., 1998) in healthy volunteers or pigs and focused on acute effects of fiber supplementation.

No clear effect of long-term sugar fiber supplementation on fasting as well as postprandial blood glucose and insulin levels has been demonstrated (Table 11). The source, processing, and physical form of the fiber in the diet but also the nature of the meal (amount of fiber, amount of lipids, sources or carbohydrates, etc.), the metabolic status of the subjects, and the duration of the experiment may explain these differences. Similarly, discrepancies in blood glucose and insulin responses in normal subjects to a single meal with added sugar beet fiber are recorded in the literature (Table 12).

No clear mechanism explains the effect of sugar beet fiber on postprandial glucose level. It is well known that soluble high molecular weight fiber, such as oat or guar gum, can significantly decrease the postprandial circulating glucose level by slowing down the gastric emptying and/or influencing the diffusion and mixing of the intestinal contents. Sugar beet fiber is only partly soluble, and it is unlikely that this soluble fiber fraction can induce a sufficient increase in the viscosity of digesta to delay starch digestion or absorption, especially in the case of a solid meal. Another mechanism suggested is by changing transit time, but again, results in the literature are discordant. Morgan et al. (1990) observed a slightly accelerated liquid gastric

Table 11 Chronic and Postprandial Responses of Plasma Insulin and Glucose in Volunteers Given Sugar Beet Fiber Supplements

Ref.	Intake (g/day/subject)	Subjects	Duration	Results
Hagander et al., 1988	8	NIDDM	8 wks	Improvement in glucose response to a standardized breakfast
Hagander et al., 1989	40	NIDDM	8 wks	Blood glucose and insulin fasting or postprandial levels were not significantly affected
				In obese NIDD patient, postprandial insulin level tended to be lower after the beet diet period
Tredger et al., 1991	20	Healthy	16 days	No changes in blood fasting glucose and insulin concentrations
Frape and Jones, 1995	18	Healthy middle aged with mild risk ischemic heart disease	3 wks	No effect on fasting plasma glucose and insulin
				Effect on the postprandial parameters:
				decrease in the area under the glucose response curves by 6.9%
				decrease in the area under insulin response curve by 9.6%, although not significant

Table 12 Postprandial Responses of Plasma Insulin and Glucose in Volunteers Given Sugar Beet Fiber Supplements

Ref.	Intake (g per meal)	Carbohydrate (g per meal)	Subjects	Results
Tredger et al., 1981	20	86	Healthy male human volunteers	No difference in the mean blood glucose and plasma insulin curves at any time between the control and fiber diets
Morgan et al., 1995	10	100	Healthy male human volunteers	An improved glucose tolerance No change in insulin level Failure of sugar beet fiber to decrease postprandial insulin secretion despite improved glucose tolerance was ascribed to increased secretion of gastric inhibitory polypeptide
Thorsdottir et al., 1998	7	51 (liquid formula)	Healthy male human volunteers	Lower postprandial blood glucose and serum insulin response compared with the formula without fiber
Leclère et al., 1993	56	653	Pigs	No effect on postprandial glycaemic and insulinemic values
Michel and Rérat, 1998	114	446	Pigs	No difference in glucose absorption between sugar beet fiber and wheat bran supplemented diets

emptying with both sugar beet fiber and guar gum supplementation, which was unexpected. Hamberg et al. (1989) and Cherbut et al. (1991) found, respectively, a decreased and an increased mouth-to-cecum transit time in subjects fed sugar beet fiber.

E. Sugar Beet Fiber and Lipid Metabolism

Sugar beet fiber, because of its significant content of water-soluble fiber, has been investigated for its effects on lipid metabolism. Studies were carried out in humans with either healthy (Lampe et al., 1991; Tredger et al., 1991; Frape & Jones, 1995), hypercholesterolemic (Israelson, 1988,), or NIDMM subjects (Hagander et al., 1988, 1989; Travis et al., 1990) and in animals, pigs (Fremont et al., 1993), or rats (Johnson et al., 1990; Mazur et al., 1992; Nishimura et al., 1993; Overton et al,., 1994; Sonoyoma et al., 1995; Hara et al., 1998). Despite the fact that the dietary pattern (daily intake of dietary fiber, high-fat, low-carbohydrate diet, and vice versa) and the duration of the experiments (from 2 to 8 weeks) differed between the studies, most concluded that sugar beet fiber is hypocholesterolemic (Tables 13, 14). In humans, it tends to reduce serum total cholesterol and apo B levels without altering or even slightly increasing high-density lipoprotein cholesterol. Only some studies reported a decrease in serum triglycerides (Hagander et al., 1989, Travis et al., 1990, Mazur et al., 1992, Overton et al., 1994).

The mechanisms sustaining such effects are still not clear (Lairon, 1996). Dietary fiber may act as an hypocholesterolemic resin, which sequesters bile acids and cholesterol, with consequent interruption of the enterohepatic bile acid cycle in the small intestine (intestinal reabsorption of bile salts in humans is 96–98% efficient) and loss of cholesterol from increased fecal bile acid excretion. This mechanism was clearly demonstrated for viscous fiber such as guar gum and oat gum. In the case of sugar beet fiber, it seems not to be valid or at least not important, as most of the studies did not find a significant increase in excretion (fecal: Lampe et al., 1991; Gallaher et al., 1992; Overton et al., 1994; ileal: Langkilde et al., 1993) of bile acids. These results are in agreement with those from Morgan et al. (1993), who did not observe changes in concentrations of circulating postprandial bile acids in humans given an acute test meal supplemented with sugar beet fiber (10 g Betafiber per meal), contrary to guar gum or cholestyramine. This also fit with in vitro data, which showed that the insoluble fraction of sugar beet fiber bound only a small quantity of glycocholate and that no bile acids were associated with the soluble fraction (Morgan et al., 1993). In a study with ileostomists (Langkilde et al., 1993) a decrease of 26% of ileal bile acid excretion was noted while cholesterol excretion increased by 52% with the sugar beet fiber diet. The excreted amount of cholesterol corresponded to half of the mean daily intake of cholesterol in this experiment. This pattern is different from the pattern generally reported for water-soluble fiber such as oat, guar gums, or pectins. The cholesterol-lowering effect of sugar beet fiber may result from its interference with lipid absorption through alteration of the digestive processes. The reduced absorption of cholesterol results in a reduced supply to the liver, which as a secondary effect could decrease excretion of bile acids as they are synthesized from cholesterol in the liver (Langkilde et al., 1993). The influence of sugar beet fiber on lipid absorption may account at least for the acute postprandial effect of dietary fiber on lipemia, but the mechanisms involved have not been explored. Moreover, the extent to which the repetition of the single meal effect can lead to a new metabolic steady state in the long run remains be further investigated. In sugar beet fiber–fed rats, hypocholesterolemia was accompanied by a reduction in hepatic cholesterol and in circulating triacylglycerol and bile acids, with no increase in bile acid fecal excretion (Overton et al., 1994). The authors pointed out another possible mechanism involving disruption of the bile acid circulation, possibly via changes in the rate of absorption patterns of triacylglycerol and its subsequent handling by circulating lipoproteins.

Table 13 Effect of Sugar Beet Fiber on Lipid Metabolism (Human Studies)

Ref.	Intake (g/day/subject)	Subjects	Duration	Results
Israelsson et al., 1998	30	Hypercholesterolemic women	2–4 wks	Significant reduction of LDL cholesterol with no change in HDL
Hagander et al., 1988	8	NIDDM	8 wks	Lower fasting blood glucose Reduction of LDL cholesterol with no change in HDL Lower fasting levels of triglycerides Improvements in glucose response to a standardized breakfast
Hagander et al., 1989	40	NIDDM	8 wks	Decrease of 8% in total cholesterol when compared with the habitual diet, but no decrease compared with the low-fiber diet
Travis et al., 1990	18	NIDDM	6 wks	Decrease of 6.2, 10.6, and 6.0% in, respectively, total cholesterol, triglycerides, and Apo B levels
Lampe et al., 1991	30	Healthy volunteers	3 wks	Decrease of 12 and 15% in total and LDL cholesterol Small changes in HDL Significant decrease in serum triglycerides
Tredger et al., 1991	20	Healthy volunteers	16 days	Decrease of 4.6% in total cholesterol; decrease more marked with subject with a high habitual fat intake No change in HDL cholesterol and triglycerides
Frape and Jones, 1995	18	Healthy middle-aged volunteers	3 wks	Decrease of 8 and 9.6% in total and LDL cholesterol in subjects in whom fasting plasma cholesterol was above normal No difference in HDL cholesterol

Table 14 Effect of Sugar Beet Fiber on Lipid Metabolism (Animal Studies)

Ref.	Level of incorporation g/kg diet	Animals	Duration	Results
Johnson et al., 1990	100 g/kg semi-synthetic diet	Rats	28 days	Significant reduction of serum cholesterol, but less than that of guar gum
Mazur et al., 1992	300 g/kg fructose-based diet	Rats	3 wks	Decrease in plasma triglyceride and cholesterol concentration in the postprandial as well as the postabsorptive period Depress of the liver triglyceride level in concert with decreased liver lipogenesis No change in liver cholesterol level Animals less fat
Overton et al., 1994	100 g/kg semi-synthetic diet	Rats	28 days	Lower circulating cholesterol, hepatic cholesterol, and circulating triacylglycerol No change in total hepatic lipid concentrations and hepatic and adipose tissue lipogenesis
Sonoyoma et al., 1994	150 g/kg a cholesterol-free diet	Rats	14 days	Lower final total plasma cholesterol Lower HDL cholesterol and Apo A-I concentrations No significant changes in hepatic cholesterol The hypocholesterolemic effect is associated with diminished expression of the hepatic apolipoprotein A-I gene
Nishimura et al., 1993	100 g/kg 25% casein diet	Rats	28 days	Lower plasma total cholesterol Lower HDL cholesterol Lower digestive tract, especially cecum, seemed to be necessary for this effect
Frémont et al., 1993	120 g/kg semi-synthetic diet	Weaning piglets	4 wks	No change in serum cholesterol and HDL cholesterol concentrations Lower fasting triacylglycerol due to reduction in VLDL synthesis

Other mechanisms of action of dietary fiber have been suggested. Modification in hormonal status, especially insulin, could influence lipoprotein lipase activity, cholesterol and bile acid synthesis, and VLDL secretion. Only a few groups (Hagander et al., 1988, 1989; Tredger et al., 1991; Frape and Jones, 1995) have investigated the effects of sugar beet fiber on gastro-intestinal hormones and cholesterol. Most of the authors reported no significant changes in the fasting levels of insulin.

It has been suggested that the hypocholesterolemic effect of dietary fiber might also be mediated through the fermentation products, which can modify the activity of regulatory enzymes involved in hepatic cholesterol synthesis. A study in rats (Nishumura et al., 1993) has demonstrated that an intact cecum and colon is necessary for the fiber to be effective. One of the SCFA, propionate, has been shown in pigs and rats to significantly lower plasma and liver cholesterol concentrations and to inhibit cholesterol synthesis in isolated rat hepatocytes. However, no such effect has been reported in humans, and the role of propionate in reducing LDL cholesterol levels is controversial. Recently, Hara et al. (1998) suggested that acetate can contribute to the reduction in plasma cholesterol concentration in rats. However, no mechanism was proposed. Moreother, this conclusion was drawn from SCFA feeding. The absorption ratio of individual SCFA ingested orally may be different from products in the large intestine, which may result in a different effect on cholesterol metabolism. SCFA reaching the liver may have modulate lipid and carbohydrate metabolism, but more comprehensive studies with human or well-validated animal models and protocols must be carried out to elucidate the mechanisms involved. It seems therefore likely that the cholesterol-lowering effect of sugar beet fiber is not dependent on increased fecal bile acid and is affected by a number of factors rather than a single mechanism.

F. Further Information

1. Growth Performance in Animals

In rats, sugar beet fiber represented 100–300 g/kg in the diet. Inclusion of fiber in the diet had no effect on food intake in five of the six rat studies. Live weight gain and feed conversion were generally similar in rats fed control or fiber-supplemented diet (Johnson et al., 1990; Mazur et al., 1992; Harland, 1993; Nishimura et al., 1993; Overton et al., 1994; Sanoyama et al., 1995). However, Dongowsky et al. (1998) reported a higher consumption of food when the diet is enriched with sugar beet. They found a reduced mean food efficiency and a significant growth retardation in animals fed the highest fiber diets.

In pig studies, semi-synthetic diet or growing pig feed was used as control diet. The levels of sugar beet fiber varied from 170 to 330 g/kg diet. No particular adverse effect was reported. Longland et al. (1993) found a slightly reduced digestibility and metabolization of energy when pigs were fed a semisynthetic diet with high levels (287g/kg diet) of sugar beet pulp. Fremont et al. (1993) in weaning piglets found a 47% increase in the apparent feed-conversion efficiency after 4 weeks of dietary treatment with sugar beet fiber (120 g/kg diet). The higher feed intake could compensate for the energy dilution by fiber.

2. Tolerance to Sugar Beet Fiber

In human studies, the daily intake varied greatly—from 7 to 40 g per subject. Generally the intake of fiber was gradually increased, in particular when large doses were concerned. The form in which fiber was ingested also differed: it was included in foods (prepared dishes, bread, biscuits, chocolate bars), pressed into tablets, or mixed as a powder in water. Generally tolerance was good. Only a few studies reported cases of discomfort, abdominal cramping, and bloating or trouble with flatulence or borborygmi. This generally occurred with the largest doses. One study (Travis et al., 1990) mentioned that subjects (five of seven) found the sugar beet fiber–supplemented bread and biscuits less palatable than normal products, which led to a reduction in compliance during the last 2 of 6 weeks of sugar beet fiber supplementation.

Three studies (Israelsson et al, 1988; Travis et al., 1990; Tredger et al., 1991) reported an increase in energy and mean daily fat intakes during the period of sugar beet fiber supplementation. In these studies, fiber was incorporated into bread, and it was suspected that the increase resulted from an increased use of high-fat spread. However, no changes in subject body weight were noticed.

3. Sugar Beet Fiber and Colon Cancer

High concentrations of bile acids in the colon, particularly secondary bile acids, are generally associated with an increased risk of colon cancer. Gallaher et al. (1992) evaluated the effect of feeding high-fiber diets on bile acid excretion in rats. They showed that sugar beet fiber slightly increased the total bile acid daily excretion, but the fecal bile acid concentration was much lower than with the fiber-free basal diet. This concentration was even lower than with oat or rye bran diets. When compared to other sources of fiber, sugar beet produced the lowest concentration of lithocholic acid but the highest lithocholic acid:deoxycholic acid ratio. Which of these parameters is the most significant is still not clear. In vitro studies (Wilpart and Roberfroid, 1986) suggested that lithocholic acid is a potent promoter of mutagenesis. However, Owens et al. (1984) postulated that lithocholic acid:deoxycholic acid ratio is an indicator of increased colorectal cancer.

Ishizuka and Kasai (1997) found that sugar beet–supplemented diet fed for 4 weeks had a suppressive effect on the formation of aberrant crypt foci induced by 1.2-dimethylhydrazine in the colon rectum of rats. They suggested that butyrate may reduce the number of initiated colonocytes by apoptosis, which would result in a decrease of aberrant crypt foci.

4. Toxic Effects

Potential toxic effects of sugar fiber supplementation have not been extensively investigated (Gallaher et al., 1992; Dongowski et al., 1998). Dongowski et al. (1998) showed in rats that enrichment of the diet with sugar beet fiber preparation up to a level 10% for 4 weeks did not substantially influence urinary, hematological, or serum parameters indicative of a toxic effect.

VI. FOOD APPLICATIONS

Sugar beet fiber is claimed to offer nutritional benefits to consumers as well as manufacturing and functional advantages to food processors. Moisture retention, good texture, and mouthfeel are the main technical properties of the beet fibers, which are proposed with a variety of particle sizes for easy blending with other ingredients. The particle size is important for applications because the ability to bind water may be affected (Auffret et al., 1994) and because it may influence the texture of the product and the mouthfeel properties (Christensen, 1989). Generally, pale fibers with pleasant flavor are preferred, although some color may be of interest for some applications, for example, in cooking where some Maillard (browning) reactions occur.

Beet fiber also has the advantage of containing no phytic acid, a substance that may be found in cereal fiber and can tighly bind minerals, and no gluten, protein from wheat to which some people are allergic (Tjebbes, 1988).

Potential applications include cereals, bakery products, pasta, processed meats, soups, and snacks. Successful recipes have been proposed for pastries, cakes, biscuits, snack foods pasta and meat products. It can be used in breads as a natural improver and to maintain freshness. In biscuits, it increases the fiber content and in meat products, it may provide chewy and juicy character.

A. Ready-to-Eat Breakfast Cereals

The properties of the sugar beet fiber make it a good candidate for fiber enrichment in high-fiber ready-to-eat cereal applications (Christensen, 1989). It has been incorporated into extruded ready-to-eat cereals at high quantities (up to 40%) without affecting the mouthfeel, flavor, or color. This property can probably be ascribed to the high water-binding properties of the beet fiber.

Nonmilled version of the fibers or flaked versions are used in rather high amounts (up to 25%) in muesli products.

B. Bakery Products

Fiber-enriched breads have had large commercial success. Beet fiber can be successfully incorporated into a large variety of products; it acts as bulking agent as well as a dietary fiber source. The high water uptake of beet fiber can enhance the qualities of baked products as a result of softer mouthfeel, less staling, and low calorie content (Christensen, 1989; Svensson, 1992). No gritty mouthfeel is encountered with this type of fiber, in contrast to cereal fibers. Beet fiber can also be used for the production of soft cookies or muffins for which fibers with a high water binding capacity are required.

Cereal bran is generally used to increase the amount of dietary fiber content in breads, but this addition influences the color, the taste, as well as the texture/consistency of the product. Beet fiber may be used as a bread improver and may be added directly to the dough. The freshness of the baked products is increased without addition of additives—the bread is softer. Beet fiber may also be used to lower the calorie content of the bread product as its content of dietary fiber and its water uptake are high.

C. Other Uses

Beet fiber (1–2%) may be incorporated into meat loaves, patés, meat products, and sausages to give a juicy character even to frozen products and to improve consistency or texture (Christensen, 1989; Svensson, 1992).

VII. CONCLUSION

Historically, beet fiber has been the most extensively studied fiber and almost all sugar companies have invested in research and efforts to produce fiber with high qualities. Beet fiber has properties such as a significant proportion of soluble dietary fiber and a high water-binding capacity, which make it advantageous for many applications. Furthermore, this fiber is extremely well documented because it has been used as a standard fiber in many studies, both nutritional as well as functional.

Sugar beet fiber may fulfill a need and is a good complement to other dietary fiber sources. It is easy to include as an ingredient in different well-accepted foods at a level ranging generally from 5 to 15% (Harland, 1993). It is therefore easy to plan palatable diets that can give dietary fiber intake of about 35–40 g/day, which is excellent from a nutritional point of view. However, the presence of ash as well as the odor and taste of the pulp require physical treatments in order to obtain acceptable fiber. The cost of the product is therefore increased, which probably explains the relatively small amount of sugar beet fiber produced.

REFERENCES

Allen MS, McBurney MI, Van Soest PJ. Cation-exchange capacity of plant cell walls at neutral pH. J Sci Food Agric 36:1065–1072, 1985.

Arslan N. Extraction of pectin from sugar-beet pulp and intrinsic viscosity-molecular weight relationship of pectin solutions. J Sci Food Technol 32:381–385, 1995.

Auffret A, Barry J-L, Thibault J-F. Effect of chemical treatments of sugar-beet fibre on their physico-chemical properties and on their in vitro fermentation. J Sci Food Agric 61:195–203, 1993.

Auffret A, Ralet M-C, Guillon F, Barry J-L, Thibault J-F. Effect of grinding and experimental conditions on the measurement of hydration properties of dietary fibres. Lebensm Wiss Technol 27:166–172, 1994.

Beale RJ, Bradbury GW, Medcaff DG, Romig WR. Sugar beet pulp bulking agent and process. U.S. Pat. 4,451,489 (1984).

Bertin C, Rouau X, Thibault J-F. Structure and properties of sugar-beet fibres. J Sci Food Agric 44:15–29, 1988.

Broughton NW, Dalton CC, Jones GC, Williams EL. Adding value to sugar beet pulp. Int Sugar J 97:57–60, 93–95, 1995.

Carpita NC, Gibeaut DM. Structural models of primary cell walls in flowering plants: consistency of molecular structure with the physical properties of the walls during growth. Plant J 3:1–30, 1993.

Champ M, Barry J-L, Hoebler C, Delort-Laval J. Digestion and fermentation pattern of various dietary fiber sources in the rat. Animal Feed Sci Technol 23:195–204, 1989.

Cherbut C. Effects of short chain fatty acids on gastrointestinal motility. In: Cummings JH, Rombeau JL, Sakata T, eds. Physiological and Clinical Aspects of Short Chain Fatty Acids. Cambridge: Cambridge University Press, 1995, pp 191–207.

Cherbut C. Fibres alimentaires: que devient l'hypothèse de Burkitt? Etat des connaissances et questions non résolues. Cah Nutr Diét 33:95–104, 1998.

Cherbut C, Salvador V, Barry J-L, Doulay F, Delort-Laval J. Dietary effects on intestinal transit in man: involvement of their physico-chemical and fermentative properties. Food Hydrocolloids 5:15–22, 1991.

Cherbut C, Aubé A-C, Mekki N, Dubois C, Lairon D, Barry J-L. Digestive and metabolic effects of potato and maize fibres in human subjects. Br J Nutr 77:33–46, 1997.

Cherbut C, Ferrier L, Roz C, Anini Y, Blottière H, Lecannu G, Galmiche J-P. Short chain fatty acids modify the colonic motility through nerves and polypeptide YY release in rat. Am J Physiol, 275: G1415–G1422, 1998.

Christensen EH. Characteristics of sugarbeet fiber allow many food uses. Cereal Foods World 34:541–544, 1989.

Clarke MA, Edye LA. Sugar beet and sugar cane as renewable resources. In: Fuller G, McKeon TA, Bills DD, eds. Agricultural Materials as Renewable Resources. Nonfood and Industrial Applications, ACS Symposium Series 647, ACS Washington, 1996, pp 229–247.

Colquhoun IJ, Ralet M-C, Thibault J-F, Faulds CB, Williamson G. Structure identification of feruloylated oligosaccharides from sugar-beet pulp by NMR spectroscopy. Carbohydr Res 263:243–256, 1994.

Cooper JM, McCleary BV, Morris ER, Richardson RK, Marrs WM, Hart RJ. Preparation, physical properties and potential foods applications of enzymatically-debranched araban from sugar-beet. In:Phillips GO, Williams PA, Wedlock DJ, eds. Gums and Stabilisers for the Food Industry 6. (Oxford):IRL Press, 1992, pp 451–460.

Cossack ZT, Rojhani A, Musaiger AO. The effect of sugar-beet fibre supplementation for five weeks on zinc, iron, and copper status in human subjects. Eur J Clin Nutr 46:221–225, 1992.

Coudray C, Bellanger J, Castiglia-Delavaud C, Rémésy C, Vermorel M, Rayssiguier Y. Effect of soluble or partly soluble dietary fibre supplementation on absorption and balance of calcium, magnesium, iron and zinc in healthy young men. Eur J Clin Nutr 51:375–380, 1997.

Dea ICM, Madden JK. Acetylated pectic polysaccharides of sugar beet. Food Hydrocolloids 1:71–88, 1986.

Dinand E. Microfibrilles de cellulose: isolement à partir de pulpes de betterave, caractérisation et propriétés. Thèse de doctorat, University Joseph Fourier, Grenoble, France, 1997.

Dinand E, Chanzy H, Vrignon MR. Parenchymal cell cellulose from sugar beet pulp: preparation and properties. Cellulose 3:183–188, 1996.

Dongowski G, Plass R, Bleyl DWR. Biochemical parameters of rats fed dietary fibre preparation from sugar-beet. Z Lebensm Unters Forsch A 206:393–398, 1998.

Dronnet VM, Renard CMGC, Axelos MAV, Thibault J-F. Characterisation and selectivity of divalent metal ions binding by citrus and sugar-beet pectins. Carbohydr Polym 30:253–263, 1996.

Dronnet VM, Renard CMGC, Axelos MAV, Thibault J-F. Binding of divalent metal cations by sugar-beet pulp. Carbohydr Polym 34:73–82, 1997.

Dronnet VM, Axelos MAV, Renard CMGC, Thibault J-F. Improvement of the binding capacity of metal cations by sugar-beet pulp. I. Impact of cross-linking treatments on composition, hydration and binding properties. Carbohydr Polym 35:29–37, 1998.

Fairweather-Taits S, Wright AJA. The effects of sugar-beet fibre and wheat bran on iron and zinc absorption in rats. Br J Nutr 64:547–552, 1990.

Fardet A, Guillon F, Hoebler C, Barry J-L. In vitro fermentation of beet fibre and barley bran, of their insoluble residues after digestion and of ileal effluents. J Sci Food Agric 75:315–325, 1997.

Frape J, Jones AM. Chronic and postprandial responses of plasma insulin, glucose and lipids in volunteers given dietary fibre supplements. Br J Nutr 73:733–751, 1995.

Fremont L, Gozzelino M-T, Bosseau AF. Effects of sugar beet fiber feeding on serum lipids and binding of low density lipoproteins to liver membranes in growing pigs. Am J Clin Nutr 57:524–532, 1993.

Fry SC. Cross-linking of matrix polymers in the growing cell walls of angiosperms. Ann Rev Plant Physiol 37:165–186, 1986.

Gallaher DD, Locket PI, Gallaher CM. Bile acid metabolism in rats fed two levels of corn oil and brans of oat, rye and barley and sugar beet fiber. J Nutr 122:473–481, 1992.

Giacosa A, Sukkar SG, Frascio F, Ferro M. Sugar-beet fibre: a clinical study in constipated patients. In: Southgate DAT, ed. Dietary Fibre—Chemical and Biological Aspects. London: Royal Society of Chemistry, 1990, pp 355–361.

Graham H, Hesselman K, Aman P. The influence of wheat bran and sugar-beet pulp on the digestibility of dietary components in a cereal based pig diet. J Nutr 116:242–251, 1986.

Guillon F, Thibault J-F. Further characterization of acid- and alkali-soluble pectins from sugar beet pulp. Lebensm Wiss Technol 21:198–205, 1988.

Guillon F, Thibault J-F. Methylation analysis and mild acid hydrolysis of the ''hairy'' fragments of sugar beet pectins. Carbohydr Res 190:85–96, 1989.

Guillon F, Thibault J-F, Rombovis FM, Voragen AGJ, Pilnik W. Enzymic hydrolysis of the hairy fragments from sugar beet pectins. Carbohyd Res 190:97–108, 1989.

Guillon F, Barry J-L, Thibault J-F. Effect of autoclaving sugar-beet fibre on its physico-chemical properties and its in-vitro degradation by human faecal bacteria. J Sci Food Agric 60:69–79, 1992.

Guillon F, Auffret A, Robertson JA, Thibault JF, Barry J-L. Relationship between physical characteristics of sugar beet fibre and its fermentability by human fecal flora. Carbohydr Polym, 37:185–197, 1998.

Haganda B, Asp NG, Efendic S, Nilsson-Ehle P, Schersten B. Dietary fiber decreases fasting blood glucose levels and plasma LDL concentration in non insulin-dependent diabetes mellitus patients. Am J Clin Nutr 47:852–858, 1988.

Haganda B, Asp NG, Ekman R, Nilsson-Ehle P, Schersten B. Dietary fibre enrichment, blood pressure, lipoprotein profile and gut hormones in NIDDM patients. Eur J Clin Nutr 43:35–44, 1989.

Hamberg O, Rumessen JJ, Gudmand-Hoyer E. Inhibition of starch absorption by dietary fibre. A comparative study of wheat bran, sugar-beet fibre, and pea fibre. Scand J Gastroenterol 24:103–109, 1989.

Hara H, Haga S, Kasai T, Kiruyama S. Fermentation products of sugar-beet fiber by cecal bacteria lower plasma cholesterol concentration in rats. J Nutr 128:688–693, 1998.

Harland JI. Beta fibre: a case history. Int J Food Sci Nutr 44:S87–S88 (1993).

Ishii T. Feruloyl oligosaccharides from cell walls of suspension-cultured spinach cells and sugar-beet pulp. Plant Cell Physiol 35:701–704, 1994.

Ishii T. Isolation and characterization of acetylated rhamnogalacturonan oligomers liberated from bamboo shoot cell-wall by Driselase. Mokuzai Gaddaishi 41:561–572, 1995.

Ishii T. O-acetylated oligosaccharides from pectins of potato tuber cell walls. Plant Physiol 113:1265–1272, 1997a.

Ishi T. Structure and function of feruloylated polysaccharides. Plant Sci 127:111–127, 1997b.

Ishii T, Matsunaga T. Isolation and characterization of a boron-rhamnogalacturonan-II complex from cell walls of sugar-beet pulp. Carbohydr Res 284:1–9, 1996.

Ishizuka S, Kasai T. Suppression of the number of aberrant crypt foci of rat colorectum by ingestion of sugar beet fiber regardless of administration of anti-asialo GM1. Cancer Lett 121:39–43, 1997.

Israelsson B, Järnblad G, Persson K. Serum cholesterol reduced with FibrexR, a sugar-beet fiber preparation. In: Moyal MF, ed. Dietetics in the 90s. Role of the Dietetian/Nutritionists. London: John Libbey Eurotext Ltd., 1990, pp 167–170.

Jezek D, Curic D, Karlovic D, Tripalo B. Production of soluble dietary fibres from sugar beet pulp with Betanaza T enzyme in the extrusion process. Chem Biochem Eng Q 10:103–106, 1996.

Johnson IT, Livesey G, Gee JM, Brown JC, Worthley GM. The biological effects and digestible energy value of a sugar-beet fibre preparation in the rat. Br J Nutr 64:187–189, 1990.

Keenan MHJ, Belton PS, Matthew JA, Howson SJ. A ^{13}C-NMR study of sugar-beet pectin. Carbohydr Res 138:168–170, 1985.

Kobayashi M, Funane K, Ueyama H, Ohya S, Tanaka M, Kato Y. Sugar composition of beet pulp polysaccharides and their enzymatic hydrolysis. Biosci Biotech Biochem 57:998–1000, 1993.

Kohn R, Malovikova A. Dissociation of acetyl derivatives of pectic acid and intramolecular binding of calcium ions to these substances. Coll Czech Chem Commun 43:1709–1719, 1978.

Lairon D. Dietary fibres: effect on lipid metabolism and mechanisms of action. Eur J Clin Nutr 50:125–133, 1996.

Lampe JW, Slavin JL, Baglien KS, Thompson WO, Duane WC, Zavoral JH. Serum lipid and fecal bile acid changes with cereal, vegetable, and sugar-beet fiber feeding. Am J Clin Nutr 53:1235–1241, 1991.

Langenhorst WTJP, Tels M, Vlugter JC, Waterman HI. Cation exchanger on a sugar-beet pulp basis. Applications for decontaminating radioactive waste water. J Biochem Microbiol Technol Eng 3:7–20, 1961.

Langkilde A-M, Andersson H, Bosaeus I. Sugar-beet fibre increases cholesterol and reduces bile acid excretion from the small bowel. Br J Nutr 70:757–766, 1993.

Leclère C, Lairon D, Champ M, Cherbut C. Influence of particle size and sources of non starch polysaccharides on postprandial glycaemia, insulinemia and triacylglycerolaemia in pigs and starch digestion in vitro. Br J Nutr 70:179–188, 1993.

Lee B. Process for cleaning sugarbeet pulp. U.S. Pat. 4,770,886 (1988).

Le Quéré J-M, Baron A, Segard E, Drilleau J-F. Modification des pectines de betteraves sucrières au cours du traitement industriel. Sci Alim 1:501–511, 1981.

Longland AC, Low AG, Quelch DB, Bray SP. Adaptation to digestion of non starch polysaccharides in growing pigs fed on cereal or semi-purified basal diets. Br J Nutr 70:557–556, 1993.

Mazur A, Gueux E, Felgines C, Bayle D, Nassir F, Demigné C, Rémésy C. Effects of dietary fermentable fiber on fatty acid synthesis and triglyceride secretion in rats fed fructose-based diet: studies with sugar beet fibre. Proc Soc Exp Biol Med 199:345–350, 1992.

McBurney MI, Thompson LU. In vitro fermentabilities of purified fibre supplements. J Food Sci 54:1457–1464, 1989.

McBurney MI, Van Soest PI, Chase LE. Cation exchange capacity and buffering capacity of neutral-detergent fibres. J Sci Food Agric 34:910–916, 1983.

Micard V, Grabber JH, Ralph J, Renard CMGC, Thibault J-F. Dehydrodiferulic acids from sugar-beet pulp. Phytochemistry 44:1365–1368, 1997.

Micard V, Renard CMGC, Thibault J-F. Enzymic saccharification of sugar beet pulp. Enzyme Microb Technol 19:162–170, 1996.

Michel P, Rérat A. Effect of adding sugar beet fibre and wheat bran to starch diet on the absorption kinetics of glucose, amino-nitrogen and volatile fatty acids in the pig. Reprod Nutr Dev 38:49–68, 1998.

Michel F, Thibault J-F, Pruvost G. Procédé de préparation de fibres alimentaires et fibres obtenues. French Pat. 85,167-48 (1985a).

Michel F, Thibault J-F, Mercier C, Heitz F, Pouillaude F. Extraction and characterization of pectins from sugar beet pulp. J Food Sci 50:1499–1500, 1502, 1985b.

Michel F, Thibault J-F, Barry J-L. Preparation and characterisation of dietary fibres from sugar-beet pulp. J Sci Food Agric 42:77–85, 1988.

Miranda Bernardo AM, Dumoulin ED, Lebert AM, Bimbenet J-J. Drying of sugar beet fiber with hot air or superheated steam. Drying Technol 8:767–779, 1990.

Morgan LM, Tredger JA, Wright J, Marks V. The effect of soluble-and insoluble-fibre supplementation on postprandial glucose tolerance, insulin and gastric inhibitory polypeptide secretion in healthy subjects. Br J Nutr 64:103–110, 1990.

Morgan LM, Tredger JA, Shavila Y, Travis JS, Wright J. The effect of non starch polysaccharides supplementation on circulating bile acids, hormone and metabolic levels following a fat meal in human subjects. Br J Nutr 70:491–501, 1993.

Nishimura N, Nishikawa H, Kiriyama S. Ileorectostomy or cecectomy but not colectomy abolishes the plasma cholesterol-lowering effect of dietary beet fiber in rats. J Nutr 123:12060–1269, 1993.

Nyman M, Asp NG. Fermentation of dietary components in the rat intestinal tract. Br J Nutr 47:357–366, 1982.

Oosterveld A. Pectic substances from sugar beet pulp: structural features, enzymatic modification, and gel formation. Ph.D. thesis, Agricultural University of Wageningen, 1997.

Oosterveld A, Beldman G, Schols HA, Voragen AGJ. Arabinose and ferulic acid rich pectic polysaccharides extracted from sugar beet pulp. Carbohydr Res 288:143–153, 1996.

Oosterveld A, Grabber JH, Beldman G, Ralph J, Voragen AGJ. Formation of ferulic acid dehydrodimers through oxidative cross-linking of sugar-beet pectin. Carbohydr Res 300:179–181, 1997.

Overton PD, Furlonger N, Beety JM, Chakraborty J, Tredger JA, Morgan LM. The effects of dietary sugar-beet fibre and guar gum on lipid metabolism in Wistar rats. Br J Nutr 72:385–395, 1994.

Owen R, Dodo M, Thompson MH, Hill MJ. The faecal ratio of lithocholate to deoxycholate acid may be an important aetiological factor in colo-rectal cancer. Biochem Soc Trans 12:861, 1984.

Özboy Ö, Sahbaz F, Köksel H. Chemical and physical characterisation of sugar beet fiber. Acta Aliment 27:137–148, 1998.

Pippen EL, McCready RM, Owens HS. Gelation properties of partially acetylated pectins. J Am Chem Soc 72:813–816, 1950.

Ralet MC, Thibault J-F, Della Valle G. Solubilization of sugar-beet pulp cell wall polysaccharides by extrusion-cooking. Lebensm Wiss Technol 24:107–112, 1991.

Ralet M-C, Thibault J-F, Faulds CB, Williamson G. Isolation and purification of feruloylated oligosaccharides from cell walls of sugar-beet pulp. Carbohydr Res 263:227–241, 1994.

Renard CMGC, Thibault J-F. Composition and physico-chemical properties of apple fibres from fresh fruits and industrial products. Lebensm Wiss Technol 24:523–527, 1991.

Renard CMGC, Thibault J-F. Structure and properties of apple and sugar-beet pectins extracted by chelating agents. Carbohydr Res 244:99–114, 1993.

Renard CMGC, Crépeau M-J, Thibault J-F. Influence of ionic strength, pH and dielectric constant on hydration properties of native and modified fibres from sugar-beet and wheat bran, Indust Crops Prod 3:75–84, 1994.

Renard CMGC, Lahaye M, Mutter M, Voragen FGJ, Thibault J-F. Isolation and characterisation of rhamno-galacturonan oligomers generated by controlled acid hydrolysis of sugar-beet pulp. Carbohydr Res 305:271–280, 1998.

Roboz E, Van Hook A. Chemical study of beet pectin. Proc Am Soc Sugarbeet Technol 4:574–583, 1946.

Roland JC, Reis D, Vian B, Roy S. The helicoidal plant cell wall as a performing cellulose-based composite. Biol Cell 67:209–220, 1989.

Rombouts FM, Thibault J-F. Feruloylated pectic substances from sugar-beet pulp. Carbohydr Res 154:177–187, 1986a.

Rombouts FM, Thibault J-F. Enzymic and chemical degradation and the fine structure of pectins from sugar beet pulp. Carbohydr Res 154:189–203, 1986b.

Rumney CJ, Henderson C. Fermentation of wheat bran or sugar beet fibre by human colonic bacteria growing in vitro in semi-continuous culture. Proc Nutr Soc 49:124A, 1990.

Sakamoto T, Sakai T. Protopectinase T: a rhamnogalacturonase able to solubilize protopectin from sugar beet. Carbohydr Res 259:77–91, 1994.

Sakamoto T, Yoshinaga J, Shogaki T, Sakai T. Studies on protopectinase-C mode of action: analysis of the chemical structure of the specific substrate in sugar beet protopectin and characterization of the enyme activity. Biosci Biotech Biochem 57:1832–1837, 1993.

Salvador V, Cherbut C, Barry JL, Bertrand D, Bonnet C, Delort-Laval J., Sugar composition of dietary fibre and short chain fatty acid production during in vitro fermentation by human bacteria. Br J Nutr 70:189–197, 1993.

Sandström B, Davidsson L, Kivistö B, Hasselblad C, Cederblad A. The effect of vegetables and beet fibre on the absorption of zinc in humans from composite meals. Br J Nutr 58:49–57, 1987.

Schweizer TF, Würsch P. Analysis of dietary fibre. J Sci Food Agric 30:613–619, 1979.

Sonoyama K, Nishikawa H, Kiriyama S, Niki R. Apolipoprotein mRNA in liver and intestine of rats is affected by dietary beet fiber or cholestyramine. J Nutr 125:13–19, 1995.

Spagnuolo M, Crecchio C, Pizzigallo MDR, Ruggiero P. Synergistic effects of cellulolytic and pectinolytic enzymes in degrading sugar beet pulp. Biores Technol 60:215–222, 1997.

Svensson S. The benefits of sugar beet fibre. Baking Ind 119–122, 1992.

Thibault J-F, Rombouts FM. Effect of some oxidizing agents, especially ammonium peroxysulfate on sugar beet pectins. Carbohydr Res 154:205–216, 1986.

Thibault J-F, Della Valle G, Ralet MC. Produits riches en parois végétales à fraction hydrosoluble accrue, leur obtention, leur utilisation et compositions les contenant. French Pat. 88–11601 (1988).

Thibault J-F, Renard CMGC, Axelos MAV, Roger P, Crépeau M-J. Studies on the length of homogalacturonic regions in pectins by acid hydrolysis. Carbohydr Res 238:271–286, 1993.

Thibault J-F, Renard CMGC, Guillon F. Physical and chemical analysis of dietary fibres in sugar-beet and vegetables. In: Linskens HF, Jackson JF, eds. Modern Methods of Plant Analysis 16. Springer-Verlag Berlin 1994, pp 23–55.

Thorsdottir I, Andersson H, Einarsson S. Sugar beet fiber in formula diet reduces postprandial blood glucose serum, serum insulin and serum hydroxyproline. Eur J Clin Nutr 52:155–156, 1998.

Tjebbes J. Utilization of fiber and other non-sugar products from sugarbeet. In: Clarke MA, Godshall MA, eds. Chemistry and Processing of Sugarbeet and Sugarcane. Amsterdam: Elsevier Science Publishers B.V., 1988, pp 139–145.

Tomlin J, Read NW. Laxative properties of plastic particles. Br Med J 297:1175–1176, 1988.

Travis JS, Morgan LM, Tredger JA, Marks V. Effects of sugar beet fibre on blood glucose, serum lipids and apolipoproteins in non insulin diabetics mellitus. In: Southgate DAT, ed. Dietary Fibre—Chemical and Biological Aspects. London: Royal Society of Chemistry, 1990, pp 366–372.

Tredger J, Sheard C, Marks V. Blood glucose and insulin levels in normal subjects following a meal with and without added sugar beet pulp. Diabetes Metabolism 7:169–172, 1981.

Tredger JA, Morgan LM, Travis J, Marks V. The effect of guar gum, sugar-beet fibre and wheat bran supplementation on serum lipoprotein levels in normocholesterolaemic volunteers. J Hum Nutr Diet 4:375–384, 1991.

Vince AJ, McNeil NI, Wager JD, Wrong OM. The effect of lactulose, pectin arabinogalactan and cellulose on the production of organic acids and metabolism of ammonia by intestinal bacteria in a faecal incubation system. Br J Nutr 63:17–26, 1990.

Vogel M. Alternative utilization of sugar beet pulp. Zuckerindustrie, 116:265–270, 1991.

Voragen AGJ, Pilnik W, Thibault J-F, Axelos MAV, Renard CMGC. Pectins. In: Stephen AM, Dea I, eds. Food Polysaccharides. New York: Marcel Dekker, 1995, pp 287–339.

Waldron KW, Ng A, Parker ML, Parr AJ. Ferulic acid dehydrodimers in the cell walls of Beta vulgaris and their possible role in texture. J Sci Food Agric 74:221–228, 1997.

Wang CCH, Chang KC. Beet pulp and isolated pectin physicochemical properties as related to freezing. J Food Sci 59:1153–1154, 1167, 1994.

Wen LF, Chang KC, Brown G, Gallaher DD. Isolation and characterization of hemicellulose and cellulose from sugar-beet pulp. J Food Sci 53:826–829, 1988.

Williams EL, Cozens AJ, Smith SK, Gay MR, Theobald TC, Cole J. Palatable compositions comprising sugar beet fibre. U.K. Pat. 2,287,636 (1994).

Williamson G, Faulds CB, Matthew JA, Archer DB, Morris JV, Brownsey GJ, Ridout MJ. Gelation of sugarbeet and citrus pectins using enzymes extracted from orange peel. Carbohydr Polym 13:387–397, 1990.

Wilpart W, Roberfroid M. Effects of secondary biliary acids on the mutagenecity of N-methyl-N-nitro-N-nitrosoguanidine, 2-acetylaminofluoren and 2 nitrofluorene towards Salmonella typhimurium strains. Carcinogenesis 7:703–706, 1986.

30

Pectin
Composition, Chemistry, Physicochemical Properties, Food Applications, and Physiological Effects

Maria Luz Fernandez
University of Connecticut, Storrs, Connecticut

The postulated role of dietary soluble fiber in human health has made the consumer aware of its potential beneficial effects in decreasing plasma cholesterol concentrations and in delaying glucose absorption. Pectin, as one of the predominant components of dietary fiber, has likewise attracted much attention.

The variability in the chemistry of pectin, including the number of esterified methoxyl groups to galacturonic acid, the differences in molecular weight among pectins, and its intrinsic properties, contribute to the interest in this soluble fiber. The food industry's main concern is to study the physicochemical properties of pectin and its potential application in food products to improve viscosity, gel consistency, and water-holding capacity, among other characteristics. These physicochemical properties have led scientists to speculate about the specific effects of pectin in the gastrointestinal tract and how they affect lipid, glucose, mineral, and vitamin metabolism. Some of the chemical and physical properties of pectin and how they relate to its physiological effects and role in human health are discussed in this review.

I. COMPOSITION AND CHEMISTRY

There is much interest in the food industry in pectin production, although some reports suggest that there might be an oversupply in the pectin market due to increased capacity and lower worldwide demand (1). Still, the worldwide consumption of pectin is 18,000–19,000 metric tons (2). Because extensive evidence suggests that pectin may reduce plasma cholesterol levels and modulate the glucose response, there is considerable concern by the general public to know which foods and food products are major sources of pectin.

The levels of pectin vary for the different plant tissues; apple pomace, sugar beet pulp, and sunflower heads are major sources of this fiber, ranging in pectin concentration from 15 to 25 g/100 g (3). The amount of pectin in citrus and other fruits varies widely and can be dependent on climate, soils, and other factors, e.g., variety, method of extraction, and fruit maturity (3). Levels in juice are too low to provide any of the claimed health benefits. Citrus fruits are one of the major sources, but it is not the fruits but the peels that manufacturers use for preparation of pectin (4). Many of the values reported in the past have overestimated the amount of pectin in fruits and vegetables due in part to technical problems (5). Some of these errors are related to inclusion of peel content, the method used for determination, the use of soluble rather than total pectin, and, occasionally, the use of unripe fruits.

For example, a pectin range of 2.8–3.0 g/100 g has been reported for lemons (6). Analysis of peeled lemons indicated a pectin content of 0.63 g/100 g (7), a more reliable number. Ross et al. (8) reported that peeled oranges contained 0.57 g/100 g pectin, thus approximately 6 g pectin could be obtained from 1 kg. The amount present in other fruits is also lower than 1 mg/100 g (9–11). Overall, citrus fruits are strongly associated with elevated concentrations of pectin, and most pectin content is actually derived from the peels. The inclusion of peels in the analysis led to an overestimation of 150% in the case of lemons, as mentioned above, and as much as 1000% in the case of grapefruit (12). Unconventional sources rich in pectin have been proposed for commercial use. One such source is sunflower heads, which must undergo two successive extractions to develop a commercial product (13). The pectin content of selected fruits and vegetables is presented in Table 1.

Pectin is located in the middle lamellae of plant cell walls and is generally associated with cellulose, forming the insoluble protopectin. During the ripening of fruit protopectin leads to the formation of pectin. There is also a solubilization of pectic compounds, which results in an increase in water-soluble and oxalate-soluble pectin. The latter has been correlated with a decrease in acid-soluble pectin in the case of cherries (14). In addition, extensive degradation of cell wall pectin associated with a decrease in molecular weight occurs due to the action of polygalacturonase, although this enzyme is apparently nonessential for pectin solubilization (15). Yet, when the production of polygalacturonase was blocked in tomatoes by a gene-wrecking technique, these food items were prevented from softening during the aging process (16).

The enzyme pectin methylesterase catalyzes the hydrolysis of methyl ester groups and is involved in the first step of the fruit-ripening process. The product of its action is a pectin with a lower degree of methylation, which in turn becomes the substrate for polygalacturonase (17). It has been reported that changes in the neutral side chains of the galacturonan backbone could modify the degree of association and the solubility of pectins (18).

Table 1 Pectin Content of Selected Fruits and Vegetables

Food	Pectin content (g/100 g)	Ref.
Apple	0.39–0.49	8
Apple pomace	15–20	3
Banana	0.55–0.68	10
Beans	0.43–0.63	8
Carrots	0.72–1.01	8
Cherries	0.40	13
Grapes	0.7	11
Grapefruits	0.65	4
Kiwifruit	0.85	9
Lemons	0.63	7
Oranges	0.57	8
Sugar beet pulp	15	3
Sunflower heads	25	3
Sweet potato	0.81	7

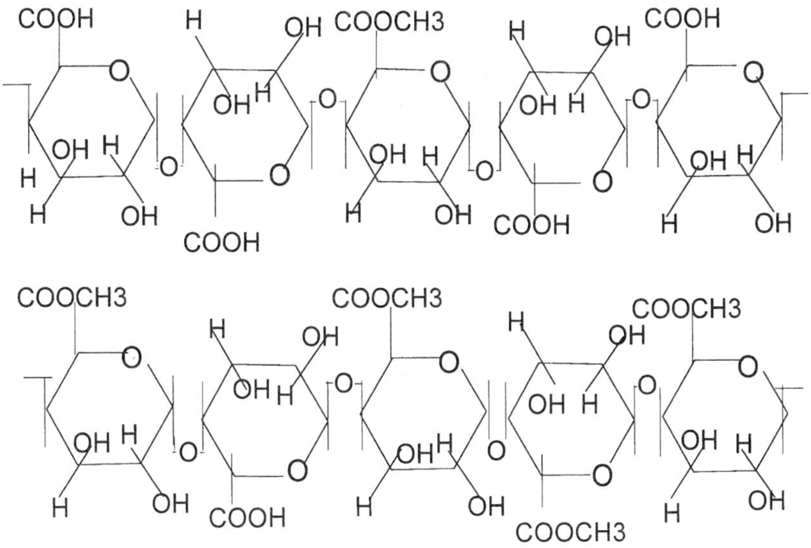

Fig. 1 Chemical structure of pectins. Upper formula corresponds to a low-methoxyl pectin with 20% esterification and lower formula to high-methoxyl pectin with 80% esterification.

Pectins are structurally composed of a linear chain of 1,4-linked α-D-galacturonic acid units, although almost all pectins contain a number of neutral sugars such as L-rhamnose, D-galactose, and L-arabinose. Some of the carboxyl groups are esterified with methyl alcohol. Chain length and degree of esterification (DE) are especially important in determining the properties of pectins. There are two types of pectins—high- and low-methoxyl pectins (Fig. 1). Most pectins have degrees of esterification of about 50–80% (high-methoxyl pectins) (19). If the degree of esterification is lower than 50% (low-methoxyl pectins), these compounds behave like a completely new family of polymers.

Pectins can form two types of gels depending on their degree of esterification. High-methoxyl pectins will form gels in acid pH and in the presence of high concentrations of sugar, while low-methoxyl pectins require a divalent cation such as calcium (19). Studies have demonstrated that calcium might be retained by absorption to the surface of pectins, indicating a weak association with this divalent cation, unlike the behavior observed for other fibers such as cellulose and lignin (20).

The primary mechanism of chain association for low-methoxyl pectins during gel formation is dimerization of polygalacturonate sequences. The calcium pectate gel strength is reduced with competitive inhibition of polygalacturonate blocks (21). The available evidence also suggests that the mechanism of crosslinking involves dimerization of chains in a twofold conformation. In contrast, the high-methoxyl pectins gel under conditions of low pH and low water activity, which suggests that the crosslinking is through aggregates of various extent rather than through junction zones (21). Pectin is an interesting example of a polysaccharide that, depending on the degree of methylation, can form gels by different mechanisms.

II. PHYSICOCHEMICAL PROPERTIES AND FOOD APPLICATIONS

Pectin has gelling capacities that are very useful for the jam industry. More than 50% of the world's pectin production is used for jellies, jams, marmalades, and confectionery products (22).

The ability of pectin to form gels is the most important property determining its commercial value. Pectins might have other applications as emulsifying agents in combination with protein (23). The emulsifying properties of protein are not always sufficient to obtain stable emulsions, thus the formation of protein-polysaccharides complexes are an alternative for the preparation of creams and mayonnaise. Dalev and Simeonova (23) reported that the emulsifying properties of protein were greatly improved by the addition of pectin. In addition, since pectin does not provide any caloric value to foods, the use of this fiber as an emulsifier can have potential applications for the use of low-calorie products with high nutritional value.

The range of food uses for pectins as thickening agents is increasing, and there are also some applications in pharmaceuticals (24) and in the preparation of biodegradable films (25). The level of methylation of pectin apparently influences the consistency of the product. High-methoxyl pectins form a gel through a combination of hydrogen bonding and hydrophobycity, which is irreversible upon heating (26). In contrast, the heat reversibility of low-methoxyl pectin gels makes it possible for these compounds to be used in bakery jams and jellies, for glazing, and for food applications such as retorting, microwaving, sterilization, or pasteurization (27).

Pectin not only has gel-forming ability, water-holding capacity (28), and thickening properties, but it can also improve the stability of emulsions (29). Sugar beet pectin is not utilized in the food industry because of its low gelling properties; however, its physicochemical characteristics are not much altered after freezing and thawing (30), and it possesses high water-holding capacity and low viscosity (31), thus it can have rather important applications in the formulation of certain products. The strength of gels with low-methoxyl pectins varies with the concentration of calcium ions in the medium as well as with the molecular characteristics of the polysaccharide. For example, sunflower head residues are high in low-methoxyl pectin and have a great potential for food applications due to their high water-holding capacity and high viscosity (32).

The molecular weight (MW) of pectin can also influence some gel strength characteristics as well as the DE. Panchev et al. (33) concluded that the optimal strength of the gel was achieved when pectins had a DE of 57–58%. However, the MW of pectins decreased as DE increased, demonstrating that low MW pectins can also form strong gels. In contrast to these observations, pectins with MW higher than 100,000 resulted in higher strength gels in dairy products (34). Low-methoxyl pectin has also been shown to be more suitable than high-methoxyl pectin for improving consistency without having drastic effects on flavor in strawberry jam (35).

From these studies it is clear that, depending on the intended product where pectins will be incorporated, the MW and DE are major characteristics determining their sensory and physical properties. How these properties are influenced depending on the chemistry of pectin becomes an important issue for obtaining adequate products with suitable shelf life and product attributes ensuring high consumer acceptability.

III. PHYSIOLOGICAL EFFECTS

Dietary soluble fiber has been postulated to have numerous physiological effects including decreasing glucose absorption and improving insulin response, lowering plasma LDL cholesterol concentrations, and binding to minerals to decrease their bioavailability. Pectin, like other soluble fibers, has been demonstrated to have some of these physiological effects, which will be discussed below. In addition, there are some reports addressing the effects of pectin on the absorption of vitamins and vitamin precursors.

A. Pectin and Mineral Absorption

Although pectin-containing fiber sources have the ability to complex with metal ions in vitro (36–38), pectin-mineral interactions have not been demonstrated in studies conducted in humans. For example, dietary pectin levels ranging from 10 to 36 g/day have not altered the balance of calcium, magnesium, phosphorus, or zinc (39,40). However, studies with ileostomy patients have shown that iron absorption may be affected by pectin (41), although no iron absorption impairment was reported in normal subjects (42). Similar to these observations in humans, animal studies also have failed to demonstrate that pectin affects mineral absorption.

Studies on the effects of pectin on mineral absorption have been carried out in rats. In one study, rats were fed with 2% pectin for 7 weeks, after which they were orally administered ^{58}Fe in combination with pectin (43). Dietary pectin at the level fed in this study had no influence on iron uptake or turnover (43). In another study in anemic rats provided an iron supplement, no differences in iron availability were observed between control supplemented rats and those fed pectins varying in DE or MW (44). The effects of these pectins on iron availability were also investigated in healthy growing rats by following erythrocyte incorporation of a dose of ^{58}Fe (45). Iron absorption was 48% in the control group and 57% in rats fed 75% esterified pectin with a MW of 89,000. Rats fed this pectin had higher serum iron and transferrin saturation in hematocrit and liver than the control group (45). These data suggest that the availability of heme iron is improved with low MW and high DE pectin.

Galibois et al. (46) tested different sources of fiber, including pectin, cellulose, oat bran, and wheat bran, to determine how mineral absorption was affected in the rat. The apparent absorption of iron, zinc, magnesium, and calcium was better with pectin than with wheat or oat bran. In the case of iron, inclusion of 5 versus 10% fiber resulted in better absorption. The authors concluded that the source rather than the amount of fiber affected absorptive parameters since pectin effects on mineral absorption were almost nonexistent compared to wheat or oat bran intake. From these studies there is no clear indication that pectin will affect mineral absorption significantly, especially in the doses used for human consumption.

B. Pectin and Vitamin Absorption

There are a few studies on the effects of pectin on vitamin E, carotenoids, and vitamin B_{12} absorption in humans and animal models. Regarding the effects of pectin on carotenoids, it was reported that individuals fed carotenoid-rich foods had lower plasma β-carotene concentrations when pectin was added to their diets (47). These data suggest that the observed reports of lower plasma β-carotene in humans after intake of foods rich in carotenoids and not in subjects taking β-carotene supplements (48) may be due to the inhibitory effect of pectin present in the consumed foods. These observations warrant further evaluation to define more clearly the role of pectin in carotenoid absorption.

The bioavailability of vitamin E was tested in rats fed different doses of pectin ranging from 0 to 8% (49). After 8 weeks, rats fed 6 and 8% pectin had lower concentrations of vitamin E in liver compared to animals fed 0 or 3%. The authors concluded that higher doses of pectin decreased vitamin E availability in rats (49). In contrast to these observations, there was more α-tocopherol present in low-density lipoprotein (LDL) isolated from guinea pigs fed pectin than from those fed a cellulose control diet (50). Both diets were identical in composition except for the type of fiber. In addition, guinea pigs fed pectin exhibited an LDL particle that was less susceptible to oxidation as measured by thiobarbituric reactive substances (TBARS) formation after incubation with copper (50). This study demonstrates a protective effect of pectin in sparing α-tocopherol concentrations in plasma and increasing LDL resistance to oxidation. A possible explanation for these controversial results could be that in this study, pectin significantly decreased plasma LDL cholesterol concentrations in guinea pigs and the LDL particles were cholesteryl ester depleted compared to those LDL derived from control animals (50). Most studies addressing the mechanisms of LDL oxidation focus on lipid (cholesteryl ester) oxidation because it is believed that it occurs prior to modifications of apolipoprotein B (51), thus a particle that contains less cholesteryl ester would be less easily oxidized. In addition, the length of time that LDL remains in circulation might be another factor associated with its potential oxidation since the longer the LDL remains in plasma, the higher the possibility of its being oxidized. Since pectin intake increased LDL apo B/E receptors in guinea pigs, the increases in LDL turnover would decrease the availability of LDL to be oxidized (50).

Negative effects of pectin on vitamin B_{12} status have been reported in vitamin B_{12}–deprived rats (52). In the pectin-fed animals the biological life of $^{57}[Co]$ vitamin B_{12} was 58 days in the fiber-free compared to 38 days in the pectin-fed rats. In addition, pectin intake increased urinary methylmalonic acid, a metabolite of vitamin B_{12} degradation (52). In a subsequent study by the same authors (53), the concentrations of methylmalonic acid in the vitamin B_{12}–deprived rats were larger than would be expected by propionate production derived from pectin, suggesting an effect of this fiber on vitamin absorption.

No conclusive statements regarding the effects of pectin on vitamin availability can be drawn from these studies. In both the clinical and the rat study, there was a negative effect of pectin on carotenoid and on vitamin E absorption. In contrast, in the guinea pig study, there was an apparent protective effect of pectin resulting in higher vitamin E concentrations in plasma LDL. For the vitamin B_{12} study, the authors used vitamin B_{12}–deprived rats, thus the effects of pectin under adequate intake of vitamin B_{12} is not defined at present.

C. Pectin and Glycemic Control

After consumption of a carbohydrate-containing meal, there is a rise in postprandial glucose levels associated with rises in serum insulin. Controlling these fluctuations in glucose and insulin becomes very important in the case of individuals with diabetes. Pectin has been shown to moderate these changes in the case of insulin-dependent and type II diabetic patients.

Reductions in plasma glucose concentrations have been reported in several clinical studies (54,55). However, the results have not been consistent since some studies have shown a lack of pectin effects on the postprandial rise of insulin and glucose concentrations (56,57). In a study by Jenkins et al. (58), different sources of fiber, including pectin, were tested in a group of normal volunteers. The addition of each fiber reduced blood glucose concentration at one or several points during a glucose tolerance test and reduced serum insulin concentrations. No such effect was observed when cholestyramine or bran was tested. The authors concluded that the effectiveness in reducing plasma glucose was directly related to the viscosity of the fiber (58).

Other studies have shown that pectin added to test meals or glucose solutions can reduce plasma glucose concentrations in healthy volunteers (59,60). While the blood glucose response was lowered by pectin in healthy volunteers, pectin had no effect when administered to a patient with total gastrectomy (61). In agreement with the former observations, Schwartz et al. (55) reported in a study of sustained pectin ingestion in type II diabetic patients that gastric emptying half-time was increased by 43% and glucose tolerance was improved. All these studies (55,59–61) suggest that increased viscosity in the gastrointestinal lumen may account in part for the reduced absorption and improved glucose response in healthy individuals and in patients with diabetes consuming pectin.

Prickly pear (*Opuntia* sp.), a plant commonly grown in Mexico, has been recognized since the Spanish conquerors for its medicinal properties against degenerative diseases (62). Prickly pear pectin has been tested in humans and demonstrated to improve glucose response and plasma lipids in nondiabetic patients (63). Individuals had significant decreases in plasma cholesterol and glucose after 8 weeks of consumption of 9 g/day pectin compared to the placebo group (63). In addition a study carried out in streptozotozin-induced diabetic rats demonstrated that at a concentration of 1 mg/kg of body weight of prickly pear pectin and in combination with insulin, blood glucose and glycosylated hemoglobin were reduced to normal levels (64). These results suggest that the pectin derived from this plant could potentially be used in the treatment of individuals with diabetes.

The effects of pectin on mucin, a high molecular weight glycoprotein responsible for the gel nature of the intestinal mucus, were examined in rats after feeding 5% citrus fiber (65). The group fed the citrus fiber had significantly greater reactivity in luminal samples from stomach and intestine to a polyclonal antibody against rat mucine (65). The results suggest that several of the reported consequences of pectin feeding, such as more rapid transit time and delayed or impaired absorption of nutrients, may be due to increments of gastrointestinal mucin (65). In addition, alterations in the intestinal loops associated with reduced glucose absorption have been reported in rats after 5 weeks of a pectin-supplemented diet (66), although the authors were unable to identify changes in the intestinal wall that could account for this reduced absorption. Adaptive changes in response to pectin feeding have also been reported in patients with non–insulin-dependent diabetes after pectin supplementation had been suspended for 3 days (55). In summary, based on these human and animal studies (55,65,66), it can be concluded that pectin may reduce the postprandial rise in blood glucose by two different mechanisms: (a) by altering the viscosity, thus delaying gastric emptying and intestinal absorption, and (b) by inducing changes in the intestinal barrier layer.

D. Pectin and Plasma LDL Cholesterol Concentrations

Increased consumption of soluble fiber is well accepted as a protective dietary habit against ischemic heart disease risk, presumably due to its intrinsic properties, which unbalance nutrient absorption in the intestinal lumen and result in plasma LDL cholesterol lowering, a response associated with decreased coronary heart disease risk (67). The focus on dietary fiber and heart disease started many years ago when evaluation of epidemiological data from a variety of studies suggested that dietary fiber might protect against coronary heart disease (68). Significant negative correlations have been established between fiber intake from vegetables, fruit, and cereals and myocardial infarction (69). Clearly, guidelines should be established to increase dietary fiber as an important dietary component to prevent coronary heart disease.

The action of fiber in the intestinal lumen (primary mechanisms) induces a reduction of hepatic cholesterol concentrations associated with important alternations in the synthesis, intravascular processing, and catabolism of lipoproteins (secondary mechanisms) (70). The response to soluble fiber differs depending on the type of fiber and the amount of dietary cholesterol. A brief description of the effects of pectin on plasma lipid levels in humans and on the mechanisms of plasma LDL cholesterol lowering using animal models will follow.

Clinical studies have demonstrated that pectin intake reduces plasma LDL cholesterol concentrations without having an effect on plasma HDL cholesterol or triglyceride concentrations (71–74). There is some controversy regarding the mechanisms of action of pectin. For example, feeding studies with ileostomy patients established that digestion of pectin in the stomach and the small intestine is fairly limited and that most of it takes place in the colon (75). This information, in addition to the absence of galacturonic acid residues in stools (76), supports the notion that pectin undergoes bacterial fermentation in the colon to yield short-chain fatty acids, which can be utilized by colonic bacteria or absorbed by the intestinal mucosa. Based on these findings, it has been suggested that propionic acid, the major short-chain fatty acid produced, could alter cholesterol biosynthesis (77). However, studies conducted in rats (78), hamsters, (79) and guinea pigs (80) with pectin or other sources of soluble fiber have failed to support this hypothesis since hepatic or whole body cholesterol synthesis is increased, not decreased, after soluble fiber intake. Levrat et al. (81) reported that pectin intake substantially increased volatile fatty acid in the cecum of the rat. However, a significant increase in the activity of hepatic HMG-CoA reductase, the regulatory enzyme of cholesterol synthesis, was also observed, which is in agreement with the previously mentioned studies (78–80) and reinforces the hypothesis that pectin fermentation in the colon to volatile fatty acids is not related to decreased cholesterol biosynthesis.

There are other potential mechanisms by which pectin acting on the intestinal lumen may reduce plasma cholesterol concentrations. One mechanism could be disruption of micelle formation. Dietary lipids can only be absorbed from the emulsion of mixed micelles, and if these disintegrate, the lipid components cannot be absorbed (82). Pectin may destabilize micelles leading to their entrapment or disintegration and therefore to reduced lipid absorption. In fact, aluminum pectate was very effective in reducing plasma cholesterol in the rat (83), and the authors postulated the formation of a complex between the positive charges in the aluminum and the negative charges in the micelle, which caused micelle disintegration.

Another mechanism may relate to the viscosity of pectin discussed above. Viscosity is associated with enlargement of the apparent thickness of the unstirred water layer, increasing resistance to diffusion and absorption (84). This phenomenon of decreased absorption of fatty acids and glucose has been observed in rats and humans fed 0–15 g/L pectin (85). Viscosities of pectin solution increased proportionally to the amount of pectin (85).

Pectin has also been shown to increase bile acid excretion, although with much less of an effect compared to bile acid–binding resins (72). This mechanism may be related to an interruption of the enterohepatic circulation of bile acids as a result of the physicochemical properties of pectin mentioned above rather than to direct binding of pectin to bile acids.

Not all clinical studies have shown a hypocholesterolemic effect of pectin. Hillman et al. (86) found no significant reduction in plasma cholesterol in healthy normolipidemic volunteers who were fed 12 g/day of pectin. The authors attributed this lack of effect to the use of normal versus hypercholesterolemic subjects or to the fact that the subjects were not consuming high cholesterol–containing diets (87). In another study Wisker et al. (88) reported an 11% decrease in plasma cholesterol concentrations in female subjects after consumption of citrus fiber for 4 weeks. However, the plasma cholesterol lowering was in the HDL cholesterol, thus, the total–to–HDL cholesterol ratio was not improved (85). Bell et al. (89) did not find significant reductions in mildly hyperlipidemic patients fed a pectin-enriched cereal for 6 weeks after the individuals had been on the step I diet for a similar amount of time. Further, Delbarre et al. (90) did not find any beneficial effects of high methoxy pectin derived from apples or lemons in patients with dyslipidemias.

In contrast, other clinical studies have demonstrated a hypolipidemic effect of pectin in concentrations ranging from 10 to 15 g/day (91–93). Judd and Truswell (94) tested low and high methoxyl pectins in 10 healthy subjects to determine whether the degree of esterification affected the physiological properties. These authors did not find any difference between low or high methoxyl pectin on their cholesterol-lowering effect or steroid secretion. They concluded that gel-forming properties of pectin are more important in determining their hypocholesterolemic effects (94). A summary of the effects of different doses of pectin on plasma cholesterol concentrations in 12 clinical studies is presented in Table 2. In the majority of these studies pectin appeared not to have an effect when fed to hyperlipidemic individuals.

Table 2 Effects of Pectin Doses on Plasma Cholesterol Reduction in 12 Human Studies

Subjects	Pectin dose	Type of pectin	Plasma cholesterol reduction (%)	Weeks	Ref.
10 healthy	15 g/day	LMP	−18	5	94
10 healthy	15 g/day	HMP	−16	5	94
9 healthy	40–50 g/day	Pectin	−13	2	72
9 healthy	15 g/day	Citrus pectin	−13	3	71
20 hypercholesterolemic	57 g/day	Pectin-EC[a]	−3.2 (NS)	6	89
12 normal	12 g/day	Pectin	−9	3	92
21 normal	15 g/day	Pectin	−8.6	6	91
7 normal	36 g/day	Pectin	−12	2	73
9 normal	15 g/day	Pectin	−15	3	74
18 normal	10 g/day	Pectin	−5	4	93
13 hyperlipidemic	6 g/day	HMP (apple)	7.5 (NS)	6	90
10 hyperlipidemic	6 g/day	HMP (lemon)	−8 (NS)	6	90
10 normal	12 g/day	Pectin	NS	4	86
10 female	24 g/day	Citrus fiber	12 (NS)[b]	4	86

LMP, low-methoxyl pectin; HMP, high-methoxyl pectin; NS, nonsignificant.
[a] Enriched cereal.
[b] Nonsignificant for LDL—only HDL cholesterol was reduced.

Studies in rats have shown no consistent effect of pectin on lowering plasma LDL cholesterol concentrations (95–97), possibly because high-density lipoprotein (HDL) is the major cholesterol carrier in this animal model. To further emphasize this point, studies by Sonoyama et al. (98) reported that rats fed beet fiber rich in pectin had lower hepatic apo A-I mRNA abundance compared to control animals, which correlated with lower concentrations of this apolipoprotein in plasma. Since pectin does not modify plasma HDL cholesterol concentrations or apo A-I levels in humans, these data from the rat studies are irrelevant with respect to the human situation.

Yet, some studies have demonstrated a hypocholesterolemic effect of pectin in the rat. Judd and Truswell (99) have shown that both the molecular weight and the extent of methylation of pectin affect the metabolic responses. High-methoxyl pectin had plasma cholesterol-lowering properties even at low doses, a phenomenon not observed with low-methoxyl pectin. Pectin has also been shown to have a more pronounced hypocholesterolemic effect than guar gum or methylcellulose in the rat (100). Interestingly, pectin did not achieve plasma cholesterol reduction when fed to vervet monkeys (101), hamsters (102), or growing pigs (103). In rhesus monkeys fed low-fat diets, pectin achieved a plasma cholesterol lowering of 18% which might be associated to the HDL fraction (104). The data from these studies suggest that there might be species differences in the hypocholesterolemic response to pectin.

The hypocholesterolemic effect of pectin has been consistently observed with high rather than with low concentrations of dietary cholesterol in rats (105–107) and in guinea pigs (71,80,108,109), although in a recent study there was no effect of different types of pectin on plasma cholesterol levels in the cholesterol-fed hamster (110). Prickly pear pectin has also been tested in guinea pigs as a hypocholesterolemic agent (109,111,112). Guinea pigs were fed hypercholesterolemic diets containing 0, 1, or 2.5% prickly pear pectin for 4 weeks, and some metabolic parameters were compared. Plasma LDL cholesterol was 33% lower compared to the control group. Hepatic apolipoprotein B/E receptor was 60% higher in guinea pigs fed the prickly pear pectin diets, which was in agreement with the twofold receptor-mediated LDL fractional catabolic rates observed in guinea pigs fed this type of fiber. Some of the effects of prickly pear pectin on cholesterol and glucose metabolism are summarized in Table 3.

Guinea pigs fed low-cholesterol diets (0.04% w/w) have been shown to have significant reductions in plasma LDL cholesterol concentrations at 10 and 12.5% pectin, and modifications in hepatic cholesterol homeostasis were observed at high pectin doses (80). In a study in which guinea pigs were fed increasing doses of pectin with 0.25% cholesterol (80), a pectin dose–related decrease in plasma total and LDL cholesterol was observed (Fig. 2, upper panel). Similarly, a pectin dose–dependent decrease in hepatic free and esterified cholesterol was reported (Fig 2, lower panel). These reductions in hepatic cholesterol concentrations were negatively correlated with the activity of hepatic acyl CoA: cholesterol acyltransferase (ACAT), the regulatory enzyme of cholesterol esterification. Further, guinea pigs fed 12.5% pectin with high-cholesterol diets had a complete reversal of hyperlipidemia since plasma LDL and hepatic cholesterol concentrations were similar to those in animals fed low-cholesterol diets (80). A significant reduction in cholesterol absorption, which might be related to pectin's ability to disrupt micelle formation, has been observed in guinea pigs. In this study, an upregulation of cholesterol 7α-hydroxylase, the regulatory enzyme of bile acid synthesis, was present (71), suggesting an interruption of the enterohepatic circulation of bile acids by pectin similar to what has been reported in human studies (72,73). This increase in cholesterol 7α-hydroxylase activity as a response to pectin feeding has also been observed in rats (113,114).

These studies suggest that the concentration of pectin in the intestinal lumen is directly related to (a) the amount of cholesterol delivered to the liver as chylomicron remnant and (b) the depletion of hepatic cholesterol (80) as a result the disruption of bile acid homeostasis (71,115).

In agreement with the previous reports, in the rat higher bile acid pool sizes have been shown after pectin consumption (116). In addition, pectin intake versus cellulose consumption resulted in lower hydrophobicity of the bile acid pool and a lower ratio of circulating 12α-hydroxylated to nonhydroxylated bile acids. This reduced hydrophobicity was shown to lower feedback inhibition of bile acid synthesis (117) and may explain in part the increases in cholesterol 7α-hydroxylase activity observed by pectin (71) and other sources of dietary fiber (118).

Gender has been shown to affect the response to pectin in studies carried out in guinea pigs (119–121). Male guinea pigs fed a hypercholesterolemic diet had lower plasma cholesterol (Fig. 3 upper panel) and higher hepatic cholesterol concentrations (Fig. 3, lower panel) than females, and the hypocholesterolemic effects of pectin were somewhat diminished in female

Table 3 Effects of Prickly Pear Pectin on Cholesterol and Glucose Metabolism

Parameter	Species	% Difference from baseline	Weeks	Ref.
Plasma LDL cholesterol	Human	−8	6	63
Triglycerides	Human	−10	6	63
Glucose	Human	−12	6	63
LDL cholesterol	Guinea pig	−33	4	111
Hepatic free cholesterol	Guinea pig	−48	4	111
LDL receptor (B_{max})	Guinea pig	+60	4	111
LDL receptor-mediated FCR	Guinea pig	+90	4	111
Glycosylated hemoglobin	Rat	−51	14	64
Glucose tolerance improvement	Rat	−31	14	64

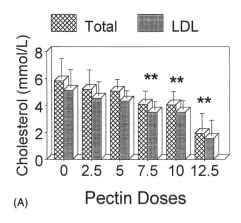

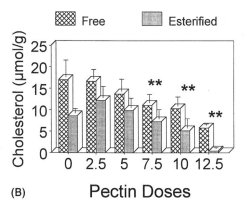

Fig. 2 (A) Plasma total (hatched bars) and LDL (gray bars) cholesterol in guinea pigs fed different doses of pectin with 0.25 g/100 g dietary cholesterol. (B) Hepatic free (hatched bars) and esterified (gray bars) cholesterol in guinea pigs fed different doses of pectin with 0.25 g/100 g dietary cholesterol. **Represents significantly different from control.

animals. These results are in agreement with human studies in which dietary fiber had less effect on females than males in lowering plasma cholesterol and apo B concentrations (122). A summary of different animal models, doses of pectin, and responses in plasma and liver cholesterol are presented in Table 4.

Effects of pectin on very low-density lipoprotein (VLDL) and LDL metabolism have been tested in female and male guinea pigs (119–121). When guinea pigs were injected with radiolabeled LDL to assess how pectin affects LDL transport in plasma, male guinea pigs had faster LDL fractional catabolic rates when compared to control animals and lower LDL apo B flux. In contrast, female animals only exhibited decreases in the flux and no changes in LDL fractional catabolic rate. Pectin did not affect triglyceride secretion rate, but apo B secretion was reduced in males while no effects were observed in female guinea pigs. These results demonstrate that the secondary mechanisms responsible for plasma cholesterol lowering are influenced by gender.

In male guinea pigs (119), the secreted VLDL was larger in size, containing more triglyceride and phospholipid than nascent VLDL from the control group. These results suggest that guinea pigs fed pectin secrete fewer VLDL molecules, larger in size and triglyceride enriched. In contrast, mature VLDL from the pectin group, as assessed by electron microscopy, were smaller in size than those VLDL from control animals, suggesting that lipoprotein lipase activity

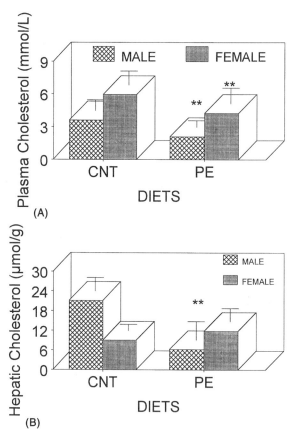

Fig. 3 (A) Differences in response in plasma cholesterol concentrations between male (hatched bars) and female (gray bars) guinea pigs fed a cellulose control (CNT) diet and a pectin (PE)-containing diet. (B) Differences in response in hepatic cholesterol concentrations between male (hatched bars) and female (gray bars) guinea pigs fed a cellulose control (CNT) diet and a pectin (PE)-containing diet. **Represents significantly different from control.

might have been enhanced by pectin intake (119). In addition, plasma cholesteryl ester transfer protein activity was 50% lower in guinea pigs fed pectin, and this was associated with a lower proportion of cholesteryl ester in VLDL and LDL. Careful analysis of these data indicate that secretion rate of apo B, compositional changes in lipoproteins occurring in the intravascular compartment, and upregulation of LDL receptors are important secondary mechanisms induced by pectin which contribute to plasma LDL cholesterol lowering (71,108,119).

In addition to lowering plasma cholesterol, pectin also reduces the amount of lipids in the heart and reduces atherosclerosis. The quantity of lipid droplets in rats fed standard or cholesterol diets (123) was lower when animals were fed pectin. In this study, significant reductions in plasma and hepatic cholesterol were also observed by pectin intake. In another study using micro-swine with sustained hypercholesterolemia, pectin intake resulted in less surface area covered by atherosclerosis and lower coronary artery narrowing compared to control animals (124). Micro-swine were fed the hypercholesterolemic diet for one year before the treatment. Although significant reductions in plasma cholesterol were not observed, the inhibition of atherosclerosis by pectin was evident.

Table 4 Effects of Pectin Intake in Reducing Plasma and Liver Cholesterol Concentrations in Different Species

Species	% Pectin	% Cholesterol	Weeks	Reduction Total/LDL	Reduction in liver (%)	Ref.
Rat						
	3	1	4	30/36	36	107
	7	—	4	27/ND	17	113
	5	0.25	4	15/ND	None	114
	8	—	2	16/none	ND	100
	8	1	2	44/59	ND	100
	10.5	—	4	13/ND	13	115
	SBF					
	5	—	3	20/none	ND	81
	2.5	1	4	22/ND	32	78
	10	2	1 1/2	32/ND	11	123
	10	—	1 1/2	12/ND	42	123
	5	1	4	19/ND	50	106
Guinea pig						
	2.5 PPP	0.25	4	30/33	48	111, 112
	1.0 PPP	0.25	4	26/34	57	109
	12.5	0.04	4	32/ND	19	71
	12.5	0.25	4	66/70	66	80
	12	0.17/low fat	4	23/25	16	108
	12	0.17/high fat	4	30/26	18	108
female	12.5	0.04	4	30/36	26	120
female	12.5	0.25	4	30/30	28	121
Hamster						
	Apples	—	4	None	66	102
	8	0.4	6	None	None	110
Swine	12 SBF	—	4	None	ND	103
Monkey						
rhesus	8 g/day	Fat P/S 2.2	3	18/ND	ND	104
vervet	14%	Western diet	34	NS	ND	101

ND, not determined; SBF, sugar beet fiber; PPP, prickly pear pectin; NS, not significant.

In summary, the majority of clinical and animal studies have shown that pectin reduces plasma cholesterol concentrations (71–73,91–94,99,100), although there may be some discrepancy associated with doses used (91–94), the inclusion of hyperlipidemic individuals (89,90), or animal model tested (98–115).

Based on the available evidence, we can conclude that the action of pectin is apparently related to some of its physicochemical properties, such as water-holding capacity (40), viscosity (54), and potential gel formation (19–22). These properties result in delayed stomach emptying (61), decreased mobilization through the ileum where lipid absorption takes place (82), and disruption of micelle formation (83). Although pectin does not bind directly to bile acids, it does disrupt the bile acid enterohepatic circulation by enhancing bile acid elimination. By the time that pectin reaches the colon, most of it has been degraded to short-chain fatty acids by colonic bacteria (55). At this point it is not clear what contribution these volatile fatty acids make to the hypocholesterolemic action of fiber. As reviewed above, studies conducted in several animal models (78–80) show that pectin upregulates hepatic cholesterol biosynthesis as a response to the depletion of cholesterol pools in the liver, precluding the notion that volatile fatty acids decrease cholesterol synthesis. Thus, it may be concluded that the main effect of pectin, which results in the lowering of plasma cholesterol, takes place in the stomach and the small intestine before pectin is degraded and fermented in the large intestine.

Whether pectin delays cholesterol absorption directly by creating a physical barrier or by disrupting micelle formation (81) or whether it interrupts the enterohepatic circulation of bile acids and promotes mobilization of hepatic cholesterol by enhancing bile acid synthesis (111–116), the net result is a decrease in hepatic cholesterol concentrations. This reduction in hepatic cholesterol pools alters cholesterol homeostasis and cholesterol is then removed from plasma by hepatic apo B/E receptors, which are upregulated by pectin (80).

Pectin is thus a type of soluble fiber that under most circumstances reduces plasma LDL cholesterol concentrations. As shown in animal studies (124), it may also have a direct effect in reducing arteriosclerosis. Since the favorable effects of pectin are numerous, intake of this soluble fiber may be beneficial for overall health and in reducing the incidence of some of the degenerative diseases, including diabetes and coronary heart disease.

REFERENCES

1. Bahner B. Pectin oversupply drives prices downward. Chem Market Rep 242:20–21, 1993.
2. Axin D. Pectin market business old niche market area. Chem Market Rep 4:16–20, 1991.
3. de Man JM. Carbohydrates. In: Principles of Food Chemistry, 2nd ed., pp. 173–175. AVI Publishers, Van Nostrand Reinhold, New York, 1990, pp 173–175.
4. Baker RA. Potential dietary benefits of citrus pectin and fiber. Food Technol 48:133–136, 1994.
5. Baker RA. Reassessment of some fruit and vegetable pectin levels. J Food Sci 62:225–229, 1997.
6. Campbell LA, Palmer GH. Pectin. In: Spiller GA, Amen RJ, eds. Topics in Dietary Fiber Research. New York: Plenum Press, 1978, pp. 105–115.
7. Vollendorf NW, Marlett JA. Comparison of two methods of fiber analysis of 58 foods. J Food Comp Anal 6:203–214, 1993.
8. Ross JK, English C, Perlmutter CA. Dietary fiber constituents of selected fruits and vegetables. J Am Diet Assoc 85:1111–1116, 1985.
9. Lodge N, Nguyen TT, McIntyre D. Characterization of a crude kiwifruit pectin extract. J Food Sci 52:1095–1096, 1987.
10. Wade NL, Kavanaugh EE, Hockley DG, Brady CJ. Relationship between softening and the polyuronides in ripening banana fruit. J Sci Food Agric 60:61–68, 1992.
11. Silacci MW, Morrison JC. Changes of pectin content of cabernet sauvignon grape berries during maturation. Am J Enol Vit 41:111–115, 1990.
12. Atkins CD, Rouse AH. Effect of arsenic spray on the quality of processed grapefruit sections-with special reference to pectin. Proc Fal State Hort 71:220–223, 1958.
13. Chang KC, Dhurandhar N, You X, Miyamoto Y. Cultivar/location and processing methods affect yield and quality of sunflower pectin. J Food Sci 59:602–605, 1994.
14. Batisse C, Fils-Lycaon B, Buret M. Pectin changes in ripening cherry fruit. J Food Sci 59:389–393, 1994.
15. Smith CIS, Watson CF, Morris PC, Bird CR, Seymour GB, Gray JE, Arnold C, Tucker GA, Schuch W, Harding S, Grierson D. Inherance and effect on ripening of antisense polygalacturonase genes in transgenic tomatoes. Plant Mol Biol 14:369–379, 1990.
16. Wilson Business Abstracts. The tomatoes of the tree of knowledge. The Economist 316:83–84, 1990.
17. Castaldo D, Quagliulo L, Servillo L, Balestrieri C, Giovane A. Isolation and characterization of pectin methylesterase from apple fruit. J Food Sci 54:653–668, 1989.
18. Gross KC. Recent development on tomato fruit softening. Postharvest News Information 1:109–112, 1990.

19. Glicksman M. Food applications for gums. In: Lineback DR, Inglett GE, eds. Food Carbohydrates Westport, CT: Avi Publishing Co., 1982, pp 270–294.

20. Torre M, Rodriguez A, Saura-Calixto F. Study of the interactions of calcium ions with lignin, cellulose and pectin. J Agric Food Chem 40:1762–1766, 1992.

21. Dea ICM. Polysaccharide conformation in solutions in gels. In: Lineback DR, Inglett GG, eds. Food Carbohydrates Westport, CT: Avi Publishing Co., 1982, pp 420–457.

22. Barford NM, Pedersen KS. Determining the setting temperature of high-methoxyl pectins. Food Technol 44:139–141, 1990.

23. Delev PG, Simeonova LS. Emulsifying properties of protein-pectin complexes and their use in oil-containing foodstuffs. J Sci Food Agric 68:203–206, 1995.

24. May CD. Industrial pectins: sources, production and applications. Carbohydr Polym 12:79–83, 1990.

25. Coffin DR, Fishman ML. Viscoelastic properties of pectin/starch blends. J Agric Food Chem 41:1192–1197, 1993.

26. DaSilva JAL, Rao MA. Rheology of structure development in high methoxyl pectin/sugar systems. Food Technol 49:70–72, 1995.

27. Li G, Chang KC. Viscosity and gelling characteristics of sunflower pectin as affected by chemical and physical factors. J Agric Food Chem 45:4785–4789, 1997.

28. Armstrong EF, Eastwood MA Brydon WG. The influence of wheat bran on the distribution of water in rat caecal contents and faeces. Br J Nutr 69:913–920, 1993.

29. Muschiolick G. Influence of xanthan gum or low methoxyl pectin on protein-stabilized emulsions. Food Hydrocoll 3:225–229, 1989.

30. Wang CCH, Chang KC. Beet pulp and isolated pectin physicochemical properties as related to freezing. J Food Sci 59:1153–1154, 1994.

31. Phatak L, Chang KC, Brown G. Isolation and characterization of pectin in sugar beet pulp. J Food Sci 53:830–836, 1988.

32. Miyamoto A, Chang KC. Extraction and physicochemical characterization of pectin from sunflower head residues. J Food Sci 57:1439–1443, 1992.

33. Panchev IN, Kirtchev NA, Kratchanov CG, Proichev T. On the molecular weight of pectin substances and its relation to gel strength. Carbohydr Polym 8:257–259, 1988.

34. Gregory DJH. The functional properties of pectins on various food systems. In: Birch GG, Lindley EG, eds. Interactions of Food Components. Barking, UK: Elsevier, 1986.

35. Guichard E, Issanchou S, Descourvieres A, Etievant P. Pectin concentration, molecular weight and degree of esterification: influence on volatile composition and sensory characteristics of strawberry jam. J Food Sci 56:1621–1627, 1991.

36. Weber CW, Kohlepp EA, Idouraine A, Ochoa L. Binding capacity of 18 fiber sources for calcium. J Agric Food Chem 41:1931–1935, 1993.

37. Idouraine A, Hassani BZ, Claye SS, Weber CW. In vitro binding capacity of various fiber sources for magnesium, zinc and copper. J Agric Food Chem 43:1580–1584, 1995.

38. Platt SR, Clydesdale FM. Mineral binding characteristics of lignin, guar gum, cellulose, pectin and neutral detergent fiber under stimulated duodenal pH conditions. J Food Sci 52:1414–1419, 1987.

39. Cummings JH, Soutgate DAT, Branch WJ, Wiggins HS, Houston H, Jenkins DJA, Jivraj T, Hill MJ. The digestion of pectin in the human gut and its effect on calcium absorption and large bowel function. Br J Nutr 41:477–485, 1979.

40. Sandberg A-S, Ahdreine R, Anderson H, Hallgreen B, Hulten L. The effect of citrus pectin on the absorption of nutrients in the small intestine. Human Nutr Clin Nutr 37C:171–183, 1983.

41. Monnier L, Collette C, Aguirre L, Mirouze J. Evidence and mechanisms for pectin-induced intestinal inorganic iron absorption in idiopahatic hemochromatosis. Am J Clin Nutr 33:1225–1232, 1980.

42. Cook JD, Noble NL, Morck TA, Lynch SR, Pettersburg SJ. Effect of fiber on nonheme iron absorption. Gastroenterology 85:1354–1358, 1983.

43. Baig MM, Burgin CW, Cerda JJ. Effect of dietary pectin on iron absorption and turnover in the rat. J Nutr 113:2385–2389, 1983.

44. Kim M, Atallah MT. Structure of dietary pectin, iron bioavailability and hemoglobin repletion in anemic rats. J Nutr 122:2298–2305, 1992.

45. Kim M, Atallah MT, Amarasiriwardena C, Barnes R. Pectin with low molecular weight and high degree of esterification increases absorption of ^{58}Fe in growing rats. J Nutr 126:1883–1890, 1996.

46. Gallibois I, Desrosier T, Guevin N, Lavigne C, Jacques H. Effects of dietary fibre mixtures on glucose and lipid metabolism and on mineral absorption in the rat. Ann Nutr Metab 38:203–211, 1994.

47. Rock CL, Swendseid ME. Plasma β-carotene response in humans after meals supplemented with dietary pectin. Am J Clin Nutr 55:96–99, 1992.

48. Brown ED, Micozzi MS, Craft NE. Plasma carotenoids in normal men after a single ingestion of vegetables or purified β-carotene. Am J Clin Nutr 49:1258–1265, 1989.

49. Schaus EE, de Lumen BO, Chow FI. Bioavailability of vitamin E in rats fed graded levels of pectin. J Nutr 115:263–270, 1985.

50. Vergara-Jimenez M, Furr H, Fernandez ML. Pectin and psyllium reduce the susceptibility of LDL to oxidation. J Nutr Biochem 10:118–124, 1999.

51. Maggi E, Marchesi E, Ravetta V, Falaschi F, Finardi G, Bellomo G. Low density lipoprotein oxidation in essential hypertension. J Hypertension 11:1103–1111, 1993.

52. Cullen RW, Oace SM. Neomycin has no persistent sparing effect on vitamin B-12 status in pectin-fed rats. J Nutr 119:1399–1403, 1989.

53. Cullen RW, Oace SM. Dietary pectin shortens the biological half life of vitamin B-12 in rats by increasing fecal and urinary losses. J Nutr 119:1121–1127, 1989.

54. Jenkins DJA, Leeds AR, Gassull MA, Cochet B, Alberti KGMM. Decrease in post-prandial insulin and glucose concentrations by guar and pectin. Ann Int Med 86:20–23, 1977.

55. Schwartz SE, Levine RA, Weistock RS, Petokas K, Mills CA, Thomas FD. Sustained pectin ingestion. Effect on gastric emptying and glucose tolerance on non-insulin dependent diabetic patients. Am J Clin Nutr 48:1413–1417, 1988.

56. Williams DRRR, James WPT, Evans IE. Dietary fibre supplementation of a ''normal'' breakfast administered to diabetics. Diabetologia 18:379–383, 1980.

57. Gardner DF, Schwartz L, Krista M, Merimee TJ. Dietary pectin and glycemic control in diabetes. Diabetes Care 7:143–146, 1984.

58. Jenkins DJA, Wolever TMS, Leeds AR, Gassull MA, Haisman P, Dilawari J, Goff DV, Metz GL, Alberti KGMM. Dietary fibres, fibre analogues, and glucose tolerance: importance of viscosity. Br Med J 1:1392–1394, 1978.

59. Gold LA, McCourt JP, Merimee TJ. Pectin: an examination in normal subjects. Diabetes Care 3:50–52, 1980.

60. Bolton RP, Heaton KW, Burroughs LF. The role of dietary fiber in satiety, glucose and insulin: studies with fruit and fruit juice. Am J Clin Nutr 34:211–217, 1981.

61. Holt S, Heading RC, Carter DC, Prescott LF, Tothill P. Effect of gel fiber on gastric emptying and absorption of glucose and paracetamol. Lancet 1:636–639, 1979.

62. Walker K. The cactus cookers. Arizona Highways 72:22–25, 1996.

63. Torres M, Posadas R, Zamora J, Trejo A, Ichazo S, Cardoso G, Posadas C. Efficacy and safety of prickly pear pectin (*Opuntia* sp) in patients with mild hypercholesterolemia. XII International Symposium on Drugs Affecting Lipid Metabolism, Houston, 1995, p 135.

64. Trejo-Gonzalez A, Gabriel-Ortiz G, Puebla-Perez AM, Huizar-Contreras MD, Munguia-Mazariegos MR, Mejia-Arreguin S, Calva E. A purified extract from prickly pear cactus (opuntia fuliginosa) controls experimentally induced diabetes in rats. J Pharm 55:27–33, 1996.

65. Satchithanandam S, Vargofcak-Apker M, Calvert RJ, Reeds AR, Cassidy MM. Alteration of gastrointestinal mucin by fiber feeding in rats. J Nutr 120:1179–1184, 1990.

66. Scwartz SE, Levine GD. Effects of dietary fiber on intestinal glucose absorption and glucose tolerance in rats. Gastroenterology 79:833–836, 1980.

67. Stamler J, Wentforth D, Neaton JD. Is relationship between serum cholesterol and risk of premature death from coronary heart disease continuous and graded? Findings in 356,222 primary screens of the Multiple Risk Factor Intervention Trial (MRFIT). JAMA 256:2823–2828, 1986.

68. Anderson JW. Dietary fiber, lipids and atherosclerosis. Am J Cardiol 60:17G–22G, 1987.

69. Rimm EB, Ascherio A, Giovannuncci E, Spiegelman D, Stampfer MJ, Willett WC. Vegetable, fruit and cereal fiber intake and risk of coronary heart disease among men. JAMA 275:447–451, 1996.

70. Fernandez ML. Distinct mechanisms of plasma LDL lowering by dietary fiber in the guinea pig: specific effects of pectin, guar gum, and psyllium. J Lipid Res 36:2394–2404, 1995.

71. Kay M, Truswell AS. Effect of citrus pectin on blood lipids and fecal steroid excretion in man. Am J Clin Nutr 30:171–175, 1977.

72. Miettinen TA, Tarpila S. Effects of pectin on serum cholesterol levels, faecal bile acids and biliary lipids in normolipidaemic and hyperipidaemic individuals. Clin Chim Acta 79:471–477, 1977.

73. Jenkins DJA, Leeds AR, Newton C. Cummings JH. Effect of pectin, guar gum and wheat fibre on serum cholesterol. Lancet 1:1116–1117, 1975.

74. Keys A, Grande F, Anderson JT. Fiber and pectin in the diet and serum cholesterol concentration in man. Proc Soc Exp Biol Med 105:55–558, 1961.

75. Holloway WD, Clifford T-J, Kerry M. Pectin digestion in humans. Am J Clin Nutr 37:253–255, 1983.

76. Werch SC, Ivy AC. A study of the metabolism of ingested pectin. Am J Dis Child 62:499–511, 1941.

77. Ullrich IH. Evaluation of a high-fiber diet in hyperlipidemia. A review. J Am Coll Nutr 6:19–25, 1987.

78. Arjmandi BH, Craig J, Nathani S, Reeves RD. Soluble dietary fiber and cholesterol influence in vivo hepatic and intestinal cholesterol biosynthesis in the rat. J Nutr 122:1559–1565, 1992.

79. Turley SD, Dietschy JM. Mechanisms of LDL-cholesterol lowering action of psyllium hydrophyllic mucilloid in the hamster. Biochim Biophys Acta 1255:177–184, 1995.

80. Fernandez ML, Sun D-M, Tosca M, McNamara DJ. Citrus pectin and cholesterol interact to regulate hepatic cholesterol homeostasis and lipoprotein metabolism: a dose-response study in guinea pigs. Am J Clin Nutr 59:869–878, 1994.

81. Levrat A-M, Texier O, Regerat F, Demigne C, Remesy C. Comparison of the effects of condensed tannin and pectin on cecal fermentation and lipid metabolism in the rat. Nutr Res 13:427–433, 1993.

82. Furda I. Interaction of dietary fiber with lipids. Mechanistic theories and their limitations. In: Furda I, Brine CJ, eds. New Developments of Dietary Fiber. New York: Plenum Press, 1990, pp 67–82.

83. Nagyvary JJ, Falk JD, Hill ML, Schmidt ML, Wilkins AK, Bradbury EL. The hypolipidemic activity of chitosan and other polysaccharides in rats. Nutr Rep Int 20:677–680, 1979.

84. Schneeman BO, Tinker LF. Dietary fiber. Ped Nutr 42:825–837, 1995.

85. Fuse K, Bamba T, Hosada S. Effects of pectin on fatty acid and glucose absorption and on thickness of unstirred water layer in rat and human intestine. Dig Dis Sci 34:1109–1116, 1989.

86. Hillman LC, Peters SG, Fisher CA, Pomare EW. The effects of the fiber components pectin, cellulose and lignin on serum cholesterol levels. Am J Clin Nutr 42:207–213, 1985.

87. Fisher H, Grimminger P, Sostman ER, Brusch MK. Dietary pectin and blood cholesterol. J Nutr 86:113, 1965.

88. Wisker E, Daniel M, Feldheim W. Effects of a fiber concentrate from citrus fruits in humans. Nutr Res 14:361–372, 1994.

89. Bell LP, Hectorn KJ, Reynolds H, Hunninghake DB. Cholesterol lowering effects of soluble-fiber cereals as part of a prudent diet for patients with mild to moderate hypercholesterolemia. Am J Clin Nutr 52:1020–1026, 1990.

90. Delbarre F, Rondier J, de Gery A. Lack of effect of two pectins in idiopathic or gout-associated hyperdyslipidemia hypercholesterolemia. Am J Clin Nutr 30:463–465, 1977.

91. Ginter E, Kubec FJ, Vozar J, Bobek P. Natural hypocholesterolemic agent: pectin plus ascorbic acid. Int J Vit Nutr Res 4:406–412, 1979.

92. Durrington PN, Manning AP, Boton CH, Hartog M. Effect of pectin on serum lipids and lipoproteins, whole gut transit time and stool weight. Lancet 2:394–396, 1976.

93. Palmer GH, Dixon DG. Effects of pectin on serum cholesterol levels. Am J Clin Nutr 18:437–442, 1966.

94. Judd PA, Truswell AS. Comparison of the effects of high- and low-methoxyl pectins on blood and faecal lipids in man. Br J Nutr 48:451–458, 1982.

95. Bond V, Ordor O, Bruckner G, Webb P, Kotchen T, Tearney RJ, Adams RG. Effects of dietary

fish oil or pectin on blood pressure and lipid metabolism in the DOCA-salt hypertensive rat. J Nutr 119:813–817, 1989.

96. Koo SI, Stanton P. Effects of cellulose, pectin and guar gum on the distribution of serum cholesterol among lipoprotein fractions. Nutr Rep Int 24:395–401, 1981.

97. Kritchevsky D, Ryder E, Fishman A, Kaplan M, Dehoff JL. Influence of dietary fiber on food intake, feed efficiency and lipids in rats. Nutr Rep Int 25:783–785, 1982.

98. Sonoyama K, Nishikawa H, Kiriyama S, Niki R. Apolipoprotein mRNA in liver and intestine of rats is affected by dietary beet fiber or cholestyramine. J Nutr 125:13–19, 1995.

99. Judd PA, Truswell AS. The hypocholesterolemic effects of pectins in rats. Br J Nutr 53:409–425, 1985.

100. Abbey M, Triantafilidis C, Topping DL. Dietary non-starch polysaccharides interact with cholesterol and fish oil in their effects on plasma lipids and hepatic lipoprotein receptor activity in the rats. J Nutr 123:900–908, 1993.

101. Kritchevsky D, Davidson LM, Scott DA, van der Watt JJ, Mendelsohn D. Effects of dietary fiber in vervet monkeys fed "western" diets. Lipids 23:164–168, 1988.

102. Sable-Amplis R, Sicart P, Bluthe E. Decreased cholesterol ester levels in tissues of hamsters fed with apple fiber enriched diet. Nutr Rep Int 27:881–889, 1983.

103. Fremont L, Gozzellino M-T, Bosseau AF. Effects of sugar beet fiber feeding on serum lipids and binding of low-density lipoproteins to liver membranes in growing pigs. Am J Clin Nutr 57:524–532, 1993.

104. Heine RJ, Schouten JA, van Gent CM, Havekes LM, Koopman PAR, van der Veen EA. The effect of dietary linoleic acid and pectin on lipoprotein and apolipoprotein A-I concentrations in rhesus monkeys. Ann Nutr Metab 28:201–206, 1984.

105. Leveille GA, Sauberlich HE. Mechanism of the cholesterol-depressing effect of pectin in the cholesterol-fed rat. J Nutr 108:630–639, 1996.

106. Kelley JJ, Tsai A. Effect of pectin, gum arabic and agar on cholesterol absorption, synthesis and turnover in rats. J Nutr 108:630–639, 1978.

107. Tinker LF, Davis PA, Schneeman BO. Prune fiber or pectin compared with cellulose lowers plasma and liver lipids in rats with diet-induced hyperlipidemia. J Nutr 124:31–40, 1994.

108. Vergara-Jimenez M, Conde K, Erickson SK, Fernandez ML. Hypolipidemic mechanisms of pectin and psyllium in guinea pigs fed high fat-sucrose diets: alterations on hepatic cholesterol metabolism. J Lipid Res 39:1455–1465, 1998.

109. Fernandez ML, Trejo A, McNamara DJ. Pectin isolated from prickly pear (*Opuntia* sp.) modifies low density lipoprotein metabolism in cholesterol-fed guinea pigs. J Nutr 120:1283–1290, 1990.

110. Trautwein EA, Kunath-Rau A, Erbersdobler F. Effect of different varieties of pectin and guar gum on plasma, hepatic and biliary lipids and cholesterol gallstone formation in hamsters fed on high-cholesterol diets. Br J Nutr 79:463–471, 1998.

111. Fernandez ML, Lin ECK, Trejo A, McNamara DJ. Prickly pear (*Opuntia* sp.) pectin reverses low density lipoprotein receptor suppression induced by a hypercholesterolemic diet in guinea pigs. J Nutr 122:2330–2340, 1992.

112. Fernandez ML, Lin ECK, Trejo A, McNamara DJ. Prickly pear (*Opuntia* sp.) pectin alters hepatic cholesterol metabolism without affecting cholesterol absorption in guinea pigs fed a hypercholesterolemic diet. J Nutr 124:817–824, 1994.

113. Garcia-Diez F, Garcia-Mediavilla V, Bayon JE, Gonzalez-Gallego J. Pectin feeding influences fecal bile acid excretion, hepatic bile acid and cholesterol synthesis and serum cholesterol in rats. J Nutr 126:1766–1771, 1996.

114. Matheson HB, Colon IS, Story JA. Cholesterol 7α-hydroxylase activity is increased by dietary modification with psyllium hydrocolloid, pectin, cholesterol and cholestyramine in rats. J Nutr 125:454–458, 1995.

115. Overton PD, Furlonger N, Beety JM, Chakkaborty J, Tredger JA, Morgan LM. The effects of dietary sugar-beet fibre and guar gum on lipid metabolism in Wistar rats. Br J Nutr 72:385–395, 1994.

116. Matheson HB, Story JA. Dietary psyllium hydrocolloid and pectin increase bile acid pool size and change bile acid composition in rats. J Nutr 124:1161–1165, 1994.

117. Heuman DM, Hylemon PB, Vlahcevic ZR. Regulation of bile acid synthesis. III. Correlation be-

tween biliary bile salt hydrophobicity index and the activities of enzymes regulating cholesterol and bile acid synthesis in the rat. J Lipid Res 30:1161–1171, 1989.

118. Horton JD, Cuthbert JA, Spady DK. Regulation of hepatic 7α-hydroxylase expression by dietary psyllium in the hamster. J Clin Invest 93:2084–2092, 1994.

119. Fernandez ML, Vergara-Jimenez M, Conde K, Behr T, Abdel-Fattah G. Regulation of apolipoprotein B-containing lipoproteins by dietary soluble fiber in guinea pigs. Am J Clin Nutr 65:814–822, 1997.

120. Fernandez ML, Vergara-Jimenez M, Romero AL, Erickson SK, McNamara DJ. Gender differences in the response to dietary soluble fiber in guinea pigs: effects of pectin, guar gum and psyllium. J Lipid Res 36:2191–2202, 1995.

121. Shen H, He L, Price RL, Fernandez ML. Dietary soluble fiber lowers plasma LDL cholesterol concentrations by altering lipoprotein metabolism in female guinea pigs. J Nutr 128:1434–1441, 1998.

122. Jenkins DJA, Wolever TNS, Rao AV, Hegele RA, Mitchell SJ, Ransom TPP, Boctor DL, Spadofora PJ, Jenkins AL, Mehling C, Relle LK, Connelly PW, Story JA, Furumoto EJ, Corey P, Wursch P. Effect on blood lipids of very high intakes of fiber in diets low in saturated fat and cholesterol. N Engl J Med 329:518–527, 1993.

123. Hexeberg S, Heseberg E, Willumsen N, Berge RK. A study on lipid metabolism in heart and liver of cholesterol- and pectin-fed rats. Br J Nutr 71:181–192, 1994.

124. Cerda JJ, Normann SJ, Sullivan MP, Burgin CW, Robbins FL, Vathada S, Leelachaikul P. Inhibition of atherosclerosis by dietary pectin in microswine with sustained hypercholesterolemia. Circulation 89:1247–1253, 1994.

31

Classification, Structure, and Chemistry of Polysaccharides of Foods

James N. BeMiller
Purdue University, West Lafayette, Indiana

I. CLASSIFICATIONS OF FOOD POLYSACCHARIDES

A. By Source

Polysaccharides can be, and are, classified in several ways. Classification by chemical structure (Sec. I.B) should be the least ambiguous. However, because of the great diversity, and in some cases complexity and uncertainty, of chemical structures, this approach is not always the most satisfactory.

Polysaccharides that are present naturally in food ingredients, such as most flours, fruits, and vegetables, and those that are isolated and added to processed foods are often classified by source (Table 1). Neither is this a precise system. For example, the carrageenans, gellan, konjac mannan, and pectins are listed as native, rather than derived, polysaccharides. However, carrageenans are converted from the native polysaccharide to the commercial gum by treatment with hot sodium hydroxide solution during extraction and/or treatment with hot potassium hydroxide solution during conversion into processed Euchema seaweed (PES, Philippine natural-grade carrageenan, alkali-modified seaweed flour); gellan and konjac mannan are often used in their deacylated forms, and modification of the native polysaccharide occurs during extraction with acidic solutions to produce commercial high-methoxyl pectins.

Most of the polysaccharide names in Table 1 are written in the plural form because most represent families of polysaccharides, with structures and properties of individual polysaccharides within a family varying with species, genotype, and environmental conditions during growth of the plant or microorganism. (Only within the family of galactomannans are individual members of the family indicated.) Starches are an example. They can be subdivided into seed/cereal starches (corn, wheat, rice, oat, barley, etc.), tuber starches (potato), root starches (tapioca/cassava, sweet potato), rhizome starch (arrowroot), and legume starches (pea, mung bean, etc.). Commercially, in addition to the modifications listed in Table 1, starches can be thinned (depolymerized), pregelatinized (made cold-water soluble), and converted into cold water–swelling starches; they are often dual, triply, and even quadruply modified, i.e., a modified food starch may be crosslinked (as a phosphate or adipate diester), stabilized (via conversion to an acetate ester or hydroxypropyl ether derivative, e.g.), acid thinned, and pregelatinized. Even the derived polysaccharide names designate families of specific products originating from different raw

Table 1 Classification of Food Polysaccharides by Source

I. Plant polysaccharides
    A. Higher plants[a]
        1. Cell-wall constituents
            a. Cellulose
            b. Native and extracted/commercial pectins
            c. Arabinans/arabans
            d. Arabinoxylans (B-type hemicelluloses and flour pentosans)
            e. Xylans
            f. Arabinogalactans
            g. Xyloglucans
            h. Beta-glucans
        2. Storage polysaccharides
            a. Starches (amyloses and amylopectins)
            b. Galactomannans (guar gum, locust bean/carob gum, tara gum)
            c. Konjac mannan
            d. Arabinogalactans
            e. Inulin and other fructans
        3. Other non–cell-wall polysaccharides
            a. Exudate gums
                i. Gum arabics
                ii. Gum tragacanths
                iii. Gum ghattis
                iv. Gum karayas
            b. Extractives
                i. Psyllium seed gums
                ii. Okra gum
    B. Algae[b]
        1. Cell-wall constituents
            a. Agars
            b. Alginates
            c. Carrageenans
            d. Furcellarans (Danish agars)
        2. Non–cell-wall constituent
            a. Laminaran
    C. Microorganisms[c]
        I. Cell constituents
            a. Yeast glucan
            b. Yeast mannan
         II. Extracellular
            a. Xanthans
            b. Gellan
            c. Curdlan
            d. Dextrans
II. Animal
    A. Crustacean
        1. Chitin[d]

Table 1 Continued

III. Derived from native polysaccharides
    A. From cellulose[e]
        1. Carboxymethylcelluloses
        2. Hydroxypropylcelluloses
        3. Hydroxypropylmethylcelluloses
        4. Methylcelluloses
        5. Microcrystalline cellulose
    B. From starch[e]
        1. Starch acetates
        2. Starch 1-octenylsuccinates
        3. Starch phosphates
        4. Starch succinates
        5. Starch adipates
        6. Hydroxypropylstarches
        7. Dextrins
    C. From native pectins
        1. Pectic acids (low-methoxyl pectins)
        2. Amidated pectins
    D. Propylene glycol alginate
    E. Chitosan
IV. Synthetic
    A. Polydextrose

[a] Land plants.
[b] Marine algae.
[c] Produced from bacteria or fungi during fermentation.
[d] Not found in food products as chitin, but rather in the deacetylated form (chitosan).
[e] Restricted to those approved and used as food additives or ingredients in the United States.

material sources, with different degrees of substitution or other modification, and with different average molecular weights.

B. By Structure

A great variety of polysaccharide structures is found in nature because of the variety of uses they are put to in the organisms that make them, because of the variety of organisms that make them, and because their monomeric units (individual sugars/monosaccharides) can be configured to make a great variety of polymeric structures. With the exception of the D-fructofuranosyl units of inulin and the L-arabinofuranosyl units of some other water-soluble gums, the sugar units of food polysaccharides are in pyranose (six-membered) rings; with the exception of the pentoses D-xylose and L-arabinose, they are hexoses; and with the exception of the D-fructose in inulin, they are aldoses. Considering only aldohexosyl units in pyranose rings linked head-to-tail by glycosidic linkages, 8 different disaccharide structures can be formed from a single sugar, and 16 different disaccharides can be formed from two different sugars. Identical aldohexopyranosyl units linked head-to-tail can form 64 different trisaccharide structures; three different aldohexopyranosyl units can form 384 different trisaccharides. As far as is known, all theoretically possible structures are not found (although all 8 head-to-tail-linked D-glucose–containing disaccharides have been found in nature), but polysaccharides contain from hundreds to hundreds of thousands of monosaccharide units, allowing the possibility of diverse structures and shapes. Eleven different kinds of monosaccharide units occur most often in the food polysaccharides of Table 1 (1). Both pyranose and furanose (the five-membered) ring forms, all possible head-to-tail linkages (i.e., $1 \rightarrow 2$, $1 \rightarrow 3$, $1 \rightarrow 4$, and $1 \rightarrow 6$ for aldohexopyranosyl units) and both anomeric configurations (α and β) of these monosaccharide units are found. Because carbohydrates are polyhydroxy compounds, branching can, and does, occur (1). In fact, several kinds of branched structures are found.

Bacterial polysaccharides (the fermentation gums) often contain regular repeating units, although postpolymerization modifications (by esterification, for example) can result in variability in the repeating-unit structure. Plant polysaccharides do not have uniform, repeating-unit–type structures; rather they are polymolecular, i.e., their fine structures vary from molecule to molecule. In addition, the average structure can vary with the specific land or sea plant source and the environmental conditions experienced by it during its growth.

Primarily because most food polysaccharides are polymolecular and, therefore, only statistical, rather than exact, structures can be written, and because even statistical structures are uncertain in some cases, classification by structure can be problematic. Several schemes can be employed. Polysaccharides can be classified by monosaccharide composition. Those containing units of a single sugar are homoglycans; those containing two different monosaccharide units are diheteroglycans; those composed of three different glycosyl units are triheteroglycans. Tetrahetero- and pentaheteroglycans round out the list because five different sugar units may be the upper limit in the polysaccharides of foods. Polysaccharides may also be classified by the specific sugar(s) contained in their structure, for example, whether a homoglycan contains D-mannosyl units (a mannan) or D-xylosyl units (a xylan). They can be classified as to whether they are linear or branched and by the overall type of architecture. They can be classified by the type of linkage, e.g., $(1 \rightarrow 4)$-linked (cellulose), $(1 \rightarrow 3)$-linked, $(1 \rightarrow 3, 1 \rightarrow 4)$-linked, and $(1 \rightarrow 3, 1 \rightarrow 6)$-linked β-glucans. Those different classification possibilities have been combined in Table 2. Some polysaccharides contain ether, ester, and/or cyclic acetal groups in addition to sugar units. For example, carrageenans contain sulfate half-ester groups, but only the basic monosaccharide units are considered in constructing Table 2; so carrageenans are listed as diheteroglycans of D-galactosyl and 3,6-anhydro-D-galactosyl units, although several sulfated forms of each basic unit may be present. In other words, derived polysaccharides (Table 1) and naturally occurring polysaccharides containing hydroxyl-group modifications are not specifically identified in Table 2, although they could be.

Polysaccharides can also be classified as to whether they are neutral, acidic, or basic (indicated in Table 2), on the basis of three-dimensional structures (2), by solubility (Table 3), and by general applications (Table 4). Table 2 could have been constructed in other ways, for example, by grouping all linear, unbranched homoglycans built with β-D-glucopyranosyl units, or simply by grouping all homoglycans, which would be the traditional way structural chemists would approach the task. However, in most cases, especially within the neutral polysaccharides, overall general shape is a more important factor in determining properties than the nature of the monomeric units, so this approach was used in constructing Table 2. Sometimes, a separate category of ''pentosans'' (especially for the arabinoxylans of cereal flours) is used (see Table 1).

Polysaccharide structures should provide the best classification scheme (Table 2), and structures should correlate with physicochemical properties and imparted functionalities. However, correlation is insufficiently possible because of the great diversity of structures and differences in interactions with other molecules of the same polysaccharide and other ingredients as a result of fine structure differences. What makes classifying polysaccharides by structure even more difficult and less than satisfactory is the fact (already mentioned) that polysaccharides are polymolecular. They are also polydisperse. And not only do fine structures, average molecular weights, and distributions of molecular weights vary with genotype, species, and growing condi-

Table 2 Classification of Unmodified Food Polysaccharides by Structure[a]

I. Linear molecules
  A. Unbranched
    1. Neutral homoglycans
      a. Cellulose, → 4)-βGlc$p$-(1 →
      b. Curdlan, → 3)-βGlc$p$-(1 →
      c. Laminarans, → 3)-βGlc$p$[b]-(1 →
      d. Yeast glucans, → 6, → 3)-βGlc$p$-(1 →
      e. Cereal β-glucans, → 3, → 4)-βGlc$p$-(1 →
      f. Amyloses, → 4)-αGlc$p$-(1 → (some molecules slightly branched)
      g. Inulins, → 1)-βFru$f$-(2 →
    2. Neutral diheteroglycans
      a. Konjac mannan, → 4)-βMan$p$-(1 →; → 4)-βGlc$p$-(1 →
      b. Agarose component of agar, → 4)-3,6-An-α-L-Gal$p$-(1 → 3)-βGal$p$-(1 →
    3. Anionic/acidic homoglycans
      a. Lambda-carrageenans, → 4)-αGal$p$ 2,6-diSO$_3^-$-(1 → 3)-βGal$p$ 2-SO$_3^-$-(1 →
      b. Pectins, pectic acids,[c] → 4)-αGal$p$A-(1 →
    4. Anionic/acidic diheteroglycans
      a. Algins/alginates, → 4)-βMan$p$A-(1 →; → 4)-α-L-Gul$p$A-(1 →
      b. Kappa-carrageenans, → 4)-3,6-An-αGal$p$-(1 → 3)-βGal$p$ 4-SO$_3^-$-(1 →
      c. Iota-carrageenans → 4)-3,6-An-αGal$p$ 2-SO$_3^-$-(1 → 3)-βGal$p$ 4-SO$_3^-$-(1 →
    5. Anionic/acidic triheteroglycan
      a. Gellan gum, → 3)-βGlc$p$-(1 → 4)-βGlc$p$A-(1 → 4)-βGlc$p$-(1 → 4)-α-L-Rha$p$-(1 →
    6. Cationic/basic homoglycan
      a. Chitosan, → 4)-βGlc$p$N-(1 →; → 4)-βGlc$p$NAc-(1 →
  B. Linear with short branches/side units
    1. Branches irregularly spaced
      a. Neutral homoglycans
        i. Arabinans/arabans, main chain: → 5)-α-L-Ara$f$-(1 →; branches: α-L-Ara$f$-(1 → 3(2))-
        ii. Fungal (mushroom) β-glucans, main chain: → 3)-βGlc$p$-(1 →; branches: βGlc$p$-(1 → 6)-
      b. Neutral diheteroglycans
        i. Galactomannans (guar gum, locust bean gum, tara gum), main chain: → 4)-βMan$p$-(1 →; branches: βGlc$p$-(1 → 6)-
        ii. Flour arabinoxylans, main chain: → 4)-βXyl$p$-(1 →; branches: α-L-Ara$f$-(1 → 2, 1 → 3, 1 → 2,3)-; α-L-Ara$f$-(1 → 5)-α-L-Ara$f$-(1 → 2 or 3)-
        iii. Larch arabinogalactan, main chain: → 3)-βGal$p$-(1 →; branches: βGal$p$-(1 → 6)-; βGal$p$-(1 → 6)-βGal$p$-(1 → 6)-; β-L-Ara$p$-(1 → 3)-α-L-Ara$f$-(1 → 6)-; α-L-Ara$f$-(1 → 6)-; βGlc$p$A- (1 → 6)-
        iv. Neutral tetraheteroglycan
          1. Xyloglucans main chain: → 4)-βGlc$p$-(1 →; branches: αXyl$p$-(1 → 6)-; βGal$p$-(1 → 2)-αXyl$p$-(1 → 6)-; βGal$p$-(1 → 2)-βGal$p$-(1 → 2)-βXyl$p$-(1 → 6)-; L-Fuc$p$-(1 → 2)-βGal$p$-(1 → 2)-βXyl$p$-(1 → 6)-
    2. Branches regularly spaced
      a. Neutral homoglycan
        i. Yeast mannan, main chain: → 6)-αMan$p$-(1 →; branches: αManp_{0-1}-(1 → 2)-αMan$p$-(1 → 2)-
      b. Anionic/acidic triheteroglycan
        i. Xanthan gum, main chain: → 4)-βGlc$p$-(1 →; branches: βMan$p$-(1 → 4)-βGlc$p$A-(1 → 2)-βMan$p$ 6-Ac-(1 → 6)-

Table 2 Continued[a]

II. Nonlinear molecules
  A. Branches in clusters, homoglycan
    1. Amylopectins, main chain: → 4)-αGlc$p$-(1 →; branch points: → 4)-αGlc$p$-(1 → 6)-
  B. Highly branched/branch-on-branch-on-branch structures, anionic/acidic
    1. Tetraheteroglycans
      a. Gum karayas, constituents: Gal, GalA, Glc, L-Rha
      b. Okra gum, constituents: Gal, GalA, Glc, L-Rha
    2. Pentaheteroglycans
      a. B-type hemicelluloses of cereal brans, etc. (arabinoxylans), constituents: L-Ara$f$, L-Ara$p$, D-Gal$p$, L-Gal$p$, Glc$p$A, Xyl$p$
      b. Gum arabic, constituents: L-Ara, Gal, GlcA, 4-O-Me-GlcA, L-Rha
      c. Psyllium seed gum: L-Ara, GalA, GlcA, L-Rha, Xyl
      d. Gum tragacanth (composed of two polysaccharides), constituents of one: L-Ara, Gal; constituents of other: GalA, L-Fuc, Xyl

[a] Abbreviations: 3,6-An-αGal$p$ = 3,6-anhydro-α-D-galactopyranosyl; 3,6-An-αGal$p$ 2-SO$_3^-$ = 2-O-sulfato-3,6-anhydro-α-D-galactopyranosyl; 3,6-An-α-L-Gal$p$ = 3,6-anhydro-α-L-galactopyranosyl; α-L-Ara$f$ = α-L-arabinofuranosyl; βFru$f$ = β-D-fructofuranosyl; L-Fuc = L-fucosyl; αGal$p$ = α-D-galactopyranosyl; βGal$p$ = β-D-galactopyranosyl; αGal$p$A = α-D-galactopyranosyluronic acid; βGal$p$ 2-SO$_3^-$ = 2-O-sulfato-β-D-galactopyranosyl; βGal$p$ 4-SO$_3^-$ = 4-O-sulfato-β-D-galactopyranosyl; αGal$p$ 2,6-diSO$_3^-$ = 2,6-di-O-sulfato-α-D-galactopyranosyl; αGlc$p$ = α-D-glucopyranosyl; βGlc$p$ = β-D-glucopyranosyl; βGlcA = β-D-glucopyranosyluronic acid; 4-O-Me-GlcA = 4-O-methyl-D-glucuronosyl; βGlc$p$N = 2-amino-2-deoxy-β-D-glucopyranosyl (β-D-glucosaminyl); βGlc$p$NAc = 2-acetamido-2-deoxy-β-D-glucopyranosyl (N-acetyl-β-D-glucosaminyl); α-L-Gul$p$A = α-L-gulopyranosyluronic acid; βMan$p$ = β-D-mannopyranosyl; βMan$p$A = β-D-mannopyranosyluronic acid; βMan$p$ 6-Ac = 6-O-acetyl-β-D-mannopyranosyl; α-L-Rha$p$ = α-L-rhamnopyranosyl; βXyl$p$ = β-D-xylopyranosyl.
[b] Some laminarans contain D-mannitol units; some contain some (1 → 6) linkages.
[c] Principal structure in commercial high- and low-methoxyl pectins. Pectins are actually complex, heterogeneous polysaccharides containing some percentage of α-L-rhamnopyranosyl units in the main chain and perhaps arabinogalactan side chains.

Table 3 Classification of Food-Ingredient Polysaccharides Based on Solubility

Class	Examples
Insoluble	Cellulose
Soluble only in hot water	Agars, algins (in the presence of Ca^{2+}), amyloses, kappa-type carrageenans (in the presence of K$^+$ or Ca^{2+}), lambda-type carrageenans (in the presence of Ca^{2+}), furcellarans (in the presence of K$^+$ or Ca^{2+}), gellan, konjac mannan, locust bean gum, LM pectins (in the presence of Ca^{2+}), granular starches and starch derivatives
Soluble in room-temperature water, insoluble in hot water	Curdlan, hydroxypropylcelluloses, hydroxypropylmethylcelluloses, methylcelluloses
Soluble in room-temperature and hot water	Alginates (as Na$^+$ salt), amylopectins, carboxymethylcelluloses, kappa-type carrageenans (as Na$^+$ salt), lambda-type carrageenans (as Na$^+$ salt), iota-type carrageenans, dextrins, furcellarans (as Na$^+$ salt), guar gum, gum arabics, gum tragacanth, HM pectins, LM pectins (as Na$^+$ salt), polydextrose, xanthan

Table 4 Classification of Food-Ingredient Polysaccharides
According to General Properties

Food gums that form gels
  Agars
  Alginates
  Carrageenans
  Curdlan
  Gellan
  Gum arabics
  Konjac mannan
  Methylcelluloses
  Hydroxypropylmethylcelluloses
  Pectins (high- and low-methoxyl types)
  Starches, including modified starches
  Locust bean gum + kappa-type carrageenans
  Locust bean gum + xanthan
Food gums used as thickeners and stabilizers
  Carboxymethylcelluloses (certain types)
  Gum arabics
  Gum tragacanths
  Hydroxypropylmethylcelluloses
  Modified starches
  Propylene glycol alginates
  Xanthan
Food gums used primarily as thickeners
  Carboxymethylcelluloses (certain types)
  Guar gum
Polysaccharide ingredients used primarily as sources of
    dietary fiber and/or fat mimetics
  Beta-glucans
  Cellulose (various forms)
  Inulin
  Polydextrose
  Psyllium seed gums
  Resistant starch

tions, major structural and compositional differences can occur, especially between species. This is especially true of the nonbacterial gums. And species differences exert profound effects on properties in individual members of families of gums such as alginates, carrageenans, other seaweed gums, starches, and the exudate gums.

C. By Properties and Applications

In Table 3, food polysaccharides are classified by solubility. With the exclusion of starch, which is generally digestible, all food polysaccharides are considered to be dietary fiber. Here also there is an exception; resistant starch, which is a primarily nondigestible form of starch, is classified as dietary fiber. Polysaccharides that are basically insoluble at human-body temperature are classified as insoluble fiber; those that are basically soluble at human-body temperature constitute soluble fiber. No polysaccharide is soluble under conditions at which its solution would gel.

In Table 4, food polysaccharides are classified by general properties. (Gelatin is also classified as a food hydrocolloid. It is a gel-forming protein. As a protein, it is digestible and, therefore, not a component of dietary fiber.)

II. CHEMISTRY OF POLYSACCHARIDES

A. Chemistry of Glycosidic Linkages

Many food gum products, particularly starch products, are polysaccharide preparations in which average molecular weights have been reduced. Depolymerization is usually accomplished with acid and heat. When a starch is depolymerized, the process is known as thinning. So-called thin-boiling starches are still granular but cook out more easily than starches that have not been acid-modified. These products form gels with improved clarity and increased strength. Hence, they are used where strong gels are desired, for example, in gum candies and in processed cheese loaves. They are also used as film formers and adhesives in coated nuts and candies. Starch dextrins are made in a similar way.

Pectins have undergone depolymerization during preparation. Some hydrolysis of glycosidic bonds occurs during extraction of high-methoxyl pectin from citrus peel with mild acid. Depolymerization via a beta-elimination mechanism occurs during saponification to produce some low-methoxyl pectins (1).

Many other gums are depolymerized purposefully to provide different viscosity grades. This is sometimes done by treatment with heat and acid, but with cellulose derivatives oxidative alkaline (beta-elimination) depolymerization is used (1). If thickening is the only attribute desired, a high-viscosity gum at low concentration is used. If binding, stabilization, or coating is desired, a low-viscosity gum at high concentration is used.

The viscosity produced by a given concentration of guar gum can be reduced by improper processing.

The extent of depolymerization is determined by the pH of the system, time, temperature, the nature of the glycosidic linkages, and, in some cases, the amount of shear. Loss of viscosity can occur during thermal processing and during product storage. It can also occur during storage of the gum powder.

Polysaccharides are also susceptible to enzyme-catalyzed hydrolysis. In food products, this happens most often with starches, since amylases are the polysaccharidases most often present. Also of concern is the presence of pectinases.

B. Chemistry of Hydroxyl Groups

Reactions of carbohydrate hydroxyl groups are no different than reactions of other primary and secondary hydroxyl groups. Naturally occurring on food polysaccharides are ester groups, ether groups, and cyclic acetal groups. Acetate ester groups are found on pectins, xanthan gum, konjac mannan, and hemicelluloses. The carrageenans and furcellaran contain sulfate half-ester groups. Native gellan gum contains glycolate ester groups. Xanthan gum contains pyruvyl cyclic acetal groups.

Modified food starch contains one or more of the following groups: (esters) distarch phosphate, distarch adipate, acetate, monostarch phosphate, 1-octenylsuccinate; (ether) hydroxypropyl. Cellulose is converted into water-soluble food gums by conversion into the following ethers: carboxymethyl, methyl, hydroxypropyl, and combinations of the latter two. Some oxidation of hydroxyl groups to carbonyl groups may occur during bleaching of a starch or gum. Greater amounts may occur via oxygen dissolved in the alkaline medium used to prepare cellulose derivatives, the introduction of carbonyl groups being followed by depolymerization via beta-elimination. Introduction of carbonyl and carboxyl groups also occurs during preparation of an oxidized starch.

C. Chemistry of Carboxyl Groups

Carboxyl groups most often occur in food polysaccharides as part of the structure of a uronic acid unit. These carboxyl groups can be converted into ester groups and are used in the preparation of propylene glycol alginates. Pectins contain naturally occurring methyl ester groups that are partially removed by saponification in the preparation of certain low-methoxyl pectins. In the preparation of so-called amidated pectins, some methyl carboxylate groups are converted into carboxamide groups.

REFERENCES

1. RL Whistler, JN BeMiller. Carbohydrate Chemistry for Food Scientists. Minneapolis, MN: Eagen Press, 1997, pp. 67, 88–89.
2. R Chandrasekaran. Advan Carbohydr Chem Biochem 52:311–439, 1997.

32

Guar Gum
Agricultural and Botanical Aspects, Physicochemical and Nutritional Properties, and Its Use in the Development of Functional Foods

Peter Rory Ellis, Qi Wang, Phillippa Rayment, Yilong Ren, and Simon B. Ross-Murphy
King's College London (University of London), London, England

I. INTRODUCTION

Guar gum, a galactomannan-rich flour extracted from a leguminous seed, has received enormous attention from nutritionists, notably as a dietary supplement in the treatment of diabetes and hyperlipidemia. There is a plethora of literature showing the effectiveness of guar gum in reducing postprandial glycemia and fasting plasma cholesterol levels in humans (Saris et al., 1998; Ellis, 1999; Leeds, 1999). It is the capacity of the galactomannan component of guar to hydrate and increase the viscosity of digesta in the gut that is now considered to be a critical determinant of its effects on carbohydrate and lipid metabolism (Ellis et al., 1996). Guar galactomannan has also been used as a model polysaccharide in studies designed to elucidate the physiological action of water-soluble, nonstarch polysaccharides (i.e., soluble dietary fiber).

There are a number of reasons why, scientifically, guar gum is a useful material to investigate. First, it can be extracted as a relatively pure form of nonstarch polysaccharide consisting almost entirely of a water-soluble galactomannan of high molecular weight. Second, its physicochemical properties have been well defined in the scientific literature. Third, these properties can be easily modified. For example, the hydration kinetics and ''viscosifying'' effect of guar galactomannan can be altered by manipulating its molecular weight as well as the particle size of the guar flour. Last but not least, guar gum is one of the most frequently tested of all the polysacccharide gums used in nutritional experiments, allowing useful comparisons to be made between different studies.

This chapter is not intended to be a comprehensive review. It focuses mainly on the nutritional and therapeutic role of guar gum and on its physicochemical properties now known to be important in influencing gut function and metabolism. This includes a discussion of how guar gum influences the rheological properties of intestinal digesta and, in turn, the digestion and absorption of available carbohydrate.* Agricultural and botanical aspects of the guar plant

---

* In this review, available carbohydrate is defined as carbohydrate that is digested by α-amylase in the

and seed and the industrial extraction and purification of guar gum flour from the seed are also dealt with in this review.

II. ORIGINS AND AGRICULTURAL ASPECTS

Guar gum is derived from the seeds of the plant *Cyamopsis tetragonoloba* (L.) Taub, a member of the Leguminosae family (Whistler and Hymowitz, 1979; Kay, 1979). The common names often used in the scientific literature for the bean, guar gum flour, and the galactomannan fraction are Indian cluster bean, guar, and guaran, respectively. There does not appear to be any general consensus of opinion as to the origins of this plant (Whistler and Hymowitz, 1979), although the concept of transdomestication was originally proposed by Hymowitz (1972). This hypothesis is an explanation of how the domesticated guar plant, *C. tetragonoloba*, developed from the drought-tolerant wild Africa species *C. senegalensis*. The latter species was originally taken from Africa to the South Asian subcontinent by Arab traders as fodder for horses, probably some time between the ninth and thirteenth centuries A.D. Thus, the domesticated species is normally associated with India and Pakistan, where the plant has been grown for centuries as a food for both humans and animals (Whistler and Hymowitz, 1979). The green bean pods have become more widely available for human consumption, even in the United Kingdom, where they are used as an ingredient for spiced vegetable stews.

The guar plant is essentially a sun-loving plant, tolerant of high environmental temperatures but very susceptible to frost (Whistler and Hymowitz, 1979; Kay, 1979). For maximum growth the plant requires a soil temperature of 25–30°C and, ideally, a dry climate with sparse but regular rainfall. Most of the guar crop produced worldwide is grown in India and Pakistan. The plant has also been cultivated in tropical areas, such as South and Central America, Africa, Brazil, and Australia, but at the present time there has been little success in cultivating the crop in the temperate regions of Europe. It was also introduced to the semi-arid regions of the southwest United States in the early 1900s, although it was not until the 1950s that guar gum was produced in commercial quantities and used in industrial applications (Whistler and Hymowitz, 1979; Kay, 1979). In the food industry, guar gum is used as a thickening and stabilizing agent in a wide variety of foods (yogurt, ice cream, salad dressing), usually in amounts of <1% of the food weight (Whistler and Hymowitz, 1979; Wielinga, 1984).

III. BOTANICAL CHARACTERISTICS

The guar plant grows as a robust, annual crop to a height usually ranging from 0.5 to 2 m (Whistler and Hymowitz, 1979; Kay, 1979). There are many cultivars of guar plant; some types are erect, others have numerous strong branches. In general, branched types are considered to be more suitable for seed production. The stems are angular, ribbed, and hollow. The leaves are alternate, trifoliolate, and borne on long petioles, at the base of which is a marked pulvinus. The leaflets are ovate and 5–10 cm in length. The flowers are small and typically papilionaceous, with white standard petal and keel and pinkish-purple wings. The pods are generally oblong, 4.0–11.0 cm in length, although there is a sickle-shaped form (Fig. 1a,b). Each pod normally contains 5–12 oval or cube-shaped seeds. The seeds are of variable size, with a diameter of

---

upper gastrointestinal tract and absorbed into the portal blood (mostly as glucose); this includes starch, dextrins, and simple sugars (e.g., sucrose, lactose).

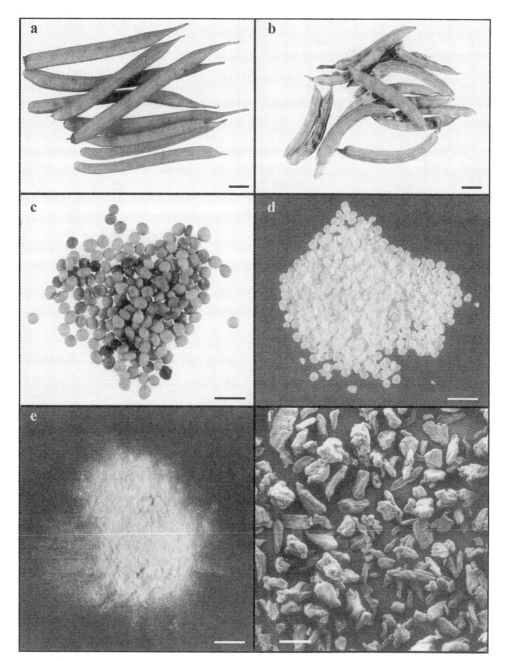

Fig. 1 Pictures of pods, seeds and endosperm extract of the guar plant (*Cyamopsis tetragonoloba* [L.] Taub.), a member of the Leguminosae family. (a) Green pods, scale bar = 1.3 cm. (b) Dried pods, scale bar = 1.6 cm. (c) Seeds, scale bar = 1 cm. (d) Endosperm halves (splits), scale bar = 1 cm. (e) Guar gum flour, scale bar = 1 cm. (f) Scanning electron micrograph of guar gum flour, scale bar = 100 μm.

approximately 6 mm when the pod is green (Fig. 1a) and about 4 mm when the pod is dried and yellow (Fig. 1b), and they are usually greyish buff or white in color (Fig. 1c).

Guar seeds consist of three major components: the testa (or hull), the endosperm, and the cotyledon (including the embryo), typically in proportions of 19–22%, 34–36%, and 43–45% by weight, respectively. Since the seeds are dicotyledonous, two endosperm halves (splits) are obtained from each seed (Fig. 1d). These endosperm halves, from which the guar gum flour is produced (Fig. 1e, f), surround the cotyledon, and they are in turn surrounded by the hull. A transverse section of the guar seed (Fig. 2) illustrates clearly the main features of the microstructure, which includes the epidermis, the characteristic hourglass cells of the hypodermis, the endosperm, and the palisade cells of the cotyledon, which are rich in protein (Saber et al., 1956).

The galactomannan fraction is the storage polysaccharide of the seed and is used for energy purposes during germination. Not surprisingly, this fraction represents the major component of the endosperm (see next section), although there appears to be some uncertainty about its location. A recent microscopic study of guar seeds stained with ruthenium red and toluidine blue, which are general stains for polysaccharide hydrocolloids (Flint, 1990), showed clear staining of the cell wall endosperm (Fig. 3a,b) (Brennan et al., 1996). This confirms the results obtained by Flint (1990) using the same technique to locate polysaccharide gums in food materials, including guar flour prepared from endosperm, and is consistent with the traditional view that the galactomannan is located in the endosperm cell walls (McClendon et al., 1976; Meir and Reid, 1982; Reid and Edwards, 1995). However, some later studies revealed the presence of large discrete inclusions in cells of the outer endosperm, which stained positively with the general

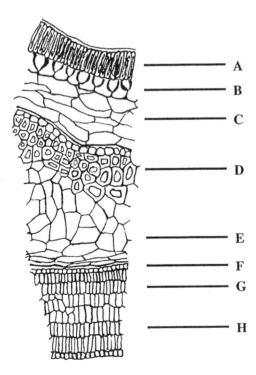

Fig. 2 Drawing of transverse section through guar seed. A = palisade cells of epidermis, B = hourglass cells of hypodermis, C = parenchyma tissue, D = outer layer of endosperm, E = inner layer of endosperm, F = epidermis of cotyledon, G = upper palisade cells of cotyledon, and H = lower palisade cells of cotyledon. Illustration not drawn to scale.

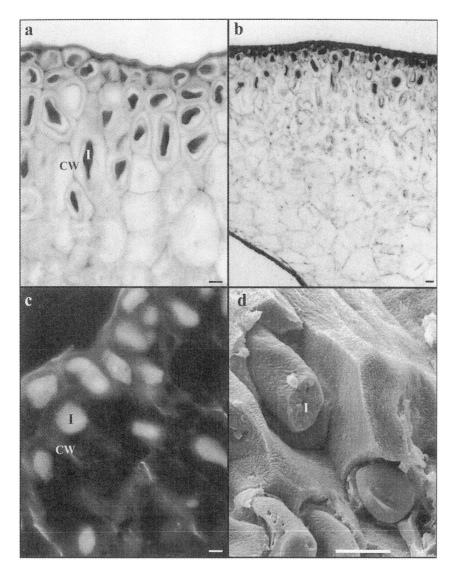

Fig. 3 (a) Transverse section of guar seed stained with ruthenium red, showing the outer layers of endosperm cells with stained intracellular inclusions (I) and stained cell walls (CW), scale bar = 20 μm. (b) Transverse section of guar seed stained with toluidine blue, showing endosperm cells with stained inclusions and cell walls, scale bar = 20 μm. (c) Transverse section of guar endosperm stained with fluorescein-labelled lectin from *Vicia faba* showing location of galactomannan in cell walls (CW) and intracellular inclusions (I), scale bar = 10 μm. (d) Scanning electron micrograph of outer layer of endosperm, showing fractured cell wall (CW) and intracellular inclusions (I), scale bar = 100 μm.

stains (Flint, 1990; Brennan et al., 1996). These inclusions were variable in size, sometimes cigar-shaped but mostly amorphous in structure, and seemed to occupy much of the intracellular space of the outer endosperm cells. Evidence to establish that galactomannan was present in these intracellular inclusions, as well as the cell walls, came from the use of fluorescein-labeled lectins (Fig. 3c). One of the lectins was specific for α-D-galactose residues and the other for D-mannose units, both of which stained positively with the endosperm cell walls and the inclusions (Brennan et al., 1996). Examination of the intracellular inclusions in the seeds and guar gum flour was also undertaken with scanning electron microscopy (SEM). These structures appeared to correspond with the images seen under the light microscope (Fig. 3a,b,c). Interestingly, SEM images revealed more detail of the inclusions, showing that they consisted of ovoid or spherical microstructures approximately 0.8–1.2 μm in diameter (Fig. 3d). Further work needs to be done to investigate the structural characteristics of these seemingly galactomannan-rich deposits and their physiological role in the germinating seed.

IV. EXTRACTION, PRODUCTION, AND COMPOSITION OF GUAR GUM FLOUR

World production of the dried guar seeds for industrial use is in the region of 0.5 million metric tons (MT) per annum, although only around 25–30% of this is processed to yield the gum (Wielinga, 2000). Thus, the world market for the guar gum is about 130,000–150,000 MT per year, with about 50,000–55,000 MT used by the food and pet food industries. Production of guar splits (endosperm halves) of variable quality is dominated by India and Pakistan, with the rest being produced mainly by the United States (Robbins, 1988).

To recover guar gum from the seed, it is necessary to separate the endosperm halves or splits from the hull and the cotyledon. Guar gum is produced from the seed endosperm splits. The production of the gum varies between different manufactures but usually involves three stages: (a) removal of the cotyledon, (b) removal of the hull, and (c) grinding of the endosperm.

On arrival at the processing plant, seeds are screened for removal of impurities. The cleaned seeds are fed into a mill, where they are cleaved into two halves and the cotyledons are freed. The cotyledons are then sifted away as finer material. The rest of the mixture is heated to soften the hull and then fed into a mill where the hull is separated away from the endosperm. Many types of mechanical grinders, such as attrition mills and special hammer and roller mills, can be utilized for this purpose. Once the endosperm has been separated from the hull and cotyledon, it is ground to a flour of fine particle size and may then be purified by repeated alcohol washings. The final product is a white or slightly off-white powder (Fig. 1e), which is similar in appearance and texture to wheat flour.

There are many systems used for grading guar gum, each gum-producing country having its own system. The most important criteria are mesh size and viscosity, which is measured under standard conditions, often using a Brookfield viscometer. Mesh size is a measure of the size of the powder particles, which is a critical determinant of the hydration kinetics of guar gum. Generally, samples of small mesh size are more expensive because a high degree of control is needed during the grinding process in order to avoid depolymerization of the galactomannan and therefore loss of viscosity in solution. When the gum is hydrated, the level of viscosity produced is dependent on the concentration and molecular weight of the galactomannan fraction of the flour. The amount and molecular weight of the galactomannan found in the endosperm extract can vary significantly, depending on the source of the seed and the growing conditions.

The *Food Chemicals Codex* specifies a standard of not less than 66% of galactomannan in food-grade guar gum in the USA (Committee on Codex Specifications, 1981), although most samples obtained commercially contain usually >80% (w/w) galactomannan (Table 1). The other components of the guar gum, including lipid and protein, which are considered to be impurities, vary between different sources (Table 1). The crude fiber value indicates the presence of cellulose originating from cell wall material, mainly from small residual hull fragments and, to a lesser extent, the endosperm. Estimates of the galactomannan content were traditionally made by analyzing the total weight of impurities and, on a percentage basis, subtracting this

Table 1 Chemical Composition of Guar Gum
Flour Available Commercially

Component	Concentration (g/100 g)
Moisture	8.0–14.0
Galactomannan	73.0–86.7
Protein	3.0–6.0
Crude fiber	1.0–4.0
Ash (total minerals)	0.8–2.0
Fat (petroleum ether extractables)	0.5–1.0
Total impurities[a]	13.3–27.0

[a] Calculated as total nongalactomannan components

value from 100. Nowadays the galactomannan fraction is often analyzed more directly, for example, by acid hydrolysis to the galactose and mannose residues followed by gas chromatography of the alditol acetate derivatives (Englyst et al., 1992; Rayment et al., 1995). Most, but not all, of the galactomannan fraction is water soluble. In addition to galactose and mannose, other monosaccharides present in the guar flour, including glucose and arabinose, account for approximately 3–5% (dry matter basis) of the total nonstarch polysaccharides, the glucose originating from the cellulose fraction (Wang, 1997). Also, a small amount of uronic acid (1.0–2.5%) is found in guar gum flour, indicating the presence of pectic substances. Deviations from the typical composition seen in Table 1 can occur when very low molecular weight grades are produced from acid, alkaline, or enzyme hydrolysis of native guar gum. Consequently, the depolymerized grades usually have a higher ash content than the native form. This increase in ash, which reflects the amount of minerals in the guar flour, is derived from a neutralization stage following the hydrolysis treatment (Ellis and Morris, 1991). On the basis of usage of guar gum, different grades are divided according to whether they are used in the food industry or for other industrial purposes.

The recognition that viscous polysaccharides can be utilized for therapeutic purposes, for example, in the dietary management of diabetes, has led to the development of various pharmaceutical preparations containing guar gum. In the United Kingdom, they are currently taken by diabetic patients in the form of a premeal drink, usually mixed with water or orange juice (British Medical Association, 1995). These include capsules or macroaggregates of guar gum, such as granules and minitablets, which have been designed to hydrate slowly in the mouth to improve their palatability. Their beneficial effects have been reported to be extremely variable, however (O'Connor et al., 1981; Ellis et al., 1986, 1991), most probably because of their lack of hydration in the proximal gut (see Sec. V.E).

V. STRUCTURE AND PHYSICOCHEMICAL PROPERTIES OF GUAR GALACTOMANNAN

A. Molecular Weight and Structure

Guar galactomannan consists essentially of a linear $(1 \rightarrow 4)$-β-D-mannopyranose backbone with heavy substitution of single-unit α-D-galactopyranosyl branches attached at O-6 (Fig. 4). The molar ratio of galactose to mannose varies with origins, but is typically in the range 1:1.5–1.8 (Dea and Morrison, 1975; Reid and Edwards, 1995; Rayment et al., 1995). The distribution of

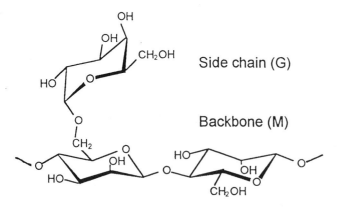

OH

OH

CH₂OH   Side chain (G)

HO   O

O

CH₂

Backbone (M)

O   OH   HO

O   O   OH   O

HO   O

CH₂OH   O

Fig. 4 Structure of guar galactomannan showing part of the mannose (M) backbone and side chain of single galactose (G) residues. Average molecular weight of native guar galactomannan is approximately in the range of 2.0–3.5 million.

D-galactosyl residues along the main chain was first believed to be at regular intervals (Baker and Whistler, 1975). Later, a block distribution was also proposed by Hall and Yalpani (1980), but the more generally accepted view is that it has a rather specific distribution of D-galactosyl residues in which there is a high proportion of substituted couplets and triplets (Hoffman and Svensson, 1978; McCleary et al., 1985). Variations in the structure are likely to occur if different methods of extracting galactomannan are used (Wielinga, 1984).

Like many polysaccharides found in nature, guar galactomannans are polydisperse, high molecular weight polymers (Dea and Morrison, 1975; Reid et al., 1987). Assuming that the galactomannan fraction hydrates to produce a viscous dispersion, the key determinants of the degree of viscosity produced in solution, measured under standard conditions, are concentration and molecular weight (and its distribution). The viscosifying effect of commercial guar gum preparations can vary enormously depending on the molecular weight of the galactomannan. Despite the importance of molecular weight, few authors in the nutrition field report this value (Ellis et al., 1986). Previous estimates of weight-average molecular weight found in the literature vary enormously, depending on what method is used, but these are typically in the range of 0.25–5 million (Dea & Morrison, 1975; Reid et al., 1987). Absolute methods have also been used to determine molecular weight, including light scattering techniques, which are also useful for providing structural information on the polysaccharide (Robinson et al., 1982; Burchard, 1994; Ross-Murphy et al., 1998; Beer et al., 1999). One relatively simple and reliable way of estimating molecular weight is to use intrinsic viscosity measurements, calibrated by light scattering or some other absolute method using the Mark-Houwink equation. Details of the intrinsic viscosity method are given in the following section. The use of such a method for native guar galactomannan samples used in human studies showed that molecular weights were in the range of 2.0–3.0 million (Ellis et al., 1991; Gatenby et al., 1996; Blake et al., 1997).

B. Solution Properties

The biological properties of guar galactomannans and other such polysaccharides are dependent on their behavior in an aqueous medium (Rees, 1977). The molecular shape or conformation of these macromolecules will determine how atoms and groups in the polymer are oriented to the outside and, therefore, interact with other molecules, solvents, or even biological surfaces. One good example here is how shape influences the relative solubility of polysaccharides in an aqueous environment, a property of critical importance in the digestion and absorption of nutrients in the human gut. Essentially, linear polymer coils in solution are typically described by the "random flight model" in which the (root mean square) size, the radius of gyration (R_g), is proportional to the square root of the molecular weight (relative molecular mass, M_r). For most linear polymers in solution, the chain "volume" (excluded volume effects) gives a slightly higher exponent $R_g \sim M_r^{0.6}$. The radius of gyration represents an average estimate of the effective size (radius) of the biopolymer molecule. The majority of water-soluble polysaccharides, including guar galactomannan, exist as fluctuating coils in solution, as opposed to a more "rigid" biopolymer material with less chain flexibility (Ross-Murphy, 1994). For spherical particles, such as globular proteins, the volume of the sphere is proportional to R_g^3 and therefore $R_g \propto M_r^{1/3}$. For rigid but infinitely thin rods, $R_g \propto M_r$.

The flow properties of guar galactomannan are dependent on molecular size and shape. A useful index of the size or hydrodynamic volume of an isolated guar galactomannan polymer coil is the limiting viscosity number or intrinsic viscosity, $[\eta]$. Intrinsic viscosity is defined as the fractional increase in viscosity per unit concentration of polymer under conditions of extreme dilution (Robinson et al., 1982). For each polymer-solvent system, viscosity increases with M_r according to the Mark-Houwink equation:

$$[\eta] = K'M_r^\alpha \tag{1}$$

where the parameters K' and α are both approximately related to the flexibility of the polymer. For flexible linear coils, sometimes referred to as "random coils," it is well accepted that α lies in the range 0.5–0.8. Robinson and coworkers elucidated the intrinsic viscosity, molecular weight, and chain flexibility of a number of guar galactomannan preparations (Robinson et al., 1982). They concluded that the variation in intrinsic viscosity with M_r followed the relationship $[\eta] \cong 3.8 \times 10^{-4}M_r^{0.72}$, which was consistent with polymer coil behavior. Recent measurements by Beer and coworkers, using a rapid method for determining the K' and α constants, are consistent with these results, producing values of 5.13×10^{-4} and 0.72, respectively (Beer et al., 1999).

Intrinsic viscosity varies with coil dimensions according to the Flory-Fox equation:

$$[\eta] = 6^{3/2}\phi R_g^3/M_r \tag{2}$$

where ϕ is a constant, 2.6×10^{26} kg^{-1}, for flexible polymers (Ross-Murphy, 1994).

By treating each polymer coil as a sphere of radius R, the hydrodynamic volume of each polymer coil varies as R_g^3. From Eq. (2), R_g^3 is proportional to $[\eta]M_r$ and the number of coils is proportional to C/M_r, where C is the concentration of the polymer. Therefore, the total volume occupied by the polymer coils can be described by the dimensionless coil overlap parameter $C[\eta]$. In order to describe accurately the behavior of guar galactomannan in solution, we have to consider the polymer in a dilute solution through semi-dilute to a concentrated regime. This requires the definition of a number of terms. A dilute polymer solution is one in which each flexible polymer chain occupies a separate domain within the solution with little or no interpenetration (see this effect at low $C[\eta]$ in Fig. 5). However, as the amount of polymer in solution increases, a polymer concentration is reached (C = C*) at which the polymer coils begin to overlap or interpenetrate. Solutions of molecules above the overlap concentration (C > C*), where significant polymer entanglement occurs, are known as semi-dilute (at high $C[\eta]$ in Fig. 5), to distinguish them from concentrated solutions, which have even higher chain density. For a guar solution, this would be at concentrations $\geq 20\%$, which is almost impossible to prepare as a solution in any case.

At low polymer concentrations, zero-shear specific viscosity (η_{sp}) increases approximately linearly with increasing concentration in a double logarithmic plot (Figs. 5,6). However, there

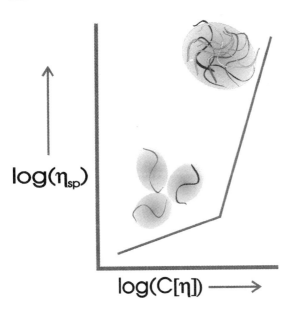

Fig. 5 Plot of dimensionless coil overlap parameter, $C[\eta]$, versus zero-shear specific viscosity, log η_{sp}, of a typical random coil polysaccharide solution. Pictures of coils on graph illustrate different concentration regimes of a random coil polymer, such as guar galactomannan, in the dilute solution region (low $C[\eta]$), where little or no interpenetration of chains occurs, and in the semi-dilute solution region (high $C[\eta]$), where significant polymer coil interpenetration or entanglement occurs.

is a marked increase in the gradient of this plot at some concentration above the specific critical concentration, the so-called C* (Fig. 6). To maintain consistency with the literature, this is defined as the critical breakpoint concentration (C_{cr}), and C* is simply approximated as $1/[\eta]$ (Ross-Murphy, 1994). The concentration at which the transition from dilute to semi-dilute solution behavior occurs varies from system to system depending on the hydrodynamic volume of the polymer coils. For very dilute solutions of random coil polymers, when a constant stress is applied, strain increases linearly with time, and they are described as Newtonian. As such, viscosity is constant over the range of shear rates measured. Here there are no complications from entanglements and the polymer molecules are sufficiently separated to move independently without much interaction. As concentration is increased the polymer chains overlap (semi-dilute region). This is characterized by a dramatic increase in the concentration dependence of viscosity (Figs. 5,6) and an increase in the pseudoplastic or shear-thinning nature of the material in solution (Fig. 7).

At concentrations above C_{cr}, the polymer coils can only exist in solution by interpenetration of neighboring chains and the formation of an "entanglement network." Hence, individual chains can only move about by wriggling or reptating through the entangled network of contiguous polymer chains (de Gennes, 1979). In a simplified discussion of the pseudoplastic behavior of semi-dilute solutions of guar gum, Morris and Ross-Murphy (1981) describe the onset of shear thinning as a situation where the rate of externally imposed movement becomes greater than the formation of new entanglements. Correspondingly, with increasing shear rate (see definition below), the extent of reentanglement decreases, with consequent decrease in the resistance to flow and viscosity (Fig. 7). In Fig. 6, when $C[\eta]$ is ≤ 1, a solution is said to be dilute, whereas when $C[\eta]$ is ≥ 1 it is said to be semi-dilute. As is well known, in the dilute regime, under steady shear conditions, specific viscosity $\eta_{sp} \approx C^{1-1.5}$, whereas when $C[\eta]$ is ≥ 10, well into

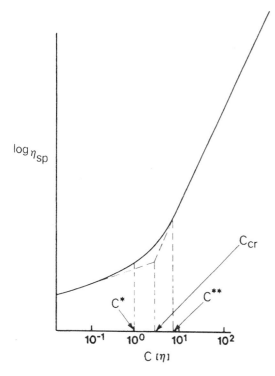

Fig. 6 Plot of the dimensionless coil overlap parameter, C[η], versus zero-shear specific viscosity (log η_{sp}) of a random coil polysaccharide solution. This corresponds to the plot seen in Fig. 5. C* marks the onset of significant coil overlap, C_{cr} is defined as the critical breakpoint concentration, and C** is the concentration where the second (higher) exponent is reached.

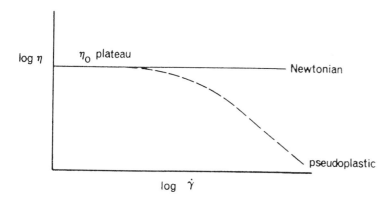

Fig. 7 Plot of log viscosity (η) versus log shear rate (γ̇) showing pseudoplastic or shear-thinning behavior of a typical random coil polysaccharide in solution. Thus, viscosity is highest at low shear rate, reaching a constant maximum at the so-called zero-shear rate (η_0 plateau) and a corresponding decrease in viscosity with increasing shear rate. For very high shear rates the pseudoplastic material reaches a second Newtonian plateau (not shown in figure).

the semi-dilute or entangled regime, $\eta_{sp} \approx C^{3.5-5}$ (Ross-Murphy, 1984). This means that for a polymer solution to be an effective thickener, $[\eta]$ has to be large for a given M_r. For solutions of guar gum, entanglement occurs when $C[\eta]$ exceeds approximately 2.5, and thereafter viscosity increases at approximately $C[\eta]^{4.3}$, so doubling the concentration or $[\eta]$ increases viscosity by a factor of about 30.

C. Rheological Methods

Rheology is defined as the flow and deformation of materials when subjected to an externally imposed force. Rheological measurements are concerned with the relationship of two physical quantities—stress and strain. Stress is the force per unit area acting upon or within a material, and strain is the amount of deformation induced by the stress. The characterization of biopolymer solutions such as guar gum depend, essentially, on the nature of the external forces applied to the materials and the time scale of their application. A relatively soft material can deform elastically like a solid when subjected to small forces for a short time, whereas a relatively hard material can flow like a liquid when subjected to large forces for a long time. Therefore, most biopolymers can be described as viscoelastic, having the properties of both a liquid and a solid. For liquids, such as solutions of guar gum, stress depends not on the amount of deformation but on the rate of change of strain with time or the *rate* of deformation. Shear viscosity is defined as $\eta = \tau/\dot{\gamma}$, where $\dot{\gamma}$ is the rate of shear strain (shear rate) and τ is shear stress.

A number of rheological techniques can be used to describe the flow properties of guar gum in solution. The intrinsic viscosity can be determined by dilute solution viscometry using a glass capillary viscometer immersed in a temperature-controlled water bath. The relative viscosity (η_r) is determined as the time taken for the dilute sample solution to pass between two defined levels marked on the glass viscometer divided by the time taken for the solvent to flow the same distance. The specific viscosity (η_{sp}) can be defined as $\eta_{sp} = \eta_r - 1$. A double log plot of η_{sp}/C and $\ln(\eta_r)/C$ versus concentration can give a determination of $[\eta]$ by extrapolation of the slopes to zero concentration. The molecular weight can then be determined using the Mark-Houwink relationship [Eq. (1)]. The flow conditions through a glass capillary are such that the polymer coils are subjected to varying, and often quite high, shear rates. However, the Newtonian nature of such dilute solutions means that these shear rate conditions are largely inconsequential. In order to describe the flow properties of such a system at concentrations where flow behavior becomes non-Newtonian in nature, techniques must be used that can accurately apply constant shear rates and operate over several decades of shear rate. This can be carried out using a controlled strain rheometer such as the Rheometrics Fluids Spectrometer (RFSII, Rheometric Scientific Inc., Piscataway, NJ) with a cone and plate geometry. With this geometry, small cone angles, say $<5°$, result in a constant shear stress and shear rate across the gap and rheological information can be obtained over approximately 5 decades of shear rate. For solutions of guar galactomannan filled with particulate inclusions, a model system that has proved useful for understanding the behavior of guar gum in the gut, a parallel plate geometry should be employed. This is due to the tendency of large particles to accumulate at the cone apex, which could result in abnormal flow conditions.

The intrinsic viscosity of commercially available native guar gum can be as high as 17 dL/g measured at 25°C, whereas some highly depolymerized products give an intrinsic viscosity of only about 0.5 dL/g under the same conditions. (Ellis et al., 1991; Blake et al., 1997; Wang, 1997). The intrinsic viscosity of a partially depolymerized guar galactomannan sample, similar to that used recently in clinical trials (Gatenby et al., 1996; Blake et al., 1997), was found to be 10.5 dL/g by extrapolation of η_{sp}/C and $\ln(\eta_r)/C$ versus C plots to zero (Fig. 8). The molecular weight was determined as 1.39×10^6 using the Mark-Houwink relationship [Eq. (1)] and

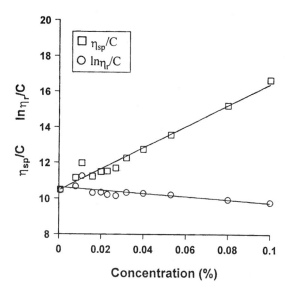

Fig. 8 Estimating intrinsic viscosity of purified guar galactomannan sample from plots η_{sp}/C versus concentration of galactomannan (%) ($\square$) and $\ln\eta_r/C$ versus concentration (%) ($\bigcirc$).

values of 3.8×10^{-4} dL/g and 0.72 from Robinson et al. (1982) for K' and α, respectively. Figure 9 shows the concentration dependence of viscosity-shear rate profiles of guar galactomannan. At concentrations of 0.2% and below, the guar galactomannan solution is Newtonian in behavior. However, as the concentration of the polymer in solution is increased, the system becomes more shear-thinning (pseudoplastic) in behavior and viscosity decreases at high shear rates.

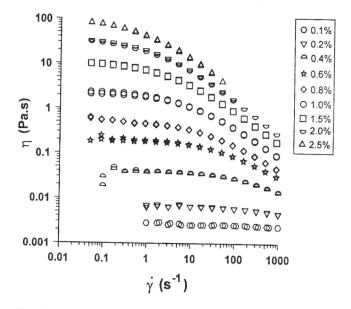

Fig. 9 Plot of viscosity (η) versus shear rate ($\dot{\gamma}$), showing shear rate and concentration dependence for viscosity of guar galactomannan solutions over a galactomannan concentration range of 0.1–2.5% (w/w). (Data taken from Rayment, 1996.)

The data plotted in Figs. 8 and 9 can be used, as discussed previously, to determine the rheological parameters C* and C_{cr}, respectively. Using these results as an example, the critical overlap concentration (C_{cr}) was calculated to be 0.24% (polymer concentration) from a double log plot of specific viscosity against the coil overlap parameter, where C[η] and η_{sp} were 2.5 and 3.8, respectively (Fig. 10), and C* was determined simply as 1/[η] ≈ 0.1%. For $\eta_{sp} < 10$, $\eta_{sp} \approx C^{1.1}$, whereas for $\eta_{sp} > 10$, $\eta_{sp} \approx C^{4.3}$, which are similar to results reported for other polysaccharides (Morris et al., 1981). The ratio C_{cr}/C* was found to be ~2.4, which is similar to the value published by Robinson et al. (1982) for other guar gum solutions. The shear-thinning nature of guar galactomannan solutions has been demonstrated previously by a number of groups (Whitcomb et al., 1980; Doublier and Launay, 1981; Richardson and Ross-Murphy, 1987; Rayment et al., 1995). This type of behavior can be described by the Cross equation (Cross, 1965), often used to describe shear-thinning behavior of other polysaccharide solutions (Doublier and Launay, 1981; Giboreau et al., 1994):

$$\eta = \eta_\infty + [\eta_{0X} - \eta_\infty]/[1 + (a\dot{\gamma})^p] \tag{3}$$

where η_{0X} and η_∞ are limiting (Cross) viscosities at zero and infinite shear rates, a and $\dot{\gamma}$ are relaxation time and shear rate, respectively, and p is an exponent. Viscosity is a constant maximum at the so-called zero-shear rate (see Newtonian plateau in Figs. 7 and 9).

Attempts have been made to characterize the shear-thinning of random coil polysaccharides by two parameters from a linear plot (Morris, 1990). The generalized shear-thinning curve for random coil polysaccharide solutions (Morris et al., 1981) showed that a single master curve could be produced irrespective of primary structure, M_r, temperature, and solvent conditions. Therefore, a two-parameter equation was produced, which attempted to match the generalized shear-thinning and allowed η_0 (zero-shear) and $\dot{\gamma}_{1/2}$ to be determined from a simple linear plot of η versus $\eta\dot{\gamma}^{0.76}$:

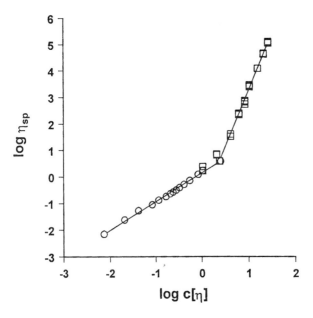

Fig. 10 Concentration dependence of zero-shear specific viscosity (η_{sp}) of a guar gum sample. The circle and square symbols represent data obtained from dilute solution viscometry and steady shear measurements on a rheometrics fluids spectrometer (RFSII), respectively. The critical breakpoint (C_{cr}) was found to be 2.5 on the x-axis (C[η]) and 3.8 on the y-axis (η_{sp}). (Data taken from Rayment, 1996.)

$$\eta = \eta_0/[1 + (\dot{\gamma}/\dot{\gamma}_{1/2})^{0.76}] \tag{4}$$

where $\dot{\gamma}_{1/2}$ is the shear rate required to reduce η to $\eta_0/2$. This can be seen to be a special form of Eq. (3) with $\eta_\infty = 0$ and $p = 0.76$.

It was envisaged that this equation would be helpful in digestive physiology studies of guar gum where only a less sophisticated viscometer was available (Morris, 1990). This approach was useful in providing an estimate of the effect of guar gum on digesta rheology in the gut lumen of experimental animals (see nutrition section). The interpretation of results from such studies however are complicated by the effects of particulate material on the shear-thinning behavior of guar gum. The effect of particulate material (i.e. filler) on the rheology of guar gum solutions has received little attention and yet this is of considerable value in facilitating our understanding the behavior of guar gum in the gastrointestinal tract of humans and other mammals (Ellis, 1994).

D.   Rheology of Guar/Starch Mixtures and Their Use in Modeling Intestinal Digesta

To study the rheological behavior of guar gum in the human gut, several factors need to be kept in mind. When ingested by humans, its effects in the proximal gut are strongly dependent on the mode of administration, dose, and characteristics of the guar gum used and on its physical state in the gut lumen (Ellis et al., 1996). Consequently, the hydration kinetics of galactomannan in the gut lumen is a critical factor (see next section). Also, intestinal motility and changes in fluid secretion and absorption will affect galactomannan concentration and flow behavior of digesta. In view of the complexity of gastrointestinal function, it is not surprising that rates of movement in the gut lumen are difficult to predict. Flow patterns in response to peristaltic movement are likely to change continually, and digesta will be subject to widely different shear rates and other modes of deformation, such as extensional flow, at different sites of the gut and at different times (Ellis et al., 1996). Moreover, the contribution of particulate material to the viscosity of digesta is of considerable importance, but it is only recently that this has been investigated.

Although digesta is an extremely heterogeneous system to investigate, it was envisaged that studying the behavior of a relatively simple model system would provide some insight into the functional properties of guar gum in vivo. Our group has recently studied the effects of increased particulate concentration (filler loadings) on the rheological behavior of a pure guar galactomannan solution (Rayment et al., 1995, 1996, 1998, 2000). In our model system, guar gum solutions were filled with increasing concentrations of rice starch. These were relatively spherical starch granules and were selected for their small size (6–10 μm) and homogeneity. Steady shear measurements of guar/rice starch mixtures were performed at 25°C using the Rheometrics Fluids Spectrometer (Rayment et al., 1995). As the amount of starch filler was increased (Fig. 11), the dispersion began to develop some additional rheological features. The effect of particulate inclusions in the guar/rice starch mixture was, primarily, to increase the steady shear viscosity above that of the pure galactomannan system. The initial Newtonian flow properties of the pure system at low shear rates became more rate dependent on increasing particulate concentration, the so-called power-law behavior. From the flow data obtained for the guar/rice starch mixtures, there was need to include an extra term, here denoted the yield stress, in the Cross model, especially for the higher filler concentrations used. This flow behavior has been described with reasonable accuracy by using a yield stress–modified Cross equation:

$$\eta = \eta_\infty + [\eta_{0X} - \eta_\infty]/[1 + (a\dot{\gamma})^p] + (\tau_X/\dot{\gamma}) \tag{5}$$

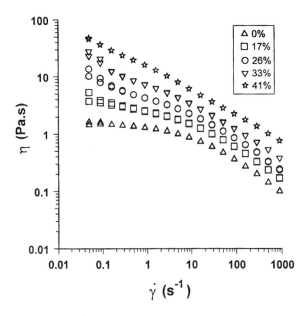

Fig. 11 Effect of increasing rice starch concentration (0–41%, w/w) on the viscosity (η)-shear rate ($\dot{\gamma}$) flow curve of a 1% (w/w) guar galactomannan solution. Duplicate data are presented to indicate good reproducibility of results. (Data taken from Rayment et al., 1995.)

Zero-shear viscosity and apparent yield stress data were determined from this equation and then fitted to a number of mathematical models, which incorporated volume fraction parameters for rice starch. By using so-called creep experiments, the experimental range can be extended to very low shear rates to verify the model applicability (Rayment et al., 1998). Using these models a new master curve was then produced, which we believe will allow us to make predictions of the rheological behavior of similar biopolymer dispersions where the volume fraction of the particulate components is known. The Landel equation (Ross-Murphy, 1984) fitted particularly well with the essentially spherical rice starch granules (Fig. 12a,b) (Rayment et al., 1995) but less so with more rod-shaped particles in the form of microcrystalline cellulose (Rayment et al., 2000). The model also worked reasonably well with a more heterogeneous food material containing wheat starch (Rayment et al., 1996). The extrapolation of this model to real food systems and even intestinal digesta is a much more complex, but not necessarily unrealistic objective. However, to achieve this, the minimum information needed is the fractional volume of particulate components at different sites of the gastrointestinal tract. One practical problem here is the recovery of representative samples of human digesta using intubation techniques in humans. As an alternative, the recovery of digesta could be achieved by using a suitable experimental animal that has been cannulated at appropriate sites of the gut (e.g., jejunum).

E. Hydration Kinetics of Guar Galactomannan

Current evidence indicates that the biological function of guar gum, when mixed into liquid foods, depends mainly on its capacity to hydrate rapidly and increase viscosity in the small intestine. The solution properties of guar gum are also likely to be important when it is mixed into a solid food such as wheat bread, but, as discussed previously, other factors may also be involved (Brennan et al., 1996). It would be reasonable to assume, therefore, that the hydration

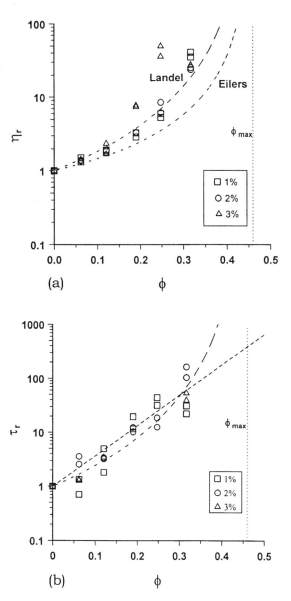

Fig. 12 (a) Relationship between normalized apparent zero-shear viscosity (η_r) and starch concentration (ϕ) (volume fraction of starch) for 1% ($\square$), 2% ($\bigcirc$), and 3% ($\triangle$) guar galactomannan solutions, fitted to the Landel and Eilers formula. The dotted line represents the maximum packing fraction (ϕ_{max}) of the system. (b) Same as (a) except that volume fraction of starch (ϕ) plotted against apparent yield stress (τ_r). (All data for (a) and (b) taken from Rayment et al., 1995.)

kinetics and rheological behavior of guar gum are useful indicators of biological function. A number of dietary supplements, which are commercially available, hydrate slowly to reduce the effect of in-mouth viscosity, but many of these have been found to be very unpalatable and therapeutically ineffective. O'Connor and colleagues (1981) investigated the rate of hydration of various preparations of guar gum used for lowering postprandial glycemia. They tested four industrial samples, including two guar gum flours and two granulate preparations, one of which was wax-coated. The results clearly showed marked differences in the rate of hydration between samples, which appeared to be dependent on the physical nature of the guar gum preparations. The two flours hydrated more quickly and produced the highest viscosity in vitro and were also equally effective in reducing the postprandial rise in blood glucose levels in human subjects.

Subsequently, our own group developed a new method for monitoring the hydration rate of a range of commercially available preparations of guar gum (Ellis and Morris, 1991). This involved hydrating each sample in turn in a standard volume of water and measuring viscosity over a 5-hour period, using a Brookfield RVT rotoviscometer (spindle 4 at 20 rpm). Marked differences in hydration rate and ultimate viscosity (measured after 24 hours) were observed between the different guar gum preparations (Fig. 13). Not unexpectedly, this was attributed mainly to differences in particle size, such that samples with a smaller particle size (<150 μm) hydrated more quickly and attained higher ultimate viscosities than those with a larger particle size (3–4 mm). Interestingly, the two preparations that were least effective in generating solution viscosity were shown in earlier studies to have little or no effect on glycemic control in experimental animals (Heppell and Rainbird, 1985) and human subjects (Holman et al., 1987; Baker, 1988). No attempt was made in our study (Ellis and Morris, 1991) to simulate in vivo conditions, on the basis that there were too many unknown factors to control for (e.g., mixing conditions, fluid secretion/absorption effects). We concluded, however, that this type of hydration method would provide a useful empirical, quantitative comparison of different preparations of guar gum. The method is also a cost-effective preliminary screening test before undertaking more costly and time-consuming clinical trials. This hydration method was later modified to allow measurements of zero-shear viscosity on the RFSII instrument and to investigate the mechanism of hydration or dissolution of guar galactomannan samples varying in polymer concentration, M_r, and particle size. From these experiments, a number of mathematical models were fitted to the

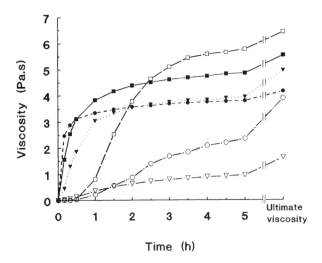

Fig. 13 Hydration rate profiles of guar gum samples presented as viscosity (Pa.s) versus time. Experimental points are mean values from measurements on four replicate solutions of native guar gum flours M150 (■) and RG30 (--●--), pharmaceutical granule preparations Guarina (···▼···), Guarem (□), and Lejguar (○), and Glucotard minitablets (▽). The ultimate viscosity is the measurement of viscosity taken after 24 hours of hydration following homogenization of the guar solution with an ultra-turrax mixer. The final viscosity is taken only when a consistent maximum reading is recorded on the viscometer (usually after homogenizing for 4–6 min). (Data taken from Ellis and Morris, 1991.)

hydration data. One of these, a logarithmic model, was found to be the best fit for describing the hydration kinetics of guar galactomannan (Wang, 1997), as seen in the following:

$$\ln(1 - \eta_t/\eta_\infty) = b + k \ln t \tag{6}$$

where b and k are hydration constants, representing the intercept and slope of the linear plot, respectively, and η_t, and η_∞ are viscosity at time t and ultimate viscosity, respectively. Consequently, the hydration process can be described simply by these two hydration constants, obtained from the linear plot. For comparative purposes, the hydration rate of different guar gum samples can then be defined in terms of a hydration index by the use of a modified version of Eq. (6):

$$t_{0.8} = (0.2/\exp(b))^{1/k} \tag{7}$$

Thus, the hydration rate index $t_{0.8}$ was defined as the time needed for the viscosity to reach 80% of the ultimate viscosity (η_∞). The smaller the $t_{0.8}$ value, the higher the hydration rate. The results of the guar study clearly showed that there was a significant inverse relationship between hydration rate and M_r, so that $t_{0.8}$ values for guar gum samples with M_rs 2.82, 1.39, and 0.75 million were 307, 103, and 29 minutes, respectively (Wang, 1997). It was also found that the hydration rate increased with increasing polymer concentration at polymer concentration (C) range 0–1.2% (w/w) but decreased when C was >1.2% (w/w). Preliminary studies by our own group (Ellis et al., 1991) and later by To et al. (1994) have also shown an inverse relationship between the particle size of guar gum and its hydration rate. A more detailed hydration kinetic study confirmed this relationship using a wide particle size range (60–500 μm) prepared from the same batch of guar endosperm (Wang, 1997). At the upper end of the particle size range, the hydration data showed a poor fit to the logarithmic relationship [Eq. (6)], but the fit was greatly improved by using a polynomial model.

Other important factors are known to influence the extent and rate of hydration of guar gum, including pH, temperature, and the presence of other solutes, such as salts and sucrose (Whistler and Hymowitz, 1979). While it is generally accepted that the hydration rate will increase with increasing temperature, it is not clear what effects pH will have on this process. Carlson et al. (1962) showed that the hydration rate of guar gum was slowest in more acidic conditions (pH 3–4), but changes in pH did not change the final viscosity. Subsequently, Maier et al. (1993) reported that the hydration rate of guar gum increased with decreasing pH. Our own recent experiments seem to be consistent with the former results (Carlson et al., 1962), indicating that lowering the pH of a 0.8% (w/w) solution from 6.5 to 3.0 significantly decreased the hydration rate, particularly during the initial stages of hydration (Wang, 1997; Wang et al., 2000). From a physiological perspective, this has an important bearing on the hydration of guar in the stomach, where gastric contents are in the acidic range, pH 1.5–5 (Rayding et al., 1984; Savarino et al., 1988).

VI. NUTRITIONAL AND PHYSIOLOGICAL EFFECTS OF GUAR GUM

It is now well established that dietary supplements of guar gum strongly influence gastrointestinal function and lipid and carbohydrate metabolism in a largely beneficial way (Truswell and Benyon, 1992; Ellis, 1994, 1999). Over 30 years ago Farenbach and coworkers demonstrated for the first time that guar gum elicited a plasma cholesterol-lowering effect in human subjects (Fahrenbach et al., 1965), a result that has been repeated many times subsequently (Gatenby, 1990; Truswell and Benyon 1992). In the mid-1970s, Jenkins and colleagues (1976a, 1977a) reported the efficacy of guar gum in attenuating the postprandial rise in blood glucose and insulin concentrations in healthy and diabetic subjects (Fig. 14). Since then, many research groups have confirmed these results, showing that guar gum, mixed into starchy foods or glucose drinks, significantly decreases postprandial glycemia and insulinemia (Morgan et al., 1979, 1985, 1990; Ellis et al., 1981, 1988a,b, 1991; O'Connor et al., 1981; Jarjis et al., 1984; Fairchild et al., 1996). These acute effects suggested that guar gum reduces the rate and/or extent of digestion and absorption of available carbohydrate in the gastrointestinal tract. Direct evidence for this is lacking in humans, however, mainly because of the problems of obtaining a quantitative estimate of glucose absorption, which requires access to the hepatic portal vein (Ellis et al., 1996).

Studies in pigs, a useful animal model for physiological studies of guar gum, provided the first direct evidence that guar gum decreases the rate of glucose absorption (Roberts et al., 1991; Simões Nunes and Malmlöf, 1992; Blake 1993a,b; Ellis et al., 1995, 1996). These studies involved measuring simultaneously the glucose concentrations in the hepatic portal vein and the peripheral blood (e.g., mesenteric artery) and also the flow rate of the portal blood. From these data, quantitative estimates of apparent glucose absorption were calculated from the arterio-venous differences and blood flow measurements. In pigs given doses of guar gum of

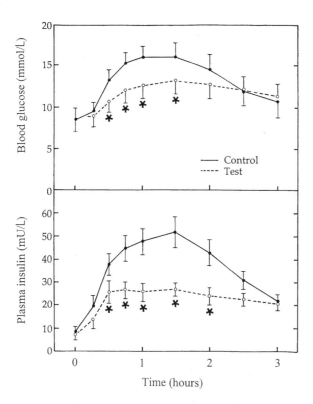

Fig. 14 Postprandial blood glucose and insulin concentrations of patients with type 2 (non–insulin-dependent) diabetes mellitus in response to control and test breakfast meals of bread and marmalade (total available carbohydrate, mainly starch and sugars, was 106 g). The test contained 16 g of guar gum (in the bread) and 10 g of pectin (in the marmalade). *Significant differences between control and test meals at each time point for glucose values: 30 min ($p < 0.01$), 45 min ($p > 0.01$), 60 min ($p < 0.01$) and 90 min ($p < 0.02$); and insulin values: 30 min ($p < 0.05$), 45 min ($p < 0.02$), 60 min ($p < 0.01$), 90 min ($p < 0.002$) and 120 min ($p < 0.01$). (Figure redrawn from data published by Jenkins et al., 1976.)

2 and 4% of the experimental diet, significant reductions in glucose absorption over 4 hours were observed (Ellis et al., 1995). At the highest concentration of guar gum, a 42% reduction in glucose absorption was seen. The doses of guar gum used in this study were equivalent to those consumed by human subjects in clinical trials where a blood glucose–lowering effect was demonstrated.

In the same pig studies, apparent insulin secretion, estimated from porto-arterial differences and blood flow measurements, was significantly decreased over 4 hours in response to the guar diet (Roberts et al., 1991; Simões Nunes and Malmlöf, 1992; Blake 1993a,b; Ellis et al., 1995, 1996). This suggests that the attenuation in the plasma insulin levels seen in human subjects is mainly due to a decrease in insulin secretion of the pancreatic islet β-cells as result of a lowered rate of glucose absorption. The insulin-lowering effect of guar gum may also be linked to a reduced stimulation of insulinotrophic hormones of the entero-insular axis, notably gastric inhibitory polypeptide (GIP) and glucagon-like peptide-1 (the GLP-1$_{(7-36)}$ amide sequence). The secretion of these gut hormones is strongly dependent on the rate and site of active absorption of glucose into the portal blood. A number of human studies have already demonstrated that guar gum decreases the postprandial rise in plasma GIP concentrations (Morgan et al., 1979, 1985, 1990; Gatenby et al., 1996). Again, quantitative data on gut hormone secretion were obtained from pig trials using the same techniques for estimating insulin secretion and showed significant decreases in total apparent GIP and GLP-1 production (Blake et al., 1993a; Ellis et al., 1995).

Another interpretation of data showing decreases in the peripheral blood insulin concentrations, in response to guar gum, is that there has been an increase in hepatic extraction of insulin. Simultaneous measurements of C-peptide and insulin concentrations in the peripheral blood can provide useful information about this process and the secretion of insulin from the islet β-cells of the pancreas (Binder, 1991). Both insulin and C-peptide are secreted into the portal blood in near-equimolar quantities from the islet β-cells. However, insulin, unlike C-peptide, is extracted from the portal blood by the liver to a large but variable degree before it reaches the peripheral blood circulation. Hepatic extraction of C-peptide is negligible under a wide variety of conditions (Binder, 1991). Also, the metabolic clearance rate of C-peptide is constant and seems to be unaffected by meal ingestion (Licioni-Paxicio et al., 1986). Thus, postprandial measurements of C-peptide in the peripheral blood reflect the secretion of the pancreas more accurately than measurements of insulin, whereas peripheral insulin levels reflect the balance between secretion and hepatic extraction. From the results of studies in healthy subjects and people with type 2 (non–insulin-dependent) diabetes mellitus, it appears that guar gum has little effect on postprandial blood C-peptide concentrations despite producing significant decreases in plasma insulin (Gatenby et al., 1996; Fairchild et al., 1996). This suggests that the insulin-lowering effect of guar gum is explained by an increase in hepatic extraction of insulin rather than a decrease in insulin secretion. However, both these studies suffered from a lack of statistical power due to low subject numbers, so the results should be treated with caution. In fact, in the study with healthy subjects there was a lowering of the C-peptide levels after guar gum ingestion, but these changes were on the borderline of statistical significance (Fairchild et al., 1996). Paradoxically, in one long-term study of healthy subjects, guar gum was reported to increase both insulin secretion and hepatic extraction of insulin (Groop et al., 1986). Overall, however, most of the metabolic data seem to support the view that guar gum improves insulin sensitivity. More direct evidence for this has come from the results of streptozotocin-induced diabetic rats (Cameron-Smith et al., 1997) and studies of healthy human subjects (Landin et al., 1992) and type 2 diabetic patients (Taglioferro et al., 1985).

Despite the large number of clinical studies carried out to assess the efficacy of guar gum, our understanding of its mechanism of action is still poor. One major reason for this is that there are profound deficiencies in our understanding of the behavior of guar galactomannan in the human gut. This is hampered by our lack of knowledge of the effects of guar gum on the physicochemical properties of digesta, an extremely complex heterogeneous material. The literature devoted to studying the nutritional effects and mechanisms of action guar gum in experimental animals and humans is extensive. No attempt is made in the following section to review all this literature, but we have endeavored to provide the reader with an overview of the work mainly related to the effects of guar gum on glucose absorption.

VII. PHYSICOCHEMICAL MECHANISMS UNDERLYING THE PHYSIOLOGICAL EFFECTS OF GUAR GUM

A. Modification of Gastrointestinal Function

There is little doubt that the ingestion of guar gum mixed into a drink or solid food can significantly modify digesta properties at all sites of the gastrointestinal tract (Read and Eastwood, 1992; Ellis et al., 1996; Johnson, 1999). One important feature, but probably not the only one, is the well-characterized behavior of guar gum for producing a highly viscous network in an aqueous solution at relatively low polymer concentrations (as described above). Early studies suggested that this property was the main determinant of its effects on postprandial glycemia (Jenkins et al., 1978; Jarjis et al., 1984), but these observations were made on aqueous solutions containing glucose and polymer only. The degree of complexity increases when the guar gum is ingested with other nutrients (e.g., animal feeds) or as part of a real food product. In such systems there is unlikely to be one unifying mechanism to explain precisely the physiological effects of guar gum in the human gut. A number of physicochemical mechanisms may be involved, but which of these predominate will depend on various factors, particularly on the type of guar gum and the form in which the gum is ingested. Accordingly, the mode of action of pharmaceutical preparations of guar gum, when administered as a premeal drink, is likely to be very different from that of a guar-enriched food product. But there is little doubt that the rheological behavior of guar gum is an important, if not critical factor, in explaining its effects on postprandial glycemia (Cherbut et al., 1990; Ellis et al., 1996). Much of the data published to date seems to indicate that guar gum decreases the rate of absorption of glucose into the hepatic portal vein mainly by inhibiting the processes associated with the digestion and absorption of available carbohydrates. These processes include gastric function, intestinal transit and mixing, α-amylase–starch interactions, and the movement of hydrolyzed products of starch.

1. Gastric Function

Several studies in experimental animals (Leeds et al., 1979; Bueno et al., 1981; Brown et al., 1988; Meyer et al., 1988) and human volunteers (Holt et al., 1979; Wilmhurst and Crawley, 1980; Blackburn et al., 1984; Torsdottir et al., 1989; Leclere et al., 1994) have demonstrated that guar gum reduces the rate of gastric emptying of a meal. However, some studies have shown that gastric emptying is unaltered (Tredger et al., 1984) or even accelerated (Morgan et al., 1990; Potkins et al., 1991). More significantly, perhaps, some of the early experiments did not indicate an association between gastric emptying rate and postprandial hyperglycemia in pigs (Rainbird and Low, 1986) and human subjects (Blackburn et al., 1984) consuming guar gum. In contrast, Torsdottir and coworkers (1989) demonstrated a strong positive correlation between the slowing of gastric emptying rate and the lowering of the postprandial rise in blood glucose. This group conducted their gastric-emptying experiments using healthy male volunteers consuming a liquid formula diet with and without guar gum.

The contradictory results from gastric-emptying experiments are probably due to differences in the types and mode of administration of guar gum being tested, the proportion of solids and liquid in the meals consumed, and the techniques used for measuring gastric emptying (Low, 1990). There are also difficulties in evaluating the pattern of gastric emptying of solid and liquid phases of digesta into the duodenum, especially when guar gum is added to the test meal (Rainbird and Low, 1986; Meyer and Doty, 1988; Low, 1990). In pig studies where this was investigated, guar gum was seen to inhibit the rate of emptying of the liquid phase, whereas the emptying of the solids was unaffected (Rainbird and Low, 1986).

The ingestion of guar gum is likely to modify gastric function in other ways (Meyer et al., 1986; Meyer and Doty, 1988; Ellis et al., 1996). In studies of gut function in dogs, guar gum was reported to impair gastric trituration and sieving by increasing the viscosity of the stomach contents. Thus, when dogs were fed guar gum mixed into a meal of meat, bread, margarine, and water, postprandial measurements showed that there was a significant increase in the proportion of large particles of food entering the small intestine (Meyer and Doty, 1988). Such an effect reduces the rate of digestibility of nutrients, as a result of a corresponding decrease in surface area of the large food particles available for enzyme hydrolysis. One possible explanation for the changes in particle size is that it may be more difficult for the stomach to sieve out and disrupt solid particles of food when the gastric contents are highly viscous.

2.   Intestinal Transit and Mixing

There is evidence from human and animal studies that guar gum delays the transit of digesta in the small intestine (Bueno et al., 1981; Blackburn et al., 1984; Brown et al., 1988; Read and Eastwood, 1992). An inhibition of the rate of flow of digesta within the small intestine will inhibit the physical mixing of nutrients and enzymes (e.g., pancreatic amylase). This reduces not only the rate of digestion, but also the movement of nutrients from the lumen to the mucosal epithelium. There is little doubt that a high level of digesta viscosity produced by guar gum in the gut severely inhibits propulsive and mixing effects of intestinal contractions (Bueno et al., 1981; Blackburn et al., 1984; Edwards et al., 1988; Cherbut et al., 1990). The effect of guar gum on mixing behavior of digesta at different sites of the gastrointestinal tract has yet to be investigated, but it is likely to be extremely complex. It has been suggested that an increase in viscosity of digesta produces laminar or "streamline" flow, rather than turbulent or disordered flow, which is characteristic of less viscous fluids and facilitates efficient mixing of digesta in the gut (Macagno et al., 1982). Laminar-type mixing under viscous conditions would probably reduce the rate at which nutrients are presented to the epithelial surface and are then absorbed into the hepatic portal vein.

B.   Measurements of Digesta Rheology

Mechanistic studies have tended to show that the biological activity of guar galactomannan is dependent largely on its capacity to increase the viscosity of digesta in the stomach and small intestine (Cherbut et al., 1990; Ellis et al., 1996; Gallaher et al., 1999). Its effects on the physical properties of digesta in the large intestine have been much less studied, although the assumption here is that the polymer has negligible effects on viscosity because it is depolymerized by bacterial enzymes. However, guar gum is likely to have significant effects on the rheology of digesta in the large bowel until such time that it is degraded by bacterial fermentation. The importance of viscosity in explaining the biological activity of guar gum in the gut has been recognized for many years (Jenkins et al., 1978a; Ebihara and Kiriyama, 1982), but surprisingly little progress has been made in understanding its rheological behavior in vivo. There are a number of reasons for this. First, attempts to measure digesta rheology in vivo are inherently problematic, because there are practical difficulties of gaining access to sites of interest in the gut, particularly in human subjects (Ellis et al., 1996). Assuming that sufficient samples of digesta can be obtained, which can be a problem in small experimental animals, there are no reliable techniques for measuring the rheological properties of whole digesta, an extremely complex heterogeneous system. Second, many factors complicate the interpretation of the rheological behavior of intestinal contents containing guar gum (Ellis et al., 1996). These include, as discussed above, a lack of information on the hydration kinetics of guar and the contribution of undissolved food particles to digesta viscosity. Also, nonstarch polysaccharides may be prone to depolymerization in the proximal gut, some evidence for this coming from studies of pigs fed oat β-glucan (Johansen et al., 1993). Consequently there is always the possibility that guar galactomannan is depolymerized in the stomach and small intestine, although evidence for this occurring in experimental animals and humans is lacking. Data from in vitro experiments suggest that the degradation of guar gum, after incubation for 5 hours at 37°C, is negligible at pH levels likely to occur in the stomach after a meal (Wang et al., 2000)

Our own research work has focused on measuring viscosity of digesta removed from the gut of pigs given diets containing guar gum (Roberts et al., 1990a,b; Ellis et al., 1995; 1996). The animals were fitted with cannulas located in the mid-jejunum region, about 2.0 m distal to the pylorus of the stomach, to allow collection of digesta. After removal of the digesta from the pig's jejunum, viscosity measurements were made at 4 or 5 shear rates on a Brookfield DV-II rotoviscometer fitted with a small sample adapter. The advantages of using the Brookfield for such studies is that it is a robust and portable instrument and small enough for use in a pig house, where space can be somewhat limited. The main disadvantage is that viscosity measurements can only be taken over a narrow shear rate range. Also, large particles of food in the digesta interfere with making reliable viscosity measurements; however, this is a limitation of viscometers in general, not just with the Brookfield. One practical solution to this problem is to remove these large particles (>0.8–1.0 mm) by gentle sieving of the digesta immediately after removal from the jejunum of the pig. As previously mentioned, the presence of particulate material in the digesta will increase not only viscosity but also the power-law behavior at low shear rates. Hence, estimates of zero-shear viscosity become increasingly more difficult as the fractional volume of particles increases (Fig. 11). Furthermore, the removal of particles > 1.0 mm, which contain starch and guar gum, will have important mechanistic implications (see next section). Estimates of zero-shear viscosity were made from the measurements of digesta viscosity using Morris's modified Cross equation [Eq. (4)] (Morris, 1990).

Given the limitations of the methods currently used for studying the rheological behavior of the digesta system, any estimates of zero-shear viscosity can only be regarded as approximate and in relative terms. The results of our feeding trials in pigs (Ellis et al., 1995) showed that native guar gum, incorporated either into a liquid semi-purified (SP) diet, at concentrations of 2 and 4 g guar gum per 100 g of diet, substantially increased the apparent zero-shear viscosity of digesta in the mid-jejunum (Fig. 15). This effect was strongly dependent on the polymer concentration in the diet. In another experiment, guar galactomannan of different M_rs were used (Roberts, 1991). The increases in digesta viscosity in the pigs were, as expected, more or less in the order of low to high galactomannan concentrations and M_rs. However, the differences in viscosity in vivo, produced by guar galactomannans of different concentrations and M_rs, were much smaller than those seen in vitro using the same grades of galactomannan. One plausible explanation is that there are likely to be large variations in the flux of fluid secretion and absorption in the gut in response to changes in digesta viscosity. Consequently, high viscosity seems to increase the amount of fluid in the digesta, possibly by increasing endogenous secretions

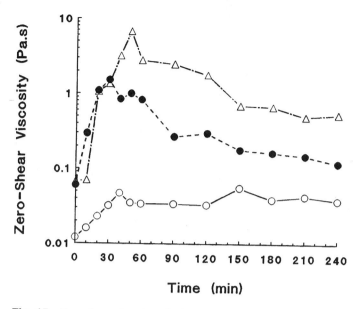

Fig. 15 Zero-shear viscosity of jejunal digesta in pigs fed control semi-purified (SP) diet (○); SP diet supplemented with 2 g guar gum/100 g of diet (--●--); and SP diet supplemented with 4 g guar gum/ 100 g of diet (−△). Viscosity measurements taken at fasting and 12 postprandial time intervals after start of consumption of experimental diets. Values are means for four pigs. (Data taken from Ellis et al., 1995.)

and/or inhibiting fluid absorption. This effect has also been seen in previous studies in which pigs were fed cereal-based diets rich in nonstarch polysaccharides (Zebrowska and Low, 1987).

The high levels of viscosity produced in the mid-jejunum of pigs given guar-containing diets (Roberts et al., 1990a,b) appeared to correspond to the decreases in postprandial glycemia seen in both pigs (Sambrook and Rainbird, 1985) and human subjects (Jenkins et al., 1978; Morgan et al., 1985; Ellis et al., 1991). To examine this relationship further, a study in which measurements of digesta viscosity and glucose absorption were recorded in the same pigs and at the same time (Ellis et al., 1995) was performed. From the results of this study, an inverse relationship was found between the amount of total glucose absorbed over 4 hours and log zero-shear viscosity (Fig. 16). This suggests that the glucose-reducing effect is proportionately more marked at relatively low viscosity levels in the small intestine. However, to evaluate fully the relationship between digesta viscosity and glucose absorption, information about the rheological changes at many other important sites of the gut are required (e.g., stomach).

C. Inhibition of Enzyme-Substrate Interactions

Guar gum is likely to influence the hydrolytic action of pancreatic amylase on starch in the gut lumen in a number of ways. An increase in viscosity produced by galactomannan will inhibit the mixing and movement of dissolved components (nutrients and enzymes) and particulate material (food particles and starch granules) in the gut lumen, thereby minimizing interactions between enzyme and substrate. If the galactomannan is part of a food matrix in an undissolved state, it may also inhibit the rate of digestion of the starch if it becomes closely associated with the substrate surface. The results of microstructural and digestibility studies do provide some evidence for this (Brennan et al., 1996). In these experiments microscopic examination of jejunal

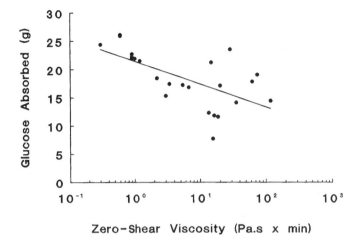

Zero-Shear Viscosity (Pa.s x min)

Fig. 16   Linear plot of glucose absorption versus log zero-shear viscosity (Pa.s $\times$ min) of jejunal digesta in pigs fed diets with and without guar gum (2 or 4 g/100 g diet). Glucose absorption data were calculated for 4-hour period and expressed as integrated values. Integrated viscosity values were estimated from 30-minute time intervals. Each experimental point in figure represents the mean value of four pigs. Correlation analysis of log-linear model: $r^2 = 0.40$, $p < 0.01$, degrees of freedom = 22. (Figure redrawn from data taken from Ellis et al., 1995.)

digesta removed from pigs given a diet of guar bread showed that the galactomannan was still closely associated with the starch granules. In the same study, in vitro digestibility data indicated that the rate of hydrolysis of guar bread was significantly decreased compared with normal wheat bread. These results suggest that guar galactomannan acts as a physical barrier to the action of amylase on starch and also, where some amylolysis has occurred, to the release of hydrolyzed products of starch (e.g., maltose).

   Early studies of amylase-starch interactions, often using pure samples of substrate, have demonstrated that guar gum can inhibit the activity of pancreatic amylase and other enzymes (Flourie, 1992). The precise mechanism by which guar gum influences the action of pancreatic amylase on starch is still unknown, however. Detailed kinetic studies are required to facilitate our understanding of this, although one important factor in attempting to answer this question will be the degree of hydration of galactomannan. Some limited in vitro experiments of everted segments of rat intestine have shown that guar gum inhibits both intestinal maltase and dipepti-dases competitively (Elsenhans et al., 1981). "Simple" competitive inhibition seems unlikely here, but further studies should be able to examine possible interactions between galactomannan, amylase, and starch and also the role played by viscosity. Many factors are likely to be important in such a highly complex system, including the availability of water, local flow conditions, diffusion of enzyme, and porosity of substrate and food matrix. One in vitro study has indicated that an entangled galactomannan network will retard the diffusion of proteins (bovine serum albumin) (Roger et al., 1991). This result suggests that in regions where amylase and starch rely solely on diffusion for interacting, the rheology of the system can have a significant effect on hydrolysis rate.

D.   Lipid Absorption and Bile Acid Metabolism

The mechanism(s) by which guar gum reduces plasma cholesterol levels is still uncertain, but the discussion about the effects of guar on viscosity and glucose absorption is also highly relevant here. Results from animal studies suggest that the level of viscosity generated in the gut is an important determinant of the hypocholesterolemic effect of guar gum (Gallaher and Hassel, 1995; Gallaher et al., 1999). The ingestion of guar gum seems to enhance fecal bile acid and neutral sterol excretion, reduce rates of digestion and absorption of lipids (including cholesterol), and inhibit hepatic synthesis of cholesterol (Ebihara and Schneeman, 1989; Johnson, 1992; Topping, 1993; Overton et al., 1994; Gallaher and Hassel, 1995; Demigne et al., 1998; Favier et al., 1998). The results of several studies indicate that the effects of viscosity on bile acid metabolism and lipid absorption kinetics are likely to be predominant mechanisms (Ebihara and Schneeman, 1989; Johnson, 1992; Topping, 1993; Gallaher and Hassel, 1995). Also, the effect of guar gum on bile acid excretion appears to be less important than that on the excretion of neutral sterols (Demigne et al., 1998; Favier et al. 1998).

The results of in vitro experiments have suggested that guar gum reduces the extent of lipid emulsification and rate of lipolysis of emulsified triacylglycerols (Pasquier et al., 1996a,b). However, the inhibitory effect of guar gum on lipid emulsification has not been confirmed in a recent rat study (Fillery-Travis et al., 1997). Previous in vitro studies have also shown that guar gum can inhibit the rate of diffusion of cholesterol mixed micelles, even at guar concentrations as low as 0.25% (Phillips, 1986). The lipid-lowering effect of guar gum has also been attributed to an inhibition of hepatic cholesterol synthesis by propionate (Chen et al., 1984), one of the short-chain fatty acids produced by bacterial fermentation of guar gum in the large intestine. The results of some in vitro and in vivo studies are not consistent with this hypothesis, however (Illman et al., 1988; Nishina and Freedland, 1990; Topping, 1993; Alvarezleite et al., 1994).

VIII. ROLE IN THE DIETARY MANAGEMENT OF DISEASE

Some problems exist in interpreting the results of clinical trials of guar gum. There are the usual problems associated with variable study design, lack of adequate controls, and heterogeneity of subject group. Another problem is the variation in characteristics of guar gum preparations, several varieties of which have been used in clinical trials. Information about the physicochemical properties of guar gum is rarely reported in the medical and nutritional literature. Sometimes it is not even known whether the guar was administered as a premeal drink or incorporated directly into the patients' diet. A good example of where this is a serious problem can be seen in a recent meta-analysis of the cholesterol-lowering effects of NSP (Brown et al., 1999). The authors attempted to evaluate all forms of guar gum, oat bran, psyllium seed, and pectin under the generic heading of soluble fiber. Given the enormous variability in the properties of these materials, the usefulness of this analysis is extremely doubtful.

The following section deals mainly with the therapeutic role of guar gum in the treatment of diabetes, hyperlipidemia and obesity. But it should also be recognized that guar may have other benefits in diet therapy, including the amelioration of symptoms associated with the dumping syndrome (Groop, 1997). This can occur in patients who have undergone gastric surgery and is characterized by rapid emptying of the hypotonic gastric contents into the duodenum. The syndrome may produce symptoms, persistent in 5–10% of cases, of hypovolemia, and/or rebound hypoglycemia and diarrhea.

A. Diabetes Mellitus and Hyperlipidemia

The plasma cholesterol-lowering properties of guar gum and similar polysaccharide gums in experimental animals and humans have been known since the 1960s (Ershof and Wells 1962; Fahrenbach et al., 1965). These and subsequent studies led to the idea of using guar gum in the treatment of hyperlipidemia (Jenkins et al., 1976b). About the same time, the concept of using guar gum in the dietary management of diabetes was introduced by Jenkins and his colleagues (Jenkins et al., 1976a). This was based on a number of pioneering studies showing that guar gum reduced the postprandial rise in blood glucose and insulin concentrations in both healthy and diabetic human subjects (Jenkins et al., 1976a, 1977a). In the studies of diabetic patients, the Jenkins group measured the postprandial blood glucose and insulin concentrations in patients given two breakfast meals (Jenkins et al., 1976a). Each meal consisted of bread and marmalade and contained a standard amount of available carbohydrate (starch and sugars). The test meal also contained 16 g of guar gum, which was incorporated into the wheat bread, and 10 g of pectin, which was mixed into the marmalade. The test meal was found to significantly reduce postprandial hyperglycemia and insulinemia in patients with type 2 diabetes (Fig. 14) and also reduce postprandial blood glucose in two subjects with type 1 (insulin-dependent) diabetes.

Studies by other research groups confirmed the early impressive acute clinical results reported by Jenkins (Morgan et al., 1979, 1985, 1990; Ellis et al., 1981, 1988a,b, 1991; O'Connor et al., 1981; Jarjis et al., 1984; Fairchild et al., 1996). Moreover, type 2 diabetes patients administered guar gum with their normal diet elicited significant long-term improvements in glycemic control and lipid metabolism using pharmaceutical preparations or guar-containing foods (Aro et al., 1981; Najemnik et al., 1984; Fuessl et al., 1987; Peterson et al., 1987; Uusitupa et al., 1989; Groop et al., 1993). The efficacy of guar gum in patients with type 1 diabetes has been much less studied, however, and there are problems in interpreting the data of those studies that have been published to date (Groop, 1997). Nevertheless, the general trend seems to show improvements in glycemic control and lipid metabolism following the administration of guar gum (Christiansen et al., 1980; Vaaler et al., 1986; Ebling et al., 1987; Vuorinen-Markkola et al., 1992; Groop, 1997). Beneficial effects have also been reported in children with type 1 diabetes (Paganus et al., 1987).

As discussed previously, some of the pharmaceutical preparations of guar gum, which are usually taken as a premeal drink, have been shown to be clinically ineffective, mainly because of their poor hydration characteristics (O'Connor et al., 1981; Heppell and Rainbird, 1985; Ellis and Morris, 1991). Results from the early clinical trials suggested that consuming guar gum as a premeal drink is less clinically effective than taking it after mixing it with foods (Jenkins et al., 1979; Wolever et al., 1979). This was substantiated by the results of acute studies (Fuessel et al., 1986; Fairchild et al., 1990) and two medium-term trials (4–6 weeks) in type 2 patients showing that guar gum is more effective when mixed into the patients' diet (Fuessel et al., 1987; Peterson et al., 1987). In the first of these trials (Fuessel et al., 1987), significant improvements in glycemic control and plasma concentrations of cholesterol, including the low-density lipoprotein (LDL) fraction, were seen in patients ingesting only 12–13 g/day of guar granules (Guarem) with their normal diet (Table 2). Improvements in glycemic control were seen as reductions in glycated hemoglobin and fasting blood glucose. In a second study (Peterson et al., 1987), wheat bread containing guar gum flour elicited significant reductions in glycated hemoglobin and total and LDL cholesterol in a group of patients with type 2 diabetes (Table 3). An important conclusion from this trial was that the metabolic improvements were achieved using a daily dose of only 7.6 g of guar gum (equivalent to 6.0 g galactomannan). Again, the critical factor in the guar bread study was that the galactomannan was intimately mixed with the food. The dose of guar gum used was significantly less than that recommended for pharmaceutical preparations, currently set at 15 g/day (British Medical Association, 1995).

In addition to the studies of diabetic patients, the plasma cholesterol-lowering effect of guar gum flour and guar granules has been investigated in other groups including those at an increased risk of coronary heart disease (Leeds, 1999). Most of these studies have shown decreases in total and LDL cholesterol concentrations in healthy, obese, and hyperlipidemic human

Table 2 Mean Values (±SEM) of Fasting Plasma Glucose, Glycated Hemoglobin (HbA_1), and Plasma Lipid Concentrations in 18 Patients with Type 2 (Non–insulin-dependent) Diabetes after Consuming a Pharmaceutical Preparation of Guar Gum (Guarem) and a Control (Placebo) for Two 4-Week Periods, Respectively[a]

	Control period		Guarem period	
	Start (0 weeks)	End (6 weeks)	Start (0 weeks)	End (6 weeks)
Fasting glucose (mmol/L)	8.74 ± 0.49	8.78 ± 0.53	9.31 ± 0.53	8.29[b] ± 0.47
HbA_1 (%)	9.27 ± 0.41	9.09 ± 0.39	9.67 ± 0.40	8.70[c] ± 0.39
Total cholesterol (mmol/L)	5.61 ± 0.24	5.61 ± 0.24	5.79 ± 0.29	5.19[b] ± 0.22
LDL cholesterol (mmol/L)	3.84 ± 0.21	3.76 ± 0.22	3.89 ± 0.23	3.49[b] ± 0.20
HDL cholesterol (mmol/L)	0.84 ± 0.07	0.81 ± 0.06	0.78 ± 0.06	0.81 ± 0.05
Triacylglycerols (mmol/L)	2.28 ± 0.37	2.45 ± 0.29	2.16 ± 0.21	2.43 ± 0.32

[a] Control and guar gum were taken by each patient in randomized order.
[b,c] Values after 4 weeks significantly different from baseline (start) at $p < 0.05$ and $p < 0.02$, respectively.
Source: Fuessl et al., 1987.

Table 3 Mean Values (±SEM) of Fasting Plasma Glucose, Glycated Hemoglobin (HbA_{1c}), and Plasma Lipid Concentrations in 16 Patients with Type 2 (Non–insulin-dependent) Diabetes after Consuming Control Wheat Bread and Bread Containing Guar Gum Flour for Two 6-week Periods, Respectively[a]

	Control period		Guar bread period	
	Start (0 weeks)	End (6 weeks)	Start (0 weeks)	End (6 weeks)
Fasting glucose (mmol/L)	9.7 ± 0.8	9.4 ± 0.7	9.7 ± 1.0	9.1 ± 0.8
HbA_{1c} (%)	11.3 ± 0.8	11.2 ± 0.8	11.5 ± 0.8	10.7 ± 0.8[b]
Total cholesterol (mmol/L)	5.7 ± 0.3	5.8 ± 0.3	5.9 ± 0.3	5.4 ± 0.2[c]
LDL cholesterol (mmol/L)	3.8 ± 0.3	3.9 ± 0.2	3.9 ± 0.2	3.5 ± 0.2[d]
HDL cholesterol (mmol/L)	1.2 ± 0.1	1.2 ± 0.1	1.2 ± 0.1	1.2 ± 0.1
Triacylglycerols (mmol/L)	1.7 ± 0.3	1.7 ± 0.3	1.8 ± 0.3	1.6 ± 0.2

[a] Control and guar bread were taken by each patient in randomized order.
[b,c,d] Values after 6 weeks significantly different from control at $p < 0.05$, $p < 0.02$, and $p < 0.01$, respectively.
Source: Peterson et al., 1987.

subjects (Tuomilehto et al., 1980, 1988; Gatenby, 1990; Todd et al., 1990; Truswell and Beynen, 1992; Blake et al., 1997; Groop, 1997), in some studies for periods of up to 1–2 years (Simons et al., 1982; Tuomilehto et al., 1988; Salenius et al., 1995; Groop, 1997). The average reductions in total and LDL cholesterol are typically 13 and 16%, respectively, but reductions within the range of 5–32% have been found in the literature (Gatenby, 1990; Truswell and Beynen, 1992). These figures should be treated as a ballpark estimate only, since the level of reductions will depend on the type and number of subjects, baseline plasma lipid concentrations of subjects, and the type, dose, and duration of feeding guar gum. In most of these studies no consistent effects on plasma high-density lipoprotein (HDL) cholesterol and triacylglycerol concentrations were reported, although decreases in the latter have been demonstrated in some hypercholesterolemic and diabetic patients (Peterson et al., 1987; Groop, 1997).

The recommended dose for pharmaceutical preparations of guar gum in diabetes therapy is usually 5 g with each meal (15 g/day). This seems to be based on the results of early clinical trials in which large doses of guar were used (Ellis, 1994; Groop, 1997). It is not known, however, what precise meal and daily doses, and indeed M_r, of guar galactomannan should be used in foods to optimize its clinical benefits. A lower and upper daily dose range of 6–15 g of native guar gum has been previously suggested for use in diabetes therapy (Ellis, 1994). This was estimated on the basis that there may be side effects, such as flatulence, at doses of >15 g/day and that there is a lack of reliable long-term studies of guar gum at doses of <6 g/day. The results of single meal or drink studies, however, show that low doses, defined here as <5 g guar gum per meal, are effective in reducing postprandial blood glucose and insulin concentrations (Wolever et al., 1979; Ellis et al., 1981, 1988; McIvor et al., 1985; Jarjis et al., 1984). This would suggest that daily doses at the lower end of the recommended range is a worthwhile target to aim for, particularly since this would facilitate the improvement in sensory qualities of guar foods (see Sec. IX).

The average M_r of native guar galactomannan samples used in clinical trials have been reported to be in the range of 2.0–3.0 million (Ellis et al., 1991; Gatenby et al., 1996). A recent study has shown that the blood glucose–lowering effect of guar bread in patients with type 2 diabetes is not diminished by an approximate fivefold decrease in M_r of galactomannan (Gatenby et al., 1996). Moreover, a partially depolymerized guar gum ($M_r \sim 1.0$ million) reduced total plasma cholesterol and LDL cholesterol by 10 and 11%, respectively, over a 3-week feeding period in hypercholesterolemic human subjects (Table 4) (Blake et al., 1997). Improvements in glycemic control and reductions in LDL cholesterol have also been observed in people with type 2 diabetes given the same depolymerized guar gum preparation for 6 weeks (Ellis et al., 1998). Further work needs to be done to define the lowest M_r and optimum dose that can be used without a loss in clinical efficacy. From a food technology standpoint there are considerable advantages in using low M_r grades of guar gum. Foods containing depolymerized grades of guar gum are significantly more palatable than those containing native guar at the same dose levels (Fig. 17) (Ellis et al., 1991). There is little doubt, therefore, that the use of partially hydrolyzed guar gum will facilitate the development of palatable low–glycemic index foods. [The glycemic index is used for ranking foods according to the incremental blood glucose they produce in healthy subjects and people with diabetes (Ellis, 1999; Leeds, 1999) (see Sec. IX).]

B. Obesity

This section will provide a brief overview of the possible role of guar gum in the dietary management of obesity. A more detailed review of this area can be found in a number of useful publications (Ryttig et al., 1990, Rossner, 1992). Obesity is associated with an increased risk of diabetes, insulin resistance, coronary heart disease (CHD), and hypertension (Saris et al., 1998). It is generally recognized that guar gum elicits clinical improvements in glycemic control, insulin

Table 4 Mean Values (±SEM) of Plasma Lipid Concentrations in 11 Moderately Hypercholesterolemic Humans After Consuming Control Wheat Bread and Bread Containing Depolymerized Guar Gum for Two 3-week Periods, Respectively[a]

	Control period		Guar bread period	
	Start (0 weeks)	End (3 weeks)	Start (0 weeks)	End (3 weeks)
Total cholesterol (mmol/L)	6.37 ± 0.21	6.53 ± 0.16	6.52 ± 0.17	5.89[b] ± 0.8
LDL cholesterol (mmol/L)	4.18 ± 0.15	4.31 ± 0.14	4.28 ± 0.19	3.81[b] ± 0.12
HDL cholesterol (mmol/L)	1.26 ± 0.05	1.31 ± 0.06	1.33 ± 0.05	1.23 ± 0.05
Triacylglycerols (mmol/L)	1.84 ± 0.25	1.86 ± 0.32	1.96 ± 0.27	1.85 ± 0.25

[a] Control and guar bread were taken by each patient in randomized order.
[b] Values after 3 weeks significantly different from control and baseline (start) values at $p < 0.001$.
Source: Blake et al., 1997.

sensitivity, and lipid metabolism in obese individuals, irrespective of whether there is a loss in body weight. However, this section will deal only with the putative effects of guar gum on satiety and weight reduction.

The idea that nonstarch polysaccharides such as guar gum could be used to facilitate weight reduction is certainly attractive, but evidence for a significant and sustained benefit in the long term has yet to be produced. Although several short-term and long-term feeding studies

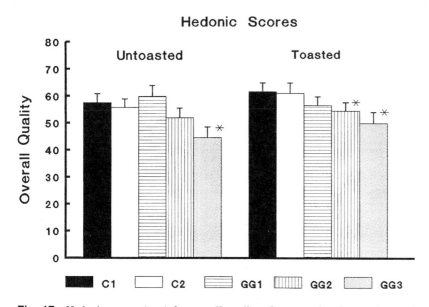

Fig. 17 Hedonic scores (mm) for overall quality of untoasted and toasted control (C1 and C2) wheat bread and wheat breads containing low molecular weight (GG1), medium molecular weight (GG2), and high molecular weight (GG3) guar gum flour. Molecular weights of GG1, GG2, and GG3 were 0.52, 1.07, and 2.38 million, respectively. Results shown for C1 and C2 show good reproducibility of method. (Data taken from Ellis et al. 1991.) *Mean values for experimental breads were significantly different from those for controls at $p < 0.05$.

have been published in this area, there are problems in interpreting the results of these experiments.

Early short-term studies in human subjects provided some evidence that oral supplements of guar gum acted as bulk-forming appetite suppressants (Evans and Miller, 1975; Wilmhurst and Crawley, 1980; Krotkiewski, 1984; Ellis et al., 1985). Some of these studies involved investigating the states and processes that influence the pattern of eating and the motivation to eat. This often involved monitoring changes in food intake and/or using visual analog scales to record changes in hunger, appetite, satiety, and satiation. Even though these terms have been described and defined by Blundell (1979), there has been considerable confusion about their use and meaning (Burley and Blundell, 1990). Despite this confusion, most short-term studies have tended to show that guar gum, either pharmaceutical preparations or flour intimately mixed with food, reduces feelings of hunger and appetite and increases feelings of satiety and satiation in normal-weight, overweight, and obese subjects (Evans and Miller, 1975, Wilmhurst and Crawley, 1980; Krotkiewski, 1984; Ellis et al., 1985; Rossner, 1992). In some of these studies guar gum also reduced energy intake and body weight (Krotkieweski, 1984; Rossner, 1992).

One problem of designing experiments to investigate feeding behavior is that it is very difficult to make the control food (placebo) look and taste like the test food, thus ensuring that the study is truly blind. It is difficult, for example, to make foods containing relatively high concentrations of native guar gum taste the same as the control (see next section). In one study, guar wheat bread elicited significantly greater feelings of satiety compared to the control in normal weight healthy subjects and also in a group of overweight patients with type 2 diabetes (Ellis et al., 1985). These results were difficult to interpret, however, because of the influence of sensory properties of guar bread on satiety scores. Breads containing a high concentration of guar gum (>5.5 g/100 g) were significantly less palatable than the control breads, which may explain why the subjects were also less hungry after consuming the guar meal. In breads containing the lowest concentration of guar gum, no effects on satiety were observed and they were also of similar palatability to that of the control. The importance of the sensory effects of foods in influencing satiety is highlighted by Burley and Blundell (1990).

In a more detailed study to monitor changes in hunger, fullness, desire to eat, and prospective consumption, Burley and coworkers (1987) showed that a high fiber breakfast meal containing guar gum flour and wheat bran had negligible effect except for increasing fullness. Moreover, the high-fiber breakfast had little effect on ad libitum food intake at lunchtime. But since the high-fiber breakfast meal contained less energy than the control, the authors reasonably concluded from these results that the presence of fiber had maintained the satiating effect of the test meal despite its lower energy content. Attempts were made in this study to produce control and guar meals with similar sensory properties.

The results of longer-term guar gum supplementation studies are contradictory. One study, using a pharmaceutical preparation of guar gum (Lejguar), showed a reduction in mean body weight in obese subjects of 4.1 kg over 8 weeks (Krotkiewski, 1984), but no placebo period was included in the experimental design. In well-controlled, randomized clinical trials using Guarem (granulated guar gum), significant reductions in body weight were also achieved in type 2 diabetes patients (Uusitupa et al., 1989) and hypercholesterolemic females (Tuomilehto et al., 1980). In contrast, other groups have reported no changes in body weight loss following the intake of guar gum (Simons et al., 1982; Fuessl et al., 1987; Peterson et al., 1987; Landin et al., 1992). It is reasonable to conclude from the results of clinical studies published so far that a therapeutic role for guar gum in weight management has yet to be established. More recent work has focused on the use of guar gum supplementation on weight maintenance in weight-reduced individuals, but here again the clinical benefits are not unequivocal (Pasman et al., 1997). One important aspect of this trial was that the guar gum tested was a highly depolymerized preparation (Benefiber), which was administered as a premeal drink. No information on galactomannan content and M_r of the guar was provided by the authors, so it is difficult to assess whether this preparation has any therapeutic potential.

IX. DEVELOPMENT OF FUNCTIONAL FOODS CONTAINING GUAR GUM

Initial attempts to incorporate foods containing guar gum were performed to overcome the serious problems of palatability associated with ingesting hydrated guar gum solutions and to test the clinical efficacy to suitable foods containing guar gum (Jenkins et al., 1977; Apling and Ellis, 1982; Ellis et al., 1985). No attempt had been made at that time to evaluate and optimize the sensory qualities of individual foods.

The first guar-containing food products to be developed for clinical use were guar wheat bread (Apling et al., 1977, 1978; Apling and Ellis, 1982) and guar crispbread (Jenkins et al., 1978b). Both products were found to be physiologically effective in healthy (Ellis et al., 1981, 1988a), diabetic (Jenkins et al., 1978b; Peterson et al., 1987), and hyperlipidemic (Jenkins et al., 1980) patients. However, data on product quality, including sensory characteristics, were only reported for the wheat bread product (Ellis et al., 1981, 1985, 1988a). These initial experiments showed that adding guar gum to the bread-making recipe produced wheat bread of inferior quality in terms of loaf characteristics. This included poor crumb structure and texture, which was excessively sticky to touch and chew and produced a gummy mouthfeel after swallowing. The decrease in bread quality was directly proportional to the amount of native guar gum added to the recipe formulation. But even at relatively high levels of guar supplementation, significant improvements in bread quality were achieved by modifications to the recipe formulation and bread-making process. For example, bread quality was improved by using high extraction wheat flour, optimizing the water absorption of the guar-wheat flour mixture and depanning during baking (Apling et al., 1978; Apling and Ellis, 1982; Ellis and Apling, 1983). In formal sensory experiments using healthy and diabetic panelists, a concentration of 3.2 g/100 g of galactomannan in bread produced an hedonic score (an index of palatability) similar to that of the control (Ellis et al., 1981, 1985, 1988a). The hedonic scores recorded by the healthy subjects suggested that the upper limit of acceptability in wheat bread was about 5.0 g/100 g of galactomannan in bread (Ellis et al., 1981, 1988a), although surprisingly this limit appeared to be higher in diabetic patients (Ellis et al., 1985). Interestingly, the blood glucose- and insulin-lowering effects of guar bread have been reported at galactomannan concentrations of 3.2 g/100 g. Based on a compromise between clinical effects and bread quality, the optimum concentration range of 3.0–5.0 g/100 g of galactomannan in the baked product seems reasonable, given also that low doses are known to be metabolically effective (see above).

The results of test-baking experiments indicated an inverse relationship between the quality of guar wheat bread and the average M_r of guar gum used in the recipe (Apling and Ellis, 1982). These results are consistent with data from a more recent sensory study showing that the hedonic ratings of toasted and untoasted guar bread were significantly improved by using depolymerized guar galactomannan (Fig. 17) (Ellis et al., 1991). Substantial improvements in the quality of guar bread, specifically texture and flavor, were observed when using guar gum grades in the M_r range of 0.5–1.1 million. Moreover, the hedonic rating given for bread containing guar gum of $M_r \sim 0.5$ million, at a galactomannan concentration of about 5.0 g/100 g, were similar to those given for control breads. The poor palatability rating of bread containing native guar gum ($M_r \sim 2.38$ million), at a similar galactomannan concentration, confirmed previous sensory data showing that this is the upper limit of acceptability for native guar gum (Ellis et al., 1981, 1988a). Guar bread products developed by other research groups were evaluated successfully in clinical trials, but little or no information was reported on the grades of guar gum used, the recipe formulation, and the sensory characteristics of the final guar products (Åckerblom et al., 1979; Pikaar et al., 1985; Vaaler et al., 1986; Sels et al., 1987; Paganus et al., 1987).

The initial studies of other guar-containing foods were broadly consistent with the data obtained for guar wheat bread products (Tredger and Ransley, 1978; Hill and Leeds, 1979). These experiments showed that native guar gum has severe deleterious effects on the quality, again mainly the textural properties, on a range of foods. However, these effects appeared to be attenuated in highly flavored foods, with strong flavors tending to mask the detrimental effects of guar gum on food texture. In the same study, the authors also noted that native guar gum was more acceptable when incorporated into low-moisture foods. Some additional evidence to support this observation comes from sensory analysis experiments of guar biscuits. The biscuits seemed to show less deterioration in palatability with increasing guar concentrations (Ellis et al., 1988b) compared with foods of higher moisture content, such as wheat bread (Ellis et al., 1981, 1985, 1988a).

A broad range of foods other than wheat bread have been developed and tested worldwide, including pasta (Gatti et al., 1984; Tagliaferro et al., 1985; Sels et al., 1994), snack bars (McIvor et al., 1985, 1986; Paganus et al., 1987), biscuits (Smith et al., 1982; Ellis et al., 1988b), marmalade (Paganus et al. 1987), and more recently breakfast cereals (Fairchild et al., 1996). Again, only a few of these studies provided information about the type of guar gum used, recipe formulation, and sensory properties of the final product, so any comparison between studies is difficult. However, most, but not all, of these products did elicit improvements in carbohydrate and lipid metabolism in healthy and diabetic subjects.

X. POTENTIAL ADVERSE EFFECTS OF GUAR GUM

In the food industry, guar gum and other such hydrocolloids are added to foods as thickening, binding, or stabilizing agents, usually in concentrations of <1 g/100 g in foods (Apling and Ellis, 1982). In the United Kingdom, such materials are a class of food additives controlled under the Miscellaneous Food Additives Regulations 1995, which implement the provisions of Directive 95/2/EC into UK law (Council of Ministers and European Parliament Directive, 1995). Guar gum (E 412 on food labels) is generally permitted for use in most processed foods, including dietetic foods, at a quantum satis level. The Food and Agricultural Organization/World Health Organization (FAO/WHO) estimate that the acceptable daily intake for guar gum is "not limited" (FAO/WHO, 1975). This is a classification that is assigned to substances of very low toxicity, especially those that are food constituents or may be considered as foods or normal metabolites in humans.

The relative benign effect of native guar gum is substantiated by the results of a number of long-term trials in human subjects. No adverse effects were reported in diabetic patients administered guar gum for periods of up to 12 months at doses of up to 30 g/day, in the form of either pharmaceutical preparations or food products (McIvor et al., 1985b; van Duyn et al., 1986; Todd et al., 1990). Accordingly, no significant changes in hepatic, renal, or hematological function were observed in patients ingesting double the daily dose recommended for pharmaceutical preparations of guar gum. Since guar gum is known to reduce the rate and possibly the extent of absorption of nutrients such as glucose and amino acids, similar effects on the absorption of minerals and electrolytes are likely to occur. There is no evidence to indicate, however, that the bioavailability of these micronutrients is influenced significantly (Todd et al., 1990; Groop, 1997). If anything, the evidence seems to suggest an improvement in the bioavailability of minerals such as zinc (Sinisalo et al., 1989) and iron (Takahashi et al., 1994). A more recent study has also shown an improvement in calcium absorption in rats fed depolymerized guar galactomannan (Hara et al., 1996).

As discussed previously, guar gum can also influence the rate and possibly the extent of lipid absorption in humans (Johnson, 1992; Topping, 1993), an effect that may, in part, explain the mechanism by which guar gum lowers blood cholesterol. It is reasonable to assume, therefore, that there is a theoretical risk of lipid-soluble vitamin deficiency in patients consuming guar gum. Uusitupa and colleagues (1989) reported a reduction in plasma concentrations of vitamins A and E in patients with type 2 diabetes given oral supplements of guar granules (Guarem) for up to 13 months with their normal diet. The authors concluded, however, that the reduction in lipid-soluble vitamins was not clinically important and that it was unlikely to alter the vitamin status of people who receive an adequate dietary intake of vitamins A and E. This does not exclude the theoretical risk to patients who are not taking a nutritionally balanced diet.

Some concern was also expressed about the possible effects of guar gum on the rate and extent of drug absorption (Todd et al., 1990; Groop, 1997). Many studies show that guar gum, usually in the form of granules taken in a premeal drink, decreases the rate of absorption of drugs (e.g., paracetamol, digoxin, various hypoglycemic agents), but the total amount of drug absorbed does not appear to be altered (Todd et al., 1990). In some studies, however, guar gum is reported to reduce the overall bioavailability of phenoxymethylpenicillin (Huupponen et al., 1984) and metformin (Gin et al., 1989). The effect of guar-containing foods, such as guar bread, on drug absorption is not known, but it may be similar to the effect of the pharmaceutical preparations.

In general, adverse effects reported in the scientific literature, in some but not all human subjects, appear to be associated with gastrointestinal events including flatulence, gastrointestinal pain or discomfort, nausea, and diarrhea (Todd et al., 1990). Some of these symptoms probably arise from the degradation of galactomannan by bacterial enzymes (e.g., *Bacteroides ovatus*) in the large intestine (Salayers et al., 1977; Nyman and Asp, 1982), leading to the formation of gas, which in some cases can result in severe abdominal pain. Increased stool frequency and bulking have also been reported in some individuals, although arguably these effects may be beneficial if subjects are suffering from chronic constipation. When adverse symptoms are carefully recorded in well-controlled clinical trials, these tend to be transient and diminish with regular consumption of guar gum. Also, adverse effects appear to be attenuated when guar gum is intimately mixed with the food and administered in moderate doses (Fuessl et al., 1987; Peterson et al., 1987). Persistent and more adverse gastrointestinal effects tend to occur only when the guar gum is consumed by individuals at doses that are now considered to be excessive—approximately 15–30 g per day (Todd et al., 1990; Ellis, 1994, 1999).

There has been concern for some time about the use of macroaggregates of guar gum that have the potential for causing obstruction in the esophagus and gastrointestinal tract (Lewis, 1992). This concern has arisen from cases of esophageal obstruction and rupture in patients ingesting guar granulate (Ahlman, 1982; Edström and Petterson, 1982). There have also been a number of reports of esophageal and small bowel obstruction in patients ingesting one type of guar-containing diet pill (Cal-Ban 3000); about 50% of these patients had preexisting esophageal and gastric disorders (Lewis, 1992). Australia and the United States have banned the use of such products. In the United Kingdom, limits were introduced in 1988 by the Ministry of Agriculture Fisheries and Food (MAFF) on the use of guar tablets or capsules intended for use as a slimming aid on the basis that there is a theoretical risk of esophageal obstruction to the consumer (Ministry of Agriculture Fisheries and Food, 1988). This regulation was superseded by EC food additives legislation (Council of Ministers and European Parliament Directive,

1995), which has been implemented into U.K. law by way of the Miscellaneous Food Additives Regulations 1995. The latter prohibits the use of guar gum and other gums for the production of "dehydrated foodstuffs intended to rehydrate on ingestion." The use of guar gum in products that are likely to swell in the esophagus has been prohibited throughout the EC. However, this legislation does not cover the use of guar products sold as medicine under license and administered to patients under medical supervision.

XI. FINAL COMMENTS AND FUTURE WORK

There is strong evidence to indicate that guar gum has therapeutic benefits for a range of metabolic disorders. At doses of guar gum that are likely to be consumed for therapeutic purposes, there is little evidence that it is detrimental to human health. On the contrary, the cholesterol-lowering property of guar gum is of benefit to those who are at an increased risk of coronary heart disease, including individuals with hyperlipidemia and diabetes. Also, the use of guar gum in decreasing the postprandial rise in blood glucose and insulin levels and improving long-term glycemic control in patients with diabetes has been well documented. Evidence from a 10-year study in the United States (DCCT Research Group, 1993) and from a more recent 20-year trial in the United Kingdom (UKPDS Group, 1998) show unequivocally that an improvement in glycemic control in patients with types 1 and 2 diabetes can reduce the risk of microvascular complications (e.g., nephropathy, retinopathy). An investigation of the potential beneficial effects of guar gum on the initiation and progression of diabetic complications is therefore warranted. The results of a rat experiment showing that guar gum inhibits the progression of diabetic nephropathy suggests that this would be worthwhile (Gallaher et al., 1992). Recent epidemiological studies have indicated also that diets comprising low–glycemic index foods may have a protective effect in the development of type 2 diabetes (Salmerón et al., 1997a,b). Guar-containing foods could play an important role in such diets and should be tested in the future for their possible prophylactic benefits. In view of putative improving effects of guar gum on insulin resistance, which in itself is a risk factor for both CHD and type 2 diabetes, the role of guar foods needs to be evaluated here also (Saris et al., 1998). The effects of guar gum on weight reduction in the long term have yet to be demonstrated, although its use in maintaining weight in weight-reduced subjects merits further study. Obese individuals are likely to benefit, however, from the effects of guar gum on glycemic control, insulin sensitivity, and lipid metabolism.

To facilitate the development of new low–glycemic index foods using guar gum as a major ingredient, it would be advantageous to have a detailed understanding of its behavior in the gut environment. Fundamental information about the way in which guar galactomannan influences the rheological behavior of digesta, either through its effects in solution, as an entangled network, or on the swelling of food particles, is of paramount importance. This would need to be linked to the effects of galactomannan on the kinetics of starch digestion and glucose absorption and to the role played by the entero-insular axis in modulating insulin secretion.

Initial attempts to produce palatable guar foods for the management of diabetes and hyperlipidemia were disappointing. However, the technological difficulties were not helped by the apparent need to use high doses of guar gum (Apling and Ellis, 1982; Ellis, 1985). More recent studies have shown that lower doses and partially depolymerized guar gum are not only clinically effective, but have significantly less detrimental effects on food quality. From a food technology perspective, it is now possible to produce guar-enriched foods that are both clinically effective and palatable. Some of these food products are at the stage of being commercially viable, but it may some time before they become available in the United Kingdom for people with diabetes and other metabolic disorders.

ACKNOWLEDGMENTS

The authors acknowledge the financial support of the British Biotechnology and Science Research Council and the Ministry of Agriculture, Fisheries and Food for some of the work described in this review. We also thank Dr. Peter Butterworth (King's College London) and Willem Wielinga [Meyhall A.G. (Rhodia Food), Kreuzlingen, Switzerland] for useful discussions during the preparation of this chapter.

REFERENCES

Åckerblom HK, Käär ML, Länkelä S. The reducing effect of guar gum bread on postprandial hyperglycemia in diabetic children. Acta Endocrinol 91:6, 1979.

Ahlman H. Total obstruction of esophagus after intake of natural products (Swedish). Lakartidningen 79: 1479, 1982.

Alvarezleite JI, Andrieux C, Ferezou J, Riottot M, Vieira EC. Evidence for the absence of participation of the microbial flora in the hypocholesterolemic effect of guar gum in gnotobiotic-rats. Comp Biochem Physiol A Physiol 109:503–510, 1994.

Apling EC, Ellis PR. Guar bread: concept to application. Chem Indust 23:950–954, 1982.

Apling EC, Leeds AR, Wolever TMS, Jenkins DJA. How to make guar bread. Lancet 1:975, 1977.

Apling EC, Khan P, Ellis PR. Guar/wheat bread for therapeutic use. Cereal Food World 23:640–644, 1978.

Aro A, Uusitupa M, Voutilainen E, Hersio K, Korhonen T, Siitonen. Improved diabetic control and hypocholesterolemic effect induced by long-term dietary supplementation with guar gum in type 2 (insulin independent) diabetes. Diabetologia 21:29–33, 1981.

Baker CW, Whistler RL. Distribution of D-galactosyl groups in guaran and locust-bean gum. Carbohydr Res 45:237–243, 1975.

Baker P. Placebo-controlled trial of guar in poorly controlled type 2 diabetes. Practical Diabetes 5:36–38, 1988.

Beer MU, Wood PJ, Weisz J. A simple and rapid method for evaluation of Mark-Houwink-Sakurada constants of linear random coil polysaccharides using molecular weight and intrinsic viscosity determined by high performance size exclusion chromatography: application to guar galactomannan. Carbohydr Polym 39:377–380, 1999.

Binder C. C-peptide and β-cell function in diabetes mellitus. In: Pickup J, Williams G, eds. Textbook of Diabetes. Vol. 1. London: Blackwell Scientific Publications, 1991:348–354.

Blackburn NA, Redfern JS, Jarjis H, Holgate AM, Hanning I, Scarpello JHB, Johnson IT, Read NW. The mechanism of action of guar gum in improving glucose tolerance in man. Clin Sci 66:329–336, 1984.

Blake DE, Hamblett CJ, Frost PG, Judd PA, Ellis PR. Wheat bread supplemented with depolymerized guar gum reduces plasma cholesterol concentration in hypercholesterolemic human subjects. Am J Clin Nutr 65:107–113, 1997.

Blake DE, Roberts FG, Canibe N, Bach Knudsen KE, Morgan LE, Ellis PR. Quantitative determination of the effect of guar gum on gut hormone secretion in the pig and use of a transit time ultra-sound flow probe. Proceedings of XV International Congress of Nutrition, Adelaide, Australia, 1993a p. 880.

Blake DE, Roberts FR, Sissons JS, Canibe N, Jones CL, Bach Knudsen KE, Ellis PR. Quantitative assessment of the effect of non-starch polysaccharides on nutrient absorption in the pig: use of a transit time, ultrasound flow probe. Proc Nutr Soc 52:200A, 1993b.

Blundell JE. Hunger, appetite and satiety–psychological constructs in search of identities. In: Turner M, ed. Nutrition and Lifestyles. London: Applied Science Publishers, 1979:21–42.

Brennan CS, Blake DE, Ellis PR, Schofield JD. Effects of guar galactomannan on wheat bread microstructure and on the in vitro and in vivo digestibility of starch in bread. J Cereal Sci 24:151–160, 1996.

British Medical Association and Royal Pharmaceutical Society of Great Britain. British National Formulary, Number 29. London: British Medical Association and The Royal Pharmaceutical Society Press, 1995:107–111.

Brown L, Rosner B, Willett WW, Sacks FM. Cholesterol-lowering effects of dietary fiber: a meta-analysis. Am J Clin Nutr 69:30–42.

Brown NJ, Worlding J, Rumsey RDE, Read NW. The effect of guar gum on the distribution of a radiolabelled meal in the gastrointestinal tract of the rat. Br J Nutr 88:223–231, 1988.

Bueno L, Praddaude F, Fioramonti J, Ruckesbusch Y. Effect of dietary fibre on gastrointestinal motility and jejunal transit time in dogs. Gastroenterology 80:701–707, 1981.

Burchard W. Light scattering. In: Ross-Murphy SB, ed. Physical Techniques for the Study of Food Biopolymers. London: Blackie Academic & Professional, 1994:151–213.

Burley VJ, Blundell JE. Action of dietary fibre on the satiety cascade. In: Kritchevsky D, Bonfield C, and Anderson JW, eds. Dietary Fiber: Chemistry, Physiology and Health Effects. New York: Plenum Press, 1990:227–246.

Burley VJ, Leeds AR, Blundell JE. The effect of high and low fibre breakfasts on hunger, satiety, and food intake in a subsequent meal. Int J Obesity (suppl)1:87–93, 1987.

Carlson WA, Ziegenfuss EM, Overton JD. Compatibility and manipulation of guar gum. Food Technol 16:50–54, 1962.

Cameron-Smith D, Habito R, Barnett M, Collier GR. Dietary guar gum improves insulin sensitivity in streptozotocin-induced diabetic rats. J Nutr 127:359–364, 1997.

Chen W-J, Anderson JW, Jennings D. Propionate may mediate the hypocholesterolemic effects of certain soluble plant fibers in cholesterol-fed rats. Proc Soc Exp Biol Med 175:215–218, 1984.

Cherbut C, Albina E, Champ M, Doublier JL, Lecannu G. Action of guar gum on the viscosity of digestive contents and on gastrointestinal motor function in pigs. Digestion 46:205–213, 1990.

Christiansen JS, Bonnevie-Nielsen V, Svendsen PA, Ronn B, Nerup J. Effect of guar gum on 24-hour insulin requirements of insulin-dependent diabetic subjects as assessed by an artificial pancreas. Diabetes Care 3:659–662, 1980.

Committee on Codex Specifications. Food Chemicals Codex. 3rd ed. Washington DC: National Academy Press, 1981:141.

Council of Ministers and European Parliament Directive. Directive 95/2/EC on Food Additives Other Than Colours and Sweeteners. Brussels: Official Journal of European Community No. L61/1, 18th March 1995.

Cross MM. Rheology of non-Newtonian fluids: a new flow equation for pseudoplastic systems. J Coll Sci 20:417–437, 1965.

Dea ICM, Morrison A. Chemistry and interactions of seed galactomannans. Advances Carbohydr Chem Biochem 31:241–312, 1975.

de Gennes PG. Brownian motion of flexible polymer chains. Nature 282:367–370, 1979.

Demigne C, Levrat MA, Behr SR, Moundras C, Remesy C. Cholesterol-lowering action of guar gum in the rat: changes in bile acids and sterols excretion and in enterohepatic cycling of bile acids. Nutr Res 18:1215–1225, 1998.

Diabetes Control and Complications Trial (DCCT) Research Group. The effect of intensive treatment of diabetes on the development and progression of long-term complications in insulin-dependent diabetes mellitus. N Engl J Med 329:977–986, 1993.

Doublier J-L, Launay B. Rheology of galactomannan solutions: comparative study of guar gum and locust bean gum. J Texture Stud 12:151–172, 1981.

Ebihara K, Kiriyama S. Comparative effects of water-soluble and water-insoluble dietary fibers on various parameters relating to glucose tolerance in rats. Nutr Rep Int 41:193–201, 1982.

Ebihara K, Schneeman BO. Interaction of bile acids, phospholipids, cholesterol and triglycerides with dietary fibers in the small intestine of rats. J Nutr 119:1100–1106, 1989.

Ebling P, Yki-Järvinen H, Aro A, Helve E, Sinisalo M, Koivisto VA. Glucose and lipid metabolism and insulin sensitivity in type 1 diabetes: the effect of guar gum. Am J Clin Nutr 48:98–103, 1987.

Edström S, Pettersson G. Oesophageal rupture after intake of natural products (Swedish). Lakartidningen 79:1478–1479, 1982.

Edwards CA, Read NW. Fibre and small intestinal function. In: Leeds AR, ed. Dietary Fibre Perspectives 2. London: John Libbey, 1990:52–75.

Edwards CA, Johnson IT, Read NW. Do viscous polysaccharides slow absorption by inhibiting diffusion or convection? Eur J Clin Nutr 42:307–312, 1988.

Ellis PR. Fibre and food products. In: Leeds AR, ed. Dietary Fibre Perspectives. London: John Libbey, 1985:83–105.

Ellis PR. Polysaccharide gums: their modulation of carbohydrate and lipid metabolism and role in the treatment of diabetes mellitus. In: Phillips GO, Wedlock DA, Williams PA, eds. Gums and Stabilisers for the Food Industry 7. Oxford: Pergamon, 1994:207–216.

Ellis PR. The effect of fibre on diabetes. In: Hill M, ed. The Right Fibre for the Right Disease. London: The Royal Society of Medicine Press Ltd., 1999:33–42.

Ellis PR, Apling EC. The development and acceptability of guar bran bread. In: Holas J, Kratochvil J, eds. Proceedings of the 7th World Cereal and Bread Congress, Prague. Amsterdam: Elsevier, 1983: 1121–1126.

Ellis PR, Morris ER. Importance of the rate of hydration of pharmaceutical preparations of guar gum; a new in vitro monitoring method. Diabet Med 8:378–381, 1991.

Ellis PR, Apling EC, Leeds AR, Bolster NR. Guar bread: acceptability and efficacy combined. Studies on blood glucose, serum insulin and satiety in normal subjects. Br J Nutr 46:267–276, 1981.

Ellis PR, Apling EC, Leeds AR, Peterson DB, Jepson EM. Guar bread and satiety: effects of an acceptable new product in overweight diabetic patients and normal subjects. J Plant Foods 6:253–262, 1985.

Ellis PR, Morris ER, Low AC. Guar gum: the importance of reporting data on its physico-chemical properties. Diabet Med 4:490–491, 1986.

Ellis PR, Burley VJ, Leeds AR, Peterson DB. A guar-enriched wholemeal bread reduces postprandial glucose and insulin responses. J Human Nutr Dietetics 1:77–84, 1988a.

Ellis PR, Kamalanathan T, Dawoud FM, Strange RN, Coultate TP. Evaluation of guar biscuits for use in the management of diabetes. Eur J Clin Nutr 42, 425–435.

Ellis PR, Dawoud FM, Morris ER. Blood glucose, plasma insulin and sensory responses to guar-containing wheat breads: effects of molecular weight and particle size of guar gum. Br J Nutr 66:363–379, 1991.

Ellis PR, Roberts FG, Low AG, Morgan LM. The effect of high-molecular-weight guar gum on net apparent glucose absorption and net apparent insulin and gastric inhibitory polypeptide production in the growing pig: relationship to rheological changes in jejunal digesta. Br J Nutr 74:539–556, 1995.

Ellis PR, Rayment P, Wang Q. A physico-chemical perspective of plant polysaccharides in relation to glucose absorption, insulin secretion and the entero-insular axis. Proc Nutr Soc 55:881–898, 1996.

Ellis PR, Blake DE, Judd PA, Frost P. Metabolic control of non-insulin-dependent diabetes using partially depolymerized guar galactomannan (abstr). Proceedings of 16th International Congress of Nutrition, Montréal, Canada, PW6.6, 1998.

Elsenhans B, Sufke U, Blume R, Caspary WF. In vitro inhibition of rat intestinal surface hydrolysis of disaccharides and dipeptides by guaran. Digestion 21:98–103, 1981.

Englyst HN, Quigley ME, Hudson GJ, Cummings JH. Determination of dietary fibre as non-starch polysaccharides by gas-liquid chromotography. Analyst 117:1707–1714, 1992.

Ershoff BH, Wells AF. Effects of guar gum, locust bean gum on liver cholesterol of cholesterol-fed rats. Proc Soc Exp Biol Med 110:580–582, 1962.

Evans E, Miller DS. Bulking agents in the treatment of obesity. Nutr Metab 18:199–203, 1975.

Fahrenbach MJ, Riccardi A, Saunders JC, Lourie IN, Heider G. Comparative effects of guar gum and pectin on human serum cholesterol level. Circulation 11:31–32, 1965.

Fairchild RM, Daniels CEJ, Ellis PR, Naqvi SHM, Kwan RMF, Mir MA. Effect of two types of guar gum in solid and liquid foods on postprandial glucose, plasma insulin and C-peptide in healthy subjects. Proc Nutr Soc 49:54A, 1990.

Fairchild RM, Ellis PR, Byrne AJ, Luzio SD, Mir MA. A new breakfast cereal containing guar gum reduces postprandial plasma glucose and insulin concentrations in normal-weight human subjects. Br J Nutr 76:63–73, 1996.

FAO/WHO. 19th Report of the Joint FAO/WHO Expert Committee on Food Additives: evaluation of certain food additives. FAO Nutrition Meeting Report Series 55A:14, 1975.

Favier ML, Bost PE, Demigne C, Remesy C. The cholesterol-lowering effect of guar gum in rats is not accompanied by an interruption of bile acid cycling. Lipids 33:765–771, 1998.

Fillery-Travis AJ, Gee JM, Waldron KW, Robins MM, Johnson IT. Soluble non-starch polysaccharides derived from complex food matrices do not increase average lipid droplet size during gastric lipid emulsification in rats. J Nutr 127:2246–2252, 1997.

Flint FO. Micro-technique for the identification of food hydrocolloids. Analyst 115:61–63, 1990.

Flourie B. The influence of dietary fibre on carbohydrate digestion and absorption. In: TF Schweizer, CA Edwards, eds. Dietary Fibre—A Component of Food. Nutritional Function in Health and Disease. London, Springer-Verlag, 1992:295–332.

Fuessl HS, Adrian TE, Bacarese-Hamilton AJ, Bloom SR. Guar in NIDD: effect of different modes of administration on plasma glucose and insulin responses to a starch meal. Practical Diabetes 3:258–260, 1986.

Fuessl HS, Williams G, Adrian TE, Bloom SR. Guar sprinkled on food: effect on glycaemic control, plasma lipids and gut hormones in non-insulin dependent diabetic patients. Diabet Med 4:463–468, 1987.

Gallaher DD, Hassel CA. The role of viscosity in the cholesterol-lowering effect of dietary fiber. In: D Kritchevsky, C Bonfield, eds. Dietary Fiber, Health and Disease. St. Paul, MN: Eagan Press, 1995: 106–114.

Gallaher DD, Olson JM, Larntz K. Dietary guar gum halts further renal enlargement in rats with established diabetes. J Nutr 122:2391–2397.

Gallaher DD, Wood KJ, Gallaher CM, Marquart LF, Engström AM. Intestinal contents supernatent viscosity of rats fed oat-based muffins and cereal products. Cereal Chem 76:21–24, 1999.

Gatenby SJ. Guar gum and hyperlipidaemia—a review of the literature. In: AR Leeds, ed. Dietary Fibre Perspectives 2. London: John Libbey, 1990:100–115.

Gatenby SJ, Ellis PR, Morgan LM, Judd PA. Effect of depolymerized guar gum on acute metabolic variables in patients with non-insulin-dependent diabetes. Diabet Med 13:358–364, 1996.

Gatti E, Catenazzo G, Camisasca E, Torri A, Denegri E, Sirtori CR. Effects of guar enriched pasta in the treatment of diabetes and hyperlipidaemia. Ann Nutr Metab 28:1–10, 1984.

Giboreau A, Cuvelier G, Launay B. Rheological behavior of three biopolymer/water systems, with emphasis on yield stress and viscoelastic properties. J Text Stud 25:119–137, 1994.

Gin H, Orgerie MB, Aubertin J. The influence of guar gum on absorption of metformin from the gut in healthy volunteers. Hormone Metab Res 21:81–83, 1989.

Groop P-H. Health benefits of guar galactomannan. In: M Yalpini, ed. New Technologies for Healthy Foods and Nutraceuticals. ATL Press, 1997.

Groop P-H, Groop L, Totterman KJ, Fyhquist F. Relationship between changes in GIP concentration and changes in insulin and C-peptide concentrations after guar gum. Scand J Clin Lab Invest 46:505–510, 1986.

Groop P-H, Aro A, Stenman S, Groop L. Long-term effects of guar gum in subjects with non-insulin-dependent diabetes mellitus. Am J Clin Nutr 58:513–518, 1993.

Hall LD, Yalpani M. A high-yielding, specific method for the chemical derivization of D-galactose-containing polysaccharides: oxidation with D-glucose oxidase, followed by reductive amination. Carbohydr Res 81:C10–C12, 1980.

Hara H, Nagata M, Ohta A, Kasai T. Increases in calcium absorption with ingestion of soluble dietary fibre, guar-gum hydrolysate, depend on the caecum in partially nephrectomized and normal rats. Br J Nutr 76:773–784, 1996.

Heppell LMJ, Rainbird AL. Effect of the physical form of dietary guar gum on nutrient absorption in the pig. In: HJ Just, H Jorgensen, A Fernandez, eds. Proceedings of the Third International Seminar on Digestive Physiology and Nutrient Absorption in the Pig. Copenhagen: National Institute of Animal Science, 1985:58–60.

Hill MA, Leeds AR. High-fibre foods: a feasibility study using guar gum. J Human Nutr 33:253–258, 1979.

Hoffman J, Svensson S. Studies of the distribution of the D-galactosyl side chain in guaran. Carbohydr Res 65:65–71, 1978.

Holman RR, Steemson J, Darling P, Turner RC. No glycaemic benefit from guar administration in NIDDM. Diabetes Care 10:68–71, 1987.

Holt S, Heading RC, Carter DC, Prescott LF, Tothill P. Effect of gel fibre on gastric emptying and absorption of glucose and paracetamol. Lancet 1:636–639, 1979.

Huupponen R, Seppälä P, Iisalo E. Effect of guar gum, a fibre preparation, on digoxin and penicillin absorption in man. Eur J Clin Pharmacol 26:279–281, 1984.

Hymowitz T. The transdomestication concept as applied to guar. Econ Bot 26:49–60, 1972.

Illman RH, Topping DL, McIntosh GH, Trimble RP, Storer GB, Taylor MN, Cheng B-Q. Hypocholesterolaemic effect of dietary propionate: studies in whole animals and perfused rat liver. Ann Nutr Metab 32:97–107, 1988.

Jarjis HA, Blackburn NA, Redfern JS, Read NW. The effect of isphagula (Fybogel and Metamucil) and guar gum on glucose tolerance in man. Br J Nutr 51:371–378, 1984.

Jenkins DJA, Leeds AR, Gassull MA, Wolever TMS, Goff DV, Alberti KGMM, Hockaday TDR. Unabsorbable carbohydrates and diabetes: decreased post-prandial hyperglycaemia. Lancet 2:172–174, 1976a.

Jenkins DJA, Leeds AR, Gassull MA, Houston H, Goff DV, Hill MJ. The cholesterol lowering properties of guar and pectin. Clin Sci Mol Med 51:8P–9P, 1976b.

Jenkins DJA, Leeds AR, Gassull MA, Cochet B, Alberti KGMM. Decrease in postprandial insulin and glucose concentrations by guar and pectin. Ann Intern Med 86:20–23, 1977a.

Jenkins DJA, Wolever TMS, Hockaday TDR, Leeds AR, Howarth R, Bacon S, Apling EC, Dilawari J. Treatment of diabetes with guar gum. Reduction of urinary glucose loss in diabetics. Lancet 2:779–780, 1977b.

Jenkins DJA, Wolever TMS, Leeds AR, Gassull MA, Haisman P, Dilawari J, Goff DV, Metz GL, Alberti KGMM. Dietary fibre, fibre analogues and glucose tolerance: importance of viscosity. Br Med J 1: 1353–1354, 1978a.

Jenkins DJA, Wolever TMS, Nineham R, Taylor RH, Metz, GL, Bacon S, Hockaday TDR. Guar crispbread in the diabetic diet. Br Med J 2:1744–1746, 1978b.

Jenkins DJA, Nineham R, Craddock C, Craig-McFeely P, Donaldson K, Leigh T, Snook J. Fibre and diabetes. Lancet 2:434–435, 1979.

Jenkins DJA, Reynolds D, Slavin B, Leeds AR, Jenkins AL, Jepson EM. Dietary fiber and blood lipids: treatment of hypercholesterolaemia with guar crispbread. Am J Clin Nutr 33:57–58, 1980.

Johansen HN, Wood PJ, Bach Knudsen KE. Molecular weight changes in the $(1\rightarrow3)(1\rightarrow4)$-β-D-glucan of oats incurred by the digestive processes in the upper gastrointestinal tract of pigs. J Agric Food Chem 41:2347–2352, 1993.

Johnson IT. The influence of dietary fibre on lipid digestion and absorption. In: TF Schweizer, CA Edwards, eds. Dietary Fibre—A Component of Food. Nutritional Function in Health and Disease. London: Springer-Verlag, 1992:167–196.

Johnson IT. The physiological mechanisms of action of different fibre classes. In: M Hill, ed. The Right Fibre for the Right Disease. London: The Royal Society of Medicine Press Ltd, 1999:33–42.

Kay DE. Crop and Product Digest No. 3—Food Legumes. London, Tropical Products Institute, 1979:72–85.

Krotkiewski M. Effect of guar gum on body-weight, hunger ratings and metabolism in obese subjects. Br J Nutr 52:97–105, 1984.

Landin K, Holm G, Tengborn L, Smith U. Guar gum improves insulin sensitivity, blood-lipids, blood-pressure, and fibrinolysis in healthy-men. Am J Clin Nutri 56:1061–1065, 1992.

Leclere CJ, Champ M, Boillot J, Guille G, Lecannu G, Molis C, Bornet F, Krempf M, Delort-Laval J, Galmiche JP. Role of viscous guar gums in lowering the glycaemic response after a solid meal. Am J Clin Nutr 59:914–921, 1994.

Leeds AR. The effect of fibre on coronary heart disease and cholesterol. In: M Hill, ed. The Right Fibre for the Right Disease. London: The Royal Society of Medicine Press Ltd., 1999:33–42.

Leeds AR, Bolster NR, Andrews R, Truswell AJ. Meal viscosity, gastric emptying and glucose absorption in the rat. Proc Nutr Soc 38:44A, 1979.

Lewis JH. Esophageal and small bowel obstruction from guar gum-containing ''diet-pills.'' Am J Gastroenterol 87:1424–1428, 1992.

Licionio-Paxicio J, Polansky KS, Given BD, Pugh W, Ostrega D, Frank BF, Rubenstein AH. Ingestion of mixed meal does not affect the metabolic clearance rate of biosynthetic human C-peptide. J Clin Endocrinol Metab 63:401–403, 1986.

Low AG. Nutritional regulation of gastric secretion, digestion and emptying. Nutr Res Rev 3:229–252, 1990.

Macagno EO, Christensen J, Lee CL. Modelling the effect of wall movement on absorption in the intestine. Am J Physiol 243:G541–G550, 1982.

Maier H, Anderson M, Karl C, Magnuson K, Whistler RL. Guar, locust bean, tara and fenugreek gums. In: RL Whistler, JN Bemiller, eds. Industrial Gums: Polysaccharides and their Derivatives. 3rd ed. London: Academic Press Inc., 1993:181–226.

McCleary BV, Clark AH, Dea ICM, Rees DA. The fine-structures of carob and guar galactomannans. Carbohydr Res 139:237–260, 1985.

McClendon JH, Nolan WG, Wenzler HF. The role of the endosperm in the germination of legumes: galacto-mannan, nitrogen, and phosphorus changes in the germination of guar (*Cyamposis tetragonoloba*; Leguminosae). Am J Bot 63:790–797, 1976.

McIvor ME, Cummings CC, Leo TA, Mendeloff AT. Flattening postprandial blood glucose responses with guar gum: acute effects. Diabetes Care 8:274–278, 1985a.

McIvor ME, Cummings CC, Mendeloff AI. Long-term ingestion of guar gum is not toxic in patients with non-insulin-dependent diabetes mellitus. Am J Clin Nutr 41:891–894, 1985b.

McIvor ME, Cummings CC, van Duyn MA, Leo TA, Margolis S, Behall KM, Michnowski JE, Mendeloff AT. Long-term effects of guar gum on blood lipids. Atherosclerosis 60:7–13, 1986.

Meir H, Reid JSG. Reserve polysaccharides other that starch in higher plants. In: FA Loewus, W Tanner, eds. Encyclopedia of Plant Physiology. Vol. 13A. New York: Springer-Verlag, 1982:418–471.

Meyer JH, Doty JE. GI transit and absorption of solid food: multiple effects of guar. Am J Clin Nutr 48: 267–263, 1988.

Meyer JH, Gu YG, Jehn D, Taylor II. Intragastric vs intraintestinal viscous polymers and glucose tolerance after liquid meals of glucose. Am J Clin Nutr 48:260–266, 1988.

Ministry of Agriculture, Fisheries & Food. Additives in food: the emulsifiers and stabilisers regulation. Amendment to regulations. SI 1980, No. 1833, London, UK, 1988.

Morgan LM, Goulder TJ, Tsiolakis D, Marks V, Alberti KG. The effect of unabsorbable carbohydrate on gut hormones. Modification of post-prandial GIP secretion by guar. Diabetologia 17:85–89, 1979.

Morgan LM, Tredger JA, Madden A, Kwasowski P, Marks V. The effect of guar gum on carbohydrate-, fat- and protein-stimulated gut hormone secretion: modification of post-prandial gastric inhibitory polypeptide and gastrin responses. Br J Nutr 53:467–475, 1985.

Morgan LM, Tredger JA, Wright J, Marks V. The effect of soluble- and insoluble-fibre supplementation on post-prandial glucose tolerance, insulin and gastric inhibitory polypeptide secretion in healthy subjects. Br J Nutr 64:103–101, 1990.

Morris ER. Shear-thinning of 'random coil' polysaccharides: characterisation by two parameters from a simple linear plot. Carbohydr Polym 13:85–90, 1990.

Morris ER, Ross-Murphy SB. Chain flexibility of polysaccharides and glycoproteins from viscosity mea-surements. Techniques Carbohydr Metab B310:1–46, 1981.

Morris ER, Cutler AN, Ross-Murphy SB, Rees DA, Price J. Concentration and shear rate dependence of viscosity in random coil polysaccharide solutions. Carbohydr Polym 1:5–21, 1981.

Najemnik C, Kritz H, Irsigler K, Laube H, Knick B, Klimm HD, Wahl P, Vollmar J, Brauning CH. Guar and its effects on metabolic control in type II diabetic subjects. Diabetes Care 7:215–220, 1984.

Nishina PM, Freedland RA. Effects of propionate on lipid biosynthesis in isolated rat hepatocytes. J Nutr 120:668–673, 1990.

Nyman M, Asp N-G. Fermentation of dietary fibre components in the rat intestinal tract. Br J Nutr 47: 357–366, 1982.

O'Connor N, Tredger J, Morgan L. Viscosity differences between various guar gums. Diabetologia 20: 612–615, 1981.

Overton PD, Furlonger N, Beety JM, Chakraborty J, Tredger JA, Morgan LM. The effects of dietary sugar-beet fibre and guar gum on lipid metabolism in Wistar rats. Br J Nutr 72:385–395, 1994.

Paganus A, Mäenpää J, Åkerblom HK, Stenman U-H, Knip M, Simell O. Beneficial effects of palatable guar and guar plus fructose diets in diabetic children. Acta Pædiatr Scand 76:76–81, 1987.

Pasman WJ, Westerterp-Plantengo MS, Muis E, Vansant G, van Ree J, Saris WHM. The effectiveness of long-term fibre supplementation on weight maintenance in weight-reduced women. Int J Obesity 21:548–555, 1997.

Pasquier B, Armand M, Castelain C, Guillon F, Borel P, Lafont H, Lairon D. Emulsification and lipolysis of triacylglycerols are altered by viscous soluble dietary fibres in acidic gastric medium in vitro. Biochem J 314:269–275, 1996a.

Pasquier B, Armand M, Guillon F, Castelain C, Borel P, Barry J-L, Pieroni G, Lairon D. Viscous soluble dietary fibres alter emulsification and lipolysis of triacylglycerols in duodenal medium in vitro. J Nutr Biochem 7:293–302, 1996b.

Peterson DB, Ellis PR, Baylis JM, Fielden P, Ajodhia J, Leeds AR, Jepson EM. Low dose guar in a novel food product: improved metabolic control in non-insulin-dependent diabetes. Diabetic Med 4:111–115, 1987.

Phillips DR. The effect of guar gum in solution on diffusion of cholesterol mixed micells. J Food Sci 37:548–552, 1986.

Pikaar NA, Wedel M, Van Dokkum W, Hermus RJ. The influence of the type of starch and of the incorporation of soluble dietary fibre in breakfast and lunch on the levels of glucose, insulin and C-peptide in plasma. Proc Nutr Soc 44:68A, 1985.

Potkins ZV, Lawrence TLJ, Thomlinson JR. Effects of structural and non-structural polysaccharides in the diet of growing pigs on the gastric emptying rate and rate of passage of digesta to the terminal ileum and through the total gastrointestinal tract. Br J Nutr 65:391–414, 1991.

Rainbird AL, Low AG. Effect of guar gum on gastric emptying in growing pigs. Br J Nutr 55:87–98, 1986.

Rayding A, Nelson A, Basted A. Influence of fibre on postprandial intragastric juice acidity, pepsin and bile acids in healthy subjects. Scand J Gastroenterol 19:1039–1044, 1984.

Rayment P, Ross-Murphy SB, Ellis PR. Rheological properties of guar galactomannan and rice starch mixtures—I. Steady shear measurements. Carbohydr Polym 28:121–130, 1995.

Rayment P, Ross-Murphy SB, Ellis PR. Rheological properties of guar galactomannan and rice starch mixtures. In: Go Phillips, PA Williams, DJ Wedlock, eds. Gums and Stabilisers for the Food Industry 8. Oxford, UK: Oxford University Press, 1996:237–246.

Rayment P, Ross-Murphy SB, Ellis PR. Rheological properties of guar galactomannan and rice starch mixtures—II. Creep measurements. Carbohydr Polym 35:55–63, 1998.

Rayment P, Ross-Murphy SB, Ellis PR. Effect of size and shape of particulate inclusions on the rheology of guar galactomannan solutions. Carbohydr Polym 43:1–9, 2000.

Read NW, Eastwood M. Gastro-intestinal physiology and function. In: TF Schweizer, CA Edwards, eds. Dietary Fibre—A Component of Food. Nutritional Function in Health and Disease. London: Springer-Verlag, 1992:103–117.

Rees DA. Polysaccharide Shapes. London: Chapman and Hall, 1977.

Reid JSV, Edwards ME. Galactomannans and other cell wall storage polysaccharides in seeds. In: Am Stephen, ed. Food Polysaccharides and their Applications. New York: Marcel Dekker, 1995:155–186.

Reid JSG, Edwards ME, Dea ICM. Biosynthesis of galactomannan in the endosperms of developing fenugreek (*Trigonella foenum-graecum* L.) and guar (*Cyamopsis tetragonoloba* [L.] Taub) seeds. Food Hydrocoll 1:381–385, 1987.

Richardson RK, Ross-Murphy SB. Non-linear viscoelasticity of polysaccharide solutions. I: Guar galactomannan solutions. Int J Biol Macromol 9:250–256, 1987.

Roberts FG, Smith, HA, Low AG, Ellis PR. Influence of wheat breads containing guar flour supplements of high and low molecular weights on viscosity of jejunal digesta in the pig. In: DAT Southgate, K Waldren, IT Johnson, GR Fenwick, eds. Dietary Fibre: Chemical and Biological Aspects. Cambridge: The Royal Society of Chemistry, 1990a:164–168.

Roberts FG, Smith HA, Low AG, Ellis PR, Morris ER, Sambrook IE. Influence of guar gum flour of different molecular weights on viscosity of jejunal digesta in the pig. Proc Nutr Soc 49:53A, 1990b.

Roberts FG, Low AG, Young S, Smith HA, Ellis PR. The effect of high viscosity guar gum flour on the rate of glucose absorption and net insulin production in the portal blood of the pig. Proc Nutr Soc 50:72A, 1991.

Robbins SRJ. A review of recent trends in selected markets for water-soluble gums. Overseas Development Natural Resources Institute Bulletin No. 2. The Scientific Unit of the Overseas Development Administration, 1988.

Robinson G, Ross-Murphy SB, Morris ER. Viscosity-molecular weight relationships, intrinsic chain flexibility and dynamic solution properties of guar galactomannan. Carbohydr Res 107:17–32, 1982.

Roger P, Hoebler C, Ficadière T, Colonna P. Bovine serum albumin diffusion in dilute and semi-dilute solutions of guar: effect of guar molecular weight. Food Hydrocoll 5:145–146, 1991.

Ross-Murphy SB. Rheological methods. In: HS Chan, ed. Biophysical Methods in Food Research. Critical Reports on Applied Chemistry. Vol. 5. Oxford: Blackwell Scientific Publications, 1984:138–199.

Ross-Murphy SB. Rheological methods. In: SB Ross-Murphy, ed. Physical Techniques for the Study of Food Biopolymers. London: Blackie Academic & Professional, 1994:343–392.

Ross-Murphy SB, Wang Q, Ellis PR. Structure and mechanical properties of polysaccharides. Macromol Symp 127:13–21, 1998.

Rössner S. Dietary fibre in the prevention and treatment of obesity. In: TF Schweizer, CA Edwards, eds. Dietary Fibre—A Component of Food. Nutritional Function in Health and Disease. London: Springer-Verlag, 1992:265–277.

Ryttig KR, Leeds A, Rössner S. Dietary fibre in the management of overweight—an update. In: AR Leeds, ed. Dietary Fibre Perspectives 2. London, John Libbey, 1990:187–199.

Saber AH, Ahmed ZF, Darwish M. A contribution to the study of guar seeds grown in Egypt. Bull Inst Desert Egypte 6:67–78, 1956.

Salayers AA, Vercellotti JR, West SEH, Wilkins TD. Fermentation of mucin and plant polysaccharides by strains of Bacteroides from the human colon. Appl Environ Microbiol 33:319–322, 1977.

Salenius J-P, Harju E, Jokela H, Riekkinen H, Silvasti M. Long term effects of guar gum on lipid metabolism after corotid endarterectomy. Br Med J 310:95–96, 1995.

Salmerón J, Ascherio A, Rimm EB, Colditz GA, Spiegelman D, Jenkins DJA, Stampfer MJ, Wing AL, Willett WC. Dietary fiber, glycemic load and risk of non-insulin-dependent diabetes mellitus in men. Diabetes Care 20:545–550, 1997a.

Salmerón J, Manson JE, Stampfer MJ, Colditz GA, Wing AL, Willett WC. Dietary fiber, glycemic load and risk of non-insulin-dependent diabetes mellitus in woman. J Am Med Assoc 277:472–477, 1997b.

Sambrook IE, Rainbird AL. The effect of guar gum and level and source of dietary fat and glucose tolerance in growing pigs. Br J Nutr 54:27–35.

Saris WHM, Asp N-GL, Björk I, Blaak F, Brouns F, Frayn KN, Fürst P, Riccardi G, Roberfroid MB, Vogel M. Functional food science and substrate metabolism. Br J Nutr 80 (suppl 1):S47–S75, 1998.

Savarino V, Mela GS, Scalabrini P, Sumberaz A, Fera G, Celle G. 24-hour study of intragastric acidity in duodenal-ulcer patients and normal subjects using continuous intraluminal pH-metry. Digest Dis Sci 33:1077–1080, 1988.

Sels JP, Flendrig JA, Postmes TJ. The influence of guar-gum bread on the regulation of diabetes mellitus type II in elderly patients. Br J Nutr 57:177–183.

Sels JP, De Bruin H, Camps MH, Postmes TJ, Menheere P, Wolfenbuttel BH, Kruseman AC. Absence of guar efficacy in complex spaghetti meals on postprandial glucose and C-peptide levels in healthy control and non-insulin-dependent diabetes mellitus subjects. Hormone Metab Res 26:52–58, 1994.

Simões Nunes C, Malmlöf K. Effects of guar gum and cellulose on glucose absorption, hormonal release and hepatic metabolism in the pig. Br J Nutr 68:693–700, 1992.

Simons LA, Gayst S, BalaSubramaniam S, Ruys J. Long term treatment of hypercholesterolemia with a new formulation of guar gum. Atherosclerosis 45:101–108, 1982.

Sinisalo M, Aro A, Ebling P, Groop PH, Koivisto VA. Effect of guar gum on zinc and magnesium status of diabetic patients. Trace Elements Med 6:12–17, 1989.

Smith CJ, Rosman MS, Levitt NS, Jackson WPU. Guar biscuits in the diabetic diet. S Afr Med J 61:196–198, 1982.

Taglioferro V, Cassader M, Bozzo C, Pisu E, Bruno A, Cavallo-Perin P, Cravero L, Pagano G. Moderate guar gum addition to usual diet improves peripheral sensitivity to insulin and lipaemic profile in NIDDM. Diabet Metab 11:380–385, 1985.

Takahashi H, Wako N, Okubo T, Ishihara N, Yamanaka J, Yamamoto T. Influence of intact and partially hydrolyzed guar gum on iron utilisation in rats fed on iron-deficient diets. Comp Biochem Physiol Comp Physiol 109:75–82, 1994.

To K-M, Mitchell JR, Hill SE, Bardon LA, Matthews P. Measurement of hydration of polysaccharides. Food Hydrocoll 8:243–249, 1994.

Todd PA, Benfield P, Goa KL. Guar gum: a review of its pharmacological properties, and use as a dietary adjunct in hypercholesterolaemia. Drugs 39:917–928, 1990.

Topping DL. Physiological aspects of food hydrocolloids. In: K Nishinari, E Doi, eds. Food Hydrocolloids: Structures, Properties and Functions. New York: Plenum Press, 1993:477–484.

Torsdottir I, Alpsten M, Andersson H, Einarsson S. Dietary guar gum effects on postprandial blood glucose and hydroxyproline in humans. J Nutr 119:1925–1931, 1989.

Tredger J, Ransley J. Guar gum—its acceptability to diabetic patients when incorporated into baked food products. J Human Nutr 32:427–432, 1978.

Tredger JA, Morgan LM, Peake J, Marks V. Effect of guar gum on the rate of gastric emptying in human subjects. Reg Peptides 9:350, 1984.

Truswell AS, Beynen AC. Dietary fibre and plasma lipids: potential for prevention and treatment of hyper-lipidaemias. In: TF Schweizer, CA Edwards, eds. Dietary Fibre—A Component of Food. Nutritional Function in Health and Disease. London: Springer-Verlag, 1992:295–332.

Tuomilehto J, Voutilainen E, Huttunen J, Vinni S, Homan K. Effect of guar gum on body weight and serum lipids in hypercholesterolemic females. Acta Med Scand 208:45–48, 1980.

Tuomilehto J, Silvasti M, Aro A, Koistinen A, Karttunen P, Gref C-G, Ehnholm C, Uusitupa M. Long term treatment of severe hypercholesterolaemia with guar gum. Atherosclerosis 72:157–162, 1988.

United Kingdom Prospective Diabetes Study (UKPDS) Group. Intensive blood glucose control with sulphonylureas or insulin compared with conventional treatment and risk of complications in patients with type 2 diabetes (UKPDS 33). Lancet 352:837–853, 1998.

Uusitupa M, Siitonen O, Savolainen K, Silvasti M, Penttila I, Parviainen M. Metabolic and nutritional effects of long-term treatment of non-insulin-dependent diabetes of poor metabolic control. Am J Clin Nutr 49:345–351, 1989.

Vaaler S, Hanssen KF, Dahl-Jørgensen K, Frøhlich W, Aaseth J, Ødegaard B, Aagenæs Ø. Diabetic control is improved by guar gum and wheat bran supplementation. Diabetic Med 3:230–233, 1986.

Van Duyn MAS, Leo TA, McIvor ME, Behall KM, Michnowski JE, Mendeloff AI. Nutritional risk of high-carbohydrate, guar gum dietary supplementation in non-insulin-dependent diabetes mellitus. Diabetes Care 9:497–503, 1986.

Vuorinen-Markkola H, Sinisalo M, Koivisto VA. Guar gum in insulin-dependent diabetes: effects on glycemic control and serum lipoproteins. Am J Clin Nutr 56:1056–1060, 1992.

Wang Q. Physico-chemical characterisation of water-soluble non-starch polysaccharides. Ph.D. thesis, University of London, 1997.

Wang Q, Ellis PR, Ross-Murphy SB. The stability of guar gum in an aqueous system under acidic conditions. Food Hydrocoll 14:129–134, 2000.

Whistler RL, Hymowitz T. Guar: Agronomy, Production, Industrial Use and Nutrition. West Lafayette, In: Purdue University Press, 1979.

Whitcomb PJ, Gutowski J, Howland WW. Rheology of guar solutions. J Appl Polym Sci 25:2815–2827, 1980.

Wielinga WC. Application of gum-based stabilization systems in ice-cream and fruit ices. In: GO Phillips, DA Wedlock, PA Williams, eds. Gums and Stabilisers for the Food Industry 2: Application for Hydrocolloids. Oxford: Pergamon Press Ltd., 1984:207–216.

Wielinga WC. Galactomannans. In: GO Phillips, PA Williams, eds. Handbook of Hydrocolloids. Cambridge: Woodhead Publishing Ltd., 2000:137–154.

Wilmhurst P, Crawley JCW. The measurement of gastric transit time in obese subjects using [24]Na and the effects of energy content and guar gum on gastric emptying and satiety. Br J Nutr 44:1–6, 1980.

Wolever TMS, Jenkins DJA, Nineham R, Alberti KGMM. Guar gum and reduction of post-prandial glycaemia: effect of incorporation into solid food, liquid food, and both. Br J Nutr 41:505–510, 1979.

Zebrowska T, Low AG. The influence of diets based on whole wheat, wheat flour and wheat bran on exocrine pancreatic secretion in pigs. J Nutr 117:1212–1216, 1987.

33

Alginate

Production, Composition, Physicochemical Properties, Physiological Effects, Safety, and Food Applications

Edvar Onsøyen
Pronova Biopolymer a.s., Drammen, Norway

I. INTRODUCTION

Populations in coastal regions have for thousands of years regarded the ocean as their most obvious source of food raw materials. In East Asia nori, wakame, and kombu, developed from seaweeds, are still a natural part of the diet. In the western world only a few coastal communities still use seaweed as a specialty food raw material. However, seaweed has occasionally been explored as a source for functional food products.

Along with the use of seaweed as a "marine vegetable," people learned to appreciate the functionality it brought to prepared foods. For example, the carrageean-containing red algae *Chondrus crispus* (Irish moss), is still in use in Bretagne and Ireland for thickening and gelforming purposes.

The first scientific studies on the extraction of alginates from brown seaweed were made by the British chemist E. C. Stanford at the end of the nineteenth century. He found that the extracted substance, which he named algin, possessed several interesting properties, including the ability to thicken solutions, make gels, and form films. From these, he proposed several industrial applications. However, large-scale industrial production of alginate was not introduced until 50 years later.

II. ALGINATE PRODUCTION

A. Biological Occurrence

Alginates occur in the cell walls and intercellular spaces of brown seaweed. The alginate molecules provide the plant with both flexibility and strength, which are necessary for plant growth in the sea. Alginates are also synthesized by some bacteria (e.g. some *Azotobacter* and *Pseudomonas* species).

B.   Raw Materials for Commercial Alginates—Geographical Occurrence

The locations for sources of brown algae industrially utilized for alginate production are shown in Fig. 1. The brown algae most widely used for industrial production include *Laminaria hyperborea*, *Laminaria digitata*, *Laminaria japonica*, *Ascophyllum nodosum*, *Macrocystis pyrifera*, and *Lessonia* and *Durvillea* species. In addition, other species of *Laminaria* (*saccharina* and *cloustoni*) as well as some *Ecklonia* species are used, but on a much smaller scale.

One of the main brown seaweed species utilized is *L. hyperborea*. This seaweed is mechanically harvested along the west coast of Norway, where large "forests" grow naturally in the clean Arctic waters. The plants are harvested in fairly shallow water, at depths of 2–15 meters. Special trawlers have been developed to harvest this seaweed. Mechanical harvesting is combined with careful monitoring of the resources to ensure regular long-term cropping of defined areas. A harvested area is regenerated within 5 years. This has been confirmed repeatedly during the 50 years of industrial utilization of *L. hyperborea*. The yearly harvested amounts of *L. hyperborea* represent less than 5% of the total yearly regrowth volume of this seaweed along the Norwegian coast.

Alginates produced from *L. hyperborea* are known for their ability to form strong gels. In order to meet other demands in terms of alginate functionality, other sources of brown seaweed are utilized. Alginate occurs in seaweed as an insoluble mix of calcium, magnesium, sodium, and potassium salts in the gelled stage. The fact that it is in the gelled stage is important, since it is the only way that alginate can contribute to the strength and suppleness of the seaweed plant. Alginate is not a fiber in itself, possessing mechanical strength like the cellulose fiber; alginate is regarded as a soluble fiber and possesses strength through its gelled network hydrated with capillary entrapped water.

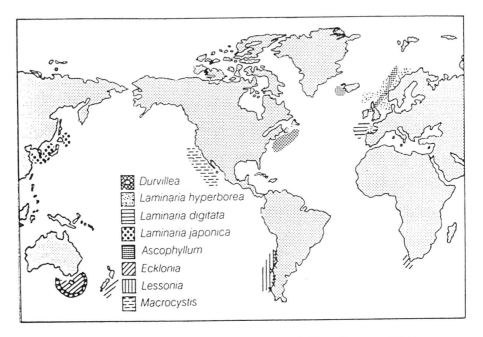

Fig. 1   Distribution of industrially utilized brown seaweed. (From Onsøyen, 1997.)

C. Alginate-Manufacturing Process

The industrial production of alginates consists of more than 20 stages. After milling of the seaweed, raw material is washed with acid to get rid of acid-soluble impurities. Then the alginate is extracted from the seaweed by an alkaline treatment, and the alginate solution is clarified and filtered to eliminate any particulate impurities.

The manufacturing process then involves precipitation to recover the product as insoluble alginic acid, either directly as alginic acid or through precipitation with calcium as calcium alginate, followed by an acid wash to transform it into alginic acid.

D. Commercial Alginates—Food and Food-Related Grades

Alginic acid has limited stability. In order to make water-soluble, functional, and stable alginate products, alginic acid is transformed into different salt forms to make commercial alginate products. The most commonly used alginates in food and food related applications are sodium alginates. Potassium and calcium alginates are also utilized to some extent.

Propylene glycol alginates (PGA) have some emulsifying properties and are therefore used as stabilizers in emulsions (e.g., salad dressings) and in beer to stabilize the beer foam. PGA has better acid functionality than alginates and is used in acid foods like yogurt and fruit juices for that reason.

III. ALGINATE COMPOSITION AND PHYSICOCHEMICAL PROPERTIES

A. Chemistry

Alginate is a polysaccharide, like starch and cellulose. It is, like cellulose, composed of several (1000–3000) building units linked together in a partly stiff and partly flexible chain. Cellulose is composed of glucose molecules, while alginate is composed of two sugars—both uronates—the salts of mannuronic and guluronic acid.

When producing alginates, uronic acid is converted into the salt forms mannuronate (M) and guluronate (G) (Fig. 2). It has been shown that the monomer M and G residues in alginates are joined together in a blockwise fashion—homopolymeric M blocks (MMMMM) and G blocks (GGGGG) or heteropolymeric blocks of altering M and G (MGMGMG). In the polymer chain the monomers will tend to find their most energetically favorable structure. For G-G it is the ${}^{1}C_{4}$ chair form linked together with an α-(1→4) glycosidic bond. For M-M it is the ${}^{4}C_{1}$ chair form linked together with a β-(1→4) glycosidic bond. The rather bulky carboxylic group is responsible for an equatorial/equatorial glycosidic bond in M-M and an axial/axial glycosidic

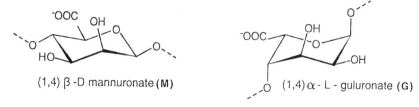

(1,4) β -D mannuronate (M)   (1,4) α - L - guluronate (G)

Fig. 2 The monomers of alginate.

bond in G-G and an equatorial/axial glycosidic bond in M-G. The result of this is a buckled and stiff polymer in the G-block regions and a flexible, ribbon-like polymer in the M-block and MG-block regions. The proportion and distribution of these blocks (Fig. 3) determine the chemical and physical properties of the alginate molecules.

The chemical composition of alginates is to a certain extent variable. It varies according to seaweed species and even within different parts of the same plant. It is also subject to seasonal changes. Nevertheless, by selecting raw materials with varying but known properties, it is possible to manufacture alginates with constant properties in a wide range of grades.

The block structure distribution of an alginate extracted from brown algae is determined by alginate biosynthesis in the brown algae and its genetical and environmental control. The pathway of alginate biosynthesis in brown algae ends up with poly(mannuronate), the homopolymer of M, as an obligate intermediate. An epimerase is then acting on the polymer level and works along the polymer chain in controlling the epimerization from M to G in certain regions of the polymer. As a rule of the thumb, one can say that the transformation from M to G will be more and more complete as the plant tissue grows older. In the stem part of *L. hyperborea*, for example, one finds the alginates with the highest gel-forming capacity. The stem region possesses tissue with old cells and hence high G content and long G blocks, and the leaf region possesses tissue that is renewed once a year and therefore with less G content. Early in the growth season of *L. hyperborea*, the plants possess a double set of leaves, before the old leaves from the previous year are rejected.

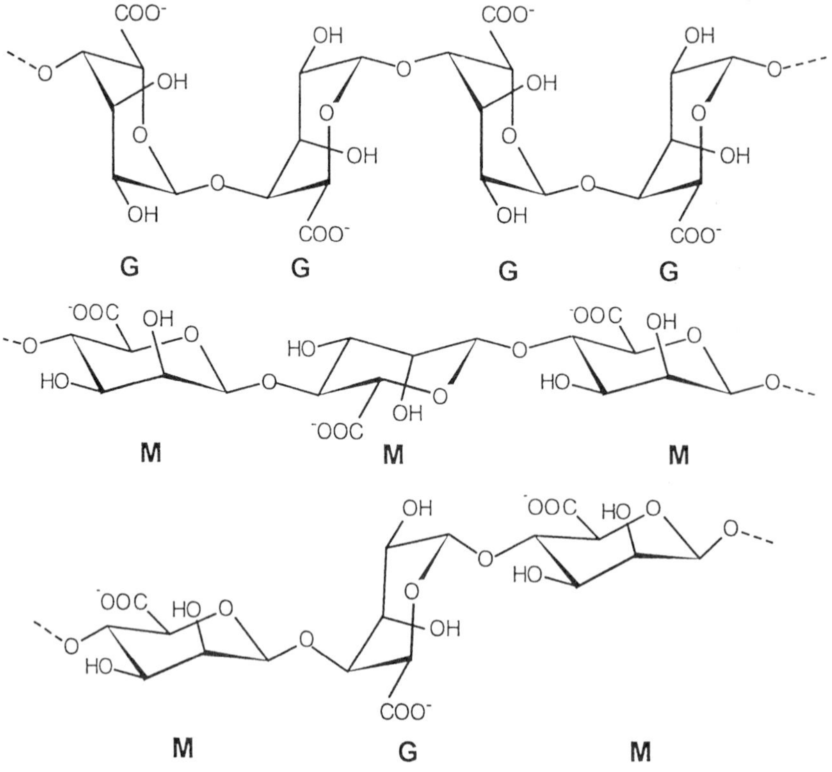

Fig. 3 Alginate block types

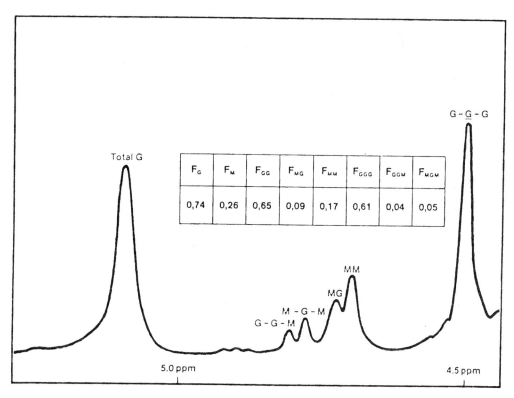

The table within the figure:

F$_G$	F$_M$	F$_{GG}$	F$_{MG}$	F$_{MM}$	F$_{GGG}$	F$_{GGM}$	F$_{MGM}$
0,74	0,26	0,65	0,09	0,17	0,61	0,04	0,05

Fig. 4 ^{1}H-NMR (400 MHz) spectrum of alginate (stipe of *Laminaria hyperborea*). (From Grasdalen, 1983.)

In recent scientific studies, information regarding the detailed chemical composition of alginate has been obtained by NMR (nuclear magnetic resonance) spectroscopy, as shown in Fig. 4.

B. Functional Properties

1. As a Thickening Agent

a. Viscosity. The viscosity of an alginate solution depends on the length of the alginate molecules, i.e., the number of monomer units in the chains. The longer the chain, the higher the viscosity at similar concentrations.

On dissolving alginates in water the molecules hydrate and the solution gains viscosity. The dissolved molecules are not completely flexible; rotation about the glycosidic linkages in the G-block regions is somewhat hindered, resulting in a stiffening of the chain. Solutions of stiff macromolecules are highly viscous.

b. Viscosity and Alginate Concentration. Many different alginate viscosities (molecular length species) are available for different applications. Additionally, one can adjust the concentration to an appropriate level to fulfill special requirements. Figure 5 shows the viscosity range of different alginate products at different concentrations.

Viscosity (mPa·s)

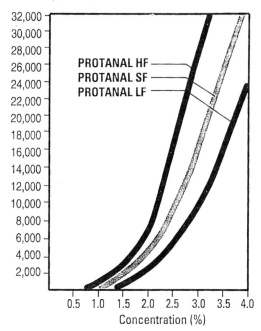

Fig. 5 Viscosity as a function of concentration of alginates in distilled water. (From Pronova Biopolymer a.s., 1995.)

c. Viscosity and Temperature.   Temperature defines the energetic state of any chemical molecule. Hence temperature influences how alginate molecules respond to shear forces. In other words, temperature contributes to a certain extent to the viscosity characteristics of an alginate molecule. As a general rule, a temperature increase of 1°C leads to a viscosity drop of approximately 2.5% (Fig. 6).

d. Rheology.   Through choice of grade and formulation, the rheology (flow characteristics) of alginates can be controlled, from free-flowing (low viscosity) to drip-free (high viscosity). Aqueous solutions of alginates have so-called shear-tinning characteristics, i.e., the viscosity decreases with increasing shear rate (stirrer speed). This property is also called pseudoplasticity, or non-Newtonian flow (Fig. 7).

e. Acid Conditions.   Standard alginate grades will precipitate or form gels in acid conditions. The pKa values for mannuronic and guluronic acid are 3.38 and 3.65, respectively. To increase the stability of alginates to acid, one may convert alginic acid to its propylene glycol ester, PGA, by reacting the free carboxylic group of the alginic acid with propylene oxide (Fig. 8).

2.   As a Gel-Forming Agent

As mentioned above, alginates contain various proportions of mannuronate and guluronate monomers, which are distributed in a variety of ways. The main property that depends on this distribution is gelling with calcium. To form a gel by reaction with calcium, alginates need to contain a sufficient level of guluronate monomer, and a certain proportion of these guluronate monomers must occur in a block.

Viscosity (mPa·s)

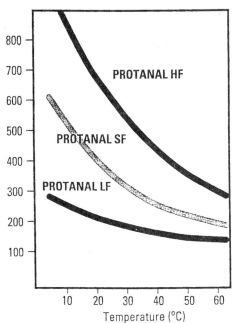

Temperature (°C)

Fig. 6 Viscosity of three 1% sodium alginate solutions at different temperatures. (From Pronova Biopolymer a.s., 1995.)

Viscosity (mPa·s)

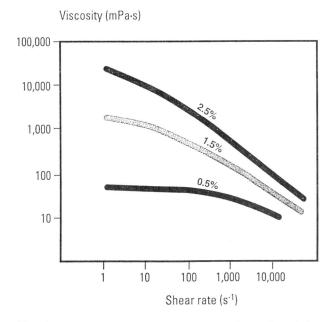

Shear rate (s⁻¹)

Fig. 7 Viscosity as a function of shear rate for sodium alginate solutions. (From Pronova Biopolymer a.s., 1995.)

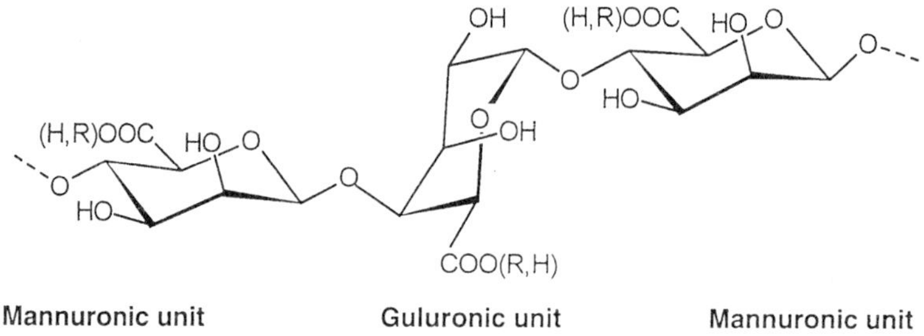

Mannuronic unit   Guluronic unit   Mannuronic unit

Fig. 8   Alginic acid chain with some acid residues esterified.

The reactivity with calcium and the consequent gelling capacity is a direct function of the average length of the G blocks. The alginates containing the highest GG fractions (i.e., stem-grade alginates from *L. hyperborea*) possess the greatest ability to form gels (see Table 1). Thus, stem-grade alginates from *L. hyperborea* are highly appreciated for high gel-strength applications.

Regions of guluronate monomers in one alginate molecule can be linked to a similar region in another alginate molecule by means of calcium or other multivalent cations (Fig. 9). The divalent calcium cation, Ca^{2+}, fits into the guluronate structures like eggs in an egg box (Fig. 10.)

Table 1   Typical M- and G-Block Profiles for Different Seaweeds as Measured by NMR

Type of seaweed	%MM	%MG + %GM	%GG
Laminaria hyperborea (stem)	18	24	58
Laminaria hyperborea (leaf)	36	38	26
Laminaria digitata	39	32	29
Eclonia maxima	38	34	28
Macrocystis pyrifera	40	40	20
Lessonia nigrescens	43	34	23
Ascophyllum nodosum	56	18	26
Laminaria japonica	48	34	18
Durvillea antarctica	58	26	16
Durvillea potatorum	69	16	15

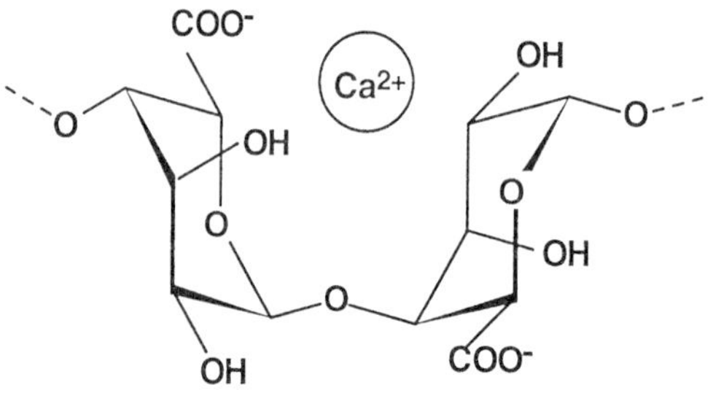

Fig. 9   Calcium-binding site in G blocks.

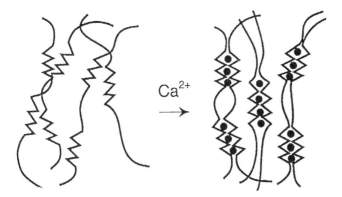

Fig. 10 ''Egg box'' model for alginate gel formation.

(Grant et al., 1973). This binds the alginate polymers together by forming junction zones, thus leading to the gelling of the solution.

An alginate gel may be considered to be partly in a solid and partly in a solution state, the junction zones representing the solid state. After gelation, the water molecules are physically entrapped by the alginate matrix but are still free to migrate. This is of great importance in many applications (e.g., alginate gels for cell immobilization/encapsulation). The water-holding capacity of the gel is a result of capillary forces.

The uniqueness of alginates as gel formers rests in their ability to form heat-stable gels, which can develop at room temperature. This is of particular interest when alginates are used as gelling agents in restructured products like canned pet food and in the preparation of bakery filling creams (custard).

It is primarily the alginate gel formation with calcium ions that is of interest in most applications. In this way, cold-prepared, thermo-irreversible, and freeze-thaw–stable mixes can be made. By manipulation of the formulation, alginate gels can be made to be firm, soft, brittle, or flexible.

The alginates extracted from different raw materials may be characterized by their gel strength. As shown in Table 2, alginates covering a broad range of gel strength can be produced from a single species of seaweed when different parts of the *L. hyperborea* plant are separated prior to alginate extraction. The FIRA values refer to gel strength measurements using a FIRA jelly tester on alginate gels with very uniform and homogeneous consistency (Toft, 1982).

At slightly acid pH levels, as in fruit and jam products, the alginate gel formed will be an acid or calcium-acid combination type. A thermo-reversible gel can be made using a combination of alginate and pectin (Toft et al., 1986).

Table 2 Alginate Gel Strength FIRA Value (mL water/30° deflection)

Alginate origin	Gel strength
L. hyperborea	
Stem	65–75
Whole plant	55–65
Double leaf	45–55
Pure leaf	40–50
A. nodosum	25–35

3. As Film-Forming Agents

When a thin layer of alginate gel or alginate solution is dried, a film or coating is formed. Alginate films are utilized in a number of applications to reduce water loss, either through the water-holding capacity of the alginate or through the more general protective character of the alginate polymeric coating.

The film-forming properties of alginates are the main reason for their use in paper-making applications. In textile-printing applications, besides controlling the flow characteristics of printing pastes, alginates contribute to successfully fixing the colors onto the fabrics. This results from the very high water-retention capacities achieved by an alginate film under the often extreme conditions of paper processing or color fixation in textile printing.

In food applications, alginate coatings are used to prevent water passing from the filling into the dry part of the cake. Alginates may also be used in icings to prevent sticking to the wrapping; they simultaneously act as anticracking agents. Alginates can be used to protect frozen fish from oxidation and loss of water by stabilizing the ice layer and making it more impermeable to oxygen and moisture. Meat carcasses and meat pieces can be protected by a calcium alginate film, which both reduces water loss and improves the bacteriological quality. The same system may be applied to poultry and to hamburger-like products.

4. As Stabilizers

Alginates are used in a wide variety of applications as stabilizers and thickening agents, often performing these two functions simultaneously. In textile making, the printing process will always be dependent upon certain rheological properties of the printing paste. The shear thinning abilities of alginates are therefore highly appreciated when used in controlling the flow characteristics of a textile printing paste.

Ice cream was the first application of alginates as stabilizers in the food industry. Alginate addition reduces the size of the ice crystals and produces a smooth product, prolonging the meltdown of the ice cream. Alginates also prevents syneresis. In systems where calcium ions are present, the alginate is usually mixed with sodium phosphate, which binds excess calcium and prevents the precipitation of calcium alginate.

IV. PHYSIOLOGICAL EFFECTS, BIOACTIVITY, AND TOXICOLOGY OF ALGINATES

A. Interference with Minerals

Alginates, when given orally as a part of the diet in humans or rodents, seem to be digested/degraded only slightly (Harmuth-Hoene and Schelenz, 1980; Manchon and Blanquat, 1986; Sandbert et al., 1994). The polyanionic character of the uronic acids in alginates makes them attract various minerals. Therefore, a concern exists that human intake of alginates may alter the mineral balance in a negative way. Mineral excretion and absorption as a result of feeding studies with alginate do not, however, directly reflect the selectivity of the alginates for different minerals, which is understandable since absorption and excretion of minerals involves complex biological systems.

There is no doubt that an ion exchange of minerals will take place in the presence of alginates, such as the documented excretion of Na in the presence of K alginate, which is advantageous as far as decreasing blood pressure values in test animals/humans (Yamori et al., 1986; Tsuji et al., 1993). Another example is th excretion of the radionucleotide Sr-90 caused by intake of Na alginates (Korzun, 1989).

From a nutritional point of view, as an overall conclusion, effects of alginates on mineral absorption or excretion in humans and rodents seem to be very weak or nonexistant. For example, absorption of elements like P, Ca, Mg, and Zn seems to be unchanged, and there is only some indication that absorption of Fe, Cr, and Co may be slightly decreased.

B. Alginate Interference with Nutrients Other Than Minerals

Studies in humans indicates that the ingestion of high levels of sodium alginate and propylene glycol alginate for 23 days resulted in no toxicological effects; in particular, the enzymatic and other sensitive indicators of adverse toxicological effects remained unchanged (Anderson et al., 1991a, b). Dietary alginate seems to have a positive effect on the fecal microbiota and fecal metabolic activity in humans (Terada et al., 1995).

The presence of alginate in the diet of rats is reported to not alter growth or the blood cholesterol level. In cholesterol-fed rats, however, both alginic acid and Na-alginate decreased elevation of the liver cholesterol level, as did various other polysaccharides and gums (Tsuji et al., 1975).

C. Safety

Based on the toxicological data available for alginic acid and alginates (sodium, potassium, calcium, and ammonium salts), the JECFA has granted an acceptable daily intake (ADI) of ''not specified.'' This is the highest possible classification for food additives.

The ADI for propylene glycol alginate has been based on the ADI for propylene glycol, which will always be present in PGA. The JECFA has allocated an ADI of 0–70 mg per kg of body weight to PGA. This limit may, however, be reevaluated at a future JECFA session, following the reevaluation of propylene glycol. Possible restrictions on use of PGA in certain applications may vary from one country to another.

V. ALGINATES IN FOOD AND FOOD-RELATED APPLICATIONS

Alginates have been used for a wide variety of applications in the food industry for over 50 years. Alginates are versatile in their basic properties and in their applications. They are soluble in cold water and will form gels with acids and with divalent cations, such as calcium ions, at room temperature.

A. As a Thickening and Stabilizing Agent

As a thickening and stabilizing agent, alginate can offer a broad spectrum of flow properties to aqueous-based food systems. The rheology of an alginate system can be controlled to produce a required effect; for example, a low molecular weight alginate or PGA produces a long syrupy flow property, a property that is exploited in flowable sauces and dressings. Alternatively, calcium or acid can be added to the alginate system to give a short, drip-free flow property, which is ideally suited to automated mechanical filling equipment. Further fine-tuning of the rheology of the system can be achieved with the inclusion of sequestrants to control the availability of calcium ions.

In terms of the rheology of alginate solutions, the most important variable is molecular weight. When molecular weight increases, viscosity increases. High-viscosity alginate solutions are more sensitive to shear than low-viscosity solutions, and the shear sensitivity can be increased by the introduction of calcium into the system. Calcium can be present in the system as residual calcium in the alginate itself, or it can be added to the aqueous system to produce the required effects. Alternatively, acid can be introduced into the system to give a similar effect. At low calcium or acid levels the viscosity increases when the level of acid or calcium increases.

Alginates are used in a wide variety of foodstuffs as stabilizers and thickening agents. One of the most important applications is in ice cream. Alginate has an excellent stabilizing effect in frozen products and is widely used in ice cream production to secure a proper viscosity in the ice cream mix. In the ready ice cream product, alginate avoids crystallization and shrinkage, secures heat-shock resistance, and gives a homogeneous meltdown without whey separation. Sodium alginate is used in ice cream sauces to give long flow properties, but an external calcium source, in this case the ice cream, sets the sauce and reduces the run-off effect.

In mustard and mustard sauces, sodium alginate or PGA can be used to perform two functions: stabilize the mustard against separation and suspend the mustard solids. It will also provide the desired rheological properties for automatic dispensers and for squeeze bottles. PGAs have a portion of their carboxylic groups esterified and hence are less acid sensitive and more lipid compatible than other alginates and possess some emulsifying power.

In beverages, alginates act as thickeners, stabilizers, and emulsifiers, giving improved body and prolonged shelf life to a variety of products. The effect obtained depends on the type of drink, whether it is neutral or acid, alcoholic or nonalcoholic, and whether it is an emulsion or a suspension. Alginates are also used in dry mix fruit drinks to give fast hydration and to provide mouthfeel. The latter is of particular value in mixes, which are sweetened by artificial sweeteners that do not provide much in the way of viscosity by themselves.

PGA is often used in combination with other gums in many types of salad dressings. The high viscosity at low shear rates gives the necessary suspension and emulsification properties for long shelf life without separation, while at the same time the lower viscosity at high shear rates produces the long flow properties required. PGA is also used in dressings that have low oil content or are free of oil. Alginates are also commonly used as stabilizers in emulsions like mayonnaise and low-fat mayonnaise, as well as in low-fat spreads, by stabilizing and thickening the water phase of the emulsions, and by producing charged films at the interfaces so the individual particles or droplet tend to repel one another.

The reaction between PGA and protein is well known. This interaction is used in beer to increase the foam level. PGA acts by fortifying the protein in the foam to give a longer-lasting foam. This effect is of particular importance in beers where the protein has been deliberately degraded to reduce the chill haze and to improve the general clarity. It is also used to reduce the foam-killing effect of detergent and grease residues transferred from a glass, from fried bar snacks, or even lipsticks.

B.   As a Gelling and Texturizing Agent

Gel formation is achieved by the carefully controlled release of the given ion/acid into an alginate solution. Thus, the gels formed are thermo-irreversible, since the setting is by a chemical crosslinking mechanism. Gel formation is also possible to achieve over a wide temperature range. Due to their greater affinity for calcium, high G alginates form strong, brittle gels with good heat stability. In contrast, high M types form weaker but significantly more tender, elastic gels with good freeze-thaw stability.

1.   Developing an Alginate Gelling System

There are three main components in a typical alginate gelling system: algiante, calcium salts, and sequestrant (usually a type of phosphate). Alginate, calcium, and the sequestering agent control the gel structure and the gel-formation rate. The alginate grade, the calcium source, and the sequestering agent or agents must be matched with the process developed to manufacture the final product.

Several different gelling systems based on alginates can be formulated. The most common are diffusion setting and internal setting. A prerequisite for successful gelling is that alginate is homogeneously distributed in a fully hydrated state throughout the mass of raw materials to be gelled.

a. Diffusion Setting. Diffusion setting is carried out by one of two alternative methods depending upon the desired pH of the final product: neutral diffusion or acid diffusion. In the neutral diffusion system, calcium ions diffuse into the alginate solution or paste from an external bath or spray. Typically, calcium chloride is applied to the surface of the mass to be gelled. The amount of time the salt solution is in contact with the mass to be gelled will determine the extent to which it is gelled. Since the rate of alginate gel formation is very fast, a short residence time will produce a skin around the mass. Longer residence time will result in a partial or complete gel throughout.

A typical example of neutral diffusion setting is the production of restructured pimiento strip used for stuffing cocktail olives. Onion rings are another example of the diffusion setting technique. In exactly the same way rice noodles can be produced in large industrial scale, by extruding the noodles into a calcium chloride setting bath.

With acid diffusion setting, a calcium salt is mixed together with the alginate in the mass to be gelled. The gel process will not start because the calcium salt used is insoluble at neutral pH. When an acid is applied to the surface the salt is solubilized, the calcium ions ar released, and the gel starts to form. Acid diffusion is used in processing many restructured fruit products, such as cherries.

b. Internal Setting. This method relies on calcium being released under controlled conditions from within the system. The process may be performed under either acid or neutral conditions. Various types of meat can be restructured in this way from soy protein or diced by-products to give an identifiable shape with uniform size for portion control.

c. Combined Setting. The diffusion and internal setting systems may also be combined, as in the production of canned restructured meat chunks.

d. Setting by Cooling. In this process the alginate is dissolved in water, together with a calcium salt and a sequestrant, and kept hot. The high temperature counteracts gelation because the alginate chains are in termal motion, which prevents from from associating. Setting will start as the solution cools. When cooled, the calcium alginate reaction will proceed, giving a heat-stable calcium alginate gel. By careful formulation gels can be made to set at temperatures ranging from 0 to 50°C. This process, however, is limited to relatively soft-textured products.

2. Alginate as a Gelling Agent in Various Foods

Several different gelling systems based on alginates can be formulated to become variously thermo-irreversible and heat-stable. These types of alginate gels are the best understood. They form gel under cold conditions and give strong, brittle gels that will not melt when heated. This property is particularly useful in systems that must be heat treated (e.g., canned pet food).

Likewise, bakery custard creams, jams, and marmalades are applications where these properties are used. With alginate cold-prepared, heat-resistant, and freeze/thaw-stable products can be made. By manipulation of the formulation, alginate gels can be made to be firm, soft, brittle, or flexible. In addition to the ability to control the set by temperature, shear, or chemical means, the alginates demonstrate real flexibility for the product developer.

A typical example of neutral diffusion setting is in the production of restructured pimiento strips used for stuffing cocktail olives. In the past a labor-intensive and expensive operation required the peppers to be cut and stuffed into the olive by hand. This process has now been almost totally replaced by the alginate gel technique with large savings in labor cost and time. The incoming peppers are washed and minced to a puree. A premix of sodium alginate and guar gum is added with water to the puree. The resulting viscous mass is fed through a series of rollers into a calcium chloride setting bath. The sheet leaving the setting bath is about 5 mm thick and requires about 20 minutes in the bath for it to be set throughout. The gelled sheet is cut into strips, which are put into a brine for several days before being filled into the pitted olives.

The same technique is used in production of restructured fruit, where the fruit strips are cut into cubes and dried or freeze-dried. This cubes are used in bakery and müsli products. A calcium chloride setting bath for restructured fruit cubes is shown in Fig. 11.

Onion rings are another example of the diffusion setting technique. Sodium alginate is mixed with flour, salt, water, and chopped onion. The mix is extruded as a ring into a calcium chloride setting bath for a few seconds. This short residence time is long enough for a coherent alginate film to be formed around the product to give it sufficient physical strength for the remainder of the production process. Rice noodles can also be produced on a large industrial scale by extruding the noodles into a calcium chloride setting bath. Sodium alginate then has the same function as the gluten in wheat noodles. Similarly, batters containing sodium alginate produce an edible coating around the product, which isolates oxygen and moisture, controls structure, and seals in the flavor.

Acid diffusion is used in many restructured fruit products. These products have been on the market for many years and have the advantage of giving properties to a fruit that it normally does not have. For example, restructured fruits can be formulated to be bake-stable or freeze/thaw-stable. Cherries can be produced by this method. An alginate solution containing sugar and a sequestrant is mixed with a cherry puree and deposited as drops of the required size into

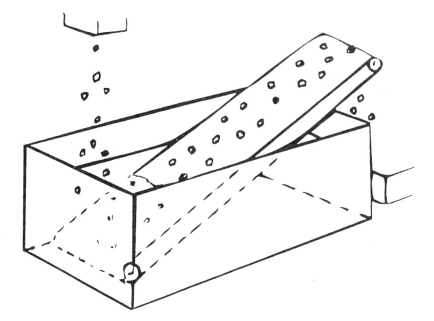

Fig. 11   Calcium chloride setting bath for alginate gel formation.

an acid setting bath. Calcium from the fruit mix will cause the gel to form. Red currants and black currants are essentially an outer skin surrounding a liquid center. These berries can also be restructured. An alginate solution is passed down the outside of two concentric tubes while a puree mix is pulsed down the center tube. As each pulse of puree falls away, it is coated with the alginate solution and drops into a setting bath of calcium lactate. Calcium from the bath and from the puree mix diffuse into the alginate skin, causing it to gel, while the center of the berry remains liquid.

Internal setting alginate gel systems require calcium to be released under controlled conditions from within the system. Generally fine particle size and low pH favor rapid calcium release, to the extent that phosphate sequestrants are used to control the reaction by competing with the alginate for calcium ions.

Internal setting is not restricted to thin layers and can be used to prepare bulk batches. Careful formulation can adjust the setting time from seconds to more than an hour. Chicken can be restructured from soy protein into an identifiable shape with uniform size for portion control. Similarly, clams can also be reformed from diced clams. Another example of internal setting is with potatoes. Processing methods vary, but the alginate system can be used to fit existing production facilities. The alginate system can be designed to give the required texture. For example, duchess potatoes should have the consistency of soft mash, while croquette needs a somewhat firmer texture. These differences are achieved when different levels of alginate, sequestrant, and calcium salt used. The process itself is simple. A dry mix of alginate, calcium salt, and seasoning is sprinkled onto the potato preparation and extruded as required. The potato raw material can be fresh mash, powder, or flake according to the prevailing economic conditions. Various product shapes can be made easily with good portion control, and novelty possibilities are limited only by the inventiveness of the product developer. These products have the advantage that they are freeze/thaw-stable, they retaini their structure on cooking, and they are easy to produce.

The diffusion and internal setting system may also be combined, as in the production of canned restructured meat chunks for pet food.

Alginate-pectin synergism is one of the very few interactions for alginate with other hydrocolloids and the only one of commercial value. High-methoxy pectins are only able to form gels at high sugar solids levels within a narrow pH range. When a sodium alginate is included, gel formation takes place at low solids, and below pH 3.8 the gel is reversible.

Recent knowledge about how to control the calcium reactivity of alginates by selecting the chemical composition may be utilized in a new range of desserts and dairy products, like cold flan, cold prepared instant puddings, and yogurt products.

VI. SUMMARY

We are still accumulating knowledge in the field of alginate food and dietary applications. Future demand for more effective utilization of the world food resources and enhanced food functionality will certainly trigger new developments in this area. Food technology process development will be targeted towards semi-continuous and continuous production and away from batch processing. This will favor alginate among the food functional hydrocolloids because alginate gel formation can take place at room temperatures and alginate gel technology is highly developed.

The market for ready-to-eat food has increased for many years and will no doubt continue to grow. This will create a general demand for hydrocolloids to control the functionality of such food products, especially for alginate technology due to its freeze-thaw and heat-stable characteristics. Alginate gel technology has also been developed for immobilization and encapsulation and other purposes in biotechnology. Many of the new developments in biotechnology can be utilized in food technology [e.g., yeast cells immobilized in alginate beads for beer and ethanol production as well as in the secondary fermentation of champagne (Onsøysen, 1990)].

REFERENCES

Anderson DM, Brydon WG, Eastwood MA, Sedgwick DM. Dietary effects of propylene glycol algiante in humans. Food Addit Contam 8(3):225–236, 1991a.

Anderson DM, Brydon WG, Eastwood MA, Sedgwick DM. Dietary effects of sodium alginates in humans. Food Addit Contam 8(3):237–248, 1991b.

Grant GT, Morris ER, Rees DA, Smith PJC, Thom D. Biological interactions between polysaccharides and divalent cations: the egg-box model. FEBS Lett 32:195, 1973.

Grasdalen H. High-field ^{1}H-NMR spectroscopy of alginate. Sequential structure and linkage confirmations. Carbohydrate Res. 118:255–260, 1983.

Harmuth-Hoene AE, Schelenz R. Effect of dietary fibre on mineral absorption in growing rats. J Nutr 110(9):1174–1784, 1980.

Korzun VN. Role of nutritive agents in the accumulation of cesium-137 and strontium-90 in the body. Vrachebnoe Delo 0(2):99–101, 1989.

Manchon P, Blanquat GD. Toxicological and nturitional evaluation of alginates 3. Nutritional and digestive aspects of alginate food intake. Aliments 6(4):495–507, 1986.

Onsøyen E. In: Voigt MN, Botta JR, eds. Advances in Fisheries Technology and Biotechnology for Increased Profitability. Lancaster, PA: Technomic Publishing Co., Inc., 1990, pp 265–286.

Onsøyen E. Alginates. In: Imeson A, ed. Thickening and Gelling Agents for Food. 2nd ed. London: Blackie Academic & Professional, 1997, pp. 22–44.

Pronova Biopolymer a.s. General information algiantes. 1995.

Pronova Biopolymer a.s. Pronova biopolymer report on the bioactivity of alginates. 1997.

Sandberg AS, Andersson H, Bosaeus I, Carlsson NG, Hasselblad K, Harrod M. Alginate, small bowel sterol excretion, and absorption of nutrients in ilestromy subjects. Am J Clin Nutr 60(5):751–756, 1994.

Terada A, Hara H, Mitsuoka T. Effect of dietary alginate on the faecal microbiota and faecal metabolic activity in humans. Microb Ecol Health Dis 8(6):259–266, 1995.

Toft K. Interactions between pectins and alginates. Prog Food Nutr Sci 6:89–96, 1982.

Toft K, Grasdalen H, Smidsrød O. Synergistic Gelation of Alginats and Pectins. In: Fishman ML, Jen JJ, eds. Chemistry and Function of Pectins. The American Chemical Society, 1986.

Tsuji E, Tsuji K, Suzuki S. Effect of polysaccharides on cholesterol metabolism, Part 6, Effects of various polysaccharides on serum and liver cholesterol levels in cholesterol fed rats. Annu Rep Natl Inst Nutr 24:83–91, 1975.

Tsuji K, Nakagawa Y, Ichikawa T. Effects of dietary potassium alginate on blood pressure, mineral balance, and serum cholesterol levels in spontaneously hypertensive rats. Nippon Kasei Gakkaishi 44(1):3–9, 1993.

Yamori Y, Nara Y, Tsubouchi T, Sogowa Y, Ikeda K, Horie R. Dietary prevention of stroke and its mechanisms in stroke-prone spontaneously hypertensive rats—preventive effect of dietary fibre and palmitoleic acid. J Hypertens Suppl 4(3):449–452, 1986.

34

Gum Arabic
Production, Safety and Physiological Effects, Physicochemical Characterization, Functional Properties, and Food Applications

P. A. Williams and G. O. Phillips
North East Wales Institute, Wrexham, Wales

I. INTRODUCTION

Gum arabic or gum acacia has been an important commercial product for thousands of years (1–3). It was used by the Egyptians in paints for hieroglyphic inscriptions and for the flaxen wrappings used to embalm mummies. It has also be found to be a constituent of the ink present on ancient Hebrew manuscripts. Eventually the gum found its way into Europe through various Arabian ports and acquired the name gum arabic after its place of origin or port of export.

The gum is the dried sticky exudation obtained from the stems and branches of certain Acacia trees, notably *Acacia senegal*, which grow principally in the semi-arid region in Africa referred to as the Sahelian belt. This area extends from the Sahara Desert in the north to the equator in the south and from Somalia in the east to Senegal in the west. As well as producing the gum, which is a valuable source of income for local farmers, the trees also protect and improve the soil, provide fodder for animals, and prevent desert encroachment (4). There are more than 1000 known species of Acacia, more than 700 of which are indigenous to Africa. A summary of their botanical classification is shown in Table 1 (5). *Acacia senegal* is classified in the Vulgares series and is believed to occur in four distinct varieties, with another 12 closely related species constituting the so-called *Acacia senegal* complex. The gum is produced by trees, 3–30 years old, and the biosynthesis process, referred to as gummosis, is most prevalent when the trees are subjected to stress conditions such as wounding, poor soil, lack of moisture, or hot temperature. The precise mechanism of gummosis is not clear, but it may occur in response to bacterial, viral, or fungal infection (6). Joseleau and Ullmann (7,8) reported that the gum was formed in a region between the tree's inner bark and the cambial zone and that gum formation may be accompanied by some wall restructuring in response to cell adaptation, as suggested by the strong hemicellulase and cellulase activities observed in tissues where the gum is produced.

Table 1 Botanical Classification of Acacia Trees

Australian species [subgenus Heterophyllum (Vassal)]
  Series *Phyllodineae Benth.*
  Series *Juliflorae Benth.*
  Series *Botryocephalae Benth.*
Indian, African, and American species
  Series *Gummiferae Benth.*—subgenus *Acacia Vassal.* (includes "*Acacia seyal*
    complex")
  Series *Vulgares Benth.*—subgenus *Aculeiferum Vassal.* (includes "*Acacia senegal*
    complex")

Source: Ref. 5.

II. PRODUCTION

Sudan has traditionally been the world's largest producer of gum arabic by far, but significant quantities also originate from Nigeria and Chad (5,9). In the Kordofan and Darfur regions in Sudan, the species grows uniformly in pure stands and occurs both wild and cultivated over a wide area. In other countries the distribution is not as uniform, and it is commonly found mixed with other species (4). Production levels have dropped from about 70,000 tons per annum in the late 1960s to less than 40,000 tons today (9). The decline has mainly been due to the fact that supplies and prices fluctuated significantly in the early 1970s and 1980s, which led many consumers to seek replacement materials. The Food and Agriculture Organization (FAO) recently commissioned a regional project to acquire information on all aspects of gum arabic production and quality control (10). Production levels reported are summarized in Table 2.

Gum production is promoted by "tapping," which involves making an incision in the bark of the trunk and branches with an axe, taking care not to damage the cambial zone. The sticky fluid that oozes from the wound dries in the sun to form glassy tears or nodules, commonly a few centimeters in diameter, which are collected 3–4 weeks after tapping (Fig. 1). The tears can range in color from pale yellow to amber to dark amber and brown. Collection is then continued every 10 days throughout the tapping season, which in Sudan usually runs from October to May. The gum is sorted according to color and size. The various types of Sudanese grades available are shown in Table 3. Following export to Europe and the United States some grades are processed before being sold. This may be by mechanical grinding, a technique known as kibbling, which breaks up the gum nodules into various specific sizes. Further processing such as spray-drying and roller-drying is also undertaken (11). This involves dissolution of the kibbled gum in water with heating and stirring. The temperature is kept to a minimum in order to avoid damaging the gum's functional characteristics (see below). The gum solution is then sieved,

Table 2 Summary of Gum Arabic
Production (tons/yr) in African Countries

Country	*Acacia senegal*	*Acacia seyal*
Sudan	17.1	3.9
Nigeria	6–10	
Chad	3.5	1.5
Other	2.7	

Source: Adapted from Ref. 10.

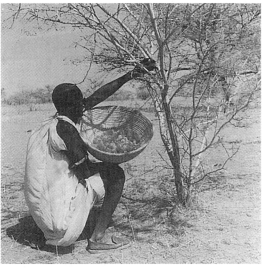

(a)

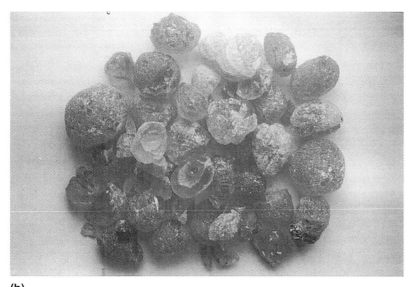

(b)

Fig. 1 (a) Collecting gum arabic from an Acacia tree; (b) nodules of gum.

decanted, or filtered to remove insoluble material and then pasteurized immediately prior to spray-drying or roller-drying. During spray-drying the solution is sprayed (atomized) into a stream of hot air, which quickly evaporates the water, and cyclones are used to separate the dry powder from the drying air. The particle size can be varied by changing the atomization conditions, and particle sizes may from 50 to 100 µm. During roller-drying, the solution is passed onto steam-heated rollers and the water is evaporated and removed by a flow of air. A knife is used to scrape the gum film continuously off the roll, and the thickness of the film is controlled by adjusting the gap between the rolls. This process produces flake-like particles,

Table 3 Various grades of Sudanese Gum

Grade	Description
Hand-picked selected	Cleanest, lightest colored, and largest pieces; most expensive
Cleaned and sifted	Material that remains after hand-picked selected and siftings are removed; comprises whole or broken lumps varying in color from pale to dark amber
Cleaned	The standard grade; varies from light to dark amber; contains siftings, but dust is removed
Siftings	Fine particles remaining following sorting of the choicer grades; contains some sand, dirt, and bark
Dust	Very fine particles collected after the cleaning process; contains sand and dirt
Red	Dark red particles

Source: Ref. 5.

which may be several hundred µm in size. Spray-dried and roller-dried gums have an advantage over kibbled and lump gum in that they are virtually free of microbial contamination and can be dissolved much more quickly.

III. SAFETY AND PHYSIOLOGICAL ASPECTS

The precise definition of gum arabic varies between the different regulatory bodies (2). The Journal Officiel of France, the Food Chemicals Codex (U.S. Academy of Sciences), and the U.S. Pharmacopoeia define it as the dried gummy exudate from stems and branches of *Acacia senegal* (L.) Willdenow or other related species (fam. Leguminosae). The European Pharmacopoeia refers to it as "*Acacia senegal* (L.) Willdenow and other species of African origin," and the U.S. Food and Drug Administration (FDA) defines it as "various species of the genus Acacia family Leguminosae." Thus, although commercial gum arabic is normally considered to consist mainly of gum from *Acacia senegal*, commonly referred to as "hashab" in Sudan, it often contains material from other species, notably *Acacia seyal* (also known as "talha"), which is also widely distributed in the gum belt. *Acacia seyal* gum is classified in the Gummiferae series (Table 1). The FAO Joint Expert Committee for Food Additives (JECFA) and the European Union (EU) have sought to achieve a more precise specification for commercial gum arabic (5). JECFA proposed that gum arabic for food use be confined to *Acacia senegal* and *Acacia seyal* only and that the phrase "closely related species" be removed from the definition. This was considered and accepted by the Codex Committee for Food Additives in 1999 (2). Identifying specifically these two species and marketing them separately, as recommended by the FAO regional project (9,10), could present industry with a serious quality control problem.

   In the United States gum arabic has been generally recognized as safe (GRAS) since 1974. In Europe the gum has been approved as E414 and classified as "acceptable daily intake (ADI) not specified" (i.e., no restriction on upper use levels was considered necessary) based on toxicological studies on commercial samples, including two long-term (2-year) studies and teratology/reproductive studies supported by biochemical data (12).

   Gum arabic is now classified as a soluble dietary fiber indigestible by humans and animals (13). Since the gum forms solutions of low viscosity, it has a very limited role in the upper gastrointestinal tract and affects the human physiology mainly by systemic effects following fermentation by anaerobic microorganisms in the large intestine. This process leads to formation of small chain fatty acids (SCFAs), which are known to be involved in many differing physiological effects. Butyrate and proprionate are produced at the expense of acetate. Phillips (14) reviewed the role of gum arabic as a nutritional fiber, its metabolism, and its caloric value. In the international standard work of Paul and Southgate (15) a caloric value of zero is assigned to gum arabic in fruit gums. However, degradation products are produced in the colon and are subsequently absorbed and metabolized. There are no usable data available for humans to serve as a basis for reproducible calculation of the utilizable energy of gum arabic. This is true for all other indigestible polysaccharides as well. The FDA current position is that only insoluble components of dietary fiber can be excluded from calculation of metabolic carbohydrate energy. Otherwise an allocation of 4 kcal/g is made unless there is specific evidence to prove otherwise. For gum arabic, values of between 0 and 4 kcal/g have been determined experimentally in animal experiments. However, the extreme differences in the anatomical and physiological characteristics of humans and test animals do not allow the transfer of the most rigorously determined results from animal studies to humans. Nevertheless, there is sufficient available information to accept a reduced caloric value for gum arabic compared to other carbohydrates for which a value of 4 kcal/g is mandatory in the United States. An upper level of 2 kcal/g for rats has been set after certain allowances were made for the energy losses from volatile fermented colonic products (16). The situation in humans is different, with greatly reduced amounts of such products and the need to adapt for periods of up to 28 days before gum arabic is attacked by the colonic bacteria. Logically, therefore, a value of significantly less than 2 kcal/g is applicable in humans.

Gum arabic has been reported to contribute to the maintenance of the mucosal wall and to produce a significant decrease in blood plasma cholesterol levels. In combination with apple fiber, gum arabic lowered total and low-density lipoprotein (LDL) cholesterol levels in men with mild hypercholesterolemia (17).

It has also been reported that gum increases the urea flux from blood to cecum and increases cecum nitrogen retention, thus reducing blood urea levels (13).

IV. PHYSICOCHEMICAL CHARACTERIZATION

Gum from *Acacia senegal* is composed of galactose, arabinose, rhamnose, glucuronic acid, and 4-O methoxyl glucuronic acid (5). The acid is normally in the mixed calcium, magnesium, and potassium salt form. The gum also contains a small proportion of protein, which is present as an integral part of the structure (18–20). A considerable body of literature now exists concerning the chemical composition of *Acacia senegal* gum from various geographical origins. Some typical analytical data for the gum obtained from various sources are given in Table 4 (21–25). The variations in sugar composition are commonly within the experimental error of the determination, however, more significant differences are often observed in the nitrogen content and molecular mass. Duvallet et al. (26), for example, reported intrinsic viscosity values ranging between 14 and 60 mL/g and nitrogen values between 0.12 and 0.57% for samples obtained from an experimental station in Senegal. Idris et al. (27) analyzed samples obtained from trees of varying age growing in both East and West Sudan where soil and climatic conditions vary. Intrinsic viscosity values ranged from 10.4 to 19.8 mL/g and nitrogen levels from 0.22 to 0.39%. The viscosity average molecular masses calculated from these latter intrinsic viscosity values indicate that the molecular mass for these particular Sudanese samples varied between 240,000 and 790,000, which was confirmed by light scattering measurements. It is interesting to note here that the latest EU specification for the gum indicates that the molecular mass is about 350,000.

Table 4 Comparative Analytical Data of *Acacia senegal* Gum from Various Sources

	Kenya	Sudan	Nigeria	Uganda
4-0-Methylglucuronic acid, %	n/a	1.5	1.5	1.0
Glucuronic acid, %	18	16	16.5	16
Galactose, %	39	44	47	48
Arabinose, %	28	25	23	22
Rhamnose, %	16	14	12	13
Ash, %	3.0	3.6	3.7	3.2
Nitrogen %	0.44	0.34	0.35	0.27
Specific rotation/degrees	-34	-30	-30	-32
Intrinsic viscosity, (dl/g)	21.9	16	18	15.0

Source: Refs. 21–25.

Anderson et al. (18) and Churms et al. (28) determined the structure of *Acacia senegal* gum by subjecting it to a series of Smith degradations involving sequential periodate oxidation and borohydride reduction. It was concluded that the gum has a highly branched structure and that the core consists of β-(1,3)-galactopyranose chains with ramified side chains linked through the 1,6 positions containing galactose, arabinose, rhamnose, and glucuronic acid. Proposed structural models (30,31) for *Acacia senegal* gum, consistent with their Smith degradation work and ^{13}C-NMR studies (29), are presented in Fig. 2. These models, however, do not take into account the proteinaceous component known to be an integral part of the structure. Akiyama et al. (32) found that the protein was covalently bound to the polysaccharide through hydroxyproline-oligoarabinoside and serine-carbohydrate linkages. These workers suggested that the gum was a kind of arabinogalactan-protein complex (AGP) because it interacted with Yariv reagent.

The gum is, in fact, a very heterogeneous material, which has been demonstrated by many techniques including fractional precipitation (20), ion exchange chromatography (IEC) (33), gel permeation chromatography (GPC) (34–38), and hydrophobic affinity chromatography (HAC) (37,38). Typical GPC elution curves are given in Fig. 3 for *Acacia senegal* (a) using UV absorption at 206nm and (b) and (c) using refractive index coupled with multiangle laser light scattering detection. Refractive index (RI) is a sensitive measure of the concentration of the gum eluting from the column, and the profile shows that the gum consists of two peaks. Light scattering indicates that the main peak, (peak A) corresponds to material with a molecular mass of ~250,000 and a radius of gyration (Rg) of ~10 nm. The smaller peak (peak B) corresponds to material with a molecular mass of 1,000,000–2,000,000 with an Rg of 20–30 nm. The Rg values are low for the molecular masses obtained, confirming that the molecules are highly branched (27). The UV elution curve is very different from that obtained by RI and shows three peaks, two corresponding to those noted by RI and a third (peak C) with a molecular mass of ~200,000. The reason for the different profiles is that UV absorption is sensitive to the chemical nature of the eluting species as well as their concentration. Following isolation of the individual fractions by semi-preparative GPC (34,37) and by HAC (38,39) it has been found that the proteinaceous moieties, which have a high molar absorptivity at the wavelength used, are not distributed evenly throughout the various molecular components present. The major fraction (peak A), which makes up about 90% of the total, contains very little protein. The second fraction (peak B), which accounts for ~10% of the total, contains about 10% protein. This fraction can be readily hydrolyzed by proteolytic enzyme yielding molecular species similar in size to the main component. It has been suggested, therefore, that this fraction has a "wattle blossom-type" structure in which large carbohydrate blocks (molecular mass ~250,000) are

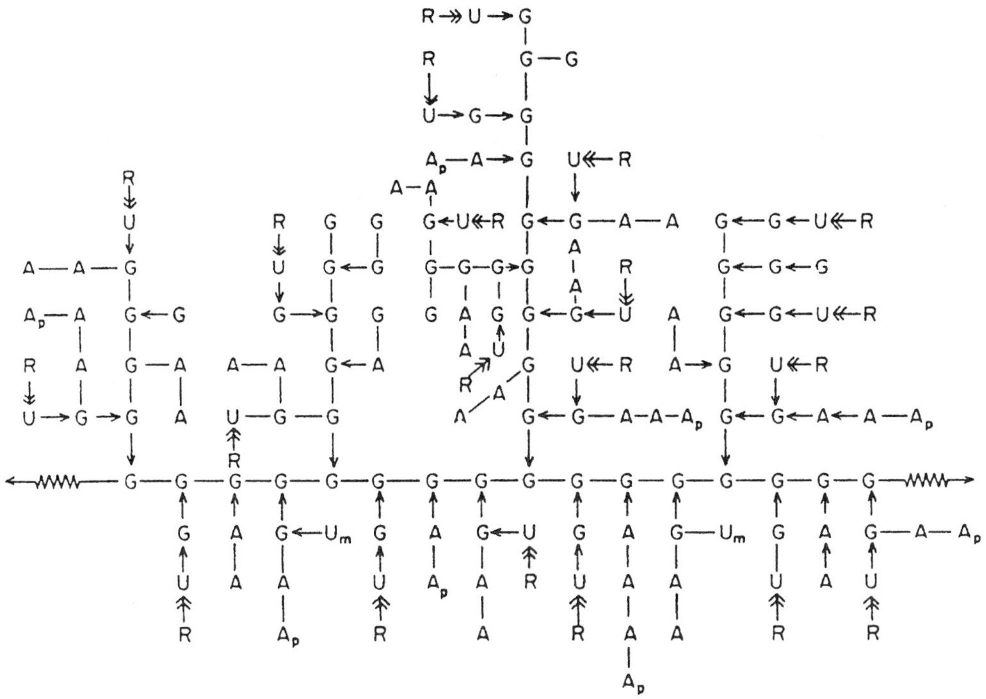

(a)

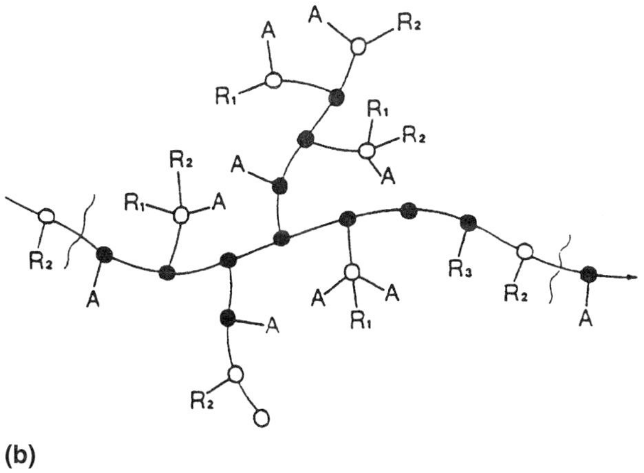

(b)

Fig. 2 (a) Illustration of a possible structural fragment of *Acacia senegal* gum. (From Ref. 31.) (b) Putative molecular structure for *Acacia senegal* gum. A = arabinosyl; O = 3-linked Gal*p* (Gal*p* attached); O = 6-linked Gal*p* (Gal*p* or GLc*p* attached), or end group; R_1 = Rha → 4GlcA (Rha occasionally absent or replaced by Me or by Ara*f*); R_2 = Gal → 3 Ara; R_3 = Ara → 3 Ara → 3 Ara. (From Ref. 30.)

linked to a common polypeptide chain (Fig. 4) (36–39). Such a structure has been suggested for AGPs generally (40). Qi et al. (41) reported that the polypetide chain consists of ~400 amino acid residues with a possible repeating sequence of [Hyp$_4$ Ser$_2$ Thr Pro Gly Leu His]. These workers, however, reported that the sugar units bound to the chain are in much smaller blocks (~30 residues) and that the structure resembles a "twisted hairy rope." The present

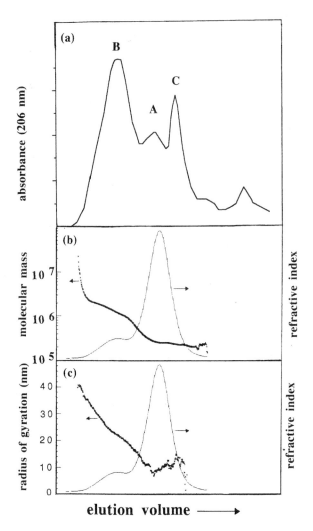

Fig. 3 Gel permeation chromatograms of *Acacia senegal* gum monitored by (a) UV absorbance at a wavelength of 206 nm, (b) and (c) refractive index and multiangle laser light scattering. GPC elution profiles (a) and (b) using refractive index and multiangle light scattering detection and (c) using UV absorption at 206 nm wavelength. (Adapted from Ref. 5.)

authors disagree with this model and have argued against it (38). The third fraction (peak C), which only represents about 1% of the total, contains between 20 and 50% protein. The amino acid composition of this third fraction differs considerably from the other two, with aspartic acid being most abundant (39). Furthermore, this fraction is not degraded by enzymes, suggesting that the protein component is within the core of the molecule and inaccessible to attack. Analysis of the fractions by NMR spectroscopy and methanolysis indicates that all fractions consist of a highly branched carbohydrate structure (42). Details of the proportions of the various sugars and their mode of linkage in each of the fractions are shown in Fig. 5 (42). All three fractions have been shown to interact with Yariv reagent and hence can be regarded as AGP complexes (38).

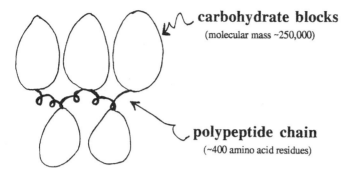

Fig. 4 Schematic representation of the "wattle blossom" structure of *Acacia senegal* gum. (Modified from Ref. 36.)

Analytical data for other important *Acacia* species are given in Table 5 (21–25) and show that, although they consist of the same sugar components, their proportions are significantly different from *Acacia senegal*. Typical amino acid compositions for various *Acacia* species, presented in Table 6 (21–25), show surprising similarities between the species, with hydroxyproline, serine, and proline being the most abundant.

The traditional means of differentiating between the various *Acacia* species has been by measurement of optical rotation often coupled with nitrogen determination. More sophisticated procedures based on, chemometric analysis (21–25), ^{13}C-NMR spectroscopy (43), and immuno-

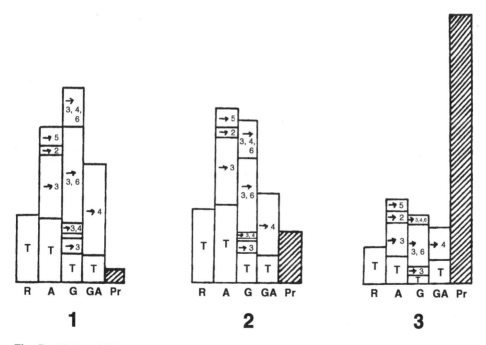

Fig. 5 Modes of linkage for the monosaccharides of fractions of *Acacia senegal* gum. T = terminal, 3 = 3-linked, etc. The unmarked modes for Gal are for fraction 1, reading up; 6, and 3,4; for fraction 2; 3,6 and 3,4; and for fraction 3; T,3 and 3,4,6.) (Adapted from Ref. 42.)

Table 5 Comparative Analytical Data of Important *Acacia* Species

	Vulgares series		Gummiferae series		
	A. senegal	*A. laeta*	*A. compylacantha*	*A. drepanolobium*	*A. seyal*
4-0-methylglucuronic acid, %	1.5	3.5	2	2.5	5.5
Glucuronic acid, %	14.5	10.5	7	6.5	6.5
Galactose, %	44	44	54	38	38
Arabinose, %	27	29	29	52	46
Rhamnose, %	13	13	8	1	4
Ash, %	3.93	3.30	2.92	2.52	2.87
Nitrogen, %	0.29	0.65	0.37	1.11	0.14
Specific rotation/degrees	−30	−42	−12	+78	+51
Molecular mass, MW × 10^3	384	725	312	950	850

Source: Refs. 21–25.

Table 6 Amino Acid Composition (residues/1000 residues) of Some *Acacia* Gums

	Vulgares series		Gummiferae series	
	Acacia senegal	*Acacia goetzii*	*Acacia gerrardii*	*Acacia seyal*
Asp	91	91	72	65
Hyp	256	215	320	240
Thr	72	62	55	62
Ser	144	121	80	170
Glu	36	56	49	38
Pro	64	64	58	73
Gly	53	41	59	51
Ala	28	56	42	38
Cys	3			
Val	35	88	60	42
Met	2		3	
Ile	11	15	36	16
Leu	70	59	52	85
Tyr	13	26	30	13
Phe	30	35	18	24
His	52	33	25	51
Lys	27	31	23	18
Arg	15	5	12	11
%N	0.365	0.89	1.86	0.147

Source: Refs. 21–25.

assays (44,45) are currently being investigated. An enzyme-linked immunosorbent assay based on monoclonal antibodies is currently under development which can detect the presence of *Acacia seyal* and *combretum* species in mixtures with gum from *Acacia senegal* at levels of less than 0.5% (46).

V. FUNCTIONAL PROPERTIES

Gum arabic has two principal properties: it readily dissolves in water to form highly concentrated solutions of relatively low viscosity and it is surface active and hence is able to effectively stabilize oil-in-water emulsions.

A. Solution Properties

Spray-dried and roller-dried samples are obtained in the form of white powders of small particle size, and hence they dissolve almost instantaneously in water. Kibbled and lump gum, however, may take up to 30 minutes and 6 hours, respectively, to dissolve completely (11). Gum arabic solutions can be prepared to a high concentration (~50%) with a relatively low viscosity (Fig. 6), which is a consequence of the gum's highly branched very compact structure (47). The viscosity only becomes significant when the concentration approaches the so-called semi-dilute regime where the molecules begin to overlap due to molecular crowding (48). A comparison of the viscosity-shear rate profiles of gum arabic, xanthan gum, and carboxymethyl cellulose (CMC) is given in Fig. 7. The viscosity of 30% solutions of the gum is seen to be less than for 1% solutions of xanthan and CMC at low shear rates, and furthermore the viscosity is not shear rate dependent. Again the highly branched compact structure of the gum reduces the possibility of intermolecular entanglements, which give rise to the shear thinning characteristics observed for solutions of xanthan gum and CMC, which have linear structures. The viscosity of the gum

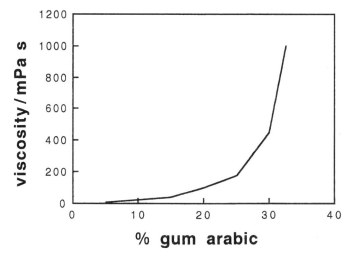

Fig. 6 Viscosity of gum arabic solutions at a shear rate of $100 \, \text{s}^{-1}$ as a function of concentration. (Adapted from Refs. 47 and 49.)

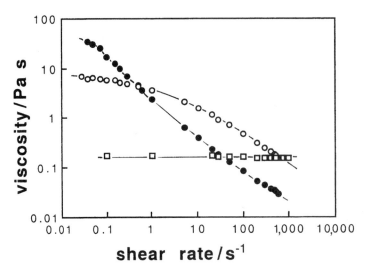

Fig. 7 Comparison of the viscosity of a 30% solution of *Acacia senegal* gum (□) and 1% solutions of sodium carboxymethylcellulose (○) and xanthan gum (●) as a function of shear rate.

decreases at low and high pH and in the presence of electrolyte (Fig. 8) (47,49). Since the molecules are highly branched it is unlikely that the viscosity decrease is due to molecular chain contraction as is commonly believed to be the case for linear polyelectrolytes under similar conditions. The reduction is probably a consequence of a decrease in the effective size of the molecules due to the compression of their electrical double layer analagous to the situation for globular proteins (50).

The viscosity of gum arabic solutions shows an irreversible decrease after heating due to denaturation and precipitation of the high molecular mass protein-rich component (51–54). On heating a 19% solution of the gum under reflux at 102°C, Williams et al. found that the viscosity measured at a shear rate of 50 s^{-1} decreased from 58 mPa·s initially to 25 mPa·s after 6.5 hours (47).

B. Emulsification Properties

Gum arabic is widely used in the food Industry as an emulsifier, but it is only recently that its mechanism of action has been effectively understood. It has been demonstrated that gum arabic is able to form thick viscoelastic films at the oil–water interface and that the surface rheological properties and emulsion stability depend on the protein content and molecular mass of the gum (55–57). Randall et al. (37) found that for 20% orange oil emulsions the minimum droplet size could only be obtained at gum arabic concentrations of >12%. (Fig. 9). Comparison of the molecular mass distribution of the initial gum solution and of the gum in the emulsion continuous phase after emulsification indicates that the high molecular mass protein-rich component adsorbs predominantly at the oil/water interface and is, therefore, responsible for the gum's emulsification properties. It has been suggested that the hydrophobic polypeptide chains adsorb onto the surface of the oil droplets while the hydrophilic carbohydrate blocks attached to the chain protrude out into solution providing a strong steric barrier preventing droplet aggregation and co-

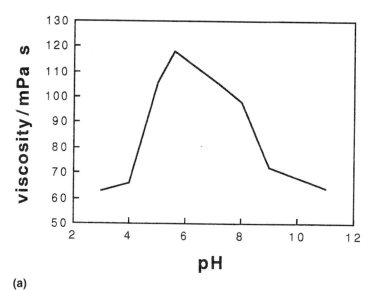

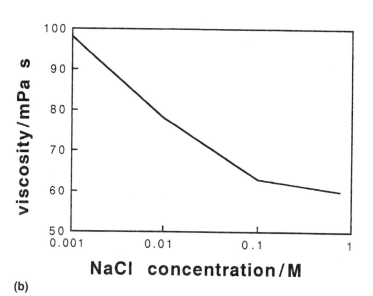

Fig. 8 Viscosity of 20% gum arabic solutions at a shear rate of 100^{s-1} (a) as a function of pH and (b) as a function of sodium chloride addition. (Adapted from Refs. 47 and 49.)

alescence (37). A schematic representation is given in Fig. 10. The bulk of the gum, which is protein deficient, has little tendency to adsorb and has little role to play in the emulsification process.

As discussed above, heating the gum at high temperatures for prolonged periods (e.g., 100°C for 6 hours) results in denaturation and precipitation of the proteinaceous gum fractions and leads to a drastic reduction in the emulsification efficiency (52–54). This is illustrated in Fig. 11, which shows that the droplet size for 20% orange oil emulsions increases when the

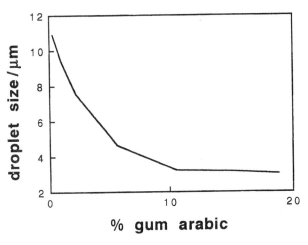

Fig. 9 Emulsion droplet size as a function of gum arabic concentration. (Adapted from Refs. 47 and 49.)

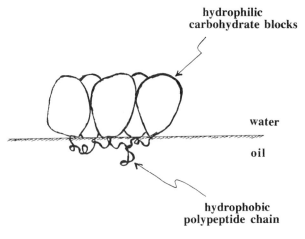

Fig. 10 Schematic representation of the high molecular mass, protein-rich fraction of *Acacia senegal* gum adsorbing at the oil–water interface. (Modified from Ref. 37.)

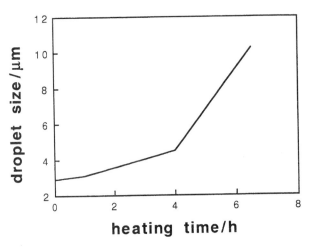

Fig. 11 Emulsion droplet size for 20% orange oil emulsions prepared with gum arabic that has been heated at 102°C for varying periods of time. (Modified from Ref. 49.)

emulsions are prepared with gum arabic that has been subjected to heat treatment (under reflux at 102°C) for increasing periods of time. Less severe heat treatment (e.g., 65°C for 24 hours) has only a minor effect.

VI. FOOD APPLICATIONS

A. Confectionery

About 80% of all gum arabic produced is used in the food Industry—about half of this in confectionery products (1,3). Since a gum arabic shortage in the early 1970s resulting in high prices, many companies have been developing alternative formulations involving other hydrocolloids such as starches, pectins, etc. for partial or total replacement of the gum (58).

The traditional hard chewy wine gums are prepared using gum arabic alone at concentrations between 40 and 55% of the total solids. The process involves dissolving the gum in water, and temperatures are kept as low as possible (~60°C) in order to avoid cloudiness. The gum solution is then added to a preboiled batch of sugar and glucose at ~70% solids, followed by coloring and flavoring. The mixture is allowed to stand in a hot room to let air bubbles rise to the surface, and any scum formed is removed. The liquid at about 60°C is deposited into starch trays, which are transferred to stoving rooms with adequate air circulation. The stoving time can be 4–6 days. The gums are then removed from the starch molds, brushed to remove starch, and then glazed with oil or wax.

Softer gums or pastilles can be obtained by reducing the stoving time to 2–3 days, by using lower gum concentrations, or by using gum arabic in combination with one or more other hydrocolloids such as starch, gelatin, pectin, and agar, which have the ability to form gels. In these mixed hydrocolloid systems there is a tendency for phase separation to occur due to the intrinsic thermodynamic incompatibility of the hydrocolloids (59). In the absence of gelation the mixtures will separate over time into two (or more) liquid layers, each enriched in one of the polymers. Phase separation competes with gelation, and the relative rates of the two processes, which will depend on many factors such as the nature of the polymers, their concentration, the presence of solutes, and the temperature, will give rise to varying gel structures and textural characteristics.

Gum arabic is also used as a fat emulsifier in caramels and toffees, as a film former for coatings for chocolates and nuts, and as a whipping agent in aerated confections such as marshmallows.

B. Beverages

Gum arabic is widely used to prepare concentrated flavor oil emulsions for use in cola and citrus-based soft drinks (3). The gum is required to inhibit droplet flocculation and coalescence not only in the concentrated emulsion but also after dilution (up to 100-fold or more) with carbonated water containing sugar prior to bottling (56). Emulsions are prepared by the controlled addition of the oil to an aqueous solution of the gum followed by high-speed mixing and homogenization. Resins are often added to the oil to act as weighting agents (60). Examples include the glycerol ester of rosin and damar gum. Such substances are employed to adjust the density of the oil phase close to that of water and hence inhibit the emulsion droplets from creaming. A typical beverage emulsion would contain 5–20% gum arabic, 4–8% flavor oil, and 4–8% weighting agent. As noted earlier the high concentration of gum is required in order to ensure complete coverage of the surface of the individual emulsion droplets.

C. Flavor Encapsulation

Gum arabic finds extensive use as an encapsulating agent for flavors that are incorporated into dry foods such as soups, dessert mixes, and beverages (3). Emulsions are prepared as described above and are then spray-dried. The gum forms a coating around the flavor particles and inhibits oxidation and evaporation of volatile material. Traditionally gum arabic was used alone, but in order to reduce costs it is now often used in conjunction with maltodextrin. Typical formulations for flavor encapsulation using gum arabic alone and in combination with maltodextrin are as follows:

Flavor	7%	10%
Gum arabic	28%	15%
Maltodextrin	NIL	25%

D. Bakery Products

Gum arabic is often used to provide glossy coatings and to seal baked goods and cereals. It is applied as a concentrated solution (30–50%) by spraying or brushing prior to baking (3).

ACKNOWLEDGMENTS

The authors are indebted to the many researchers at the North East Wales Institute whose efforts have yielded a far greater understanding of the structural characteristics and functional properties of gum arabic.

REFERENCES

1. RL Whistler. Exudate gums. In: RL Whistler, ed. Industrial Gums. 3rd ed. Academic Press, London, 1993.
2. PA Williams, GO Phillips. In: GO Phillips & PA Williams, eds. Handbook of Hydrocolloids. Cambridge: Woodhead Publishing Ltd, 2000, pp 155–168.
3. A Imeson. Exudate gums. In: A Imeson, ed. Thickening and Gelling Agents for Foods. Glasgow: Blackie Academic and Professional, 1992, pp 66–97.
4. EI Hag Makki Awouda. Outlook for gum arabic production and supply. In: GO Phillips, DJ Wedlock, PA Williams, eds. Gums and Stabilisers for the Food Industry 4. Oxford: IRL Press, 1988, pp 425–434.
5. AM Islam, GO Phillips A Sljivo, MJ Snowden, and PA Williams. A review of recent developments on the regulatory, structural and functional aspects of gum arabic. Food Hydrocoll 11:493, 1997.
6. J Vassal. Gum bearing acacias and gummosis. In: Gums and Hydrosoluble Natural Vegetal Colloids. Marseilles: ranex S.A. Publishers, 1976.
7. JP Joseleau, G Ullmann. Relation between starch metabolism and the synthesis of gum arabic. Bull Int Group Study Mimosideae 13:46, 1985.
8. JP Joseleau, G Ullmann. Biochemical evidence for the site of formation of gum arabic in *Acacia senegal*. Phytochemistry 29:3401, 1990.

9.   E Casadei. FAO Regional Project on gum arabic specifications and quality control. In: PA Williams, GO Phillips, eds. Gums and Stabilisers for the Food Industry 9. Cambridge: Royal Society of Chemistry Publishers, 1998, pp 69–75.

10. BN Chikamai. A Review of Production, Markets and Quality Control of Gum Arabic in Africa. Rome: FAO, 1996.

11. GR Williams. The processing of gum arabic. In: GO Phillips, DJ Wedlock, PA Williams, eds. Gums and Stabilisers for the Food Industry 5. Oxford: IRL Press, 1990, pp 37–40.

12. DMW Anderson, MA Eastwood. The safety of gum arabic as a food additive and its energy value as an ingredient: a brief review. J Human Nutr Diet 2:137, 1989.

13. TP Kravtchenko. The use of gum arabic as a source of soluble dietary fibre. In: PA Williams, GO Phillips, eds. Gums and Stabilisers for the Food Industry 9. Cambridge: Royal Society of Chemistry Publishers, 1998, pp 413–420.

14. GO Phillips. Acacia gum (gum arabic): a nutritional fibre; metabolism and calorific value. Food Add Contam 15:251, 1998.

15. AA Paul, DA Southgate. The Composition of Foods. 4th ed. Amsterdam: Elsevier, 1978.

16. G Livesey. The energy values of dietary fibre and sugar alcohols for man Nutr Res Revs 5:61, 1992.

17. KA Mee. Apple fiber and gum arabic lowers total and low density lipoprotein cholesterol levels in men with mild hypercholesterolemia. J Am Diet Assoc 97:422, 1997.

18. DMW Anderson, EL Hirst, JL Stoddart. Studies on uronic acid materials XV11. Some structural features of *Acacia senegal* gum. J Chem Soc C 1959, 1966.

19. DMW Anderson, JF Stoddart. Studies on uronic acid materials Part XV. The use of molecular sieve chromatography in studies on *Acacia senegal* gum (gum arabic). Carbohydr Res 2:104, 1966.

20. DMW Anderson, EL Hirst, S Rahman, G Stainsby. Studies on uronic acid materials Part XVIII. Light scattering studies on some molecular weight fractions from *Acacia senegal* gum. Carbohydr Res 3:308, 1967.

21. BN Chikamai, WB Banks. Analysis of Kenyan *A. senegal* gum. Food Hydrocoll 7:521, 1993.

22. DMW Anderson, and W Weiping. Gum arabic from Uganda. Food Hydrocoll 5:297, 1991.

23. P Jurasek, M Kosik, GO Phillips. A chemometric study of the Acacia (gum arabic) and related natural gums. Food Hydrocoll 7:73, 1993.

24. P Jurasek, M Kosik, GO Phillips. The classification of natural gums. Part II. Characterisation of the gum arabic of commerce based on a chemometric study of amino acid compositions. Food Hydrocoll 7:157, 1993.

25. P Jurasek, M Kosik, GO Phillips. The classification of natural gums. III Acacia senegal and related species (gum arabic). Food Hydrocoll 7:255, 1993.

26. S Duvallet, JC Fenyo, MC Vandevelde, The characterisation of gum arabic from an experimental field of Ferlo (North Senegal). Food Hydrocoll 7:319, 1993.

27. OHM Idris, PA Williams, GO Phillips. Physicochemical characterisation of *Acacia senegal* gum from trees of different age and location using multidetection gel permeation chromatography. Food Hydrocoll 12:379, 1998.

28. SC Churms, EH Merrifield, AM Stephen. Some new aspects of the molecular structure of *Acacia senegal* gum (gum arabic). Carbohydr Res 123:267, 1983.

29. J Defaye, E Wong. Structural studies of gum arabic, the exudate polysaccharide from *Acacia senegal*. Carbohydr Res 150:221, 1986.

30. AM Stephen, SC Churms. Gums and mucilages. In: AM Stephen, ed. Food Polysaccharides and Their Applications. New York: Marcel Dekker, 1995, p 377.

31. CA Street, DMW Anderson. Refinement of structures previously proposed for gum arabic and other Acacia gum exudates. Talanta 30:887, 1983.

32. Y Akiyama, S Eda, and K Kato. Gum arabic is a kind of arabinogalactan protein. Agric Biol Chem 48:235, 1984.

33. ME Osman, AR Menzies, B Albo Martin, PA Williams, GO Phillips, TC Baldwin. Characterisation of *Acacia senegal* fractions obtained by anion exchange chromatography using DEAE cellulose. Phytochemistry 38:409, 1995.

34. MC Vandevelde, JC Fenyo. Macromolecular distribution of *Acacia senegal* (gum arabic) by size exclusion chromatography. Carbohydr Polym 5:251, 1985.

35. S Connolly, JC Fenyo, MC Vandevelde. Heterogeneity and homogeneity of an arabinogalactan protein: *Acacia senegal* gum. Food Hydrocoll 1:477, 1987.

36. S Connolly, JC Fenyo, MC Vandevelde. Effect of a proteinase on the macromolecular distribution of *Acacia senegal* gum. Carbohydr Polym 8:23, 1988.

37. RC Randall, GO Phillips, PA Williams. The role of the proteinaceous component on the emulsification properties of gum arabic. Food Hydrocoll 9:123, 1988.

38. ME Osman, PA Williams, AR Menzies, GO Phillips, TC Baldwin. The molecular characterisation of the polysaccharide gum from *Acacia senegal*. Carbohydr Res 246:303, 1993.

39. RC Randall, GO Phillips, PA Williams. Fractionation and characterisation of gum from *Acacia senegal*. Food Hydrocoll 3:65, 1989.

40. GB Fincher, BA Stone, AE Clarke. Arabinogalactan—proteins; structure, biosynthesis and function. Ann Rev Plant Physiol 34:47, 1983.

41. W Qi, C Fong, DTA Lamport. Gum arabic glycoprotein is a twisted hairy rope. Plant Physiol 96: 848, 1991.

42. PA Williams, GO Phillips, AM Stephen. Spectroscopic and molecular comparisons of three fractions for *Acacia senegal* gum. Food Hydrocoll 4:305, 1990.

43. DMW Anderson, JRA Millar, W Weiping. Gum arabic (*Acacia senegal*): unambiguous identification by ^{13}C NMR spectroscopy as an adjunct to the revised JECFA specifications and application of ^{13}C NMR spectra for regulatory/legislative purposes. Food Add Contam 8:405, 1991.

44. PA Williams, AR Menzies, GO Phillips, CJ Smith. Specific identification and assessment of emulsification properties of gum arabic by ELISA. In: MRA Morgan, CJ Smith, PA Williams, eds. Food Safety and Quality Assessment: Application of Immunoassay Systems. London: Elsevier Applied Science Publishers, 1992, pp 385–392.

45. ME Osman, PA Williams, AR Menzies, GO Phillips. Characterisation of commercial samples of gum arabic. J Agric Food Chem 4:71, 1993.

46. MI Thurston, GA Bonwick, PA Williams, JHH Williams, QCB Cronk, FM Dewey. Detection of gum from *Acacia seyal* and species of combretum in admixtures with *A. senegal* using monoclonal antibodies. J Food Agric Immunol 10:237–247, 1998.

47. PA Williams, GO Phillips, RC Randall. Structure-function relationships of gum arabic. In: GO Phillips, DJ Wedlock, PA Williams, eds. Gums and Stabilisers for the Food Industry 5. Oxford: Oxford University Press 1990, pp 25–36.

48. FM Goycoolea, ER Morris, RK Richardson, AE Bell. Solution rheology of mesquite gum in comparison with gum arabic. Carbohydr Polym 27:37, 1995.

49. RC Randall. Molecular characterisation and functional properties of gum arabic. Ph.D. thesis, University of Salford, 1992.

50. C Rha, P Pradipasena. Viscosity of proteins. In: JR Mitchell, DA Ledward, eds. Functional Properties of Food Macromolecules. London: Elsevier Applied Science Publishers, 1985.

51. JC Fenyo, MC Vandevelde. Physicochemical properties in relation to structure. In: GO Phillips, DJ Wedlock, PA Williams, eds Gums and Stabilisers for the Food Industry 5. Oxford: Oxford University Press, 1990, pp 17–23.

52. RC Randall, GO Phillips, PA Williams. Effect of heat on the emulsifying properties of gum arabic. In: E Dickinson. Food Colloids. Cambridge: Royal Society of Chemistry, 1990, pp 386–390.

53. MJ Snowden, GO Phillips, PA Williams. Adsorption and stabilising properties of gum arabic samples of different origin. In: GO Phillips, DJ Wedlock, PA Williams, eds. Gums and Stabilisers for the Food Industry 4. Oxford: IRL Press, 1988, pp 489–496.

54. BN Chikamai, WB Banks, DMW Anderson, W Weiping. Processing of gum arabic and some new opportunities. Food Hydrocoll 10:309, 1996.

55. E Dickinson, BS Murray, G Stainsby, DMW Anderson. Surface activity and emulsification behaviour of some Acacia gums. Food Hydrocoll 2:477, 1988.

56. E Dickinson, DJ Elverson, BS Murray. On the film forming and emulsion stabilising properties of gum arabic: dilution and flocculation aspects. Food Hydrocoll 3:101, 1989.

57. E Dickinson, VB Galazka, DMW Anderson. Emulsifying behaviour of gum arabic. Part 2. Effect of the gum molecular weight on the emulsion droplet size distribution. Carbohydr Polym 14:385, 1991.

58. P Lawson, M Gonze, F Van Der Schueren, K Rosenplanter. Gum arabic replacement in confectionery applications. In: PA Williams, GO Phillips, eds. Gums and Stabilisers for the Food Industry 9. Cambridge: Royal Society of Chemistry Publishers, 1998, pp 76–83.

59. AS Whitehouse, P Ashby, R Abeysekera, AW Robards. Phase behaviour of biopolymers at high solids content. In: GO Phillips, PA Williams, DJ Wedlock, eds. Gums and Stabilisers for the Food Industry 8. Oxford: IRL Press Publishers, 1996, pp 287–295.

60. F Thevenet. Acacia gums. Stabilizers for flavor encapsulation. A.C.S. Symposium Series 370:37, 1988.

35
Gellan Gum

Raymond C. Valli and Frank J. Miskiel
CP Kelco, San Diego, California

I. INTRODUCTION

Fermentation has long been used in the production of foods. In products such as cheese, yogurt, and beer, bacterial fermentation plays an important role in developing both flavor and texture. In more recent years, bacteria has played an important role in the production of food polysaccharides. Polysaccharides are commonly used as stabilizers, texturizers, and gel formers. Dextran, xanthan gum, and gellan gum are all polysaccharides produced commercially by bacterial fermentation. Other food polysaccharides, such as those derived from seaweed, seeds, and plant exudates, are often subject to the uncertainty of nature or the political instability of the producing countries. Quality, price, and continued availability are major concerns for users of these gums. Producing polysaccharides by fermentation is advantageous because fermentation can produce gums on demand and with consistent quality.

CP Kelco pioneered the commercial development of bacterial polysaccharides. After their success with xanthan gum in the 1970s, Kelco undertook an extensive research program isolating more than 900 gum-forming bacteria from all over the world. In 1978, *Sphingomonas elodea* (ATCC 31461, formally called *Pseudomonas elodea*) was found growing on a lily pond in Pennsylvania. The bacteria produced the extracellular polysaccharide gellan gum.

II. MANUFACTURING PROCESS

Gellan gum is produced commercially by inoculating *S. elodea* into a specially formulated fermentation media. The media contains a carbon source such as glucose, organic and inorganic nitrogen sources, and a number of inorganic salts. The fermentation proceeds under sterile conditions with strict controls over agitation, temperature, and pH. When the fermentation is complete, the viscous broth is pasteurized to kill all viable cells prior to recovering the gum.

The broth can be recovered in different ways to produce two different types of gellan gum (Fig. 1). If the gum is recovered directly from the broth using alcohol precipitation, it will retain its native, high-acyl chemical structure. Solutions of high-acyl gellan gum are viscous, and the gels exhibit a cohesive and elastic nature. Alternatively, the gum can be treated with alkali to remove acyl constituents, creating a deacylated structure. Deacylated gellan gum exhibits comparatively low solution viscosities, while the gels are quite firm and brittle. The deacyla-

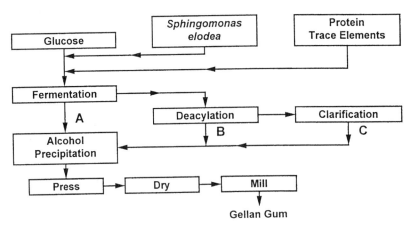

Fig. 1   Gellan gum manufacturing process. Gellan gums produced include (A) high-acyl unclarified product (KELCOGEL LT 100), (B) low-acyl unclarified product (KELCOGEL LT), and (C) low-acyl clarified product (KELCOGEL, KELCOGEL F, GELRITE).

tion can be controlled, yielding intermediate acyl levels, but such gums are not currently commercially available.

Optionally, the deacylated gellan gum can be clarified to remove cellular debris before the alcohol precipitation. KELCOGEL, a food grade gellan gum, and GELRITE, a microbiological media gellan gum, are both deacylated and clarified. KELCOGEL LT is nonclarified, deacylated gellan gum, while KELCOGEL LT100 is a high acyl, native gellan gum.

III. COMPOSITION

Gellan gum is a linear polysaccharide with a tetrasaccharide repeat unit of glucose, glucuronic acid, and rhamnose in the molar ratio of 2:1:1 (Fig. 2) (1,2). In its native form, there are approximately 1.5 O-acyl groups per repeating unit. The O-acyl groups have been identified as O-acetyl and O-L-glycerate. Both substituents are attached to the 3-linked glucose at the 6 and 2 positions, respectively. There is one acetate per every two repeat units, while the glycerate appears on every repeat unit (3).

In the deesterified form of gellan gum, the acyl groups are stripped off, resulting in a simple linear chain. Light scattering and intrinsic viscosity give a molecular mass of approximately 0.5×10^6 daltons for the deacylated form of gellan gum (4).

Side chains play an important role in defining the properties of gellan gum. For example, both rhamsan and welan gum, polysaccharides produced by different species of *Sphingomonas*, share the same backbone as gellan but have different mono- and disaccharide side chains and share no similarity to native gellan gum in solution behavior (5). The presence of the acyl groups in gellan gum also differentiates its properties from the deacylated forms of the gum.

Molecular modeling studies examined the effect of acyl substituents on the conformational properties of gellan gum. The relative extension of the polymer chains, as measured by the characteristic ratio, was determined for native and deacylated forms of gellan gum using Rotational Isomeric State–Metropolis Monte Carlo calculations (16). The native gellan gum goes from a more extended molecule to a much more coiled molecule than deacylated gellan gum as the strength of hydrogen bonding increases (Fig. 3). The tendency of the gellan molecules

(a)

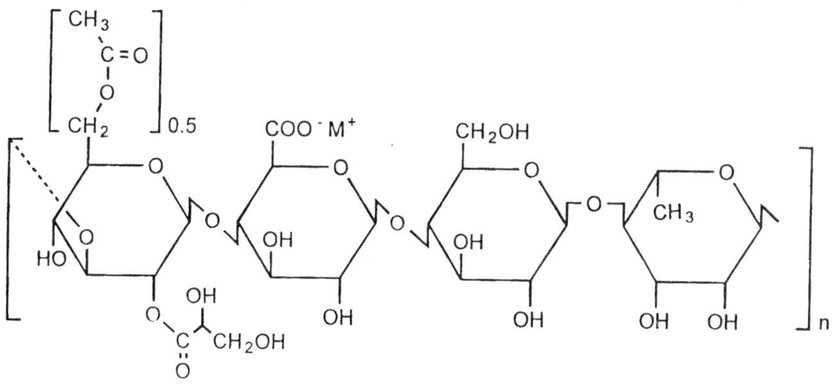

(b)

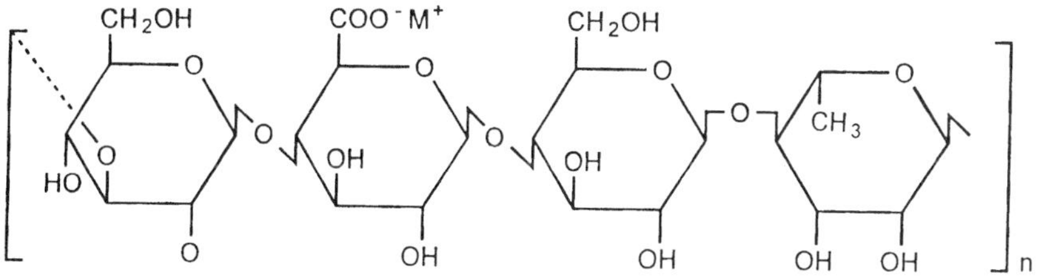

→3)–β–D–Glcp–(1→4)–β–D–GlcpA–(1→4)–β–D–Glcp–(1→4)–α–L–Rhap–(1→

Fig. 2 Primary structure of gellan gums: (a) native or high-acyl gellan gum; (b) low-acyl gellan gum (Kelcogel, Gelrite).

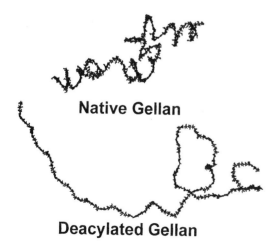

Native Gellan

Deacylated Gellan

Fig. 3 Relative extension of native and deacylated gellan gum chains determined by computational molecular modeling.

to coil is due to a shift in the conformational space available to rotations about the α-L-Rha$p$-(1 → 3)-β-D-Glc$p$ backbone linkage. The modeling results provide an explanation for the different physical properties of the different forms of gellan gum.

The structural properties of gellan gum have been extensively investigated. X-ray diffraction studies of deacylated gellan fibers showed that the ordered form adopts a left-hand, three-fold, double-helical strand organized in a parallel fashion in an intertwined duplex (Fig. 4) (7). The pair of molecules that constitutes the helix is stabilized by hydrogen bonds at the carboxylate group. In the potassium salt form, the potassium ion is coordinated to the carboxylate group,

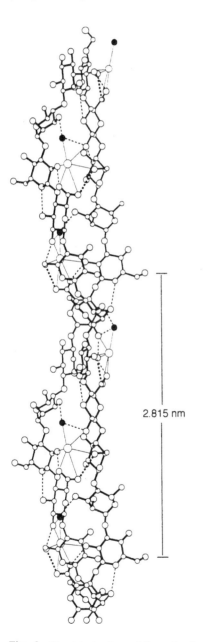

2.815 nm

Fig. 4 Crystal structure of the potassium salt of deacylated gellan gum (From Ref. 8.)

which is then involved in interchain hydrogen bonding. The potassium ions are located on the outside of the helix so that, besides stabilizing the helix formation, they also allow the helices to aggregate. This aggregation results in the formation of a gel. In the calcium salt form, the model is similar, but calcium replaces two potassium ions and one molecule of water (8). The side chains of native gellan gum do not interfere with helix formation, but the glycerate groups interfere with the helix aggregation, resulting in a softer, elastic gel rather than the firm, hard texture associated with deacylated gellan gum.

Commercially available forms of gellan gum are mixed salts containing sodium, potassium, calcium, and magnesium, although both commercial forms are predominantly potassium salts. Unclarified forms of gellan gum will contain residual cellular debris including proteins and cell wall materials.

IV. PHYSIOCHEMICAL PROPERTIES

The physical properties of gellan gum are strongly influenced by the presence and level of acyl group side chains. In theory, gellan gum can elicit a wide range of physical properties based on the acyl content and on the ratio of acetate to glycerate side chains. However, only the fully acylated native gum and fully deacylated gum are currently commercially available, so the properties of gellan gum are conveniently covered by an examination of fully acylated and fully deacylated versions of gellan gum.

A. Properties of Deacylated Gellan Gum

1. Hydration

A pure sodium salt of deacylated gellan gum will dissolve in deionized water at room temperature. The presence of divalent salts in the commercially available forms of deacylated gellan gum inhibit the gum's hydration. In cold deionized water, commercial gellan gum will only partially hydrate. Hydration is further inhibited by divalent ions that are present in most water supplies. Suppression of hydration is often useful to attain a good gum dispersion and eliminate lumping that can occur with more readily soluble hydrocolloids. In soft water, standard gum dispersion techniques such as dry blending with other ingredients and using good agitation can improve the dispersion.

Monovalent ions also suppress hydration, but to a much smaller degree than divalent ions. While calcium levels of 180 ppm are sufficient to inhibit gellan hydration even on boiling, the gum hydrates in a 1% solution of sodium ions at approximately 90°C. In simple food systems, monovalent ions are not usually high enough to inhibit hydration. The effects of dissolved ions on hydration temperature is shown in Table 1.

To attain complete hydration, the gellan gum dispersion in water should be heated. In deionized water, hydration occurs around 70°C, but higher calcium levels will require higher temperatures for full hydration. Just as added calcium drives the hydration temperature higher, removal of calcium through the use of sequestrants lowers the hydration temperature. Sequestrants, such as sodium citrate, potassium citrate, and phosphates, bind calcium in a competitive equilibrium with gellan gum. Sequestrants are able to remove calcium from both the water and the gum itself. As the concentration of sequestrant is increased, the calcium that inhibits hydration is removed from the system and the hydration temperature falls accordingly. With sufficient sequestrant, deacylated gellan gum can be hydrated at room temperature even in relatively hard water. Since the level of sequestrant needed for hydration is typically less than 0.3%, the added

Table 1 Hydration Temperature of 0.25%
Gellan Gum as a Function of Ion
Concentration

% Dissolved Ca^{2+}	% Dissolved Na^+	Hydration temperature (°C)
0.004	—	88
0.008	—	>100
0.012	—	>100
—	0.046	50
—	0.092	52
—	0.184	60
—	0.276	70
—	0.368	82
—	0.460	89

sodium or potassium ions are not sufficient to inhibit hydration. Table 2 shows how sodium citrate can be used to manipulate the hydration temperature in the presence of calcium. At the practical level, the hydration temperature of deacylated gellan gum can occur from below room temperature to over 100°C by controlling the divalent ion levels.

Gellan gum displays poor hydration in mildly acidic (pH > 4.0) systems. When the pH is below 4.0, the hydration temperature starts to increase dramatically and the effect of mono- and divalent ions becomes more pronounced. With careful use of sequestrants, the gum can still be hydrated at low pH, but if the pH is 3.2 or lower, gellan gum hydration is completely inhibited.

Soluble solids can also inhibit gellan gum hydration. In a solution that contains greater than 45% sucrose, gum hydration is inhibited and the effect of ions becomes greater. Seques- trants must be used judiciously because the effect of added sodium from the sequestrant is no longer trivial. With careful use of a sequestrant, however, it is possible to hydrate gellan gum in solutions up to 80°Brix. Typically, sequestrant levels are reduced to 0.1% or less when solids are very high. The source of the soluble solids is an important consideration. It is easier to hydrate gellan gum in corn syrups, especially high-fructose corn syrups, than it is to hydrate in a sucrose solution of equivalent brix.

2. Solution Properties

Hydrated in cold water with the aid of sequestrants, gellan gum solutions are highly viscous. At a concentration of 1% (w/v) gellan gum is less pseudoplastic or shear-thinning than xanthan

Table 2 Influence of the Sequestrant, Sodium Citrate, on the
Hydration Temperature of 0.25% Gellan Gum

% Dissolved Ca^{2+}	Corresponding water hardness (ppm $CaCO_3$)	% Sodium citrate	Hydration temperature (°C)
0.008	200	—	>100
0.008	200	0.3	24
0.016	400	—	>100
0.016	400	0.3	35
0.040	1000	0.3	78

gum but more pseudoplastic than high molecular weight sodium alginate (9). The viscosity is highly temperature dependent in that a large decrease occurs when the temperature is raised. The viscosity change reflects a conformational change in the gellan molecule as it transforms from an ordered, nonaggregated double helix to a random coil (10). The conformational change is reversible and the temperature of the transition is ion dependent, typically occurring between 25 and 50°C. The temperature dependence of viscosity allows high concentrations of gum to be used without the handling problems of high viscosity.

The flow behavior and dynamic viscoelasticity of deacylated gellan gum solutions was studied by Tako et al. (11). In deionized water, gellan gum showed Newtonian behavior at concentrations under 0.9% but plastic flow behavior above 1.0% at 25°C, with an estimated yield value of 10 dyn/cm^2. Gelation occurred during further cooling when the gum concentration was over 0.8%. With no added calcium, the gels melted when reheated. With the addition of calcium (6 mM CaCl$_2$), the dynamic modulus of a 0.2% gellan gum solution showed high values at low temperatures and increased with increasing temperature to approximately 80°C, then decreased rapidly, exhibiting a higher melting temperature with calcium.

Under neutral conditions, gellan gum solutions are highly stable, capable of being held at 80°C for several hours without degradation (5). If high temperatures are combined with acidic conditions, hydrolytic degradation occurs resulting in a subsequent loss of gel strength. While subject to acid degradation, gellan gum is more stable than many other gums such a carrageenan, gelatin, and agar.

3.   Gelation

Several studies suggest that the initial step of gellan gelation occurs through the formation of double helices, followed by their ion-induced association (9). Heating and cooling solutions of gellan gum allow the fibrils to form as neighboring molecules form a double helix (12). In the presence of ions, these fibrils aggregate into a three-dimensional structure, forming a gel (Fig. 5).

Because gellan gum can be hydrated in the cold with the use of sequestrants, the controlled addition of divalent ions can be used to form gels. Presumably, the gellan gum fibrils were never melted into random coils and only require ions to induce aggregation. However, cold set gels exhibit syneresis unless further stabilized with other gums (9). More coherent stable gels can be made by heating and cooling solutions of gellan gum in the presence of gel-inducing ions. Optimally, the solution is heated and the cations added before the solution is cooled.

Deacylated gellan gum is commercially available in both clarified and unclarified forms. Clarified gellan gum has exceptional clarity at low ion concentrations. At higher ion concentrations birefringence develops, creating a slight whitish haze. The addition of sugar eliminates

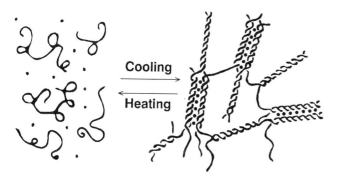

Cooling

Heating

Fig. 5 Proposed model for mechanism for gelation of gellan gum.

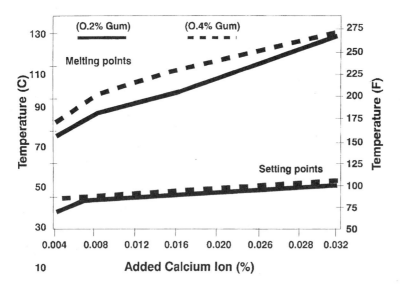

Fig. 6 Setting and melting points of deacylated gellan gum gels versus calcium ion concentration.

birefringence and gels develop a sparkling clarity. The unclarified form of gellan gum forms translucent to opaque white gels.

Set and melt temperatures of deacylated gellan gum are highly dependent on ion type and ion concentration. To a lesser extent, gum concentration, pH, and soluble solids also affect the set and melt temperatures. Increased concentrations raise both the set and melt temperatures. The setting behavior of calcium-gellan gels has been studied using rheological measurements, light spectroscopy, and direct observation. A mathematical model based on the van't Hoff equation was used to predict gelling temperatures from calcium level and gum concentration information (13). Figures 6 and 7 show that calcium gels set between 25 and 40°C, while sodium gels

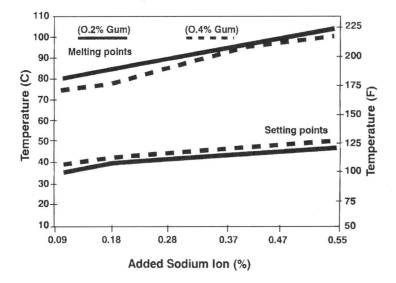

Fig. 7 Setting and melting points of deacylated gellan gum gels versus sodium ion concentration.

set between 40 and 50°C. The differences in ion levels illustrate the relatively higher efficiency of divalent versus monovalent ions. The gels exhibit considerable hysteresis, melting at temperatures considerably higher than the set temperatures. As the ion concentration increases, the gels become more difficult to melt. At higher ion concentrations, the gels do not melt at 100°C, a property useful for applications requiring heat stability.

The texture of deacylated gellan gum gels is commonly described as firm and brittle. However, food texture is a complex perception, and this basic description is not adequate to fully characterize the texture of the gels. Texture profile analysis (TPA) was first developed by General Foods in their work correlating instrumental measurements to sensory perceptions (14–16). An adaptation of the original technique was used to quantify and study the textural aspects of gums (17). The technique uses two successive compressions while the force-deformation data are captured and evaluated with the help of a computer. Using TPA, a number of textural measurements are collected (Fig. 8). Hardness, the maximum force during the first compression, is a measure of the force needed to rupture the gel. Modulus, the initial slope of the force-deformation curve, is a nondestructive measurement of firmness. Brittleness is a measurement of how far the gel can be squeezed before it breaks. Elasticity is a measure of how much the gel springs back after the first compression.

Typical values for the TPA textural parameters are shown in Figs. 9 and 10. The gels were made by dispersing the gum in distilled water, heating the water to 75°C, adding ions, then cooling. Hardness increased rapidly as the concentration of calcium ions increased. As more calcium was added, the increase in hardness passed through a peak at 0.04% added calcium. The modulus increases very rapidly with small amounts of calcium, but quickly peaks and falls

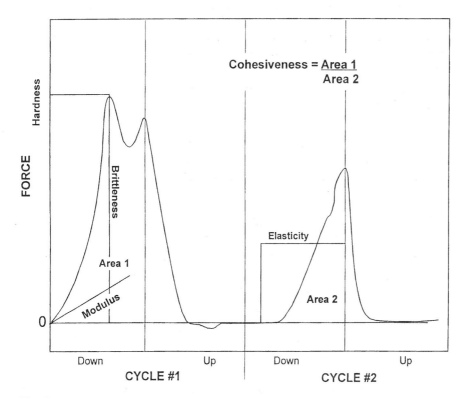

Fig. 8 Idealized texture profile (TPA) for a gel.

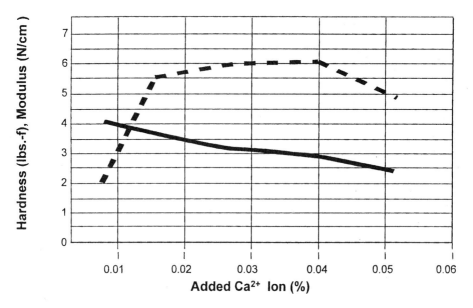

Fig. 9 Deacylated gellan gum (0.25%): hardness (solid line) and modulus (dashed line) versus calcium ion concentration.

slowly. Brittleness and elasticity are also sensitive to ions, decreasing as added calcium increases. However, between 0.016 and 0.04% added calcium, the gel texture parameters are fairly constant.

Magnesium and other divalent ions have similar effects on the gel textural parameters. Monovalent ions also promote gelation, but less efficiently, so that higher concentrations are needed. Maximum hardness and modulus occur at 1% sodium salt and falls off until the concentration reaches 7%. Interestingly, a second peak occurs as the concentration approaches 15% sodium chloride, as shown in Fig. 11.

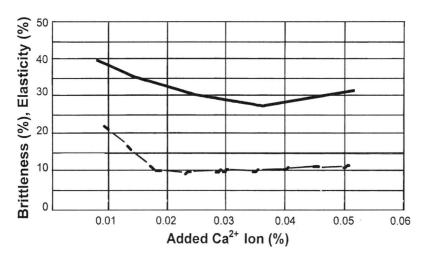

Fig. 10 Deacylated gellan gum (0.25%): brittleness (solid line) and elasticity (dashed line) versus calcium ion concentration.

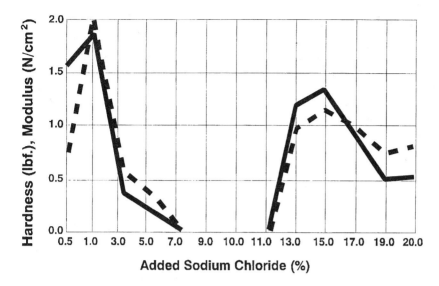

Fig. 11 Deacylated gellan gum (0.25%): hardness (solid line) and modulus (dashed line) versus sodium ion concentration.

Both hardness and modulus increase with gum concentration, but brittleness and elasticity remain essentially constant over the typical use range of deacylated gellan gum, namely 0.1–0.5%. Gels can be prepared at levels up to 5%. At high gum levels, the gum becomes self-gelling due to the ions in the gum and the gels develop a texture similar to candle wax.

The textures of agar, kappa carrageenan, and gellan gum were compared using TPA (Fig. 12). All gels were prepared at the ion level providing optimal hardness for each particular gum. Gellan gum gels had higher hardness and modulus than the other gels at equivalent use levels.

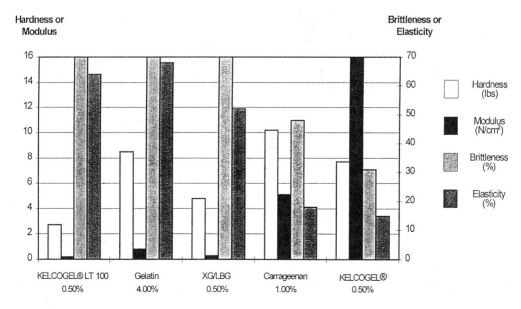

Fig. 12 Comparison of the typical gel textures of several gelling agents.

The texture of deacylated gellan gum gels is largely unaffected by pH in the range of 4–7. However, since some sequestrants, such as sodium citrate, are highly sensitive to pH, lowering the pH can free ions and strengthen gels. At a pH lower than 3.2, deacylated gellan gum forms an acid gel. Acid gels are extremely brittle giving them a mushy texture unless plasticized by high levels of sugars or polyols.

At low levels, sugars and polyols have little effect on gellan gum textures. However, when formulations contain greater than 30% sugar, the gel strength becomes more sensitive to ions in the system. In excess of 40% sugar, gel strength drops rapidly as sugar increases, and calcium in excess of 2 mM brings a reduction of gel strength and brittleness. Several studies have investigated gellan gum in high-solids systems (18,19). The studies confirmed that gellan gum gelation is a two-step process consisting of helix formation followed by an aggregation. In low-solids systems, these steps are closely linked in time, giving gellan gum a "snap" set depending on temperature only. In high-solids system, however, these processes become separated in time. Sugars stabilize the formation of helices so the transition temperature increases as the solids increase, but the aggregation process is slowed so the set has a time element as well as a temperature dependence. Low pH, which creates very brittle acid gels in low solids, can be used very effectively to form firm gels in high-solids systems where the plasticizing effects of sugars reduce excessive brittleness.

4. Fluid Gel

Gels occur when hot gellan gum solutions are allowed to cool and set under quiescent conditions. However, if the hot solution is sheared while setting, the ordering of helices is forced to occur within small spatial areas determined by the shear field. The solution separates into polymer-rich and polymer-poor regions. The polymer-rich phase forms microparticles, while the polymer-poor phase forms the interstitial space between the particles. The overall rheology of the system comes from particle/particle interactions, which can be disrupted by low shear rates and shear stresses (20). These systems, commonly known as fluid gels, can have a wide range of textures including a light pourable gel and a thicker spreadable paste.

The viscosity and structure in fluid gels correlates with the gel strength of an unsheared gel. To form smooth homogeneous gellan gum fluid gels, systems must be formulated to give a weak gelation using low gum concentrations or manipulating ion concentration. Not surprisingly, the heat stability of fluid gels correlates with the melting temperatures of quiescently set gels. Gellan gum also provides good acid stability to fluid gels. Over the pH range of 3–6, gellan gum fluid gels exhibit little structural change. If clarity is desired, a clarified gellan gum can be used to create a fluid gel that is invisible to the eye.

Rheologically, gellan gum fluid gels have a high low shear viscosity, providing remarkable suspending properties at low gum concentrations. With highly pseudoplastic flow properties, suspension can be achieved while maintaining a desirable mouthfeel (21).

5. Films

Gellan gum solutions can be cast and dried into a film. The gellan solution can be prepared hot or cold (using sequestrants) with little difference in film tensile strength. Ions are not needed to form films and can interfere with film formation by crystallizing during the drying process. Plasticizers, such as glycerol, are used in hydrocolloid films to make them less brittle. Deacylated gellan gum is unique in that plasticizers increase the film tensile strength rather than decrease it. Gellan films are particularly tolerant of plasticizers and can tolerate up to 50% glycerol by weight with no reduction in gel strength.

The barrier properties of films are as important as the mechanical properties in applications. Oil, oxygen, and moisture barrier properties are common considerations in film technology. Gellan films have excellent resistance to oil as measured by the contact angle of several common oils, including corn oil and mineral oil. The films exhibit relatively low oxygen transmittance with a 1.6 mm gellan gum film with 25% glycerol plasticizer transmitting 12.1 $cc/m^2/$ day at 25°C. Since gellan gum is extremely hydrophilic, gellan gum films are not good moisture barriers. The addition of hydrophobic additives such as paraffin wax or stearic acid generally cause problems with the film formation, and the resulting properties do not approach the transmittance values of better moisture barriers.

6. Compatibilities and Interactions

Gellan gum is compatible with most other hydrocolloids. Common thickeners, including xanthan gum, guar, locust bean gum, and carboxymethylcellulose, can be used advantageously with deacylated gellan gum to provide extra protection against syneresis due to adverse storage conditions. At typical levels in the range of 0.1–0.3%, these gums do not strongly affect the texture of the gels. Gellan gum is also particularly suited for use with starch. Other thickening gums can build excessive viscosity as starches are cooked, but deacylated gellan hydrates at a higher temperature with little contribution to viscosity. Deacylated gellan gum can be used to improve texture, stability, and flavor release of starch gels.

In high-moisture systems, deacylated gellan gum gels tend to be very brittle. In some applications, a less brittle gel is needed and deacylated gellan gum can be blended with more elastic gums, such as carrageenan, alginate, and xanthan gum/locust bean gum combinations. As more elastic gums are combined with deacylated gellan gum, the textures become less brittle as the concentration of the elastic component increases. Fully acylated gellan gum is particularly useful in this regard as labeling is short and straightforward. Alginates can also be used with gellan gum and since both will gel with calcium ions, interesting textural effects can be created by altering the levels of ions.

The interaction between gellan gum and konjac glucomannan has been studied in the presence of various cations (22). Thermal scanning rheological measurements indicated that konjac glucomannan lowered the order-disorder transition of gellan gum molecules. Rheological results indicated that synergism occurred at low temperatures where gellan gum molecules were sufficiently aggregated. With the progressive addition of monovalent cations, the elastic modulus and the loss modulus gradually increased. With divalent cations, the synergistic interaction increased up to a certain concentration, but excessive divalent cations promoted phase separation.

Gellan gum can be used in a wide variety of formulations, but there are some noted incompatibilities. Gellan gum is degraded by strong oxidizing agents and mixtures of oxidizing and reducing agents. Cationic surfactants will cause precipitation through associations with the negative charged carboxyl group on the polymer. Water-miscible organic solvents such as alcohols will precipitate the gum from solutions, but low levels of alcohol are tolerated.

The compatibility of gellan gum with proteins depends on a number of factors including concentrations, pH, ionic conditions, temperature, and time. At neutral pH, deacylated gellan is compatible with milk proteins, soy, egg albumen, whey, and sodium caseinate. In model systems, gellan gum will precipitate with these proteins when the pH is lowered to 4, but formulation variables including protective colloids such as guar and carboxymethylcellulose allow acidified milk products to be produced. Gelatin/gellan combinations can also be incompatible, forming coacervates, but with careful manipulation of formulation variables, gellan gum can be used to prevent toughening on storage, improve flavor release, and improve heat stability of gelatin gels.

B. Properties of Native Gellan Gum

1. Hydration Process

The acyl side chains on the native form of gellan gum alter the properties described above for the deacylated form of gellan gum. Deacylated gellan gum, for example, is relatively easy to disperse in deionized water. Native gellan gum, however, will swell in deionized water forming a very thick particulate system. On heating, the thick paste loses viscosity suddenly when the hydration temperature is reached at around 70°C. The swelling behavior of native gellan gum is very dependent on ions. Small amounts of sodium or calcium raise the swelling temperature so that native gellan gum can be easily dispersed in most tap water. On heating, the gum will then pass through the swelling phase before it hydrates with a subsequent loss of viscosity.

The hydration temperature of native gellan gum climbs sharply with very small amounts of sodium or calcium (Figs. 13,14), but climbs slowly as ions are increased further. The acylated gum is much less sensitive to ions than the deacylated form. In 0.04% calcium solutions, native gellan gum hydrates at approximately 80°C, where deacylated gellan gum would be insoluble. Native gellan gum is more sensitive to sodium ions than deacylated gellan gum. With deacylated gellan gum, sequestrants can be used to make the gum soluble in cold water by binding calcium. With native gellan gum, sequestrants are less effective because the added sodium from the sequestrant offsets the benefits of calcium removal. Therefore, native gellan gum requires heat for hydration.

The hydration temperature also increases with soluble solids (Fig. 15). However, the type of solid is an important consideration. Monosaccharides like dextrose and fructose have less of an effect than sucrose or polydextrose.

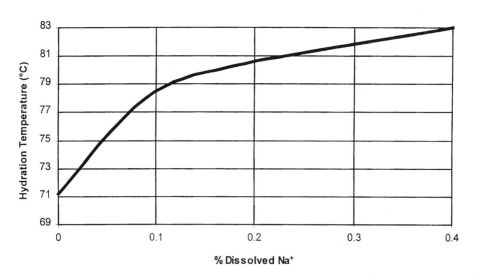

Fig. 13 Hydration temperature of native gellan gum versus sodium ion concentration.

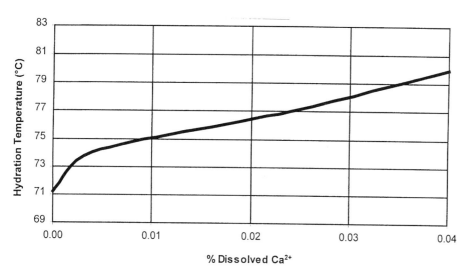

Fig. 14 Hydration temperature of native gellan gum versus calcium ion concentration.

2. Viscosity

The cold dispersions of native gellan provide extremely high viscosities. The solutions seem to be highly thixotropic, apparently the result of a gel-like structure. However, native gellan gum is very sensitive to salt. Xanthan gum, although much less viscous at equivalent concentrations in low-salt systems, provides a stable viscosity over a broad range of salt, whereas native gellan gum viscosity falls rapidly as salt increases.

When native gellan gum dispersions are heated, the viscosity falls suddenly as the gum hydrates. Comparatively, however, hot native gellan gum solutions are much more viscous than deacylated gellan solutions. At neutral pH, native gellan gum solutions are very stable, with little loss in functionality when heated to 95°C for 180 minutes. While acid hydrolysis occurs

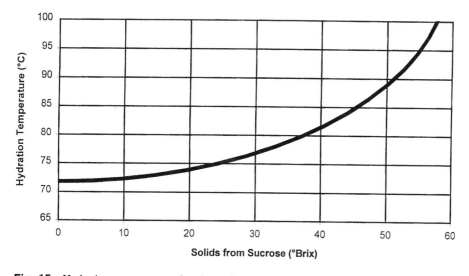

Fig. 15 Hydration temperature of native gellan gum versus solids level.

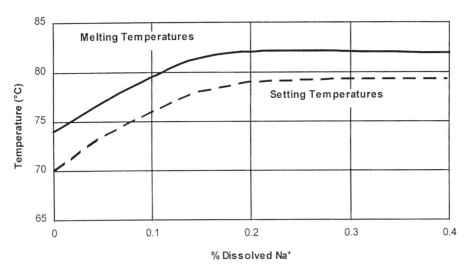

Fig. 16 Setting and melting points of native gellan gum gels versus sodium ion concentration.

in low-pH hot solutions, native gellan gum is relatively stable when compared to other hydrocolloids.

3. Gelation

The set and melt behavior of native gellan gum contrasts sharply with the deacylated form of the gum (Figs. 16–18). Native gellan gum exhibits a higher set temperature with comparatively less hysteresis. The gels are thermoreversible even at higher calcium concentrations.

The texture of native gellan gum gels also contrasts sharply with the brittle gels made with deacylated gellan gum. While deacylated gellan gum displays textural similarity to κ-carrageenan and agar, the native product is more like xanthan/locust bean gels. Texture profile

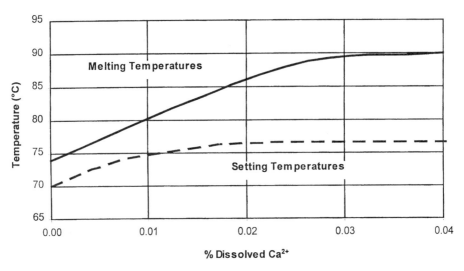

Fig. 17 Setting and melting points of native gellan gum gels versus calcium ion concentration.

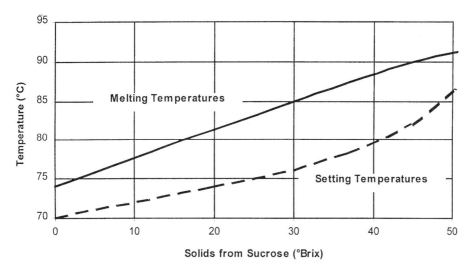

Fig. 18 Setting and melting points of native gellan gum gels versus solids level.

analysis data are more difficult to interpret for native gellan gum than for the deacylated gum. The elastic gels do not break even at a compression of 85% of the original height of the gel.

Like deacylated gellan gum, native gellan gum is strengthened by ions (Figs. 19–22). Sugar solids also increase the strength of these gels up to 50 °Brix, but higher sugar solids gradually weaken the gel. The gels are relatively stable over a wide range of pH. There is a very gradual increase in gel strength as the pH is lowered to 4.0, followed by a rapid decrease as the pH is lowered further.

4. Fluid Gel

At concentrations of less than 0.03% (w/w), native gellan gum does not form a cohesive gel. Shearing this system either before or after cooling will result in a fluid gel. Shearing before or

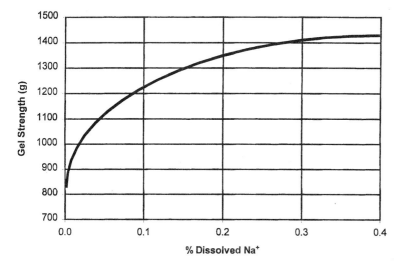

Fig. 19 Gel strength of native gellan gum gels versus sodium ion concentration.

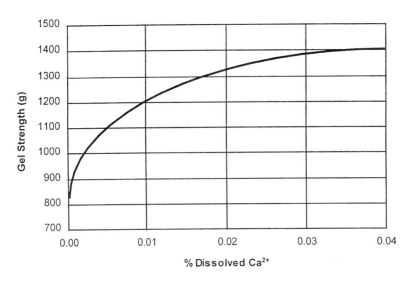

Fig. 20   Gel strength of native gellan gum gels versus calcium ion concentration.

after cooling has little effect on the viscosity, but solutions that were sheared after cooling will have a higher elastic modulus and will exhibit a slightly higher degree of thixotropy.

Like fluid gels made from deacylated gellan gum, the fluid gels from native gellan gum are sensitive to ions. The highest elastic modulus occurs at 10 mM sodium or 2mM calcium ions. Beyond these levels the modulus decreases. For either ion, increasing the level of salt slows the thixotropic recovery of elastic modulus. Soluble solids and pH also affect the fluid gel properties. The addition of solids increases the elastic modulus. The effect of pH depends on the level of solids. At 20% solids, lowering the pH to 3.2 lowered the elastic modulus, but at 60% solids, pH had little effect.

Fluid gels made from native gellan gum have significantly higher yield stress than ones made from deacylated gellan gum. Because of this high yield stress, native gellan gum can provide suspension with less viscosity than either xanthan gum or deacylated gellan gum.

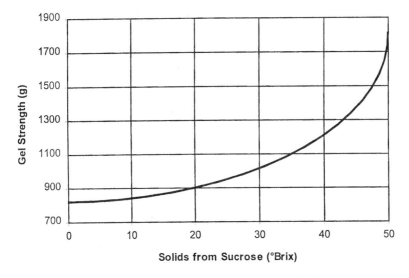

Fig. 21   Gel strength of native gellan gum gels versus solids level.

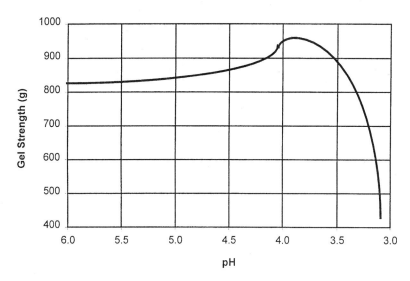

Fig. 22   Gel strength of native gellan gum gels versus pH.

5.   Films

Native gellan gum solutions can be cast and dried into a film similarly to the deacylated form of gellan gum. The noticeable difference between the two gellan gums forms is the difference in their rheologies. Native gellan gum exhibits a higher viscosity than comparable concentrations of deacylated gellan gum, making the film formation process more difficult. Other than this processing issue, native and deacylated gellan gum films produce films with very similar properties.

6.   Compatibilities and Interactions

Like deacylated gellan gum, native gellan gum is compatible with a wide range of other hydrocolloids. While native gellan gum is not particularly prone to syneresis, thickening hydrocolloids

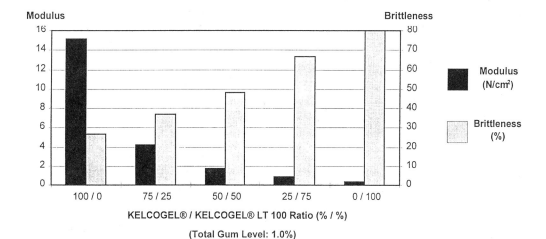

Fig. 23   Textural variations using native gellan gum (KELCOGEL® LT 100) in combination with deacylated gellan gum (KELCOGEL®).

such as guar or locust bean gum can be used to further bind water. However, its compatibility with other gelling hydrocolloids is probably more important. It is useful to blend native gellan gum with brittle gels to develop intermediate textures. It is particularly advantageous to blend native gellan gum with deacylated gellan gum because only gellan gum is declared on the food label (Fig. 23). By varying the ratio of the two forms of gellan gum, a wide variety of textures can be obtained.

Native gellan gum has an interaction with starch. This interaction can delay native gellan gum hydration if high amounts of starch are present. However, when used properly with starch, the gum can be used advantageously to produce fast gelling food products with high shear stability and low rigidity (23).

V. PHYSIOLOGICAL EFFECTS

A. Nutrition

It has long been established that an increase in dietary fiber intake is beneficial to health, but the perceived negative organoleptic properties of insoluble fiber such as wheat bran have induced general resistance to increasing consumption of such fibers. In both animal and human feeding studies, including gellan gum in the diet increased the volume of the excreted fecal matter with effects similar to that caused by ingestion of wheat bran (24). Additional feeding studies indicated that ingestion of gellan gum at high doses had no perceptible effects on the concentrations of HDL cholesterol, phospholipids, or triglycerides, but serum cholesterol concentrations decreased perceptibly ($p < 0.1$)—13% on average in females and 12% on average in males (25). Increased fecal volume and reduced serum cholesterol levels can be considered desirable from a dietetic viewpoint.

Generally, most nonstarch polysaccharides are resistant to naturally occurring enzymes in the human metabolic pathways and pass through the small intestine unaffected. Studies using a range of polysaccharides have shown that when nonstarch polysaccharides are included in the diet, they can be recovered quantitatively at the terminal ileum (26). Animal feeding studies using radioactively labeled gellan gum showed that the majority of administered gellan gum was excreted in the fecal matter, suggesting that no endogenous enzymes, which enable breakdown of gellan gum in the small intestine, are present.

B. Flavor

By itself, gellan gum is essentially tasteless to bland in terms of flavor perception. When using the deacylated form, gellan gum makes gels that are very brittle and that release entrained water rapidly when fractured. Usage levels are generally less than 0.25% in most applications. The combination of all of these factors results in excellent flavor release profiles in food systems that incorporate gellan gum as the gelling agent. Flavor masking by some polysaccharides such as starch can be minimized or eliminated by replacing the starch with gellan gum or by decreasing the usage level of such polymers and replacing the portion removed with sufficient gellan gum to provide the desired rheological characteristics.

Studies of flavor release in polysaccharide gels have related sweetness and flavor intensity to yield strain, which correlates well with brittleness (27). In polysaccharide gels, the perceived intensities of sweetness and flavor decreased with increasing yield strain. At equivalent firmness levels, gellan gum exhibited particularly good release characteristics versus other gums.

VI. SAFETY

As of November 25, 1992, gellan gum is approved in the United States under CFR 172.665 as a stabilizer and thickener in foods generally in accordance with good manufacturing practice where Standards of Identity do not preclude such use. Gellan gum is also approved for use in foods in Argentina, Australia, Belgium, Canada, Chile, Colombia, Costa Rica, France, Hong Kong, Indonesia, Israel, Mexico, Norway, Philippines, Singapore, South Africa, South Korea, Sri Lanka, Taiwan, and Thailand.

Gellan gum appears as E418 in Annex 1 (the list of generally permitted additives) of the European Community proposal for a Council Directive on food additives other than colors and sweeteners. Both the Joint FAO/WHO Expert Committee on Food Additives (JECFA) and the European Community Scientific Committee for Food have given gellan gum an Acceptable Daily Intake (ADI) of ''not specified.''

In Japan, gellan gum has been considered a ''natural food additive'' since 1988. Petitions for approval are under active review in other countries. CP Kelco is committed to a proactive policy of working with potential customers to seek regulatory approvals internationally wherever they are needed.

VII. FOOD APPLICATIONS

Gellan gum has broad application in foods. Its versatility provides food processors a unique hydrocolloid, which, used by itself or in combination with other food hydrocolloids, provides functionality in gelling, texturizing, stabilizing, suspension, film forming, and adhesion.

A. Water-Based Gels

Water-based applications of gellan gum include dessert gels, ready-to-eat dessert gels, and savory aspics. Also included in this category are Asian foods such as mitsumame (gelled cubes in a fruit cocktail) and tokoroten (gel noodles in a sweet syrup). These applications are typically made by dissolving a gelling agent in water and adding the appropriate color and flavors. Historically, gelatin, agar, carrageenan, and locust bean gum have been used in these applications, but gellan gum's unique properties are particularly useful for water-based gels.

Gellan gum is a highly efficient gelling agent capable of forming gels at concentrations as low as 0.05% gum. Gellan gum contributes clarity, sheen, structure, texture, stability, and flavor release. For dessert gels, deacylated gellan gum is usually recommended for its clarity and thermal stability, but this form of gellan gum is rather brittle. Brittleness is not completely undesirable because the rapid breakdown of the gel and subsequent syneresis creates a refreshing burst of flavor during mastication. In applications such as mitsumame, brittleness is needed to match a traditional agar texture. For most dessert gels, however, gellan gum is usually blended with other hydrocolloids to reduce excessive brittleness. Algins or blends of xanthan gum and locust bean gum have been used with gellan gum to make heat-stable RTE dessert gels.

In water jellies and mitsumami, where clarity is not always an issue, the native form of gellan gum can be blended with deacylated gellan gum to provide a more elastic texture with the added benefit of having a brief label declaration. Gellan gum can also be used with other gelling agents such as agar, gelatin, and carrageenan/locust bean gum to provide added acid and thermal stability or to improve the flavor release and texture of products such as dessert gels and aspics.

B. Fruit Products

In the United States, jams and jellies are covered by a standard of identity. All products labeled as jams and jellies must contain pectin. Outside the standard of identity, however, are imitation jams, low- or no-sugar spreads, and all-fruit spreads. High-methoxyl pectin will not work in many of these systems because both low pH and high sugar solids are required to form a gel. Traditionally, κ-carrageenan or low-methoxyl pectin have been used to work around these requirements. Gellan gum, requiring only added calcium to form a gel, avoids these restrictions. Additionally, gellan gum exhibits improved acid and heat stability over carrageenan and pectin. Therefore, gellan gum significantly improves the processing tolerance during the manufacture of fruit products. Also beneficial are gellan gum's sparkling clarity, low use level, and exceptional flavor release.

Typically, the deacylated form of gellan gum is used in fruit products, although it can be combined with the native gum if clarity is not critical and a more elastic texture is needed. In high-solids formulations, additional elasticity is rarely needed because sugars plasticize the gel creating a softer texture. In low-solids or artificially sweetened fruit products, the deacylated gellan gum can be blended with other gums. When portion-packed, xanthan gum and guar are used with gellan gum to reduce syneresis, which can occur in the transport and handling of the low-solids jellies.

C. Starch-Based Products

Starch is a common stabilizer for bakery fillings, puddings, and fruit yogurt preparations. When used at low levels with starch, gellan gum is able to add structure and stability to fillings without compromising the traditional textures provided by starch. Often gellan gum is used as a partial starch replacement to increase flavor release.

Commercial bakery fillings cover a wide range of fruit levels, pH, acidity, and soluble solids. Gellan gum provides a needed flexibility in formulating fruit fillings because of its functionality in a broad range of pH and solids. The stability of gellan gum also makes it very tolerant to different processing conditions so it fits well with most standard procedures for cook-up starches. The low cook-up viscosity is also an advantage for processing. For pastry and pie fillings, deacylated gellan gum is usually preferred. After cook-up, the filling sets into a soft gel that can be sheared and deposited onto the baked goods where it will partially recover structure. In low-solids fillings, gellan gum binds water to reduce syneresis and reduce moisture loss. While syneresis is less of a concern in higher-solids fillings, gellan gum is used to improve bake stability. Because gellan gum can be formulated not to melt by adding calcium, fillings do not "boil out" and foul ovens.

Since gellan gum is compatible with milk, its use can be extended to puddings and milk-based fillings. In puddings, deacylated gellan gum is used to improve moisture retention, flavor release, and storage stability and to reduce syneresis or weeping.

D. High Solids Applications

Gelled confections can be made with a wide number of hydrocolloids. Such products include starch jellies, gummy candies, pastilles, pectin jellies, and marshmallows. High-solids jellies made with deacylated gellan gum have sparkling clarity, good flavor release, and good storage stability. Low hot viscosity and rapid set are processing advantages. It can also be used with more traditional gums. In starch jellies, deacylated gellan gum can replace some starch to speed the gel set and improve flavor and storage stability. In gummy candies, deacylated gellan gum is used with other gums such as xanthan/locust bean gum or native gellan gum to provide a more elastic texture. Products made with gellan gum contain no animal products and can be consumed without concern for religious dietary restrictions. Deacylated gellan gum is also used with gelatin to improve the heat stability of gummy candy. In marshmallow, native gellan gum can replace gelatin if an appropriate foaming agent is used for air incorporation. The marshmallows have improved heat stability and contain no animal products. Gellan gum's compatibility with polyols also make it useful in confections targeting the dietetic market.

The ability of gellan gum to tolerate high solids also enables it to work as a stabilizer for icings and frostings. Stabilizers provide structure and set to icings and frostings and they slow moisture loss and prevent graininess. Many hydrocolloids are used in this application area, including agar, gelatin, starch, algin, and xanthan gum. Each gum has its own processing requirements. Gellan gum's processing requirements are closest to agar, requiring heating to hydrate the gum. Icings made with deacylated gellan have a glossy sheen and good flavor release. Gellan gum breaks down smoothly without developing a slimy texture or off-flavor as can happen with agar. Gellan gum can be used alone, but the industry often combines different stabilizers into a blend. Guar and locust bean gums are useful in gellan gum icings if the baked good is to be wrapped (for example, a snack cake).

E. Dairy Foods

Compatibility with milk proteins is an important concern for dairy stabilizers. Additionally, since many dairy products are delicately flavored, it is important that stabilizers have clean flavors. Gellan gum has both of these properties and so it finds use in products like flan, custard, ice cream, cheese, yogurt, and sour cream.

In flan or custards, deacylated gellan gum can be used alone or in combination with native gellan gum to provide an egg-like texture. The product may be a instant dry mix or a fluid-gel that will melt and set on heating and cooling.

In cultured dairy products, gellan gum binds water to reduce weeping and provides body, texture, and mouthfeel. These features are especially important in low-fat or fat-free products, which can lack the organoleptic properties provided by fat. In yogurts and sour cream, traditional stabilizers have included gelatin, pectin, and starch. Gellan gum is an excellent alternative to these stabilizers, particularly when producers want to avoid gelatin for religious dietary reasons. Typically, low levels of deacylated gellan gum are used with starch in these applications. The use of native gellan gum for these products, however, is expanding as more producers are looking at gelatin alternatives. Gellan gum can be used in the production of cheese to increase yield and in the production of fat-free cheese to provide texture, binding, and mouthfeel.

F. Beverages

Gellan gum fluid gels are useful in various beverage suspensions. Deacylated gellan gum is used in citrus beverages to suspend pulp or clouding agents. Both deacylated and native gellan gum are used to suspend cocoa in chocolate milk beverages. One such beverage is a total meal replacement beverage. It demonstrates gellan gum's ability to tolerate the ionic environment caused by the high usage levels of vitamins and minerals in the product. Native gellan gum has also been used to suspend tea and herbs. Gellan gum's compatibility with residual proteins is important for this application.

Clarified, deacylated gellan gum is also used to make beverage novelties with gel bead inclusions. The gellan gum is used both in the clear beverage to provide suspension without excessive viscosity and to make the colored beads that are suspended in the beverage. Other unique beverage applications include textured beverages. One such beverage includes small transparent gel cubes in an apple juice. The cubes are invisible to the eye, but provide a unique mouthfeel. Gellan gum is also used in the production of drinking jellies. Drinking jellies are soft gels that break down when shaken. The resulting beverage is then consumed as a textured beverage.

G. Baked Goods

The use of gums in baked goods to improve perceived moistness is well established. Typical gums used in baking include xanthan gum, guar, and carboxymethyl cellulose (CMC). However, these gums hydrate during mixing, and high use levels can add too much viscosity to the batter. Gellan gum avoids this problem, since the gum hydrates only during the baking cycle. Therefore, the deacylated form of gellan gum finds use in cakes and brownies to provide moistness to the cakes and chewiness to the brownies. Gellan gum has also been used in fried products, such as churros, as a structuring agent to reduce breakage.

H. Film Forming

Gellan gum's film-forming properties are used in a variety of applications. Since gellan gum is an effective oil barrier, it can be used in batters, breading, and other coating systems. Gellan gum also enhances crispness in these applications. Gellan gum can be added to a dry mix, but its oil barrier properties are strongest when the substrate is dipped in a hot solution of gellan gum and the film is allowed to set.

Another use of gellan gum's film forming is in the area of nonfat adhesion systems. Typically, spices are adhered to snack foods with specialty oils, but gellan gum can be used to provide a fat-free adhesion system. Since hot deacylated gellan gum solutions have little viscosity, they can be finely sprayed over crackers, pretzels, and other snack foods. Spices and flavors can be incorporated in the solution or added immediately after spraying. The spices are then incorporated into the film as the solution dries and the spices and flavors are adhered to the food.

VIII. OTHER APPLICATIONS

In addition to the varied applications for gellan gum in food systems, utility for this polysaccharide has been found in a number of nonfood applications. In pharmaceutical applications, gellan gum has been used as a novel drug-delivery vehicle, in film formation for transdermal drug delivery, and as a component in controlled-release systems. In personal care products, such as sunscreens and lotions, gellan gum has been used as a structuring rather than a gelling agent, providing body, stability, and exceptional handfeel. Novel personal care products, which have inclusions of botanicals or microparticles, utilize the fluid gel technology described previously.

In gelled systems, gellan gum has been utilized in a number of application areas. The transparent deacylated form of gellan gum demonstrates a high tolerance for fragrances and superior thermal stability. The recent trend toward high-end transparent, concentrated products, as well as the move of air freshener gels out of the bathroom and into other areas of the home, office, and automobile, has made reformulation of existing formulations necessary and presents an opportunity for alternative gelling technology to be evaluated. The clarified deacylated product has also been used for many years as a microbiological and plant tissue medium.

The interaction that gellan gum elicits in combination with starch has been employed in the surface sizing of paper (28). The low viscosity of gellan gum solutions at higher temperatures has made this surface sizing system easier to work with than those currently utilized and allows for faster running of the paper machine.

REFERENCES

1. O'Neil MA, Selvendran RR, Morris VJ. Structure of the acidic extracellular gelling polysaccharide produced by *Pseudomonas elodea*. Carbohydr Res 124:123–133, 1983.
2. Jansson PE, Lindberg B, Sanford PA. Structural studies of gellan gum, an extracellular polysaccharide elaborated by *Pseudomonas elodea*. Carbohydr Res 124:135–139, 1983.
3. Kuo M-S, Dell A, Mort AJ. Identification and location of L-glycerate, an unusual acyl substituent in gellan gum. Carbohydr Res 156:173–178, 1986.
4. Grasdalen H, Smidsrod O. Gelation of gellan gum, Carbohydr Polymers 7:371–393, 1987.
5. Sanderson GR. Gellan gum. In: Nussinovitch A, ed. Hydrocolloids Applications. London: Blackie Academic and Professional, 1997, pp 63–82.
6. Talasheck T. The effect of acyl substituents on the conformational properties of gellan, Presented at the National ACS Spring Meeting, Dallas, 1998.
7. Chandrasekaran R, Millane RP, Arnot S. Crystal structure of gellan. Carbohydrate Res 175:1–15, 1988.
8. Chandrasekaran R, Puigjaner LC, Joyce KL. Cation interactions in gellan: an x-ray study of the potassium salt. Carbohydrate Res 181:23–40, 1988.
9. Gibson W. Gellan gum. In: Imeson A, ed. Thickening and Gelling Agents for Food. London: Chapman and Hall, 1992, pp 227–249.
10. Robinson G, Manning CE, Morris ER. In: Phillips GO, Wedlock DJ, Williams PA, eds. Gums and Stabilizers for the Food Industry. Vol 4. Oxford: IRL Press, 1987, pp 173–181.
11. Tako M, Sakae A, Nakamura S. Rheological properties of gellan gum in aqueous media, Agric Biol Chem 53(3):771–776, 1989.
12. Gunning AP, Morris VJ. Light scattering studies of tetramethylammonium gellan. Int J Biol Macromol 12:338–341, 1990.
13. Tang J, Tung MA, Zeng Y. Gelling temperature of gellan solutions containing calcium ions. J Food Sci 62(2):276–280, 1997.
14. Szczesniak AS. Classification of textural characteristics. J Food Sci 28:385–389, 1963.
15. Friedman HH, Whitney JE, Szczesnial AS. The texturometer—a new instrument for objective texture measurement. J Food Sci 28:390–396, 1963.
16. Szczesniak AS, Brandt MA, Friedman HH. Development of standard rating scales for mechanical parameters of texture and correlation between the objective and the sensory methods of texture evaluation. J Food Sci 28:397–403, 1963.
17. Sanderson GP, Bell VL, Ortega D. Comparison of gellan gum, agar, κ carrageenan, and alginate. Cereal Foods World 34:991–999, 1989.
18. Willoughby LE, Kasapis S. The influence of sucrose upon the gelation of gellan gum in large deformation compression analysis. Food Sci Technol Today 8:227–228, 1994.
19. Sworn G, Kasapis S. The use of Arrhenius and WLF kinetics to rationalize the mechanical spectrum in high sugar gellan systems. Carbohydr Res 309:353–361, 1998.
20. Norton I. Unilever Research Website, http://research.unilever.com/examples/colloid.htm, (1997).
21. Sworn G, Sanderson GR, Gibson W. Gellan gum fluid gels. Food Hydrocolloids 9(4):265–267, 1994.
22. Miyoshi E, Takaya T, Willimas PA, Nishinari K. Rheological and DSC studies of mixtures of gellan gum and konjac glucomannan. Macromol Symp 120:271–280, 1997.
23. Clark RC, Burgum DP. Blends of high acyl gellan gum with starch. U.S. Patent 4,869,916 (1989).
24. Edwards CA, Adiotomre J, Eastwood MA. Dietary fibre: the use of in-vitro and rat models to predict action on stool output in man. J Sci Food Agric 59:257–260, 1992.
25. Adiotomre J, Eastwood MA, Edwards CA, Brydon WG. Dietary fiber: in vitro methods that anticipate nutrition and metabolic activity in humans. Am J Clin Nutr 52:128–134, 1990.

26. Englyst HN, Cummings JH. Digestion of the polysaccharides of some cereal foods in the human small intestine. Am J Clin Nutr 42:778–787, 1985.

27. Morris M. Rheological and organoleptic properties of food hydrocolloids. In: Nishinari K, Doi E, eds. Food Hydrocolloids: Structures, Properties and Functions. New York: Plenum Press, 1994, p 201–210.

28. Winston PE, Dial H, Clare K, Ortega TM. Paper surface sizing composition—contains gellan gum and chemically modified starch, cellulose derivatives or PVA, in water, used as a binder for pigmented paper coating. U.S. Patent 5,112,445 (1990).

36

Inulin and Oligofructose

Paul Coussement and Anne Franck
ORAFTI Active Food Ingredients, Tienen, Belgium

I. DEFINITIONS

Inulin was identified by Rose in the early 1800s as the carbohydrate substance that he isolated from the root of *Inula helenum* (Rose, 1804). We now know that it is present in a wide range of plants, including common vegetables, fruits, and cereals (Van Loo et al., 1995). Inulin is a polydisperse substance. It is a mixture of oligomers and polymers of β-(2-1)-fructose from the fructan family (Fig. 1) (Phelps, 1965; De Leenheer et al., 1994) with a structure that can be represented by the formula GF_n, in which G = the glucosyl unit, F = the fructosyl unit, and n = the number of fructosyl units linked ($n \geq 2$) by β(2-1) linkages. Inulin also contains minor amounts of F_n fructans ($n \geq 2$), in which the glucosyl end unit is not present. The degree of polymerization (DP) of chicory inulin ranges mainly from 2 to 60.

Today, only inulin from chicory roots is commercialized as a purified food ingredient. The chicory roots that are used are of the same species (*Cichorium intybus*) that has long been used to produce a coffee substitute. At the moment, no GMO-derived chicory roots are used.

About 70% of chicory inulin molecules have a DP of > 10. Oligosaccharides are defined as having a DP between 2 and 10 (IUB-IUPAC, 1982). Therefore, inulin is a mixture of oligo- and polysaccharides but contains mainly polysaccharides.

Several commercial inulin types are available, all of which have a very high purity and differ with regard to their powder characteristics and carbohydrate composition (Table 1). Standard inulin, as it is extracted from chicory roots, always contains a small amount of sugar (up to 10%). The sugars are present in the root—they are not a result of processing. Low-sugar and high-performance inulin are obtained by chromatographic or physical removal of the mono-, di-, and oligosaccharide fractions.

Oligofructose was introduced as a synonym for fructo-oligosaccharides by ORAFTI in 1989. Oligofructose is a mixture of β-(2-1)-fructans with the general structure GF_n or F_n, in which G = the glucosyl unit, F = the fructosyl unit, and n = the number of fructosyl units linked. The DP of oligofructose ranges in principle from 2 to 10. The DP of oligofructose in RAFTILOSE® products ranges from 2 to 8. One would expect oligofructose or fructo-oligosaccharides to consist of only fructose-based oligomers. In practice, it is generally accepted that molecules that start with one glucose moiety, followed by fructose moieties, are also called oligofructose or fructo-oligosaccharides.

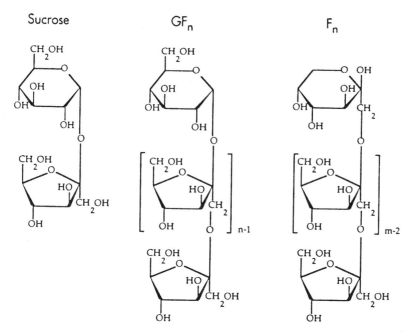

Fig. 1 Chemical structures of sucrose, inulin, and oligofructose.

Oligofructose can be obtained by partial enzymatic hydrolysis of inulin or by enzymatic synthesis from sucrose. Partial hydrolysis of inulin leads to a mixture of GF$_n$- and F$_n$-type molecules. Enzymatic synthesis from sucrose leads to GF$_n$ molecules only.

In most cases the word oligofructose refers to the partial hydrolysate of inulin. For this process, an endo-inulinase enzyme is used (Norman and Hojer-Pedersen, 1989). The resulting products can have different carbohydrate compositions, as reflected in Table 2.

All of these industrial products are free of gluten, fat, protein, and phytic acid and contain only very small (negligible) amounts of some minerals and salts. They are also free of pesticides, toxins, and allergens. Thanks to their plant origin, together with the use of modern processing techniques, the commercial inulin and oligofructose products can easily meet today's high microbiological standards for food ingredients.

Table 1 Typical Composition of Some Commercial Inulin Powders

	RAFTILINE®ST(%)	RAFTILINE®LS(%)	RAFTILINE®HP(%)
Dry substance (d.s.)	≥95	≥95	≥95
Inulin on d.s.	~92	~99.5	~100
Sugars[a] on d.s.	~8	~0.5	~0
Oligosaccharides on d.s.	~30	~30	<3
Dietary fiber[b] on d.s.	~92	~99.5	~100
Carbohydrates on d.s.	>99.5	>99.5	>99.5
Ash (sulfated) on d.s.	<0.2	<0.2	<0.2

[a] Glucose, fructose, and sucrose.
[b] As determined by AOAC Fructan method 997.08.

Table 2 Typical Compositions of Some Commercial Oligofructose Products

	RAFTILOSE®L60(%)	RAFTILOSE®L95(%)	RAFTILOSE®P95(%)
Form	Syrup	Syrup	Powder
Dry substance (d.s.)	≥75	≥75	≥95
Oligofructose on d.s.	~60	~95	~95
Sugars[a] on d.s.	~40	~5	~5
Oligosaccharides on d.s.	~60	~95	~95
Dietary fiber[b] on d.s.	~60	~95	~95
Carbohydrates on d.s.	>99.5	>99.5	>99.5
Ash (sulfated) on d.s.	<0.2	<0.2	<0.2

[a] Glucose, fructose, and sucrose.
[b] As determined by AOAC Fructan method 997.08.

II. NATURAL OCCURRENCE AND HISTORY OF USE

Both inulin and oligofructose are present in the daily diet of many of the world's populations (Van Loo et al., 1995). This presence is not a matter of trace amounts: several grams per day may be ingested through the normal diet (Table 3). This fact is the cornerstone of the safety evaluation of both inulin and oligofructose. On the one hand, it shows that humans have been exposed daily to both substances for centuries. On the other hand, the fact that specific meals and even some diets can contain considerable amounts of inulin or oligofructose (up to 20 g) provides a history of exposure to such high amounts through the diet.

As far as we know, the historical literature provides no specific reports questioning the safety of inulin-containing vegetables. Although this is no proof of safety, it is a comforting fact to know that, throughout so many centuries, the safety of inulin-containing foods has not been questioned. On the contrary, many of these foods (e.g., chicory, garlic, leeks) have been hailed as stimulants of good health, especially for diabetic patients (Külz, 1874; Strauss, 1911; Lewis, 1912).

III. NUTRITIONAL PROPERTIES

A. Nondigestibility

It has been confirmed with ileostomy patients that inulin and oligofructose are not digested in the small intestine (Knudsen and Hessov, 1995; Ellegård et al., 1997). The β-(2-1) bonds linking the fructose molecules cannot be hydrolyzed by the human (mammal) small intestinal sucrase-maltase complex. They enter the colon almost quantitatively, where they are metabolized mostly to short-chain fatty acids and lactate by the intestinal bacteria (Roberfroid, 1993).

Table 3 Estimations of the Average Inulin Consumption

	g/day per capita	50th percentile	90th percentile
Europe	3–11		
North America	1–4	0.8–3	2–8

Source: Van Loo et al., 1995.

B. Caloric Value

The nondigestibility of inulin and oligofructose is at the basis of their reduced caloric value compared with their component monosaccharide moieties. Inulin and oligofructose, furthermore, are only marginally affected during their passage through the mouth and stomach. This has been demonstrated by means of ileostomy studies. This means that the ingested inulin or oligofructose almost quantitatively reaches the colon.

In the colon, the fructans are completely metabolized by the intestinal bacteria. Even at high intakes, no significant amounts have been detected in the feces.

Inulin and oligofructose are completely converted, mainly to short-chain fatty acids (SCFA)—acetate, propionate, and butyrate—lactate, bacterial biomass, and gases. Only the SCFA and lactate contribute to the host's energy metabolism. This corresponds to only a fraction of the original energy content of the component sugars. The SCFA and lactate, moreover, are less effective energy substrates than sugars. All these facts together explain the reduced caloric value of inulin and oligofructose.

Based on ^{14}C studies in humans, the caloric value of fructo-oligosaccharides was calculated by Hosoya et al. (1988) to be 1.5 kcal/g. Experimental in vitro data (fermentation) and in vivo data (rat experiments), allowed Roberfroid et al. (1993) to calculate the caloric value of oligo-fructose according to basic biochemical principle. When 1 mole of fructose is completely fermented into CO_2, 40 moles of ATP are produced. When the fructose is bound as in oligofructose, it is 40% converted into bacterial biomass, 5% into CO2, 40% into SCFA, and 15% into lactate. Only 90% of these metabolites are absorbed in the blood. Metabolism of these compounds in the liver produces 14 moles of ATP, which is 35% of the caloric content of free fructose. This gives a caloric value of 1.4 kcal/g oligofructose.

Other scientific observations have suggested even lower caloric values (Delzenne et al., 1995a; Ellegård et al., 1997). Consequently, a caloric value between 1 and 1.5 kcal/g for inulin and oligofructose is currently used for food labeling.

C. Improvement of Lipid Metabolism

In rats, distinct effects on lipid metabolism have been observed. Mainly, the serum triglycerides are affected. The observed metabolic changes originate at the level of the liver (Bhattathiry, 1971; Hata, 1982; Oku and Tokunaga, 1984; Delzenne et al., 1993; Levrat et al., 1994; Fioraldiso et al., 1995; Delzenne and Kok, 1998).

Biochemical studies with isolated hepatocytes have demonstrated that inulin or oligofruc-tose consumption reduces the activity of key hepatic enzymes related to lipogenesis (de novo synthesis of fatty acids or assembling of triglycerides from acyl groups and glycerol) (Kok et al., 1996a, b; Kok et al., 1998a). Further research revealed that altered gene expression is at the basis of the downregulation. It is hypothesized that inulin and oligofructose, or their bacterial metabolites, affect the hormone status (insulin and/or glucose-dependent insulinotropic polypep-tide) of rats (Kok et al., 1998b). Recently, a dose-effect study in golden Syrian hamsters also showed a significant decrease in serum triglycerides and cholesterol (VLDL-C) (Trautwein et al., 1998).

Human volunteer studies indicate that inulin and oligofructose have a modulating effect. It has been reported that the consumption of fructans reduces serum triglycerides and cholesterol (mostly LDL cholesterol) in healthy volunteers who are (slightly) hyperlipidemic. The optimal lipid parameters of healthy normolipidemic young adults, on the contrary, were not affected. Recent studies indicate that the triglyceride-lowering effect might take some time to establish (about 8 weeks) (Hata et al., 1983; Canzi et al., 1995; Davidson et al., 1998).

A new line of thought, involves checking the impact of inulin or oligofructose on an unbalanced diet in normolipidemic subjects, a chronic problem of western society. Rat experiments demonstrated that the addition of 10% inulin or oligofructose to a fat-rich diet reduced the postprandial serum triglyceride contents, as well as the serum cholesterol content, by more than 50% compared with control groups. Enhanced triglyceride-rich lipoprotein catabolism seems to be at the basis of this observation (Kok et al., 1998a).

D. Effects on Gut Function

Inulin and oligofructose have a fecal bulking effect similar to that of pectin and guar gum (Roberfroid, 1993). Each gram of ingested inulin or oligofructose increases the fecal wet weight by 1.5–2 g. This is also reflected by an increased fecal dry weight excretion. The latter is mainly caused by an increased excretion of bacterial biomass (Gibson et al., 1995).

The stimulation of gut function also results in increased stool frequency. The increase is higher in volunteers with a low initial stool frequency. Relief of constipation has been reported with both oligofructose and inulin (Gibson et al., 1995; Kleessen et al., 1997; Menne et al., 1997; Den Hond et al., 1997). The effects on intestinal transit time are more contradictory; some researchers observed an increased and others a decreased transit time.

E. Modulation of Gut Flora Bifidogenicity

Because they are nondigestible, inulin and oligofructose reach the colon almost untouched. The colon is an energy-deficient ecosystem: the import of easily fermentable carbohydrates has a major impact on the composition and metabolic activity of its complex microflora. The latter is composed of more than 400 different kinds of bacteria and represents over 50% of the dry solids content of the colon.

Both inulin and oligofructose selectively promote the growth and metabolic activity of bifidobacteria (Fig. 2). Their bifidogenicity has been demonstrated in in vitro models and in several in vivo rat studies (Djouzi and Audrieux, 1997) and human volunteer studies (Bouhnik et al., 1994; Buddington et al., 1996; Gibson et al., 1995; Menne et al., 1997; Kleessen et al., 1997; Roberfroid et al., 1998).

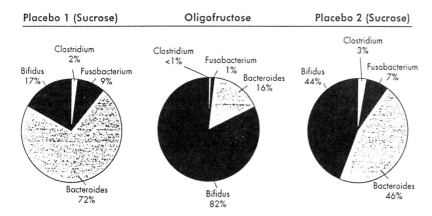

Fig. 2 Significant changes in gut flora composition after intake of oligofructose. (From Gibson et al., 1995.)

By means of in vitro experiments, the bifidogenicity of the high-DP fractions of inulin (DP > 10) has been confirmed. This fraction is fermented twice as slowly as the low-DP fraction (DP < 10). So the long-chain inulin fraction has an interesting potential for the stimulation of the metabolic activity in the distal part of the colon.

In fermentation studies, no distinction in the fermentation pattern has been observed between GF_n- and F_n-type molecules. The bifidogenic effect of an F_n-type oligofructose was confirmed by means of an in vivo study with human volunteers who were administered 8 g/day of the preparation (Menne et al., 1997).

A compilation of all the data available suggested that in the range of 4–20 g/day there is no dose effect of the administered inulin or oligofructose. However, the increase in the numbers of bifidobacteria appears to be inversely correlated with their counts at the start of the studies. A daily intake of 4 g of inulin or oligofructose is sufficient to enhance bifidobacteria (Roberfroid et al., 1998).

Many possible beneficial effects have been attributed to Bifidobacteria. Recent objective observations in the most recent years tend to support their potential health-promoting activity.

As bifidobacteria counts increased in several human feeding studies with inulin or oligofructose, a concomitant decrease in potentially pathogenic populations was observed in some studies (*Clostridium* spp., *E. coli*, and *Bacteroides* in human studies; *Salmonella* in poultry and in in vitro models; *Veillonella*, *Shigella*, and *Listeria* in in vitro models).

In experiments with gnotobiotic quails (a model for premature babies) in an isolated environment, different flora were administered. Quails administered a necrotizing enterocolitis inducing flora (comprising *Clostridium butyricum*) died. In contrast, the groups administered bifidobacteria made a complete recovery. This is a first objective demonstration of a health effect of bifidobacteria in living beings (Butel et al., 1998).

In the same set of experiments it was observed that oligofructose can enhance the effect of bifidobacteria. This effect became even more pronounced when the intestinal flora of the quails was made more complex by exposing them to normal environmental conditions (Catala et al., 1998). In addition to this, it has been recently observed that patients suffering from Crohn's disease systematically have low counts of bifidobacteria (Favier et al., 1997).

Inulin and oligofructose, being able to stimulate probiotic strains, are considered prebiotics. It appears that the combination of the two (synbiotic) has synergistic effects. Recent observations indicate that synbiotics can contribute to the health food concept (Gibson and Roberfroid, 1995).

F. Suitability for Diabetics

Both inulin and oligofructose are hydrolyzed to a negligible extent during their passage through the human mouth, stomach, and small intestine. As a consequence, both inulin and oligofructose have no influence on blood glucose level when ingested orally. This has been confirmed by many researchers, e.g., in humans by Beringer and Wenger (1955) and Sanno et al. (1984) and in rats by Takeda and Niizato (1982) and Brichard (1989).

The potential use of inulin as a food for diabetics has been known since the beginning of the twentieth century: Persia in 1905 (Lewis, 1912) recommended inulin to diabetics and stated that the product was well digested and assimilated by those people in large doses and for long periods of time. Strauss (1911) reported the feeding of 40–100 g/day of pure inulin to be very beneficial for the patient. This was also confirmed by Root and Baker (1925), McCance and Lawrence (1929), and Wise and Heyl (1931). Since then, many more applications for diabetics have been described in the literature, e.g. inulin-based diabetic bread and pastry

(Beringer and Wenger, 1955; Kuppers-Sonnenberg, 1971) and inulin-based diabetic jam (Birch and Soon, 1973).

G. Cancer Prevention

Very recent research indicates that inulin and oligofructose have a significant chemopreventive potential (Koo and Rao, 1991; Roland et al., 1994a, b, 1995, 1996; Delzenne et al., 1995b; Taper et al., 1995, 1997, 1998; Gallaher et al., 1996; Reddy et al., 1997; Rowland et al., 1998). They can prevent to a significant extent the formation of chemically induced colonic precancerous lesions in rats. They obviously delay the initiation phase of carcinogenesis.

Long-chain inulin (RAFTILINE®HP) may be more effective than the shorter-chain fructans in preventing lesion formation in the distal part of the colon. This is the place with the highest cancer incidence in humans. This may be due to slower fermentation of the long-chain molecules and hence stimulated bacterial activity in the distal part of the colon (Fig. 3) (Reddy et al., 1997).

Other experiments indicate that long-chain inulin is also able to delay the propagation phase of colon carcinogenesis in rats. Synergistic effects were observed when inulin and bifidobacteria were administered together. This is the first experimental observation of a synbiotic effect in vivo (synergistic physiological effect obtained by combining a probiotic with a prebiotic) (Fig. 4) (Rowland et al., 1998).

It was furthermore demonstrated that inulin and oligofructose inhibit the development of cancer cells transplanted in the thigh and peritoneum of mice (Taper et al., 1997, 1998). They also can reduce the development of chemically induced breast cancer in rats.

H. Increase in Mineral Absorption

Inulin and oligofructose significantly increase the intestinal absorption of calcium, iron, and magnesium in rats. This has been demonstrated and confirmed by several authors (Shimura et al., 1991; Ohta et al., 1993, 1995a, b, 1998; Delzenne et al., 1995a; Scholz-Ahrens et al., 1998).

Rat experiments revealed that the increased calcium absorption results, moreover, in increased bone mineral density (Taguchi et al., 1995; Lemort and Roberfroid 1997; Scholz-Ahrens et al., 1998). This means that the increased absorption effectively results in building up the body's calcium reserve. It was demonstrated in ovariectomized rats (a model for postmenopausal

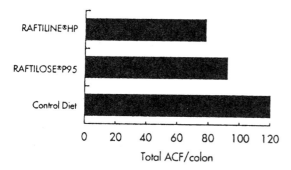

Fig. 3   Reduction in chemically induced colonic aberrant crypt foci (ACF) in rats administered either RAFTILINE®HP or RAFTILOSE®P95. ACF are biomarkers for future tumor incidence. (Adapted from Reddy et al., 1997.)

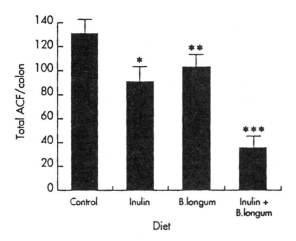

Fig. 4 Reduction in chemically induced colonic ACF by oral intake of RAFTILINE®HP and/or *Bifido-bacterium longum*. The combination of both shows synergistic effects (synbiotic effect). *p < 0.05; **p < 0.01; ***p < 0.001. (Adapted from Rowland et al., 1998.)

women) that the calcium uptake from food is improved and that bone mineral density is increased by oligofructose (Scholz-Ahrens et al., 1998).

Recently a method using stable isotopes of Ca and Mg has been validated for use in human volunteers. In analogy with rat experiments, where data on increased mineral absorption were obtained with growing animals, the experiments in humans were repeated with adolescents. This stage of life is characterized by increased mineral absorption. It was observed that the intake of 15 g/day of oligofructose (RAFTILOSE®P95) significantly increases the absorption of Ca in teenagers ($n = 11$). The magnesium absorption seemed to be modified accordingly (Van den Heuvel et al., 1998).

This is an important finding because it is in this particular period of life that humans build up their Ca reserve. The higher the peak bone mass becomes at this period of life, the more the probability of occurrence of osteoporosis in future life is reduced. In a study where healthy adult volunteers were given 40 g/day of inulin, a significant increase in Ca absorption was observed as well (Coudray et al., 1997).

These results give promising evidence that inulin and oligofructose increase Ca absorption in humans and could therefore actively contribute to the prevention of osteoporosis.

I. Intestinal Acceptability

Intestinal acceptability of nondigestible components is mainly determined by two phenomena. First, the osmotic effect leads to an increased presence of water in the colon. Smaller molecules exert a higher osmotic pressure and bring more water into the colon. This is probably the reason why sorbitol, for example, has a higher laxative potential than oligofructose (Hata and Nakajima, 1984). Second, the fermentation effect is caused by the fermentation products, mainly short chain fatty acids and gases. Slowly fermenting compounds appear to be more easily tolerated than their fast-fermenting analogs. This can explain why inulin is easier to tolerate than oligofructose.

It is difficult to distinguish between an acceptable and an unacceptable side effect of fermentation. Flatulence, for instance, is a well-known and often accepted side effect of the intake of vegetables. Dietary fibers, in general, are known and rewarded for their properties of stool softening; the progression to a laxative effect is thus small.

ORAFTI's tests and experience show that 2–6 g daily of inulin or oligofructose are easily tolerated by most people. At higher doses, flatulence may cause discomfort. Daily doses of 10–15 g cause no significant discomfort. Inulin rarely causes diarrhea (Absolonne et al., 1995). Little or no general information is available concerning the acceptability of indigestible carbohydrates in children. A test with oligofructose (Cadranel et al., 1995) has shown that daily doses of 3, 6, and 9 g of oligofructose in drinks or confectionery products cause no significant undesirable side effects in children 10–13 years old.

J. Other Nutritional Side Effects

Dietary fibers can have other unwanted side effects, such as a negative influence on vitamin or mineral absorption, allergic reactions, and an undesirable influence on the gut flora and its metabolism. No such negative effects have been found for inulin and oligofructose. On the contrary, recent research suggests that the effects on mineral absorption and gut flora are positive.

IV. USE AS FOOD INGREDIENT

Inulin and oligofructose are macronutrients. They are used either as supplements to foods or as macronutrient substitutes.

As supplements, they are added mainly for their nutritional properties. Adding inulin or oligofructose increases the dietary fiber content of the food. Such additions are usually in the range of 3–6 g/portion, in extreme cases up to 10 g. In other applications, inulin or oligofructose are added to allow a specific nutritional claim, such as regarding bifidogenic activity. In these foods, typical levels are 1–6%, leading to about 3–8 g per portion. As a macronutrient substitute, inulin is mainly used to replace fat and oligofructose to replace sugars.

The fat-replacing potential of inulin was discovered and patented by ORAFTI in 1992. Using a specific processing technique, inulin is combined with water to produce the same texture and mouthfeel as fat. This is only possible in water-based foods, such as dairy products and table spreads, and not in dry foods, such as most snacks, bakery, and confectionery products. Typically, one gram of fat is replaced by a quarter gram of inulin. Consequently, fat replacement in most foods will lead to inulin concentrations of around 2–6 g per portion.

Oligofructose has technical properties that are comparable to sugar and glucose syrups, yet nutritionally speaking it has totally different properties. The sweetness of (pure) oligofructose is about 30% that of sugar. Consequently, it is difficult to use oligofructose alone as a sugar substitute: most often it must be combined with intense sweeteners to obtain the desired sweetness level. The use of oligofructose (and inulin) is further not possible in most soft drinks and fruit jams. In such acid foods with a long shelf life, both substances are slowly hydrolyzed into fructose. Therefore oligofructose is used as a sugar substitute mainly in dairy and bakery products at levels that cause no intestinal discomfort. In practice, amounts of 2–6 g per portion are used frequently.

Based on these considerations, a committee of experts (Kolbye et al., 1992) concluded that even for a consumer at the 90th percentile, increased exposure to inulin and oligofructose is likely to be of negligible biological significance. Several hundred different food products containing inulin or oligofructose are on the market today. The most successful applications are in dairy products such as fermented milk, milk, milk drinks, and cheeses, desserts, bakery products, spreadable products, chocolate, meal replacers, bars, cereals, ice creams. This provides a solid base of experience. Most foods contain doses of 2–4 g inulin or oligofructose per portion. Others contain higher amounts. In none of these cases have acceptability problems with consumers caused the manufacturers to reconsider the formulation or labeling of the products.

V. LEGAL STATUS

A. Food Ingredients

Inulin and oligofructose are legally classified as food or food ingredients, and not as additives, in all countries where they are used. Although this seems evident if one considers the nutritional properties and the use of both substances, it has not been easy to have this legal status confirmed by many of the legal authorities in the world.

     As a consequence, neither inulin nor oligofructose is listed as an accepted food additive in the standard lists from the European Union or Codex Alimentarius. In the United States, a committee of experts convened by ORAFTI declared both inulin and oligofructose as generally recognized as safe (GRAS) in 1992 (Kolbye et al., 1992). The evaluation took all the elements shown in Table 4 into account.

B. Labeling: Ingredient List

The food laws of most countries require that a specific name be used for the ingredients list. For chicory inulin, the name inulin is a logical and legally accepted choice. For oligofructose, either fructo-oligosaccharide or oligofructose can be used, the latter being a more consumer-friendly choice.

     About 70% of chicory inulin molecules have a DP of >10. Oligosaccharides are defined as having a DP of between 2 and 10 (IUB-IUPAC, 1982). Oligofructose was defined by the AOAC as having a DP of between 2 and 10 (Hoebregs, 1997). Therefore, it is not acceptable to label inulin as oligofructose.

Table 4 Elements Taken into Consideration in the Safety Evaluation of Inulin and Oligofructose

Definitions
Production process data
Food application data
History of long-term use prior to 1958
Estimates of intake in the United States
Estimated consumption of added inulin and oligofructose by the U.S. population
Metabolism, nutritional and physiological effects
Safety of comparable carbohydrates
Food intake data
Human studies
Animal toxicity data

C. Analytical Determination

Inulin and oligofructose can be analyzed using the AOAC "fructan method" 997.08 (Hoebregs, 1997). This method measures the total of inulin plus oligofructose in any food product. The method is very specific for both substances and has proven to be both accurate and reliable. Oligofructose can be measured separately using HPLC or GC techniques (Coussement, 1995).

D. Nutrition Labeling

Inulin and oligofructose behave as dietary fibers in the human body, and therefore it is logical to classify these substances as dietary fiber. This principle has already been accepted by almost all European countries and is now being evaluated in most other countries.

   Both substances comply with the Codex Alimentarius definition of dietary fiber, which is "edible plant and animal material not hydrolyzed by the endogenous enzymes of the human digestive tract as determined by the agreed upon method" [Codex Guidelines on Nutrition Labelling CAC/GL 2-1985 (Rev. 1—1993)]. They also meet the AOAC definition of "remnants of plant cells resistant to hydrolysis by the alimentary enzymes of man" (Trowell, 1974).

   In many countries, dietary fiber is defined for labeling purposes as substances measured by a specifically prescribed analytical method. Most often, the AOAC methods are the standard. These methods do not measure inulin or oligofructose, and neither do the Englyst methods (Coussement, 1995). Therefore, the specific AOAC fructan method must be used. This method can be combined with the AOAC total dietary fiber methods (Fig. 5). It seems most logical to include inulin and oligofructose in the soluble dietary fiber group.

   The caloric value of inulin and oligofructose has been evaluated as between 1 and 1.5 kcal/g (Roberfroid et al., 1993). This scientific value, however, is often in conflict with the legal caloric values as they are prescribed for dietary fiber, e.g., in Europe (0 kcal/g) or the United States (4 kcal/g for soluble fiber, 0 kcal/g for insoluble fiber). Requests have been submitted to adapt the food laws to the scientific and nutritional values for inulin and oligofructose.

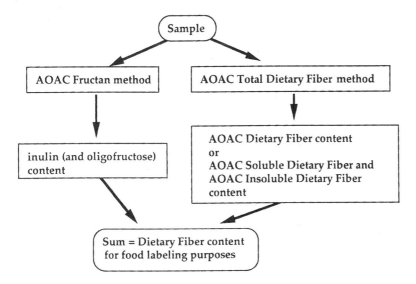

Fig. 5 Schematic presentation of AOAC methods for dietary fiber determination including inulin and oligofructose.

E. Health Claims

In Europe and Japan and several other countries, the nutritional properties of inulin and oligofructose are used to formulate health claims for food products and food supplements. An overview of these is given by Coussement (1997). In most countries, including the United States and European countries, such claims should not suggest the cure or prevention of disease, should not be misleading, and should be based on sound science.

At the moment, claims regarding the dietary fiber effects and the stimulation of bifidobacteria, by inulin or oligofructose are legally being made in many countries. In some countries, a specific authorization from the legal authorities has been obtained for specific claims. Such claims are also called nutrient-function claims or positive claims. In the United States, the Dietary Supplement Health and Education Act allows four ''statements of nutritional support'' under certain conditions. The stimulation of bifidobacteria by inulin or oligofructose can be classified among such claims.

F. Future Labeling

Inulin and oligofructose as ''novel'' dietary fibers might have significant consequences on nutrition labeling systems. In most countries these substances have caused experts to reconsider the definitions of, among others, carbohydrates, complex carbohydrates, and dietary fiber (Lee and Prosky, 1995). Furthermore, the standard nutrition labeling might not be able to cope adequately with the appearance of these nondigestible oligosaccharides. Suggestions have been made that the classification of carbohydrates be reconsidered (Cummings et al., 1997).

In the United States, the Nutrition Labeling and Education Act in principle allows ''disease-related'' claims if a substance has obtained an official authorization from FDA or a confirmation from a National Institutes of Health. This might allow more claims to be made for inulin and oligofructose relating to, e.g., osteoporosis, heart disease, or colon cancer, under the condition that the present research indications are confirmed by further research. In Europe, such claims on food products would require a fundamental change in the labeling directives.

REFERENCES

Absolonne J, Jossart M, Coussement P, Roberfroid M. Digestive acceptability of oligofructose, in Proc. First ORAFTI Research Conference, Brussels, 1995, pp 151–160.

Beringer A, Wenger R. Inulin in der Ernährung des Diabetikers. Dtsch. Zeitschr. f. Verdauungs-u. Stoffwechselkrankh., 15:268–272, 1955.

Bhattathiry EPM. Effects of polysaccharides on the biosynthesis of lipids in adult rats. Far East Med J 7(6):187–190, 1971.

Birch GG, Soon EBT. Composition and properties of diabetic jams. Confect Prod 39(2):73–76, 1973.

Bouhnik Y, Flourié B, Ouarne F, Riottot M, Bisetti N, Bornet F, Rambaud J. Effects of prolonged ingestion of fructo-oligosaccharides on colonic bifidobacteria, fecal enzymes and bile acids in humans. Gastroenterology 106(4):A598, 1994.

Brichard S. Influence de mesures nutritionnelles sur l'homéostasie glucidique du rat diabétique: Effets bénéfiques des fructo-oligosaccharides et du vanadium. UCL thesis, Brussels, 1989.

Buddington R, Williams C, Chen S, Witherly S. Dietary supplement of Neosugar alters the fecal flora and decreases activities of some reductive enzymes in human subjects. Am J Clin Nutr 63(5):709–716, 1996.

Butel M, Roland N, Hibert A, Papot F, Favre A, Tessedre A, Bensaada M, Rimbault A, Szylit O. Clostridial pathogenicity in experimental necrotising enterocolitis in gnotobiotic quails and protective role of bifidobacteria. J Med Microbiol 47:391–399, 1998.

Cadranel S, Coussement P. Tolerance study with oligofructose for school children. Proc. First ORAFTI Research Conference, Brussels, 1995, pp 217–218.

Canzi E, Brighenti F, Casiraghi M, Del Puppo E, Ferrari A. Prolonged consumption of inulin in ready-to-eat breakfast: effect on intestinal ecosystem, bowel habits and lipid metabolism. COST'92 Workshop on Dietary Fibre and Fermentation, Helsinki, 1995.

Catala I, Butel M, Bensaada M, Popot F, Tessedre A, Rimbault A, Szylit O. Oligofructose contributes to the protective role of bifidobacteria in experimental necrotising enterocolitis in quails. J Med Microbiol 48:89–94, 1999.

Coudray C, Bellanger I, Castiglia-Delavaud C, Rémésy C, Vermorel M, Rayssignuier Y. Effect of soluble or partly soluble dietary fibres supplementation on absorption and balance of calcium, magnesium, iron and zinc in healthy young men. Eur J Clin Nutr 51(6):375–380, 1997.

Coussement P. Inulin and oligofructose as dietary fiber: analytical, nutritional and legal aspects. In: Complex Carbohydrates in Foods, New York: Marcel Dekker, 1999.

Coussement P. Powerful Products. The World of Ingredients, August 1997, pp 12–17.

Cummings JH, Roberfroid MB, and members of the Paris Carbohydrate Group. Review—a new look at dietary carbohydrate: chemistry, physiology and health. Eur J Clin Nutr 51:417–423, 1997.

Davidson M, Maki K, Synecki C, Torri SA, Drennan KB. Effects of dietary inulin on serum lipids in men and women with hypercholesterolemia. Nutrition Res 18(3):503–517.

De Leenheer L, Hoebregs H. Progress in the elucidation of the composition of chicory inulin. Starch 46(5): 193–196, 1994.

Delzenne N, Kok N. Effect of non-digestible fermentable carbohydrates on hepatic fatty acid metabolism. Biochem Soc Trans 26:228–230, 1998.

Delzenne N, Kok N, Fiordaliso MF, Deboyser DM, Goethals FM, Roberfroid MR. Dietary fructo-oligosaccharides modify lipid metabolism in rats. Am J Clin Nutr 57:820s, 1993.

Delzenne N, Aertssens J, Verplaetse N, Roccaro M, Roberfroid M. Effect of fermentable fructo-oligosaccharides on energy and nutrients absorption in the rat. Life Sci 57(17):1579–1587, 1995a.

Delzenne N, Taper H, Allaeys V, De Hertogh H, Roberfroid MR. Effect of oligofructose on MNU induced mammary tumorogenesis in rats. Proc. First ORAFTI Research Conference, Brussels, 1995b, pp 275–278.

Den Hond E, Geypens B, Ghoos Y. Long-chain chicory inulin positively affects bowel habits in healthy subjects with a low stool frequency. Abstracts of NDO Symposium, Wageningen, 1997.

Djouzi Z, Andrieux C. Compared effects of three oligosaccharides on metabolism of intestinal microflora in rats inoculated with a human faecal flora. Br J Nutr 78(2):313–324, 1997.

Ellegård L, Andersson H, Bosaeus I. Inulin and oligofructose do not influence the absorption of cholesterol, and the excretion of cholesterol, Fe, Ca, Mg, and bile acids but increase energy excretion in man. A blinded, controlled cross-over study in ileostomy subjects. Eur J Clin Nutr 51:1–5, 1997.

Favier C, Neut C, Mizon A, Cortot A, Colombel J-F, Mizon J. Fecal β-D-galactosidase production and bifidobacteria are decreased in Crohn's disease. Dig Dis Sci 42:817–822, 1997.

Fiordaliso M, Kok N, Desager JP, Goethals F, Deboyser D, Roberfroid M, Delzenne N. Dietary oligofructose lowers triglycerides, phospholipids and cholesterol in serum and very low density lipoproteins of rats. Lipids 30(2):163–167, 1995.

Gallaher DD, Stallings WH, Blessing LL, Busta FF, Brady LJ. Probiotics, cecal microflora and aberrant crypts in the rat colon. J Nutr 126(5):1362–1371, 1996.

Gibson GR, Roberfroid MB. Dietary modulation of the human colonic microbiota—introducing the concept of prebiotics. J Nutr 125:1401–1412, 1995.

Gibson GR, Beatty ER, Wang X, Cummings JH. Selective stimulation of bifidobacteria in the human colon by oligofructose and inulin. Gastroenterology 108:975–982, 1995.

Hata A. The influence of Neosugar on the lipid metabolism of experimental animals. Proc. 1st Neosugar Research Conference, Tokyo, 1982.

Hata H, Nakajima K. Fructo-oligosaccharides intake and effect on digestive tract. Proc. 2nd Neosugar Research Conference, Tokyo, 1984.

Hata Y, Hara T, Oikawa T, Yamamoto M, Hirose N, Nagashima T, Torihama N, Nakajima K, Watanabe A, Yamashita M. The effect of fructo-oligosaccharides (Neosugar) on lipidemia. Geriatr Med 21: 156–167, 1983.

Hoebregs H. Fructans in foods and food products, ion-exchange chromatographic method: collaborative study. J AOAC Int 80(5):1029–1037, 1997.

Hosoya N, Dhorranintra B, Hidaka H. Utilisation of U-14C fructo-oligosaccharides in man as energy resources. J Clin Biochem Nutr 5:67–74, 1988.

IUB-IUPAC. Abbreviated terminology of oligosaccharide chains. J Biol Chem 257(7):3347–3351, 1982.

Kleessen B, Sykura B, Zunft HJ. Effect of inulin and lactose on fecal microflora, microbial activity, and bowel habit in elderly constipated persons. Am J Clin Nutr 65:1397–1402, 1997.

Knudsen KEB, Hessov I. Recovery of inulin from Jerusalem artichoke (*Helianthus tubersosus* L.) in the small intestine of man. Br J Nutr 74(1):101–113, 1995.

Kok N, Roberfroid M, Delzenne N. Dietary oligofructose modifies the impact of fructose on hepatic triacyl-glycerol metabolism. Metabolism 45(12):1547–1550, 1996a.

Kok N, Roberfroid M, Robert A, Delzenne N. Involvement of lipogenesis in the lower VLDL secretion induced by oligofructose in rats. Br J Nutr 76(6):881–890, 1996b.

Kok N, Taper HS, Delzenne NM. ''Oligofructose modulates lipid metabolism alterations induced by a fat-rich diet in rats. J Appl Tox 18(1):47–53, 1998a.

Kok N, Morgan L, Williams C, Roberfroid M, Thissen JP, Delzenne N. Insulin, glucagon-like peptide 1, glucose-dependent insulinotropic polypeptide and insulin-like growth factor I as putative mediators of the hypolipidemic effect of oligofructose in rats. J Nutr 128(7):1099–1103, 1998b.

Kolbye AC, Blumenthal H, Bowman B, Byrne J, Carr CJ, Kirschman JC, Roberfroid MB, Weinberger MA. Evaluation of the food safety aspects of inulin and oligofructose—GRAS determination. ORAFTI internal report, 1992.

Koo M, Rao V. Long-term effect of bifidobacteria and Neosugar on precursor lesions of colonic cancer in CF1 mice. Nutr Cancer 16:249–257, 1991.

Külz E. Beiträge zur Path. Therapie der Diabetes. Jahrb Tierchem 4:448, 1874.

Kuppers-Sonnenberg GA. ''Topinambur in der Diabetiker-Diät. Selecta 37:2836–2840, 1971.

Lee SC, Prosky L. International survey on dietary fiber: definition, analysis and reference materials. J AOAC Int 78(1):22–36, 1995.

Lemort C, Roberfroid M. Effect of chicory fructo-oligosaccharides on Ca balance. Abstracts of NDO Symposium, Wageningen, 1997, p. 163.

Levrat M-A, Favier M-L, Moundras C, Rémésy C, Demigné C, Morand C. Role of dietary propionic acid and bile acid excretion in the hypocholesterolemic effects of oligosaccharides in rats. J Nutr 124(4): 531–538, 1994.

Lewis HB. The value of inulin as a foodstuff. J Am Med Assoc 58:1176–1177, 1912.

McCance RA, Lawrence RD. The carbohydrate content of foods—inulin and the fructosans. Medical Research Council, Special Report Series 35, 1929, p. 58.

Menne E, Guggenbühl M, Absolonne J, Dupont A. Prebiotic effect of the (fructosyl-fructose) Fm-type inulin hydrolysate in humans. Abstracts of NDO Symposium, Wageningen, 1997, p. 164.

Norman BE, Hojer-Pedersen B. The production of fructo-oligosaccharides from inulin or sucrose using inulinase or fructosyltransferase from *Aspergillus ficuum*. Denpun Kagaku 36(2):103–111, 1989.

Ohta A, Osakabe N, Yamada K, Saito Y, Hidaka H. The influence of fructo-oligosaccharides and various other oligosaccharides on the absorption of Ca, Mg and P in rats. J Jpn Soc Nutr Food Sci 46(2): 123–129, 1993.

Ohta A, Ohtsuki M, Baba S, Adachi T, Sakata T, Sakaguchi E. Calcium and magnesium absorption from the colon and rectum are increased in rats fed fructo-oligosaccharides. J Nutr 125(9):2417–2424, 1995a.

Ohta A, Ohtsuki M, Baba S, Takizawa T, Adachi T, Kimura S. Effects of fructo-oligosaccharides on the absorption of iron, calcium and magnesium in iron deficient anemic rats. J Nutr Sci Vit 41(3):281–291, 1995b.

Ohta A, Motohashi Y, Ohtsuki M, Hirayama M, Adachi T, Sakuma K. Dietary fructo-oligosaccharides change the concentration of calbindin-D9k in the mucosa of the small and large intestine of rats. J Nutr 128:934–939, 1998.

Oku T, Tokunaga R. Improvement of metabolism: Effect of fructo-oligosaccharides on rat intestine. Proc. 2nd Neosugar Research Conference, Tokyo, 1984.

Phelps CF. The physical properties of inulin solutions. Biochem J 95:41, 1965.

Reddy DS, Hamid R, Rao CV. Effect of dietary oligofructose and inulin on colonic preneoplastic aberrant crypt foci inhibition. Carcinogenesis 18(7):1371–1374, 1997.

Roberfroid M. Dietary fiber, inulin and oligofructose: a review comparing their physiological effects. Crit Rev Food Sci Nutr 33(2):103–148, 1993.

Roberfroid M, Gibson GR, Delzenne N. (1993) Biochemistry of oligofructose, a non-digestible fructooligo-saccharide: an approach to estimate its caloric value. Nutr Rev 51(5):137–146, 1993.

Roberfroid M., Van Loo J, Gibson G. The bifidogenic nature of chicory inulin and its hydrolysis products. J Nutr 128(1):11–19, 1998.

Roland N, Nugon-Baudon L, Szylit O. Influence of dietary fibres on two intestinal transferases in rats inoculated with a whole human faecal flora. R Soc Chem 123:369–373, 1994a.

Roland N, Nugon-Baudon L, Flinois JP, Beaune P. Hepatic and intestinal cytochrome P450, glutathion-S-transferase and UDP-glucuronyltransferase are affected by six types of dietary fibre in rats inoculated with a human whole faecal flora. J Nutr 124(9):1581–1587, 1994b.

Roland N, Nugon-Baudon L, Andrieux C, Szylit O. Comparative study of the fermentative characteristics of inulin and different types of fiber in rats inoculated with a human whole fecal flora. Br J Nutr 74(2):239–249, 1995.

Roland N, Rabot S, Nugon-Baudon L. Modulation of the biogenical effects of glucosinolates by inulin and oat fibre in gnotobiotic rats inoculated with a whole human flora. Food Chem Toxicol 34:671–677, 1996.

Root H, Baker M. Inulin and artichokes in the treatment of diabetes. Arch Intern Med 36:126–145, 1925.

Rose. Neues Allg J Chem 3:217–219, 1804.

Rowland IR, Rummey CJ, Coutts JT, Lievense L. Effects of *Bifidobacterium longum* and inulin on gut bacterial metabolism and carcinogen-induced aberrant crypt foci in rats. Carcinogenesis 19(2):281–285, 1998.

Sanno T, Ishikawa M, Nozawa Y, Hoshi K, Someya K. Application of Neosugar P for diabetic subjects. The effect of Neosugar P on blood glucose. Proc 2nd Neosugar Research Conference, Tokyo, 1984.

Scholz-Ahrens K, Van Loo J, Schrezenmeir J. Oligofructose stimuliert die Femurmineralisation in Abhängigkeit von der Calciumzufuhr bei der ovariektomisierten Ratte. Symposium Deutsche Gesellschaft für Ernährungsforschung, Karlsruhe, 1998.

Shimura S, Saeki Y, Ito Y, Suzuki K, Shiro G. Effects of galacto-oligosaccahrides and fructo-oligosaccharides on mineral utilisation in rats. J Nutr Food Sci 44(4):287–291, 1991.

Strauss H. Zur verwendung inulinreicher Gemüse bei Diabetikern. Ther Gegenwart III:347–351, 1911.

Taguchi A, Ohta A, Abe M, Baba S, Ohtsuki M, Takizawa T, Yuda Y, Adachi T. Effects of fructo-oligosaccharides on bone and mineral absorption in the rat model with ovariectomized osteoporosis. Meiji Seika Kenkyu Nenpo Vol. 1994: 33, 37–43, 1995.

Takeda U, Niizato T. Metabolic effects of fructo-oligosaccharides on normal and diabetic rats. Proc. 1st Neosugar Research Conference, Tokyo, 1982.

Taper HS, Delzenne N, Tshilombo A, Roberfroid M. Dietary fructo-oligosaccharides (FOS) protect young rats against the atrophy of exocrine pancreas induced by high fructose and partial copper deficiency. Food Chem Toxicol 33(8):631–639, 1995.

Taper H, Delzenne N, Roberfroid MB. Growth inhibition of transplantable mouse tumours by non digestible carbohydrates. Int J Cancer 71:1109–1112, 1997.

Taper H, Lemort C, Roberfroid M. Inhibition effect of dietary inulin and oligofructose on the growth of transplantable mouse tumor. Anticancer Res 18:4123–4126, 1998.

Trautwein EA, Rieckhoff D, Erbersdobler HF. Dietary inulin lowers plasma cholesterol and triacylglycerol and alters biliary bile acid profile in hamsters. J Nutr (in press).

Trowell HC. Lancet 1:503, 1974.

Van den Heuvel E, Muys T, Van Dokkum W, Schaafsma G. Oligofructose stimulates calcium absorption in adolescents. Am J Clin Nutr 69:544–548, 1999.

Van Loo J, Coussement P, De Leenheer L, Hoebregs H, Smits G. On the presence of inulin and oligofructose as natural ingredients in the western diet. Crit Rev Food Sci Nutr 35(6):525–552, 1995.

Wise E, Heyl F. Failure of a diabetic to utilize inulin. J Am Pharm Soc 1931; 20(1):26–29.

37
Curdlan

Fumio Yotsuzuka
Takeda Chemical Industries, Ltd., Tokyo, Japan

I. INTRODUCTION

Curdlan is a polysaccharide produced by microbial fermentation having thermal gelling properties. This neutral and nonionic polysaccharide was incidentally discovered by Dr. Tokuya Harada during his screening process of acidic polysaccharides (1). Shortly thereafter the primary structure of the substance was found to be a linear chain of D-glucose monomers linked exclusively by β-1,3 glucosidic linkages. Because of its "curdling" property when heated in water, it was given the name curdlan (2).

Since that time the basic properties, usage, and production of curdlan have been studied by many scientists (3–6), and it was put into commercial production by Takeda Chemical Industries, Ltd. of Osaka, Japan, in 1989. Currently curdlan is approved in Japan for use as a food hydrocolloid and is listed in the "List of Existing Food Additives." Outside of Japan it is also approved for food use in South Korea and Taiwan. In December 1996 the U.S. Food and Drug Administration (FDA) approved curdlan as a direct food additive (7).

The use of curdlan has been studied in areas other than food, e.g., pharmaceutical and industrial chemical applications. In Japan, curdlan is being used as a concrete additive due to its ability to improve flowability (8–10).

II. PROPERTIES OF CURDLAN

A. Structure

Curdlan is a β-1,3 glucan. It consists of D-glucose monomers linked by β-glucosidic bonds at C_1 and C_3 to form a linear chain with no branching, as shown in Fig.1 (2,11). Curdlan molecules are reported to exist as a single chain in its dry form (12).

B. Production Method

The current commercial production of curdlan starts with the culture of *Agrobacterium biovar I* (identified as *Alcaligenes faecalis* var. *myxogenes* at time of discovery) in a medium containing glucose, nitrogen sources, and trace minerals. The first phase of the fermentation mainly involves the growth and multiplication of the cells. As this process slows down, the second phase begins, as produced curdlan accumulates in the medium. The fermentation ends when glucose is to-

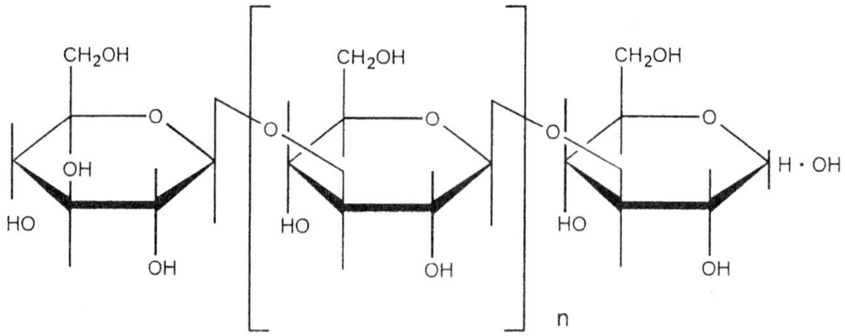

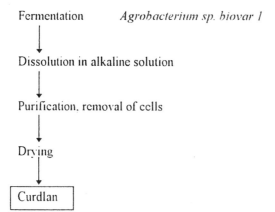

Fig. 1 Chemical structure of curdlan. (From Refs. 2, 11.)

tally consumed. Alkali is then added to the fermentation broth to dissolve curdlan before the cells are removed. The alkaline solution is purified and then dried to obtain curdlan powder (Fig. 2) (13).

C. Quality Standards

Upon approval of curdlan, FDA established its specifications as follows (7):

1. Identification: positive for curdlan
2. Assay for curdlan (calculated as anhydrous glucose): not less than 80%
3. pH of 1% aqueous suspension: 6.0–7.5
4. Lead: not more than 0.5 mg/kg
5. Heavy metals as Pb: not more than 0.002%
6. Total nitrogen: not more than 0.2%
7. Loss on drying: not more than 10%
8. Residue on ignition: not more than 6%
9. Gel strength of 2% aqueous suspension: not less than 600×10^3 dyne per cm^2
10. Aerobic plate count: not more than 10^3 per gram
11. Coliform bacteria: not more than 3 per gram

Fermentation   *Agrobacterium sp. biovar 1*

↓

Dissolution in alkaline solution

↓

Purification, removal of cells

↓

Drying

↓

Curdlan

Fig. 2 Outline of curdlan production.

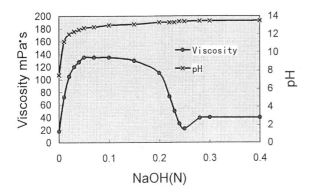

Fig. 3 Influence of sodium hydroxide concentration on viscosity of curdlan aqueous suspension.

D. Physicochemical Properties

1. Solubility

Curdlan is insoluble in water, alcohol, and most organic solvents. Curdlan is soluble in aqueous systems having a pH of 12 and higher due to dissociation of hydroxyl groups within the molecule. Alkaline solutions of curdlan are viscous, and their viscosity is dependent on the concentration of the alkali source (Fig. 3) (14,15). Curdlan is also soluble in formic acid and dimethyl sulfoxide (Table 1). Solubility of curdlan in less common solvents such as cadoxen and *N*-methyl-morpholene-*N*-oxide have been reported as well (15–16).

2. Aqueous Suspensions

Stable aqueous suspensions of curdlan can be obtained by suspending curdlan in water followed by vigorous mechanical mixing with high shear. A stable suspension is viscous under room temperature conditions. At approximately 54°C its viscosity sharply increases and reaches the maximum at 60–70°C, as shown in Fig. 4 (11,18). In the food industry, aqueous suspensions are prepared using high shear mixing devices such as cutter mixers and bowl mixers.

Table 1 Solubility of Curdlan in Various Solutions

Substance	Concentration (%)	Solubility
NaOH	0.05	+++
KOH	0.05	+++
Na_3PO_4	0.05	++
HCOOH	100	++
$OS(CH_3)_2$	100	++
$CO(NH_2)_2$	Saturated	+
$SC(NH_2)_2$	Saturated	+
KSCN	25	+
KI	25	+

Source: Ref. 15.

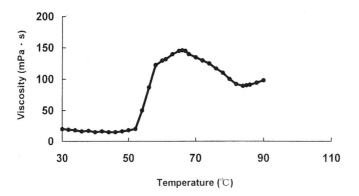

Fig. 4   Effect of temperature on viscosity of curdlan aqueous suspension.

3.   Gels

Gelation of curdlan occurs by heating its aqueous suspension. There are two types of thermally induced curdlan gels. The high-set gel, formed by heating the suspension to $\geq 80°C$, is a thermo-irreversible gel (19). The low-set gel is created by heating a curdlan suspension to approximately $60°C$ and then cooling it to below $40°C$. This gel is reversible, similar to agar-agar and gelatin gels (20). A schematic diagram of the thermal gelation of curdlan is shown in Fig. 5.

Two types of curdlan gels are formed by way of alkali solution. When an alkali solution of curdlan is either neutralized by acid or dialyzed, a gel forms. This type of gel is called a neutralized gel. The other type of gel—not utilized in the food industry—forms when calcium or magnesium ions are added to an alkali solution (11,14,21,22). Figure 6 shows the various pathways of gelation of curdlan. The low-set gel and neutralized gel are transformed to irreversible high-set gels once they are heated to $\geq 80°C$.

In most food applications, curdlan exists in the high-set gel form. Hereafter, the properties of curdlan gel are assumed to be those of the high-set gel, unless otherwise indicated.

The low-set curdlan gel has been reported to be a result of hydrogen bonds between curdlan micelles, while the ultra structure of the high-set gel results from water entrapment

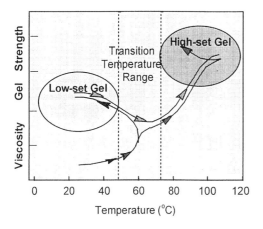

Fig. 5   Schematic diagram of thermal viscosity increase and gelation of curdlan. (Modified from Ref. 15.)

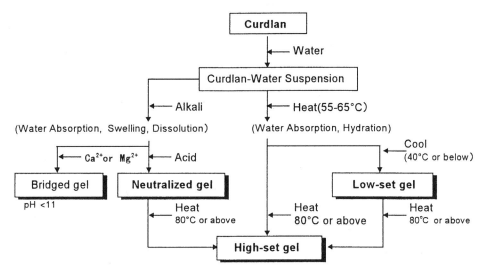

Fig. 6 Various pathways of curdlan gelation.

within a three-dimensional network consisting of curdlan micelles linked by hydrophobic bonds (15,20–24).

The texture of curdlan gel is often described to be intermediate in character between the firm and brittle agar-agar gel and the soft and elastic gelatin gel (Fig. 7) (25). A 1–2% curdlan gel produced by heating a deaerated stable suspension in water at 100°C has a firmness similar to that of gelatin desserts. Higher concentrations of curdlan yield firmer gels.

4. Parameters Affecting Gel Formation

a. Heating Temperature and Time. Gel strength measurements of gels obtained by heating aqueous curdlan suspension reveal that the gel becomes noticeably stronger when the heating temperature is $\geq 80°C$ (Fig. 8) (19). Gel strength is measured as breaking stress at 20°C. This trend is observed for heating temperatures of up to 130°C. Longer heating times produce stronger gels, especially as heating temperature increases (Fig. 9) (25).

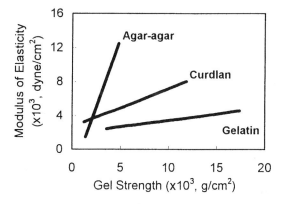

Fig. 7 Comparison of texture properties of gels of agar-agar, curdlan, and gelatin. (From Ref. 25.)

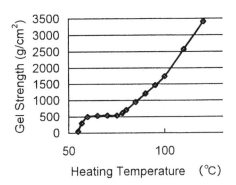

Fig. 8 Effect of heating temperature on curdlan gel strength (3% curdlan, 10 min heating time). (From Ref. 19.)

b. Curdlan Concentration. Up to approximately 5%, gel strength increases almost proportionately to the curdlan concentration (Fig. 10) (18,24,25).

c. Effect of pH. Curdlan is capable of producing strong gels within a wide pH range of 2–10 (11,18,19,26). The gel strength of curdlan within pH 4–10 is relatively consistent, while at a pH <4 it becomes stronger (Fig. 11). Exposing a gel prepared at neutral pH to buffer solutions having different acidity quickly renders the pH of the gel to that closer to the buffer solution. However, no decrease in gel strength is observed.

d. Influence of Coexisting Ingredients. In general, curdlan gel formation is negatively influenced by the presence of competing ingredients in the system, especially when the ingredients are present at higher levels. Sucrose, for instance, at ≥30% has a detrimental effect on gel strength. The influence of glucose or fructose is significantly smaller (Fig. 12) (18). The influence of salt is small when present at levels typically found in food systems. However, at higher levels it reduces the curdlan gel strength significantly; at 4% it lowers the gel strength to almost one third (Fig. 13) (18). The effect of other inorganic salts has been studied quite extensively, but

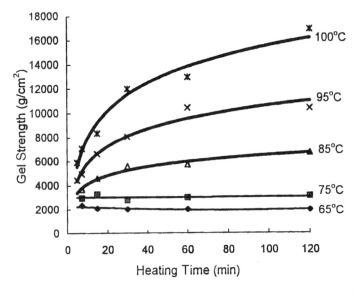

Fig. 9 Effect of heating time on curdlan gel strength (4% curdlan). (From Ref. 25.)

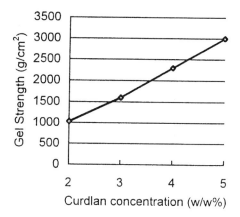

Fig. 10 Effect of curdlan concentration on gel strength (10 min, 100°C).

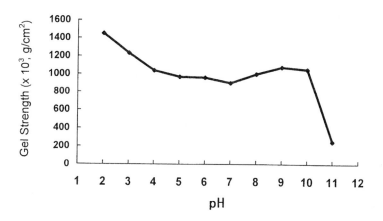

Fig. 11 Effect of pH on gel strength (2% curdlan).

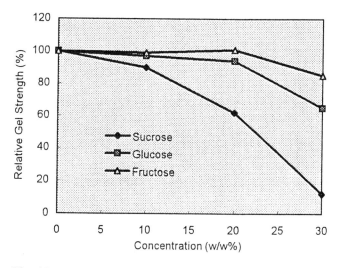

Fig. 12 Effects of sugars on gel strength (2% curdlan).

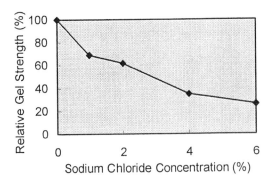

Fig. 13 Effect of salt (NaCl) on gel strength (2% curdlan).

other than borate, which substantially increases gel strength, their effects are not as significant (11,19).

Starches contribute, to weaker gels but they are the most effective in reducing syneresis of curdlan gels (18,26–28).

Curdlan is very compatible with fats and oils. A curdlan gel having a high fat or oil content can be produced utilizing the thermal gelation properties. For instance, a system consisting of 3% curdlan, 24% refined corn oil, and 73% water can be gelled without a problem. This gel can be dried to obtain a dry system having 85% oil, which can be reconstituted to regain its gel state (29). An emulsified system with up to 30% fat or oil and 2–3% curdlan can be stored frozen if starch is added for prevention of syneresis during the freeze-thaw cycle. Curdlan aqueous systems with other gelling substances or hydrocolloids, such as proteins and gums, normally produce gels weaker than those of pure curdlan systems. This is postulated to be due to mutual interference of the gel network.

5. Freeze-Thaw Stability

The strength and structure of the curdlan gel is maintained even after the freeze-thaw cycle, even though some syneresis is observed. This property is not found with similar gelling agents such as agar-agar, konjac mannan, and carrageenan (Table 2) (26).

6. Prevention of Syneresis of Gels

Syneresis must be controlled in food systems relying on the gel structure of curdlan. Syneresis is severe, especially after a freeze-thaw cycle. The amount of water released increases with higher heating temperatures and decreases with increasing curdlan. Starch is most effective in preventing syneresis of curdlan gels (18,26,28). Addition of starch at a 10% level reduces the release of water to a negligible level, but at the expense of altered texture and mouthfeel. Typically 4–7% starch is added. All types of starch, including native starch, are capable of effectively controlling syneresis. However, in order to avoid retrogradation during storage and processing, waxy corn starch (Table 3) or modified starches are more appropriate choices. Addition of these starches can also be utilized to control syneresis of the curdlan gel upon retort processing. Tannin is also known to reduce syneresis of curdlan gels (22).

E. Physiological and Biological Properties

Like agar-agar, curdlan is nutritionally inert. On an anhydrous basis curdlan contains 96% total dietary fiber when determined according to the AOAC enzymatic-gravimetric method.

Table 2 Influence of One Freeze-Thaw Cycle on Syneresis and Strength of Gels of Curdlan, Carrageenan, Agar-Agar, and Konjac

Gelling agent	Concentration (w/w%)	Storage at 4°C for 20 hours before freezing		After freezing and thawing	
		Breaking stress (g/cm^2)	Syneresis (%)	Breaking stress (g/cm^2)	Syneresis (%)
Curdlan	2	493	20.6	504	35.0
	4	2190	10.3	2496	20.6
Carrageenan	2	810	1.5	163	na
	3.5	2307	1.4	509	na
Agar-agar	1	463	3.6	0	na
	3	2409	0.6	188	na
Konjac	2	688	8.9	1434	18.6
	3.5	2312	10.3	6010	21.0

Source: Ref. 26.

na = syneresis could not be measured due to excessive release of water from gels.

There remains a lot to be clarified about the physiological functions of curdlan in animals and humans. One can assume that it functions quite differently from the most common fiber, cellulose, as its structure is a β-1,3 glucan, a well-known immune stimulant. A recent study reported that when curdlan was combined at 5% in a high-cholesterol diet and fed to rats, increased excretion of fecal neutral sterols and fecal bile acids were observed. In the same study, rats fed with curdlan had increased cecum weight and cecal content having significantly lower pH. Curdlan was also found to selectively increase bifidobacterium in the cecum, suggesting the possibility of improved microbial flora in the later part of the digestive tract (30,31). The same research group demonstrated low-density lipoprotein (LDL) cholesterol reduction when acid-hydrolyzed curdlan is orally administered to rats (J. Shimizu, unpublished).

Antitumor activity of curdlan or its derivatives has been reported in a number of studies. In 1978, Sasaki et al. (32) reported that curdlan administered through daily intraperitoneal injections of 5–50 mg/kg for 10 days demonstrated inhibitory activity against subcutaneously implanted sarcoma 180. It also exhibited very high activity at doses of 60 and 100 mg/kg as a single intraperitoneal injection 7 days after the initial subcutaneous implantation of sarcoma 180. The mechanism of the curdlan activity was reported to be host mediated (32). In a further study by Sasaki et al. (33) it was found that in vitro incubation of mice serum treated with curdlan rendered peritoneal macrophages from untreated mice cytotoxic to tumor cells. Two

Table 3 Effect of Waxy Corn Starch on Syneresis of Curdlan Gels

Waxy corn starch(%)	2% curdlan gel stored at 4°C for 20 hours	4% curdlan gel stored at 4°C for 20 hours	2% curdlan gel after freeze-thawing	2% curdlan gel after freeze-thawing
0	20.6(%)	17.3(%)	35(%)	20.6(%)
2.5	5.61	8.7	8.68	8.42
5	2.12	3.99	1.39	2.58
10	0.09	0.21	0.32	0.27

Source: Ref. 26.

direct activators, a peptide and a peptidoglycan, were isolated from the mice serum (33). A similar effect of curdlan has been reported on shorter-chain curdlan obtained by acid hydrolysis (32).

Morikawa et al. (34) confirmed that curdlan administration to mice activates polymorphonuclear (PMN) leukocytes, rending them cytotoxic against mammary carcinoma cells in vitro. Kasai et al. (35) reported that, in the presence of curdlan, mice PMN had a strong cytotoxic effect against sarcoma 180 cells and inhibited the growth of tumor cells both in vitro and in vivo.

At least two studies so far indicate that oral administration of curdlan enhances the immune functions of fish. A study by Yano et al. (36) involved oral administration of curdlan to carp prior to infecting the fish with *Edwardsiella tarda* and *Aeromonas hydrophilia*. The study reported that when curdlan was fed at 100 mg/kg in the diet for 3 days, the survival rate of fish infected with *E. tarda* increased significantly compared to the control. Curdlan was also found to be responsible for an increase in the phagocytic activity of head kidney phagocytes and in complement activation capability. Complement activation was found to be greater than for fungus derived β-1,3 glucans with β-1,6 glucosidic side chains, such as scleroglucan and schyzophyllan (37). Amemura et al. (37) conducted a similar study using flounder. Their study involved the oral administration of curdlan prior to infection by *E. tarda* as well as the oral administration of curdlan with formalin-killed *E. tarda* cells (FKC). The study reported that the survival rate of the fish increased when curdlan is fed prior to infection and that FKC enhanced the effect of curdlan.

III. SAFETY OF CURDLAN

For the most part, toxicity studies conducted to assess the safety of curdlan are not publicized but are submitted to FDA during the food additive–petitioning process. Upon approval of curdlan as a direct food additive, the FDA concluded as follows: "Curdlan lacks specific toxicity and the producing organism, *Alcaligenes faecalis* var. *myxogenes*, is non-pathogenic and non-toxicogenic, and there is a history of safe consumption of similar glucose polymers in food. Based on this information, the agency concludes that the proposed food use in curdlan is safe" (7). The safety of curdlan is also confirmed by the Joint FAO/WHO Expert Committee on Food Additives of the United Nations.

IV. FOOD APPLICATIONS OF CURDLAN

The applications of curdlan in food systems can be categorized in two types. One application involves the usage of curdlan in regular food systems, where it is added directly as is at low usage levels (<1%). The other is involved in the creation of new types of food products requiring higher usage levels and careful preparation of curdlan gel, which is the building block of the food structure in this type of application.

A. Curdlan Usage in Conventional Food Systems

When used in common food systems, curdlan is added directly in its powder, predispersed, or dissolved form in order to improve texture, water-holding capacity, thermal stability, yield, and freeze-thaw stability. This type of usage does not involve special techniques, nor does it require modification of the existing manufacturing process of the food product because curdlan can be added along with other ingredients. In addition, when curdlan is used for this purpose, the amount used in the food is low, with addition levels often being 0.5% or less (Table 4). This type of application does not call for the prior preparation of the curdlan gel. In food systems, however, curdlan particles are evenly dispersed throughout and develop as tiny gel particles after heat processing. These gel particles are deemed to behave similarly to prepared curdlan

Table 4 Usage of Curdlan in Conventional Food Products

| Applications | Objective of adding curdlan | | Use level and method |
	Direct function	Advantages	
Major			
Processed meat and poultry	Texture modification	Maximum moisture retention at processing temperature	0.1–1%
	Water binding	Minimized cook and processing loss(yield increase)	Added dry or predispersed in pickling or marinade
	Emulsion stabilization	Consistent firmness, juiciness, and clasticity	
	Fat replacement and mimicking	Heat and freeze-thaw stability	
Batter and coating systems	Texture modification	Consistent tender and juicy texture of substrate	0.1–1%
	Water holding and entrapment	Improved batter pickup and cook loss	Added dry or predispersed
	Film formation (water and oil barrier)	Heat and freeze-thaw stability	
	Viscosity agent		
Noodles and pasta	Texture modification	Improved firmness and clasticity	0.2–1%
		Minimized cook loss and softening	Added dry or predispersed/dissolved in alkali (oriental noodles)
		Improved processing and shaping qualities	
Other			
Sauces and dressings	Texture modification	Fuller mouthfeel	0.2–1%
	Viscosity agent	Heat and freeze-thaw stability(retort stable)	Can be added as powder but predispersion is preferred
	Taste and flavor modification	Adds thixotropic property, less stickiness	
	Fat replacement	Delayed release of sharp acid and saltiness	
Baked goods	Texture modification	Added moistness	0.2–1%
	Fat replacement	Improved shaping and processing qualities	Added dry or predispersed in water

gels. The water absorption and holding capacities of curdlan upon thermal gelation contributes to benefits such as tender texture, fuller mouthfeel, and increased processing and cooking yield.

1. Processed Meat and Poultry Products

Curdlan is capable of improving the quality of injected meat and poultry products, such as bacon, ham-type products, and turkey breasts. The viscosity of curdlan aqueous suspension increases significantly between 50 and 60°C and reaches a maximum at 65°C due to water absorption and swelling of the curdlan particles. In a model system using ground pork and water or pickling solution, it was confirmed that pork meat starts to release water when the temperature goes beyond 40°C, while curdlan starts to absorb the moisture coming from meat at 50°C up to around 70°C (Fig. 14) (39,40). Upon rheological measurements on the model system, firmness, springiness, and chewiness increased with curdlan addition, while cohesiveness did not seem to be influenced (Fig. 15). This demonstrates that curdlan is capable of improving texture and production yield of commercial injected or marinated meat products (40). Curdlan has also been successfully used in substrates of deep fat fried poultry and meat products.

2. Batters and Breadings

The thermal gelling property of curdlan can be used effectively in batter systems. In this application, curdlan can contribute to improved texture, increase batter pick-up and yield, and minimize texture alteration due to freeze-thawing and reheating. It is also capable of forming a barrier and minimizing oil pick-up during deep fat frying. Curdlan can be combined with other ingredients prior to the addition of water, but in a high-solid system it is recommended to prehydrate

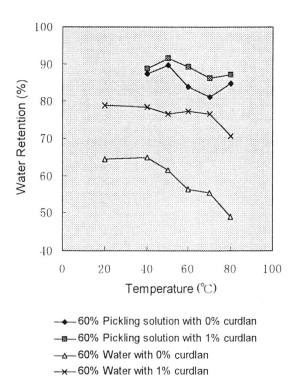

—◆— 60% Pickling solution with 0% curdlan
—▣— 60% Pickling solution with 1% curdlan
—△— 60% Water with 0% curdlan
—✕— 60% Water with 1% curdlan

Fig. 14 Effect of curdlan on the holding capacity of ground pork. (From Ref. 39.)

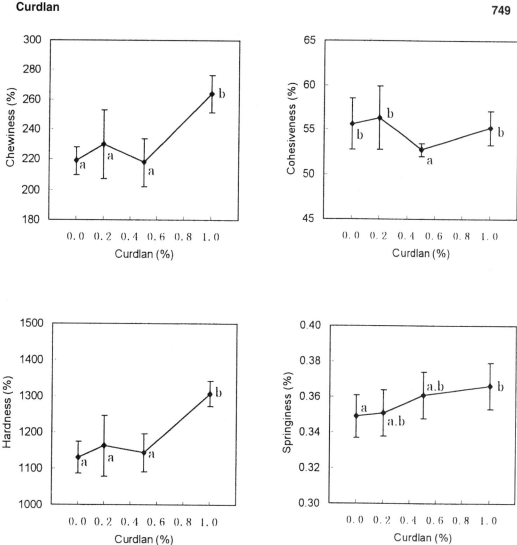

Fig. 15 Effects of curdlan on the textural parameters of meat gel heated at 75°C for 60 minutes. (From Ref. 39.)

curdlan to avoid competition for water with other ingredients. It can be used as an ingredient in pre–dust coatings as well.

3. Fat Replacement

Because of the ability of curdlan to produce thermo-irreversible gels having firmness, elasticity, and lubricity resembling those of fat, it is being studied as an ingredient in fat-replacement systems (41,42). A formulation and processing method for a frankfurter-type cooked sausage are shown in Table 5 and Fig. 16. In this prototype formulation, the fat-replacement system consists of 10% modified tapioca starch, 8% maltodextrin, 2% curdlan, and 80% water. The system can be used to replace the fat added during production of sausage. The fat-replacement ingredients either can be combined before addition to the main system to mimic the appearance of fat or can be added together with other ingredients. The incorporation technique does not

Table 5 Formulation for Pork Sausage Using Curdlan as a Key Fat-Replacing Ingredient

	Low-fat formulation	Full-fat formulation
Fresh chopped pork (lean)	50.0 parts	50.0 parts
Pork fat	na	20.0
Water	36.0	20.0
Potato starch	2.5	2.5
Modified tapioca starch	2.0	na
Salt	2.0	2.0
Dextrose	2.0	2.0
Sodium caseinate	1.8	1.8
Maltodextrin	1.6	na
Curing agent[a]	0.6	0.6
Spices	0.6	0.6
Smoke flavor	0.5	0.5
Curdlan	0.4	na
Total	100.0	100.0
Total fat(%)	2–3%	18 to 19%
Calories per 100 g	95	227

[a] Curing agent: sodium phosphates, 87%; sodium ascorbate, 11%; sodium nitrite, 2%.
Source: Ref. 39.

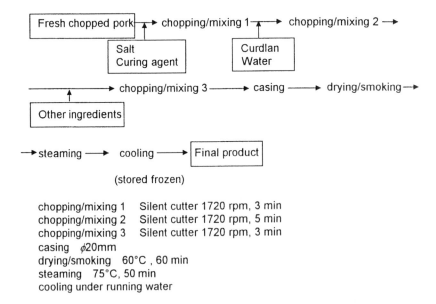

chopping/mixing 1   Silent cutter 1720 rpm, 3 min
chopping/mixing 2   Silent cutter 1720 rpm, 5 min
chopping/mixing 3   Silent cutter 1720 rpm, 3 min
casing ϕ20mm
drying/smoking   60°C , 60 min
steaming   75°C, 50 min
cooling under running water

Fig. 16 Production of low-fat sausages using curdlan.

influence the textural and organoleptic properties of the end product, which were very similar in the two cases. Curdlan was found to be an effective fat replacer in meat patties as well. For this application, one-to-one replacement of the fat results in an excessively moist product. It was found that addition of 0.25% curdlan and 5% water to lean meat is sufficient to replace fat present at 20% in the full-fat meat patty formulation. Low- or nonfat processed meat products formulated with curdlan as a key ingredient were found to have similar texture and mouthfeel properties to their full-fat counterparts. Currently in the United States curdlan is not approved for use in meat and poultry products according to Standards of Identity but can be used in nonstandardized products or those having reduced-fat claims covered by USDA Policy Memo 123 and 121B.

4. Noodles

In Japan, curdlan is actively used in noodle products as a texture modifier. The benefits of curdlan are increased firmness and elasticity as well as prevention of overcooking and starch loss. Curdlan can be added in powder form at levels ranging between 0.1 and 1.0% (flour weight). Recently it was found that the effect of curdlan is even greater when it is added predissolved in alkali. Tribasic sodium phosphate or tribasic potassium phosphate are the alkali sources typically used for this purpose.

5. Surimi-Based Formed Seafood

Curdlan can be used in surimi-based seafood products to improve texture or to partially replace the surimi. Alkaline solutions or suspensions (pH $\geq$ 11) with relatively high concentration of curdlan ($\sim$5%) have the appropriate viscosity to directly replace surimi. Advantages of replacing surimi include higher product yield, minimization of surimi cost fluctuations, and production of high water-added products without starch. Starch-free surimi products have a tender and elastic texture and longer shelf life, since the shelf life of surimi products is often dictated by starch degradation.

6. Freeze-Dried Foods

Curdlan has been demonstrated to be effective in improving freeze-dried foods. It improves the rehydration time and also the textural qualities of freeze-dried meat and seafood products at 0.5–1.0% levels added along with other ingredients. This is thought to be due to the capacity of the curdlan gels to retain their network structure even after loss of water.

7. Sauces and Gravies

Curdlan adds thixotropic properties to fluids in which viscosity is based on pseudoplastic viscosity agents such as xanthan and guar gum. It is also effective in providing body to starch- or flour-based sauces and gravies. The recommended addition level for this usage is 0.3–0.5%.

B. Foods Using Curdlan Gels

Curdlan gels are irreversible and tolerant to freeze-thawing and extreme heating conditions. These characteristics make curdlan suitable to create various types of foods relying on its gel structure. Another advantage of the curdlan gel is that it has no taste, odor, or color of its own and therefore can be easily flavored and colored as needed. Also, curdlan gels can be used to reinforce the strength of weakly structured systems, such as tofu products (Table 6). In this type of application where curdlan is used as the building block of the food, the usage level is relatively

Table 6 Food Products Relying on Curdlan Gels

Application	Benefit of adding curdlan	Usage level
Imitation meat and poultry products and seafood delicacies	Gels mimic meat structure (vegetarian sausage and ham) and texture	3–10%
	Gels also mimic texture of seafood delicacies such as crabmeat and abalone	
	Provides stability under extreme temperature conditions	
	Partial or complete functional replacement of protein sources such as egg whites and soy	
	Products can be used in vegetarian diets	
Tofu products	Products can be frozen or retorted	0.5–5%
	Improved textural attributes	
	Improved shaping qualities	
Jelly-type desserts	Texture can have both resilient and spreadable characteristics	0.5–3%
	Freeze-thaw stable	
	Can be served both hot or cold	
Fillings and sheet-film type foods	Can be made heat stable, without boil-out during cooking or processing (bake stability)	0.5% or above
	Gelation of spreads	
	Freeze-thaw stable	

Table 7 Formulation for Meatless Sausages Using Curdlan (based on 100 parts water)

1. Curdlan Suspension	
Warm water(70 to 72°C)	60 parts
Water(30 to 32°C)	40
Ice	17.8
Curdlan	7.5
Modified corn starch	4
Calcium carbonate	0.7
Subtotal	130 parts
2. Flavor and other ingredients	
Egg white powder	6 parts
Modified corn starch	5
Salt	2.8
Skimmed milk powder	2
Apple vinegar	2
Curdlan	1
Sugar	1
Soy sauce	1
Flavor enhancers	0.76
Sausage flavor	0.3
Smoke powder	0.3
Carmine color	0.3
Spice blend	0.2
Onion powder	0.1
Caramel	0.05
Subtotal	22.81
Total	152.81

high, ranging between 1 and 10%. Special procedures for preparation of curdlan suspensions and gels are required.

1. Vegetarian Meat and Seafood Substitutes

The popularity of vegetarian foods has increased rapidly as a result of growing consumer demand for more healthful foods and ethnic eating habits. Curdlan can be processed to form gels mimicking the texture and mouthfeel of meat or seafood (Table 6).

The formulation and procedure for the manufacture of meatless sausages are shown in Table 7 and Fig. 17. The process involves the preparation of a stable curdlan suspension, developing high viscosity through heating to 50°C and then cooling to 35°C. The entrapped air is removed under vacuum so that a uniform structure can be obtained after heating. The heating temperature should be high enough to maximize the gelling capabilities of curdlan at the given

(In silent cutter type equipment)

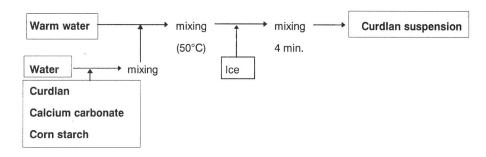

(in mixer, preferably with vacuum)

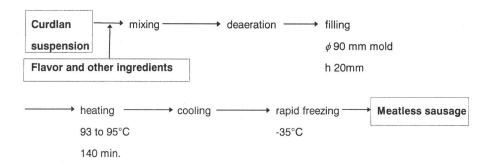

Content of key ingredients in finished product

Curdlan　　　　　　: 5.6%

Modified corn starch : 5.9%

Egg white powder　 : 3.9%

Fig. 17 Production method of meatless sausages.

concentration. In this case, the curdlan concentration in the final product is 5.5%. Because curdlan does not contribute any calories, the product is also low in calories—approximately 50 kcal/100 g.

By combining gels having different degree of gelation and coarseness, texture can be adjusted to match the texture of various types of meat or poultry products. Curdlan gels can be also used to mimic the texture of seafood, such as abalone, squid, and crab meat. Shown in Table 8 and Fig. 18 are the formulation and manufacturing procedure for a crab substitute using curdlan. This product can be manufactured using a regular production line for surimi-based imitation crab meat. The key in this application is to bring the rheological properties of the curdlan suspension close to those of surimi, and therefore textural adjustments are necessary using ingredients such as other gums and cellulose. Curdlan is incorporated predispersed in an aqueous alkaline condition to obtain the desired viscosity.

2. Tofu Products

Tofu cannot be frozen or retorted due to protein denaturation. Replacing part of the soy milk with a curdlan aqueous suspension results in tofu products that are freeze-thaw and retort stable. Curdlan can also be used to reinforce the fragile structure of tofu, which enables shaping of products in unique ways, such as tofu noodles. Tofu noodles using curdlan are currently commercially produced in Japan and Korea.

Table 8 Formulation for a Vegetarian Crabmeat Substitute Using Curdlan

	Percent
1. Main structure	
Water	50.82
Ice	25
Microcrystalline cellulose preparation	6.0
Modified starch	4.7
Curdlan	4.1
Tribasic sodium phosphate dodecahydrate	0.6
10% lactic acid solution	1.85
Calcium carbonate	1.0
Sugar	2.4
Crab flavor	2.2
Salt	1.0
Flavor enhancers	0.33
Total	100.0
2. Coloring structure	
Water	55.3
Ice	30
Curdlan	2.8
Modified starch	2.0
Microcrystalline cellulose preparation	2.0
Tribasic sodium phosphate dodecahydrate	0.4
10% lactic acid solution	1.3
Beta-carotene colorant	6.2
Total	100.0

Main structure (to be done using a high-shear mixer under vacuum)

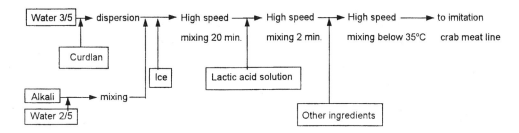

Colored structure (to be done using a high-shear mixer under vacuum)

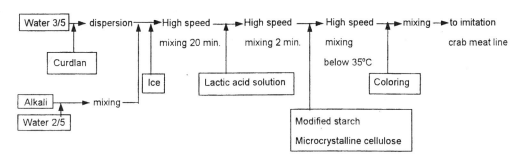

Fig. 18   Production method of vegetarian crabmeat substitute.

3.   Jelly-Type Confectionery

Curdlan gels can be directly utilized and flavored to create jelly-type food products. They can be produced using the thermal gelling process alone or by combining neutralized gelling and heat. Neutralized gels have a smoother texture than heat-induced gels. Jelly-type food products made with curdlan can be served either hot or cold and can also be stored frozen.

   In addition to the food products mentioned above, the gel structure of curdlan can be used in various types of unique applications, such as edible films and packaging, sheeted foods, and edible coolants.

REFERENCES

1.   T Harada, M Masada, K Fujimori, I Maeda. Production of a firm, resilient gel-forming polysaccharide by a mutant of *Alcaligenes faecalis* var. *myxogenes* 10C3. Agric Biol Chem 30:196–198, 1966.
2.   T Harada, A Misaki, H Saito, Curdlan: a bacterial gel-forming β-1,3-glucan. Arch Biochem Biophys 124:292–298, 1968.
3.   T Harada. Special bacterial polysaccharides and polysaccharases. Biochem Soc Symp 48:97–116, 1983.
4.   KR Phillips, HG Lawford. Curdlan: its properties and production in batch and continuous fermentation. Prog Ind Microbiol 18:201–229, 1983.
5.   HG Lawford, KR Phillips, JE Keenan, W Orts. The effect of agitations and mixing on curdlan production: Proc Bio Expo 305–320, 1986.
6.   T Harada, M Terasaki, A Harada. Curdlan: Industrial Gums, 3rd ed. Academic Press, Inc., 1993, pp 427–445.

7. Fed. Reg. 61, No. 242, 65941–65942 (Dec. 16, 1996).

8. J Sakamoto, Y Matsuoka, T Shindoh, S Tangtermsirikul, an application of super workable concrete to construction of actual structures. Trans Jpn Concrete Inst 13:41–48, 1991.

9. M Hayakawa, Y Matsuoka, K Yokota. Application of super-workable concrete in the construction of 70 story building in Japan: Second CANMET-ACI International Conference on Advances in Concrete Technology, 1995, pp 381–397.

10. Y Matsuoka, T Shindoh, K Yokota, S Kusui. Property of β-1,3-glucan (curdlan) as a viscosity agent for super-workable concrete. Fifth CANMET-ACI International Conference on Superplasticizers and Other Chemical Admixtures in Concrete, 1997, pp 475–483.

11. I Nakanishi, S Kusui, K Kimuru, K Ohnishi, T Kanamaru. Studies on curdlan-type polysaccharide. II. Physical and chemical properties of curdlans 13140 and 13127. J Takeda Res Lab 51:99–108, 1992.

12. H Saito, M Yokoi. High resolution ^{13}C NMR study of (1-3)-β-D-glucans in the solid state: DMSO-induced conformational change and conformational characterization by spin-relaxation measurements. Bull Chem Soc Jpn 62:392–398, 1989.

13. I Nakanishi, K Kimura, T Kanamaru. Studies on curdlan-type polysaccharide I. Industrial production of curdlan-type polysaccharide. J Takeda Res Lab 51:99–108, 1992.

14. A Konno, H Kimura. Gel formation of curdlan and Ca^{++} in aqueous alkaline solution. Kinran Junior College Kenkyu Shi 1992, pp 173–182.

15. S Sato, K Okumura, T Harada. Properties of curdlan and food applications (in Japanese). New Food Ind 20:49–57, 1978.

16. I Hirano, Y Einaga, H Fujita. Curdlan (bacterial β-1,3-glucan) in a cadoxen-water mixture: Polym J 11:901–904, 1979.

17. H Chanzy, B Chmpitazi, A Pegny. Solutions of polysaccharides in N-methylmorpholine N-oxide(MMNO). Carbohydr Polym 2:35–42, 1982.

18. Y Nakao, K Suzuki. Curdlan, properties and applications to food. Inte Food Ingredients 5:35–39, 1994.

19. I Maeda, H Saito, M Masada, A Misaki, T Harada. Properties of gel formed by heat treatment of curdlan, a bacterial β-1,3 glucan. Agric Biol Chem 31:1184–1188, 1967.

20. A Konno, H Kimura, T Nakagawa, T Harada. Gel Formation of curdlan (in Japanese). Nippon Nogeikagaku Kaishi 52(6):247–250, 1978.

21. T Harada, S Sato. Curdlan, properties, production and applications (in Japanese). Hakko Kogyo 36: 86–97, 1978.

22. T Harada, S Sato, A Harada. Curdlan. Bull Kobe Women's Univ 20(2):143–164, 1987.

23. T Harada. Curdlan, conformation and physical properties (in Japanese). New Food Ind 29:79–87, 1987.

24. A Konno, Y Azechi, H Kimura. Properties of curdlan gel. Agric Biol Chem 43:101–104, 1979.

25. H Kimura, S Moritaka, M Misaki. Polysaccharide 13140: a new thermo-gelable polysaccharide. J Food Sci 38:668–671, 1973.

26. Y Nakao, A Konno, T Taguchi, T Tawada, H Kasai, J Toda, M Terasaki. Curdlan: properties and application to foods. J Food Sci 56(3):769–776, 1991.

27. K Ishida, I Shiga, Y Yokoo. Textural characterization of curdlan 13140-starch gel (in Japanese). Nippon Shokuhin Kogyo Gakkaishi 25:673–676, 1978.

28. K Ishida, T Takeuchi. Starch to repress syneresis of curdlan gel. Agric Biol Chem 45:1409–1412, 1981.

29. Y Kanzawa, F Takahashi, T Harada, A Harada. Ability of curdlan gel to hold hydrophobic substance (in Japanese). Kasei-gaku Zasshi 38:363–368, 1987.

30. J Shimizu, S Innami. Effects of curdlan and gellan gum on lipid concentrations of serum and liver, fecal steroid excretion and gastrointestinal function in rats fed a hypercholesterolemic diet (in Japanese). J Agric Sci Tokyo Nogyo Daigaku 42(1):41–47, 1997.

31. J Shimizu, N Dobashi, K Kudo, M Wada, K Takita, S Innami. Effects of curdlan administration on cecum microbial flora in rats (in Japanese). Abstr 51st Annual Conf Jpn Soc Nutr Food Sci 51:139, 1997.

32. T Sasaki, N Abiko, Y Sugino, K Nitta. Dependence on chain length of antitumor activity of (1-3)-

b-D-glucan from *Alcaligenes faecalis* var. *myxogenes* IFO13140, and its acid-degraded products. Cancer Res 38:379–383, 1978.

33. T Sasaki, M Tanaka, H Uchida. Effect of serum from mice treated with antitumor polysaccharide on expression of cytotoxicity by mouse peritoneal macrophages. J Pharm Dyn 5:1012–1016, 1982.

34. K Morikawa, R Takeda, M Yamazaki, D Mizuno. Inductions of tumoricidal activity of polymorphonuclear leukocytes by a linear β-1,3-D-glucan and other immunomodulators in murine cells. Cancer Res 45:1496–1501, 1985.

35. S Kasai, S Fujimoto, K Nitta, H Baba, T Kunimoto. Antitumor activity of polymorphonuclear leukocytes activated by a β-1,3-D-glucan. J Pharm Dyn 14:519–525, 1991.

36. K Fujiki, M Nakao, M Kajikawa, M Asai, T Yano. Enhancement of resistance to bacterial infection in carp *Cyprinus carpio* L., by oral administration of curdlan (in Japanese). Abstracts 1997 Autumn Conf. Japanese Society of Scientific Fisheries, 1997.

37. T Ashida, M Kajikawa, E Okimasu, M Asai, A Amemura. Augmentative effect of curdlan on host defense and superoxide anion production in leukocytes of Japanese flounder *Paralichtys olivaceus* (in Japanese). Abstracts 1997 Autumn Conf. Japanese Society of Scientific Fisheries, 1997.

38. T Funami, Y Nakao. Properties of curdlan and application to processed meat (in Japanese). Gekkan Food Chem 11(8):51, 1995.

39. T Funami, Y Nakao. Effect of curdlan on thermo-gelation of minced pork gel (in Japanese). Nippon Shokuhin Kogyo Gakkaishi 43:21, 1996.

40. T Funami, H Yada, Y Nakao. Curdlan properties for application in fat minetics for meat. J Food Sci 63(2):283–287, 1998.

41. T Funami, M Takeuchi, H Yada, Y Nakao. Curdlan: gelling characteristics and its application to food products. Institute of Food Technologists 1997 Annual Meeting, Orlando, FL: Book of Abstracts, 77.

38
Dietary Fiber in Childhood

Christine L. Williams
Columbia University, New York, New York

Laura Boccia Tolosi
American Health Foundation, Valhalla, New York

Marguerite C. Bollella
New York Presbyterian Hospital, New York, New York

I. INTRODUCTION

The importance of dietary fiber (DF) has been recognized by leading U.S. health organizations, but most have addressed their recommendations to adults, rather than to children and adolescents (1–6). The National Cancer Institute recommended that adults consume 20–30 g of dietary fiber daily to reduce the risk of certain kinds of cancer (1). The Surgeon General and the National Academy of Science also recommended increased intake of DF (2,3). The American Health Foundation recommended that adults consume at least 25 g/d of dietary fiber (4). Each set of guidelines also included recommendations for reducing intake of total fat, saturated fat, and cholesterol and increasing intake of complex carbohydrates (2).

All of the above recommendations for dietary fiber target adults and reflect the fact that the bulk of scientific evidence linking DF and good health concerns adults. There is growing evidence, however, that dietary fiber is important in childhood and may contribute to significant present and future health benefits.

II. BACKGROUND

Since the 1950s the term ''dietary fiber'' has been used to describe the structural parts of plant foods that are resistant to digestion by humans. A mixture of polysaccharides and lignin, DF is usually divided into two major categories based on water solubility. The physical properties of soluble and insoluble DFs in food determine their physiological effects, which in turn are related to their known and potential health benefits (7).

Interest in DF was stimulated during the 1970s by Burkitt et al. (8), who reported markedly lower prevalence rates for chronic disease in Africa as compared with Western industrialized countries. They proposed a ''dietary fiber hypothesis,'' in which common gastrointestinal diseases, such as colon cancer, diverticulosis, and appendicitis, were due in part to insufficient intake of DF (8).

In recent years, knowledge of the chemistry, physiology, epidemiology, and health effects of DF has been significantly expanded by new basic, clinical, and epidemiological research. Reviews of scientific information have prompted leading health organizations to formally recognize the health benefits of DF in the diet and to recommend that adults consume 25–35 g/d.

Interest in and research on DF and health have focused primarily on adults, and less is known about the physiology and health effects of DF in childhood. As a result, few quantitative pediatric recommendations have been proposed for DF intake. The known or potential health benefits of DF in childhood, however, include promotion of normal laxation and prevention of GI disorders; prevention and treatment of childhood obesity; reduction of blood cholesterol; modulation of postprandial hyperglycemia and glucose intolerance; and possible effects on reducing risk of future chronic diseases, such as cancer, cardiovascular disease (CVD), and adult-onset diabetes.

III. LAXATION AND GASTROINTESTINAL HEALTH BENEFITS

The physiological effects of DF depend on the type of fiber ingested, the part of the gastrointestinal (GI) tract involved, and other factors. In the stomach, DF tends to delay gastric emptying time, whereas in the small intestine the effects of DF are more variable. DF delays the absorption of many nutrients, and this increases or decreases intestinal transit time depending on the specific effects of the malabsorbed nutrients.

In the large intestine, insoluble DF softens and enlarges the stool by absorbing water, increasing bacterial proliferation, and increasing gas production. This results in decreased stool transit time and increased frequency of bowel movements. Both effects are influenced by the type of DF and the circumstances of ingestion (9). Soluble fiber in the large intestine may also increase stool volume and water content and decrease stool transit time. Soluble fibers fermented by intestinal bacteria, as well as the proliferating bacteria themselves, increase fecal mass. Fermentation also produces other byproducts, which have a laxative effect.

The net effect is that high levels of DF tend to result in larger stools, which are softer and passed easily and more frequently, while low levels of DF favor hard, dry stools, which are passed less frequently and with greater difficulty. Of interest is the fact that even Hippocrates recognized the beneficial laxative effects of dietary fiber (10).

Constipation is a common clinical problem in childhood (11). Children with this problem tend to pass stools of extremely large size as a result of chronic overdistention and insensitivity of the colon (12). Incomplete rectal emptying results in chronic overdistension with retention of huge fecal masses. The internal rectal sphincter is chronically held open, and overflow diarrhea (encopresis or fecal soiling) occurs. Treatment is aimed at reestablishing normal colonic muscular tone and instituting a plan of therapy that promotes the frequent passage of softer, more normal-sized stools. The latter often includes a dietary recommendation for increased intake of DF and fluid, which together promote the regular passage of softer stools and slowly allows the return of normal rectal function and tone.

Both soluble and insoluble fibers have value in treating childhood constipation (13). Consumption of a variety of fruits, vegetables, and complex carbohydrates provides a mixture of both types of fiber, with about 25–35% of the total as soluble (14).

IV. DIETARY FIBER AND CHILDHOOD OBESITY

An inverse relationship between DF intake and obesity has been suggested from observations that obesity is rare in developing countries where a high proportion of calories come from complex carbohydrates rich in DF (15). Conversely, in Western countries, where less DF is consumed, obesity is more prevalent (15).

Dietary fiber may influence the development of obesity through effects on food intake, digestion and absorption of nutrients (especially energy), and carbohydrate metabolism (16). There is usually an inverse relationship between the dietary fiber and dietary fat, so that fiber-rich diets tends to have lower caloric density compared with fiber-poor diets. Fiber is bulky and displaces fat in the diet, thus providing fewer calories per unit of food consumed. The stomach fills sooner with fiber-rich bulkier foods, and satiety is reached with lower caloric consumption. Foods rich in DF require more chewing, which may help trigger satiety signals and tend to slow gastric emptying, which helps reduce hunger and prolong the feeling of fullness.

High-fiber diets may also have a negative effect on metabolized energy since the digestibility of protein and carbohydrate (but not fat) is reduced (17). Increased bulk also shortens transit time, allowing less time for digestion and adsorption. Increased loss of fecal energy due to high intake of DF has also been reported (18,19). Foods rich in soluble fiber also modulate the insulin response to carbohydrate, resulting in a blunted postprandial glucose and insulin response (20). Lower serum levels of insulin may influence satiety, since insulin is an appetite stimulant.

With respect to children, there is little published information on the association between a low-fiber diet and increased risk for obesity. Kimm reported preliminary data suggesting that DF may be a negative risk factor for obesity in childhood (21). In this study, preadolescent girls in the upper quartile of adiposity by skinfold measure tended to consume less DF than girls in the lowest quartile of adiposity. There was also a strong negative correlation between DF and dietary fat intake (21). Thus, a high-fiber diet, which is almost always accompanied by high carbohydrate and lower fat, may help decrease risk for childhood obesity.

Dietary fiber has also been used in the treatment of obesity, and studies suggest a beneficial effect on weight reduction, although the magnitude of effect is relatively small (about 2 kg added weight loss with fiber supplementation) (22–32). Most of the clinical studies involved adults (Table 1). One study with obese children added 15 g/d DF to a reduced-calorie diet (26).

Table 1 Summary of Clinical Studies on the Effect of a Fiber-Enriched Diet in Hypercholesterolemic Children

Study (Ref.)	N	Age (yr)	Base T-chol (mmol/L)	Type of trial	Fiber dose (g/day)	LDL-C change (%)
Gold et al. (34)	49	10	5.46	4	Oat bran, 38 g	−6
			5.53	wkpar	vs. Step I	−2
Williams et al. (35)	48	2–11	5.66	12 wk	Psyllium, 6 g	−16
			5.38	par	vs. Step I	−6
Dennison and Levine (36)	20	5–18	5.22	20 wk	Psyllium, 6 g	nc
				x-over	Wheat, 5 g	nc
Glassman et al. (37)	36	3–17	6.44	32 wk FU	Psyllium, 5–10 g	−23
Blumenschein et al. (38)	20	5–12	6.39	20 wk FU	Oat bran 1g/kg vs. Soy Pro 1g/kg	−7 nc
Taneja et al. (39)	11	16–18	4.71	3 wk x-over	Psyllium 25g Low fiber	−7 (TC)
Zavoral et al. (40)	11	10–18	8.20	16 wk x-over	Locust bean gum 10–20 g	−19%

par = parallel trial; x-over = crossover design; FU = follow-up study; Soy Pro = soybean protein (Cholsoy brand); T-chol = total cholesterol; nc = no change. *Note:* To convert mmol/L to mg/dL, multiply by 38.7.

Mean weight loss was greater during the high-fiber versus low-fiber treatment periods in this crossover study, but the difference between treatments was not statistically significant.

Thus, while limited, these studies provide some evidence that increasing DF intake could potentially play a useful role in treating obesity, probably by modifying energy intake. DF intake can be increased by a general increase in higher fiber foods or through the use of supplements. The former is preferable, since concomitant calorie dilution per unit volume of food occurs.

There is general consensus that prevention rather than treatment is far preferable as a strategy for reducing childhood obesity. Since U.S. children are at increased risk for obesity, increasing DF may be an attractive population approach to this problem. Increasing fiber in children's diets could result in slightly lower energy intake by decreasing the caloric density of the diet and perhaps maintaining satiety between meals to help avoid excessive snacking.

In summary, DF may play a useful role both in the prevention and treatment of childhood obesity. However, because of the limited amount of data available, there is a need for more research in order to further evaluate the safety and efficacy of this approach in childhood.

V. DIETARY FIBER AND BLOOD CHOLESTEROL IN CHILDHOOD

Based upon pathological, epidemiological, and genetic evidence that atherosclerosis begins in youth, the National Cholesterol Education Program (NCEP) Expert Panel on Blood Cholesterol Levels in Children and Adolescents (33) recommended a dual approach to prevent coronary artery disease and other complications of atherosclerosis: (a) a population approach for all healthy children above 2 years of age, which included a Step One diet moderately reduced in total and saturated fat and cholesterol but increased in complex carbohydrates, along with general attention to other risk factors; (b) a high-risk approach in which children from families with early CAD (≤ 55 years of age) and/or a high blood cholesterol in a parent (≥ 240 mg/dL), or those with two or more other CAD risk factors, undergo cholesterol screening (33).

After screening, children are classified as having a high, borderline high, or acceptable level of total and low-density lipoprotein (LDL) cholesterol. High levels include total cholesterol > 5.17 mmol/L and LDL cholesterol > 3.36 mmol/L. Treatment is primarily dietary through initiation of a Step One Diet emphasizing decreased consumption of total and saturated fat and cholesterol and increased intake of complex carbohydrates, many rich in DF. A possible adjunct to the dietary management of such children is the addition of water-soluble fiber to the diet in an effort to lower LDL cholesterol further without the use of drug therapy. A small number of studies have evaluated the effect of soluble fiber (primarily from oat bran and psyllium) on hypercholesterolemia in children. They have generally involved relatively small sample sizes of moderately hypercholesterolemic children (Table 1).

Gold et al. (34) studied 49 hypercholesterolemic children who were treated with a Step One diet or an oat bran–supplemented Step One diet and reported an additional 6% lowering of LDL cholesterol for those on the fiber-supplemented diet. Although this was not statistically significant, the mean difference of 9 mg/dL in apoB levels for the fiber-supplemented group was significant.

Williams et al. (35) compared a fiber-enriched Step One diet with a regular Step One diet in 48 hypercholesterolemic children. The decrease in LDL cholesterol was significantly greater for the fiber-supplemented group (6.4 g/d psyllium) compared with controls (24% vs. 8.5%). In addition, the ratio of total to high-density lipoprotein (HDL) cholesterol was significantly decreased for the fiber-supplemented group (5.7 to 4.6) compared to controls (4.3 to 4.1).

Dennison and Levine (36) also studied the effects of psyllium on lowering elevated LDL cholesterol levels in children. After 3 months on a strict Step Two low-fat diet, added psyllium did not result in additional lowering of plasma total or LDL cholesterol. This study may suggest that in individuals already consuming a diet significantly reduced in total fat, saturated fat, and cholesterol, addition of water-soluble DF has less of an effect than in individuals consuming a regular, higher fat American diet.

Glassman et al. (37) added soluble fiber to the Step One diet of 36 hypercholesterolemic children for 8 months and reported a 5–10% decrease in LDL cholesterol levels. This study was not randomized, blinded, or controlled, and dietary data was not reported, so interpretation of the data is more difficult. Blumenschein et al. (38) compared the effects of oat bran or soy protein (Cholsoy) with wheat bran in 20 hypercholesterolemic children and found more favorable lipid and lipoprotein effects of oat bran compared with wheat bran or Cholsoy. Taneja et al. (39) added 25 g/d of isobgol husk to the diet of hypercholesterolemic girls and noted a greater decrease in serum cholesterol compared with controls. Zavoral et al. (40) studied the effect of locust bean gum in markedly hypercholesterolemic children with heterozygous familial hypercholesterolemia (FH) and found that fiber decreased LDL cholesterol by an additional 19% compared with the low fat diet alone.

In summary, a diet low in total fat, saturated fat, and cholesterol is the primary treatment for hypercholesterolemia in childhood and adolescence. The addition of water-soluble fiber may provide added benefit when used in conjunction with such a diet, since fiber contains no cholesterol, is very low in saturated fat, and is quite useful as a substitute for foods high in saturated fat and/or cholesterol. Several studies have suggested a small to moderate effect of the addition of water-soluble fiber to a Step One diet, but additional clinical trials in larger numbers of well-defined children are needed to further assess the effectiveness of this treatment.

VI. CURRENT DIETARY FIBER INTAKE IN U.S. CHILDREN

Prior to the 1990s, information on dietary fiber intake in the U.S. population was very limited and available primarily for adults (41–44). In addition, estimates of DF intake were based on analyses using a variety of different measurement protocols and methods of food analysis. Until 1991, the U.S. Department of Agriculture (USDA) food composition tables provided values only for crude fiber, which underestimated total DF due to the analytical procedure used (45). In 1991 the USDA released version 4 of their nutrient database, which included DF values for foods that could then be used in other nutrient databases and dietary analyses.

Analysis of data from the 1976–80 National Health and Nutrition Examination Survey (NHANES II) estimated the average DF intake of 4- to 19-year-olds about 12 g/d or 6 g/1000 kcal (46). Nicklas et al. (47) also reported an average DF intake of 12 g/d for children in Louisiana.

Saldanha et al. (48) examined trends in DF intake among U.S. children (2–18 years) from 1977–78 to 1987–88 using USDA's Nationwide Food Consumption Survey (NFCS) data and reported significant decreases in DF consumption during this decade. Preschool children dropped from 9 to 5.5 g/d; 6 to 11-year-old children dropped from 12 to 7 g/d, and 12 to 18-year-old males dropped from 15 to 14 g/d. Fiber intake among adolescent girls was unchanged (Table 2). Primary sources of DF shifted away from fruits and vegetables to bread, cereals, and combination foods (Table 3). Children who regularly ate breakfast tended to consume 1–3 gd more DF than breakfast skippers.

Nicklas et al. (47) reported that total DF intake remained unchanged from 1976 to 1988 among Louisiana children, even after adjusting for energy intake (mean 12 g/d or 5 g/1000 kcal). Blacks had higher DF intakes per 1000 kcal than whites from ages 10–17 years. Dinner contributed the greatest percent of total daily DF (34–44%), followed by lunch (26–33%),

Table 2 Changes in Dietary Fiber Consumption for Children, 1977–78 vs. 1987–88, Nationwide Food Consumption Surveys

Group	Age (yr)	1977–78 NFCS, mean ± SD (g)	1987–88 NCFS, mean ± SD (g)
Children	2–5	8.9 ± 5.5	8.2 ± 4.7[a]
Children	6–11	12.1 ± 6.9	11.5 ± 6.4[a]
Males	12–18	15.2 ± 9.5	14.0 ± 9.0[a]
Females	12–18	11.0 ± 7.1	10.6 ± 6.6

[a] $p < 0.001$.

snacks (24–29%), and breakfast (12–19%). NHANES II data was similar with one third of DF derived from snacks and 13% from breakfast (Fig. 1) (46). Vegetables, soups, breads, and cereals accounted for 50–75% of total DF consumed by 10- to 13-year-olds. For adults (44), vegetables are the leading source of fiber (27%), followed by breads (19%). For 10-year-old Louisiana children, milk and fruit contributed about 25% of total DF intake. Milk was a major source of DF due to addition of chocolate flavoring containing carrageenan, a thickener containing DF. Children in the highest quartile of fiber intake consumed significantly less fat than children in the lowest fiber quartile (34 vs. 40% of calories from fat) (47). Children with high DF intakes consumed more fruit, fruit juice, vegetables, soup, bread, and grains, while children with low DF intakes consumed more high-fat foods like cheese, pork, beef, eggs, and oils. Mean DF intake of 12 g/d or 5 g/1000 kcal reported by Nicklas et al. (47) is similar to the NHANES II DF intake for children reported by Fulgoni and Mackey (46). Among preschool children, the Healthy Start Project, a 3-year cardiovascular risk-reduction program for 3- to 5-year-old pre-school children begun in 1995, reported a mean baseline daily fiber intake of almost 11 g/d (49). Data from the CATCH (Child and Adolescent Trial for Cardiovascular Health) study, a school- and family-based intervention study to reduce the risk of cardiovascular disease in a group of third- to fifth-students, reported that children in this study met the American Health Foundation recommendation for dietary fiber (50).

In a recent U.S. national survey, the Continuing Survey of Food Intake in Individuals (CSFII)–1995 shows slightly higher fiber intake for children and adolescents compared with the Nationwide Food Consumption Survey (NFCS) of 1987–88 (51,52). The NHANES III,

Table 3 Sources of Dietary Fiber in Rank Order for U.S. Children: Comparison of 1977–78 and 1987–88 Dietary Intake Data from USDA Nationwide Food Consumption Surveys

All: 2–5 yr		All: 6–11 yr		Male: 12–18 yr		Female: 12–18 yr	
'77–78	'87–88	'77–78	'87–88	'77–78	'87–88	'77–78	'87–88
Veg	Bread	Veg	Bread	Veg	Bread	Veg	Bread
Fruit	Cer	Fruit	Cer	Bread	Starch	Bread	Combo
Bread	Fruit	Bread	Fruit	Starch	Cer	Starch	Cer
Nut/L	Veg	Starch	Starch	Nut/L	Veg	Fruit	Veg
Starch	Starch	Cer	Veg	Fruit	Combo	Nut/L	Fruit
Cer	Combo	Combo	Combo	Combo	Nut/L	Combo	Nut/L

Veg = Vegetables; Cer = cereals; Nut/L = nuts and legumes; Combo = combination foods (e.g., pizza, taco, etc.).
Source: Adapted from Ref. 48.

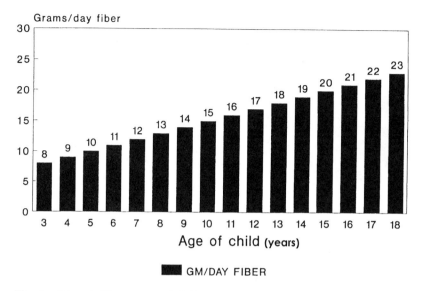

Grams/day fiber

Fig. 1 ''Age + 5''-recommended fiber intake for children: age of child plus 5 rule. (From Ref. 55.)

phase 1 (1988–91) survey data also reported an increase in fiber intake for both boys and girls in the 16–18 years of age compared to NHANES II data (1976–80), although there was little change for younger children and teens (53,54).

The most recent estimate of dietary fiber intake for 3- to 18-year-old U.S. children and adolescents is 12.4 g/d, based on data derived from the National Health and Nutrition Examination Survey (NHANES III, phase 1—1988–91) (53). NHANES III and the Continuing Survey of Food Intakes by Individuals (CSFII-95) classify mean fiber intake according to age and sex categories (see Table 4). When actual dietary fiber intake in the CSFII-95 and NHANES III surveys is compared with recommended intake based on the Age + 5 guideline, fiber intake is minimally adequate in both boys and girls through age 11 (based onmean intake in the 6-/11-year-old category) (53,55). This is consistent with previous data on fiber intake in young children as well as data from the Healthy Start Project and the CATCH studies (49,50). After age 11, however, fiber goals based on either the Age + 5 formula or the 0.5 g/kg/d AAP guideline are not met, despite the modest increase in fiber intake in the 16- to 18-year-old category for both boys and girls reported in the NHANES III survey (53,56).

VII. THE SAFETY OF HIGH DIETARY FIBER INTAKES IN CHILDHOOD

Although DF is associated with important health benefits in childhood, there have been concerns that very high-fiber diets could result in adverse health effects. Some have urged caution in the use of high-fiber foods for children, although a prudent diet emphasizing increased consumption of complex carbohydrates rich in DF has been recommended by American Academy of Pediatrics (AAP) since 1986 (57).

In 1991, NCEP's Expert Panel on Cholesterol in Children and Adolescents, in collaboration with the AAP, recommended a fat-modified Step One diet for all children over 2 years of age (Table 2) (58). Although this diet recommends that 50–60% of calories be derived from carbohydrate, no specific levels of DF intake have been specified (58–60).

Those concerned about the safety of high DF in childhood caution that high-fiber diets

Table 4 Selected Fiber Intake for Children, Ages 3–18 years, Compared with Current Levels of Dietary Fiber Intake (*CSFII-95* and NHANES-III)

Age (yr)	AAP (0.5g/kg)	10 g/1000 kcal	"Age + 5" recommendation Age + 5 (min)	Age + 10 (max)	Current intake (g/day) CSFII-95	NHANES-III
Boys						
3y	7	14	8	13		
4y	8	17	9	14	11.2	11.2
5y	9	17	10	15		
6y	10	18	11	16		
7y	11	18	12	17		
8y	13	19	13	18		
9y	14	19	14	19	14.0	13.1
10y	16	22	15	20		
11y	18	22	16	21		
12y	20	27	17	22		
13y	23	27	18	23	17.4	15.1
14y	25	27	19	24		
15y	29	27	20	25		
16y	32	27	21	26		
17y	33	27	22	27	17.4	17.4
18y	35	28	23	28		
Girls						
3y	7	14	8	13		
4y	8	17	9	14	11.2	10.2
5y	9	17	10	15		
6y	10	18	11	16		
7y	11	18	12	17		
8y	13	19	13	18		
9y	14	19	14	19	12.7	11.8
10y	16	22	15	20		
11y	18	22	16	21		
12y	21	22	17	22		
13y	23	22	18	23	12.7	11.5
14y	25	23	19	24		
15y	27	23	20	25		
16y	29	23	21	26		
17y	29	28	22	27	12.7	12.6
18y	29	23	23	28		

Numbers have been rounded. Dietary fiber recommendations are for g/kg/day; 10 g/1000 kcal; or as g of fiber equal to child's age plus 5 or plus 10 range (55). AAP = American Academy of Pediatrics (67). Fiber intake is based on median weight at each age on NCHS growth charts. CSFII = Continuing Food Consumption Survey in Individuals; NHANES III: National Health and Nutrition Examination Survey-III (1988–93).

could limit caloric intake and reduce the bioavailability of minerals and other nutrients. High-fiber diets could reduce caloric intake in small children since they have a smaller stomach capacity than adults, and high-fiber foods are bulkier and lower in caloric density than low-fiber foods. Thus, a high-fiber diet could result in inadequate caloric intake for normal growth. Food fiber may displace available nutrients in the diet, slow down the intake of food by requiring more chewing, and reduce the absorptive efficiency of the small intestine (61). Refined products stripped of DF are easier to digest, more completely absorbed, and have a higher energy-to-satiety ratio. While providing a ready source of energy for children, such refined products may promote obesity. On the other hand, reverting to more natural, higher-fiber products could result in decreased caloric intake. The question is, how much of a reduction in energy intake occurs when DF is increased, and is this decrease likely to be beneficial or harmful with respect to the present nutritional status of U.S. children?

Studies among adults have reported some loss of energy as DF is increased. Southgate and Durnin (62) fed young British women 23 g/d DF for 7 days and observed an increase in fecal loss of energy (4%), nitrogen (8%), and fat (4%). Energy absorption was reduced about 1% for every 6 g of added DF, a decrease unlikely to be biologically significant unless intake of major nutrients was frankly deficient.

Levine et al. (63) reported a 10% decrease in calories consumed during breakfast and lunch after adults consumed a very high-fiber (20 g/DF serving) breakfast cereal. Stevens et al. (64) reported decreased energy intake and increased fecal energy loss when young women consumed an added 23 g/d DF. Since DF intake of adult U.K. women is about 18 g/d, DF intake in this study may have been >40 g/d (much higher than recommended adult intake of ~25 g/d).

Far fewer data are available for children. In Hummel et al.'s classic 1943 study (65), 18 preadolescent children consumed diets containing 4–6 g/d of crude fiber for 1–6 months. Good health and normal bowel function was reported with no evidence of adverse effects on absorption of nitrogen or mineral balance. They also noted an age-dependent increase in ability to ferment DF.

Hamaker et al. (66) reported an increase in fecal energy loss (52 to 118 kcal/d) when Peruvian toddlers were fed 9–22 g/d of DF from maize, amaranth, or cassava flours. It is difficult to extrapolate these findings to industrialized countries such as the United States, however, since these undernourished children had weight-ages and length-ages half or less their chronological ages, suggesting significant chronic malnourishment.

In summary, dietary fiber tends to increase dietary bulk, decrease caloric density, and reduce caloric intake. Fecal energy loss may increase as intestinal transit time decreases, leaving less time for digestion and absorption of nutrients (67). These effects may be beneficial for most U.S. children who usually consume a calorically dense, highly refined, high-fat diet. On the other hand, increasing DF in malnourished children from underdeveloped countries with inadequate nutrient intake could further reduce available energy (68–72).

A second safety concern has been that high-fiber diets in childhood may reduce the bioavailability of minerals. This reflects the fact that some foods high in DF contain phytate (inositol hexaphosphate), which may form insoluble compounds with minerals, rendering them unavailable for normal absorption and metabolism. Other plant foods contain oxalic acid, which can also interfere with iron absorption (73).

Studies of the effects of DF on mineral balance have generally been acute, short-duration, high-dose feeding studies. A gradual dietary increase in DF containing added phytate that bound minerals and decreased bioavailability would trigger a compensatory physiological response to increase in intestinal absorption (74,75). Thus, decreased bioavailability of minerals is likely to be a chronic problem only when the mineral intake is inadequate and absorption cannot be increased (74,76,77). In the United States and other industrialized countries, vitamin/mineral intake is generally adequate, and DF intake is moderately low.

There are special segments of the population in which caution is prudent, such as in preschool children, adolescents with mineral-deficient diets, impoverished children with inadequate nutritional support, and some vegetarian chlidren who have nutritionally inadequate diets. Although DF intake may be very high (2–4 times recommended intake) and may be accompanied by poor growth, the high-DF may not be the cause of the latter (78). The growth stunting has been linked to lack of essential nutrients, low energy intake, and underutilization of health care services.

In reviewing studies of DF and mineral deficiencies in childhood, it is important to compare the actual concentration of DF and phytate in the study population with levels of intake among U.S. children. Cooking and baking processes must also be considered. Phytate is destroyed by leavening, thus mineral deficiencies due to phytate binding are rare in countries where leavened bread is consumed.

In the 1970s, poor physical growth was reported for rural Iranian children for whom unleavened whole grain pita bread provided 75% of energy intake and was the main dietary source of zinc (79). For U.S. children, however, only about 20% of zinc intake comes from bread and cereal, intake of animal protein is high, and the majority of bread consumed is leavened. Phytate intake in Iran was 2 g/d, compared to an estimated intake of 0.4 g/day in the United States (80). One third of the rural Iranian children had iron-deficiency anemia compared with about 5% of U.S. children (81). Bioavailability of iron is significantly enhanced by calcium and magnesium in the U.S. diet, which competitively form salts with phytic acid and neutralize the phosphate in phytic acid. U.S. children also consume more animal foods, which are a source of highly bioavailable heme iron. Vitamin C also increases iron absorption and is generally abundant in U.S. diets.

More recent studies have evaluated the effects of DF on mineral balance. Drews et al. (82) fed 14 g/d of DF to adolescent males for 4 days, and although fecal zinc, copper, and magnesium increased, serum levels were unchanged. Kawatra et al. (83) found that 25 g/d of psyllium increased fecal excretion and decreased serum levels of zinc, copper, and manganese in adolescent Indian girls, but anemia was not present. Dennison and Levine (36) found that children's growth and serum vitamin (A, D, E and folic acid) and mineral (iron, zinc and calcium) levels were not affected when 12 g/d DF was added to their usual diet for 1–2 months, suggesting that a doubling of usual DF intake for U.S. children with adequate intake of essential vitamins and minerals may not adversely affect growth, serum vitamin, or mineral levels.

McClung et al. (84) treated constipated children with a doubling of DF to 0.6 g/kg (about 18 g/d) and found no decrease in serum vitamin, mineral, or hemoglobin levels during 6 months of treatment. Kelsay (85) reviewed the effects of DF on mineral bioavailability and concluded that up to 32 g/d of DF and 2 g/d of phytic acid had no adverse effect on mineral balance. Even among U.S. vegetarian children with very high DF intake, anemia is not common, perhaps because higher vitamin C intake enhances iron absorption (86, 87).

The ability of DF to bind to compounds may also be beneficial since it could inactivate carcinogens and prevent cancer. The Finns, who consume a high-fat, high-DF diet, have less colon cancer than in the United States, where high-fat, low-DF diets are the rule. These findings have been duplicated in rats under controlled laboratory conditions (88–90).

In summary, studies suggest that although a small loss of energy may occur with a high intake of DF, this small decrease is unlikely to be significant for children with adequate nutrient intake. Increases in DF up to a doubling of current intake are not likely to adversely effect growth or serum vitamin and mineral levels in healthy U.S. children on adequate diets. Thus, for U.S. children, a moderate increase in DF would be more healthful than harmful.

VIII. RECOMMENDATIONS FOR DIETARY FIBER INTAKE IN CHILDHOOD

Pediatric dietary guidelines have recently been established for recommended intake of total fat and fatty acids, protein, carbohydrate, and cholesterol in U.S. children over 2 years of age (Table 5) (10,33,59,75,90–92). While these guidelines suggest that U.S. children increase con-

Table 5 Summary and Comparison of Dietary Fat and Cholesterol Guidelines From Major U.S. Health Organizations for Children >2 Years of Age

Organization, year of guideline	Guideline for childhood dietary intake of fat and cholesterol	Notes on differences
American Academy of Pediatrics, Committee on Nutrition: Statement on Cholesterol, 1992	Recommends an average daily intake of ≤30% kcal from total fat (but more than 20% kcal); <10% kcal from saturated fat, and <300 mg of cholesterol per day, with gradual adoption of guidelines between 2 and 5 years of age	Sets lower limit for total fat intake at 20% kcal Recommends transition period for preschool children <age 5 years
Healthy People 2000: National Health Promotion & Disease Prevention Objectives, 1991	Objective 2.5: Reduce dietary fat intake to an average of 30% of energy or less and average saturated fat intake to <10% of energy among people 2 years and older	No transition period
American Heart Association, Council on Cardiovascular Disease in the Young: 1991, 1983	Recommends total fat intake at ≤30% kcal, saturated fat <10% kcal, and cholesterol intake <300 mg/day	No transition period
United States Department of Agriculture; U.S. Dept of Health and Human Services; Dietary Guidelines for Americans, 4th ed. 1995	Recommends an average daily intake of ≤30% kcal from total fat; <10% kcal from saturated fat, and <300 mg of cholesterol per day, with transition period between 2 and 5 years of age	Transition period for children 2–5 years old
National Cholesterol Education Panel: Report of the Expert Panel on Blood Cholesterol Levels in Children & Adolescents, 1992	Recommends total fat intake at ≤30% kcal, saturated fat <10% kcal; and cholesterol intake <300 mg/day; transition period for children 2–3 years old	Transition period for children 2–3 years old
National Institutes of Health Consensus Development Panel, 1985	Recommended total fat intake at ≤30% kcal, and saturated fat <10% kcal for all Americans over 2 years of age	No transition period

sumption of complex carbohydrate, which includes a variety of foods rich in dietary fiber, no quantitative level of fiber intake was proposed.

NCEP dietary goals and the USDA Food Pyramid guide apply to children over age 2, with 2–3 a transition year (33). The need for DF earlier in life is debated. Some suggest that DF may not be needed during the first year of life (93), while others recommend that weaning diets include at least 5 g/d of DF (94).

The AAP, Committee on Nutrition, has recommended a DF intake of 0.5 g/kg of body weight (75). Based on this recommendation and NCHS median weight for age, DF intake would range from 6.8 to 34.5 g/d for 3- to 19-year-old average-weight boys and 6 to 28.5 g/d for 3- to 19-year-old average-weight girls. In contrast, current DF intake plateaus at 12–15 g/d for U.S. adolescents (Table 4). The AAP recommended DF intake for older, heavier adolescents whose body weight is significantly above the median weight-for-age, could well approach 40 g/d, however, the AAP guideline places a cap on recommended daily DF intake at 35 g/d. From a safety perspective, DF intake of >30 g/d for adolescents with inadequate intake of minerals (calcium, iron, zinc) could potentially lead to deficiencies (67). Up to 25 g/d during adolescence should not be deleterious, however, even with suboptimal mineral intake (67,95).

The FDA food label bases DF recommendations on calories consumed and does not distinguish between adults and children. At 2000 kcal/d, 25 g/d DF is recommended (12.5 g/1000 kcal) and at 2500 kcal/d, 30 g/d DF (~12 g DF/1000 kcal). DF intake based on 12g/1000 kcal is lower than AAP recommended levels for most adolescents, especially girls. On the other hand, DF intake based on this formula may be too high for young preschool children. At the RDA recommended caloric intake of 1800 kcal/d (range 1300–2300) for 4-to 6-year-olds, 16–28 g/d (mean 22) of DF would be recommended based on the 12 g/1000 kcal formula (91).

The USDA Food Pyramid does not specify a recommended amount of DF per day, but estimates may be made based on number of servings and usual serving size (92). At caloric intakes of 2200 and 2800 kcal/d, DF intake may be estimated at 32–40 g/d (2 g DF per serving of bread group, small fruit, or half cup of vegetables). For preschool children who consume 1600 kcal/d and half-size servings of vegetables, DF intake could be about 19 g/d.

A new recommendation by Williams et al. (55) proposes that a reasonable goal for DF intake during childhood and adolescence may be approximately equivalent to the age of the child plus 5 g/d (Age + 5) (Fig. 1) (87). Based on Age + 5, minimal DF intake would range from 8 g/d at age 3, to 25 g/d by age 20, the lower level of adult recommended intake (55). Based on current levels of DF intake, 55–89% of 2- to 18-year-old U.S. children consume less than the Age + 5 goal (Fig. 3).

The Age + 5 level of DF intake for children is similar to the AAP (67) recommendation (0.5 g/kg/d) up to the age of 10, but it is lower for older adolescents (Figs. 2,3). The Age + 5 level of DF intake is felt to represent a level that would provide health benefits, such as normal laxation, without compromising mineral balance or caloric intake in children over 2 years of age. In addition, the Age + 5 recommendation is consistent with current guidelines for adult DF intake (25–35 g/d) (1–6), since the mineral adult DF intake of 25 g/d would be reached by age 20 applying the Age + 5 rule.

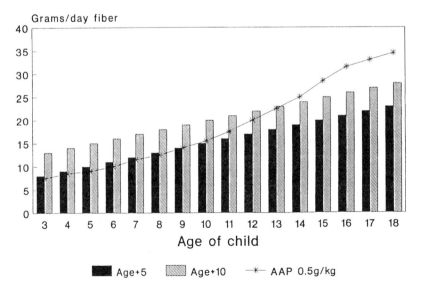

Fig. 2   Recommended fiber for boys Age + 5 to Age + 10 range vs. AAP (0.5 g/kg). (From Ref. 55.)

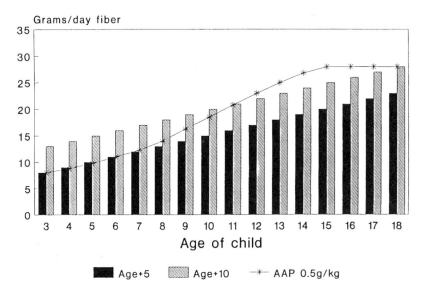

Fig. 3 Recommended fiber for girls: Age + 5 to Age + 10 range vs. AAP (0.5 g/kg). (From Ref. 55.)

Williams's recommendation also suggests that a range of DF intake between Age + 5 and Age + 10 (g/day) may represent a safe and tolerable level for most children based on current knowledge (67). The Age + 10 upper level of DF intake is similar in some respects to levels based on 10–12 g/1000 kcal. These levels have been suggested as safe even for Japanese adolescents, who have low levels of calcium intake (95).

Dietary fiber may be increased gradually in childhood by encouraging greater consumption of a variety of fiber-rich fruits, vegetables, legumes, cereals, and whole grain products (Table 6). Fiber supplements for children are not recommended as a means of meeting DF requirements. Supplements may be clinically useful, however, as an adjunct to the dietary treatment of constipation, hypercholesterolemia, and obesity in childhood.

At the present time, there is little scientific information on which to base additional recommendations for specific proportions of intake of soluble versus insoluble fiber in childhood. Both types of fiber are associated with important health benefits, and both are consumed in generous amounts by following the Food Pyramid Guide. A ratio of 1:4 or 1:3 (soluble:insoluble DF) has been recommended for adults (96). Very young children consume more soluble fiber than insoluble (especially from fruits), with consumption of the latter increasing gradually with age (94).

Since DF increases water retention in the colon, resulting in bulkier, softer stools, recommendations for water intake should be increased commensurate with increases in DF. The amount of water needed for children to produce soft bulky stools is estimated to be 6–8 cups/day (97). Others have recommended 6 cups per day for children weighting 26 pounds, increasing up to 10.5 cups per day for children weighing 100 pounds (mean weight of a 13-year-old boy) (93). Water intake for older adolescents with higher DF intakes should be higher.

IX. SUMMARY

Dietary fiber has important health benefits in childhood, especially in promoting normal laxation. In addition, research suggests that DF in childhood may be useful in preventing and treating

Table 6 High-Fiber Foods Commonly Included in the Diets of U.S. Children

Food source	Approximate serving size	Grams dietary fiber
Beans	1 cup, baked	13
Chili w/beans	1 cup	7
Almonds	2 oz, dry roasted	7
Peanuts	2 oz, dry roasted	4
Peanut butter	2 tbsp	2
Cereal	1 cup	>2[a]
Whole wheat bread	2 slices	4
Broccoli	0.5 cup	2
Corn	0.5 cup	3
Popcorn	2 cups, popped	2
Potato	1 medium, baked	2 (3.5 w/skin)
Sweet potato	1 medium	3
Carrot	medium (raw)	3
Strawberries	1 cup	4
Pear	1 medium	4
Banana	1 large	3
Blueberries	1 cup	3
Apple	1 medium	3
Apricots	10 dried halves	3
Kiwi	1 large	3
Apple sauce	0.5 cup	2

[a] Dietary fiber content of cereal varies widely from very low to very high. Best "fiber choice" for children has 3 or more g/serving (e.g., raisin bran type, oatmeal, etc). Other suggestions: "trail mix" of raisins, peanuts, dates, and cereal; whole grain crackers with 2–3 g of fiber/1/2 oz. serving; and brown rice with 4 g dietary fiber/cup.

obesity and in lowering blood cholesterol levels, both of which may help reduce the risk of future cardiovascular disease. Among adults, a high-fiber, low-fat diet has been linked to reduced rates of colon and other human cancers, and while it seems highly likely that this benefit would be even greater if begun in childhood, epidemiological and experimental confirmation is lacking at present.

Children currently consume amounts of DF that may not be adequate to maintain good health and prevent disease. It would be prudent, therefore, to recommended that children over 2 years of age increase DF intake. Dietary fiber intake should be increased gradually in childhood by increasing consumption of a variety of fruits, vegetables, legumes, cereals, and other whole grain products, along with a concomitant increase in water consumption. A safe range of dietary fiber intake for children may be between Age + 5 and Age + 10 g/d. After age 20, adult levels of 25–35 g/d of DF are recommended. This range of DF intake is felt to be safe even for children and adolescents with marginal intake of some vitamins and minerals. It should provide enough DF for normal laxation and may provide enough added DF to help prevent future chronic disease. Although there are some potential adverse effects of very high fiber intake in childhood, the potential health benefits of a moderate increase in dietary fiber in childhood are felt to significantly outweigh the potential risks, especially in highly industrialized countries such as the United States.

REFERENCES

1. Diet, Nutrition & Cancer Prevention: A Guide to Food Choices. Health and Human Services. Public Health Service, National Institutes of Health. NIH Publ. No. 87-2878. Washington, DC: U.S. Government Printing Office, 1987.
2. The Surgeon General's Report on Nutrition and Health. U.S. Department of Health and Human Services. Public Health Service. Publ. No. 88-50210. Washington, DC: U.S. Government Printing Office, 1988.
3. Diet and Health. Implication for Reducing Chronic Disease Risk. Washington, DC: National Academy of Sciences. National Research Council. National Academy Press, 1989.
4. Live Well: The Low-Fat/High Fiber Way. New York: American Health Foundation, 1990.
5. U.S. Department of Agriculture. Dietary Guidelines for Americans. 3rd ed. U.S. GPO Pub. NO. 1990-273-930. U.S. Department of Health and Human Services, Washington, D.C., 1990.
6. National Research Council, Committee on Diet, Nutrition, and Cancer. Diet, Nutrition, and Cancer. Washington, DC: National Academy Press, 1990.
7. Gurr MI, Asp NG. Dietary Fibre. Washington, DC: International Life Science Press, 1994.
8. Burkitt DP, Walker ARP, Painter NS. Effect of dietary fibre on stools and transit times and its role in the causation of disease. Lancet 1972; 2:1408–1412.
9. Eastwood MA, Kay RM. An hypotheses for the action of dietary fiber along the gastrointestinal tract. Am J Clin Nutr 1979; 32:364–367.
10. Adams F. The Genuine Works of Hippocrates. Baltimore, MD: Williams and Wilkins, 1939.
11. Hatch TF. Encopresis and constipation in children. Pediatr Clin North Am 1988; 35:257–280.
12. Loening/Baucke VA. Sensitivity of the sigmoid colon and rectum in children treated for chronic constipation. J Pediatr Gastroent Nutr 1984; 3:454–459.
13. Eastwood MA, Smith AN, Brydon WG, et al. Comparison of bran, ispaghula and lactulose on colon function in diverticular disease. Gut 1978; 19:1144–1147.
14. Anderson JW, Bridges SR. Dietary fiber content of selected foods. Am J Clin Nutr 1988; 47:440–447.
15. Van Italie TB. Dietary fiber and obesity. Am J Clin Nutr 1978; 31S43–S52.
16. Ali R, Staub H, Leveille GA, Boyle PC. Dietary fiber and obesity: a review. In: Vahouny GV, Kritchevsky D, eds. Dietary Fiber in Health and Disease. New York: Plenum Press, 1982, pp. 139–149.
17. Southgate DAT, Durnin JUGA. Caloric conversion factors. An experimental reassessment of the factors used in the calculation of the energy value of human diets. Cr J Nutr 1970; 24:517–535.
18. Farrell DJ, Girliel AJ. Effects of dietary fibre on the apparent digestibility of major food components and on blood lipids in men. Aust J Exp Biol 1978; 56:469–479.
19. Kelsay JL, Behall KM, Pratner ES. Effect of fiber from fruits and vegetables on metabolic responses of human subjects. 1. Bowel transit time, number of defecations, fecal weight, urinary excretion of energy and nitrogen and apparent digestibilities of energy, nitrogen, and fat. Am J Clin Nutr 1978; 31:1149–1153.
20. Jenkins DJA, Wolever TMS, Leeds AR, et al. Dietary fibers, fibre analogues and glucose tolerance, importance of viscosity. Br Med J 1978; 1:1392–1394.
21. Kimm SYS. Dietary fiber and childhood obesity. Pediatrics 1995; 96(5)S:1010–1014.
22. Mickelsen O, Makdani DD, Cotton RH, Titcomb ST, Colmey JC, Gatty R. Effects of a high fiber bread diet on weight loss in college-age males. Am J Clin Nutr 1979; 32:1703–1709.
23. Tuomilehto J, Voutilainen E, Huttunen J, Vinni S, Homan K. Effect of guar gum on body weight and serum lipids in hypercholesterolemic females. Acta Med Scand 1980; 208:45–48.
24. Walsh DE, Yaghoubian V, Behforooz A. Effect of glucomannan on obese patients: a clinical study. In J Obese 1984; 8:289–293.
25. Solum TT, Ryttig KR, Solum E, Larsen S. The influence of a high-fibre diet on body weight, serum lipids and blood pressure in slightly overweight persons. Int J Obese 1987; 11(suppl. 1):7–71.
26. Gropper SS, Acosta PB. The therapeutic effect of fiber in treating obesity. J Am Coll Nutr 1987; 6(6):533–535.
27. Rossner S, Zweigbergk DV, Ohlin A, Ryttig K. Weight reduction with dietary fibre supplements: results of two double-blind randomized studies. Acta Med Scand 1987; 222:83–88.

28. Rossner S, Anderson IL, Ryttig K. Effects of fietary fibre supplements to a weight reduction programme on blood pressure: a randomized, double-blind placebo-controlled study. Acta Med Scand 1988; 223:353–357.

29. Ryttig KR, Tellnes G, Haegh L, Boe E, Fagerthun H. A dietary fibre supplement and weight maintenance after weight reduction: A randomized, double-blind placebo-controlled long-term trial. Int J Obese 1989; 13:165–171.

30. Rigaud D, Ryttig KR, Angel LA, Apfelbaum M. Overweight treated with energy restriction and a dietary fibre supplement: a 6-month randomized, double-blind, placebo-controlled trial. Int J Obese 1990; 14:763–769.

31. Astrup A, Vrist E, Quaade F. Dietary fiber added to very low calorie diet reduces hunger and alleviates constipation. Int J Obese 1990; 14:105–112.

32. Stevens J. Does dietary fiber affect food intake and body weight? JADA 1988; 88(8):939–945.

33. National Cholesterol Education Program Report of the Expert Panel on Blood Cholesterol Levels in Children and adolescents. Pediatrics 1992; 89(suppl):525–584.

34. Gold K, Wong N, Tong A, et al. Serum apolipoprotein and lipid profile effects of an oat-bran supplemented, low-fat diet in children with elevated serum cholesterol. Ann NY Acad Sci 1991; 623:429–431.

35. Williams CL, Bollella M, Spark A, Puder D. Effectiveness of a psyllium-enriched Step 1 diet in hypercholesterolemic children. JACN 1991; 14(3):251–257.

36. Dennison BA, Levine DM. Randomized, double-blind, placebo-controlled, two-period crossover clinical trial of psyllium fiber in children with hypercholesterolemia. Pediatrics 1993; 123:24–29.

37. Glassman M, Spark A, Berezin S, Schwartz S, Medow M. Treatment of type IIa hyperlipidemia in childhood by a simplified American Heart Association diet and fiber supplementation. Am J Dis Child 1990; 144:193–197.

38. Blumenschein D, Torres E, Kushmaul E, Crawford J, Fixler D. Effect of oat bran-soy protein in hypercholesterolemic children. Ann NY Acad Sci 1991; 623:413–415.

39. Taneja A, Bhat CM, Arora A, Kaur AP. Effect of incorporation of isabgol husk in a low fibre diet on faecal excretion and serum levels of lipids in adolescent girls. Eur J Clin Nutr 1989; 43:197–202.

40. Zavoral JH, Hannan P, Fields DJ. The hyperlipidemic effect of locust bean gum food products in familial hypercholesterolemic adults and children. Am J Clin Nutr 1983; 38:285–294.

41. Lanza E, Jones Y, Block G, Kessler L. Dietary fiber intake in the US population. Am J Clin Nutr 1987; 46:790–797.

42. Anderson JW, Bridges SR, Tietyen J, Gustafson NJ. Dietary fiber content of a simulated American diet and selected research diet. Am J Clin Nutr 1989; 49:352–357.

43. Thomson FE, Sowers MF, Frongillo EA. Sources of fiber and fat in diets of U.S. women aged 19 to 50. Implications for nutrition education and policy. AJPH 1992; 82:695–702.

44. Block G, Lanza E. Dietary fiber sources in the United States by demographic group. JNCI 1987; 79(1):83–91.

45. Slann JL. Dietary fiber: classification, chemical analyses, and food sources. J Am Diet Assoc 1987; 87(9):1164–71.

46. Fulgoni VL, Mackey MA. Total dietary fiber in children's diets. Ann NY Acad Sci 1989; 623:369–379.

47. Nicklas TA, Farris R, Myers L, Berenson GS. Dietary fiber intake of children and young adults: The Bogalusa Heart Study. JADA 1995; 95:209–214.

48. Saldanha LG, Yagalla MV, Keast DR. Trends in dietary intake among children 2–18 years of age: Comparison of 1977–78 versus 1987–88 Nationwide Food Consumption Surveys. Pediatrics 1995; 96(5):S884–997.

49. Bollella MC, Boccia LA, Nicklas TA, Lefkowitz KB, Pittman BP, Zang EA, Williams CL. Assessing dietary intake in preschool children: The Healthy Start Project—New York. Nutr Res 1999; 19(1) 37–48.

50. Lytle LA, Stone EJ, Nichaman MZ, Perry CL, Montgomery DH, Nicklas TA, Zive MM, Mitchell P, Dwyer JS, Ebzery MK, Evans MA, Galati TP. Changes in nutrient intakes in elementary school children following a school-based intervention: Results from the CATCH Study. Prev Med 1996; 25:465–477.

51. U.S. Department of Agriculture. Food and Nutrient Intakes by Individuals in the United States, 1 Day, 1989–91. Riverdale, MD: Agricultural Research Service; NFS Report N. 91-2 (NTIS Accession No. PB95-272746), 1995.

52. Wright HS, Guthrie HA, Wang MQ, Bernardo V. The 1987–88 Nationwide Food Consumption Survey: An update on the nutrient intake of respondents, Nutr Today 1991; 25:21–27.

53. Alaimo K, McDowell MA, Briefel RR, Bischof AM, Caughman CR, Loria CM, Johnson CL. Dietary intake of vitamins, minerals and fiber of persons ages 2 months and over in the United States: Third National Health and Nutrition Examination Survey, Phase 1, 1988–91, Advance data from vital and health statistics; no 258. Hyattsville, MD: National Center for Health Statistics, 1994.

54. National Center for Health Statistics, Dietary Source Data: United States 1976–1980. Vital and Health Statistics. Hyattsville, MD: U.S. Department of Health and Human Services; NCHS publication (PHS) 83-1681, series II, No. 231, 1983.

55. Williams CL, Bollella M, Wynder EL: A new recommendation for dietary fiber in childhood. Pediatrics 1995; 96(5)S:985–988.

56. Mueller S, Keast DR, Olson BH. Intakes and food sources of dietary fiber in children (abtr). FASEB J 1997; 11:A187.

57. Committee on Nutrition, American Academy of Pediatrics. Cholesterol in children. Pediatrics 1998; 101:141.

58. National Cholesterol Education Program. Report of the Expert Panel on Blood Cholesterol Levels in Children and Adolescents. USDHHS, PHS, NIH, USDHHS Publ. No. (NIH) 91-2732, 1991.

59. American Heart Association, Task Force Committee of the Nutrition Committee and Cardiovascular Diseases in the Young Council. Diet in the healthy child. Circulation 1986; 74:1411A–1414A.

60. Wynder EL, Berenson GC, Strong WB, Williams CL. Coronary artery disease prevention: cholesterol—a pediatric perspective. Prev Med 1989; 18(3):323–409.

61. Heaton KW. Food fiber—an obstacle to energy intake. Lancet 1973; ii:1418–1421.

62. Southgate DAT, Durnin JVGA. Calorie conversion factors. An experimental reassessment of the factors used in the calculation of the energy value of human diets. Br J Nutr 1970; 23:517–535.

63. Levine AS, Tallman JR, Grace MK, Parker SA, Billington CJ, Levitt MD. Effect of breakfast cereal on short-term food intake. A. J Clin Nutr 1989; 50:1303–1307.

64. Stevens J, Levitsky DA, Van Soest PJ. Effect of psyllium gum and wheat bran on spontaneous energy intake. Am J Clin Nutr 1987; 46:812–817.

65. Hummel FC, Shepherd ML, Macy IG. Disappearance of cellulose and hemicellulose from the digestive tracts of children. J Nutr 1943: 25:59–70.

66. Hamaker BR, Rivera K, Morales E, Graham GG. Effect of dietary fiber on fecal composition in preschool Peruvian children consuming maize, amaranth, or cassava flours. J Ped Gastroenterol Nutr 1991; 13:59–66.

67. Williams CL, Bollella M. Is a high fiber diet safe for children? Pediatrics 1995; 96(5):S 1014–1019.

68. Cummings JH, Southgate DAT, Branch W, Houston H, Jenkins DJA, James WPT. Colonic response to dietary fiber from carrot, cabbage, apple, bran and guar gum. Lancet 1978; i:5–9.

69. Karlsson A, Svanberg U. Dietary bulk as a limiting factor for nutrient intake in preschool children. IV. Effect of digestive enzymes on the viscosity of starch-based weaning foods. J Trop Ped 1982; 28:230–234.

70. Hellstrom A, Hermansson AM, Karlsson A. Dietary bulk as a limiting factor for nutritient intake—with special reference to the feeding of pre-school children. II. Consistency as related to dietary bulk. J Trop Ped 1981; 27:127–135.

71. Brandtzaeg B, Melleshi NG, Svanberg U, Desikachar HSB, Mellander O. Dietary bulk as a limiting factor for nutrient intake in preschool children. III. Studies of malted flour. J Trop Ped 1981; 27: 184–189.

72. MacDonald I. The effects of dietary fiber: Are they all food? In: G. Spiller, R Amen, eds. Fiber in Human Nutrition. New York: Plenum Press, 1976, pp 263–269.

73. Committee on Nutrition, American Academy of Pediatrics. Plant fiber intake in the pediatric diet. Pediatrics 1981; 67(4):572–575.

74. Walker ARP, Fox FW, Irving JT. Studies in human mineral metabolism. I. The effect of bread rich

in phytate on the metabolism of certain mineral salts with special reference to calcium. Biochem J 1948; 42:452–462.

75. Barness LA, ed. Committee on Nutrition, American Academy of Pediatrics. Pediatric Nutrition Handbook. 3rd ed. Elk Grove Village, IL: American Academy of Pediatrics, 1993, p. 104.

76. Ekvall S. Constipation and fiber. In: Ekvall S, ed. Pediatric Nutrition in Chronic Diseases and Developmental Disorders: Prevention and Treatment. New York: Oxford University Press, 1994, pp 301–309.

77. Cullumbine H, Basnayake V, Lemottee J. Mineral metabolism of rice diets. Br J Nutr 1950; 4:101–111.

78. Dwyer J. Dietary fiber for children: How much? Pediatrics 1995; 96(5):S1019–1023.

79. Haghshensas M, Mahloudji M, Reinhold JG, Mahammad N. Iron-deficiency anemia associated with high intakes of iron. Am J Clin Nutr 1972; 25:1143–1146.

80. Thompson FE, Sowers MF, Frongillo EA, Parpia BJ. Sources of fiber and fat in the diets of women aged 19–50: implications for nutrition education and policy. AJPH 1992; 82:695–702.

81. Weihang B, Dalferes ER, Srinivasan SR, Webber LS, Berenson GS. Normative distribution of complete blood count from early childhood through adolescence: *The Bogalusa Heart Study*. Prev Med 1993; 22:825–837.

82. Drews LM, Kies C, Fox HM. Effect of dietary fiber on copper, zinc, and magnesium utilization by adolescent boys. Am J Clin Nutr 1979; 32:1893.

83. Kawatra A, Bhat CM, Arora A. Effects of isobgol husk supplementation in a low-fibre diet on serum levels and calcium, phosphorus and iron balance in adolescent girls. Eur J Clin Nutr 1993; 47:297–300.

84. McClung HJ, Boyne LJ, Linsheid T, Heitlinger LA, Murray RD, Fyda J, Li Buk. Is combination therapy for encopresis nutritionaly safe? Pediatrics 1994; 91(3):591–594.

85. Kelsay JL. Effects of fiber, phytic acid, and osalic acid in the diet on mineral bioavailability. Am J Gastroenterol 1987; 82(1):893–97.

86. Sanders TAB, Reddy S. Vegetarian diets and children. Am J Clin Nutr 1994; 59:1176S–1181S.

87. Jacobs C, Dwyer JT. Vegetarian children: appropriate and inappropriate diets. Am J Clin Nutr 1988; 43(suppl 3):S811–818.

88. Reddy BS. Overview of diet and colon cancer. Prog Clin Biol Res 1988; 279:111–121.

89. Reddy BS, Engle A, Katsifis S, Simi B, Bartram H, Perrino P, Mahan CL. Biochemical epidemiology of colon cancer: effect of types of dietary fiber on fecal mutagens acid, and neutral sterols in healthy subjects. Cancer Res 89; 49:4629–4635.

90. Weisburger JH, Reddy BS, Rose D, Cohen L,l Kendall MD, Wynder EL. Protective mechanisms of dietary fibers in nutritional carcinogenesis. In: Bronzetti G, ed. Antimutagenesis and Anticarcinogenesis Mechanisms III. New York: Plenum Press, 1993, pp 45–63.

91. National Academy of Sciences. Recommended Dietary Allowances. 10th ed. Washington, DC: National Academy Press, 1989.

92. U.S. Department of Agriculture. The Food Guide Pyramid. Hyattsville, MD: Human Nutrition Information Service, 1992.

93. Hendricks K, Walker A. Manual of Pediatric Nutrition. 2d ed. Philadelphia: BC Decker, 1990.

94. Agostoni C. Dietary fiber in weaning foods of young children. Pediatrics 1995; 96(5):S1002–S1005.

95. Nishimune T, Sumimoto T, Konishi Y, Yakushiji T, Komachi Y, Mitsuhashi Y, Okazaki K, Tsuda T, Ichihashi A, et al. Dietary fiber intake of Japanese younger generations and the recommended daily allowance. J Nutr Sci Vitaminol 1993; 39(3):263–278.

96. Pilch SM, ed. Physiologic effects and health consequences of dietary fiber. Center for Food Safety, DA, DHHS. Washington, DC: FASEB, 1987.

97. Ekvall, SW. Constipation and fiber. In: Pediatric Nutrition in Chronic Diseases and Developmental Disorders: Prevention, Assessment and Treatment. New York: Oxford University Press, 1993, pp 301–309.

39
Dietary Fiber Intake in Spain: Recommendations and Actual Consumption Patterns

Isabel Goñi Cambrodón
University Complutense of Madrid, Madrid, Spain

I. THE SPANISH DIET: MEDITERRANEAN DIET PATTERN

Spain may be considered a typical Mediterranean country. This term is not a geographic concept, rather it refers to dietary pattern found in olive-growing areas of the Mediterranean region described in the 1960s as having an abundance of plant foods that are minimally processed, seasonally fresh, and locally grown. The variety of foods, cooking procedures, and exceptional palatability of the diet and the pleasure taken in eating are the distinctions of this healthy dietary pattern.

The Mediterranean and Spanish diet pattern can be described as healthful in relation to diseases, the incidence of which is supposed to be strongly influenced by diet. Mediterranean regions are characterized by low incidence of coronary heart disease and several cancers, and an etiological link with some components of the diet, such as fruit and green and yellow vegetables, has been postulated.

Generally, the Mediterranean diet may have a regulatory role in relation to human antioxidant potential and, hence, the risk of cancer and cardiovascular diseases. Nutritionally, it contains specific nutrient and nonnutrient components, antioxidant vitamins, dietary fiber, and a variety of phenolic compounds that have been identified as being protective against major chronic diseases. This could help explain the health-promoting qualities associated with the Mediterranean way of eating (1). The Mediterranean pattern constitutes a centuries-old tradition that contributes to excellent health, provides a sense of pleasure and well-being, and forms a vital part of the world's collective cultural heritage. The pyramid model designed as a dietary guide by the U.S. Department of Agriculture (USDA) in 1992 corresponds to the relative proportions and frequency of servings of foods and food groups consumed traditionally in Mediterranean regions. Therefore, the Mediterranean diet is now defined as the most healthy dietary pattern.

A. Foods Consumed

The consumption of Spanish food has been estimated from national food consumption data obtained annually from household budget questionnaries, which are carried out daily in three national sectors: 2500 private family households, 500 hotels and restauration establishments,

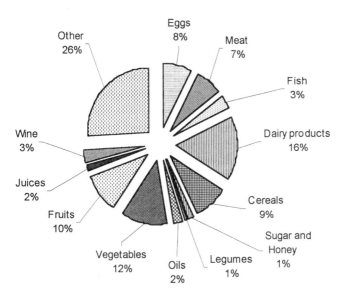

Fig. 1 Food consumption in the Spanish diet.

and significant official institutions are surveyed. National consumption data were collected and published every year up to 1987 (3). The data include 130 foods bought and sold in Spain at home and outside the home and give the average consumption at a national level. There is no correction for waste, therefore, the data provide information on food items purchased but are not a direct measure of what has been eaten.

The average Spanish diet includes great amounts of vegetables, fruits, cereals, legumes, fish, and vegetable oils. The consumption of dairy products and meat is moderate, poultry being the more consumed meat. Also, wine is consumed in low to moderate amounts—normally with meals (Fig. 1).

Vegetables and fruits are frequently eaten raw in salads. Fresh fruits constitute the typical daily dessert. Olives are included in the fruit group, but normally they are consumed as an appetizer, and olive oil is the first source of dietary fat in Spain. Fish is eaten in large quantities, frequently fried in olive oil. Garlic, onions, and herbs are frequently used as condiments.

B. Nutritional Status

Figure 2 shows contributions of macronutrients and energy to recommended intakes (= 100). Nutritional analysis data show a higher energy consumption than Spanish dietary allowances (2650 vs. 2360 kcal/person/day) (4). Energy provided by protein and, particularly, by fat has increased at the expense of that contributed by carbohydrates. The daily intake of alcoholic drinks in Spain is high (80 g of wine, 174 g of beer, 3.4 g of cider, and 15 g of spirits), therefore, to obtain the dietary calorie profile we have calculated calories percentages provided by macro-nutrients and total alcohol, (Fig. 3). Relative caloric values indicate elevated protein and fat intakes, low consumption of carbohydrates, and a moderate amount of calories from alcohol (5% of total diet energy).

Although some studies support the hypothesis that wine may play a cardioprotective role, there is not sufficient evidence to conclude that wine per se is responsible for lower rates of

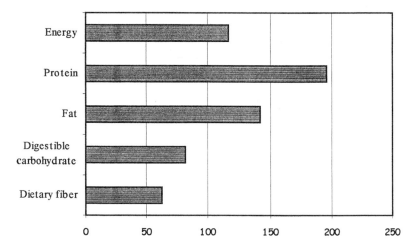

Fig. 2   Nutritional analysis of the Spanish diet. Contribution to dietary recommendations (100).

cardiovascular disease, and moderate alcohol consumption can be considered only one component of a healthy Mediterranean lifestyle.

Protein and fat intakes are high, but they are of good quality. In the last 30 years, the protein quality index has improved appreciably because animal food consumption has increased. This fact is associated with other adverse consequences, because fat intake has been increased.

Although incidence of cardiovascular disease is high, it is not as much as expected considering the high level of fat intake. This may be a consequence of the healthful proportions of monounsaturated, polyunsaturated, and saturated fatty acids and of the moderate alcohol intake, mainly from wine (5). Of total fat intake, 76% consists of vegetable oils (Fig. 4). Olive and sunflower oils represent 88% of total vegetable oils. Olive oil is consumed in two very common ways in the Mediterranean world, in the dressing of foodstuffs consumed raw, and in deep frying, which results in special organoleptic characteristics.

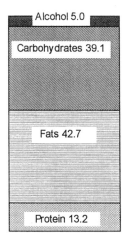

Fig. 3   Calorie profile. Macronutrients and alcohol contribution.

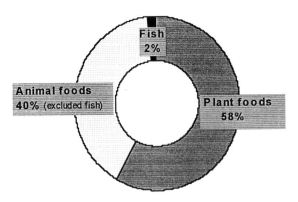

Fig. 4 Dietary fat sources in the Spanish diet.

C. Dietary Evolution

Dietary modifications are considered to be among the most important of the lifestyle changes resulting from industrialization and technical and economic development. These changes affected the eating habits of the population and, in turn, its nutritional status. Some aspects of this trend have been positive, but others related to food consumption pattern and lifestyle have been associated with an increase in degenerative diseases, which is a characteristic of the developed societies.

In addition, there has been a significant decrease in consumption of foods rich in complex carbohydrates, such as bread, beans, potatoes, pasta, and rice. An increase in the consumption of all meats, particularly poultry, fish, and dairy products, as well as a rise in the consumption of vegetables and a decline in fruit, wine, and sugar consumption have been the main changes observed. Potatoes, bread, and legumes are foods that have experienced more decreased intakes. These changes in eating habits may result from the perception of the foods as fattening. This lower consumption may be partially offset by an increased intake in processed products that often contain more salt and fat and fewer carbohydrates.

Dietary patterns are changing rapidly—generally in an undesirable direction. The results of such changes is a diet with a higher levels of saturated fat and cholesterol and lower levels of digestible and nondigestible carbohydrates content than a few years ago (6). Since 1990, olive oil intake in Spain has decreased by 4.8 g/person/day. Olive oil has been partially replaced by other vegetables oils, mainly sunflower oil. Nowadays vegetable oils account for 76% of total edible oils and fats and sunflower oil represents 41% of vegetable oils; olive oil continues to be the oil most consumed in the Spanish diet, accounting for 47%. Unfortunately, changes in diets of Mediterranean countries are unhealthful, and efforts are needed to persuade people to preserve the healthful dietary traditions within the Mediterranean region and to encourage greater consumption of plant foods, mainly vegetables and fruits, that were the base of the Spanish diet just a few years ago.

II. INDIGESTIBLE CARBOHYDRATES INTAKE: RESISTANT STARCH AND DIETARY FIBER

Dietary guidelines for Western countries encourage a considerable increase in carbohydrate intake (7), but nowadays more precise recommendations distinguishing between available and unavailable carbohydrates is necessary. Digestibility in the small intestine is the nutritionally most important property of food carbohydrates. Digestible carbohydrates provide glucose to the tissues, whereas indigestible carbohydrates reach the colon and are fermented to short-chain fatty acids, enhancing colon health (8).

Determination of carbohydrate intake in often not precise because of errors in the analysis of protein, fat, ash, and moisture and minor components, such as lignin, tannins, phytate, and organic acids, that are included in carbohydrate value. Indigestible carbohydrates constitute the main fraction of dietary fiber (DF), but DF does not constitute a defined chemical group, because it is a combination of chemically heterogeneous substances. The most widely accepted definition of DF is a physiological one in which it is assumed that nonstarch polysaccharides and lignin are the components of the DF residues obtained using enzymatic-gravimetric analytical methods, which are resistant to enzymatic hydrolysis in the small intestine. It is clearly necessary to reevaluate the definition of DF with regard to inclusion of resistant plant components that escape digestion in the human upper gastrointestinal tract (9). Moreover, definition, classification, and analytical methodology to quantify all small intestine indigestible components of foods should proceed at the same time.

A. Carbohydrate Intake

The total amount of available carbohydrates in the Spanish diet is 259 g/person/day, which represents 39% of total calorie intake. The main contributors to carbohydrate intake are cereal products (42.3%), vegetables, including potatoes (8%), sugar and honey (9.28%), and fresh fruits (7.69%) (3). The most important aspect of this macronutrient in the Spanish diet is its constant decline over the years (421 g in 1964 to 288 g in 1991), mainly due to the large drop in the consumption of bread, potatoes, and legumes, mentioned below. Considering that carbohydrates are an excellent source of energy in the diet, it would be desirable to increase their consumption in order to modify the present calorie profile.

B. Resistant Starches

A significant proportion of starch from a large range of foods is indigestible in the small intestine, but it reaches the colon and becomes an available substrate for bacterial fermentation (10,11) and is defined as resistant starch (RS) (12). RS and DF have been established as the principal substrates controlling the pattern of fermentation in the colon. Resistant starches usually ferment with a profile rich in butyrate, which could be beneficial in colonic disease prevention. Similar properties and physiological implications of both dietary components suggest that RS could be considered a DF constituent. It is therefore of interest to be able to determine the RS content in foods. There are some methods to analyze resistant starches in foods and food products, but they are not uniform. A key question in RS research and epidemiological studies is how to develop a homogeneous analytical method to quantify RS and compare results.

Table 1 shows the values of resistant starch in the principal Spanish starchy foods prepared in the Spanish manner. The analytical method used to determine RS is a modification of Berry's method (13) assayed in an interlaboratory study into the EURESTA program of the European Union (14). The analysis of RS involves mimicking the enzymatic hydrolysis that takes place in the upper part of the digestive tract. The quantification of RS is made by direct analysis of the residual starch after hydrolysis. The course of starch hydrolysis is unique for each product. There is a wide variation between food products in α-amylase susceptibility, from the lowest for lentils to the highest for boiled potatoes. Cooked legumes also produce a much lower metabolic glycemic response than do cereals and potato in both healthy and diabetic individuals (15).

Table 1 Resistant Starch Intake in the Spanish Diet

	Food consumption (g)	Resistant starch content (% dry matter)	Resistant starch intake (g)
Bread	159.13	2.49	2.95
Pasta (boiled)	12.24	2.92	0.33
Rice (boiled)	15.57	2.53	0.34
Biscuits	32.54	1.59	0.49
Lentils (boiled)	5.24	7.56	0.36
Chickpeas (boiled)	5.34	4.35	0.21
Beans (boiled)	4.39	4.96	0.19
Potatoes			
Boiled	78.21	1.00	0.20
Fried	78.21	4.02	0.82
Total			5.89

Therefore, they exhibit a lower glycemic index (16), thereby helping in the dietary control of diabetes.

Legumes shows the highest RS content, followed by fried potatoes and cereals. The mean value of Spanish RS intake is 5.9 g/person/day, which is the highest value in Europe (17), and it has remained stable on the last years. One difference between Spain and other countries is the traditional frying process, which increases RS content in starchy foods (18), as observed for boiled (1% RS) and fried (4% RS) potatoes. Approximately half of the potatoes eaten are fried in olive oil, accounting for 11.67% of RS in the diet, while boiled potatoes account for only 3.48%.

Although the present RS intake in Europe seems low, there is considerable potential to increase RS content in manufactured products if it is proved to be beneficial to the consumer. It should be stressed that studies on the impact of RS on human health require reliable data about both the nature and the amount of RS in the diet.

C. Dietary Fiber Intake

Dietary fiber is found in vegetables, fruits, grains, seeds, nuts, and legumes. Two broad categories of dietary fibers, soluble and insoluble, are defined analytically, depending on their chemical solubility in water and buffer solution or on physiological conditions. The soluble fraction is mainly contained in fruits, vegetables, and legumes, and it is associated mainly with cholesterol lowering and more rapid colonic degradation and with high fermentability. While insoluble fiber is thought to affect primarily the function of the large bowel, and it is predominant in cereals and legumes. As described below, the Spanish diet is rich in these foods: cereals, vegetables, legumes, fruits, and nuts account for 35% of total food consumption.

Total dietary fiber intake is currently 18.9 g/person/day, which is equivalent to 7.13 g/1000 kcal. Intake of the soluble fraction is 5.2 g/person/day. Both total and soluble dietary fiber intakes are lower than dietary allowances. Soluble DF could be increased if RS intake could be added, in which case the value would be increased to 11 g/person/day.

To estimate dietary fiber intakes in the Spanish diet, we used the DF content reported by MacCance and Widdowson (19), which include nonstarch polysaccharides and substances measured as lignin and some enzymatically resistant starches in the DF residue. Therefore, the results obtained by this methodology were overestimated due to the presence of appreciable

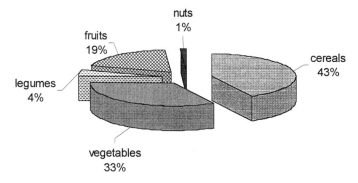

Fig. 5 Food contribution (%) to total dietary fiber intake.

amounts of RS and condensed tannins plus a small fraction of extractable polyphenols that constitute a part of DF residue. Soluble DF values were not indicated in the above reference, therefore they have been obtained from data reported by Englyst et al. (20,21). Contribution of different groups of foods to total DF intake are shown in Fig. 5. Overall, 43% of DF is derived from cereals, 33% from vegetables, including potato, 19% from fruit, 4% from pulses, and 1% from nuts.

Total DF intake at the beginning of the 1960s was >32 g/person/day. In 1991 it had decreased to 22.4 g/person/day, and the present average intake is 18.9 g—a 16% decrease since 1991 (Fig. 6). Figure 7 shows the trend of consumption of plant foods in the Spanish diet. Legumes are associated with many typical Mediterranean dishes, and they contain both soluble and insoluble dietary fiber. Moreover they contain other indigestible compounds, such as oligosaccharides, resistant starch, and bioactive polyphenols, which may be considered as associated components in the dietary fiber fraction in foods. However, despite their benefits, the intake of these foodstuffs is now decreasing, particularly in the western Mediterranean countries. In Spain, a great decrease occurred between the 1960s and the 1980s. At this time, consumption remains

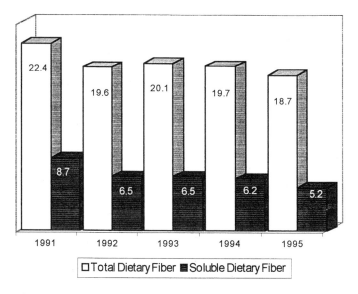

Fig. 6 Trend of total and soluble dietary fiber intake (g).

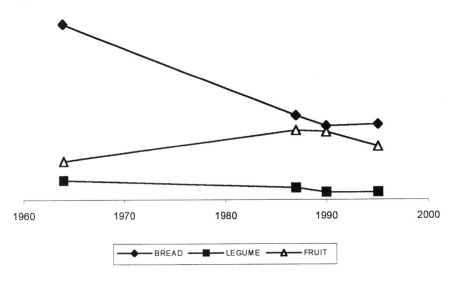

Fig. 7 Trend of bread, legume, and fruit consumption in the Spanish diet.

stable at 15 g/person/day. A similar decrease in bread consumption has occurred and seems to have stabilized. Fruit intake decreased significantly in a few years, probably due a sharp increase in price, and this fact directly affects the quality of DF intake.

Both insoluble and soluble DF intakes are decreasing, with that of the soluble fraction decreasing more significantly (40% since 1991), indicating a lower consumption of foods containing soluble DF, such as fresh fruits and legumes. It is evident that both the quantity and the quality of DF content in foods has decreased in recent years. Educational efforts are needed to reverse those changes and return to what was originally a very healthy dietary pattern.

REFERENCES

1. Steinmetz KA, Potter JD, Vegetables, fruit and cancer 1. Cancer Causes Control 2:325–357, 1991.
2. U.S. Department of Agriculture. The Food Guide Pyramid. Hyattsville, MD: Human Nutrition Information Service, Publication HG252, 1992.
3. Secretaría General Técnica, ed. Ministerio de Agricultura, Pesca y Alimentación. Madrid, 1996.
4. National study on nutrition and food consumption. Household budget survey, Spain, 1990–91. Madrid: Instituto Nacional de Estadística, 1996.
5. Renaud S, Lorgeril M. Wine, alcohol, platelets, and the French paradox for coronary heart disease. Lancet 339:1523–1526, 1992.
6. Saura-Calixto F, Goñi I. In: Cummings KH, Frolich W, eds. Dietary Fibre Intakes in Europe. Luxembourg: Commission of the European Communities, 1993.
7. Diet, nutrition, and prevention of chronic diseases. Technical Report Series 797. Geneva: World Health Organization, 1990.
8. M Roberfroid. Dietary fiber, inulin, and oligofructose: a review comparing their physiological effects. Food Sci Nutr 33(2):103–148, 1993.
9. Lee SS, Prosky L. International survey on dietary fiber: Definition, analysis, and reference materials. J AOAC Int 78(1):22–36, 1995.
10. Stephen AM. Mechanism of action of dietary fibre in the human colon. Nature 284:283–284, 1980.
11. Cummings JH, Englyst HN. Measurement of starch fermentation in the human large intestine. Can J Physiol Pharmacol 70:443–459, 1991.

12. Asp NG. Proceedings from the second plenary meeting of EURESTA. Physiological implications of the consumption of resistant starch in man. Eur J Clin Nutr 46(2):S1, 1992.

13. Goñi I, García-Diz L, Mañas E, Saura-Calixto F. Analysis of resistant starch: a method for food and food products. Food Chem 56(4):445–449, 1996.

14. Champ M. Determination of resistant starch in foods and food products: interlaboratory study. Eur J Clin Nutr 46(2):S51–S62, 1992.

15. Jenkins DJ, Wolever TMS, Kalmusky J, Giordano C, Wong SG, Bird JN, Pattern R, Hall M, Buckley G and Little JA. Low glycemic index carbohydrate foods in the management of hyperlipidemia. Am J Clin Nutr 42:604–617, 1985.

16. Goñi I, García-Alonso A, Saura-Calixto F. A starch hydrolysis procedure to estimate glycemic index. Nutr Res 17(3):427–437, 1997.

17. Drysseler P, Hoffem D, Estimation of resistant starch intake in Europe. In: Asp NG, Amelsvoort JMM, Hautvast JGAJ, eds. Proceedings of the concluding plenary meeting of EURESTA, European Commission, Wageningen, Netherlands, 1995, pp 84–86.

18. Goñi I, Bravo L, Larrauri JA and Saura-Calixto F. Resistant starch in potatoes deep-fried in olive oil. Food Chem 59(2):269–272, 1997.

19. In: Holland B, Welch AA, Unwin ID, Buss DH, Paul AA, Southgate DAT, eds. McCance and Widdowson's. The composition of foods, 5ᵃ Ed. Royal Society of Chemistry and Ministery of Agriculture, Fisheries and Food, Cambridge, UK, 1993.

20. Englyst HN, Bingam SA, Runswick SA, Collison E, Cummings JH. Dietary fibre (non-starch polysaccharides) in fruit, vegetables and nuts. J Hum Nutr Diet (1):247–286, 1988.

21. Englyst HN, Bingam SA, Runswick SA, Collison E, Cumming. Dietary fibre (non-starch polysaccharides) in cereal products. J Hum Nutr Diet (2):253–271, 1989.

40

Dietary Fiber in Israel: Recommendations, Consumption, and Research

Aliza H. Stark and Zecharia Madar
The Hebrew University of Jerusalem, Rehovot, Israel

Dorit Nitzan Kaluski
Ministry of Health, Jerusalem, Israel

I. INTRODUCTION

Established only 50 years ago, Israel is a melting pot for Jews from numerous countries, cultures, and ethnic backgrounds. Israel is a unique case study with a heterogeneous population that is growing and changing. Each ethnic group has brought its traditional dietary habits from its native country and contributed to the local cuisine. A thriving agricultural industry produces a wide variety of local produce that is of high quality and inexpensive. High fruit and vegetable consumption is characteristic of the Israeli diet along with ethnic foods that commonly contain legumes and whole grains (1). Hummus, falafel, tabouli, and majadara are just a few foods commonly eaten in Israel that are rich in dietary fiber.

Food consumption data for the Israeli population are sparse, and few studies have evaluated fiber consumption in healthy individuals. Much of the data is out of date or does not report total dietary fiber intake. To further complicate the issue, eating patterns are in transition in Israel. In the past 10 years, close to one million individuals from the former Soviet Union have taken residency in Israel (2). This represents approximately 15–20% of the present population of Israel. Nutritional assessments have not been carried out in this sector of the population. These new immigrants have brought nutritional habits native to their country of origin. Furthermore, many Western fast-food chains have entered the Israeli market. This has had a significant impact on food consumption, as individuals who in the past chose a high-fiber falafel (ground chick peas, a traditional Middle Eastern food) for a snack have new options such as pizza or a hamburger. Although precise data are not available, the worldwide trend of increased consumption of high-fat, low-fiber fast food is also occurring in Israel.

II. RECOMMENDATIONS

Dietary fiber consumption plays an important role in maintaining good health and preventing disease. The U.S. Department of Agriculture (USDA) currently recommends 12.5 g of dietary fiber per 1000 calories consumed (3), a range of approximately 20–35 g/day for adults. Recent recommendations of the American Health Foundation suggest that the goal of minimal intake of dietary fiber for children and young adults 3–20 years of age be equal to age plus 5 g of dietary fiber per day (Age + 5). This recommendation suggests that 3-year-old children consume no less than 8 g/day of dietary fiber and that a 20-year-old consume 25 g/d (4). The Israeli Ministry of Health advocates high fiber intake, but no official recommended daily intake has been established.

III. EVALUATION OF DIETARY FIBER CONSUMPTION IN ISRAEL

No single large-scale randomized analytical study has been carried out to assess nutrient consumption in Israel. Food balance sheets from the Central Bureau of Statistics have been published annually since 1949, but these data reflect per capita disappearance of foods and levels of nutrients available in the food supply. Although this provides interesting information on the foods generally eaten in Israel, it is not an accurate source for assessing dietary fiber intake by the population. In order to provide an overall picture of dietary fiber intake in Israel, data from epidemiological case-control studies, ecological studies, and cross-sectional studies have been collected. Extrapolating from the these studies and making generalizations within the limitations of available data, it appears that most of the Israeli population consume levels of dietary fiber consistent with the USDA guidelines—approximately 12.5 g/1000 kcal.

Lubin et al. (1) reported dietary fiber intake in a retrospective nutritional case-control study using a quantified dietary food history. The study collected information of dietary habits prior to disease onset in 196 cases of colon adenomas and in the same number of matched controls (total of 382 individuals). One third of the population consumed a mean daily intake of <24 g of dietary fiber, while two thirds consumed greater than this amount. The highest tertile of the population reported the daily mean intake of fiber to be >34 g/day, levels considered to constitute high fiber consumption. A second case-control study using similar methodologies was carried out in Israel and investigated the role of nutrition in brain cancer (5). Using a semi-quantitative food frequency questionnaire, it was found that two thirds of the controls reported >19 g/day of fiber consumption, with the highest tertile having an intake of 29 g/d or more. Data from both these studies provide a similar picture of daily dietary fiber consumption in Israel.

Two small studies have been carried out in the elderly population. Abraham (6) interviewed healthy subjects of high socioeconomic status (70 women, 40 men) of average age 80.3 ± 0.6 years; mean daily dietary fiber intake was calculated to be 19.6 ± 0.7 g/day, with women consuming 1735 ± 56 kcal/day and 18.2 ± 0.8 g of fiber and men consuming 1796 ± 45 kcal/day and 22.0 ± 1.3 g/day of fiber. Data was collected using a food frequency questionnaire and was analyzed for a wide range of nutrients, including calories and dietary fiber. A second study (7) was carried out in a home for the aged and looked at 21 healthy individuals of average age 81.4 ± 5.1 years. Using a food frequency questionnaire, daily fiber intake in this group was assessed as 16.1 ± 5.9 g/day.

The most comprehensive data available on dietary fiber consumption in Israel is a survey carried out in 1985, which represents the only large-scale study of food intake in a healthy adult population. The random sample was stratified by sex, age, and ethnic background. The study included detailed analyses of food-consumption patterns of different ethnic groups in Israel divided geographically into four groups: Yemenites, Middle Eastern (Iraqi, Syrian, Lebanese, etc.), North African (Moroccan, Algerian, Tunisian, Egyptian, etc.), and European/American. Data is reported for 632 participants in the age range of 41–70 years using a quantified dietary history questionnaire. Approximately half of those interviewed were female (52%; n = 329)

Table 1 Summary of Nutritional Studies Carried out in Israel that Included Measurement of Dietary Fiber Intake

Study (ref.)	Participants	Dietary fiber intake
Abraham, 1997	n = 110 Age: 80.3 ± 0.6 years	11.1 g/1000 kcal 19.6 ± 0.7 g/day
Dror et al., 1996	n = 21 Age: 65–87 years x = 81.4 ± 5.1	8.6 g/1000 kcal 16.1 ± 5.9 g/day
Kaplan, 1994	278 controls Age 50 ± 15 125 males, 153 females	Intermediate tertile: 19–28 g/day 66% of control subjects consumed >19 g/day
Lubin et al., 1997	382 individuals (matched pairs) Age: 21–74 years 222 males, 170 females	Intermediate tertile: 24–34 g/day 66% of population consumed >24 g/day
Lubin et al., 1997	n = 632 Age: 41–70 years 303 males, 329 females	Average 29.8 g/day 77% report intake of >20 g/day

and each ethnic group included a minimum of 100 individuals. Average daily dietary fiber consumption was 29.8 g/day, with 77% of participants reporting a daily intake of >20 g/day. The highest fiber consumption was found in Yemenite men (88.7%; > 20 g/d), and the lowest consumption was in European/American females, only 55% of whom consumed 20 g/day.

Lubin et al. (8) also examined food-consumption patterns by food group and compared Israeli fruit and vegetable intake to that in the United States. The traditional Israeli diet is rich in fruits and vegetables, with approximately 14–18% of daily caloric intake derived from fruits and vegetables. In the United States it has been estimated that only 3–4% of the daily calories consumed are derived from fruit and vegetable sources (9). In comparison to the high fiber intake in the Israeli population, Posner et al. reported that fewer than 3% of subjects in the Framingham study met the guidelines for dietary fiber intake (10).

The Israeli Ministry of Health, Department of Nutrition, and the Israel Center for Disease Control, in conjunction with the Central Bureau of Statistics and the Ben-Gurion University of the Negev, collected data for the first large-scale nutritional study in Israel. The project, called the Israel National Nutrition Survey (INNS), provides information on food and nutrient intake, dietary habits, physical activity, smoking habits, anthropometric measurements, socioeconomic status, health status, and nutrition knowledge, attitudes, and practices. The survey commenced in November 1998 and continued through December 2000 and included a representative sample of Israelis aged 25–65 years. The study assessed the nutritional needs of the population and identified public health issues. It also provides a basis for "country-specific food-based guidelines" and identifies areas for intervention through nutrition education and national public health policy.

IV. DIETARY FIBER RESEARCH IN ISRAEL

Basic research on the metabolic and physiological roles of dietary fiber has been carried out in both animal studies and human intervention trials. Development of new sources of dietary fiber with therapeutic benefits has also been an important aspect of fiber research in Israel. Fenugreek, a legume commonly eaten in Asia and Africa, has been widely researched and the biologically active fiber component isolated and investigated (11–13). Soybean dietary fiber, cottonseed dietary fiber, lupin bean dietary fiber, and spent grain dietary fiber have all been used in human intervention studies (14–17). Recently a corncob fiber treated with the fungus *Pleurotus ostreatus* was investigated as a new source of concentrated insoluble dietary fiber and its effects on 1,2-dimethylhydrazine (DMH)-induced colon cancer evaluated (18).

A. Studies with New Sources of Dietary Fiber

Fenugreek (*Trigonella foenum-graecum*) was fed to normal and diabetic subjects as part of a meal tolerance test (11). When fenugreek was added to the meal, postprandial plasma glucose levels were reduced at 30, 60, and 120 minutes. The endosperm of fenugreek seeds is rich in soluble fibers composed of galactomannans (12). These highly viscous gelforming fibers are considered responsible for the potent antidiabetic activity of fenugreek. The use of fenugreek has been limited due to its bitter taste and pungent odor. A patented method has been developed to isolate an odorless, tasteless fraction from the whole fenugreek seeds (13). This new product, rich in galactomannans, may be useful in both the treatment and prevention of diabetes.

The physiological effects of cottonseed dietary fiber have also been studied in Israel (14). In streptozotocin-induced diabetic rats, a diet containing 15% of this fiber tended to reduce postprandial glucose levels. In diabetic subjects, a daily supplementation of 16.5 g of dietary fiber over a 1-month period led to significant decreases in glucose excursions following a meal tolerance test containing the cottonseed fiber.

The efficacy of soybean fiber to improve glycemic profiles in Type II diabetic subjects has also been investigated (15). The fiber was highly palatable and was consumed either in a powdered form or added into bread. In long-term studies, dietary fiber added to bread was more effective in lowering postprandial glucose levels than when consumed in the powdered form. In addition, individuals with fasting plasma glucose levels of >130 mg% had significantly lower blood glucose levels at baseline and at 30 and 60 minutes following a meal tolerance test. This study showed that both the form in which the fiber was consumed and the severity of diabetes determine the effectiveness of dietary fiber supplementation.

The role of dietary fiber in colon cancer prevention has been investigated using animal models of DMH-induced colon cancer. Zusman et al. (18) fed rats dietary fiber derived from corncobs and treated with the fungus *Pleurotus ostreatus*. In comparison with animals fed crude corncob fibers or a diet of 3% cellulose, administration of the fungus-treated fibers led to a significantly lower rate of tumor incidence (26% vs. >44%). In addition, increased levels of p53 tumor-supressor proteins were measured in the cell cytoplasm and serum of tumor-bearing rats fed the treated corncob fiber. It appears that consumption of highly insoluble dietary fiber from corncobs treated with fungus may have potential use in colon cancer prevention.

B. Glycemic Index of Ethnic Foods Commonly Eaten in Israel

One of the projects undertaken in our laboratory was to establish the glycemic response to consumption of various foods commonly eaten by different ethnic groups in Israel (19). Four food items were chosen for this research project: melawach (Yemenite bread), majadra (a Syrian lentil and rice dish), kugel (a Polish noodle casserole), and couscous (Moroccan semolina with chickpeas and vegetables). A meal tolerance test was carried out in normal and diabetic subjects and the results were compared to both a standard breakfast and a 50 g glucose load. All meals were isocaloric and contained 1660 J (400 kcal) and 50 g of carbohydrate. The glycemic index was calculated by comparing the postprandial glucose excursions of each food to the 50 g

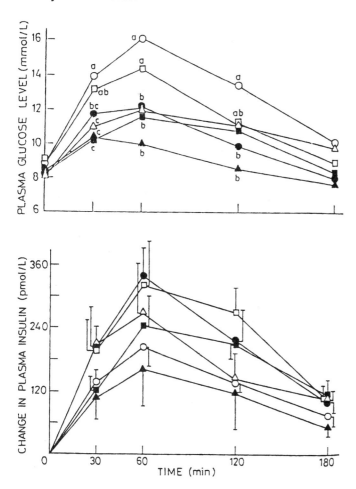

Fig. 1 Glucose and insulin responses to various kinds of ethnic foods eaten in Israel given to NIDDM subjects: (●) standard meal, (△) melawach, (▲) majadra, (□) kugel, (■) couscous, (○) glucose. For each time, values not sharing a common letter were significantly different, $p < 0.05$. (Adapted from Ref. 19.)

glucose load (scored as 100). As illustrated in Fig. 1, the glycemic response in type II diabetic subjects was greatest for the Polish dish and lowest for the Syrian dish (66 ± 5.5 vs. 24 ± 5.1, respectively). In healthy individuals, the area under the glucose curve following each test meal was less than the area of the glucose load. However, only majadera and the test meal significantly decreased glucose excursions. This clearly demonstrates the ability of healthy individuals to maintain a tight control over glucose uptake and prevent increased blood glucose levels despite rapid rates of glucose absorption from the intestine.

Possible explanations for the differences in glycemic response in diabetic subjects may be the high dietary fiber content of majadara (7.6 g) and low fiber content of the kugel (2.0 g). In addition to its high fiber content, majadera contains lentils, which are rich in amylose. In comparison to other carbohydrate sources, amylose is broken down slowly in the digestive tract and the rate of glucose absorption is contingent on the efficiency of amylase in breaking down the starch molecules. Overall, this study illustrates the physiological response to various ethnic foods eaten in Israel and the great variability in potential health benefits related to diet.

Based on data collected concerning the glycemic index of ethnic foods eaten in Israel, melawach (Yemenite bread) was chosen to be enriched with 15 g of dietary fiber from three different sources (16). This was an attempt to improve the relatively high glycemic index of melawach, which is made of white flour and fat (butter). Diabetic subjects were given melawach with added locust bean gum, corncob fiber, or dietary fiber isolated from lupin beans. Of the three fiber varieties, only locust bean gum significantly decreased the glycemic index of the melawach. This may be explained by the high galactomannan content of this particular fiber. As seen with fenugreek fiber, the galactomannans found in locust beans have physicochemical properties that include high water-binding capacity and the formation of very viscous gels at relatively high dilutions (13). This may account for the ability to inhibit or delay nutrient absorption in the digestive tract, resulting in a lower glycemic index. Lupin fiber is produced from a legume and contains mainly pectic materials, which had little effect in lowering plasma glucose levels when incorporated into the melawach. Corncob fiber is predominately cellulose and hemicellulose and is considered largely insoluble (20). It is well accepted that the presence of insoluble fiber in foods influences intestinal function and has little or no affect on carbohydrate metabolism.

V. CONCLUSION

All available data indicate that the Israeli population, on the whole, consumes dietary fiber at levels similar to guidelines set by the USDA. Information on food consumption in children and new immigrants does not exist; therefore, no conclusions concerning dietary fiber intake can be made regarding these large sectors of the population. It is of interest to note that despite reports of relatively high fiber consumption in Israel, colon cancer incidence is higher than in most Western countries with the exception of the United States and Germany (21).

A wide variety of research in the field of dietary fiber has been carried out and continues in Israel. Ongoing studies include development of additional sources of dietary fiber with nutraceutical properties and achieving a better understanding of the mechanisms of action of dietary fiber in the body.

REFERENCES

1. Lubin F, Rozen P, Arieli B, Farbstein M, Knaani Y, Bat L, Farbstein H. Nutritional and lifestyle habits and water-fiber interaction in colorectal adenoma etiology. Cancer Epidemiol Biomarkers Prev 6:79–85, 1997.
2. Statistical Abstract of Israel 1997. Vol. 48. Jerusalem: Central Bureau of Statistics, 1997.
3. U.S. Department of Agriculture. Food Guide Pyramid: A Guide to Daily Food Choices. Washington, DC: U.S. Department of Agriculture, 1992.
4. Willians CL, Bollella M, Wynder WL. A new recommendation for dietary fiber in childhood. Pediatrics 96:985–988, 1995.
5. Kaplan S. Role of exposure to nitroso compounds in the development of primary brain tumors. Ph.D. dissertation. Ramat Aviv, Israel: Tel Aviv University, 1994.
6. Abraham S. Relation between nutritional status and cellular immunity in independent elderly people living in protected housing. Masters thesis. Rehovot, Israel: The Hebrew University of Jerusalem, 1997.
7. Dror Y, Stern F, Nemish L, Hart J, Grinblat J. Macronutrient consumption and nutritional status in a selected well-established group of elderly people in a home for the aged in Israel. J Am Coll Nutr 15:475–480, 1996.

8. Lubin F, Lusky A, Chetrit A, Modan M. Differential nutritional habits and weight in distinct ethnic groups in Israel. Proceedings of the 3rd Abraham Conference on Preventive Nutrition: Dietary Assessments in Populations, Beer Sheba, Israel, 1997.

9. Block G, Dresser CM, Hartman AM, Carroll MD. Nutrient sources in the American diet. Am J Epidemiol 122:27–40, 1985.

10. Posner BM, Cupples LA, Gagnon D. Healthy people 2000. Arch Intern Med 153:1549–1556, 1993.

11. Arad Y, Abel R, Madar Z. Fenugreek as a means of reducing glucose levels in diabetic type II subjects. Advances Diet Nutr 2:121–125, 1988.

12. Shomer I, Madar Z. Polysaccharide compostition of a gel fraction derived from fenugreek and its effect on starch digestion and bile acid absorption in rats. J Agr Food Chem 38:1535–1539, 1990.

13. Garti N, Madar Z, Aserin A, Sternheim B. Fenugreek galactomannans as food emulsifiers. Food Sci Technol 30:305–311, 1997.

14. Madar Z, Nir M, Trostler N, Norenberg C. Diabetes. Effect of cottonseed dietary fiber on metabolic parameters in diabetic rats and non-insuling dependent diabetic humans. J Nutr 118:1143–1148, 1988.

15. Madar Z, Arieli B, Trostler N, Norynberg C. Effect of consuming soybean dietary fiber on fasting and postprandial glucose and insulin levels in Type II diabetes. J Clin Biochem Nutr 4:165–173, 1988.

16. Feldman N, Norenberg C, Voet H, Manor E, Berner Y, Madar Z. Enrichment of an Israeli ethnic food with fibres and their effect on the glycaemic and insulinaemic responses in non-insulin-dependent diabetes mellitus subjects. Br J Nutr 74:681–688, 1995.

17. Odes H, Madar Z, Trop M, Namir S, Gross J, Cohen T. A pilot study of the efficacy of spent grain dietary fiber in the treatment of constipation. Isr J Med Sci 22:12–15, 1986.

18. Zusman I, Reifen R, Livni O, Smirnoff P, Gurevich P, Sandler B, Nyska A, Gal R, Tendler Y, Madar Z. The role of apoptosis, proliferation cell nuclear antigen and p53 protein in chemically induced colon cancer in rats fed corncob fiber treated with the fungus *Pleurotus ostreatus*. Anticancer Res 17:2105–2114, 1997.

19. Indar-Brown K, Norneberg C, Madar Z. Comparison of glycemic and insulinemic response following ingestion of ethnic foods by NIDDM and healthy subjects. Am J Clin Nutr 55:89–95, 1992.

20. Madar Z, Timar B, Nyska A, Zusman I. Effects of high fiber diets on pathological changes in DMH-induced rat colon cancer. Nutr Cancer 20:87–96, 1993.

21. Health Status in Israel. Israeli Center for Disease Control, Publication #202, 1997.

41

Dietary Fiber Intake in China: Recommendations and Actual Consumption Patterns

Guangya Wang
Chinese Academy of Preventive Medicine, Beijing, China

I. INTRODUCTION

Data on the dietary fiber intake of the Chinese population are meager. The term ''crude fiber'' was widely used in China until the insoluble fiber content of food items was included in the Chinese Food Composition Tables in 1991 (1). Thus, the total dietary fiber intake was not available from the recent national dietary survey (2). In this chapter, the information on dietary fiber intake in the Chinese population has been obtained from two primary sources: a comprehensive ecological survey of Chinese rural countries in 1983 designed to examine the relationships among diet, lifestyle, and mortality in China (3), and the 1992 National Nutrition Survey designed to assess the dietary and nutritional status of the Chinese population (2). In the first study in 1983, the 65 survey counties are widely distributed in 24 out of 30 provinces in mainland China, which covered the most populous areas and different dietary patterns, as well as geographical variations. Foods samples representative of cereals and vegetables consumed in the counties were collected and analyzed by direct laboratory methods (4–6) to estimate contents of dietary fiber and its components. In the second study in 1992, a total of 27,000 households was surveyed. City residents and rural residents accounted for one and two thirds of the study participants, respectively. The intakes of insoluble dietary fiber from foods were calculated based on the food composition table (1).

II. METHODS

A. The 1983 Ecological Survey

1. Food Sample Collection and Preparation

Cereals and vegetables most commonly consumed in significant amounts were collected in the uncooked state from selected households and markets in each county to yield a total of 600 samples of approximately 40 foods. After removal of the nonedible portion, vegetables were washed and air-dried in the shade, then transferred to the county laboratory where they were dried in a ventilated oven at 55–65°C until a constant weight was reached. Cereal samples (as consumed) were also dried and sent in sealed plastic bags to Cornell University, (Ithaca, NY), where they were ground by a Tecator Cyclotec mill fitted with a 1 mm screen.

2. Analytical Methods

Dry matter and ash were estimated by drying a 1.5–2.0 g sample overnight in a 105°C oven, weighing, then ashing at 525°C overnight and weighing. Crude protein (N $\times$ 6.25) was determined using the Kjeldahl procedure. Total dietary fiber (TDF) was estimated by an enzymatic-gravimetric procedure (AOAC method 43.A14–43.A20) and the detergent system of analysis (4,5) with the following modification: sample size was reduced to 0.75 g with proportional concentration reduction in buffers, NaOH, H_3PO_4 solution, but maintaining original concentration of enzymes. Analysis was done in quadruplicate.

Insoluble fiber or neutral detergent fiber (NDF) was determined using the amylase method with some modification (6). The neutral detergent residue was sequentially treated with acid-detergent solution and 72% H_2SO_4 to estimate hemicellulose (HE), cellulose (CE), and lignin (LS). Residual cell wall protein was measured to allow an estimate of soluble fiber (SF) since the total dietary fiber was corrected for residual nitrogen. Soluble fiber was estimated as the difference between total dietary fiber and NDF corrected for residual protein (SF = TDF − NDF-cell wall protein).

3. Dietary Survey Methods

The 3-day household food intake measurements (weighing and recording) were used to collect information on the pattern of food consumption among Chinese households. Using these food consumption data and the calculation of the proportion of foods, each individual food in the diet, a representative mixed-plant diet sample, including cereals and vegetables, was made from each of the 65 counties for determination of dietary fiber components. The intakes of the dietary fiber components were calculated by the fiber contents of mixed diet per person. Because the composition was originally formulated on the basis of per capita intake, the calculations were straightforward.

B. The 1992 National Nutrition Survey

1. Source of Data

The food samples were prepared and analyzed in 15 local laboratories according to a unified methodology with proper quality control procedures, after which the data of insoluble fiber (neutral detergent fiber) were included in *The Composition of Chinese Foods*, published in 1991 (1). Food samples were collected in 15 provinces representing most of the populated area of China. The sampling procedures, estimation methods, and analytical methods used in the different regions were conducted using the same instruction manual prepared by the Department of Food Chemistry at the Institute of Nutrition and Food Hygiene in Beijing, China. The analytical method for neutral detergent fiber of foods is the same as that used at Cornell University.

2. Dietary Survey Methods

The National Nutrition Survey in 1992 was a nationwide household sampling survey using combined weighing and recording methods to collect household food consumption data over 3 days. At the same time, food intake data for individual members of the household were collected using the 24-hour recall method for 3 consecutive days. The survey data were analyzed separately by food consumption of households and individual household members. The dietary fiber intakes were calculated using *The Composition of Chinese Food* (1). The estimation of average dietary fiber intake for China was derived as a weighted average of values for all provinces or autonomous regions and municipalities in China.

III. RESULTS AND DISCUSSION

A. Dietary Fiber Intake for the Rural Population—1983 Survey

1. Dietary Fiber Composition of Selected Food Groups

Table 1 presents the fiber content and its constituents of 38 individual foods grouped into six groups: cereals, starchy tubers, legumes(dry), legumes(fresh), cucurbits and fruits, and roots and leafy vegetables (7). Cereals contain substantially less TDF than dry beans and higher TDF than tubers and vegetables (except beans). TDF values for starchy tubers, such as potatoes and sweet potatoes, are close to those for roots and vegetables. On the basis of consumption, however, vegetables contribute much less fiber to the average Chinese diet than do cereals. Soluble fiber constitutes approximately 40–50% of the total dietary fiber of these foods. Hemicelluloses are the major component of insoluble fiber in cereals. In beans and tubers, hemicelluloses represent about one third of the insoluble fiber. In leafy vegetables, roots, gourds, and fruits, cellulose makes up 75% of the insoluble fiber. Although lignin is a relatively minor component of cereals and tubers, there is a substantial amount of lignin in cucurbits, fruits, and fresh beans. For cereals, variation in fiber content is attributable in large part to the climate, time of harvest, storage conditions, and processing and preparation techniques. There were substantial variation in the contents of dietary fiber and its components for the same foods collected in different parts of China. For example, there was a threefold range between the maximum and minimum fiber contents for corn meal, long grain rice, etc. Assay measurement error on repeat analysis was only 3–4%.

2. Dietary Fiber Intake

The average dietary fiber intake value for rural populations in 65 counties was calculated using data from Ref. 3 (Table 2). The mean dietary fiber intake in the rural population was 33.3 g/day for total dietary fiber, 24.4 g/day for NDF, 11.6 g/day for hemicellulose, 9.5 g/day for cellulose, 2.22 g/day for lignin, and 9.45 g/day for pectin, which is the main component of the soluble fiber fraction. Total soluble fiber (SF) was estimated as SF = TDF − NDF = 33.3 − 24.4 = 8.9 g/day. This value is close to the 9.45 g/d for pectin, because the residual cell wall protein (undigested protein) was included in the value of NDF. Thus, the mean value for total dietary fiber (TDF) was 12.6 g/1000 kcal and for NDF was 9.2 g/1000 kcal (using the average dietary energy intake of 2641 kcal).

B. Dietary Fiber Intake in Chinese Population—1992 Survey

1. Food Consumption Pattern

The 1992 National Nutrition Survey, (2) food consumption pattern of the Chinese population is presented in Table 3. The results show that although the food consumption patterns of rural and urban residents are similar, rural residents consumed more cereals and starch tubers and fewer fruits than urban residents. The consumption of cereals was 485.8 g/d for rural and 405.4 g/d

Table 1 Dietary Fiber Composition (g/100 g edible portion) of Selected Food Groups in 1983 Survey

	Cereals	Starch tubers	Legumes, dry	Legume products	Cucurbits fruits	Root	Leafy vegetables
No. of samples	145	57	47	32	77	34	135
DM							
Mean ± SD	89.1 ± 1.36	18.6 ± 6.05	92.2 ± 2.16	11.4 ± 4.56	7.8 ± 3.6	7.2 ± 3.05	7.5 ± 3.11
Min~Max	82.7–92.8	4.8–32.9	84.9–94.6	5.5–24.1	2.5–18.9	2.4–16.2	1.6–18.8
TDF							
Mean ± SD	4.5 ± 3.15	2.2 ± 0.73	20.2 ± 3.56	4.3 ± 0.59	2.7 ± 0.67	2.1 ± 0.34	2.7 ± 0.36
Min~Max	1.1–15.6	1.4–6.1	14.2–27.2	2.9–5.9	1.6–4.4	1.2–2.6	2.0–4.1
SF							
Mean ± SD	1.8 ± 1.07	1.1 ± 0.36	10.0 ± 2.96	1.8 ± 0.37	1.1 ± 0.34	1.1 ± 0.22	1.4 ± 0.22
Min~Max	0.2–8.7	0.7–3.2	2.3–3.0	1.0–2.7	0.5–1.9	0.5–1.6	0.9–2.4
NDF							
Mean ± SD	3.4 ± 3.22	1.3 ± 0.52	11.2 ± 2.3	2.8 ± 0.54	1.8 ± 0.66	1.1 ± 0.23	1.5 ± 0.30
Min~Max	0.4–14.5	0.6–3.1	7.3–15.7	1.6–4.0	0.8–3.9	0.7–1.6	0.9–2.5
HC							
Mean ± SD	2.3 ± 2.64	0.4 ± 0.21	4.0 ± 1.22	0.6 ± 0.17	0.3 ± 0.09	0.2 ± 0.06	0.3 ± 0.09
Min~Max	0.2–12.0	0.1–1.0	1.8–6.8	0.3–1.0	0.1–0.6	0.2–0.3	0.2–0.8
CE							
Mean ± SD	0.7 ± 0.59	0.7 ± 0.30	6.4 ± 1.58	1.7 ± 0.32	1.0 ± 0.26	0.8 ± 0.14	1.0 ± 0.16
Min~Max	0–3.0	0.4–2.2	4.6–11.1	1.1–2.7	0.5–1.7	0.4–1.1	0.6–1.6
LS							
Mean ± SD	0.3 ± 0.14	0.1 ± 0.10	0.7 ± 0.50	0.4 ± 0.20	0.5 ± 0.45	0.1 ± 0.06	0.2 ± 0.17
Min~Max	0–0.6	0–0.4	0–1.6	0.2–0.9	0.1–1.7	0.04–0.3	0.1–0.9
TDF/NDF	4.5/3.4=	2.2/1.3=	20.2/11.2=	4.3/2.8=	2.7/1.8=	2.1/1.1=	2.7/1.5=
	1.32	1.69	1.80	1.54	1.54	1.91	1.80

DM = Dry matter; TDF = total dietary fiber; SF = soluble fiber; NDF = neutral detergent fiber; HC = hemicellulose; CE = cellulose.

Table 2 Dietary fiber intake of Rural Residents (g/day/person)

	TDF	NDF	HC	CE	Lignin	Cutin	Pectin
Median	28.9	20.1	9.3	9.3	2.04	0.85	8.87
Mean	33.3	24.4	11.6	9.5	2.22	1.01	9.45
SD	17.8	12.3	7.9	5.0	1.19	0.74	3.98
CV%	53	50	68	53	54	74	42
Min.	7.7	3.7	0.3	0.5	0.5	0.1	1.3
Max.	76.6	57.7	30.0	25.9	6.46	3.49	17.96

TDF = Total dietary fiber; NDF = neutral detergent fiber (or insoluble dietary fiber); HC = hemicellulose; CE = cellulose.
Source: Data from Ref. 7.

Table 3 Food Consumption (g/day/person) Pattern in 1992 Dietary Survey

	Cereals	Starch tubers	Legume	Vegetable	Fruit
National average	439.9	86.6	11.2	320.3	49.2
Rural	485.8	108.0	10.2	317.5	32.0
Urban	405.4	46.0	13.3	327.3	80.1

Table 4 Dietary Fiber Intake in Chinese Population

National urban and rural income level	NDF (g/day)	NDF (g/1000 kcal)	TDF (g/day)	TDF (g/1000 kcal)
Average	13.3 ± 9.9	5.7 ± 4.2	19.8 ± 14.6	8.5 ± 6.3
low	15.1 ± 11.7	6.6 ± 5.1	22.5 ± 17.3	9.7 ± 7.6
middle	13.2 ± 9.3	5.8 ± 4.1	19.7 ± 13.8	8.5 ± 6.0
high	11.5 ± 8.1	4.8 ± 3.4	17.1 ± 12.0	7.0 ± 5.0
Urban	11.6 ± 8.7	4.8 ± 3.6	17.4 ± 13.0	7.2 ± 5.4
Rural	14.1 ± 10.4	6.1 ± 4.5	20.9 ± 15.4	9.0 ± 6.7

TDF is calculated using the factors such as 1.49 for national average, 1.48 for rural, 1.50 for urban; factors showed in Table 5.
Energy intake (X $\pm$ SD, kcal): National total average 2328 $\pm$ 735, low income 2289 $\pm$ 719, middle income 2284 $\pm$ 721, high income 2410 $\pm$ 755, urban average 2394 $\pm$ 793, rural average 2294 $\pm$ 700.
Data of NDF intakes cited from Ref. 2.

Table 5 Calculation of Factors for Estimating TDF Intakes (g/day)

		Cereals	Tubers	Legumes	Vegetables	Fruits	Total	Conversion factor
National	TDF	11.6	1.5	1.1	6.8	1.0	22.0	1.49
Average	NDF	8.8	0.9	0.6	3.8	0.7	14.8	
Rural	TDF	12.8	1.8	0.9	6.8	0.8	23.1	1.48
	NDF	9.7	1.1	0.5	3.8	0.5	15.6	
Urban	TDF	10.7	0.8	1.3	7.0	1.8	21.6	1.50
	NDF	8.1	0.5	0.7	3.9	1.2	14.4	

for urban residents (Table 3). These figures are much higher than those of American residents (8).

2. Dietary Fiber Intake

Dietary fiber intake values for the survey population were calculated based on NDF content (1). Mean dietary fiber intakes for the Chinese population are shown in Table 4. The TDF intake was calculated from NDF intake using the ratio of TDF to NDF for selected food groups (Table 1) and using the food consumption pattern and TDF/NDF ratio for rural and urban populations. The conversion factors for estimating TDF intake were 1.49 for the national average, 1.48 rural, and 1.50 urban (Table 5). Table 4 shows that the intake values of TDF were 19.8 and 8.5 g/1000 kcal for the national average, 17.4 and 7.2 g/1000 kcal urban, and 20.9 and 9.0 g/1000 kcal rural. The NDF intake values were 13.3 and 5.7 g/1000 kcal for the national average, 11.6 and 4.8 g/1000 kcal urban, and 14.1 and 6.1 g/1000 kcal rural. When the income was lower, the fiber intake was higher. The rural intake values in the 1992 survey were much lower than those in the 1983 survey.

The dietary fiber intake estimate is usually strongly influenced by the data source. Here we have reported dietary fiber intakes of Chinese population obtained from two large studies, which resulted in different estimates. As indicated in Table 6, the TDF and NDF intakes from the 1992 National Nutrition Survey were significantly lower than the intakes from the 1983 ecological study. The main reason for this discrepancy is using the difference in fiber contents of the same group of foods rather than differences in food consumption. Using the same fiber contents for foods, the estimates of fiber intake from these two studies are quite close (TDF 35.7 vs. 33.3 g/day; NDF 24.4 vs. 24.4 g/day). The differences in fiber content for the same food groups are not caused by difference in analytical methods, since these two database were developed by the same analytical methods, but by geographical variations in the food-producing areas. For example, the TDF of corn meal, short grain rice, and wheat flour ranged from 5.4 to 17.4, 1.2 to 3.4, and 3.0 to 7.9 g/100 g dry matter (7). These differences could be geographical variations but they could also reflect the degree of milling of the product. The variation in vegetables would reflect variety, time of harvest (storage), and type of preparation. For potatoes, the TDF contents ranged from 7.7 to 13.1 g/100 g dry matter with a moisture contenting range from 75 to 95%; all other tubers had a wide range of moisture and fiber contents. The water and fiber contents in roots and leafy vegetables varied as widely as the tubers.

Table 6   Difference of Dietary Fiber Intake (g/day) for Rural Residents

Fiber	TDF	NDF
Source 1[a]	20.9	14.1
Source 2[b]	35.7	24.4
Source 3[c]	33.3	24.4

[a] Data cited from 1992 survey, indicated in Table 4.
[b] Data calculated using the food consumption in 1992 survey, but the fiber intakes are calculated using fiber contents of selected food groups analyzed in 1983 at Cornell.
[c] Data cited from 1983 survey, showed in Table 2.

Table 7 Comparison of Dietary Fiber Composition (g/100 g edible portion) of Selected Food Groups

Food groups[a]	Cereals	Starch tubers	Legumes	Vegetables	Fruits
Dry matter, %[b]	89.1	18.6	92.2	7.5	—
Dry matter, %[c]	87.2	22.8	88.3	7.7	16.8
TDF[b]	4.1	2.2	18.7	2.7	—
TDF[c]	2.6	1.7	17.8	2.2	2.2
NDF[b]	2.8	1.3	10.7	1.7	—
NDF[c]	2.0	1.0	9.9	1.2	1.5

[a] Food groups: Cereals including rice, wheat flour, corn meal, and millet; legumes including mung bean, red bean, and soy bean; vegetables including leafy, root, and fruit bearing vegetables; starch tubers including sweet potato, potato and taro; fruits including apple, Chinese date, peach, pear, and orange. There is no datum for fruit in Ref. 7.
[b] Data analyzed in Cornell University 1983 survey, cited from Ref. 7.
[c] Data collected from *The Composition of Chinese Foods* (Ref. 1) and the TDF content of food is calculated using factors showed in Table 1.

IV. RECOMMENDATIONS FOR DIETARY FIBER INTAKE

It is difficult to make fully informed recommendations on the basis of these somewhat limited data. The lack of data on total dietary fiber contents of foods in *The Composition of Chinese Foods* only allows for the estimation of NDF intake using food intake data from the Chinese National Nutrition Survey in 1992. For comparing the data, we use the factors (TDF/NDF) listed in Table 1 for calculating TDF intakes. A recommended food guide and food guide pagoda was suggested by the Chinese Nutrition Society in 1998.

First it is necessary to determine a dietary fiber composition of selected food groups according to the pattern of food consumption in 1992 survey. Then the TDF and NDF contents of the food groups are estimated (Table 7). Using the dietary fiber composition of selected food groups in the 1983 survey for calculating the recommendation, a comparison of dietary fiber composition of selected food groups is also presented in Table 7. A recommendation for fiber intake for achieving the Chinese food guide pagoda estimated using the data in Table 7 is shown in Table 8.

Table 8 Recommended Fiber Intake for Achieving Chinese Food Guide Pagoda (g/day)

Food intake[a]	Cereals[b]	Vegetables	Fruits	Legumes[c]	Total intake g/d	g/1000 kcal
Low energy (1800 kcal)	300	400	100	50	850	
TDF	7.8	8.8	2.2	4.4	23.2	12.9
NDF	6.0	4.8	1.5	2.5	14.8	8.2
Median energy (2400 kcal)	400	450	150	50	1050	
TDF	8.0	9.9	3.3	4.4	25.6	10.7
NDF	8.0	5.4	2.2	2.5	18.1	7.5
High energy (2800 kcal)	500	500	200	50	1250	
TDF	12.0	11.0	4.4	4.4	31.8	11.4
NDF	10.0	6.0	3.0	2.5	21.5	7.7

[a] Food intakes are recommended by Chinese Food Guide.
[b] Cereals including starch tubers.
[c] Legumes and its products: for calculating the fiber content of legumes/products, 25 g dry beans is used as 50 g legumes/products.

Table 9 Relationship Between NDF Intake and Grain and Animal
Food Consumption (g/day)

Area	NDF	Energy	Grain[a]	Meat[b]
Hainan rural	6.6	1852	395	136
Guangxi urban	6.6	2108	338	301
Shanghai urban	9.0	2432	381	256
Shanghai rural	9.1	2271	443	144
Beijing urban	11.1	2503	405	207
Beijing rural	12.5	2475	476	111
Xinjiang urban	12.9	2491	548	122
Shandong urban	15.0	2339	460	206
Anhui rural	18.0	2806	782	51
Xinjiang rural	18.4	2800	658	58
Shandong rural	19.4	2312	599	59
Xizang rural	22.4	3127	605	120

[a] Grains including cereals and starch tubers.
[b] Meats including animal meats, fish, and egg.
Source: Ref. 2.

We propose recommended dietary fiber intakes for the general Chinese population based on the recently developed food pagoda (Table 8) and the dietary fiber content of plant food groups (Table 7) derived from the Chinese food composition table (1). These recommended dietary fiber intake values are in general consistent with the recommended values from other countries. Cummings et al. demonstrated that a dose-response relationship exists between the intake of nonstarch polysaccharides and stool weight up to an intake of 32 g/day (9). It was suggested that an intake of 18 g/day of nonstarch polysaccharides is required for a healthful diet (10). These values are similar to the estimate of 10 g/1000 kcal of dietary fiber recommended by the Life Sciences Research Office Expert Panel and to the recommended dietary fiber intake of 25–35 g/d or 10–13 g/1000 kcal in the United States made by the AHF (11). In comparison with the results from the 1992 National Nutrition Survey, populations with relatively poor diets (higher grain and lower animal food consumption) have higher NDF intakes (Table 4), which are usually close to or exceed the above recommended values (Table 8). In contrast, the populations with relatively affluent diets (lower grain and higher animal food consumption) have lower NDF intakes (Table 9), which are usually lower than the above recommended values (Table 8).

According to this approach, the recommended daily total dietary fiber intakes are 23.2 g or 12.9 g/1000 kcal for a low energy intake population, 25.6 g or 10.7 g/1000 kcal for a medium energy intake population, and 31.8 g or 11.4 g/1000 kcal for a high energy intake population. The recommended value of 23.2–31.8 g or 10.7–12.9 g/1000 kcal is quite close to the recommendation in the United States, which is approximately 10–13 g/1000 kcal or 20–35 g/day (11). This recommendation will allow for a more scientifically justified recommendation for the Chinese population. Until that time, the preliminary recommendations presented here will serve as an adequate interim benchmark for China.

ACKNOWLEDGMENTS

The author is very grateful for the constructive comments of Dr. Junshi Chen of the Institute of Nutrition and Food Hygiene, Chinese Academy of Preventive Medicine, and Dr. Banoo Parpia of the Division of Nutritional Sciences, Cornell University.

REFERENCES

1. (a) GY Wang. The Composition of Chinese Foods. Beijing: People's Medical Publishing House, 1991, pp 2–27; (b) GY Wang, Parpia B, Wen ZM. The Composition of Chinese Foods. Washington, DC: ILSI Press, 1997, pp 10–82.
2. KY Ge. The Dietary and Nutritional Status of Chinese Population (1992 National Nutrition Survey). Beijing: People's Medical Publishing House, 1996, pp 107–109, 195–197.
3. JS Chen, TC Campbell, JY Li, P Richard. Diet, Life-style and Mortality in China. Oxford University Press, Cornell University Press, and People's Medical Publishing House, Beijing, China, 1991, pp 506–514, 520, 606–624.
4. AOAC. Changes in official methods. J Assoc Off Anal Chem 68:399, 1985.
5. L Prosky N-G ASP, I Furda, JW Drvries, TF Schweizer, B Harland. Determination of total dietary fiber in foods, food products and total diets: Inter-laboratory study. J Assoc Off Anal Chem 67: 1044–1052, 1984.
6. JB Robertson, PJ VanSoest. The detergent system of analysis and its application to human foods. In: WPT James, O Theander, eds. The Analysis of Dietary Fiber in Food. New York: Marcel Dekker, 1981, pp 123–158.
7. GY Wang, J Robertson, B Parpia, JS Chen, TC. Campbell. Dietary composition of selected foods in the People's Republic of China. J Food Comp Anal 4(4):293–303, 1991.
8. JW Aderson, SR Bridges, J Tietyen, NJ Gustafson. Dietary fiber content of a simulated American diet and selected research diet. Am J Clin Nutr 49:352–357, 1989.
9. JH Cummings, SA Bingham, MA Eastwood. Fecal weight, colon cancer risk and dietary intake of non-starch polysaccharides (dietary fiber). Gastroenterol 103:1783–1789, 1992.
10. DM Klurfeld. The role of dietary fiber in gastrointestinal disease. J Am Diet Assoc 87:1172–1177, 1987.
11. SM Pilch. Physiological effects and health consequences of dietary fiber. Life Sciences Research Office, Federation of American Societies for Experimental Biology, 1987, p 163.

42

Dietary Fiber Intake in Poland: Recommendations and Actual Consumption Patterns

Elżbieta Bartnikowska and Adam Niegodzisz
Meat and Fat Research Institute, Warsaw, Poland

I. INTRODUCTION

In various countries humans consume different types of food products. The structure of food consumption is influenced by the natural and economic conditions as well as by industrial development and local traditions. With an increase in industrial development, we observe a rise in the consumption of highly processed products of animal origin and also highly purified products of plant origin, which are low in dietary fiber and other compounds bound to plant cell walls, e.g., phenolic compounds. This leads to a significant elevation of caloric density in the daily food ration and affects the balance of nutrient intake of both animal and plant origin to which the human organism has been adapted for several thousand years (1,2).

Acceptance of these types of nutritional standards have resulted in the massive increase in overweight and obesity, which in turn causes non–insulin-dependent diabetes mellitus, cholelithiasis, and diseases of cardiovascular and bone systems (3,4). This type of diet per se also increases the risk of coronary heart disease, development of diseases of digestive tract (e.g., constipation and diverticulosisis), as well as some cancers (5–7).

Dietary fiber has a significant impact on the function of digestive tract, and a diet rich in fiber prevents the development of various functional diseases of digestive tract as well as disorders of lipid and carbohydrate metabolism. Moreover, a diet rich in whole grain products, vegetables, and fruits or supplemented with a dietary fiber preparation helps in the pharmacological treatment of many metabolic disorders and diseases, such as hyperlipidemia or diabetes mellitus. This fact has encouraged many research workers to develop various methods for the determination of fiber in food products (8–11). However, dietary fiber consists of various compounds, both soluble and insoluble in water. Their amounts and proportions change depending on plant species, variety, and maturity rate. Therefore, one universal method for fiber determination in any type of dietary product would be ideal, but such a method is extremely difficult to prepare. In addition, the elaboration of such a method is not easy because starch present in plant products may interfere with the determination of dietary fiber. Moreover, during some technological processes (e.g., purification of grain seeds or peeling of fruit and vegetables), some parts of the fiber are removed, and some technological processes, such as extrusion, affect the ratio of water-soluble to insoluble fiber in the final product as compared with the raw material. Therefore, dietary fiber should be determined not only in the raw material but also in processed food products.

Due to the lack of any established method for dietary fiber determination in food products, in Poland, like other countries, little research has been done concerning the direct determination of dietary fiber content in daily diet.

Daily dietary fiber consumption could also be estimated indirectly based on anticipating the level and structure of food consumption using balance methods and evaluation of family budgets. In Poland results concerning the level of consumption of the ground groups of food products based on the balance method and household budget surveys are published annually by Central Statistical Office (CSO) in Statistical Yearbook. Consumption rate of the ground groups of food products according to such balances is estimated in the following manner:

$$\text{Consumption} = \text{domestic production} + \text{import}$$
$$- \text{export and losses during production and marketing}$$

taking also into account the movement of reserves in plant production and the number of inhabitants.

Data generated through the balance method do not include food losses in households, food consumption by pets, etc. These values are not precisely known and usually are calculated using the estimation method. Therefore, they do not represent real food intake, but rather give information about food available for the average inhabitant. The consumption of food products calculated by the balance method is usually overestimated. It is assumed that this overestimation in some cases may be 25% (12).

Another source of information regarding the level and structure of food consumption is the analysis of family budgets, namely the comparison of income and expenses, both monetary and natural, within households in a given time interval, divided by the number of persons in one common household. In addition to data published by the Central Statistical Office since 1991, the results of such studies are published annually in the reports of the Institute of Agricultural and Food Economics (IAFE). The knowledge concerning both the level and structure of food consumption of various socioeconomic groups leads to more detailed estimation of dietary fiber intake.

Consumption estimated by such a method is usually increased by 15% in order to include food consumed in other places. One should remember, however, that information collected using this method can have a 20% error factor due to the fact that respondents participating in such studies estimate the structure of their income and expenses as well as consumption rate and structure themselves (13).

Data based on the balance method, like household budget surveys, are useful in revealing trends and changes in dietary habits. More detailed estimations of dietary fiber intake, however, should include questionnaire studies, for example, 24-hour dietary recalls in randomly selected groups of consumers as well as chemical analysis of dietary fiber and its constituents in daily food rations. Calculations based on the questionnaire formula concerning 24-hour recalls are very popular because they reflect actual consumption levels and mode of nutrition; moreover they are not as expensive and time consuming as chemical analysis of whole food rations. Studies concerning the level and structure of consumption using the questionnaire formula have been conducted by several research institutes in Poland. Those studies usually cover shorter periods of time and include limited groups of participants, selected according to the aim of study.

II. CHANGES IN THE CONSUMPTION OF GRAIN PRODUCTS, VEGETABLES, AND FRUITS IN POLAND, 1950–1996

For monitoring of the changes in fiber consumption, an attempt has been undertaken in the present work to estimate the mass of the average daily food ration in Poland as well as the mass of plant products containing fiber (without oils) consumed daily by an average Pole. For this purpose the results of balance studies published annually by CSO in Statistical Yearbooks (14) were utilized together with the reports from the National Food and Nutrition Institute (NFNI) in Warsaw (15,16). Figure 1 shows the mass of the average food ration and the average daily intake of plant products in Poland for the years 1950–1996. Data concerning the total consumption various food products in earlier or later years cannot be included because they have not been published yet.

As mentioned earlier, data concerning the level and structure of food consumption using the balance method are collected from estimations and therefore vary significantly. Figure 2 depicts a comparison of the average mass of daily food ration in Poland for selected years, and Fig. 3 shows the average contribution of products of plant origin to the daily food ration in Poland for selected years. The calculations are based on data from Statistical Yearbooks of CSO (14) and data published by NFNI (15,16) as well as FAO reports (17).

The mass of daily food ration depends on age, sex, and physical activity as well as the health status of all members of the investigated population. Although the mass of a daily ration varies even for the same person from day to day, the approximate average mass of daily food ration for an average inhabitant calculated for whole year should not change significantly. The average mass of daily food ration in Poland in the years 1950–1996 varied from 1481 g in 1985 to 1654 g in 1979 (average 1565 ± 41 g). Average values calculated from balance studies are very similar to the values obtained from 24-hour monitoring of diets. For example, our calculations from the balance studies indicate that the average mass of daily food ration in Poland in

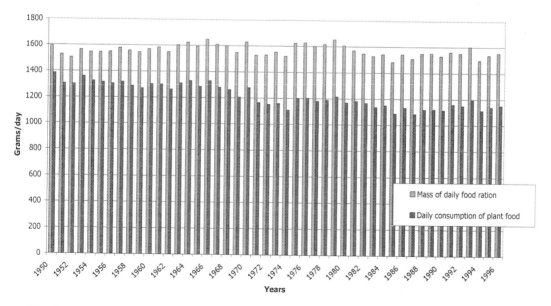

Fig. 1 Mass of the average daily food ration and average daily consumption of plant food in Poland, 1950–1996, based on CSO and NFNI data.

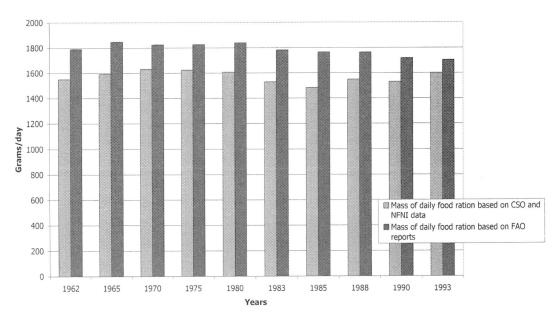

Fig. 2 Comparison of the mass of daily food ration in Poland in selected years based on CSO, NFNI, and FAO data.

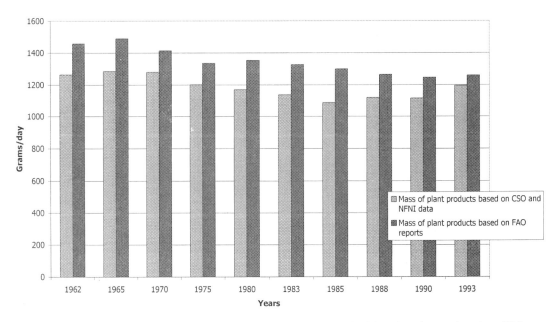

Fig. 3 Comparison of daily consumption of plant products in Poland in selected years based on CSO, NFNI, and FAO data.

1996 amounted to 1536 g. Data from 24-hour dietary recalls used to calculate the average mass of daily food ration in the same year indicated daily intakes of 1133 g among working women and 2095 g among working men; average intake for a group of clerks was 1120 and 1893 g for women and men, respectively (18).

Economic conditions, technical and technological progress, and the knowledge concerning nutrients have had a substantial impact on the change of nutritional habits and the structure of food consumption. Products of plant origin predominate in the food ration of poor societies, especially developing countries, while in highly industrialized countries the contribution of processed animal products to the diet is higher. In other words, the intake of dietary fiber in poor societies is higher than in rich countries. According to calculations of Bright-See (19), based on FAO reports for 38 selected countries, daily fiber intake in the years 1972–74 fluctuated widely from 22.1 g/person/day in Sweden and Holland to 88.1 g/person/day in Romania to 93.6 g/person/day in Mexico. It is also interesting to note that in Romania and Mexico grain products provided 81% and 84% of dietary fiber, respectively, whereas in Sweden and Holland grain products supplied only 44% and 35% of dietary fiber, respectively.

These general observations from the world epidemiological nutritional studies confirm the data collected in Poland. After the Second World War, the agricultural sector predominated in Poland, and the share of food products of plant origin in the mass of daily food ration reached 87%, whereas in the 1990s it declined to 75% (Fig. 4). Changes in the level and structure of plant products consumed in Poland in the second half of this century are shown in Table 1.

Sekula and coworkers, analyzing changes in the levels and structure of food consumption in Poland over many years, distinguish three periods: 1950–1980, 1981–1982, and 1983–1989 (20). In the first and third period the changes in the food consumption were typical for prosperous societies, where in the daily food ration the contribution of food products of animal origin is increasing. In the period 1982–1983 during the economic crisis in Poland, the system of food rationing was introduced, first for meat and its products, followed by butter, wheat flour, groats,

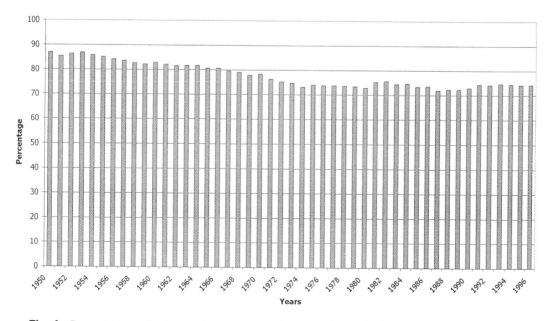

Fig. 4 Percentage contribution of plant products in the mass of daily food ration in Poland, 1950–1996, based on CSO and NFNI data.

Table 1 Comparison of Plant Product Consumption in Poland in the 1950s and 1990s

	1950s		1990s		Change
	g	%	g	%	(%)
Mass of daily food ration	1551 ± 25	100	1547 ± 32	100	−0.3
Mass of plant products in daily food ration	1317 ± 31	85	1146 ± 28	74	−12.9
Consumption of grain products (g/day)	432 ± 25	27.9	326 ± 7	21	−24.7
Consumption of potatoes (g/day)	653 ± 37	42.1	385 ± 14	25	−41.0
Consumption vegetables (g/day)	193 ± 25	12.4	327 ± 10	21	+69.3
Consumption of fruits (g/day)	38 ± 13	2.4	109 ± 19	7	+188.1

grain flakes, rice, sugar, and sweets. During that time the mass of daily food ration did not decrease significantly because of increased consumption of potatoes, vegetables, and fruits, which were not rationed at that time.

Grain products are a staple food for humans. The position of grains, different kinds of grain products, and the form of their consumption depend on their varieties and gradual changes of cultivated grain species. Climate and culture as well as tradition are also important factors. In Poland, belonging to a cooler zone of moderate climate, potatoes and various grain products have the highest share in the total consumption of foods of plant origin. Vegetables and fruits are more expensive, since their production requires more funds and in addition has a seasonal character. Therefore, their contribution to the daily food ration changes in an opposite direction compared to that observed for grain products and potatoes. Figure 5 shows changes in the consumption of grain products and potatoes in Poland in the years 1950–1996. Figure 6 depicts changes in the consumption of vegetables and fruits during the same period of time. Calculations are based on the data from Statistical Yearbooks of CSO (14) and from reports of NFNI (15,16).

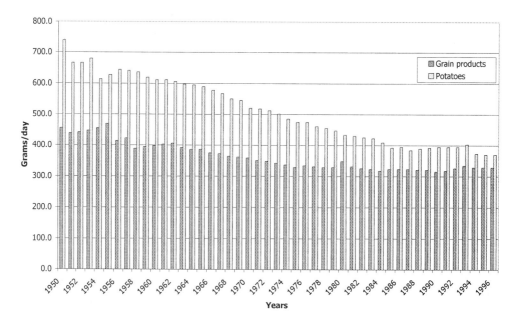

Fig. 5 The contribution of grain products and potatoes in the daily food ration in Poland, 1950–1996, based on CSO and NFNI data.

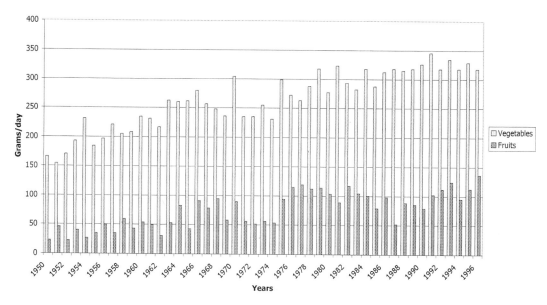

Fig. 6 The contribution of vegetables and fruits in the daily food ration in Poland, 1950–1996, based on CSO and NFNI data.

Bread has the highest share in the consumption of total grain products in Poland. With an increase in economic development, the consumption of grain products decreases, especially that of bread, whereas the consumption of highly processed grain products for breakfast increases. In Poland in 1934 bread consumption per capita was estimated to be around 390 g/person/day, in 1994 it was estimated at around 270 g/person/day (21). Poland holds a leading position in terms of rye production calculated per capita; in fact, rye used to be called "the Polish grain." In the past, rye bread production and consumption was very popular in Poland. In 1934 rye bread accounted for 80% of total bread consumption. In 1952 rye bread constituted half of the total bread consumption. During the following years, the consumption of rye bread slowly but steadily decreased with a concomitant rise of mixed (wheat-rye) bread (21). In Poland today, rye bread is practically not produced. At present, the annual consumption of bread is estimated to be around 100 kg per capita per year, of which almost 60% is mixed bread (wheat-rye) and around 25% wheat bread. The remaining bakery products consist of rye bread, special bread made from whole grains, or bread enriched with bran or fiber preparations, minerals, or impoverished in some minerals, e.g., low-sodium bread (22,23).

The production and consumption of rye bread in Poland has decreased mainly because of the belief that rye bread is a product of lesser quality appropriate only for lower-income groups. The drastic decline in the consumption of rye bread is mainly responsible for the observed decrease in dietary fiber in the pool of grain products.

For more precise evaluation of the consumption structure of products of plant origin, an analysis of household budgets published by the Institute of Agricultural and Food Economics (IAFE) was used (24). Figure 7 presents the structure of grain product consumption in Poland in the 1990s based on data from IAFE (24). From that comparison one could notice that at present the highest contribution to the total consumption of grain products belongs to products made from wheat, rye, and barley. The share of oat and corn in the pool of grain products is marginal.

Until the mid-1980s barley and oat flakes and groats were widely used in the preparation of breakfast cereals. In recent years a variety of breakfast products rich in fiber have become

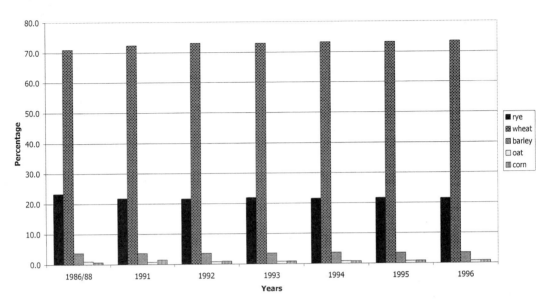

Fig. 7 Structure of the consumption of grain products in Poland in the 1990s based on IAFE data.

available: these include oat and barley bran, corn, wheat, and rye flakes, and muesli with dried fruits, raisins, and nuts. However, in spite of the recommendations of nutrition specialists, the total consumption of breakfast foods rich in fiber is still too low.

Only a few locally grown vegetable species dominate the Polish market. These are cabbages, carrots, beet roots, onions, tomatoes, and cucumbers. (Poland is the highest European producer of cabbage and carrots per capita.) These vegetables together account for over 80% of total consumption of fresh vegetables. Vegetable consumption in Poland in the 1990s is shown in Fig. 8. The calculations are based on data from IAFE (24).

Processed vegetables contribute somewhat less to the total consumption of vegetables. In 1991–1996 their share of total vegetable consumption fluctuated between 10.7 and 14.1% (24). Among all processed vegetables, sauerkraut accounts for >50%, whereas frozen vegetables intake is still very low.

Poland is recognized as a major producer of fruits, but fruit consumption in Poland is relatively low. So-called stone fruits, especially apples, as well as berries play an important role in the structure of fruit consumption in Poland, in contrast with countries with warmer climates, where consumption of citrus fruits, grapes, apricots, peaches, and tropical fruits is common. The structure of fruit consumption in Poland in the 1990s is presented in Fig. 9. The calculations are based on data from IAFE (24).

In industrialized countries, populations living in big cities consume significantly less vegetables than those living in the country. In Poland in 1960–1985, agricultural populations consumed on average 59% more vegetables and 73% more fruits than those living in cities (25, 26).

Seasonal fluctuation has an influence on the profile of fruit consumption. Since 1960 we have observed a slow decline in the annual fluctuation of fruit consumption. Two factors are responsible: (a) a decrease in the fluctuation of fruit production and (b) the compensatory effect of fruit imports in bad years. In the 1990s the consumption of fruits significantly increased, mainly due to the rise of import of citrus fruits. At present, citrus fruits amount to over 20% the total pool of consumed fruits, whereas in the 1950s their share was marginal (24).

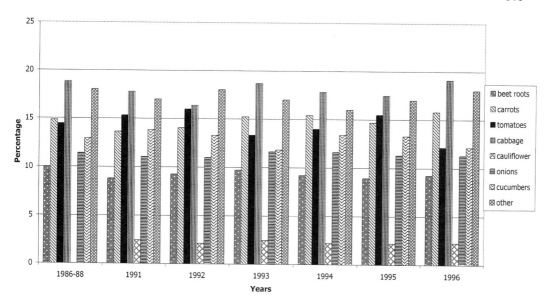

Fig. 8   Structure of the consumption of vegetables in Poland in the 1990s based on IAFE data.

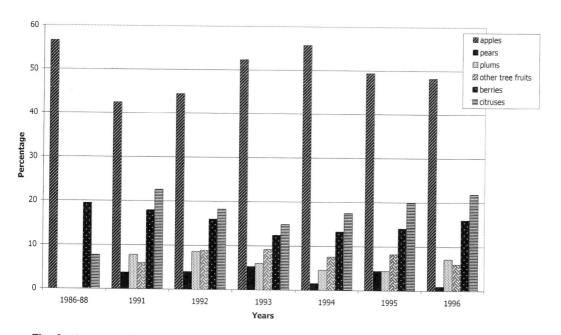

Fig. 9   Structure of the consumption of fruits in Poland in the 1990s based on IAFE data.

In the 1990s the consumption of fruits and vegetables in Poland increased by 188% and 63%, respectively, compared with the 1950s (Table 1). Nevertheless, it is believed that the consumption of fruits and vegetables in Poland is still too low. It is estimated that the inhabitants of European Union consume approximately 3 times more fruits and 2 times more vegetables (27). This situation is heightened by seasonal variations in consumption and a lack of dietary supplementation during winter/spring with processed fruits and vegetables. Dried vegetable and fruits as well as vegetables and fruit juices play a marginal role in daily food intake. The main reason for this situation according to questionnaire studies is that most Polish citizens see no need to increase their consumption of fruits and vegetables. Another factor is, of course, the high price of fresh and processed fruits and vegetables.

III. CONSUMPTION OF DIETARY FIBER IN POLAND

Information concerning the level and structure of food consumption during selected time intervals allows the estimation of changes in dietary fiber consumption. However, the accuracy of that estimation depends mainly on the method used for the determination of fiber content in the food products. Table 2 shows the comparison of the content of dietary fiber in white wheat bread and cabbage depending on the methods of determination.

In the present review, values of dietary fiber content in selected foods given by Kunachowicz and coworkers in *Nutritive Value of Selected Food Products and Typical Meals* (1997) were used for the calculation of the consumption of dietary fiber in Poland (32). The authors did not provide information about the method used for the determination of dietary fiber, but this reference was selected because it is adapted to the composition of Polish meals.

Figure 10 presents the level and structure of the dietary fiber consumption in Poland for the years 1950–1996. The calculations are based on data from the Statistical Yearbooks of CSO (14) and from reports of the NFNI (15,16). Figure 11 depicts the percentage contributions of grain products, potatoes, vegetables, and fruits to the daily dietary fiber pool in Poland during 1950–1996. In these calculations data concerning fiber content in grain products, potatoes, vegetables, and fruits according to Kunachowicz and coworkers (32) were used.

Results of studies estimating the consumption structure in Poland in the past and at present indicate the same pattern of change, but the rate of change is different depending on the method of calculation and investigated population group (25,26,33). Table 3 presents a comparison of dietary fiber consumption in the 1950s and 1990s using our calculations and calculations made by the NFNI (15,16).

Table 2 Total Dietary Fiber Content of White Wheat Bread and Cabbage

Method (ref.)	Total dietary fiber (g/100 g fresh weight)	
	White wheat bread	Cabbage
Hellendorn et al. (28)	2.4	2.1
Southgate et al. (29)	2.7	3.4
van Soest (30)	1.5	1.1
Englyst and Cunnings (31)	1.6	3.3
Kunachowicz et al. (32)	2.1	2.5

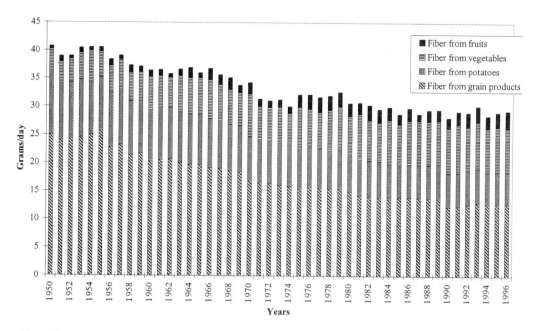

Fig. 10 Level and structure of dietary fiber consumption in Poland, 1950–1996, based on CSO and NFNI data.

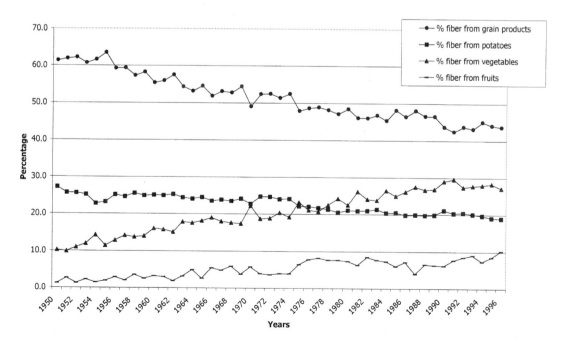

Fig. 11 Percentage contribution of grain products, potatoes, vegetables, and fruits in daily dietary fiber intake.

Table 3 Comparison of Dietary Fiber Consumption
in Poland in the 1950s and the 1990s

	Dietary fiber consumed (g/person/day)	
	1950s	1990s
Authors' calculations	39.9 ± 1.3	29.0 ± 0.7
Calculations of NFNI[a]	37.2 ± 1.5	31.8 ± 0.7

[a] National Food and Nutrition Institute.

Bright-See and McKeown-Eyssen (19), in work concerning the consumption of dietary fiber in 38 countries in 1972–1974, elaborated based on FAO report estimates that the average dietary fiber consumption in Poland amounted to 37.2 g per capita per day. According to reports from NFNI, dietary fiber consumption in Poland in 1972–1974 was 32 g per capita per day; our calculation for this period is almost the same—31.3 g per person per day. Calculations concerning the level of food consumption in Poland based on FAO food balance sheets are higher than calculations based on the balance method published by CSO in Statistical Yearbooks and reports of NFNI (Fig. 2). This is the main reason for the higher estimation of dietary fiber intake by Bright-See and McKeown-Eyssen than by Polish authors. [Similar discrepancies between statistics published by the Organization for Economic Cooperation and Development and FAO were also observed (34).]

In addition, Bright-See and McKeown-Essen estimated that grain products accounted for 59.6%, vegetables 17.2%, and fruits 5.6% of daily dietary fiber intake (19). Our calculations indicate that in this period of time grain products provided around 51%, potatoes around 24%, vegetables 21%, and fruits 4% of daily dietary fiber intake. Potatoes contribute to a great extent to the mass of daily food ration in Poland (Fig. 5), and their share in the daily fiber pool is significant (Fig. 10). Therefore, we subtract this product from the estimations concerning food product contribution to the daily fiber pool. It is most probable that this is the main reason for the discrepancy between the results of these studies.

Calculations based on the balance method and on the household budget analysis differ significantly. For example, in 1994, according to the data of NFNI, dietary fiber consumption in Poland amounted to 31.9 g/person/day; according to our calculations, also based on the balance method, it was 28.4 g/person/day. Based on the household budget analysis it was estimated that dietary fiber consumption in 1994 fluctuated from 14.4 to 21.2 g/person/day (35).

Calculations based on the balance method are usually overestimated. On the other hand, calculations based on the household budget surveys are underestimated (12). Most likely, this is the reason for the discrepancy between cited results. Data based on household budget surveys underline, however, that dietary fiber intake ranges significantly according to socioeconomic group and the level of household income. It was surprising that the highest consumption of dietary fiber occurred in pensioners' households. Limited data suggest that dietary fiber intake per 1000 kcal may be higher among elderly than among adolescents and adults. However, caloric requirements of the elderly are usually lower than in adults. On the other hand, consumption of fruits and vegetables also increases with an increase in household income. Income in pensioner households in Poland is usually lower than in workers' households. Therefore, it is difficult to interpret the results of studies indicating that consumption of dietary fiber in pensioners' household is significantly higher than in workers' households and simultaneously that the structure of fiber consumption in pensioners' household is similar to that in workers' household (35,36).

Although it is assumed that studies based on the questionnaire formula are useful for research, the results are often difficult to compare. For example, in the studies based on 24-hour dietary recall conducted in various regions of Poland in 1991–1994, Szponar and Rychlik (37) estimated that daily consumption of dietary fiber in groups of boys aged 11–12 years was 25.2–29.2 g/day. Duda and coworkers (38), in similar studies conducted in the same period of time in the Wielkopolska region, calculated that consumption of dietary fiber by boys aged 11–12 years was 16.2–17.8 g/day. A similar discrepancy was observed for groups of girls of the same age. Szponar and coworkers (39) estimated that consumption of dietary fiber by girls aged 11–12 years amounted to 26.2–25.8 g/day, and Gertig and coworkers estimated intakes at 14.3–14.8 g/day (38). Results of cited studies concerning the consumption of dietary fiber by boys and girls in Poland in the 1990s are difficult to compare because the authors did not indicate which socioeconomic groups the investigated children belonged to. It is likely that socioeconomic status of investigated children could explain the differences in fiber intake.

In the Polish literature, data comparing the consumption of dietary fiber by different age groups are rather scarce. Szponar and coworkers demonstrated that although dietary fiber intake varied significantly in groups of boys and men as well as girls and women, the highest intake of dietary fiber was in younger persons. Thereafter the consumption of dietary fiber steadily declined with age (37,39).

In prospective studies in Poland within an international program of MONICA (MONItoring of Trends and Determinants in Cardiovascular Disease—a WHO project), it was estimated that dietary fiber consumption in the years 1984–1993 decreased by 9.7%, from 30.4 to 27.4 g/day, in men and by 10.9%, from 20.9 to 18.6 g/day, in women (40). Other results from pol-MONICA studies showed that in the year 1993 the main source of dietary fiber for men was grain products, which supplied about 48% of that substance, followed by vegetables, potatoes, and fruit. In daily food intake by women, the structure of dietary fiber consumption differed. Cereal products provided 40%, but the contribution of other products decreased as follows: vegetables, fruits, and potatoes (41,42). Different levels and structure of dietary fiber intake by men and women probably results from different organoleptic preferences of men and women. Our calculation indicate that in 1993 the average Pole consumed 30.1 g dietary fiber daily, and the main source of this compound was grain products followed by vegetables, potatoes, and fruits.

Changes in the level and structure of grain product consumption affect not only total dietary fiber intake, but also the intake of its soluble and insoluble components. Our calculations indicate that in the 1950s grain products provided on average 23.8 g dietary fiber per day and in the 1990s 13.8 g, which amounted 60% and 44% of daily dietary fiber intake, respectively. The ratio of soluble to insoluble components of dietary fiber in grain products differs significantly from 0.16 in wheat to 1.11 in husked oat (43). The proportion of soluble to insoluble components of dietary fiber varies in vegetables from 0.06 in cabbage to 0.2 in cucumber, and in fruits from 0.11 in apple to 0.42 in banana (44). Taking into account the ratio of soluble to insoluble fiber in grain products and the structure of grain product consumption, it could be calculated that in Poland in the 1950s grain products provided 7.2 g/person/day of soluble and 16.6 g/person/day of insoluble fiber. However, in the 1990s grain products provided 3.3 and 10.5 g/person/day of soluble and insoluble fiber, respectively. Based on similar patterns it is possible to calculate that in the 1990s in Poland, vegetables provided 1.0 g of soluble and 7.1 g of insoluble fiber components in the daily food ration, whereas fruits provided 0.8 and 1.6 g of soluble and insoluble dietary fiber, respectively. However, the proportion of soluble to insoluble fiber in the daily food ration (around 1:3) did not change significantly in 1950–1996. Daily intake of soluble and insoluble fiber in Poland in 1950–1996 is presented in Figs. 12 and 13, respectively.

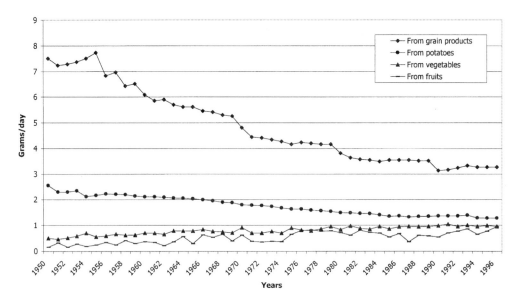

Fig. 12 Daily intake of soluble fiber from grain products, potatoes, vegetables, and fruits in Poland, 1950–1996.

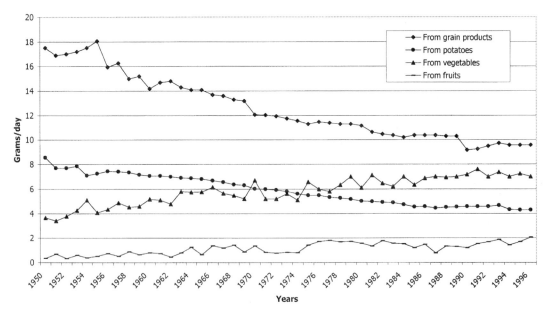

Fig. 13 Daily intake of insoluble fiber from grain products, potatoes, vegetables, and fruits in Poland, 1950–1996.

Polish dietary allowances of 1980 and 1994 do not contain the precise amounts of dietary fiber that should be consumed in the daily food ration of various population groups (45,46). In the Polish nutritional literature it is most often assumed that for the maintenance of good health, the intake of dietary fiber should be from 20 to 40 g/day (46). For adult patients with disorders of lipid or carbohydrate metabolism, higher consumption of dietary fiber—30–40 g/day, particularly soluble fiber—is recommended (47,48). However, in the Polish literature there is no recommendation concerning the intake of dietary fiber by children or elderly persons. On the basis of comparison of recommended intake and calculated levels of consumption, it may be stated that estimated consumption of dietary fiber in Poland is too low.

Data from questionnaire studies concerning dietary fiber consumption in Poland in 1992–1993 by healthy people, patients with obesity, and patients with clinical symptoms of atherosclerosis are of interest (49). According to these studies, dietary fiber consumption varied significantly, being in the range of 7.9–28.7 g/person/day. Healthy people consumed more dietary fiber than unhealthy patients. Moreover, results of this study confirmed that the main sources of dietary fiber in the diet of both healthy people and patients were vegetables and grain products (~90%). It is also characteristic that healthy people preferred products with higher fiber content, whereas patients preferred products with low fiber content.

The results from questionnaire studies regarding the reason for low consumption of vegetables and fruits as well as preferences of patients with atherosclerosis for products with low fiber content indicate lack of awareness of the advantages of consumption of whole grain products, fruits, and vegetables (27).

In the pyramid of nutrition that is the model of optimal nutrition, it is recommended that the numbers of servings from fruits and vegetables be five or more daily. This recommendation was made primarily because these food products provide micronutrients that have been associated with a protective role in cancer and increasing dietary fiber consumption was not a major factor in this recommendation. However, we should remember that the most of these micronutrients are bound to the plant cell wall with dietary fiber components.

Dissemination of knowledge concerning this issue is the main objective of many programs going on in Poland, including the National Program of Cholesterol Prevention and the National Program of the Defense Against Neoplastic Diseases (27,50).

Nutritional education, especially regarding the principles of healthy nutrition based on whole grain products, fruits, and vegetables, may take a long time. It is hoped that during the coming years, the consumption of grain products, fruits, and vegetables will increase, especially among patients with lipid and carbohydrate metabolism disorders. This hope is supported by the observations that fiber consumption in Poland is changing in a positive manner. Until now attention has been focused on the level and structure of fat consumption. More attention is now being focused on consumption of grain products, fruits, and vegetables, which are rich sources of dietary fiber, vitamins, and flavonoids with antioxidative properties as well as minerals. As a result of nutritional education, the supply of plant products has increased. This in turn has caused some changes in the nutritional habits of the society and led to the slow decrease in mortality rate from cardiovascular diseases observed in Poland since 1992 (50).

REFERENCES

1. DD Gallaher, BO Schneeman. Dietary fiber. In: E Ziegler, LJ Filer, eds. Present Knowledge in Nutrition. Washington, DC: ILSI Press, 1996, pp 87–97.
2. Simopoulos AP. Omega 3 fatty acids in health and disease and in growth and development. Am J Clin Nutr 54:438–463, 1991.

3. Dietary fiber. In: Diet and Health: Implications for Reducing Chronic Disease Risk. Committee on Diet and Health Food and Nutrition Board, Commission on Life Sciences National Research Council. Washington, DC: National Academy Press, 1989, pp 291–309.
4. Obesity and overweight; diabetes mellitus; ischaemic heart disease; gall stones. In: Medical Aspects of Dietary Fibre. Summary of a Report of the Royal College of Physicians of London. Pitman Medical Ltd., 1980, pp 63–103.
5. Anderson JW, Chen WJL. Plant fiber, carbohydrate and lipid metabolism. Am J Clin Nutr 32:346–363, 1979.
6. Burkitt DP, Walker ARP, Painter, NS. Dietary fiber and disease. J Am Med Assoc., 229:1068–1074 (1974).
7. Trowell H. Definition of dietary fiber and hypothesis that it is a protective factor in certain diseases. Am J Clin Nutr 29:417–427, 1976.
8. Southgate DAT, Hudson GJ, Englyst H. The analysis of dietary fibre. The choices for the analyst. J Sci Food Agric 29:978–988, 1978.
9. Asp N. Critical evaluation of some methods suggested for assay of dietary fibre. In: KW Heaton, ed. Dietary Fibre: Current Developments of Importance to Health. London: Libbey, 1978, pp 21–26.
10. Prosky L, Asp NG, Furda I, DeVries JW, Schweizer TF, Harland BF. Determination of total dietary fiber in foods and food products: collaborative study. J Assoc Off Anal Chem 68:677–679, 1985.
11. Monro JA. Dietary fiber. In: LML Nollet, ed. Handbook of Food Analysis. Vol. 1. Physical Characterization and Nutrient Analysis. New York: Marcel Dekker Inc., 1996, pp 1051–1088.
12. Bingham S. Definition and intakes of dietary fiber. Am J Clin Nutr 45:1226–1231, 1987.
13. Bingham S. The assessment of individual risk from diet in large bowel cancer epidemiology. In: GV Vahouny, D Kritchevsky, eds. Dietary Fiber, Basic and Clinical Aspects. New York: Plenum Press, 1986, pp 457–465.
14. Statistical Yearbooks of Central Statistical Office in Poland. Warsaw: Central Statistical Office, 1951–1997 (in Polish).
15. Sekula W, Niedzialek Z, Figurska K, Morawska M, Boruc T. Intake of Food Products in Poland in the Years 1950–1991 Calculated as Intake of Energy and Nutrients. Warsaw: National Food and Nutrition Institute, 1992 (in Polish).
16. Sekula W, Niedzialek, Z, Figurska K, Morawska M, Boruc T. Intake of Food Products in Poland in the Years 1950–1996 Calculated as Intake of Energy and Nutrients. Warsaw: National Food and Nutrition Institute, 1997 (in Polish).
17. FAO Food Balance Sheets 1992–1994. Rome: FAO, 1996, pp 362–363.
18. Wojtasik A, Barylko-Pikielna N, Jabłońska B, Gajlzer M, Szponar L. Degree of potential risk connected with intake of heavy metals with daily food ration by working men and women. Pol J Human Nutr Metabol 24(suppl 2):35–46, 1997 (in Polish).
19. Bright-See E, McKeown-Eyssen GE. Estimation per capita crude and dietary fiber supply in 38 countries. Am J Clin Nutr 39:821–829, 1984.
20. Sekula W, Szostak WB, Niedzialek Z. Development in the dietary pattern and CHD mortality in Poland. Pol J Human Nutr Metabol 18:175–187, 1991 (in Polish).
21. Gasiorowski H. Rye—old and new possibilities its utilization. Cereal Milling-Rev 42:2–4, 1998 (in Polish).
22. Piesiewicz H. Consumption of bakery products in Poland. I. Energetic value and importance of protein, dietary fiber and vitamins. Bakery Confectionery Rev 44:8–9, 1996 (in Polish).
23. Ambroziak Z. Trends in bakery industry development and stock condition. Cereal Milling Rev 38:2–6, 1994 (in Polish).
24. Institute of Agricultural and Food Economics: Situation and Outlook Reports for Different Agricultural Products (Grains, Potatoes, Vegetables, Fruits) on Polish Market (1992–1998). Warsaw: Institute of Agricultural and Food Economics in Poland, 1992–1998 (in Polish).
25. Majcher G, Niedzialek Z. Changes in the level and structure of consumption of vegetables and fruits in Poland in the years 1960–1973. Pol J Human Nutr 2:131–143, 1975 (in Polish).
26. Sekula W, Niedzialek Z, Świstak E. Changes in food consumption by socio-economic groups of the households in Poland in 1975–1983. Pol J Human Nutr Metabol 12:80–94, 1985 (in Polish).

27. Mitek MK, Przewoźniak K, Kuźma I, Zatoński WA. Fruit and vegetable intake in Poland in 1996–1997. Food Indust 52:10–13, 1998 (in Polish).
28. Hellendorn EW, Nordhoff MG, Slagman J. Enzymatic determination of indigestible residue (dietary fibre) content of human foods. J Sci Food Agric 26:1461–1468, 1975.
29. Southgate DAT, Bailey B, Collinson E, Walker AF. A guide to calculating intakes of dietary fibre. J Hum Nutr 30:303–313, 1976.
30. Van Soest PJ. Fiber analysis tables. Am J Clin Nutr 31(suppl):S284, 1978.
31. Englyst HN, Cunnings JH. Simplified method for the measurement of total NSP by GLC of constituent sugars as alditol acetates. Analyst 109:937–942, 1984.
32. Kunachowicz H, Nadolna I, Iwanow K, Przygoda B. Nutritive Value of Selected Food Products and Typical Meals. Warsaw: Wydawnictwo Lekarskie PZWL, 1997 (in Polish).
33. Berger S, Dobrzańska A, Kowrygo B, Monka E, Maciejewska M. Quantitative and qualitative transformations in the domain of population nutrition in Poland 1950–1975. Ann Agric Sci, Series D, Monographs, Vol. 175. Warsaw: Państwowe Wydawnictwo Naukowe (PWN), 1978 (in Polish).
34. Dietary sources and intake of complex carbohydrates. In: Complex Carbohydrates in Foods. The Report of the British Nutrition Foundation's Task Force. Chapman and Hall, 1990, pp 22–25.
35. Kunachowicz H, Nadolna I, Paczkowska M, Sekuła W. Effect of dietary fiber on estimation of energetic value of food products and daily food ration. Proceedings of International Symposium on Dietary Fiber, Its Chemical Composition and Biological Effects. Radzików, 1997, pp 195–199 (in Polish).
36. Majchrzak D, Gronowska-Senger A, Morawiec K. The consumption of dietary fibre in Poland. Ann Natl Inst Hygiene 38:392–400, 1987 (in Polish).
37. Szponar L, Rychlik E. Nutrition mode and nutritional status of boys and men in Poland. Pol J Human Nutr Metabol 23(suppl 2):3–37, 1996.
38. Duda G, Gertig H, Maruszewska M, Przysławski J. Nutritional value of daily food ration of school children. Pol J Human Nutr Metabol 24:427–436, 1997 (in Polish).
39. Szponar L, Rychlik E, Respondek W. Nutrition mode and nutritional status of girls and women in Poland. Pol J Human Nutr Metabol 23(suppl 2):38–70, 1996.
40. Pardo B, Jasiński B, Sygnowska E, Waśkiewicz A. Nutritional mode and risk factors of cardiovascular diseases in the Warsaw Pol-MONICA population during 10 years observation. Risk Factors (4): 55–62, 1996 (in Polish).
41. Sygnowska E, Waśkiewicz A, Pardo B. Changes in habitual nutritional mode in the Warsaw Pol-Monica population in the years 1984-1993. Pol J Human Nutr Metabol 24:234–248, 1997 (in Polish).
42. Sygnowska E, Jasiński B, Waśkiewicz A, Pardo B, Broda G. Sources of energy and nutrients in the diet of the urban population studied in the Pol-MONICA programme. Pol J Human Nutr Metabol 23:110–127, 1996 (in Polish).
43. Bartnik M, Rothekaehl J. Oat. Food Indust 51:17–19, 1997 (in Polish).
44. Marlett JA. Content and composition of dietary fiber in 117 frequently consumed foods. J Am Diet Assoc 92:175–186, 1992.
45. Szczygieł A, Bułhak-Jakimczyk B, Nowicka L, Szostak WB. Polish Dietary Allowances. Parts I and II. Warsaw: National Food and Nutrition Institute, 1980 (in Polish).
46. Ziemlański Ś, Bułhak-Jakimczyk B, Budzyńska-Topolewska J, Panczenko-Kresowska B, Wartanowicz M. Polish dietary allowances (energy, protein, fats, vitamins and mineral compounds). Pol J Human Nutr Metabol 21:303–338, 1994 (in Polish).
47. Bartnikowska E. Lipid metabolism as influenced by dietary fiber. Pol J Human Nutr Metabol 21:1–17, 1994 (in Polish).
48. Bartnikowska E. Dietary fiber in health and diseases. Proceedings of International Symposium on Dietary Fiber, Its Chemical Composition and Biological Effects. Radzików, 1997, pp 101–118. (in Polish).
49. Gawęcki J, Czarnocińska J, Wróblewska D. Food preferences and dietary fiber intake in health subjects or subjects with obesity and atherosclerosis. Pol J Human Nutr Metabol 21:117–123, 1994 (in Polish).
50. Szostak WB, Cybulska B. The role of treatment of hyperlipidemia in the prevention of cardiovascular diseases. Risk Factors (2/3):4–10, 1996 (in Polish).

43

Dietary Fiber Intake in Chile: Recommendations and Actual Consumption Patterns

Nelly Pak
University of Chile, Santiago, Chile

I. INTRODUCTION

Chile is a country located in the southwest of South America, bordering the Pacific Ocean with more than 4000 km of coastline and a mainland area of 756,626 km^2. The total population of Chile in 1992 (last census) was estimated to be 13,559,441 inhabitants. A high proportion of the population (83.5%) lives in urban areas. The metropolitan area, where Santiago—the nation's capital—is located, accomodates 40.5% of the population. In the last 20 years a number of important demographic, social, and economic changes have taken place in Chile, which have contributed to the modification of the morbility and mortality patterns (1).

An aging of the population, a decrease in the prevalence of transmissible diseases, and changes in lifestyles (dietary changes, increase in alcohol and cigarette consumption, decrease in physical activity) have worked in favor of the prevalence of nontransmissible chronic diseases. Among these, the most notorious are the high prevalence of obesity, diabetes, dislipidemias, high blood pressure, and cancer (1,2).

In Chile close to 60% of deaths are due to three main causes: cardiovascular disease, cancer, and accidents (2,3). In a period of epidemiological transition such as the one Chile is currently going through, international experience advises that efforts must be made toward the furthering of good health habits and healthier lifestyles.

A team of experts called on by the Ministry of Public Health defined the intervention priorities in terms of the current epidemiological profile—dislipidemias, obesity, cancer, high blood pressure, diabetes, osteoporosis, and anemia. Taking these priorities into account, a number of nutrients and dietary components were defined as critical or having a major impact as risk or prevention factors in relation to these pathologies. Among these components, dietary fiber was identified as a preventive factor that must be included as part of the strategy of promotion of good health and must be taken into account in nutritional education (4).

II. RECOMMENDATIONS FOR DIETARY FIBER

During the last 3 years, considerable research has been conducted on the role of dietary fiber in health and disease. Interest was stimulated by epidemiological studies that associated a low intake of dietary fiber with the incidence of colon cancer, heart disease, and other diseases and disorders.

In recent years, different national and international agencies have provided recommendations of dietary fiber for the population segment of healthy adults with the object of promoting good health and minimizing the risk of contracting these diseases. In general, all these recommendations are aimed at increasing fiber consumption as much as possible by means of natural food products. Following is a description of these recommendations.

In 1987, in regard to the U.S. population, a panel of experts on dietary fiber concluded that fiber consumption must be provided by the diet itself—whole grains, vegetables, and fruit—more than by means of specific supplements (5). Consumption should ideally provide an insoluble fiber-to-soluble fiber ratio of 3:1. Intake based on conditions related to the desired stool weight and transit time would be 20–35 g/day, or close to 10–13 g/1000 kcal. This intake was suggested for a normal adult. Additional factors must be taken into account when prescribing for children, elders, or people with special diets (5).

Although fiber may be important, in its latest 1989 report (6), the National Research Council indicated that it is not feasible to recommend a specific amount of fiber consumption. Because of a possible decrease in the absorption of nutrients that could be induced by a high fiber consumption, strong increases in dietary fiber should be avoided. For the population in general, moderate increases in fiber consumption are desirable through the intake of vegetables, fruit, legumes, and whole grains.

In 1991, the World Health Organization (WHO) set low and high limits (27 and 40 g of dietary fiber a day) (7). In 1990, the Dietary Guidelines for the American population recommended an increase in the consumption of dietary fiber by eating a larger variety of foods that naturally contained fiber (8).

In 1991 the Department of Health of the United Kingdom pointed out that diets should contain an average of 18 g/day (range of 12–24) of nonstarch polysaccharides of a wide variety of foods whose composition includes them as a naturally integrated component (9). It is noteworthy to mention that recommendations for nonstarch polysaccharides are lower than those for total dietary fiber, because these do not take into account neither lignin nor resistant starch (10).

In Chile, the current recommendation is included in the Dietary Guidelines for the Chilean population (4) of 1997, which suggest an increase in the consumption of fruit, vegetables, and legumes. These recommendations are valid for the adult population. Fiber consumption in childhood is associated with important health benefits, especially those related with fomenting normal bowel movements. Dietary fiber can also help reduce the future risk of cardiovascular disease, certain cancers, and diabetes. Currently there are few guidelines concerning the consumption of dietary fiber during childhood. Consequently, the Nutritional Committee of the American Pediatric Academy suggests 0.5 g/kg of weight (11) or 10 g/1000 kcal (12). The American Health Foundation recommends a minimum dietary fiber intake equivalent to age + 5 g for children between ages 3 and 20 years old. According to this general principle, fiber intake goes from 8 g/day for 3-year-old children to 25 g/day for 20-year-olds. A safe range of consumption for children is suggested as being between age + 5 g/day and age + 10 g/day. This is deemed a safe range of fiber consumption even if intake of vitamins and minerals is marginal. It would provide enough fiber to foment normal bowel movements and could help prevent future chronic diseases (12).

III. ENRICHMENT, REGULATION, AND LABELING OF FOOD PRODUCTS AS RELATED TO FIBER

The cornerstone for promoting healthy nutrition is providing the consumer with accurate and up-to-date information about the health and nutritional values of food products and projecting it towards the achievement of a healthy lifestyle (13). In Chile, nutritional labeling involves a system of guidelines included in the Sanitary Food Regulations, recently developed by the Ministry of Public Health (14). It promotes healthy nutrition.

Food product labeling must act as a guideline for the consumer regarding his or her choice of a high-fiber diet, which is recommended in the nutritional guides (4). According to the current Sanitary Food Regulations, the daily reference value for adults and children 4 years old and older to be used on nutritional labels in Chile is a minimum of 25 g of dietary fiber. In said regulations, the following articles are included as related to fiber.

Article 120: A product is to be classified as fortified or enriched with dietary fiber when 10% or more of the daily reference value (25 g/day of dietary fiber) per serving has been added to it. Good source of dietary fiber: When a serving contains between 10 and 19% of the daily reference value. High in dietary fiber: when a serving contains 20% or more of the daily reference value.

Article 502: In commercially prepared children's foods to be consumed directly (beikost), the total amount of dietary fiber must be a maximum of 2% in the product when ready for consumption.

Article 509: In processed children's foods based on cereals, the total amount of dietary fiber must be a maximum of 5% in the dry base.

Article 525: Products for weight control as substituted for an entire day's meals, which provide an energy intake between 300 and 1200 kcal, must provide a minimum dietary fiber intake of 13 g.

IV. INTAKE OF DIETARY FIBER: DIETARY METHODOLOGY

Three main methods for obtaining dietary fiber data have been used (15):

1. Food balance sheets: Food balance is calculated by taking into account the quantity of foodstuffs produced in the country added to the quantity imported and adjusted for any changes in stocks that may have occurred. In order to determine availability for human consumption, the quantity exported, fed to livestock, used for seed and for nonnutritional purposes, and losses during storage and transportation are all taken into account. In general, it is felt that such surveys overestimate consumption by individuals. They are incapable of determining waste at a variety of levels, including the home. In countries with little food waste, they are closer to actual consumption. Nutrients derived this way should be viewed with caution.
2. Household surveys: These are carried out at intervals by many governments. These usually record spending on food and need to be corrected for waste in the home, meals consumed outside of the home, and adjusted for household size and composition.
3. Individual assessments: Studies of the dietary fiber intakes of individuals should more accurately approach true dietary fiber intakes. Many countries, particularly in the developing world, do not have the resources to mount large nutrition surveys, and even

small studies on specific groups can be hard to find. There are always questions about the representativeness of each group as regarding the entire population.

V. CONSUMPTION AND SOURCES OF DIETARY FIBER IN CHILE

Information available in Chile regarding the consumption of dietary fiber is scarce. The values that we outline correspond to the most recent data about fiber intake, which are derived from a research project on the 1992–1994 food balance sheet of the Food and Agriculture Organization (FAO), from a family budget survey conducted in the period between December 1987 and November 1988, and from individual assessments of adults, the elderly, and preschool children conducted in 1995, 1996, and 1996, respectively.

A. FAO Food Balance Sheet for 1992–1994

Through this information we estimate the possible dietary fiber intake in terms of g/person/ day. It is necessary to emphasize that data of supply per person that appear on the food balance sheets only represent the average available supply for the population and are not necessarily indicative of what we actually eat. Since the FAO expresses the supply of foodstuffs per person/ day in terms of weight of the primary product (16), it was necessary to obtain the net weight as it is ingested. For that purpose, values were adjusted utilizing percentages of loss for a particular food product. This information was obtained mainly from the tables of the Institute of Nutrition of Central America and Panama (17), or from the tables of composition of foods of the FAO for international use (18) and from national sources (19).

  The supply of total, soluble, and insoluble dietary fiber was obtained mainly from national sources (20–22) by means of enzymatic-gravimetric methods (23–24), and the rest from the literature with equivalent techniques. The apparent intake of dietary fiber in terms of g/person/ day amounted to 22.1, of which 68% is attributable to insoluble fiber and 32% to soluble fiber. Expressed as energy density, dietary fiber yields a figure of 8.1 g/1000 kcal (Table 1).

  It is noteworthy to mention that the average intake of dietary fiber of nine European countries obtained using this same methodology is 23 g/day, with a range of 21–25.3 g (15). While food balance data may be subject to considerable error in terms of absolute consumption, it can give a reasonable picture of the distribution of sources contributing to the overall intake of a nutrient.

  Table 2 shows the contribution of foodstuffs as sources of dietary fiber. Cereals stand out (54.4% of the supply), followed by vegetables (30.1%) and a lower preponderance of fruit and legumes (2.1%).

  Among the cereals, it is noteworthy that the main source is wheat and that it is ingested mainly through bread produced with processed flour with 78% of extraction. Integral wheat

Table 1 Food Balance Sheet 1992–1994 in Chile: Total Dietary Fiber and Percentage of Insoluble and Soluble Dietary Fiber

Total dietary fiber		Insoluble fiber	Soluble fiber
g/person/day	g/1000 kcal	(%)	(%)
22.1	8.1	68	32

Table 2 Food Balance Sheet 1992–1994 in Chile: Dietary Fiber by Food Group and as % of Total Dietary Fiber

Food group	Dietary fiber	
	g/person/day	%
Cereals	12.0	54.4
Fruit	3.0	13.4
Vegetables	6.6	30.1
Legumes	0.5	2.1
Total	22.1	100

flour is also used, although in low quantities. A high overestimation of availability of fiber can be incurred if wheat is taken into account with a 100% extraction, such as was the case with the Bright-See and Mckeown-Eyssen paper, which, based on calculations from the 1972–1974 FAO balance sheets, obtained a supply of dietary fiber of 55.9 g/day for Chile (25). This value was later corrected to 35 g/day (26).

Among vegetables, potatoes stand out as a source of fiber—36.5%—which, added to tomatoes, onions, squash, carrots, corn, and tender beans, account for 80.1% of the total vegetable supply of fiber. Among fruit, peaches and nectarines, oranges, bananas, and apples account for 61.2% of dietary fiber. Among legumes, beans account for 40% of the amount supplied, although the total amount of supply is very low.

In general, the main sources of dietary fiber provided by cereals, vegetables (including potatoes), legumes, and fruit, as found in this study, are to a large extent equivalent to recent data from 13 European countries (15).

B. Household Food Survey

Research was based on the IV Family Budget Survey in Greater Santiago conducted by the National Statistics Institute (INE) from December 1987 to November 1988 (27) (the fifth survey is being conducted this year). The INE survey was carried out in order to obtain data for seasonal variations experienced by household expenditures throughout the year. The geographical area is that of the Greater Santiago district. The study was based on a sample of 5076 homes with population from all the different socioeconomic strata of society. Homes were put in order according to their level of expenditures in quintile groups, in which the first quintile was that of the lowest income bracket.

Conversion of expenditures to food in terms of quantities of food per person/day, according to the quintile group, was obtained from a study published by the labor Economy Program in order to estimate the basket of foods based on INE data (28). Foodstuffs obtained through governmental and nongovernmental aid programs were not taken into account, which obviously have a bearing on the low-income bracket. As was the case with the study on food balance sheets, foodstuffs as a source of fiber based on an edible portion were estimated taking into account national data on total dietary fiber—soluble and insoluble—using enzymatic-gravimetric techniques (20–24) and in very few products foreign data with equivalent techniques.

The supply of dietary fiber in g/person/day increases from 14.8 to 32.5 in the higher socioeconomic levels. The percentages of soluble and insoluble fiber are relatively similar in the different quintiles, with an average of 66.8% insoluble fiber and 33.2% soluble fiber. The

Table 3 Household Food Surveys: Average Total Dietary Fiber Intake and Percent of Insoluble and Soluble Dietary Fiber According to Income in the Population of Santiago[a]

Income quintile	Total dietary fiber		Insoluble fiber (%)	Soluble fiber (%)
	g/person/day	g/1000 kcal		
1	14.8	12.3	66.9	33.1
2	20.2	11.9	66.8	33.2
3	23.4	11.1	66.7	33.3
4	27.0	10.8	66.7	33.3
5	32.5	10.2	67.1	32.9

[a] December 1987–November 1988.
Source: Ref. 21.

supply of dietary fiber per 1000 kcal of diet decreases from 12.3 to 10.2 in the higher-income bracket (Table 3).

Foodstuff contribution to the supply of dietary fiber according to the quintile groups in the Santiago population shows that cereals are the most important source, followed by vegetables. In the higher socioeconomic strata the percentage supplied by cereals and legumes decreases and that of fruit and vegetables increases. Legumes are the third supplier group for quintiles 1 and 2, and in quintiles 3, 4, and 5 are displaced by fruit (Table 4).

C. Individual Assessments

Only one nutritional survey has been conducted on a nationwide sample basis in Chile during the period 1974–1975 (29). Consequently, dietary fiber is not taken into account. Neither is it expedient to reassess the compiled information in order to determine the intake of dietary fiber, as it would not be valid today.

Later, a number of studies were conducted about certain physiological or age groups (e.g., pregnant women, nursing women, children, adolescents, senescents) in small samples and with a lower representation (30–35). Most of these prioritized the assessment of energy and nutrient deficit (minerals and vitamins), and there was less concern about other aspects of the diet that have more relevance in terms of the current epidemiological profile, such as the consumption

Table 4 Household Food Surveys: Sources of Dietary Fiber and Percent Contribution to Total Dietary Fiber Intake According to Income in the Population of Santiago, Chile[a]

Food group	Quintile				
	1	2	3	4	5
	Dietary fiber (%)				
Cereals	57.4	53.5	49.6	46.7	40.3
Fruit	6.1	8.4	10.6	14.1	19.7
Vegetables	24.3	28.7	32.5	33.3	35.7
Legumes	12.2	9.4	7.3	5.9	4.3
Total dietary fiber (%)	100	100	100	100	100

[a] Period December 1987–November 1988.
Source: Ref. 21.

of fiber. The following information corresponds to recent data of fiber intake compiled in our country, in adults, elders and pre-schoolers, obtained in individual assessments.

1. Adults

The object of this study (36) was to assess the adult intake of foods and nutrients in the metropolitan region (Santiago). This information was deemed essential in order to support the Dietary Guidelines recently developed by the Public Health Ministry, as part of a good health-promotion strategy (37). With that in mind, a study was conducted in a group of 859 adults (412 men, 447 women) who attended 120 primary medical assistance facilities of the National Healthcare System.

Information on food intake was obtained through a nutritional survey by means of a 24-hour recall conducted by trained nutritionists. The supply of energy, nutrients, and fiber of each food product was estimated using the American "Food Processor II" chemical composition food table program (38).

Table 5 shows the average dietary fiber intake ±SD in g/day and in g/1000 kcal, in men and women, and in total, the percentage of that recommended (12 g/1000 cal), and the percentage of people with lower than 75% of the recommended intake (9 g/1000 kcal). The percentage of adequacy observed was 74.5% greater in women than in men, and there was a large segment of people with lower than 75% of the recommended intake, with men being more affected than women.

Estimation of sources of dietary fiber as percentage of intake of dietary fiber points to cereals as the main source (Table 6), followed by an equal supply of fruit and vegetables, with legumes as a source of less importance.

2. The Elderly

Chile is experiencing an accelerated process of population aging. Those over 60 years old currently represent 10.5% of the population, 10.8% of whom are poor (39). Government agencies are interested in defining and implementing policies oriented toward improving the quality of life of the elderly. There is no updated information available concerning the nutritional standard for this segment of the population. Consequently, a study was conducted with the object of assessing the nutritional standard of those citizens over 65 years living in the more vulnerable districts within the metropolitan area.

Table 5 Individual Assessment: Dietary Fiber Intake and Adequacy to Recommendations of Adults—Santiago, Chile

	Males (n = 412)	Females (n = 447)	Total (n = 859)
Dietary fiber intake (g/day)[a]	18.9 ± 10.2	16.8 ± 9.3	17.8 ± 9.9
Energy intake (kcal/day)[a]	2436.5 ± 880.0	1811.0 ± 765.3	2111.2 ± 880.5
Dietary fiber intake (g/1000 kcal)[a]	8.0 ± 3.8	9.8 ± 4.6	8.9 ± 4.3
Adequacy (%)[a]	66.8 ± 31.5	81.5 ± 38.4	74.5 ± 36.0
Number of persons with intakes < 75% recommendations (%)	69.2	51.0	59.7

[a] Mean ± SD.
Method of dietary assessment = 24-hour recall questionnaire.
Method of fiber analysis = various.
Source: Adapted from Ref. 36.

Table 6 Sources of Dietary Fiber and Percent Contribution to Total
Dietary Fiber Intake of Adults—Santiago, Chile

	Dietary fiber (%)		
Food group	Males (n = 412)	Females (n = 447)	Total (n = 859)
Cereals	44.0	38.7	41.0
Fruit	23.8	27.3	25.8
Vegetables	28.0	29.2	28.7
Legumes	4.2	4.8	4.5
Total dietary fiber (%)	100	100	100

Source: Adapted from Ref. 36.

An assessment was made of a random and representative sample of 254 elders. A previously standardized 24-hour recall nutritional survey was applied by nutritionists. The survey was conducted in the homes; the amount of energy, nutrients, and fiber of each food product was estimated using the American "Food Processor II" chemical composition food table program (38). The adequacy of the recommendations was estimated for each nutrient (adequate intake of dietary fiber was estimated at 12 g/1000 kcal) as was the percentage of people with a lower than 75% of the recommended intake. The assessed group was made up of 66 men and 188 women with an average age of ±SD of 72.1 ± 6.7 years and a range between 65 and 97. The intake for all nutrients was set at lower ranges than the recommended amounts. Table 7 shows the average ±SD dietary fiber intake given in g and g/1000 kcal and its adequacy to the recommended amounts and the percentage of people with a lower than 75% of the recommended intake in men, in women, and in total.

Fiber intake is low, but so is energy intake, making it valid to estimate the adequacy in this segment of population only in terms of g/1000 kcal, which yields 79.4% for the entire segment. The percentage of people with a lower than 75% of the recommended intake is high (50% of the surveyed population).

Cereals are the main source of dietary fiber, followed very closely by vegetables, then fruit, and legumes with a very low incidence (Table 8).

Table 7 Individual Assessment: Dietary Fiber Intake and Adequacy to Recommendations of the Elderly Living in Poor Communities of Santiago, Chile

	Males (n = 66)	Females (n = 188)	Total (n = 254)
Dietary fiber intake (g/day)[a]	12.9 ± 6.0	11.2 ± 5.5	11.6 ± 5.7
Energy intake (kcal/day)[a]	1547 ± 510	1171 ± 406	1268 ± 465
Dietary fiber intake (g/1000 kcal)[a]	8.5 ± 3.3	9.8 ± 4.7	9.5 ± 4.4
Adequacy (%)[a]	71.2 ± 27.2	82.3 ± 39.0	79.4 ± 36.6
Number of persons with intakes < 75% recommendations (%)	56.1	48.4	50.4

[a] Mean ± SD.
Method of dietary assessment = 24-hour recall questionnaire.
Method of fiber analysis = various.
Source: Adapted from Ref. 39.

Table 8 Sources of Dietary Fiber and Percent Contribution to Total Dietary Fiber Intake in the Elderly Living in Poor Communities of Santiago, Chile

	Dietary fiber (%)	
Food group	Male (n = 66)	Female (n = 188)
Cereals	42.5	39.3
Fruit	18.9	19.6
Vegetables	33.9	36.6
Legumes	4.7	4.5
Total dietary fiber (%)	100	100

Source: Adapted from Ref. 39.

3. Preschoolers

The following information is part of a study on the prevention and control of obesity in preschoolers that attend the Fundación Integra Day Care Centers (National Foundation for the Integral Development of Children) (40). This foundation maintains a network of day care centers throughout the country for poor children aged 0–6 years old. In these centers children receive comprehensive care throughout the day in facilities opened to that effect 10 months of the year.

An assessment was conducted of the daily intake of energy, macronutrients, dietary fiber, and some critical micronutrients in preschool children (average age $\pm$ SD = 47.6 $\pm$ 4.0 months) that attend 4 day care centers of the Fundación Integra in Santiago. They receive their meals 5 days a week at the center (breakfast, lunch, and evening snack), and the rest at their homes. The meals they ingested at home (2 days a week) were also recorded. Nutritional intake was determined by a 24-hour recall survey, and the supply of energy, nutrients, and fiber was estimated using the American ''Food Processor II'' chemical composition food table program (38).

Table 9 shows the average dietary fiber intake sample $\pm$SD in g and in g/1000 kcal. If the recommended intake is deemed equivalent to 10 g/1000 kcal (12), the adequacy percentage was 72%, with similar patterns at home and at the day care center. The percentage of children with <75% of the recommended intake was high—roughly about 60% of the children.

Table 9 Individual Assessment: Dietary Fiber Intake and Adequacy to Recommendations of Preschool Children

	Day care center (n = 73)	Home (n = 26)	Total (n = 99)
Dietary fiber intake (g/day)[a]	11.2 $\pm$ 4.9	9.6 $\pm$ 5.2	10.8 $\pm$ 5.0
Energy intake (kcal/day)[a]	1573 $\pm$ 254.5	1257 $\pm$ 383.4	1490 $\pm$ 324
Dietary fiber intake (g/1000 kcal)[a]	7.0 $\pm$ 2.9	7.5 $\pm$ 3.1	7.2 $\pm$ 3.0
Adequacy (%)[a]	70.9 $\pm$ 26.3	74.6 $\pm$ 30.9	71.9 $\pm$ 26.0
Number of persons with intakes < 75% recommendations (%)	58.9	57.7	58.6

[a] Mean $\pm$ SD.
Method of dietary assessment = 24-hour recall questionnaire.
Method of fiber analysis = various.
Source: Adapted from Ref. 40.

D. Comments

Based on the outlined results, we must emphasize that the estimation of fiber consumption based on the food balance sheets and family budget surveys was conducted taking into account national dietary fiber data, with the recommended enzymatic-gravimetric techniques, in which both soluble and insoluble dietary fibers were included, which, as we know, play different physiological roles. Most of the studies conducted on dietary fiber only include data related to total dietary fiber.

In the individual assessments, studies conducted within the same country vary greatly as to the estimates of dietary fiber intake due to the specific groups assessed. This happened when analyzing the dietary fiber intake in adults, elders, and preschoolers. It is noteworthy to mention that the yielded values for the different groups correspond to current data and are comparable, since the same database was used in all surveys to estimate the fiber intake, and a similar methodology was used to calculate the adequacy of the intake and the sources of fiber of the food groups.

According to the assessment conducted on the studies in relation to the consumption of dietary fiber, we must emphasize the scarcity of information regarding this matter. It is necessary to encourage further studies at the national level in order to obtain information on dietary fiber intake.

E. Conclusions

The apparent intake of dietary fiber amounted to 22.1 and 23.6 g/person/day according to the food balance sheet and the family budget survey, respectively. The percentage of insoluble and soluble fiber was similar in both cases, approximately 67.5% and 32.5%. The average intake of dietary fiber $\pm$SD of adults, elders, and preschoolers was 17.8 ± 9.9, 11.6 ± 5.7, and 10.8 ± 5.0 g, respectively. The average percentage of adequacy in relation to the recommended intake (12 g/1000 kcal in adults and elders and 10 g/1000 kcal in preschoolers) was low in all three groups (72% to 79%), and the percentage of people with <75% of the recommended intake amounted to 60% in adults and preschoolers and 50% in elders.

Taking into account the sources of fiber, the various studies indicate cereals as the main source, followed by vegetables and fruit; in all cases legumes were the source that provided the lowest amount.

Due to the importance of fiber regarding prevention of nontransmissible chronic diseases, it is clear that there is a need to promote its consumption according to current nutritional guidelines.

ACKNOWLEDGMENTS

I am indebted to Dr. Eduardo Atalah Samur for making it possible to acquire the pertinent information about dietary fiber in the individual assessments done in adults, elders, and preschoolers.

REFERENCES

1. C Albala, F Vio. Epidemiological transition in Latin America: the case of Chile. Public Health 109: 431–442, 1995.

2. F Vio, C Castillo. Diagnóstico de la situación nutricional en Chile. In: C Castillo, R Uauy, E Atalah, eds. Guías de Alimentación para la Población Chilena. Santiago, Chile: Ministerio de Salud, Universidad de Chile, 1997, pp 23–42.

3. E Atalah, H Amigo. Situación nutricional en Chile. In: M Ruz, H Araya, E Atalah, D Soto, eds. Nutrición y Salud. Santiago, Chile: Universidad de Chile, 1996, pp 381–394.

4. C Castillo, M Báez, X Benavides. Validación de guías alimentarias para la población mayor de dos años. In: C Castillo, R Uauy, E Atalah, eds. Guías de Alimentación para la Población Chilena. Santiago, Chile: Ministerio de Salud, Universidad de Chile, 1997, pp 43–61.

5. SM Pilch. Physiological Effects and Health Consequences of Dietary Fiber. Bethesda, MD: Federation of American Societies for Experimental Biology, 1987.

6. Food and Nutrition Board. Commission on life Sciences, National Research Council. Recommended Dietary Allowances. 10th ed. Washington, DC: National Academy Press, 1989.

7. World Health Organization. Study Group in Diet, Nutrition and Prevention of Noncommunicable Diseases. Nutr Rev 49:291–301, 1991.

8. U.S. Departments of Agriculture and Health and Human Services: Dietary Guidelines for Americans N°232. Washington, DC: U.S. Government Printing Office, 1990.

9. Department of Health: Dietary Reference Values for Food Energy and Nutrients for the United Kingdom. London: HMSO, 1991, pp 61–71.

10. JH Cummings, GI Hudson, ME Quigley, HN Englyst. The classification and measurement of dietary carbohydrates. Proceeding of a workshop: recent progress in the analysis of dietary fiber, Luxembourg: Office for Official Publications of the European Communities, 1995, pp 17–36.

11. American Academy of Pediatrics, Committee on Nutrition. Carbohydrate and dietary fiber. In: L Barness, ed. Pediatric Nutrition Handbook. Elk Grove Village, IL: American Academy of Pediatrics, 1993, pp 100–106.

12. CL Williams, M Bollella, EL Wynder. A new recommendation for dietary fiber in childhood. Pediatrics 96 (suppl):985–988, 1995.

13. H Araya, G Vera, I Zacarias. Etiquetado nutricional en la promoción de una alimentación saludable. In: C Castillo, R Uauy, E Atalah, eds. Guías de Alimentación para la Población Chilena. Santiago, Chile: Ministerio de Salud, Universidad de Chile, 1997, pp 151–164.

14. Reglamento Sanitario de los Alimentos, Ministerio de Salud, Santiago, Chile, 1997.

15. JH Cummings. Dietary fiber intakes in Europe: An overview. Food and Agriculture Organization of the United Nations. In: JH Cummings, W Frolich, eds. Dietary Fiber Intakes in Europe. Luxembourg: Commission of the European Communities, 1993, pp 11–19.

16. Food and Agriculture Organization of the United Nations, Food Balance Sheets average 1992–1994, Rome.

17. Instituto de Nutrición de Centro América y Panamá. Comité Interdepartmental de Nutrición para la Defensa Nacional. Tabla de Composición de Alimentos para uso en America Latina. Editorial Interamericana SA, 1960.

18. Organización de las Naciones Unidas para la Agricultura y la Alimentación. Tabla de Composición de Alimentos para Uso Internacional. Washington, DC: 1949.

19. C Urteaga, C Gaete. Valor nutricional de preparaciones culinarias habituales en Chile. Santiago: Universidad de Chile, 1995.

20. N Pak, C Ayala, G Vera, I Pennacchiotti, H Araya. Fibra dietética soluble e insoluble en cereales y leguminosas cultivadas en Chile. Arch Latinoamer Nutr 40:116–125, 1990.

21. N Pak. Fibra dietética: concepto, contenido en alimentos y consumo en Chile. Rev Chil Nutr 20: 124–135, 1992.

22. N Pak. Por publicar.

23. NG Asp, CG Johansson, H Hallmer, M Siljestrom. A rapid enzymatic assay of insoluble and soluble dietary fiber. J Agric Food Chem 31:476–482, 1983.

24. SC Lee, L Prosky, JW De Vries. Determination of total, soluble and insoluble dietary fiber in foods. Enzymatic-Gravimetric method, MES-TRIS buffer; Collaborative study. J AOAC Int 75:395–416, 1992.

25. E Bright-See, G McKeown-Eyssen. Estimation of per capita crude and dietary fiber supply in 38 countries. Am J Clin Nutr 39:821–829, 1984.

26. E Bright-See. Reply to letter by Rutishauser. Am J Clin Nutr 41:825–826, 1985.

27. Instituto Nacional de Estadística. IV Encuesta de Presupuestos Familiares, Diciembre 1987, Noviembre 1988, Santiago, Chile, 1989.

28. B Teitelboin. Canasta de Alimentos y Salarios Minimos de Satisfacción de Necesidades Básicas. Documento de trabajo N°77, Santiago, Chile: PET, 1990.

29. República de Chile, Ministerio de Salud. Encuesta continuada sobre el estado nutricional de la población chilena, Julio 1974, Junio 1975, Santiago-Chile, 1982.

30. T Boj. El consumo alimentario de las familias y niños beneficiarios del programa Nacional de Alimentación Complementaria en Chile. Rev Chil Nutr 22:109–114, 1994.

31. MT Oyarzún, D Sanjur. Dieta de mujeres pobres urbanas en Chile Central. Rev Chil Nutr 21:87–97, 1993.

32. C Albala, P Villarroel, S Olivares. Mujeres obesas de alto y bajo nivel socioeconómico: composición de la dieta y niveles séricos de lipoproteinas. Rev Méd Chile 117:3–9, 1989.

33. CL Villanueva, A Arteaga, A Maiz, A González-Koch, C Descouvieres. Lípidos séricos como factor de riesgo coronario: influencia de la dieta en 358 hombres sanos. Rev Chil Nutr 17:175–181, 1989.

34. P Bustos, E Atalah, A Rebolledo. Efecto de la suplementación con tiamina, riboflavina y piridoxina en embarazadas del área Norte de Santiago. Rev Chil Nutr 20:28–37, 1992.

35. D Ivanovic, R Ivanovic, MC Durán, J Hasbún. Ingesta alimentaria de escolares rurales de la Región Metropolitana de Chile. Arch Latinoamer Nutr 42:374–388, 1992.

36. C Castillo, E Atalah, X Benavides, C Urteaga. Patrones alimentarios en adultos que asisten a consultorios de atención primaria en la Región Metropolitana. Rev Méd Chile 125:283–289, 1997.

37. C Castillo, R Uauy, E Atalah. Guías de Alimentación para la Población Chilena. Santiago, Chile Ministerio de Salud, Universidad de Chile, 1997.

38. ESHA Research. The Food Processor: User Guide. Salem, EEUU, 1995.

39. E Atalah, X Benavides, L Avila, S Barahona, R Cárdenas. Características alimentarias de adultos, mayores de comunas pobres de la Región Metropolitana. Rev Méd Chile 126:489–496, 1998.

40. Departamento de Nutrición, Facultad de Medicina, Universidad de Chile. Prevención y Control de la Obesidad en preescolares de la Fundación integra. Segundo Informe: Evaluación de un programa piloto en la Región Metropolitana, Santiago, Abril de 1997.

44

Dietary Fiber Intake in Mexico: Recommendations and Actual Consumption Patterns

Jorge L. Rosado
National Institute of Nutrition, Mexico City, and University of Queretaro, Queretaro, Mexico

I. DIETARY PATTERNS IN MEXICO

In Mexico it has been reported (1–4) that 80–85% of Mexicans, representing a significant part of the suburban population and most of the rural population, consume diets based on corn tortillas, beans, vegetables, and fruit. Tortillas and beans provide most of the dietary energy and protein for this population, whereas inclusion of animal products is only occasional and highly variable. In contrast, the population in the cities consume diets similar to those found in developed countries. These diets include more animal foods, greater amounts of refined cereals and sugar, and fewer foods of plant origin, thus they consume lower amounts of complex carbohydrates, including dietary fiber (5). This discrepancy in dietary pattern may be involved in the etiology of disease. Table 1 shows the composition of typical average diets consumed in rural and urban areas. As can be observed, concentration of dietary fiber is about four times higher in rural than in urban diets.

II. DIETARY FIBER INTAKE IN MEXICO

A. Dietary Fiber Intake in the Rural Population

In an initial study (6), we used both the information for food consumption in the different regions of the country obtained from the two National Nutrition surveys carried out in the country in 1979 and 1989 and the information on the dietary fiber composition of Mexican foods to obtain habitual dietary fiber intake. Accordingly, dietary fiber intake was expressed in grams per person per day. The information was reported as consumption of soluble dietary fiber (SDF), insoluble dietary fiber (IDF), as well as total dietary fiber (TDF) for the different regions studied. The contribution of different foods or food groups to dietary fiber intake was also analyzed in both of the surveys.

Average dietary fiber intake expressed in grams per person per day is shown in Table 2. Average per capita intake of TDF ranged from 19.8 to 34.0 g/d in 1979 and from 17.5 to 27.1 g/d in 1989, depending on the region of the country. In 1979, average consumption of TDF in

Table 1 Nutrient Content of Typical Average Rural and Urban Diets[a]

Nutrient	Rural Mexican diet	Urban Mexican diet
Energy (kcal/d)	1588 ± 326	1849 ± 360
Protein (g/d)	42.1 ± 8.9	66.1 ± 13.4
Animal	2.2 ± 0.4	40.5 ± 7.7
Vegetable	40.0 ± 8.5	25.5 ± 5.8
Fat (g/d)	34.0 ± 7.3	64.4 ± 12.9
Carbohydrate (g/d)	292 ± 58	252 ± 53.2
Calcium (mg/d)	869 ± 185	545 ± 120
Iron (mg/d)	30.8 ± 6.6	21.4 ± 5.5
Sodium (mg/d)	43.6 ± 11.1	1187 ± 238
Vitamin A (μg retinol/d)	1490 ± 458	707 ± 205
Riboflavin (mg/d)	0.9 ± 0.1	1.2 ± 0.2
Thiamine (mg/d)	1.6 ± 0.3	1.3 ± 0.2
Niacin (mg/d)	18.3 ± 3.7	28.0 ± 5.4
Vitamin C (mg/d)	324 ± 69	128 ± 59
Cholesterol (mg/d)	10.8 ± 2.3	434 ± 120
Crude fiber (g/d)	18.3 ± 4.3	3.8 ± 1.0
NDF (g/d)[b]	40.2 ± 10.4	12.1 ± 3.6
Phytic acid (mmol/d)	1.62 ± 0.14	0.09 ± 0.02
(g/d)	1.07 ± 0.09	0.07 ± 0.01

[a] $\bar{x}$ ± SD, n = 16. Values calculated from data in Mexican food composition tables.
  Adapted from Ref. 5.
[b] Neutral detergent fiber determined from blended, lyophilized diet samples.

the 19 regions into which the country was divided was 27.2 ± 3.3 g/d. Of this, 87.2% (23.7 ± 2.9 g/d) was insoluble fiber and 12.8% (3.5 ± 0.5 g/d) was soluble fiber. In 1989, average consumption of TDF decreased to 22.5 ± 2.2 g/d, of which 87.6% (19.7 ± 2.1 g/d) was insoluble and 12.8% (2.9 ± 0.2 g/d) was soluble fiber. As can be observed from the table, all regions of the country showed a decrease in dietary fiber intake from 1979 to 1989, with only one exception—region 18, encompassing to the states of Veracruz, Tabasco, and Campeche. The decrease in consumption is highly significant ($p < 0.0001$). This suggests that dietary fiber intake in rural Mexico is decreasing, which may be associated with an increase in fat and sugar consumption (7). Some studies (8,9) have suggested an increase in the incidence of obesity in rural areas as well as an increase in blood lipids and cardiovascular disease (10); reduction in dietary fiber intake might be contributing to such observations.

B. Dietary Fiber Intake in the Urban Population

Consumption of dietary fiber in urban areas was calculated from the food consumption data obtained from a survey carried out in urban areas (11) and the information on dietary fiber composition of Mexican foods (12). Table 3 shows the results of such calculations; dietary fiber intake is given as per capita intake in grams per person per day. Intake of soluble, insoluble, and total dietary fiber of populations from different socioeconomic status is included (SES). Total dietary fiber intake in urban Mexico varied from 14.2 g/d in the medium high SES to 16.6 g/d in the very low SES. On average, including urban populations from all SES, dietary fiber intake was 15.4 ± 0.9 g/d, and it was about 7 g/d lower than intake from rural population

Table 2 Per Capita Intake (g/day) of Dietary Fiber in Rural Mexico[a]

Region[b]	1979 survey			1989 survey			TDF (1989–1979)
	IDF	SDF	TDF	IDF	SDF	TDF	
1	21.01	4.03	25.04	15.04	2.51	17.55	−7.49
2	21.28	4.08	25.36	17.12	2.90	20.02	−5.34
3	23.06	3.90	26.96	17.51	2.81	20.32	−6.64
4	28.62	4.52	33.14	23.61	3.50	27.11	−6.03
5	23.38	3.66	27.04	17.92	2.81	20.73	−6.31
6	22.40	3.48	25.88	16.65	2.42	19.07	−6.81
7	28.29	4.25	32.54	19.76	2.98	22.74	−9.80
8	21.14	2.84	23.98	19.27	2.74	22.01	−1.97
9	25.19	3.67	28.86	19.18	2.83	22.01	−6.85
10	24.40	3.35	27.75	21.31	2.98	24.29	−3.46
11	23.02	3.11	26.13	20.75	2.81	23.56	−2.57
12	22.07	3.06	25.13	21.46	3.10	24.56	−.057
13	22.57	2.86	25.43	20.72	2.75	23.47	−1.96
14	30.04	3.94	33.98	21.08	2.93	24.01	−9.97
15	24.79	3.28	28.07	19.96	2.95	22.91	−5.16
16	23.04	3.04	26.08	21.91	2.97	24.88	−1.20
17	23.72	3.20	26.92	21.29	3.16	24.45	−2.47
18	17.35	2.43	19.78	19.43	2.85	22.28	2.50
19	25.19	3.56	28.75	20.38	2.88	23.26	−5.49
Average	23.71	3.49	27.02	19.07	2.89	22.60	−4.61[a]
SD	2.97	0.54	3.34	2.10	0.23	2.29	3.22

[a] Average difference is statistically significant ($p < 0.001$). Adapted from Ref. 6.
[b] Numbers indicate different regions in which the country was divided for the nutrition surveys (1,2).

Table 3 Per Capita Dietary Fiber Intake of Population in Urban Areas According to Socioeconomic Status

Socioeconomic status	Dietary fiber intake (g/d)		
	SF	IF	TDF
High SES	2.2	14.2	16.1
Medium-high SES	2.0	12.4	14.2
Medium-low SES	2.1	14.2	16.2
Low SES	1.9	13.0	14.8
Very low SES	2.1	14.6	16.6
Peri-urban population	1.8	12.7	14.4
Average	2.0	13.5	15.4
SD	0.1	0.8	0.9

from the survey of 1989 ($p < 0.05$) and about 12 g/d lower than the intake in rural areas from the survey of 1979 ($p < 0.01$).

III. SOURCES OF DIETARY FIBER INTAKE IN RURAL AND URBAN POPULATIONS

The contribution of the different foods to dietary fiber intake in the rural population of different regions of Mexico in 1989 is shown in Table 4. Cereals were the major source of dietary fiber in all regions of the country. Of the different cereals, maize was the major single source of dietary fiber. The contribution of maize to TDF intake varied from 24.1 to 62.4%. For wheat, the variation was from 2.0 to 24.7%, for rice 0.1 to 0.7%, for legumes 11.8 to 29.6%, for fruit 0.6 to 13.4%, for roots and tubers 0.6 to 7.3%, and for other vegetables 10.8 to 27.3%.

The contribution of different foods to total dietary fiber intake in the urban population of different SES is shown in Table 5. The contribution of total cereals to dietary fiber intake in the different SES of urban population varied from 34.5 to 60.3%, maize being the main source, which varied from 30.4 to 57%. For roots and tubers the variation was from 2.4 to 3.4%, for legumes from 11.2 to 16.6%, for fruits from 7 to 33%, and for other vegetables from 13.2 to 21.3%. As for the rural population, maize is the most important single source of dietary fiber

Table 4   Source of Dietary Fiber Intake in Rural Areas

Region[a]	Total cereals	Wheat	Rice	Maize	Roots and tubers	Legumes	Fruits	Other vegetables
1	49.2	24.7	0.3	24.2	7.3	16.0	4.5	23.0
2	42.8	18.2	0.5	24.1	4.5	19.0	13.4	25.3
3	55.2	21.6	0.3	33.3	4.5	23.3	2.1	15.0
4	52.9	6.3	0.3	46.3	2.5	25.3	1.3	18.0
5	49.5	13.7	0.3	35.5	3.0	22.8	3.6	21.1
6	58.7	7.9	0.5	50.3	2.3	19.8	3.7	15.4
7	53.8	4.9	0.3	48.6	1.4	14.9	13.3	16.6
8	59.3	4.2	0.4	54.7	1.4	20.4	4.3	14.6
9	54.8	6.6	0.2	48.0	1.5	17.7	6.5	19.5
10	61.3	6.1	0.3	54.5	1.6	16.6	2.5	18.0
11	65.9	3.2	0.2	62.4	1.4	17.1	2.5	13.0
12	53.7	7.9	0.2	45.6	1.6	11.8	5.6	27.3
13	67.0	4.6	0.2	62.3	1.1	14.2	1.5	16.2
14	60.6	4.8	0.1	55.8	1.6	12.5	4.5	20.7
15	56.0	4.3	0.4	46.3	1.2	17.0	6.1	19.6
16	63.0	2.7	0.2	60.1	0.6	20.1	0 .6	15.8
17	54.4	2.0	0.1	52.4	1.4	29.6	3.8	10.8
18	56.3	4.4	0.7	51.2	1.1	14.4	11.6	16.7
19	66.3	7.7	0.1	58.4	0.7	14.8	6.9	11.4
Average	56.9	8.2	0.3	48.1	2.1	18.2	5.1	17.8
SD	6.3	6.5	0.1	11.5	1.6	4.5	3.8	4.3

[a] Numbers indicate different regions in which the country was divided for the nutrition survey (2).
Source: Adapted from Ref. 6.

Table 5 Contribution of Different Foods to Dietary Fiber Intake of Urban Population

Socioeconomic status	% of total dietary fiber intake							
	Total cereals	Wheat	Rice	Maize	Roots tubers	Legumes	Fruits	Other vegetables
High SES	34.5	3.5	0.6	30.4	3.4	11.2	33.2	17.6
Medium-high SES	39.9	4.8	0.7	34.4	3.3	11.3	24.1	21.3
Medium-low SES	53.7	4.5	0.5	48.7	3.1	10.3	16.4	16.3
Low SES	59.5	3.6	0.4	55.5	3.1	12.2	10.2	14.9
Very low SES	60.3	3.1	0.2	57.0	2.5	15.7	7.0	14.5
Peri-urban population	59.8	3.8	0.4	55.6	2.4	16.6	8.0	13.2
Average	51.28	3.90	0.47	46.95	2.96	12.89	16.48	16.31
SD	10.31	0.58	0.16	10.68	0.39	2.39	9.50	2.64

intake, but total intake of fiber from maize varied in the urban areas depending on SES. The contribution of dietary fiber intake from maize in populations from very high and medium high SES was lower than that in populations from lower SES. The contribution of maize to dietary fiber intake in the lower SES of urban population was similar to that in rural population. This demonstrates that total consumption of dietary fiber as well as the contribution from different foods is affected by SES. In general, diets of the lower SES in urban areas and of populations in rural areas contain more dietary fiber, and the main source of dietary fiber intake is corn tortillas. The contribution of fruits to total dietary fiber intake in the different SES has an opposite trend compared with maize: while the proportion of fiber from maize and therefore from total cereals increases as SES decreases, the fiber intake from fruits increases as SES increases. In the high SES 33% of fiber intake come from fruits and only 30% from maize or 34% from total cereals; in the very low SES only 7% of fiber comes from fruits and 57% from maize and 60% from total cereals. Dietary fiber from fruits in rural areas was lower than in urban areas. Intake of dietary fiber from legumes was higher in the lower SES than in the higher SES (Tables 4 and 5).

IV. DIETARY FIBER INTAKE AND UTILIZATION OF RURAL AND URBAN MEXICAN DIETS

The amount of fiber in typical rural and urban Mexican diets that is utilized or bioavailable has been measured (5). Table 6 shows the result of a metabolic study carried out with 16 women who ingested average rural and urban diets. Subjects ingested 3.3 times more dietary fiber (measured as neutral detergent fiber) with the rural than with the urban diet. All fractions of dietary fiber—hemicellulose, cellulose, and lignin—were significantly higher in the rural diet. Significantly more dry matter was excreted with the rural diet by a factor of 2.8. Fecal excretion of fiber was about five times higher with the rural diet, affecting all fractions in about the same proportion. Significantly more fiber (22.7 g/d, 56%) was digested from the rural diet than from the urban diet (8.9 g/d, 70%). Of the 40.2 g/d of dietary fiber ingested with the rural diet, 23 g/d (56%) was digested and presumably used as a source of energy, thus contributing to energy intake. The fact that a higher proportion of fiber was digested from the diet containing less fiber suggests that the human colon has a threshold for fermentation of ingested dietary fiber.

Table 6 Intake, Fecal Excretion, and Digestion of Neutral Detergent
Fiber, Acid Detergent Fiber, Hemicellulose, Cellulose, and Lignin by
16 Women Consuming Rural and Urban Mexican Diets[a]

Intake (g/d)			
Dry matter	406.3 ± 24.8	386.3 ± 17.6	NS[b]
NDF	40.2 ± 2.6	12.1 ± 0.9	<0.0001
ADF	28.7 ± 1.8	8.2 ± 0.5	<0.0001
Hemicellulose	11.4 ± 1.6	3.7 ± 1.0	<0.0003
Cellulose	17.4 ± 1.4	5.5 ± 0.7	<0.0001
Lignin	11.3 ± 1.3	2.6 ± 0.2	<0.0001
Fecal excretion (g/d)			
Dry matter	36.6 ± 3.5	13.3 ± 1.0	<0.0001
NDF	17.5 ± 1.5	3.6 ± 0.4	<0.0001
ADF	10.9 ± 0.9	2.3 ± 0.3	<0.0001
Hemicellulose	6.8 ± 0.7	1.2 ± 0.3	<0.0001
Cellulose	6.4 ± 0.5	1.3 ± 0.1	<0.0001
Lignin	4.5 ± 0.4	1.0 ± 0.1	<0.0001
Digestibility (g/d)			
NDF	22.7 ± 2.3	8.9 ± 1.0	<0.0001
ADF	17.8 ± 1.7	5.9 ± 0.5	<0.0001
Hemicellulose	4.6 ± 1.3	2.7 ± 1.1	NS
Cellulose	11.0 ± 1.2	4.3 ± 0.7	<0.0001
Lignin	6.8 ± 1.1	1.7 ± 0.2	<0.0002
Digestibility (%)			
NDF	55 ± 4	70 ± 4	<0.0166
ADF	61 ± 3	70 ± 5	NS
Hemicellulose	40 ± 5	73 ± 7	<0.0012
Cellulose	63 ± 2	75 ± 2	<0.0451
Lignin	53 ± 7	58 ± 5	NS

[a] ± SEM.
[b] Difference not statistically significant at $p < 0.05$.
Source: Adapted from Ref. 5.

V. NUTRIENT DEFICIENCIES ASSOCIATED WITH HABITUAL INTAKE OF HIGH-FIBER DIETS

A. Dietary Fiber Intake and Nutrient Bioavailability

Nutrient deficiencies are caused by (a) poor ingestion of a nutrient, (b) a decrease in nutrient bioavailability, and/or (c) an increase in the requirement for the nutrient. High-fiber diets are less energy dense and may also contain less protein. The information of the National Nutrition Survey (1) carried out in rural areas in Mexico shows that deficient energy and protein intake occurs only in the most marginal regions of the country among the poorest groups of the population. The ingestion of some vitamins, especially vitamin A, riboflavin, and ascorbic acid, is reported to be low in several groups of Mexicans associated with the ingestion of the rural Mexican diet (13). Intake of minerals is not deficient, even though iron deficiency anemia is the most common nutritional deficiency in the country (14); high-fiber diets like the rural Mexican diet contain more iron than other diets. Thus, the habitual ingestion of high-fiber, plant-based diets might lead to low ingestion of some nutrients, especially some vitamins.

High-fiber diets like the diet typical of rural areas in Mexico are high in substances that may interfere with the absorption of several nutrients. Of relevance to this potential effect is a

Table 7 Absorption as Percent of Intake of Energy, Nitrogen, Zinc, Iron, and Calcium (mean + SEM) of 16 Women Consuming Rural and Urban Mexican Diets

	Rural diet	Urban diet	p-value
Energy	89 ± 0.9	95 ± 0.3	<0.001
Nitrogen	67 ± 3.0	90 ± 0.4	<0.001
Zinc	4 ± 1.0	16 ± 2.2	<0.05
Iron	14 ± 1.2	32 ± 2.8	<0.05
Calcium	-18 ± 2.9	4 ± 0.9	<0.05

Source: Adapted from Refs. 4, 15.

study (15) in which we evaluated the effect of an average rural diet on the absorption of nutrients. The average rural diet contained 1.1 ± 0.1 g/d of phytic acid and 40.2 ± 2.6 g/d of dietary fiber (Table 1). The absorption of nutrients with this diet was evaluated by balance studies using polyethylene glycol (PEG) as quantitative marker, and it was compared with the absorption of the same nutrients with an average urban diet that contained more animal foods. In average the urban diet contained only 0.07 g/d of phytic acid and 12.1 ± 0.9 g/d of dietary fiber. A summary of the results of this study is presented in Table 7. The apparent absorption of all nutrients studied was significantly reduced with the rural diet. Specially there was a very high reduction in the absorption of iron, zinc, and calcium with the rural diet. This study and the large body of information about the negative effect of plant food constituents on the absorption of minerals suggest that the low bioavailability of nutrients might be an important mechanism responsible for the high incidence of nutrient deficiencies in a population that habitually consumes high-fiber plant-based diets in Mexico.

B. Dietary Fiber Intake and Micronutrient Deficiencies

In a recent study we found the existence of several nutrient deficiencies in a group of 219 children from a rural area of Central Mexico (16). The children studied, 102 boys and 117 girls ranging in age from 18 to 36 months, consumed a typical high-fiber rural diet. Indicators of the nutritional status of iron, zinc, vitamin A, vitamin E, vitamin B_{12}, and riboflavin were included in the analysis. The percentage of children that presented low or deficient values with each indicator studied as well as cut-off criteria used in the definition are shown in Table 8. Of the

Table 8 Micronutrient Deficiency in 219 Preschoolers of a Rural Community in Mexico

	% of children with deficiency	Cut-off criteria
Hemoglobin	72	<11.7 g/dL
Plasma ferritin	51	<12.0 ng/mL
Plasma zinc	25	<70.0 µg/dL
Erythrocyte riboflavin	9	≥ 1.4 SI
Plasma vitamin B_{12}	10	<200 pg/mL
Plasma retinol	29	<200 ng/mL
Plasma vitamin E	64	<500 ng/mL

SI = Stimulation index.
Source: Adapted from Ref. 4.

219 preschoolers, 203 (93%) had a deficiency of at least one nutrient and 149 (68%) had a deficiency of two or more nutrients. Nutritional deficiencies of riboflavin, vitamin B_{12}, and vitamin E had not been previously reported to occur in the Mexican population (13,14). The high incidence of Holo transcobalamin II deficiency associated with vitamin B_{12} deficiency suggests that vitamin B_{12} deficiency in these children is mainly due to low absorption of the vitamin (17) (Holo transcobalamin II is an indicator of recently absorbed vitamin B_{12}). The high incidence of multiple micronutrient deficiencies associated with the habitual intake of high-fiber, plant-based diets suggests that chronic ingestion of such diets may be contributing somehow to the deterioration in the nutritional status of some micronutrients.

VI. CONCLUSION

Dietary fiber intake in Mexico is highly associated with socioeconomic status. Populations of lower SES in the less "developed" rural areas consume diets that are based on plant foods and consequently consume significantly higher amounts of dietary fiber than populations in the cities, especially of the higher SES. Unfortunately there is a trend to decreasing dietary fiber intake in both rural and urban areas of the country. Corn tortillas, the most important staple food, contributes about 30–60% of the total dietary fiber intake, the lower level of the range being for the higher SES and the higher level for the high SES. High-SES populations include less dietary fiber in their diet, with fruits and vegetables being more important sources than in the lower SES. The intake of plant-based diets in Mexico in the poor regions of the country is associated with micronutrient deficiencies. Deficiency of some micronutrients, such as iron, zinc, and vitamin B_{12}, occur mainly due to the lower absorption commonly found with high-fiber foods and diets. The risk of deficiency is exacerbated by the fact that the ingestion of a plant-based diet, associated with poverty, is accompanied by a lack of variety, and in some instances it is also insufficient. It is well known that when an adequate number of plant foods are mixed, the result could be a highly nutritious diet with the additional benefits of being low in fat especially low in saturated fat, and a good source of fiber and other plant food constituents that have been associated with a lower risk of developing chronic diseases. The beneficial effects of such diets have been the subject of many recent investigations.

REFERENCES

1. Instituto Nacional de la Nutrición. Encuesta nacional de alimentación 1979. Resultados de la encuesta rural analizada por ponderación, presentada por entidad federativa y desagregada según zonas nutricionales. INNSZ L-46, México, 1982.
2. Instituto Nacional de la Nutrición. Encuesta nacional de alimentación en el medio rural, 1989. INNSZ L-86, México DF, 1990.
3. Madrigal H, Chávez A, Moreno-Terrazas C, García T, Gutierrez V. Consumo de alimentos y estado nutricional de la población del medio rural mexicano. Rev Inv Clin (Méx), 1986; 38 suppl:9–19
4. Rosado JL. Vegetarian diets in Mexico: an evaluation of its potential risks and benefits. Invited comment. Nutr Rev 1987; 55:s65–s67.
5. Rosado JL, López P, Morales M, Allen LH. Digestibility and breath hydrogen excretion in subjects consuming rural and urban Mexican diets. Am J Clin Nutr 1991; 53:55–60.
6. Rosado JL, López P, López G, Madrigal H, Huerta Z. Consumption of dietary fiber in rural Mexico. Ecol Food Nutrition 1995; 34:129–136.
7. Flores M, Melgar H, Cortés C, Rivera M, Rivera J, Sepúlveda J. Consumo de energía y nutrimentos en mujeres mexicanas en edad reproductiva. Salud Pub Mex 1998; 40:161–171.

8. Sepulveda J. Estado nutricional de los preescolares y las mujeres en Mexico. Resultados de una encuesta nacional probabilistica. Gac Med Mex 1990; 26:207–225.

9. Quibrera-Infante R, Hernandez-Rodriguez HG, Aradillas-Garcia C, Gonzalez-Rodriguez S, Callers-Escandon J. Prevalencias de diabetes mellitus, intolerancia a la glucosa, hiperlipidemia y factores de riesgo en funcion del nivel socioeconomico. Rev Inv Clin 1994; 46:25–38.

10. Batrouni L, Chávez A. Modernización de la dieta urbana y enfermedades cardiovasculares. Rev Inv Clin (Méx) 1986; 38 (suppl):21–26.

11. Instituto Nacional de la Nutrición. Encuesta Urbana de Alimentación y Nutrición en la zona metropolitana de la Ciudad de México, 1995.

12. Rosado JL, López P, Huerta Z, Muñoz E, Mejía L. Dietary fiber in Mexican foods. J Food Comp Anal 1993; 6:215–222.

13. Rosado JL, Bourges H, Saint-Martin B. Deficiencia de vitaminas y minerales en Mexico. Una revisión crítica del estado de la información. II. Deficiencia de vitaminas. Salud Pub Mex 1995; 37:452–461.

14. Rosado JL, Bourges H, Saint-Martin B. Deficiencia de vitaminas y minerales en México. Una revisión crítica del estado de la información. I Deficiencia de minerales. Salud Púb Mex 1995; 37:130–137.

15. Rosado JL, López P, Morales M, Muñoz E, Allen LH. Bioavailability of energy, nitrogen, fat, zinc, iron and calcium from rural and urban Mexican diets. Br J Nutr 1992; 68:45–58.

16. Allen LH, Rosado JL, Casterline JE, López P, Muñoz E, Martinez H. Lack of hemoglobin response to iron supplementation in anemic Mexican preschoolers with multiple micronutrient deficiencies. Am J Clin Nutr 2000; 71:1485–1494.

17. Allen LH, Rosado JL, Casterline JE, et al. Vitamin B_{12} deficiency and malabsorption are prevalent in rural Mexican communities. Am J Clin Nutr 1995; 62:1013–1019.

45

Dietary Fiber and Resistant Starch Intake in Brazil: Recommendations and Actual Consumption Patterns

Franco Maria Lajolo and Elizabete Wenzel de Menezes
University of São Paulo, São Paulo, Brazil

I. BRAZILIAN DATA ON DIETARY FIBER AND RESISTANT STARCH CONTENT IN FOODS

Food composition tables presently available in Brazil are outdated and incomplete in terms of foods and nutrients. Most of these tables include data only on crude fiber (1); others show neutral and acid detergent fractions (2) or simply do not include this component (3). There are only a few isolated published articles dealing with dietary fiber (DF) composition obtained using the enzymatic-gravimetric method in specific foods (4–6).

Computerized programs employed in Brazil for estimating the nutritional value of diets usually use crude fiber and not DF or they use data from foreign tables that do not totally correspond to the values of foods consumed in Brazil, which can lead to considerable errors.

For this reason, the estimate of DF intake for preventive or diet-therapeutic purpose in specific groups—children, the elderly, expectant mothers, and the general population—suffers from a lack of data regarding our daily eating habits. Similarly, the same problem arises when specific products rich in fiber or diets are attempted.

A. Collaborative Study of Dietary Fiber Analysis

Taking into account the lack of Brazilian data on DF and the composition of foods in general, an Integrated Program of Food Composition has been formed to foster initiatives to update data on food composition reflecting the reality of our country and to improve information quality and interlaboratory communication (7,8). The program has coordinated a national/international laboratory network since 1989 and has been carrying out several common activities.

An initial interlaboratory collaborative study was carried out to identify suitable analytical techniques and methods for validation of results. Studies then were undertaken to analyze contents of DF, carotenoids, amino acids, and some complex B vitamin in foods.

The need for adequate analytical methods for the analysis of DF, taking into account the importance of the analytical quality of data and the lack of proper information not only in Brazil but in several Latin American countries, a collaborative study was also undertaken under the sponsorship of CYTED (Programa Iberoamericano de Ciencia y Tecnología para el Desarrollo).

Nineteen research laboratories from eight countries took part in the first stage of the study. Standard samples of different fiber sources were evaluated by the enzymatic-gravimetric method as routinely used by laboratories. Among them, 37% did not obtain results acceptable within the control limits statistically established (9,10).

Some procedures in use in different laboratories could account for the results found. Most of the laboratories experienced problems related to residual protein analysis. Furthermore, several laboratories did not perform enzyme control or analytical control by means of reference material or standard reference material (SRM). This is not uncommon, as was stated in an international survey that reported that only 20% out of 147 respondents used reference materials for dietary fiber analysis. (11). All the problems were corrected, and a technique based on the procedure of Lee et al. (12) was proposed to obtaining data for food composition tables and for nutritional labeling purposes.

B. Quality Evaluation of Analytical Data

Adequate analytical quality criteria are important. They are crucial for data gathering (compilers), for exact analysis of nutrients (analysts), and for effective and correct reading of data (users).

Considering the importance of DF in human food, the international concern about data quality assurance, and the lack of Brazilian data on DF, a first effort to publish a reliable dietary fiber database was started (13–15). The compiled figures had their quality evaluated to guarantee the data to be used for this purpose were accurate and precise by analytical standards.

Analytical quality evaluation of DF data to construct the database was based on studies carried out by the U.S. Department of Agriculture (USDA) with other nutrients, such as selenium and vitamin A (16–18). According to parameters and criteria set forth by Holden et al. (17) and Mangels et al. (18), adaptations were introduced so as to be suitable when applied to data referring to fiber (15,19).

Data quality parameters usually include suitable number of samples, sampling plan, sample handling procedures, analytical method, and analytical quality control. Each parameter permits the evaluation and rating of data quality to produce an accurate and representative estimate. The rating scale ranged from 0 to 3, 3 being the optimum possible score for each parameter (source, food, and value). Ratings for individual parameters were combined to yield a single indicator of data quality per source—the quality index—which ranged from 0.6 to 3.0. Quality indices for various acceptable sources were combined to yield a single confidence code (A, B, or C).

Only foods analyzed by enzyme-gravimetric methods or by nonenzyme-gravimetric (20), in the case of fruits with little or no starch, were included in the database. Food evaluated using other methods (crude fiber and acid/neutral-detergent) that did not express acceptable qualities were excluded.

The compilation was based on many Brazilian sources, such as published scientific papers, doctoral and masters theses, and research reports from government and private laboratories and the food industry. As a result of this information-gathering process, a total of 545 vegetal foods were checked. The first rating criteria used, analytical technique, showed the following distribution: enzymatic-gravimetric (33%), neutral and acid detergent (32%), crude fiber (13%), and nonanalyzed fiber (22%) (15,19).

The result achieved in the quality evaluation of data from the remaining 180 foods was 29% under codes A and B. Foods that were awarded credibility code A were those for which users can have considerable confidence in the value presented. Code B implies that the users can have confidence in the value, but some problems exist regarding the data on which the value is based. The remaining foods (71%) were classified under code C, meaning that the users should have less confidence because of limited quantity and/or quality of data. For 244 food items it was not feasible to establish a credibility code due to an unsuitable methodology used in the fiber analysis (15,19).

Looking at the more frequently consumed foods in the Brazilian diet (21–23), it can be observed that of the 43 most common vegetal foods, DF was not analyzed for 10; 31 were rated C, 2 rated B, and none A (15,19).

The high number of foods graded C was in part due to the lack of detailed information about the analytical procedures, insufficient numbers of sample, or poor description of the analytical quality control used. Another factor is related to the nonusage of adequate reference material. Holden (16), assessing the quality of USDA food composition data, found difficulties in achieving the highest score—3. For instance, analytical reference materials, one of the prerequisites for a rating of 3, is not available for many components in foods. However, the use of reference material is recommended, and within the next few years more material is expected to be available for analysis.

Keeping in mind the goal of making Brazilian researchers more aware of and advising them regarding to the importance of adequate procedures for the production of food composition data, a specific form was developed (14,24). This form supplies detailed instructions about number of samples, sampling plan, sample description handling, analytical method, analytical quality control, and food identification. It was made available to all laboratories interested in obtaining analytical data or sending data to be included in the dietary fiber database.

In summary, the analytical quality evaluation of DF allowed the real assessment of analytical data and determined which were the highest priority foods for future analysis. The evaluated DF data were then included in the Brazilian Table of Food Composition–USP (14).

It is important to note that energy intake can be miscalculated depending on the data on fiber, since it is usually obtained by difference. Comparing the energy intake of the Brazilian population calculated using fiber contents obtained by different analytical methods an 11% overestimation was observed. For instance, a typical Brazilian woman between 18–30 years of age and performing moderate activity eating a diet containing rice, beans, meat, vegetables, and fruits would have a fiber intake of 7g using crude fiber but 27 g using the enzymatic-gravimetric method. The real energy intake would therefore be 2100 kcal, not 2350 kcal (19).

C. Dietary Fiber and Resistant Starch Contents of Brazilian Foods

Table 1 shows the DF content of foods commonly eaten by Brazilians. Some of these data were used in the assessment of DF intake by the Brazilian population, as will be discussed further in this chapter. These data are taken from the Brazilian Table of Food Composition—USP (14) for which DF content was analyzed by the enzymatic-gravimetric method (25) except for fruits with little or no starch (20), which were analyzed using the nonenzymatic-gravimetric method.

DF information regarding manufactured foods is scarce. A possible reason is the lack of interest among some Brazilian food industries in using labeling for nutritional information and education.

In Brazil, Ministry of Health guidelines 234 (26) and 41 (27), related, respectively, to special purpose foods and to food labeling, determined inclusion of specification for DF data. The amount (in grams) must be obtained by an enzymatic-gravimetric technique. As a consequence it is expected that data on manufactured foods will increase in the near future.

Another initiative that has helped to obtain data on DF in Latin America is the Project CYTED XI.6 for the identification and characterization of dietary fiber for application in dietetic foods. The aim of this project is to gather as much information as possible (basic, technological,

Table 1   Fiber Content of Common Brazilian Foods

Foods	n	Moisture (%)	TDF (%)	IDF (%)	SDF (%)
Cereals					
Bread, gluten, loaf	4	38.36	2.75		
Bread, oat, loaf, diet	4	34.69	3.58		
Bread, rye, loaf	3	37.98	5.24		
Bread, wheat, black, loaf	6	36.85	5.56		
Bread, wheat, French	1	24.50	3.20	1.90	1.30
Bread, wheat, loaf	6	35.50	2.79		
Bread, wheat, wholemeal, loaf	12	35.03	4.48		
Breakfast cereal, All Bran	2	4.69	21.53		
Breakfast cereal, corn, Corn Flakes	4	7.00	3.55	3.18	0.37
Breakfast cereal, oat	2	6.00	4.90		
Breakfast cereal, rice, Rice Krispies	4	4.26	1.38		
Cereals, meal, Neston	2	6.05	1.81		
Corn, green, canned	2	78.80	3.40	3.24	0.16
Corn, meal, cooked	2	73.10	1.40	1.30	0.10
Corn, meal, raw	2	10.52	3.68	1.91	1.76
Oat, bran	4	9.60	15.98	9.90	6.08
Oat, flakes	12	9.70	9.42	5.75	3.67
Oat, meal	4	9.80	10.26	5.94	4.32
Rice, white, cooked	4	77.00	0.90	0.70	0.20
Rice, white, raw	2	12.90	1.65		
Rice, whole, raw	2	12.85	3.00		
Rye, wholemeal	2	7.90	21.90	17.4	4.50
Spaghetti, cooked	2	71.50	1.40	0.80	0.40
Fruits					
Acerola	2	92.00	2.49		
Apple	2	85.20	2.20	1.50	0.70
Banana	1	77.30	1.80	1.20	0.60
Banana, green	20	69.65	3.10		
Cashew	2	87.80	3.17		
Grape	2	87.46	2.27		
Guava, red	2	85.81	4.95		
Guava, white	2	86.07	5.63		
Jabuticaba	2	87.85	2.06		
Mango	2	82.11	3.28		
Orange	2	91.00	2.20	1.70	0.50
Soursop	2	87.12	4.31		
Sugar apple	2	79.80	5.62		
Surinam cherry	6	90.96	2.18		
Uvaia	2	85.53	2.04		
Vegetables					
Bean, black, cooked	2	76.60	6.00	4.40	1.60
Bean, brown, cooked	4	72.35	5.90	4.10	1.80
Bean, brown, raw	7	12.15	21.58		
Beet, cooked	2	92.85	2.24	1.70	0.54
Broccoli, cooked	2	92.19	2.86		
Broccoli, raw	2	94.10	2.17	1.74	0.43
Cabbage, white, raw	2	95.44	1.34	1.10	0.24

Table 1 Continued

Foods	n	Moisture (%)	TDF (%)	IDF (%)	SDF (%)
Carrot, raw	2	96.40	1.54		
Cauliflower, raw	2	93.86	2.05	1.60	0.45
Chayote, raw	2	95.10	1.33	1.00	0.33
Chickpea, raw	4	10.80	20.72	19.94	0.94
Cucumber, raw	2	97.10	1.11	0.88	0.23
Eggplant, raw	2	93.96	2.51	1.60	0.91
Green bean, cooked	12	93.90	1.99		
Green bean, raw	12	91.30	2.78		
Lettuce	2	96.80	1.20	1.10	0.10
Manioc, cooked	2	72.10	1.80		
Manioc, meal, raw	1	7.60	6.20	5.00	1.20
Manioc, yellow, raw	2	71.30	1.94	1.43	0.51
Okra, raw	2	91.00	3.60		
Onion, raw	2	87.80	1.60	1.30	0.30
Pepper, sweet, raw	2	94.60	0.62	0.50	0.12
Potato, cooked	2	85.40	1.90	1.30	0.60
Pumpkin, raw	2	95.14	1.94	1.41	0.53
Spinach, cooked	2	94.76	1.60	1.24	0.36
Squash, raw	2	95.32	1.21	0.91	0.30
Sweet potato, cooked	2	61.00	3.90		
Sweet potato, raw	2	65.90	3.87	3.13	0.74
Swiss chard, cooked	2	95.80	1.25	0.90	0.35
Tomato, raw	4	95.50	1.10	0.80	0.30
Turnip, raw	2	96.30	1.11	0.80	0.31
Yam, cooked	2	71.16	2.58		
Yam, raw	2	73.80	2.34	1.74	0.60

TDF = Total Dietary Fiber; IDF = Insoluble Dietary Fiber; SDF = Soluble Dietary Fiber.
Source: Adapted from Ref. 14.

and physiological) on potential regional vegetable sources for DF. One of the specific aims is to set up a Spanish-American Dietary Fiber Database and disseminate information on research projects going on in the field (13).

Starch is the major ingredient of our diet, responsible for the supply of energy to be either used or stored by the human body. It was traditionally believed that starch was digested almost entirely in the small intestine. However, it is now known that there are different stages of starch digesting, producing compounds with several physiological effects (28–30).

These starch fractions are called resistant starch (RS), defined as the sum of starch and products of starch degradation not absorbed in the small intestine of healthy individuals (31). RS is made up of four subcategories: RS1—physically inaccessible starch; RS2—native starch granules; RS3—retrograded starch (product of processing); and RS4—chemically modified starches. The ubiquitous distribution of RS in most processed foods means that they are important in many societies.

Starch digestibility can be changed through processing and storage, at both the industrial as well as domestic levels. Many factors can alter the technological characteristics of starch, causing changes in RS content (32–36).

Table 2 Resistant Starch Content of Common Brazilian Foods

Foods	n	Moisture (%)	Resistant starch (%)
Cereals			
Bread, wheat, French	3	24.50	1.34 ± 0.04
Bread, wheat, loaf	4	35.70	1.02 ± 0.20
Bread, wheat, wholemeal, loaf	3	34.24	1.15 ± 0.08
Breakfast cereal, corn, flakes	10	5.07	2.69 ± 0.31
Breakfast cereal, oat, honey, nut	2	5.15	0.33 ± 0.04
Corn, cooked	2	68.68	1.19 ± 0.03
Corn, meal, cooked	2	67.20	1.26 ± 0.00
Oat, bran	2	9.60	1.19 ± 0.05
Oat, flakes	7	9.70	1.41 ± 0.56
Rice, white, cooked	3	77.35	0.48 ± 0.03
Rice, whole, cooked	2	75.10	0.61 ± 0.05
Spaghetti, cooked	2	66.48	0.33 ± 0.00
Wheat bran	2	9.26	0.73 ± 0.03
Wheat, whole	3	5.17	1.10 ± 0.13
Vegetables			
Bean, black, cooked	3	69.17	1.54 ± 0.09
Bean, brown, cooked	10	72.61	1.37 ± 0.28
Bean, white, cooked	3	76.96	0.89 ± 0.64
Chickpea, cooked	4	69.65	2.08 ± 0.15
Corn, meal, yellow	2	2.54	2.46 ± 0.05
Lentil, cooked	2	68.29	1.36 ± 0.00
Manioc, cooked	2	70.57	0.31 ± 0.00
Manioc, fried	2	25.34	1.31 ± 0.04
Manioc, meal, raw	3	7.60	0.55 ± 0.15
Pea, cooked	3	62.67	1.52 ± 0.05
Potatoes, cooked	3	85.67	0.45 ± 0.01
Potatoes, sweet, raw	3	65.90	2.23 ± 0.11
Fruits			
Apple	2	83.43	0.12 ± 0.00
Banana, ripe	2	74.34	3.75 ± 0.02
Banana, unripe, meal	3	8.94	29.23 ± 2.86
Manufactured products			
Biscuit, sweet	2	3.60	1.74 ± 0.00
Biscuit, water	3	5.19	1.20 ± 0.08
Cake, orange	2	20.89	0.00
Pudding, coconut	2	72.15	0.28 ± 0.00
Snacks, corn	2	0.00	1.80 ± 0.09

Source: Adapted from Ref. 13.

One example of the effect of the cooking process is what happens to potatoes. When cooked and immediately eaten, almost 99% of its starch is digested; when fired in oil, there is an increase of 4% in RS (37). Storage of beans under high-humidity conditions leads to an increase of cooking time concomitant with an increase of RS (38). Menezes et al. (39) observed that the storage of starchy foods under low temperatures (-20 or $+5°C$) induced the formation of RS in some of them. Thus low-temperature storage, an habitual storage procedure for keeping food, results in formation of RS and could significantly contribute to an increase in the intake of this component by population.

The determination of RS content of Brazilian foods has been carried out at Sao Paulo University. Initially, the technique described by Faisant et al. (40) was used (41,42). Due to its simplicity and improved accuracy and precision, the method proposed by Goñi et al. (43) was adopted (13). Table 2 shows the RS content in some common Brazilian foods.

II. DIETARY FIBER AND RESISTANT STARCH INTAKE IN BRAZIL

Brazil is a large country with marked regional characteristics, especially eating habits. In spite of the need for information about food consumption, such information is scarce, and there are no data expressing a real profile of the foods actually consumed by Brazilians (44,45). The few surveys of food consumption conducted (21,23) did not assess DF intake.

In this chapter, estimates of intake of dietary fiber and resistant starch were based on data about food purchased over a period of three decades. In the 1970s and 1980s, data were gathered in 1974/75 (23) and 1987/88 (22), respectively. The 1990 consumption estimate was projected based on partial data of the Pesquisa de Orçamento Familiar (POF) in 1995/96 (46).

To estimate the average food consumption and to observe regional differences, six metropolitan areas were chosen. They included states of the northern region (Belem—PA), northeast (Recife—PE), southeast (São Paulo—SP, Rio de Janeiro—RJ, and Belo Horizonte—MG) and south (Porto Alegre—RS). The average values found are indicative of an individual from this population, regardless of sex or age, since the IBGE data are based on intrafamily distribution and not an individualized form for each family member.

The intake of DF by Brazilians may be indirectly evaluated using the amounts of white rice, French bread, and beans eaten. Beans represent a considerable source of DF and are eaten in all regions. White rice and French bread, even if not having high amounts of DF, are eaten in large quantities, and thus their contribution becomes relevant. These three foods represented 65% of total DF intake during the three decades examined. Other food sources of DF, such as vegetables and fruits, accounted for, respectively, 7 and 12% of the total DF.

Table 3 shows the average consumption of beans, white rice, and French bread in Brazil during the 1970s, 1980s, and 1990s. It can be seen that between the 1970s and 1990s the ingestion of beans fell 36%, of rice 32%, and of bread 42%. The reduction of consumption of these foods had an immediate effect on the total DF intake. During the 1970s, for example, beans accounted for an average of 9.1 g of a daily total of 19.3 g/day, falling to 6.8 g/day and 5.8 g/day during the 1980s and 1990s, respectively. White rice and French bread followed the same pattern (Table 3).

Table 3 Important Sources of Dietary Fiber and Resistant Starch in the Average Brazilian Diet (g/day)

	Food ingestion			Dietary fiber			Resistant starch		
	70	80	90	70	80	90	70	80	90
Beans	42.1	31.6	26.9	9.1	6.8	5.8	1.2	0.9	0.8
Rice	91.8	71.9	62.7	1.5	1.2	1.0	1.2	1.0	0.8
Bread	81.4	55.2	47.4	2.4	1.7	1.4	1.1	0.7	0.6

   The average DF intake of Brazilians in the 1970s was 19.3 g/day, 16.0 g/day in the 1980s, and 12.4 g/day in the 1990s (Fig. 1). These results reflect a significant and constant drop in global ingestion during the last 30 years, possibly due to changes in eating habits followed by changes in lifestyles in accordance with the socioeconomic profile of the country.

   Considering each region of Brazil separately, we can observe that this downward trend was greater in the regions of São Paulo and Porto Alegre, with a drop of 50% between the 1970s and the 1990s (Table 4). These regions underwent significant changes in their socioeconomic profiles, going from a mixed structure (agricultural and urban) to mainly an urban one with a high degree of industrialization. The recent globalization of the country's economy is turning the typical Brazilian diet into a diet more like that found in developed countries.

   On the other hand, fewer changes in intake of DF in the north and northeastern regions were observed, with percentage changes of 16 and 29%, respectively, which can be explained by the same factors but occurring more slowly, allowing the continuation of regional eating habits.

   Considering that these DF foods are also sources of carbohydrates, it would be natural to presume that the intake of total energy by the people would also drop. What is observed is a substitution for these more traditional starch foods by other energy sources, especially fats and manufactured products. Major sources of energy, such as white rice, beans, roots, and tubers

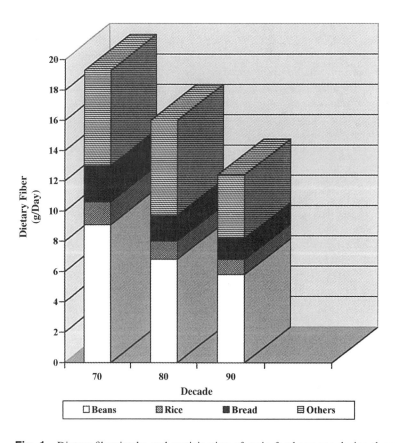

Fig. 1   Dietary fiber intake and participation of main food sources during three decades.

Table 4 Estimated Intake of Carbohydrate, Resistant Starch, and Dietary Fiber in Six Brazilian Metropolitan Areas (g/day) .

	Carbohydrate			Resistant starch			Dietary fiber		
	70	80	90	70	80	90	70	80	90
São Paulo	276	235	158	4.8	4.0	2.8	18.8	15.3	9.3
Rio de Janeiro	285	234	238	5.3	4.2	3.5	20.8	16.7	15.0
Porto Alegre	301	228	183	5.9	3.6	2.7	17.9	13.4	8.5
Belo Horizonte	284	277	210	4.8	4.4	3.5	17.8	15.9	10.3
Recife	286	228	250	5.2	4.4	4.3	21.7	17.7	15.3
Belem	273	234	225	4.1	3.7	3.4	18.7	16.9	15.7
Mean	284	239	211	5.0	4.1	3.4	19.3	16.0	12.4

were in part replaced by animal foods and vegetable oils and fats, with an observable increase in the consumption of milk and eggs (21,44,45,47).

Nutritional recommendations for Brazilians (4) suggest a DF intake of >8 g/1000 kcal or at least 20 g/day for both adolescents and adults. During the 1970s the ingestion of DF was within acceptable levels according to the minimum suggested above, falling to 80% and to 62% of adequacy in the following decades.

It must be remembered that these data do not consider consumption of food outside the house. Some people may have a balanced meal at a restaurant; on the other hand, most eat snacks and certain ready-made and manufactured products that do not alter the ingestion of DF significantly. A 1990 study carried on in the Cotia region of São Paulo showed that only 19% of the adult population had an adequate intake of DF (48).

The DF intake inadequacy of Brazilians is relevant considering the physiological benefits of their habitual ingestion for the prevention of several chronic diseases (29,49–52). This inadequate consumption tends to worsen with greater industrialization and a resultant larger number of people living in urban areas. The problem of lack of food has been replaced by excess, with overweight people found in all income classes; it is now a public health problem in Brazil (47).

In Brazil, 7.6% of the population suffers from diabetes mellitus, and a significant increase of this disease for all of Latin America is expected until 2010 (53). The increase of diabetes exceeds demographic growth; it can be associated to several factors, such as urbanization and industrialization, changes in lifestyle and eating habits, and increased percentage of obesity, among others.

In large cities (e.g., São Paulo) diabetes mellitus incidence is 9.7%; in Porto Alegre incidence is 8.9% (53). These high percentages can be inversely correlated to a drop in the consumption of sources of complex carbohydrates (Table 4).

The proportional mortality rate due to cancer according to deaths registered in Brazil during 1984 and 1994, increased somewhat for colon, pancreas, lung, rectum, breast, and prostate cancer (54). It was observed that neoplasic diseases contributed to mortality more in economically developed regions.

Demographic and epidemic trends suggest that if these conditions prevail, more than 85% of Brazilians will be living in urban areas within 30 years. The number of elderly will double and 12% of citizens will be over 60 years old. Cardiovascular diseases, cancer, and its external causes will together be responsible for 75% of deaths (55).

Colon cancer is a type of cancer associated with western eating habits and is considered to be responsive to preventive measures (56). Nonstarch polysaccharide could be important in preventing colon and breast cancer. Vegetables and fruits seem to lower the risk of colon, rectum, stomach, lung, esophageal, and mouth cancer and also probably lower the risk of breast, pancreas, bladder, and larynx cancer (57).

Cardiovascular disease in Brazil is the major cause of death, accounting for one third of the total; its role has increased in the past 50 years. In 1950 it accounted for 14.2% and in 1989 32% of deaths in some state capitals. Although many factors contributed to the increase of cardiovascular disease, healthy eating habits are a significant prevention factor (58,59).

A prospective study of healthy men in the United States suggested that the insoluble component of fiber is significantly associated with a decreased risk of diverticular disease and that this inverse association was particularly strong for cellulose (60). A Brazilian study evaluated the dietary fiber intake and the dietary habits of children (78 months) with and without chronic constipation. The daily intake of insoluble dietary fiber was statistically lower in the constipation group (6.3 g) than in the control group (9.4 g), while the intake of soluble fiber was similar. The low intake of insoluble fiber suggests that it plays an important role in the pathogeneses of chronic constipation in children (61).

Due to the different physiological effects that each component of fiber can have, it is interesting to know the level of intake of each. In Brazil it was found that the proportions were 70% insoluble fiber and 30% soluble fiber, which has remained steady for the last three decades. The ratio of insoluble to soluble fiber in the food supply commonly consumed in the United States is on average approximately fourfold greater for the insoluble fraction (62). To help in food selection, part of our database (Table 1) supplies information regarding soluble and insoluble fiber contents of some of the foods commonly consumed by Brazilians.

Dietary fiber has been studied since the 1970s and has been recognized as responsible for many physiological effects in the prevention of degenerative diseases. In the 1980s, it was observed that a significant amount of starch escaped from digestion in the small intestine, reaching the large intestine to be fermented there. This fraction, called resistant starch (RS), was then deemed responsible for determined physiological effects attributed earlier to DF (28–30).

Resistant starch associated with insoluble fiber has physiological effects such as increase in fecal volume, dilution of potentially carcinogens (28), lowering of postprandial plasma glucose, insulin, triglycerides, and low-density lipoproteins (LDL) (28,30), and production of short-chain fatty acids (SCFA), important for intestinal cell metabolism and cancer prevention (28,63).

Because RS and DF may have complementary roles in the prevention of chronic diseases, the consumption of this component has been evaluated in Brazil compared to several other countries (28,29,64). The present intake of RS in European countries is 4.1 g/day, ranging from 3.2 g/day in Norway to 5.7 g/day in Spain (28,64). In Australia the average is higher, around 5.5 g/day, and in Asia RS intake is significantly greater, reaching 8.0 g/day in Japan and 18.5 g/day in China (value obtained assuming that 5% of total carbohydrate ingested are RS) (29). In Brazil, the estimated intake of RS has dropped over the last three decades from 5.0 g/day during the 1970s to 3.4 g/day in the 1990s. This followed a lowering of total carbohydrate intake estimated as 26%. (Table 4).

White rice, beans, and French bread, which represent good DF sources due to the frequent consumption by Brazilians, also supply large amounts of RS. The consumption of these foods has dropped over the last three decades, contributed to the decrease in RS intake (Table 3). At the same time, some regional foods contribute a great deal to RS intake. For instance, bananas are consumed in all regions of Brazil, corn meal in the central and northeast regions, tapioca meal in the north, biscuits, spaghetti, and potatoes in all regions.

RS is closely related to DF in its analytical (28,65) and physiological aspects (28–30,51,63,66). The ingestion of RS in conjunction with DF has been correlated to lower risk of diseases of the large intestine (66). Nutrition guidelines from several countries suggest increased intake of complex carbohydrate from vegetal sources (4,67,68) but are not recommendations for RS intake so far. A daily intake of around 20 g/day has been suggested as beneficial for gastrointestinal function (29,30).

III. CONCLUSION

The estimates of average intake of DF and RS by the Brazilian population, based on food purchasing data, in six metropolitan regions and over three decades showed a marked reduction in intake. During the 1970s the average DF intake was 19.3 g/day, decreased to 16.0 g/day during the 1980s, and 12.4 g/day in the 1990s. Changes in eating habits followed by changes in lifestyle account for these changes. The reduction in DF ingestion was markedly higher in regions where industrialization was more intense, such as São Paulo-SP and Rio Grande do Sul-RS.

Evaluating the adequacy of DF intake according to nutritional recommendations set for Brazilians (a minimum of 20 g/day for both adolescent and adults), we can observe that during the 1970s, ingestion was adequate, falling to 80% and 62% during the following decades.

The estimated average intake of RS has dropped during the last three decades, from around 5.0 g/day during the 1970s to 3.4 g/day in the 1990s. This followed a 26% decrease of the ingestion of total carbohydrates. The intake of RS in Brazil is similar to that in Europe (3.2 g/day). Considering that RS and DF may have a complementary role for prevention of determined chronic diseases, the intake of these components could be beneficial.

To guarantee adequate intake of DF and RS, considering prevention and/or control of chronic disease, it would be necessary to maintain healthy eating habits, including an adequate consumption of vegetable foods (rice and beans), and increase ingestion of complex carbohydrates.

REFERENCES

1. Fundação Instituto Brasileiro de Geografia e Estatística (IBGE), ed. Tabelas de Composição de Alimentos. 2 ed. Rio de Janeiro-IBGE, 1977.
2. Mendez MHM, Derivi SON, Rodriguez MCR, Fernandez ML, eds. Tabela de Composição dos Alimentos. Niterói, EDUFF, 1995.
3. Franco G ed. Tabela de Composição Química dos Alimentos. 9 ed. Rio de Janeiro: Atheneu, 1997.
4. Vannucchi H, Menezes EW, Campana AO, Lajolo FM, eds. Aplicação das Recomendações Nutricionais Adaptadas à População Brasileira. Ribeirão Preto, Legis Suma. Cadernos de Nutrição-SBAN 2, 1990.
5. Fillisetti-Cozi TMCC, Lajolo FM. Fibra alimentar insolúvel, solúvel e total de alimentos brasileiros. Rev Farm Bioquím Univ São Paulo 27:83–99, 1991.
6. Lajolo FM, Menezes EW, Filisetti-Cozzi TMCC. Considerações sobre carboidratos e fibra. In: JM Bengoa, B Torún, M Behar, N Scrimshaw, eds. Metas Nutricionales y Guias de Alimentación para América Latina. Bases para su Desarrollo. Caracas: Fundación Cavendes, 1988, pp 147–170.
7. Lajolo FM, Menezes EW. Uma análise retrospectiva e contextualização da questão. Bol Soc Bras Ciênc Technol Aliment 31:90–92, 1997.
8. Lajolo FM. Grupo de trabalho: composição de alimentos. Bol Soc Bras Ciênc Technol Aliment 29: 57–69, 1995.
9. Filisetti TMCC. Estudo colaborativo para análise de fibra alimentar. Bol Soc Bras Ciênc Technol Aliment 31:112–113, 1997.
10. Filisetti TMCC, Colloca MJ, Lajolo FM. Estudo colaborativo Ibero-americano: análise de fibra alimentar. XI Congresso Sociedad Latinoamericana de Nutrición. Guatemala, SLAN, 1997.

11. Lee SC, Prosky L. International survey on dietary fiber: definition, analysis, and reference materials. J AOAC Int 78:22–36, 1995.

12. Lee SC, Prosky L, De Vries LW. Determination of total, soluble and insoluble dietary fibre in foods. Enzimatic-gravimetric method, MESTRIS Buffer: Colaborative Study. J AOAC Int 7:395–416, 1992.

13. Menezes EW, Lajolo FM, eds. Contenido en Fibra Dietética y Almidón Resistente en Alimentos y Productos Iberoamericanos [Proyecto CYTED XI.6 Obtención y caracterización de fibra dietética para su aplicación en regímenes especiales]. São Paulo: Docuprint, 2000, p. 121.

14. Universidade de São Paulo (USP), ed. Tabela Brasileira de Composição de Alimentos-USP. São Paulo: FCF-USP, 1998. (http://www.fcf.usp.br/tabela).

15. Menezes EW, Caruso L, Lajolo FM. An application of criteria to evaluate quality of dietary fibre data in Brazilian foods. J Food Comp Anal 13(4):4555–4473, 2000.

16. Holden JM. Assessment of the quality of data in nutritional databases. Bol Soc Bras Ciênc Technol Aliment. 31:105–108, 1997.

17. Holden JM, Schubert A, Wolf WR, Beecher GR. A system for evaluating the quality of published nutrient data: selenium, a test case. In: WM Rand, CT Windham, BW Wyse, VR Young, eds. Food Composition Data: A User's Perspective. Tokyo: UNU, 1987, pp 177–193.

18. Mangels AR, Holden JM, Beecher GR, Forman MR, Lanza E. Carotenoid content of fruits and vegetables: an evaluation of analytic data. J Am Diet Assoc 93:284–296, 1993.

19. Caruso L. Avaliação da qualidade analítica dos dados sobre fibra alimentar-um modelo. Dissertação de mestrado, Universidade de São Paulo, Faculdade de Ciências Farmacêticas, São Paulo, 1998.

20. Li BW, Cardozo MS. Determination of total dietary fiber in foods and products with little or no starch, nonenzymatic-gravimetric method: collaborative study. J AOAC Int 77:687–698, 1994.

21. Galeazzi MAM, Domene SMA, Sichieri R. Estudo Multicêntrico sobre Consumo Alimentar INAN/MS/NEPA. In: Cadernos de Debate. Campinas, UNICAMP, 1997.

22. Fundação Instituto Brasileiro de Geografia e Estatística (IBGE), ed. Pesquisa de Orçamentos Familiares, 1987/1988. Consumo Alimentar Domiciliar ''per capita''—Regiões Metropolitanas, v.2. Brasília. IBGE, 1991.

23. Fundação Instituto Brasileiro de Geografia e Estatística (IBGE), ed. Consumo Alimentar, Despesa Familiar. (ENDEF–Estudo Nacional da Despesa Familiar, v.3, Publicações Especiais, t.2). Rio de Janeiro: IBGE, 1978.

24. Menezes EW, Caruso L, Lajolo FM. Uniformização internacional de dados brasileiros de composição de alimentos. Bol Soc Bras Ciênc Technol Aliment 31:93–104, 1997.

25. Prosky L, Asp NG, Schweizer TF, DeVries JW, Furda I. Determination of insoluble, soluble, and total dietary fiber in food products: interlaboratory study. J Assoc Off Anal Chem 71:1017–1023, 1988.

26. Brasil. Ministério da Saúde, Secretaria de Vigilância Sanitária. Portaria n. 234-DETEN/MS de 21 de maio de 1996. Alimentos para fins especiais. Diário Oficial [da República Federativa do Brasil], Brasília, 1996.

27. Brasil. Ministério da Saúde, Secretaria de Vigilância Sanitária. Portaria n. 41-DETEN/MS de 14 de janeiro de 1998. Rotulagem nutricional para alimentos embalados. Diário Oficial [da República Federativa do Brasil], Brasília, 1998.

28. Asp N-G, van Amelsvoort JMM, Hautvast JGAJ, eds. EURESTA Physiological Implication of the Consumption of Resistant Starch in Man (European FLAIR—Concerted Action n.11-COST 911). [Proceedings of the concluding plenary meeting of EURESTA, Wageningen] FLAIR, 1994.

29. Baghurst PA, Baghurst KI, Record SJ, eds. Dietary Fibre, Non-starch Polysaccharides and Resistant Starch. A Review. Australia, CSIRO. Food Australia 48 (suppl):1–35, 1996.

30. Muir JG, Young GP, O'Dea K, Cameron-Smith D, Brown IL, Collier GR. Resistant starch-the neglected dietary fiber? Implications for health. Dietary Fiber Bibliogr Rev 1:33–47, 1993.

31. Champ M. Definition, analysis, physical and chemical characterization of RS. In: N-G Asp, JMM van Amelsvoort, JGAJ Hautvast, eds. EURESTA Physiological Implication of the Consumption of Resistant Starch in Man (European FLAIR–Concerted Action n.11-COST 911). [Proceedings of the concluding plenary meeting of EURESTA, Wageningen] FLAIR, 1994, pp 1–14.

32. Escarpa A, González MC, Morales MD, Saura-Calixto F. An approach to the influence of nutrients and other constituents on resistant starch formation. Food Chem 60:527–532, 1997.

33. Escarpa A, González MC, Mañas E, García-Diz L, Saura-Calixto F. Resistant starch formation: standardization of a high-pressure autoclave process. J Agric Food Chem 44:924–928, 1996.

34. Menezes EW, Lajolo FM, Seravalli EAG, Vannucchi H, Moreira EA. Starch availability in Brazilian foods: "in vivo" and "in vitro" assays. Nutr Res 16:1425–1436, 1996.

35. Tovar J, Velasco Z. Available and resistant starch content in some Venezuelan foods. Acta Cient Venez 46:208–209, 1995.

36. Galvani ACR, Camargo A, Ciacco CF. Efeito de lipídios, açúcares, sais e ácidos nas propriedades de gelatinização e retrogradação do amido. Ciênc Tecnol Aliment 14:3–13, 1994.

37. Goñi I, Bravo L, Larrauri JA, Saura-Calixto F. Resistant starch in potatoes deep-fried in olive oil. Food Chem 59:269–272, 1997.

38. Garcia E, Lajolo FM. Starch alteration in hard-to-cook beans (*Phaseolus vulgaris*). J Agric Food Chem 42:612–615, 1994.

39. Menezes EW, Canzio AE, Lajolo FM. Formação de amido resistente em alimentos armazenados em baixas temperaturas. In: FM Lajolo, EW Menezes, eds. Fibra Dietética. Temas en Tecnología de Alimentos. [Anais do Simpósio Iberoamericano sobre fibra dietética em alimentos—projeto CYTED XI.6, São Paulo, 1997] México: IPN, v.2, 1998, pp 191–198.

40. Faisant N, Planchot V, Kozlowski F, Pacouret M-P, Colonna P, Champ M. Resistant starch determination adapted to products containing high level of resistant starch. Sci Aliment 15:85–91, 1995.

41. Menezes EW, Cordenunsi BR, Lajolo FM. Determinação do conteúdo de amido resistente em alimentos brasileiros. In: J Ruales, ed. Conferencia Internacional de Almidón-Propriedades Físico-químicas, Funcionales y Nutricionales. Usos. Quito: Escuela Politecnica Nacional, 1996, pp 267–274.

42. Menezes EW, Lajolo FM, Leite MS. Determinação do conteúdo de amido resistente no feijão: comparação de métodos. I Internacional Symposium of Latin American and Caribbean Section—AOAC International. São Paulo: FCF/USP, 1995.

43. Goñi I, García-Diz L, Mañas E, Saura-Calixto F. Analysis of resistant starch: a method for foods products. Food Chem 56:445–449, 1996.

44. Tartaglia JC. Industrialização, alimentação e segurança alimentar no Brasil. In: JE Dutra-de-Oliveira, Marchini JS, eds. Ciências Nutricionais. São Paulo: Sarvier, 1998, pp 322–349.

45. Mondini L, Monteio CA. Mudanças no padrão de alimentação da população urbana brasileira (1962–1988), Rev Saúde Pública 28:433–439, 1994.

46. IBGE (Fundação Instituto Brasileiro de Geografia e Estatística), ed. Pesquisa de Orçamentos Familiares, 1995/1996—Regiões Metropolitanas. Rio de Janeiro: IBGE, 1997.

47. Monteiro CA, Mondini L, Souza ALM, Pokin BM. Da desnutrição para a obesidade: a transição nutricional no Brasil. In: CA Monteiro, ed. Velhos e Novos Males da Saúde no Brasil. São Paulo: Hugitec, NUPENS/USP, 1995, pp 247–255.

48. Matos LL. Consumo de fibras alimentares em população adulta de região metropolitana de São Paulo. Dissertação de Mestrado, Universidade de São Paulo, Faculdade de Saúde Pública, São Paulo, 1997.

49. Steinhart CE, Doyle ME, Cochrane BA, eds. Food Safety. New York: Marcel Dekker, 1996.

50. Walker ARP. Fibre in health/disease-what now? Nutr Res 18:607–614, 1998.

51. Schneeman BO. Dietary fiber and gastrointestinal function. Nutr Res 18:625–632, 1998.

52. Williams CL. Importance of dietary fiber in childhood. J Am Diet Assoc 95:1140–1146, 1995.

53. Malerbi DA, Franco LJ. Multicenter study of the prevalence of diabetes mellitus and impaired glucose tolerance in the urban Brazilian population aged 30–69 yr. The Brazilian cooperative group on the study of diabetes prevalence. Diabetes Care 15:1509–1516, 1992.

54. Ministério da Saúde. Datasus, eds. Sistema de Informações sobre Mortalidade. Brasília, MS, 1998 (http://www.datasus.gov.br).

55. Ministério da Saúde. Instituto Nacional do Câncer. Coordenação de programas de controle de câncer, eds. O Problema do Câncer no Brasil. Rio de Janeiro, 1997.

56. Alabaster O, Tang ZC, Shivapurkar N. Dietary fibre and chemopreventive modulation of colon carcinogenesis. Mutat Res 350:185–197, 1996.

57. World Cancer Research Fund. American Institute for Cancer Research, eds. Food, Nutrition and the Prevention of Cancer: a Global Perspective (Summary). Washington, DC: WCRF, 1997.
58. Lotufo PA, Lolio CA. Tendências de evolução da mortalidade por doenças cardiovasculares: o caso do Estado de São Paulo. In: CA Monteiro, ed. Velhos e Novos Males da Saúde no Brasil. São Paulo: Hugitec, NUPENS/USP, 1995, pp 279–288.
59. Jenkins DJA, Kendall CWC, Ransom TPP. Dietary fiber, the evolution of human diet and coronary heart disease. Nutr Res 18:633–652, 1998.
60. Aldoori WH, Giovannucci EL, Rockett HRH, Sampson L, Rimm EB, Willett WC. A prospective study of dietary fiber types and symptomatic diverticular disease in men. J Nutr 128:714–719, 1998.
61. Morais MB, Vítolo MR, Aguirre ANC, Medeiros EH, Antoneli EM, Fagundes-Neto U. Teor de fibra alimentar e de outros nutrientes na dieta de crianças com e sem constipação intestinal crônica funcional. Arq Gastroenterol 33:93–99, 1996.
62. Marlett JA. Content and composition of dietary fiber in 117 frequently consumed foods. J Am Diet Assoc 92:175–186, 1992.
63. Hylla S, Gostner A, Dusel G, Anger H, Bartram H-P, Christl, SU, Kasper H, Scheppach W. Effects of resistant starch on colon in healthy volunteers: possible implications for cancer prevention. Am J Clin Nutr 67:136–142, 1998.
64. Goñi I, García-Alonso A, García-Diz L. Almidon resistente, componente indigestible de la dieta. Alimentaria (abril):31–34, 1995.
65. Cho S, DeVries JW, Prosky L, eds. Dietary Fiber Analysis and Applications. AOAC International, 1997.
66. Birkett AM, Jones GP, de Silva AM, Young GP, Muir JG. Dietary intake and faecal excretion of carbohydrate by Australians: importance of achieving stool weights greater than 150 g to improve faecal markers relevant to colon cancer risk. Eur J Clin Nutr 51:625–632, 1997.
67. Achterberg C, McDonnell E, Bagby R. How to put the food guide pyramid into practice. J Am Diet Assoc 94:1030–1035, 1994.
68. Bengoa JM, Torún B, Behar M, Scrimshaw N. Metas nutricionales y guias de alimentación para América Latina. Bases para su desarrollo. Arch Latinoam Nutr 38:375–426, 1988.

Index